HANDBOOK OF DEPRESSION

HANDBOOK OF DEPRESSION

Second Edition

Edited by
IAN H. GOTLIB
CONSTANCE L. HAMMEN

THE GUILFORD PRESS
New York   London

The authors have checked with sources believed to be reliable in their efforts to provide information
that is complete and generally in accord with the standards of practice that are accepted at the time
of publication. However, in view of the possibility of human error or changes in medical sciences,
neither the authors, nor the editor and publisher, nor any other party who has been involved in the
preparation or publication of this work warrants that the information contained herein is in every
respect accurate or complete, and they are not responsible for any errors or omissions or the results
obtained from the use of such information. Readers are encouraged to confirm the information
contained in this book with other sources.

Library of Congress Cataloging-in-Publication Data

Handbook of depression / edited by Ian H. Gotlib, Constance L. Hammen. — 2nd ed.
   p. ; cm.
Includes bibliographical references and index.
ISBN 978-1-59385-450-8 (hardcover : alk. paper)
1. Depression, Mental—Handbooks, manuals, etc.   I. Gotlib, Ian H.   II. Hammen, Constance L.
[DNLM: 1. Depressive Disorder.   2. Depression.   3. Risk Factors.   WM 171 H2367 2008]
RC537.H3376 2009
616.85′27—dc22
                                                                         2008010575

About the Editors

Ian H. Gotlib, PhD, is Professor of Psychology at Stanford University and Director of the Stanford Mood and Anxiety Disorders Laboratory. In his research, which is supported by the National Institute of Mental Health, Dr. Gotlib examines information-processing styles of children, adolescents, and adults suffering from depression; patterns of brain activation of depressed patients in response to emotional stimuli; and genetic and biological aspects of risk for depression in young children of depressed parents. Dr. Gotlib has published over 200 scientific articles and is the author or coauthor of several books in the areas of depression and stress.

Constance L. Hammen, PhD, is Distinguished Professor of Psychology at the University of California, Los Angeles, and also has an appointment in the Department of Psychiatry and Behavioral Sciences. She served as chair of the Clinical Psychology Program at UCLA for 13 years. Dr. Hammen's research interests include risk factors for depression and bipolar disorders, with a particular focus on family, social, and stress processes in depression, as well as genetic and neuroendocrine factors. Her current work involves offspring at risk due to parental depression. Dr. Hammen has written and coauthored numerous articles, books, and textbooks, and has developed widely used interview methods for assessment of acute and chronic life stress.

Contributors

Alinne Z. Barrera, PhD, Department of Psychiatry, San Francisco General Hospital, University of California, San Francisco, California

Steven R. H. Beach, PhD, Institute for Behavioral Research, University of Georgia, Athens, Georgia

Alan L. Berman, PhD, American Association of Suicidology, Washington, DC

Dan G. Blazer MD, PhD, Department of Psychiatry, Duke University Medical Center, Durham, North Carolina

Robert J. Boland, MD, Residency Training Office, Butler Hospital, Brown Medical School, Providence, Rhode Island

Sarah R. Brand, MA, Department of Psychology, Emory University, Atlanta, Georgia

Robert M. Carney, PhD, Department of Psychiatry, Washington University School of Medicine, St. Louis, Missouri

Yulia E. Chentsova-Dutton, PhD, Department of Psychology, Georgetown University, Washington, DC

Gregory N. Clarke, PhD, Kaiser Permanente Center for Health Research, Portland, Oregon

Amy K. Cuellar, PhD, Department of Psychiatry and Behavioral Sciences, Baylor College of Medicine, and Michael E. DeBakey VA Medical Center, Houston, Texas

Richard J. Davidson, PhD, Departments of Psychology and Psychiatry, University of Wisconsin, Madison, Wisconsin

Joanne Davila, PhD, Department of Psychology, Stony Brook University, Stony Brook, New York

Shane P. Davis, PhD, Department of Psychiatry and Behavioral Sciences, Emory University School of Medicine, Atlanta, Georgia

Sona Dimidjian, PhD, Department of Psychology, University of Colorado, Boulder, Colorado

C. Emily Durbin, PhD, Department of Psychology, Northwestern University, Evanston, Illinois

Sarah A. Frankel, MA, Department of Psychology and Human Development, Vanderbilt University, Nashville, Tennessee

Kameron J. Franklin, MS, Department of Psychology, University of Georgia, Athens, Georgia

Kenneth E. Freedland, PhD, Department of Psychiatry, Washington University School of Medicine, St. Louis, Missouri

Jill Friedman, MS, Department of Psychology, Drexel University, Philadelphia, Pennsylvania

Catherine M. Gallerani, MA, Department of Psychology and Human Development, Vanderbilt University, Nashville, Tennessee

Judy Garber, PhD, Department of Psychology and Human Development, Vanderbilt University, Nashville, Tennessee

Katholiki Georgiades, PhD, Department of Psychiatry and Behavioral Neurosciences and Offord Centre for Child Studies, McMaster University, Hamilton, Ontario, Canada

Michael J. Gitlin, MD, Department of Psychiatry and Mood Disorders Clinic, University of California, Los Angeles, California

Sherryl H. Goodman, PhD, Department of Psychology, Emory University, Atlanta, Georgia

Ian H. Gotlib, PhD, Department of Psychology, Stanford University, Stanford, California

Constance L. Hammen, PhD, Department of Psychology, University of California, Los Angeles, California

Lori M. Hilt, MPhil, Department of Psychology, Yale University, New Haven, Connecticut

Steven D. Hollon, PhD, Department of Psychology and Human Development, Vanderbilt University, Nashville, Tennessee

Celia F. Hybels, PhD, Department of Psychiatry, Duke University Medical Center, Durham, North Carolina

Rick E. Ingram, PhD, Department of Psychology, University of Kansas, Lawrence, Kansas

Sheri L. Johnson, PhD, Department of Psychology, University of Miami, Coral Gables, Florida

Thomas E. Joiner, Jr., PhD, Department of Psychology, Florida State University, Tallahassee, Florida

Deborah J. Jones, PhD, Department of Psychology, University of North Carolina, Chapel Hill, North Carolina

Jutta Joormann, PhD, Department of Psychology, University of Miami, Coral Gables, Florida

Nadine J. Kaslow, PhD, ABPP, Department of Psychiatry and Behavioral Sciences, Emory University School of Medicine, Atlanta, Georgia

Martin B. Keller, MD, Department of Psychiatry and Human Behavior, Butler Hospital, Brown Medical School, Providence, Rhode Island

Ronald C. Kessler, PhD, Department of Health Care Policy, Harvard Medical School, Boston, Massachusetts

Daniel N. Klein, PhD, Department of Psychology, Stony Brook University, Stony Brook, New York

Huynh-Nhu Le, PhD, Department of Psychology, George Washington University, Washington, DC

Minsun Lee, MA, Department of Psychology, Drexel University, Philadelphia, Pennsylvania

Douglas F. Levinson, MD, Department of Psychiatry and Behavioral Sciences, Stanford University School of Medicine, Stanford, California

David J. Miklowitz, PhD, Department of Psychology, University of Colorado, Boulder, Colorado

Christopher Miller, MS, Department of Psychology, University of Miami, Coral Gables, Florida

Scott M. Monroe, PhD, Department of Psychology, University of Notre Dame, Notre Dame, Indiana

Ricardo F. Muñoz, PhD, Department of Psychiatry, San Francisco General Hospital, University of California, San Francisco, California

Arthur M. Nezu, PhD, ABPP, Departments of Psychology, Medicine, and Community Health and Prevention, Drexel University, Philadelphia, Pennsylvania, and Department of Forensic Mental Health, University of Nottingham, Nottingham, United Kingdom

Christine Maguth Nezu, PhD, ABPP, Departments of Psychology and Medicine, Drexel University, Philadelphia, Pennsylvania, and Department of Forensic Mental Health, University of Nottingham, Nottingham, United Kingdom

Jack B. Nitschke, PhD, Departments of Psychiatry and Psychology, University of Wisconsin, Madison, Wisconsin

Susan Nolen-Hoeksema, PhD, Department of Psychology, Yale University, New Haven, Connecticut

Diego A. Pizzagalli, PhD, Department of Psychology, Harvard University, Cambridge, Massachusetts

Karen D. Rudolph, PhD, Department of Psychology, University of Illinois at Urbana–Champaign, Champaign, Illinois

Stewart A. Shankman, PhD, Departments of Psychology and Psychiatry, University of Illinois at Chicago, Chicago, Illinois

Greg J. Siegle, PhD, Department of Psychiatry, Western Psychiatric Institute and Clinic, University of Pittsburgh Medical Center, Pittsburgh, Pennsylvania

George M. Slavich, PhD, Department of Psychiatry, University of California, San Francisco, California

Chaundrissa Oyeshiku Smith, PhD, Department of Psychiatry and Behavioral Sciences, Emory University School of Medicine, Atlanta, Georgia

Lisa R. Starr, MA, Department of Psychology, Stony Brook University, Stony Brook, New York

Catherine B. Stroud, MA, Department of Psychology, Stony Brook University, Stony Brook, New York

Michael E. Thase, MD, Department of Psychiatry, Western Psychiatric Institute and Clinic, University of Pittsburgh Medical Center, Pittsburgh, Pennsylvania

Katherine A. Timmons, MS, Department of Psychology, Florida State University, Tallahassee, Florida

Leandro D. Torres, PhD, Department of Psychiatry, San Francisco General Hospital, University of California, San Francisco, California

Jeanne L. Tsai, PhD, Department of Psychology, Stanford University, Stanford, California

Philip S. Wang, MD, DrPH, Division of Services and Intervention Research, National Institute of Mental Health, National Institutes of Health, Bethesda, Maryland

Contents

PART II. VULNERABILITY, RISK, AND MODELS OF DEPRESSION

PART IV. PREVENTION AND TREATMENT OF DEPRESSION

Introduction

Ian H. Gotlib *and* Constance L. Hammen

Depression is among the most prevalent of all psychiatric disorders. Recent estimates indicate that about 20% of the American population, primarily women, will experience a clinically significant episode of depression at some point in their lives, a significant increase over rates reported two decades ago and earlier. In fact, the rates of depression are so high that the World Health Organization (WHO) Global Burden of Disease Study ranked depression as the single most burdensome disease in the world in terms of total disability-adjusted life years among people in midlife (Murray & Lopez, 1996). In epidemiological studies, depression has been found to be associated with poor physical health, in particular, with fibromyalgia, high rates of cardiac problems, and higher rates of smoking (e.g., Nicholson, Kuper, & Hemingway, 2006; Wulsin & Singal, 2003). There is also a significant economic cost of depression. In a recent analysis of depression in the workplace, Kessler and colleagues (2006) estimated that the annual salary-equivalent costs of depression-related lost productivity in the United States exceeds $36 billion. And because this figure does not take into account the impact of depression on factors such as the performance of coworkers, turnover, and industrial accidents, it is likely to be an underestimate.

In addition to these findings concerning the impact of depression on health and workplace productivity, there is now mounting evidence that depression adversely affects the quality of interpersonal relationships and, in particular, relationships with spouses and children. Not only is the rate of divorce higher among depressed than among nondepressed individuals (e.g., Wade & Cairney, 2000), but also the children of depressed parents have themselves been found to be at elevated risk for psychopathology (for reviews of this literature, see Joormann, Eugène & Gotlib, in press; Hammen, Chapter 12, this volume).

Depression is a highly recurrent disorder. Over 75% of depressed patients have more than one depressive episode (see Boland & Keller, Chapter 2), often developing a relapse of depression within 2 years of recovery. This high recurrence rate in depression suggests that specific factors serve to increase people's risk for developing repeated episodes of this disorder. In this context, therefore, in trying to understand mechanisms that increase risk for depression, investigators have examined biological and genetic factors and psychological and environmental characteristics that may lead individuals to experience depressive episodes.

The enormous costs of depression, combined with the recent documentation of increasing rates of depressive disorders, have led to an exponential increase in research examining factors involved in the onset, course, and maintenance of depression, and the effectiveness of psychological and biological treatments for depression, which has resulted in significant advances in our understanding of virtually all its aspects. Because there was not a single source to which scientists and other interested readers could turn to learn about recent important developments in different areas of depression research, we began to assemble the first edition of this *Handbook* in 2000. The rapid development of research and theory in depression since then provided the impetus for us to update and expand this *Handbook*. In particular, we have added new chapters on depression and health, on the functioning of offspring of depressed parents, and on pharmacological and psychosocial treatments for bipolar disorder.

We have organized this book into four broad sections; we believe that these domains are the major areas of depression research in which significant advances have been made over the past decade, and in which research will continue to increase our understanding of the nature of this disorder. The authors of the chapters in the first section discuss descriptive and definitional aspects of depression, including epidemiology, course and outcome, assessment, methodological issues in the study of depression, personality, health, and the relation between unipolar and bipolar depression. The second section contains chapters dealing with vulnerability, risk, and models of depression. Some describe advances in the genetics, biology, and neurobiology of depression, arguably the three areas of research in depression that have experienced the greatest growth over the past decade. Others discuss developments in our understanding of cognitive and interpersonal aspects of depression, the nature of the functioning of offspring of depressed parents, and the importance of stress and of early adverse experiences. The third section of this *Handbook* describes advances in our understanding of depression as it occurs in specific populations. The authors of these chapters discuss the presentation of depression in different cultures; depression in couples and families; gender differences in depression; depression in children, adolescents, and older adults; and issues in assessing the relation between depression and suicide. The final section of the volume is devoted to issues involving the prevention and treatment of depression. Here the authors describe recent developments in the prevention of major depression and advances in pharmacotherapy, cognitive-behavioral therapy, marital and family therapy, and interpersonal therapy for depression. This section also includes important chapters describing pharmacological and psychosocial interventions for bipolar disorder and innovations in the treatment of depression in children and adolescents. As in the previous edition, we asked all of the authors in this edition of the *Handbook* to conclude their chapters with a section describing what they think are the most important directions for future research in this field. These comments give the reader a sense of not only the advances that have been made in each area of research in depression but also the important issues that are likely to take center stage over the next few years. As you will see from the chapters in this *Handbook*, we have clearly made progress over the past decade in our quest to understand, treat, and prevent the onset of depression. And more important, the coming decade promises to be even more exciting than the last.

REFERENCES

Joorman, J., Eugène, F., & Gotlib, I. H. (in press). Parental depression: Impact on offspring and mechanisms underlying transmission of risk. In S. Nolen-Hoeksema (Eds.), *Handbook of adolescent depression*. New York: Guilford Press.

Kessler, R. C., Akiskal, H. S., Ames, M., Birnbaum, H., Greenberg, P., Hirschfeld, R. M., et al. (2006). Prevalence and effects of mood disorders on work performance in a nationally representative sample of U.S. workers. *American Journal of Psychiatry, 163*, 1561–1568.

Murray, C. J., & Lopez, A. D. (1996). *The global burden of disease*. Cambridge, MA: Harvard University Press.

Nicholson, A., Kuper, H., & Hemingway, H. (2006). Depression as an aetiologic and prognostic factor in coronary heart disease: A meta-analysis of 6362 events among 146,538 participants in 54 observational studies. *European Heart Journal, 27*, 2763–2774.

Wade, T. J., & Cairney, J. (2000). Major depressive disorder and marital transition among mothers: Results from a national panel study. *Journal of Nervous and Mental Disease, 188*, 741–750.

Wulsin, L. R., & Singal, B. M. (2003). Do depressive symptoms increase the risk for the onset of coronary disease?: A systematic quantitative review. *Psychosomatic Medicine, 65*, 201–210.

PART I

DESCRIPTIVE ASPECTS OF DEPRESSION

Depression is one of the most common psychiatric disorders and, from a societal perspective, is perhaps the most costly. Depression is also a highly recurrent disorder with an increasingly younger age of onset for the initial episode. In the seven chapters in this section, the authors discuss issues concerning the onset and course of depression, its prevalence and societal costs, and important factors involved in studying this disorder. Kessler and Wang (Chapter 1) describe epidemiological aspects of depression—its prevalence and its economic cost. Boland and Keller (Chapter 2) discuss the course and outcome of this disorder, describing the results of several large-scale longitudinal investigations that have monitored the course of depression over many years. Nezu, Nezu, Friedman, and Lee (Chapter 3) describe the most widely used interview-based and self-report measures of depression, and discuss important issues involved in the assessment of this disorder. Extending this discussion, Ingram and Siegle (Chapter 4) describe a number of methodological issues in the study of depressive disorders, and make several noteworthy recommendations concerning how research in this area might proceed most fruitfully. Klein, Durbin, and Shankman (Chapter 5) then describe the nature of the relation between depression and various aspects of personality functioning. Freedland and Carney (Chapter 6) examine links between depression and medical illness, and delineate controversies and challenges in the assessment and treatment of depression in medically ill individuals. Finally Johnson, Cuellar, and Miller (Chapter 7) discuss similarities and differences in the clinical phenomenology and psychosocial predictors of unipolar and bipolar depression.

CHAPTER 1

Epidemiology of Depression

Ronald C. Kessler *and* Philip S. Wang

The first modern, North American general population epidemiological surveys that included information about depression were carried out in the late 1950s in the Midtown Manhattan Study (Srole, Langner, et al., 1962) and the Stirling County Study (Leighton, Harding, et al., 1963). Researchers in these early surveys used dimensional screening scales of nonspecific psychological distress to pinpoint respondents with likely mental disorders, then administered clinical interviews to the respondents. The outcome of primary interest was a global measure of mental disorder rather than individual diagnoses. No prevalence estimates of depression were reported. The screening scales in these studies, however, included a number of items that assessed depressed mood and other symptoms that have subsequently become part of the depressive syndrome. It is possible to make rough estimates about the prevalence and correlates of depressive disorders from these data (Murphy, Laird, et al., 2000).

In later surveys, variants on the screening scales used in the Midtown Manhattan and Stirling County studies were generally used without clinical follow-up (see Link & Dohrenwend, 1980, for a review). Scale scores were sometimes dichotomized to define "cases" of mental disorder based on some external standard of a clinically relevant cut point, although there was ongoing controversy about the appropriate decision rules for defining cases (Seiler, 1973). To resolve this controversy, structured diagnostic interviews appropriate for use in community surveys were developed in the late 1970s. The Diagnostic Interview Schedule (DIS; Robins, Helzer, et al., 1981) was the first of these instruments. Dimensional screening scales continued to be widely used to screen for mental illness in primary care (Goldberg, 1972), and to assess symptom severity and treatment effectiveness among patients in treatment for mental disorders (Derogatis, 1977) even after the introduction of the DIS. However, psychiatric epidemiologists, influenced by the widely published results of the Epidemiologic Catchment Area Study (ECA; Robins & Regier, 1991), which was based on the DIS, largely abandoned the study of dimensional distress measures in favor of dichotomous case classifications in general population surveys.

We now have had three decades of experience with community epidemiological surveys using fully structured diagnostic interviews like the DIS and the more recently developed Composite International Diagnostic Interview (CIDI; Robins, Wing, et al., 1988), the Primary Care Evaluation of Mental Disorders (PRIME-MD; Spitzer, Williams, et al., 1994), and the Mini-International Neuropsychiatric Interview (MINI; Sheehan, Lecrubier, et al., 1998). It is clear from this experience that fully structured diagnostic interviews, although useful, in and of themselves are inadequate to provide the information needed by health policy planners concerning the magnitude of the problem of untreated depression. The reason for this is that the DSM and ICD criteria are so broad that close to one-half of people in the general population receive one or more diagnoses on a lifetime basis (Kessler, Berglund, et al., 2005a) and close to one-fifth at any one point in time (Kessler, Chiu, et al., 2005; Kessler & Frank, 1997). With prevalence estimates as high as these, the dichotomous case data provided in diagnostic interviews need to be supplemented with dimensional information on severity to be useful to health policy planners (Regier, Kaelber, et al., 1998).

Only the most recently available adult general population epidemiological data on the prevalence of major depression include dimensional measures of severity. This is an important expansion of previous research in light of the suggestion by some commentators that the majority of community cases meeting criteria for major depression have fairly mild disorders (Regier, Narrow, et al., 2000). The first part of this chapter presents a broad overview of the main findings in the literature on the descriptive epidemiology of major depression, including the most recent evidence on clinical severity. The second part of the chapter expands the discussion of severity by reviewing available data on the consequences of depression as assessed in community surveys. The third section reviews epidemiological data on patterns of help seeking for depression. We conclude the chapter by describing promising directions for future research.

DESCRIPTIVE EPIDEMIOLOGY

Point Prevalence

Community surveys that assess depression with symptom screening scales find that up to 20% of adults and up to 50% of children and adolescents report depressive symptoms during recall periods between 1 week and 6 months (Kessler, Avenevoli, et al., 2001). There is a U-shaped distribution of mean scores in these surveys in relation to age, with the highest scores found among the youngest and the oldest respondents and the lowest among people in midlife (Kessler, Foster, et al., 1992). Point prevalence estimates for DSM major depression (MD) in surveys that use structured diagnostic interviews are considerably lower. Rates of current MD are typically less than 1% in samples of children (reviewed by Merikangas & Angst, 1995), as high as 6% in samples of adolescents (reviewed by Kessler, Avenevoli, et al., 2001), and in the range 2–4% in samples of adults (WHO International Consortium in Psychiatric Epidemiology, 2000).

The discrepancy between the high prevalence of symptoms in screening scales and the comparatively low prevalence of depressive disorders means that many people have subsyndromal depressive symptoms. Recent epidemiological studies have started to investigate these subsyndromal symptoms using the diagnostic criteria for minor depression (mD) and recurrent brief depression (RBD) stipulated in DSM-IV (American Psychiatric Association, 1994). MD requires 2 weeks of clinically significant dysphoria or anhedonia (or irritability among children), along with a total of five symptoms. mD, in comparison, requires two to four symptoms with the same severity and duration requirements as MD, whereas RBD requires the repeated occurrence of the same number and severity of symptoms as MD for several days each month over the course of a full year. These recent studies have documented rates of subsyndromal depression among both adolescents (Kessler & Walters, 1998a) and adults (Judd, Akiskal, et al., 1997) that are as high as, if not higher than, the rates of MD. In addition, a longitudinal study of adolescents followed into adulthood found that subsyndromal depression is a powerful predictor of the subsequent onset of MD (Angst, Sellaro, et al., 2000).

Twelve-Month Prevalence

Many community surveys report 12-month prevalence of depression (i.e., percentage of respondents who had an episode of depression some time in the 12 months before the interview), based on the fact that public health planning efforts are typically made on an annual basis. The most recent national estimate comes from the National Comorbidity Survey Replication (NCS-R; Kessler & Merikangas, 2004), a nationally representative household survey carried out in 2001–2003. Twelve-month prevalence of DSM-IV major depressive disorder (MDD) was 6.6%, equivalent to a national population projection of approximately 13 million adults in the United States with 12-month MDD (Kessler, Berglund, et al., 2003). These estimates are intermediate between those in earlier large-scale U.S. surveys (Blazer, Kessler, et al., 1994; Weissman, Livingston, et al., 1991) and very similar to estimates in a separate national survey carried out at about the same time as the NCS-R (Hasin, Goodwin, et al., 2005). The NCS-R estimates are likely to be more accurate than those in these other surveys in that the concordance between CIDI diagnoses and independent clinical diagnoses in the NCS-R is higher than in earlier community epidemiological surveys. However, the 12-month prevalence estimate is lower in the NCS-R than that a decade earlier in the baseline NCS (Blazer, Kessler, et al., 1994) due to the fact DSM-IV criteria for MDD are stricter than the DSM-III-R criteria used in the earlier survey.

Lifetime Prevalence

Epidemiological surveys that administer diagnostic interviews generally assess lifetime prevalence of MD and estimate age-of-onset distributions from retrospective reports. Lifetime prevalence estimates of MD in U.S. surveys have ranged widely, from as low as 6% (Weissman, Livingston, et al., 1991) to as high as 25% (Lewinsohn, Rohde, et al., 1991). The estimate in the NCS (Kessler, McGonagle, et al., 1994), which interviewed people in the 15–54 age range, was 15.8% using DSM-III-R criteria. The estimate in the NCS-R, which interviewed people in the age range 18+, was 16.6% using DSM-IV criteria (Kessler, Berglund, et al., 2005a). Clinical reappraisal data confirm the validity of the NCS-R estimate (Haro, Arbabzadeh-Bouchez, et al., 2006), which suggests that more than 30 million adults in the United States have met criteria for MDD at some time in their life.

Age of Onset

It is important to recognize that the lifetime prevalence estimates represent prevalence to date rather than lifetime risk. Some of the survey respondents who never had an episode of MDD will have one at some later date. Lifetime risk can be estimated with actuarial methods that use retrospective age-of-onset (AOO) reports among lifetime cases to project risk throughout the life course for respondents who have not yet passed through the risk period for first onset. This type of analysis was carried out in the NCS-R (Kessler, Berglund, et al., 2005a). Projected lifetime risk of MDD was estimated at 23.3% compared to the observed lifetime prevalence to date of 16.6%. The roughly 40% higher risk than prevalence is due to the fact that the AOO distribution of MDD is quite wide, with a median estimated AOO of age 32 and an interquartile range (i.e., 25th to 75th percentiles) between ages 19 and 44, and an estimated 10% of all lifetime cases not having first onsets until after age 55.

In considering these results, it is important to recognize that the NCS-R lifetime risk projections are based on the assumption that conditional risk of first onset at given ages is constant across cohorts. This assumption is clearly incorrect, as shown by the fact that the AOO curves differ substantially by cohort, with estimated risk successively higher in each younger cohort (Kessler, Berglund, et al., 2005a). This pattern of intercohort variation could be due to the risk of depression increasing in successively more recent cohorts, to various methodological possibilities involving cohort-related differences in willingness to admit depression or to recall past episodes of depression (Giuffra & Risch, 1994), or to some combination of substantive and methodological possibilities.

There is no way to adjudicate among these contending interpretations definitively with cross-sectional data. Longitudinal data are needed. One published report that presented such data made a comparison of depression prevalence estimates in two national surveys administered in 1991–1992 and 2001–2002 that used similar (but not identical) assessments of 12-month episodes (Compton, Conway, et al., 2006). The comparison suggested that the prevalence of depression increased significantly over the decade of the 1990s. This result can be called into question, however, based on the fact that the baseline prevalence estimate (3.3%) was implausibly low due to methodological limitations in the assessment method that were corrected in the second survey. Researchers would have expected these corrections to result in a substantial increase in the prevalence estimate. The prevalence estimate in the second survey was very similar to that obtained in the NCS-R. A global comparison of 12-month prevalence in the NCS-R and the NCS, using identical measures, showed no evidence of an increase in 12-month prevalence over the decade of the 1990s (Kessler, Demler, et al., 2005). A similar result was found in a comparison of the 12-month prevalence of suicidal ideation, plans, and attempts, none of which changed between the early 1990s and the early 2000s in the NCS-R compared to the NCS (Kessler, Berglund, et al., 2005b).

Subtypes

A number of proposals have been made to subtype the diagnosis of MD based on symptom profiles (reviewed by Kendell, 1976). The most consistent suggestion concerns a distinction between depression with vegetative symptoms (e.g., weight loss, insomnia, appetite loss) and with reverse-vegetative symptoms (e.g., weight gain, hypersomnia, appetite increase) (Eaton, Dryman, et al., 1989). Between one-third and one-fourth of people with MD have a reverse-vegetative symptom profile, with some evidence that this atypical depression is more common among women than men, and more strongly associated than is vegetative depression with a family history of depression. There is little evidence, in comparison, that atypical depression is more persistent or severe than typical depression. Indeed, in one analysis of depression subtyping, typicality and severity emerged as separate and largely independent subtyping dimensions (Sullivan, Kessler, et al., 1998).

Another important subtyping distinction concerns the existence of cyclical depression. Two cycling depressive subtypes have been identified exclusive of those associated with bipolar disorder: seasonal affective disorder (SAD; Rosenthal, Sack, et al., 1984) and premenstrual mood disorder (Halbreich, 1997). Community surveys find that 10% or more of people in the general population report seasonal variations in depressed mood and related symptoms (e.g., Booker & Hellekson, 1992). Seasonal depression is typically most common in the winter months and more prevalent in northern than in southern latitudes. However, the prevalence of DSM narrowly defined SAD, which requires a lifetime diagnosis of recurrent MD or mD and at least two-thirds of all episodes following a seasonal pattern, is much less common. Indeed, Blazer, Kessler, and colleagues (1998) found that only 1% of the population meet narrowly defined criteria for SAD, representing only about 5% of all people with mD or MD. Among people with clinical depression, Blazer, Kessler, and colleagues found that SAD was somewhat more common among men than among women, and among older than among younger respondents.

Community surveys show that the majority of women report experiencing some symptom changes associated with their menstrual cycles (Pearlstein & Stone, 1998). Only between 4 and 6% of women, however, report what appears to be a premenstrual mood disorder (PMD; Sveindottir & Backstrom, 2000). A diagnosis of PMD requires a clear and recurring pattern of onset and offset of five or more mood and related symptoms at specific points in the majority of menstrual cycles over the course of a full year. Assessments with daily mood diaries over two or more menstrual cycles (Freeman, DeRubeis, et al., 1996) typically show that only about half of the women who report cyclical mood problems actually have PMD. The others have more chronic syndromal or subsyndromal mood disorders that are sometimes exacerbated by menstrual symptoms. There is currently a great deal of interest in PMDs among depression researchers based on evidence of family aggregation with MD and responsiveness to selective serotonin reuptake inhibitors but not tricyclic antidepressants (Freeman, Rickels, et al., 1999). There is also controversy, however, regarding appropriate diagnostic and assessment criteria (Severino, 1996). Community epidemiological data are scant due to the logistic complications created by the fact that a definitive diagnosis requires the collection of daily mood diaries across two or more menstrual cycles. Such diaries are typically collected only in clinical samples, although a few small community surveys have collected diary data as well (e.g., Sveindottir & Backstrom, 2000). Given the existence of so many uncertainties in this area of investigation, a large, representative epidemiological survey of PMD using diary data would be very valuable.

Another potentially important subtyping distinction that has received less empirical attention concerns the presence of irritability. Clinical studies of depressed children and adolescents show that irritability is the single most frequently reported symptom in moderate depression (Crowe, Ward, et al., 2006). This observation is consistent with the DSM-IV stipulation that irritability is a core symptom of MD in children and adolescents. However, DSM-IV does not include irritability as a symptom of MDD among adults, despite the fact that irritability is commonly found in clinical samples of adults with MDD (Perlis, Fraguas, et al., 2005). The clinical literature also suggests that irritability might be a meaningful subtyping variable in MDD, with irritable cases more likely than nonirritable cases to be female, young, unemployed, more severely depressed, lower in functional status and quality of life, and to have a history of at least one suicide attempt (Perlis, Fraguas, et al., 2005). These differences are of considerable importance in light of evidence that irritability with anger attacks might be present in more than one-third of patients with MDD (Fava, Nierenberg, et al., 1997).

Course

Little longitudinal research has studied the course of depression in general population samples (but for important exceptions, see Angst & Merikangas, 1997; Lewinsohn, Rohde, et al., 2000). Cross-sectional surveys, however, consistently find that the prevalence ratio of 12-month MD versus lifetime MD is in the range between .5 and .6 (Kessler, McGonagle, et al., 1993). This means that between one-half and two-thirds of people who have ever been clinically depressed will be in a MD episode in any given year over the remainder of their lives. At least three separate processes contribute to the size of this ratio: the probability of a first episode becoming chronic; the probability of episode recurrence among people with a history of MD who are not chronically depressed; and speed of episode recovery among people with recurrent MD episodes.

Epidemiological studies show that the first of these three processes is quite small, with only a small fraction of 1% of people in the population reporting a single lifetime depressive episode that persists for many years (Kessler, McGonagle, et al., 1993). The prevalences of dysthymia and chronic mD are somewhat higher, but still only in the range of 3–4% combined in the total population (Kessler, McGonagle, et al., 1994). Episode recurrence, in contrast, is very common, with more than 80% of people with a history of MD having recurrent episodes (Kessler, Berglund, et al., 2003). In the NCS, the median number of episodes was seven among respondents with an age of first onset more than a decade prior to the interview, and over 90% of all episodes in the year prior to the interview were recurrences rather than first onsets. Finally, speed of episode recovery appears to be highly variable, although the epidemiological evidence is slim. Only two large community surveys have studied speed of episode recovery. One found that 40% of cases of MDD recovered by 5 weeks and over 90% by 1 year (McLeod, Kessler, et al., 1992). The other found that the median time to recovery was 6 weeks, with over 90% recovered within a year (Kendler, Walters, et al., 1997). Very few of the people with short episodes ever come to clinical attention, which means that time to recovery is considerably longer in clinical samples (Brugha, Bebbington, et al., 1990).

Comorbidity

Studies of diagnostic patterns in community samples show that there is substantial lifetime and episode comorbidity between depression and other mental disorders and substance use disorders (Kessler, Berglund, et al., 2003). Indeed, comorbidity is the norm among people with depression. In the NCS-R, nearly three-fourths of respondents with lifetime MDD also met criteria for at least one of the other DSM-IV disorders assessed in the survey (Kessler, Berglund, et al., 2003). This includes 59% with at least one lifetime comorbid anxiety disorder, 31.9% with at least one lifetime comorbid impulse control disorder, and 24.0% with at least one lifetime comorbid substance use disorder. Lifetime comorbidity is even higher among respondents with 12-month MDD, implying that comorbid MDD is more persistent (i.e., more likely to be either chronic or recurrent) than pure MDD. Approximately two-thirds (65.2%) of respondents with 12-month MDD meet criteria for at least one other 12-month disorder, with comorbid anxiety disorders (57.5%) again more common than either comorbid substance use disorders (8.5%) or comorbid impulse control disorders (20.8%). Comparison of retrospective AOO reports shows that MDD is temporally primary (i.e., reported to have started at an earlier age) in relation to all other comorbid disorders in only 12.4% of lifetime cases and 12.2% of 12-month cases, although temporal priority is much more common in cases of comorbidity with substance use disorders (41.3–49.2%) than with either anxiety disorders (13.7–14.6%) or impulse control disorders (17.9–20.9%).

Controversy exists about the extent to which high comorbidity of this sort is an artifact of changes in the diagnostic systems used in almost all recent studies of comorbidity (Frances, Manning, et al., 1992). Beginning with DSM-III and continuing through DSM-IV-TR, these systems dramatically increased the number of diagnostic categories and reduced the number of exclusion criteria, so that many people who would have received only a single diagnosis in previous systems now receive multiple diagnoses. The intention was to retain potentially important differentiating information that could be useful in refining understanding of etiology, course, and likely treatment response (First, Spitzer, et al., 1990). However, it can also be argued that it had the unintended negative consequence of artificially inflating the estimated prevalence of comorbidity. This uncertainty will presumably be resolved in the future by use of established criteria to determine the validity of diagnostic distinctions (Cloninger, 1989). Until that time, though, we are left with a situation in which depression appears to be highly comorbid with a number of other disorders.

The majority of comorbid depression is temporally secondary in the sense that the first onset of depression occurs subsequent to the first onset of at least one other comorbid disorder. Survival analysis of the cross-sectional NCS data using retrospective AOO reports to determine temporal priority shows that a wide range of temporally primary anxiety, substance, and other disorders predict the subsequent first onset of depression (Kessler, Nelson, et al., 1996). Time-lagged effects are strongest for generalized anxiety disorder (7.6) and simple phobia (4.2). There is little evidence of change in these odds ratios as a function of time since onset of the primary disorder. Most of these odds ratios are confined to effects of active primary disorders as opposed to remitted primary disorders. This means that people who currently have these other disorders are at risk of developing depression. The fact that history of remitted anxiety is generally not associated with risk of depression suggests indirectly that anxiety is a risk factor rather than a risk marker. Two important exceptions, though, are early-onset simple phobia and panic, both of which appear to be markers rather than risk factors. The key evidence here is that people with a history of these disorders have elevated risk of subsequent first onset of depression, even when the primary disorders are no longer active (Kessler, Nelson, et al., 1996).

Clinical Severity

The NCS-R is the only large-scale epidemiological survey of which we are aware that assessed the clinical severity of depression. Respondents who met criteria for 12-month MDD in the NCS-R were administered the Quick Inventory of Depressive Symptomatology Self-Report (QIDS-SR; Rush, Carmody, et al., 2000) to assess symptom severity in the worst month of the past year. The QIDS-SR, a fully structured measure, is strongly related to the Hamilton Rating Scale for Depression (HRSD; Hamilton, 1960). Transformation rules developed for the QIDS-SR were used to convert scores into clinical severity categories mapped to conventional HRSD ranges of *none* (i.e., not clinically depressed), *mild*, *moderate*, *severe*, and *very severe*. Over 99% of respondents with 12-month MDD were independently classified by the QIDS-SR as being clinically depressed during the worst month of the year, with 10.4% of persons with mild, 38.6% with moderate, 38.0% with severe, and 12.9% with very severe depression. QIDS-SR mild through severe cases had average episode durations of 13.8–16.6 weeks, whereas very severe cases had average episode duration of 23.1 weeks during the year. Symptom severity was also strongly related to both role impairment and comorbidity. These results speak directly to the concern that prevalence estimates in community surveys might be upwardly biased due to the inclusion of clinically insignificant cases (Narrow, Rae, et al., 2002). This concern is clearly misplaced with respect to MDD, because close to 90% of 12-month NCS-R cases were classified as moderate, severe, or very severe according to standard HRSD symptom severity thresholds.

CONSEQUENCES OF DEPRESSION

Psychiatric epidemiologists have traditionally been much more interested in discovering modifiable risk factors (e.g., Eaton & Weil, 1955) than in studying the consequences of mental illness (e.g., Faris & Dunham, 1939). This situation has changed in the past two decades, though, because the managed care revolution and the rise of evidence-based medicine have made it necessary to document the societal costs of illness (Gold, Siegel, et al., 1996). Depression has emerged as an important disorder in this new work. Indeed, the WHO Global Burden of Disease (GBD) study ranked depression as the single most burdensome disease in the world in terms of total disability-adjusted life years among people in the middle years of life (Murray & Lopez, 1996). This top ranking was due to a unique combination of high lifetime prevalence, early AOO, high chronicity, and high role impairment.

Role Impairment

The Medical Outcomes Study (Wells, Stewart, et al., 1989) was one of the first population-based studies to collect data on role impairment caused by depression by screening primary care patients for a small number of sentinel conditions, including major depression, and following these patients over time to evaluate their medical costs and role functioning. The role impairments caused by depression were comparable to those caused by seriously impairing, chronic physical disorders. Similar results were subsequently found in the nationally representative general population sample assessed in the MacArthur Foundation's Midlife Development in the United States (MIDUS) survey (Kessler, Mickelson, et al., 2001) and several other large, population-based surveys (Merikangas, Ames, et al., 2007; Stewart, Ricci, et al., 2003; Wang, Beck, et al., 2003). In the NCS-R, MDD was associated with the second largest number of days out of role impairment in the United States of all the chronic physical and mental disorders studied (386.6 million days per year), second only to chronic back/neck pain, and exceeding the number of days of role impairment associated with disorders such as arthritis, cancer, and heart disease (Merikangas, Ames, et al., 2007).

A substantial part of the role impairment caused by depression involves reduced work performance. A recent economic analysis of the costs of depression in the workplace estimated that the annual salary-equivalent costs of depression-related loss of productivity in the United States exceeds $36 billion, including $11.7 billion due to excessive absenteeism, and $24.5 billion due to reduced performance on the job (Kessler, Akiskal, et al., 2006). This is an underestimate of overall workplace costs, because it excludes effects of depression on the performance of coworkers, industrial accidents, turnover, and hiring–training costs. It is important to note that these effects of depression on work performance disappear among remitted cases (Kessler & Frank, 1997), suggesting that effective depression treatment would reduce workplace costs.

Simulations suggest that employers could have a positive return on investment (ROI) in the expanded treatment of depression due to improved work performance (Wang, Patrick, et al., 2006). A definitive effectiveness trial to determine the accuracy of these simulated results is underway (Wang, Simon, et al., 2003), but the results have not yet been reported. Other depression treatment trials, however, have consistently documented significant effects of treatment on work outcomes (Mintz, Mintz, et al., 1992; Rost, Smith, et al., 2004; Wells, Sherbourne, et al., 2000).

Role Transitions

We noted in the discussion of the GBD study that depression has a unique constellation of characteristics that led to its rating by the WHO as the single most burdensome chronic condition in the world among people in the middle years of life. One of the most important of these characteristics is that a sufficiently substantial proportion of people with depression have onsets in childhood, adolescence, and early adulthood that influence life course trajectories in an important way. A series of analyses based on the NCS used retrospectively dated AOO reports to estimate the effects of depression and other mental disorders on early life role transitions. One analysis (Kessler, Foster, et al., 1995) found that early-onset depression prior to completing high school significantly predicted (odds ratio) high school dropout (1.5) and, among high school graduates, predicted failure to enter college (1.6). Depression at the age of high school completion powerfully predicted college dropout among respondents who went to college (2.9). Early-onset depression is also associated with a 2.2 relative odds (2.2) of teenage pregnancy among both girls and boys, as well as elevated rates of failure to use contraception (Kessler, Berglund, et al., 1997). A history of depression prior to marriage predicts both poor marital quality and divorce (1.7; Kessler, Walters, et al., 1998b). Welfare-to-work experiments have documented significant adverse effects of depression on making a successful transition from welfare to work (Danziger, Carlson, et al., 2001).

Other Adverse Consequences of Depression

We noted in the previous subsection that the financial savings to the employer due to increased work productivity with the remission of employee depression are likely to have a positive ROI. Although results of the critical experiment needed to test this hypothesis have not yet been published, another type of published experimental result documents a cost saving of depression treatment for managed care. Specifically, services research shows that people with untreated depression are often heavy users of primary care medical services for vaguely defined physical complaints. This observation has led some clinical researchers to speculate that systematic screening, detection, and treatment of primary care patients with depression might lead to an overall reduction in primary care costs. A series of experiments has shown that a partial offset effect of this sort exists (Katon, Robinson, et al., 1996; Katzelnick, Simon, et al., 2000). The vast majority of depressed patients detected in primary care screening accept treatment for their depression. The average total treatment cost to the managed care system, exclusive of the cost of depression treatment, decreases significantly after these patients' depression is treated. This reduction partially offsets the cost of depression treatment over a follow-up period of 1 year. It is conceivable that the total costs of depression treatment are recovered over a longer time period, but long-term follow-up studies have not yet been carried out to determine whether this is the case.

EPIDEMIOLOGICAL STUDIES OF HELP SEEKING

Speed of Initial Treatment Contact

The findings we reviewed earlier concerning the adverse effects of early-onset depression on role transitions raise an obvious question: Would timely treatment substantially reduce these effects? We do not know the answer. The critical experiment has never been carried out. We do know, though, that timely treatment is the exception rather than the rule, and that this is especially true for early-onset cases. This evidence comes from parallel studies of speed of initial treatment contact based on analysis of the NCS (Kessler, Olfson, et al., 1998), the Mental Health Supplement to the Ontario Health Survey (Olfson, Kessler, et al., 1998), and the NCS-R (Wang, Berglund, et al., 2005). All these surveys asked respondents with a history of depression whether they had ever sought treatment and, if so, their age when first obtaining treatment. Comparisons of reported AOOs with ages of first obtaining treatment were used to study patterns and correlates of delay in seeking treatment. The results showed consistently that delays in initial help seeking are pervasive. Only about one-third of the people who ever sought treatment did so in the same years as the first onset of their MD, whereas the median delay among those who did not seek immediate treatment was more than 5 years. Even more striking was the consistent finding that speed of contact was strongly related to AOO. The vast majority of respondents who reported first onsets of depression in middle age or later sought treatment soon after the onset. Respondents with first onsets in early adulthood, in comparison, were much slower to seek treatment. Respondents with child or adolescent onsets, finally, were by far the slowest of all, with median delays of more than a decade. It is not clear why this is the case, but one plausible hypothesis is that youngsters must rely on adults to initiate a treatment referral. Whatever the case may be, this is an especially disturbing pattern for two reasons. First, early-onset depression is often more severe than later-onset depression. Second, as noted earlier, early-onset depression has powerful effects on critical developmental transitions that affect well-being throughout life. These results strongly suggest that special efforts are needed to reach out to children and adolescents with depression.

Current Service Use

Turning from speed of initial lifetime help seeking to treatment at a point in time, the most recent data from the NCS-R reveal that 56.7% of respondents with 12-month MDD received some type of treatment in the 12 months before interview. The specialty sector was involved in the highest proportion of these cases (54.9%) and the human services sector in the lowest proportion (16.4%) (Kessler, Berglund, et al., 2003). Treatment met conventional criteria for adequacy based on minimal concordance with published treatment guidelines, however, in only 41.7% of cases. This means that no more than 20.9% of all people with 12-month MDD (i.e., 36.9% of the 56.7% in treatment) received adequate treatment. Although a higher proportion of serious-to-severe (72.4%) than mild-to-moderate (47.1%) 12-month NCS-R cases received treatment, severity was not significantly related to either the sector in which treatment was received or the adequacy of treatment. Sector of treatment, however, was found to be related to treatment adequacy, with a significantly higher 62.3% of patients treated in the specialty mental health sector versus 42.4% of patients treated in the general medical sector receiving treatment that conformed with published guidelines. There is clear evidence that depression treatment that fails to conform with treatment guidelines is associated with incomplete recovery and increased risk of recurrence (Melfi, Chawla, et al., 1998).

These results document serious problems in the treatment of people with depression in the United States. Increasing use of some modalities, most notably pharmacotherapies and physician-administered psychotherapies (Olfson, Marcus, et al., 2002), over the past decade has generated hope that depression might now be treated much more effectively than in the past. The NCS-R results suggest that such optimism is premature. Mental health service use for depression remains disturbingly low, both because a substantial proportion of cases do not receive any care in the prior year, and because many of those who successfully access health care fail to get adequate treatment according to established treatment guidelines. These results are broadly consistent with previous studies of treatment quality for mood disorders (Blanco, Laje, et al., 2002; Wang, Berglund, et al., 2000; Wang, Demler, et al., 2002; Young, Klap, et al., 2001).

The frequent use of treatments with uncertain benefit is striking. This is especially worrisome for complementary–alternative medicine (CAM) treatments (e.g., energy healers, massage therapists) that account for a substantial minority of all visits for the treatment of depression despite a paucity of data supporting their efficacy (Eisenberg, Davis, et al., 1998). A challenge for the providers of conventional services is to determine why CAM has such great appeal and whether legitimate aspects related to this appeal (e.g., a greater orientation to patient-centered care) can be adopted by conventional mental health care providers to increase the attractiveness of evidence-based treatments.

On the positive side, the proportion of NCS-R respondents with depression who reported 12-month mental health service use is considerably higher than that found a decade earlier in the baseline NCS (Kessler, Zhao, et al., 1999) and a decade before that in the ECA study (Regier, Narrow, et al., 1993). By far the greatest part of this expansion, though, occurred in the general medical sector. General medical doctors act as gatekeepers responsible for initiating mental health treatments themselves and for deciding whom to triage for specialty care (Forrest, 2003; Trude & Stoddard, 2003). Increasing awareness of mental disorders on the part of primary care physicians, coupled with an increase in consumer demand stimulated by direct-to-consumer advertising, has probably also played a role in this growth (Kroenke, 2003). Nevertheless, the fact that only a small minority of patients treated in the general medical sector receives even minimally adequate care makes these trends concerning. Reasons for the low rate of treatment adequacy are unclear, but they presumably involve both provider (e.g., competing demands, inadequate reimbursements for treating depression, less training and experience in treating depression) and patient factors (e.g., worse compliance with treatments than in mental health specialty sectors) (Pincus, Hough, et al., 2003).

CONCLUSIONS AND FUTURE DIRECTIONS

The epidemiological evidence reviewed here shows clearly that MDD is a commonly occurring, seriously impairing, and often undertreated disorder. MDD occurs in the context of a very high prevalence of depressed mood and a high prevalence of subsyndromal depressive episodes that include mD and RBD. It is also important to recognize that a fairly high proportion of the episodes in existence at any one point in time in the population are associated with bipolar spectrum disorder rather than with MDD. MDD is often recurrent. It is typically comorbid with other mental disorders, and it is usually temporally secondary in the sense that first lifetime onset of MDD usually occurs after the onset of at least one other lifetime comorbid anxiety disorder or impulse control disorder. The structural impairments that occur subsequent to the onset of MDD include low educational attainment, poor marital outcomes (bad marriages, marital disruptions), and poor socioeconomic outcomes (bad jobs, unemployment, low family income). The day-to-day role impairments that occur in conjunction with MDD include high numbers of days out of role and poor performance in both productive and social roles. Although treatments can be effective, there are pervasive delays in initially seeking treatment for depression after first onset. When treatment is obtained, it is often of poor quality when judged against published treatment-quality guidelines. Treatment dropout is common. Treatment-quality improvement programs can correct many of these problems, but such programs are as yet uncommon.

Increased efforts are needed to document the cost-effectiveness of expanded depression treatment and of treatment-quality improvement initiatives. Because employers play such a large part in driving health insurance benefit design in the United States, it is especially important to document the ROI of expanded depression outreach–treatment from the employer perspective. We also need to expand research on modifiable barriers to help seeking for depression and to evaluate the effectiveness of systematic depression screening and outreach programs designed to increase the proportion of depressed people who seek treatment.

In addition, we need to know much more than we currently do about time–space variation in the prevalence and correlates of depression. The WHO World Mental Health (WMH) Survey Initiative, an exciting new undertaking that addresses this issue, is carrying out coordinated nationally representative surveys such as the NCS-R in over 30 countries throughout the world (*www.hcp.med.harvard.edu/wmh*). Although a number of WMH analyses deal with depression, perhaps the most fascinating of these is the attempt to study time–space variation in the association between gender and major depression. The goal here is to determine whether the female preponderance in depression that is found consistently in Western countries exists throughout the world, and whether the magnitude of this association changes over time in specific countries as the roles of women change with the modernization of the country.

We also need to increase our understanding of the epidemiology of depression using genetically informative epidemiological study designs. Important work along these lines has been carried out in regional studies (Kendler & Prescott, 2006), but this needs to be expanded both geographically and conceptually. Epidemiological studies in which DNA is collected also hold great promise (Caspi, Sugden, et al., 2003) and will almost certainly be used more often in the future. Indeed, in a number of the WMH surveys mentioned earlier, DNA is being collected from all respondents to create a repository for future genetic epidemiological studies.

There is currently a great deal of interest in using epidemiological research to help refine the diagnostic criteria for the upcoming DSM and ICD revisions (Zimmerman, McGlinchey, et al., 2006). Epidemiological data can be of great value in evaluating the implications of proposed changes in diagnostic criteria, if they include questions and skip pattern rules to facilitate the analysis of proposed diagnostic changes.

Finally, as we learn more about social consequences and risk factors for depression, we need to increase the extent to which epidemiological studies are blended with quasi-experimental and experimental policy interventions. Kling, Liebman, and colleagues (2007), for example, evaluated the effects of neighborhood disorganization on the mental health of residents by carrying out an epidemiological survey of low-income, single mothers who applied for Department of Housing and Urban Development (HUD) housing vouchers allocated on the basis of a lottery. A random half of the applicants were awarded the vouchers, creating a unique opportunity to study neighborhood effects on the mental health of high-risk children. Experimental manipulations of this sort embedded in larger epidemiological surveys have enormous potential to expand our understanding of the correlates of depression, as well as of other mental disorders. Experiments of nature can be used in this same way. For example, Costello, Mustillo, and colleagues (2003) used the opening of a casino on a Native American reservation midway between the two waves of an epidemiological survey to evaluate the impact of increased parental income on child mental health. Many experiments of nature exist that could be used in a similar way to expand our understanding of the environmental determinants of mood disorders. It is important that we remain alert to the existence of such opportunities and capitalize on them to expand our understanding of environmental influences on the onset and course of depression.

ACKNOWLEDGMENTS

Portions of this chapter have appeared previously in Kessler, Berglund, et al. (2003) and Wang and Kessler (2005). Copyright 2003 by the American Medical Association. All rights reserved. Copyright 2005 by the American Psychiatric Publishing, Inc. All rights reserved. Reprinted by permission. We appreciate the helpful comments of Kathleen Merikangas, Ellen Walters, and the editors on earlier versions of this chapter. Preparation of this chapter was supported by grants from the U.S. Public Health Service (Nos. MH46376, MH49098, MH528611, MH061941, U01-MH060220, and R01-MH070884) and the W.T. Grant Foundation (No. 90135190).

REFERENCES

American Psychiatric Association. (1994). *Diagnostic and statistical manual of mental disorders* (4th ed.). Washington, DC: Author.

Angst, J., & Merikangas, K. (1997). The depressive spectrum: Diagnostic classification and course. *Journal of Affective Disorders, 45,* 31–39; discussion 39–40.

Angst, J., Sellaro, R., et al. (2000). Depressive spectrum diagnoses. *Comprehensive Psychiatry, 41,* 39–47.

Blanco, C., Laje, G., et al. (2002). Trends in the treatment of bipolar disorder by outpatient psychiatrists. *American Journal of Psychiatry, 159,* 1005–1010.

Blazer, D. G., Kessler, R. C., et al. (1994). The prevalence and distribution of major depression in a national community sample: The National Comorbidity Survey. *American Journal of Psychiatry, 151,* 979–986.

Blazer, D. G., Kessler, R. C., et al. (1998). Epidemiology of recurrent major and minor depression with a seasonal pattern: The National Comorbidity Survey. *British Journal of Psychiatry, 172,* 164–167.

Booker, J. M., & Hellekson, C. J. (1992). Prevalence of seasonal affective disorder in Alaska. *American Journal of Psychiatry, 149,* 1176–1182.

Brugha, T. S., Bebbington, P. E., et al. (1990). Gender, social support and recovery from depressive disorders: A prospective clinical study. *Psychological Medicine, 20,* 147–156.

Caspi, A., Sugden, K., et al. (2003). Influence of life stress on depression: Moderation by a polymorphism in the 5-HTT gene. *Science, 301,* 386–389.

Cloninger, C. R. (1989). Establishment of diagnostic validity in psychiatric illness: Robins and Guze's method revised. In L. N. Robins & J. Barrett (Eds.), *Validity of psychiatric diagnosis* (pp. 9–18). New York: Raven Press.

Compton, W. M., Conway, K. P., et al. (2006). Changes in the prevalence of major depression and comorbid substance use disorders in the United States between 1991–1992 and 2001–2002. *American Journal of Psychiatry, 163,* 2141–2147.

Costello, E. J., Mustillo, S., et al. (2003). Prevalence and development of psychiatric disorders in childhood and adolescence. *Archives of General Psychiatry, 60,* 837–844.

Crowe, M., Ward, N., et al. (2006). Characteristics of adolescent depression. *International Journal of Mental Health Nursing, 15,* 10–18.

Danziger, S. K., Carlson, M. J., et al. (2001). Post-welfare employment and psychological well-being. *Women's Health, 32,* 47–78.

Derogatis, L. R. (1977). *SCL-90 administration, scoring and procedures manual for the revised version.* Baltimore: Johns Hopkins University.

Eaton, J. W., & Weil, R. J. (1955). *Culture and mental disorders.* Glencoe, IL: Free Press.

Eaton, W. W., Dryman, A., et al. (1989). DSM-III major depressive disorder in the community: A latent class analysis of data from the NIMH Epidemiologic Catchment Area programme. *British Journal of Psychiatry, 155,* 48–54.

Eisenberg, D. M., Davis, R. B., et al. (1998). Trends in alternative medicine use in the United States, 1990–1997: Results of a follow-up national survey. *Journal of the American Medical Association, 280,* 1569–1575.

Faris, R., & Dunham, H. (1939). *Mental disorders in urban areas.* Chicago: University of Chicago Press.

Fava, M., Nierenberg, A. A., et al. (1997). A preliminary study on the efficacy of sertraline and imipramine on anger attacks in atypical depression and dysthymia. *Psychopharmacology Bulletin, 33,* 101–103.

First, M. B., Spitzer, R. L., et al. (1990). Exclusionary principles and the comorbidity of psychiatric diagnoses: A historical review and implications for the future. In J. D. Maser & C. R. Cloninger (Eds.), *Comorbidity of mood and anxiety disorders* (pp. 83–109). Washington, DC: American Psychiatric Press.

Forrest, C. B. (2003). Primary care in the United States: Primary care gatekeeping and referrals: Effective filter or failed experiment? *British Medical Journal, 326,* 692–695.

Frances, A., Manning, D., et al. (1992). Relationship of anxiety and depression. *Psychopharmacology, 106*(Suppl.), S82–S86.

Freeman, E. W., DeRubeis, R. J., et al. (1996). Reliability and validity of a daily diary for premenstrual syndrome. *Psychiatry Research, 65,* 97–106.

Freeman, E. W., Rickels, K., et al. (1999). Differential response to antidepressants in women with premenstrual syndrome/premenstrual dysphoric disorder: A randomized controlled trial. *Archives of General Psychiatry, 56,* 932–939.

Giuffra, L. A., & Risch, N. (1994). Diminished recall and the cohort effect of major depression: A stimulation study. *Psychological Medicine, 24,* 375–383.

Gold, M. R., Siegel, J. E., et al. (1996). *Cost-effectiveness in health and medicine.* New York: Oxford University Press.

Goldberg, D. P. (1972). *The detection of psychiatric illness by questionnaire: A technique for the identification and assessment of non-psychotic psychiatric illness.* London: Oxford University Press.

Halbreich, U. (1997). Premenstrual dysphoric disorders: A diversified cluster of vulnerability traits to depression. *Acta Psychiatrica Scandinavica, 95,* 169–176.

Hamilton, M. (1960). A rating scale for depression. *Journal of Neurology, Neurosurgery, and Psychiatry, 23,* 56–62.

Haro, J. M., Arbabzadeh-Bouchez, S., et al. (2006). Concordance of the Composite International Diagnostic Interview Version 3.0 (CIDI 3.0) with standardized clinical assessments in the WHO World Mental Health surveys. *International Journal of Methods in Psychiatric Research, 15,* 167–180.

Hasin, D. S., Goodwin, R. D., et al. (2005). Epidemiology of major depressive disorder: Results from the National Epidemiologic Survey on Alcoholism and Related Conditions. *Archives of General Psychiatry, 62,* 1097–1106.

Judd, L. L., Akiskal, H. S., et al. (1997). The role and clinical significance of subsyndromal depressive symptoms (SSD) in unipolar major depressive disorder. *Journal of Affective Disorders, 45,* 5–17; discussion, 17–18.

Katon, W., Robinson, P., et al. (1996). A multifaceted intervention to improve treatment of depression in primary care. *Archives of General Psychiatry, 53*, 924–932.

Katzelnick, D. J., Simon, G. E., et al. (2000). Randomized trial of a depression management program in high utilizers of medical care. *Archives of Family Medicine, 9*, 345–351.

Kendell, R. E. (1976). The classification of depressions: A review of contemporary confusion. *British Journal of Psychiatry, 129*, 15–28.

Kendler, K. S., & Prescott, C. A. (2006). *Genes, environment, and psychopathology: Understanding the causes of psychiatric and substance use disorders.* New York: Guilford Press.

Kendler, K. S., Walters, E. E., et al. (1997). The prediction of length of major depressive episodes: Results from an epidemiological sample of female twins. *Psychological Medicine, 27*, 107–117.

Kessler, R. C., Akiskal, H. S., et al. (2006). Prevalence and effects of mood disorders on work performance in a nationally representative sample of U.S. workers. *American Journal of Psychiatry, 163*, 1561–1568.

Kessler, R. C., Avenevoli, S., et al. (2001). Mood disorders in children and adolescents: An epidemiologic perspective. *Biological Psychiatry, 49*, 1002–1014.

Kessler, R. C., Berglund, P., et al. (2003). The epidemiology of major depressive disorder: Results from the National Comorbidity Survey Replication (NCS-R). *Journal of the American Medical Association, 289*, 3095–3105.

Kessler, R. C., Berglund, P., et al. (2005a). Lifetime prevalence and age-of-onset distributions of DSM-IV disorders in the National Comorbidity Survey Replication. *Archives of General Psychiatry, 62*, 593–602.

Kessler, R. C., Berglund, P., et al. (2005b). Trends in suicide ideation, plans, gestures, and attempts in the United States, 1990–1992 to 2001–2003. *Journal of the American Medical Association, 293*, 2487–2495.

Kessler, R. C., Berglund, P. A., et al. (1997). Social consequences of psychiatric disorders: II. Teenage parenthood. *American Journal of Psychiatry, 154*, 1405–1411.

Kessler, R. C., Chiu, W. T., et al. (2005). Prevalence, severity, and comorbidity of 12-month DSM-IV disorders in the National Comorbidity Survey Replication. *Archives of General Psychiatry, 62*, 617–627.

Kessler, R. C., Demler, O., et al. (2005). Prevalence and treatment of mental disorders, 1990 to 2003. *New England Journal of Medicine, 352*, 2515–2523.

Kessler, R. C., Foster, C., et al. (1992). The relationship between age and depressive symptoms in two national surveys. *Psychology and Aging, 7*, 119–126.

Kessler, R. C., Foster, C. L., et al. (1995). Social consequences of psychiatric disorders: I. Educational attainment. *American Journal of Psychiatry, 152*, 1026–1032.

Kessler, R. C., & Frank, R. G. (1997). The impact of psychiatric disorders on work loss days. *Psychological Medicine, 27*, 861–873.

Kessler, R. C., McGonagle, K. A., et al. (1993). Sex and depression in the National Comorbidity Survey: I. Lifetime prevalence, chronicity and recurrence. *Journal of Affective Disorders, 29*, 85–96.

Kessler, R. C., McGonagle, K. A., et al. (1994). Lifetime and 12-month prevalence of DSM-III-R psychiatric disorders in the United States: Results from the National Comorbidity Survey. *Archives of General Psychiatry, 51*, 8–19.

Kessler, R. C., & Merikangas, K. R. (2004). The National Comorbidity Survey Replication (NCS-R): Background and aims. *International Journal of Methods in Psychiatric Research, 13*, 60–68.

Kessler, R. C., Mickelson, K. D., et al. (2001). The association between chronic medical conditions and work impairment. In A. S. Rossi (Ed.), *Caring and doing for others: Social responsibility in the domains of family, work, and community* (pp. 403–426). Chicago: University of Chicago Press.

Kessler, R. C., Nelson, C. B., et al. (1996). Comorbidity of DSM-III-R major depressive disorder in the general population: Results from the U.S. National Comorbidity Survey. *British Journal of Psychiatry, 168*(Suppl.), 8–21.

Kessler, R. C., Olfson, M., et al. (1998). Patterns and predictors of treatment contact after first onset of psychiatric disorders. *American Journal of Psychiatry, 155*, 62–69.

Kessler, R. C., & Walters, E. E. (1998a). Epidemiology of DSM-III-R major depression and minor depression among adolescents and young adults in the National Comorbidity Survey. *Depression and Anxiety, 7*, 3–14.

Kessler, R. C., Walters, E. E., et al. (1998b). The social consequences of psychiatric disorders: III. Probability of marital stability. *American Journal of Psychiatry, 155,* 1092–1096.

Kessler, R. C., Zhao, S., et al. (1999). Past-year use of outpatient services for psychiatric problems in the
National Comorbidity Survey. *American Journal of Psychiatry, 156,* 115–123.

Kling, J. R., Liebman, J., et al. (2007). Experimental analysis of neighborhood effects. *Econometrica, 75,*
83–119.

Kroenke, K. (2003). Patients presenting with somatic complaints: Epidemiology, psychiatric comorbidity
and management. *International Journal of Methods in Psychiatric Research, 12,* 34–43.

Leighton, D. C., Harding, J. S., et al. (1963). *The character of danger: Vol. 3. The Stirling County Study of
psychiatric disorder and sociocultural environment.* New York: Basic Books.

Lewinsohn, P. M., Rohde, P., et al. (1991). Age and depression: Unique and shared effects. *Psychology
and Aging, 6,* 247–260.

Lewinsohn, P. M., Rohde, P., et al. (2000). Natural course of adolescent major depressive disorder in a
community sample: Predictors of recurrence in young adults. *American Journal of Psychiatry, 157,*
1584–1591.

Link, B. G., & Dohrenwend, B. P. (1980). Formulation of hypotheses about the true relevance of demoralization in the United States. In B. P. Dohrenwend, B. S. Dohrenwend, M. S. Gould, B. Link, R.
Neugebauer, & R. Wunsch-Hitzig (Eds.), *Mental illness in the United States: Epidemiological estimates* (pp. 114–132). New York: Praeger.

McLeod, J. D., Kessler, R. C., et al. (1992). Speed of recovery from major depressive episodes in a community sample of married men and women. *Journal of Abnormal Psychology, 101,* 277–286.

Melfi, C. A., Chawla, A. J., et al. (1998). The effects of adherence to antidepressant treatment guidelines
on relapse and recurrence of depression. *Archives of General Psychiatry, 55,* 1128–1132.

Merikangas, K. R., Ames, M., et al. (2007). The associations of mental and physical conditions with role
disability in the U.S. adult household population. *Archives of General Psychiatry, 64,* 1108–1180.

Merikangas, K. R., & Angst, J. (1995). The challenge of depressive disorders in adolescence. In M. Rutter
(Ed.), *Psychosocial disturbances in young people: Challenges for prevention* (pp. 131–165). Cambridge, UK: Cambridge University Press.

Mintz, J., Mintz, L. I., et al. (1992). Treatments of depression and the functional capacity to work. *Archives of General Psychiatry, 49,* 761–768.

Murphy, J. M., Laird, N. M., et al. (2000). A 40-year perspective on the prevalence of depression: The
Stirling County Study. *Archives of General Psychiatry, 57,* 209–215.

Murray, C. J. L., & Lopez, A. D. (Eds.). (1996). *The global burden of disease: A comprehensive assessment of mortality and disability from diseases, injuries, and risk factors in 1990 and projected to
2020.* Cambridge, MA: Harvard University Press.

Narrow, W. E., Rae, D. S., et al. (2002). Revised prevalence estimates of mental disorders in the United
States: Using a clinical significance criterion to reconcile two surveys' estimates. *Archives of General
Psychiatry, 59,* 115–123.

Olfson, M., Kessler, R. C., et al. (1998). Psychiatric disorder onset and first treatment contact in the
United States and Ontario. *American Journal of Psychiatry, 155,* 1415–1422.

Olfson, M., Marcus, S. C., et al. (2002). National trends in the use of outpatient psychotherapy. *American Journal of Psychiatry, 159,* 1914–1920.

Pearlstein, T., & Stone, A. B. (1998). Premenstrual syndrome. *Psychiatric Clinics of North America, 21,*
577–590.

Perlis, R. H., Fraguas, R., et al. (2005). Prevalence and clinical correlates of irritability in major depressive disorder: A preliminary report from the Sequenced Treatment Alternatives to Relieve Depression Study. *Journal of Clinical Psychiatry, 66,* 159–166.

Pincus, H. A., Hough, L., et al. (2003). Emerging models of depression care: Multi-level ("6 P") strategies. *International Journal of Methods in Psychiatric Research, 12,* 54–63.

Regier, D. A., Kaelber, C. T., et al. (1998). Limitations of diagnostic criteria and assessment instruments for
mental disorders: Implications for research and policy. *Archives of General Psychiatry, 55,* 109–115.

Regier, D. A., Narrow, W. E., et al. (1993). The de facto U.S. mental and addictive disorders service system: Epidemiologic catchment area prospective 1-year prevalence rates of disorders and services.
Archives of General Psychiatry, 50, 85–94.

Regier, D. A., Narrow, W. E., et al. (2000). The epidemiology of mental disorder treatment need: Community estimates of "medical necessity." In G. Andrews & S. Henderson (Eds.), *Unmet need in psychiatry: Problems, resources, responses* (pp. 41–58). Cambridge, UK: Cambridge University Press.

Robins, L. N., Helzer, J. E., et al. (1981). *NIMH Diagnostic Interview Schedule: Version III*. Rockville, MD: National Institute of Mental Health.

Robins, L. N., & Regier, D. A. (Eds.). (1991). *Psychiatric disorders in America: The Epidemiologic Catchment Area study*. New York: Free Press.

Robins, L. N., Wing, J., et al. (1988). The Composite International Diagnostic Interview: An epidemiologic instrument suitable for use in conjunction with different diagnostic systems and in different cultures. *Archives of General Psychiatry, 45*, 1069–1077.

Rosenthal, N. E., Sack, D. A., et al. (1984). Seasonal affective disorder. A description of the syndrome and preliminary findings with light therapy. *Archives of General Psychiatry, 41*, 72–80.

Rost, K., Smith, J. L., et al. (2004). The effect of improving primary care depression management on employee absenteeism and productivity: A randomized trial. *Medical Care, 42*, 1202–1210.

Rush, A. J., Carmody, T., et al. (2000). The Inventory of Depressive Symptomatology (IDS): Clinician (IDS-C) and Self-Report (IDS-SR) ratings of depressive symptoms. *International Journal of Methods in Psychiatric Research, 9*, 45–59.

Seiler, L. H. (1973). The 22-item scale used in field studies of mental illness: A question of method, a question of substance, and a question of theory. *Journal of Health and Social Behavior, 14*, 252–264.

Severino, S. K. (1996). Premenstrual dysphoric disorder: Controversies surrounding the diagnosis. *Harvard Review of Psychiatry, 3*, 293–295.

Sheehan, D. V., Lecrubier, Y., et al. (1998). The Mini-International Neuropsychiatric Interview (M.I.N.I.): The development and validation of a structured diagnostic psychiatric interview for DSM-IV and ICD-10. *Journal of Clinical Psychiatry, 59*(Suppl. 20), 22–33.

Spitzer, R. L., Williams, J. B., et al. (1994). Utility of a new procedure for diagnosing mental disorders in primary care: The PRIME-MD 1000 study. *Journal of the American Medical Association, 272*, 1749–1756.

Srole, L., Langner, T. S., et al. (1962). *Mental health in the metropolis: The Midtown Study*. New York: McGraw-Hill.

Stewart, W. F., Ricci, J. A., et al. (2003). Lost productive work time costs from health conditions in the United States: Results from the American Productivity Audit. *Journal of Occupational and Environmental Medicine, 45*, 1234–1246.

Sullivan, P. F., Kessler, R. C., et al. (1998). Latent class analysis of lifetime depressive symptoms in the National Comorbidity Survey. *American Journal of Psychiatry, 155*, 1398–1406.

Sveindottir, H., & Backstrom, T. (2000). Prevalence of menstrual cycle symptom cyclicity and premenstrual dysphoric disorder in a random sample of women using and not using oral contraceptives. *Acta Obstetricia et Gynecologica Scandinavica, 79*, 405–413.

Trude, S., & Stoddard, J. J. (2003). Referral gridlock: Primary care physicians and mental health services. *Journal of General Internal Medicine, 18*, 442–449.

Wang, P. S., Beck, A., et al. (2003). Chronic medical conditions and work performance in the health and work performance questionnaire calibration surveys. *Journal of Occupational and Environmental Medicine, 45*, 1303–1311.

Wang, P. S., Berglund, P., et al. (2000). Recent care of common mental disorders in the United States: Prevalence and conformance with evidence-based recommendations. *Journal of General Internal Medicine, 15*, 284–292.

Wang, P. S., Berglund, P., et al. (2005). Failure and delay in initial treatment contact after first onset of mental disorders in the National Comorbidity Survey Replication. *Archives of General Psychiatry, 62*, 603–613.

Wang, P. S., Demler, O., et al. (2002). Adequacy of treatment for serious mental illness in the United States. *American Journal of Public Health, 92*, 92–98.

Wang, P. S., Patrick, A., et al. (2006). The costs and benefits of enhanced depression care to employers. *Archives of General Psychiatry, 63*, 1345–1353.

Wang, P. S., Simon, G., et al. (2003). The economic burden of depression and the cost-effectiveness of treatment. *International Journal of Methods in Psychiatric Research, 12*, 22–33.

Weissman, M. M., Livingston, B. M., et al. (1991). Affective disorders. In L. N. Robins & D. A. Regier (Eds.), *Psychiatric disorders in America: The Epidemiologic Catchment Area study* (pp. 53–80). New York: Free Press.

Wells, K. B., Sherbourne, C., et al. (2000). Impact of disseminating quality improvement programs for depression in managed primary care: A randomized controlled trial. *Journal of the American Medical Association, 283,* 212–220.

Wells, K. B., Stewart, A., et al. (1989). The functioning and well-being of depressed patients: Results from the Medical Outcomes Study. *Journal of the American Medical Association, 262,* 914–919.

WHO International Consortium in Psychiatric Epidemiology. (2000). Cross-national comparisons of the prevalences and correlates of mental disorders. *Bulletin of the World Health Organization, 78,* 413–426.

Young, A. S., Klap, R., et al. (2001). The quality of care for depressive and anxiety disorders in the United States. *Archives of General Psychiatry, 58,* 55–61.

Zimmerman, M., McGlinchey, J. B., et al. (2006). Diagnosing major depressive disorder introduction: An examination of the DSM-IV diagnostic criteria. *Journal of Nervous and Mental Disease, 194,* 151–154.

CHAPTER 2

Course and Outcome of Depression

Robert J. Boland *and* Martin B. Keller

In the past several decades, we have gained an increasing understanding of the course of depression. Previously viewed as an acute and self-limiting illness, it is now clear that, for many individuals, depression is a lifelong illness. Furthermore, we now increasingly appreciate the importance of course in affecting associated psychosocial outcomes, comorbidities, and treatment. This understanding is a result of a number of important investigations, including long-term naturalistic studies of depression that have been conducted over the last several decades. This chapter reviews these studies and their implications for understanding depression.

DEFINITION OF TERMS: THE CHANGE POINTS IN DEPRESSION

For longitudinal studies to be useful, some agreement had to be reached in defining the key change points in a depressive course. Early studies were hindered by the lack of any such consensus, making the results difficult to compare. Terms such as *remission* or *recovery* were used inconsistently and sometimes interchangeably. For this reason, a MacArthur Foundation task force (Frank et al., 1991) recommended that the change points be described with the following terms: *episode, remission, response, relapse,* and *recurrence.*
An *episode* is defined as having a certain number of symptoms for a certain duration. Although the exact values for these variables may differ depending on the study, researchers have generally followed the standards of the *Diagnostic and Statistical Manual of Mental Disorders,* currently in its fourth edition (DSM-IV; American Psychiatric Association, 1994).
A *remission,* conceptually, is the point at which an episode ends. It is defined by a period of time in which an individual no longer meets criteria for the disorder. Such a remission can be partial or full. In *partial remission,* an individual still has more than minimal symptoms. *Full remission* is defined as the point at which an individual no longer meets criteria for the disorder and has no more than minimal symptoms (it should be noted that full remission does not necessarily imply the absence of any symptoms).

A remission may or may not be related to an intervention. A *response*, however, is a remission that is due to a treatment intervention. Response is, in reality, an "apparent" response, due to the inherent difficulty in establishing causality between treatment and response. The assumption is that a remission occurring at or near the time of a treatment intervention is most likely causally related. Such an assumption is difficult to prove.

Episode, *response*, and *remission* are all acute phenomena. Of concern to the investigator of disease course is the point at which an illness has ended: When has the patient *recovered*? Such a definition is important in differentiating *relapse* from *recurrence*.

Recovery is defined as a full remission that lasts for a defined period. Conceptually, it implies the end of an episode of the illness, not the end of the illness itself. A *relapse* is defined as the early return of symptoms following an apparent response. Treatment that occurs during this interval is referred to as *continuation treatment* and conventionally is defined as lasting from 4 to 6 months after the initial response. Episodes that occur during this period are relapses.

A *recurrence* refers to a new episode occurring after recovery from a previous episode. During continuation treatment, one expects a relapse to occur soon after discontinuation of treatment, because the treatment has presumably suppressed rather than eradicated the disease. For recurrence, reemergence of symptoms does not necessarily occur soon after stopping treatment, because the patient presumably has been brought into a state of well-being. The change points of a course of major depression are illustrated in Figure 2.1.

These definitions rely on a number of assumptions that cannot be proven, because we lack valid biological markers for major depression. The definitions instead rely on statistical likelihoods, and one must decide where to place symptomatic and duration cutoffs. One must also consider whether such cutoffs should be conservative or liberal, and what type of error one is willing to accept. Although not independently validated, these definitions represent reasonable working definitions and are used in some form by most of the studies that are reviewed here.

Beyond these change points, certain other terms are relevant when considering the course of depression. DSM-IV defines *chronic depression* as lasting more than 2 years. Within the general category of chronic depression are a number of subtypes. *Chronic major depressive disorder* describes the continuation of full major depressive symptoms for 2 years

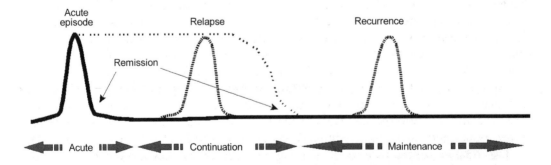

FIGURE 2.1. The change points of depression. The course is divided into the acute, continuation, and maintenance periods. The triple-dotted line (... ... ...) illustrates the acute and continuation course of an untreated episode; the solid line, a treated episode. The points at which relapse and recurrence would occur are illustrated with dotted lines. If conceptualized as a graph, the *x* axis would be *time* and the *y* axis would be *number of depressive symptoms*.

or more. *Dysthymic disorder,* or *dysthymia,* is a less severe form of chronic depression, in which the symptoms do not reach the level of major depression. *Double depression* describes the presence of dysthymia interspersed with major depression episodes. *Major depressive disorder with poor interepisodic recovery* describes a type of recurrent depression characterized by incomplete remission. Although currently classified independently in DSM-IV, there is some debate as to whether these are distinct subtypes of depression. McCullough and colleagues (2003) looked at 681 outpatients with various forms of chronic depression and found little difference in demographic or clinical variables; they also found that treatment response was similar across the groups, suggesting that differences between the subtypes of chronic depression may be more dimensional than categorical.

STUDYING THE COURSE OF DEPRESSION

Researchers in the 1970s and 1980s suggested that after patients were successfully treated for depression, then discontinued from that treatment, many relapsed back into depression (National Institute of Mental Health [NIMH] Consensus Development Conference Statement, 1985). It seemed that although the symptoms were being controlled by medication, the disease state persisted. By the mid-1980s, the general wisdom was to continue a patient on medications for a certain duration following symptomatic improvement (the *continuation period*). Although the proper length of continuation treatment was not clear, it seemed likely that it should be as long as a usual episode of untreated depression. Recommendations for the continuation period varied widely. For example, the U.S. Department of Health's Clinical Practice Guidelines for the treatment of depression in primary care (Depression Guideline Panel, 1993) recommended a continuation interval of 4 to 9 months—a rather wide range.

Even with adequate continuation treatment, it was clear that some patients had a recurrence of symptoms when treatment was discontinued, even though the discontinuation was well beyond the period assumed for a single episode. Other patients never seemed to recover fully. Understanding the likelihood of such outcomes, and the risk factors for them, became paramount for guiding treatment recommendations.

To shed light on these questions, one had to understand the natural course of depression. Treatment studies alone were not adequate; that is, although treatment studies could establish the effectiveness of a medication at various stages of the illness, one had to understand the natural course of the illness before investigating the effect of interventions on that course. In natural studies of the course of depression patients are followed, often for many years. Because these are "natural studies," there is no systematic intervention; patients may receive treatment in the community, and information about that treatment is collected. However, the investigators generally do not influence the treatment; thus, treatment is considered as one potential variable among many. This approach is called *natural* because the behavior of depression in these studies is presumably more akin to the real-world behavior of the disorder than that in intervention studies with carefully controlled treatment.

The groundwork for such research was laid in the pioneering work of Angst (1986) and his colleagues in Zurich. Beginning in the early 1960s, they identified 173 patients originally hospitalized with major depression, and evaluated this group every 5 years for up to 21 years. This study provided some of the first information regarding the relation between the course and outcome of depression, a good deal of which has been supported by subsequent studies.

Much of the information informing our current understanding of the course of depression is from the Collaborative Depression Study (CDS; Katz & Klerman, 1979). The CDS is a prospective, long-term, naturalistic study of depression that built on the work of Angst, using a larger sample from multiple centers and more up-to-date diagnostic methods. Subjects in the CDS were recruited from patients with depression seeking outpatient or inpatient psychiatric treatment at one of five sites (university or teaching hospitals in Boston, Chicago, Iowa City, New York, and St. Louis) from 1978 to 1981. This study included programs in biological and clinical studies. The data presented here are from the clinical studies program. In the clinical studies program, 555 subjects had an index episode of unipolar major depression. Subjects were examined at 6-month intervals for 5 years, then annually for a minimum of 18 years.

Other studies have added important information on the course of depression. The Medical Outcomes Study (Wells et al., 1989) provided a good deal of information on the relationship of depression to other medical illnesses. It examined the course of five major diseases (myocardial infarction, congestive heart failure, hypertension, diabetes, and depression) in a variety of health care settings (ranging from large medical group to solo practices) and specialties (including psychiatry). More than 20,000 patients from three cities (Los Angeles, Boston, and Chicago) were evaluated annually for 3 years.

Several international studies have added important data as well, including survey data from England (Blacker, Thomas, & Thompson, 1997), France (Limosin et al., 2004), the Netherlands (Ormel, Oldehinkel, Brilman, & van den Brink, 1993), Scandinavia (Kendler, Gatz, Gardner, & Pedersen, 2006; Rytsälä et al., 2006), Poland (Rybakowski, Nowaka, & Kiejna, 2004), New Zealand (Mental Health and General Practice Investigation [MaGPIe] Research Group, 2003), and Australia (Andrews, Henderson, & Hall, 2001). Several large-scale studies have surveyed populations in multiple countries, including the Longitudinal Investigation of Depression Outcomes in Primary Care (LIDO; Simon, Fleck, Lucas, & Bushnell, 2004) study and the World Health Organization (WHO) Collaborative Project on Psychological Problems in General Health Care study (Barkow et al., 2003). The latter study, begun in the early 1990s, is the largest primary care survey to date, involving 15 cities across the world, screening over 25,000 subjects, and conducting Stage II interviews on more than 5,000 persons. Additional studies have examined the course of depression in special populations, including adolescents and the elderly, and these are discussed later in this chapter.

We should emphasize from the start that there are limitations to even the largest of these studies. Most conduct their investigations in clinical settings and may not be representative of the community at large. They are not random samples, and they generally lack control groups. However, as a group, these studies have been successful in observing large numbers of individuals over long periods and are the cornerstone of our expanding knowledge on the course of depression.

RESULTS OF NATURAL STUDIES

Recovery

Early studies suggested that, for many patients, the course of depression might extend beyond the normally accepted periods for an acute major depressive episode. Kerr, Roth, Shapira, and Gurney (1972), following initially hospitalized patients, found that 6% remained ill for the 4 years of the study (again, investigators collected information about treatment but were not directly involved in the treatment). In a prospective follow-up of 96 patients with major depression, Rounsaville, Prusoff, and Padian (1980) found that 12% of subjects had not recovered after 16 months. Other studies show comparable data. In the Zurich study, Angst and colleagues (1973) reported that during the follow-up evaluations, about 13% of patients did not recover from their episode of major depression.

In the CDS, approximately 70% of patients recovered from the index episode of major depression within the first year (Keller, Shapiro, Lavori, & Wolfe, 1982). However, most patients who did not recover in the first year still had not recovered after a much longer time. By 2 years, about one-fifth of the original sample was still depressed; thus, two-thirds of those who remained depressed at 1 year were still in their index episode of depression at 2 years. At 5 years, 12% of patients had not recovered (Keller et al., 1992); by 10 years, 7% had not recovered (Mueller et al., 1996). By 15 years, the number seemed to have leveled off at 6% (Keller & Boland, 1998). The probability of recovery from an index episode is illustrated in Figure 2.2.

The long duration of the CDS allowed the investigators to observe subsequent episodes of major depression that began during the study. This was particularly useful for identifying the onset of symptoms more accurately than with retrospective judgment. Researchers found that, for each new episode of depression, the rates of recovery were similar to those seen during the index episode. For the second episode (the first prospectively observed episode), approximately 8% of the subjects did not recover after 5 years. An analysis of subsequent episodes (the second, third, and fourth prospectively observed episodes) showed similar findings. By the fifth episode, the rate decreases, but not significantly so (Solomon et al., 1997). The probability of recovery after each subsequent episode is illustrated in Figure 2.3.

It appears that for each episode of depression, some individuals—about 10%—remain ill for at least 5 years.

Because the CDS was a naturalistic study, treatment data were collected but not controlled. In a subsequent analysis, investigators did look at a subsample of patients that did not receive any somatic therapy during the illness course. They found that the mean time to recovery in this group was 13 weeks (Posternak, Solomon, & Leon, 2006).

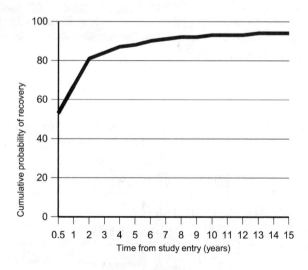

FIGURE 2.2. Collaborative Depression Study (CDS): Recovery from the index episode of depression.

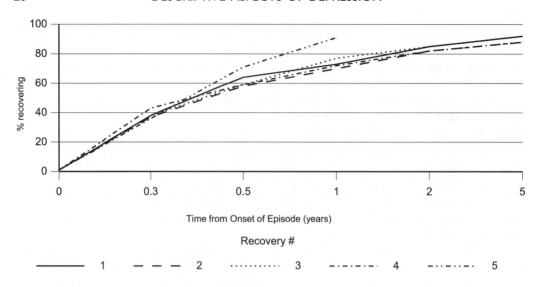

FIGURE 2.3. CDS: Proportion of subjects' recovery from subsequent episodes of depression.

International studies have had varied results, some better and some worse than the CDS. In the Groningen Primary Care Study (Ormel et al., 1993) conducted in the Netherlands, 93% of depressed patients had remitted from their index episode by 1 year. In France, Limosin and colleagues (2004) found a recovery rate of 65% by 6 months, and the WHO study (Barkow et al., 2003) reported that 67% of patients had recovered by 12 months. Perhaps most surprising was the LIDO study (Simon et al., 2004), in which only 35% of patients reported a complete remission by 1 year. The authors of that study did not offer any reason for these lower-than-expected remission rates; it is notable, however, that their definition of *recovery* was complete remission of all depressive symptoms, a more conservative criterion than most other studies.

In general, longitudinal studies suggest that the majority of patients with a major depressive episode recover within a year. However, a substantial number do not recover, and many of these individuals still do not have a remission after 5 years. Once the individual has recovered, each new episode of depression contains the disturbing chance that, this time, he or she may develop a chronic disorder.

Relapse

For the 141 patients in the CDS who recovered from their index episode of major depression, 22% relapsed within 1 year of follow-up (Keller, Lavori, Lewis, & Klerman, 1983). Two international studies have included data on relapse rates. Limosin and colleagues (2004) in France reported that after 6 months of follow-up, 11% of their patients had relapsed after recovery. The Groningen Primary Care Study (Ormel et al., 1993) reported a relapse rate of 30% within that 1-year period.

Various factors have been reported to predict relapse. The CDS found that multiple episodes of major depression, older age, and a history of nonaffective psychiatric illness were predictive (Keller, Lavori, Lewis, et al., 1983). The number of previous episodes of depression was a particularly strong predictor of a relapse. When the characteristics of this relapsed group were also examined, researchers found that the likelihood of remaining depressed for at least a year after a relapse was 22%. Predictors of prolonged time to recovery included a longer length of the index episode, older age, and a lower family income.

Limosin and colleagues (2004) also found recurrent depression to be predictive of relapse, as have most other studies examining relapse. One curious exception was a study based in Australia. Parker, Holmes, and Manicavasagar (1986) found that patients with recurrent depression were more likely to improve at 20 weeks than those with other patterns of depression. The relatively small sample size and short follow-up time of this particular study limit the conclusions, however.

The overall message appears to be that, again, a sizable minority of patients experience a relapse of symptoms after initial recovery. For some of these patients, achieving a subsequent remission will be more difficult.

Recurrence

A number of early studies found high rates of recurrence of depression. Weissman and Kasl (1976) found that two-thirds of women seen for more than 1 year had a recurrence of depression. Rao and Nammalvar (1977), examining more than 100 cases of depression in India for a follow-up of between 3 and 13 years, found that only about 25% of the original group reported no recurrence of symptoms. Angst (1992), reporting on a 10-year follow-up of patients in the Zurich study, found that 75% of the sample had one or more recurrences of depression. Though Angst examined a number of sociodemographic variables, none significantly predicted the recurrence.

In the CDS, there was a 25–40% rate of recurrence after 2 years. These rates of recurrence in the CDS group increased over time: 60% after 5 years (Lavori, Keller, Mueller, & Scheftner, 1994), 75% after 10 years, and 87% after 15 years (Keller & Boland, 1998). This increase in rate continues as long as patients are observed, and at 20 year follow up, 91% of patients have relapsed (Keller, unpublished data, 2007). This suggests that, in contrast to

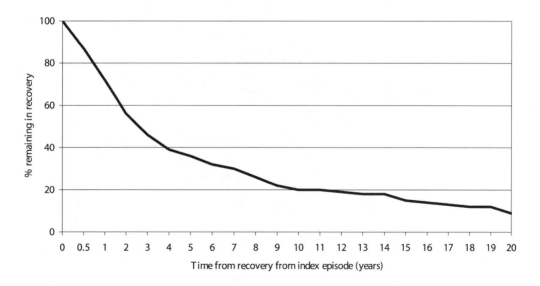

FIGURE 2.4. CDS: Risk of recurrence following recovery from the index episode.

rates of recovery (which level off after 5–10 years), individuals continue to be at a high risk for recurrence after 5, and even 10 years.

These rates of recurrence risk are illustrated in Figure 2.4.

The rates of recurrence tended to increase with subsequent episodes. In a 10-year follow-up to the CDS, nearly two-thirds of individuals who were depressed at the beginning of the study had suffered at least one recurrence (Solomon et al., 1997). The risk of recurrence increased by 16% with each subsequent episode; thus, a patient with five lifetime episodes of major depressive disorder was more than twice as likely to suffer a recurrence as a patient with 1 lifetime episode. These different rates of recurrence are illustrated in Figure 2.5.

The mean time to recurrence decreased with subsequent episodes: 150 weeks for the first prospective recurrence, 83 weeks for the second recurrence, 77 weeks for the third, 68 weeks for the fourth, and 57 weeks for the fifth recurrence (Solomon et al., 2000). However, interepisode duration between individuals was highly variable.

The rate and timing of recurrence seem most dependent on the type of recovery. Patients in the CDS who fully recovered had a much lower rate of recurrence (66%) than did those who had some residual symptoms (87% recurrence rate). The time to recurrence was much longer in the asymptomatic group: The mean was 180 weeks in the asymptomatic group and 33 weeks in the group with residual symptoms.

The predictors for recurrence seemed to change with time. For example, secondary depression, older age at intake, and three or more prior episodes of major depressive disorder predicted recurrence within the first 2 years of follow-up, whereas after 15 years of follow-up, the predictors were female sex, longer episode prior to intake, greater number of prior episodes, and never marrying (Solomon et al., 2000).

The potential risk factors for recurrent depression found in the CDS are summarized in Table 2.1.

Most other large-scale studies are of shorter duration. For example, the LIDO (Simon et al., 2004) and WHO (Barkow et al., 2003) studies followed patients for 1 year—not long

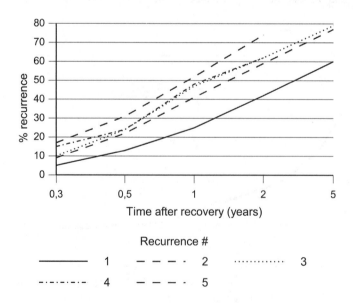

FIGURE 2.5. CDS: Probability of recurrence following recovery from the index episode and subsequent episodes of depression.

TABLE 2.1. Collaborative Depression Study: Risk Factors for Recurrent Depression during Prospective Follow-Up

- History of three or more prior episodes
- Double depression (major depression plus dysthymia)
- Long duration of individual episodes
- Poor symptom control during continuation therapy
- Comorbid anxiety disorder or substance abuse
- Onset after 60 years of age
- Family history of affective disorder
- Female gender
- Never married

enough for meaningful information on recurrence. Other studies that went beyond a year, such as the Groningen study (Ormel et al., 1993), focused on time to remission as the endpoint. Some studies that have looked at recurrence in special populations, such as adolescents and older adults, are discussed separately.

It appears that although the risk of nonrecovery and relapse is of concern, recurrence is a particularly oppressive problem. Most patients experience a recurrence by 5 years, and the rate of recurrence continues upward beyond that time. Thus, although most patients can expect to recover from an episode of depression, the same patients should expect eventually to have a recurrence of their depression.

Subsequent Episodes

It has long been suggested that the risk factors for depressive episodes change with subsequent episodes. Specifically, the depression of earlier episodes has been thought to be more susceptible to environmental stress triggers, whereas later episodes are thought to be more autonomous. A version of this was proposed by Post (2002), who used the "kindling" model associated with seizure activity to suggest that an analogous process underlies recurrent depression. Lewinsohn, Allen, Seeley, and Gotlib (1999) tested this hypothesis, prospectively examining more than 1,700 adolescents who were part of the Oregon Adolescent Depression Project. They found that the number of stressful events was strongly related to first episodes of depression but not to recurrent episodes. Many other studies have had similar findings. For example, Kendler, Thornton, and Gardner (2000), studying female–female twin pairs from the Virginia Twin Registry, reported that the odds ratio between major stressful events and an episode of major depression was high in the case of the first onset of depression but lower for recurrences. Similar relationships have been reported by Ormel, Oldehinkel, and Brilman (2001) and Maciejewski, Prigerson, and Mazure (2001).

This finding has not been consistent, and the reasons may relate to the type of stress being studied. For example, Daley, Hammen, and Rao (2000), in their longitudinal study of adolescent women, found that chronic stress was a more potent trigger of first episode depression than subsequent episodes, but that episodic stress continued to be a predictor for subsequent episodes.

Some of these inconsistencies in findings might also be explained by ambiguities in understanding the potential effect of stress on depression. As discussed by Monroe and Harkness (2005), there is some confusion about the fundamental relationship between stress and depression: Is it that individuals become desensitized to stress over time, or do they become overly sensitized? In the first case, referred to as the *autonomy model*, after the initial few episodes, stress no longer plays a significant role in the etiology of depression, which is instead brought on by other, presumably neurobiological mechanisms. In the latter case, called the *stress sensitivity model*, individuals become overly sensitive to stress, such that even minor events can trigger an episode of depression. Although there are data to support either assumption, the definitive studies are yet to be performed. Monroe and Harkness point out that the different assumptions are testable, because they do predict different observable findings. Longitudinal studies that follow patients through several recurrences and carefully measure stressful events during the course of depression would shed important light on this question.

Rates of Chronicity

As noted in studies such as the CDS, a small but significant number of individuals—approximately 10%—did not recover from a given episode of depression (Keller & Boland, 1998). This seemingly high rate of chronicity was surprising. A reasonable concern about this result was that this patient population may have been unusually treatment resistant. This group of patients sought treatment at one of five major medical centers and, as such, may not truly have represented the general population.

However, other studies have reported similar rates of chronicity; the Groningen study (Ormel et al., 1993), for example, reported a 25% rate of chronicity, and some studies, such as the LIDO study (Simon et al., 2004), have reported much worse rates of recovery than did the CDS.

FACTORS MODERATING COURSE

Age of Onset

Early-Onset Depression

Early-onset depression appears to be associated with poorer outcomes of depression, including a longer time to remission, a lower likelihood of remission, and poorer symptomatic improvement (Keitner, Ryan, Miller, & Norman, 1992). Not all studies have been consistent on these points, and the difference may explained by the variations across studies, including different definitions of depression and of "early onset," different populations examined, and different outcome measures. Results may differ depending on whether investigators concentrate on symptomatic versus functional outcomes. Moses, Leuchter, Cook, and Abrams (2006), for example, found that earlier age of illness onset was predictive of a poorer overall quality of life, even when symptomatic improvement was comparable to that of persons with an older age of onset. This may relate to the longer time spent being depressed, developmental difficulties relating to early-onset depression, or the better social environment that is likely found in individuals with previously good functioning.

Rao, Hammen, and Daley (1999) undertook a study of the course of early-onset depression, examining 155 high school volunteers (average age at entry, ~18 years old) chosen to be demographically representative of their region (Los Angeles County). They found a high risk for depression: Almost half of the group had one or more episodes of major depression during the 5-year study. The risk for recurrence was high as well: Approximately one-fourth of the patients had a relapse in the first year after recovery. Depression in the group had a significantly negative effect on psychosocial functions such as school performance and intimate relationships. Predictors of depression in this group included having witnessed family violence before age 16, having a parent with a psychiatric disorder, and having a nonmood Axis I disorder (Daley et al., 2000). Age of onset was not predictive of the rate of recurrence. This study underscores both the frequency of depression in adolescent women and the fact that the disorder is as highly recurrent in this group as in adult populations.

The similarity of childhood and adolescent depression to adult depression has been found by other groups as well. Birmaher and colleagues (2004), who followed prepubertal children and postpubertal adolescents with no history of depression for 5 years, found that episodes of depression experienced during the study were similar for both groups, both in phenomenology and course of illness. They then divided the group into high- and low-risk depression groups (Williamson, Birmaher, Axelson, Ryan, & Dahl, 2004); this distinction was determined by the presence or absence of a significant family history of a mood disorder. They found that the high-risk group had three times the depression risk of the low-risk group.

Late-Onset Depression

Depression that occurs in old age also carries some risk. The CDS found that older subjects (age 65+) experiencing acute depression had a time to recovery similar to that of younger patients (Mueller et al., 2004); however, they tended to have a more rapid time to recurrence than other groups. The data were most striking for elderly patients who had their first onset of depression in later life.

In this group with late-onset depression, the evidence of increased risk of recurrence and associated treatment resistance may be explained by a number of studies finding that neuroanatomic abnormalities are more likely to play a role in the pathophysiology of this subgroup. Alexopoulos (2006) has described *vascular depression*, a subtype of depression resulting from cerebrovascular disease, and this has been supported by other investigators. For example, Lavretsky and colleagues (2002) found that the risk of chronic depression in older adult patients was directly associated with the severity of cerebrovascular risk factors. In addition, they found that those men with late onset depression were more likely to have cerebrovascular-related neuroradiological abnormalities; in patients with early-onset depression, there was no gender difference (Lavretsky, Lesser, Wohl, & Miller, 1998).

The presence of cognitive decline may also have a deleterious effect on depression. Using data from the IMPACT (Improving Mood: Promoting Access to Collaborative Treatment for Late-Life Depression) study, a large multisite trial, Steffens and colleagues (2006) found that subjects with ongoing cognitive decline over 2 years had a worse course of depression.

Symptoms

Certain symptoms may predict a more chronic course of depression. For example, Moos and Cronkite (1999) followed a population of 313 depressed patients over a 10-year period. They found that symptoms such as severe fatigue, loss of interest, insomnia, suicidal ideation, and social withdrawal were predictive of a more chronic course of depression. Suicidal thoughts as a risk factor has been found in other studies (Gilchrist & Gunn, 2007), and the presence of certain physical complaints (e.g., abdominal pain) was found to be predictive of nonremission in the WHO Collaborative Project (Barkow et al., 2003).

Comorbidity

The presence of comorbid illnesses has a negative effect on outcome. This was demonstrated in a study by Keitner, Ryan, Miller, Kohn, and Epstein (1991), who examined inpatients with major depression who also had a comorbid, nonaffective psychiatric or medical illness. They referred to patients with one of these comorbid disorders as having *compound depression*. They found that patients with compound depression had both significantly poorer function during the 12-month follow-up of the study and lower recovery rates than patient with "pure" depression.

These findings are important for several reasons. As the population ages, physicians deal increasingly with geriatric depression, and medical–psychiatric comorbidity is common in this group. Some specific types of comorbidity are considered below.

Double Depression

Double depression, the concurrent presence of dysthymia and major depression (Keller & Shapiro, 1982), appears to be an important course modifier. By definition, patients with this disorder have a chronic course. The effect on major depressive episodes is notable as well: Patients with double depression seem to recover more rapidly from episodes of major depression than do patients with major depression alone. This was observed dramatically in the CDS. A large percentage of patients in the study—approximately 25%—had double depression. On 1-year follow-up, 88% of the patients with double depression had recovered from their index episode of depression, whereas only 69% of patients with major depression alone had recovered. This pattern continued through 2 years of follow-up, in which researchers found that 97% of patients with double depression had recovered from the index episode of major depression, whereas only 79% of the group with major depression alone had recovered (Keller, Lavori, Endicott, Coryell, & Klerman, 1983). Klein, Shankman, and Rose (2006) examined 97 adults recruited in a clinical setting, and found that patients with double depression had significantly worse depressive symptoms at 10-year follow up than patients with nonchronic major depression.

Patients with double depression do not appear to experience a full recovery, but rather return to a level of dysthymia. In the CDS, of the subjects with double depression who recovered from their major depressive episode, 58% had not recovered from their underlying dysthymia by the second year of follow-up (Keller, Lavori, Endicott, et al., 1983). Klein and colleagues (2006) reported that patients with dysthymia had a much slower rate of improvement from major depressive symptoms.

Patients with double depression are also more likely to relapse into major depression. In the CDS, relapse was twice as likely for patients with double depression compared to other depressed patients (Keller, Lavori, Endicott, et al., 1983). Klein and colleagues (2006) similarly found high relapse rates in patients with dysthymia: Almost three-fourths of patients with dysthymia had a relapse into depression, and appeared just as likely to relapse into dysthymia as into chronic major depression.

Subthreshold Depression

Even when not reaching the level of a dysthymic disorder, the presence of any lingering depressive symptoms following an episode of major depression can have a deleterious effect on a patient's course. The CDS found that the majority of patients who recover from

TABLE 2.2. Completeness of Recovery from First Lifetime Episode of Unipolar Major Depression as a Predictor of 12-Year Clinical Course

	Remained free of any depressive episodes (%)	Mean number of subsequent episodes of depression
Complete recovery ($n = 70$)	34*	1.5**
Residual symptoms ($n = 26$)	8*	2.5**

*$p < 0.01$; **$p < 0.0001$.

major depression still have substantial subsyndromal symptoms and associated impairment in functioning. This degree of lingering impairment predicts subsequent relapse of major depression (Judd, Akiskal, & Zeller, 2000). The relevance of incomplete recovery from a major depressive episode to the course of depression is described in Table 2.2. Similarly, Ormel and colleagues (1993) reporting results from the Groningen Primary Care Study found that at 1- and 3.5-year follow-up, partial remission was the rule, and was associated with residual disability.

Anxiety Disorders

Coryell, Endicott, and Andreasen (1988) found that depressed patients with panic disorder were more likely to have been depressed for longer periods. They also noted that the symptoms of depression were more severe in patients with comorbid anxiety disorders. Similarly, in the CDS, Clayton, Grove, and Coryell (1991) found that patients with major depression and a high anxiety rating had a longer time to recovery.

Traditionally, it has been thought that anxiety disorders precede depressive disorders, and may in fact be harbingers of them. This has been investigated specifically with generalized anxiety disorder. A number of studies have found that when anxiety and depression are comorbid, the anxiety precedes the depression. This has been found in large-scale community samples, such as the National Comorbidity Survey (NCS; Kessler et al., 1996) and in clinical studies (Fava et al., 2000). However, as pointed out by Moffitt and colleagues (2007), the majority of studies finding this relationship have significant biases, including reliance on retrospective recall and clinical populations. There are few long-term prospective studies that examine this question directly. The existing studies (Moffitt et al., 2007) tend to show that anxiety precedes depression; however, there is inadequate consensus between studies. More recently, Moffitt and colleagues investigated this question using the Dunedin (New Zealand) Multidisciplinary Health and Development Study, which followed more than 1,000 infants born in 1972 or 1973 for 32 years. Their study did not support the assumption of a sequence from anxiety to depression, and patients were as likely to have depression and then anxiety, as the reverse. Similar to other studies, they did find the relationship between major depressive disorder and generalized anxiety disorder to be strong: 72% of patients with lifetime generalized anxiety disorder also had major depressive disorder, and 48% of patients with lifetime major depressive disorder also had generalized anxiety disorder. Perhaps more important, virtually all of the patients with a recurrent form of one of the disorders also developed the other disorder.

The high comorbidity between depression and anxiety may be a particular problem in certain subgroups of patients. For example, Steffens and McQuoid (2005) found that patients with late-life depression had a worse course when it was comorbid with generalized anxiety disorder. This association was found even when researchers controlled for medication use, stressful life events, social support, and functional status. Schoevers, Deeg, van Tilburg, and Beekman (2005), examining a community sample of over 2,000 older adult patients, found that remission rates for patients with comorbid major depression and generalized anxiety disorder were dramatically poorer than those for either disorder alone (27% for the comorbid group vs. 41% for depression alone and 48% for anxiety alone).

Personality Disorders

There is a commonly held belief that personality disorders adversely affect the outcome of depression. Although this impression is based more on clinical experiences than on actual data, most relevant studies tend to confirm this belief. Reich and Green (1991) reviewed a number of inpatient and outpatient studies, and reported that all of the studies found outcomes to be poorer in patients with comorbid depression and a personality disorder. However, these studies were mostly naturalistic in design, and the patients with comorbid illness tended to be more depressed than were the "pure" depressed patients. More recently, Morse and colleagues (2005) looked at specific clusters of personality disorders, and found that patients with Cluster C (fearful, anxious) personality disorders had a longer time to response during acute treatment, and more nonresponse in continuation and maintenance treatment.

It may be, however, that the relationship between personality disorders and course of depression is not a direct one, but is instead mediated by some other factor. One potential candidate is early childhood trauma (Shea, 1996), which may independently lead to both depression and a personality disorder. Though trauma and violence are compelling potential mediators, the underlying cause may simply be any source of chronic interpersonal stress (Kessler & Magee, 1994). This is supported by the previously discussed study of adolescent women in which Rao and colleagues (1999) also found a relationship between chronic stress and depression (Daley et al., 2000).

Absent a personality disorder, certain personality traits may play a key role in influencing the course of a depressive disorder. For example, Hirschfeld and colleagues (1998) found that although a personality disorder did not predict a poorer course of depression, the presence of certain personality traits (labeled as *depressive personality traits*) did do so. Other investigators have suggested that personality characteristics such as "negative self-complexity" (Woolfolk, Gara, & Ambrose, 1999), neuroticism, external locus of control, hostility, and submissiveness (McCullough et al., 1994) may predispose an individual to a worse course of depression.

Substance Abuse

The presence of comorbid alcoholism can exert a deleterious effect on the course of major depression. Mueller and colleagues (1994), examining the CDS cohort, found that depressed subjects with alcoholism, as defined by Research Diagnostic Criteria, were half as likely as other patients to recover from their episode of major depression. This toxic relationship between substance abuse and depression has been found in most studies examining the relationship, and in various special populations, including adolescents and young adults (Rao et al., 1999), and older adults (Oslin, Katz, Edell, & Ten Have, 2000).

Comorbidity of depression and other substance abuse is common as well. Overall, individuals with any type of drug abuse (not including alcohol or nicotine) have an almost fivefold risk of depression compared with the general population (Volkow, 2004). Depression is relatively common in persons using nicotine (Zimmerman, Chelminski, & McDermut, 2002), opiates, or cocaine (Regier et al., 1990), and the course (of both the substance use disorder and the depression) is worse for individuals with any of these comorbidities than for those with only one of the disorders (Volkow, 2004).

In considering the relationship between comorbid substance abuse and depression, the question inevitably arises as to which disorder is primary. There are various possible relationships between the two disorders; most commonly cited are the *secondary depression* and *self-medication hypotheses.* In the first, the depressive symptoms are considered secondary to the direct effects of alcohol, with the presumption that the depressive symptoms will improve, without antidepressant treatment, once the substance is removed (a variant of this theory posits direct neurobiological effects of chronic use, which may not entirely reverse on cessation of the substance). Conversely, the self-medication hypothesis suggests that patients use substances in response to their depression, with the presumption that if the depressive symptoms resolve, then the patients' substance use concurrently decreases.

A full discussion of the potential mechanisms of comorbidity is beyond the scope of the chapter (the reader is referred to a review by Swendsen & Merikangas, 2000). However, an understanding of the course of the disorders, alone and in cases of comorbidity, can help to clarify the relationship. Perhaps most frequently cited is the work of Brown and Schuckit (1988) at the San Diego Veterans Administration Medical Center, who detoxified male alcoholics with comorbid depression. They found that the depressive symptoms spontaneously remitted within 4 weeks of abstinence from alcohol. The assumed cause and effect of the intervention, coupled with the unusual course of the depressive symptoms, argued for secondary depression as an explanation. Other investigators (Swendsen & Merikangas, 2000) have reported similar findings. However, conflicting data exist; some investigators have found depressive symptoms to be stable in alcoholics, and unrelated to the current pattern of drinking (Merikangas & Gelernter, 1990). Similarly, other investigators have reported that depressive symptoms precede substance use (Bovasso, 2001; Kokkevi & Stefanis, 1995). However, this finding has not been consistent.

It is likely that a number of factors are confounding attempts to make a broad statement about the relationship between substance abuse and depression. Most longitudinal investigations are in clinical populations, often recruited during an inpatient hospitalization, and as such are not reflective of the general population. Furthermore, substance abuse itself is a heterogeneous disorder, and not all studies have sufficiently accounted for subtypes of the disorder. In studies that have accounted for this, different patterns of comorbidity emerge. For example, Brown and colleagues (1995) found that spontaneous remission of depression was true only in patients whose alcohol dependence preceded their depression (and depression only occurred in the context of drinking). In cases in which the mood disorder preceded the onset of alcohol dependence, the depressive symptoms remained elevated during the length of the study.

Clearly, clinical studies are not adequate to decide the question of causal direction. Additional data from epidemiological and genetic studies are necessary as well. It should not be surprising that such studies have underscored the complexity of the potential relationships (Swendsen & Merikangas, 2000). In addition, genetic studies point to other potential relationships, such as the possibility that rather than causing the other, the two disorders may have shared risk factors, be they genetic or environmental (Volkow, 2004).

Comorbid Medical Illness

Comorbid medical illness may predispose patients with major depression to a more chronic course of disease. Several studies have suggested this, but little research has examined this question directly. The Medical Outcomes Study (Wells et al., 1989) found that medical and psychiatric illnesses have a combined effect on patient functioning, suggesting a worse overall outcome for patients with medical–psychiatric comorbidity. Similarly, Schmitz, Wang, Malla, and Lesage (2007), using data from a large Canadian survey, found that physical illness and depression exert a joint effect on functional disability.

Certain types of comorbid physical illness have deserved special scrutiny. For example, it has long been known that depression can worsen morbidity in patients with coronary heart disease. The relationship between these disorders is clearly complex and interrelated. Koenig, Johnson, and Peterson (2006), for example, examining the course of illness in patients with major depression and heart failure and/or chronic pulmonary disease, found that the courses of the medical and psychiatric illness are interdependent and tend to improve either conjointly, or not at all. It follows that in cases of comorbid medical and psychiatric illness, it is likely crucial to treat both illnesses with equal vigor. The comorbidity of depression and medical illness is discussed in more detail by Joiner and Timmons, Chapter 14, this volume.

FUTURE DIRECTIONS

The field has been helped greatly by natural studies of the course of depression that have encouraged us to view depression in longitudinal terms, with different stages of disease. We also now appreciate that depression for many is a lifelong illness. Although we understand this for large populations, we need more information to apply this to our individual patients. We still cannot adequately predict who will develop what type of depression: who will get only a single episode; who will go on to experience recurrent episodes, with interepisode recovery; and who will become chronically depressed. Consequently, many patients are fated to suffer the morbidity of major depressive episodes because of premature treatment withdrawal and inadequate treatment. Clearly, we need to target better which patients should have long-term treatment, then understand which treatments will best prevent future episodes.

If we hope to improve the course of major depression in our patients, we also need to understand other factors, apart from natural history and traditional treatment efficacy data. One potential barrier to treatment efficacy is patient adherence; yet most of the studies discussed in this review do not collect data on adherence, or on variables that may explain problems with adherence. To understand how adherence affects the long-term course of depression we need to incorporate this data into long-term intervention and natural history studies.

Even less is understood about the behaviors of physicians. What little information there is on the decision-making processes of physicians suggests that more than mere education is needed to improve the process of initiating and maintaining treatment in patients with depression.

The problems of comorbidity and its effects on the course of depression are also important areas in need of investigation. Although there is a growing literature in this area, more work is needed to clarify the nature of the interaction among depression, comorbid nonaffective psychiatric disease, and comorbid medical disease.

The role of the environment in depression, particularly the importance of adverse life events and their effect on depression, is another important area of study. As discussed, there is currently some controversy regarding the role that stress plays in the etiology and maintenance of depression, and more work needs to be done to clarify these relationships.

We have much to learn; however, some things seem clear. Patients with recurrent or chronic depression have worse outcomes than other depressed patients. This is true even when the symptoms of depression are not severe. Furthermore, patients with recurrent or chronic depression have an increased risk of becoming treatment unresponsive. Identifying and preventing depression is of utmost importance. It appears that early and intensive interventions using both medication and psychotherapy may be the most effective strategy to improve the outcome of a depressive illness. Beyond that, social interventions, including improvement of home and community environments for children, may be crucial for preventing the onset of depression. Effecting such changes will be difficult and expensive, and we hope that future studies will direct our understanding of how our resources should best be spent.

REFERENCES

Alexopoulos, G. S. (2006). The vascular depression hypothesis: 10 years later. *Biological Psychiatry, 60,* 1304–1305.

American Psychiatric Association (1994). *Diagnostic and statistical manual of mental disorders* (4th ed.). Washington, DC: Author.

Andrews, G., Henderson, S., & Hall, W. (2001). Prevalence, comorbidity, disability and service utilisation: Overview of the Australian National Mental Health Survey. *British Journal of Psychiatry, 78,* 145–53.

Angst, J. (1986). The course of major depression, atypical bipolar disorder, and bipolar disorder. In H. Hippius, G. L. Klerman, & N. Matussek (Eds.), *New results in depression research* (pp. 26–35). Berlin/Heidelberg: Springer-Verlag.

Angst, J. (1992). How recurrent and predictable is depressive illness? In S. Montgomery & F. Rouillon (Eds.), *Long-term treatment of depression* (pp. 1–15). New York: Wiley.

Angst, J., Baastrup, P., Grof, P., Hippius, H., Poldinger, W., & Weis, P. (1973). The course of monopolar depression and bipolar psychoses. *Psychiatria, Neurologia, Neurochirurgia, 76,* 489–500.

Barkow, K., Maier, W., Ustun, T. B., Gansicke, M., Wittchen, H. U., & Heun, R. (2003). Risk factors for depression at 12-month follow-up in adult primary health care patients with major depression: An international prospective study. *Journal of Affective Disorders, 76,* 157–169.

Birmaher, B., Bridge, J. A., Williamson, D. E., Brent, D. A., Dahl, R. E., Axelson, D. A., et al. (2004). Psychosocial functioning in youths at high risk to develop major depressive disorder. *Journal of the American Academy of Child and Adolescent Psychiatry, 43,* 839–846.

Blacker, C. V., Thomas, J. M., & Thompson, C. (1997). Seasonality prevalence and incidence of depressive disorder in a general practice sample: Identifying differences in timing by caseness. *Journal of Affective Disorders, 43,* 41–52.

Bovasso, G. B. (2001). Cannabis abuse as a risk factor for depressive symptoms. *American Journal of Psychiatry, 158,* 2033–2037.

Brown, S. A., Inaba, R. K., Gillin, J. C., Schuckit, M. A., Stewart, M. A., & Irwin, M. R. (1995). Alcoholism and affective disorder: Clinical course of depressive symptoms. *American Journal of Psychiatry, 152,* 45–52.

Brown, S. A., & Schuckit, M. A. (1988). Changes in depression among abstinent alcoholics. *Journal of Studies on Alcohol, 49,* 412–417.

Clayton, P. J., Grove, W. M., & Coryell, W. (1991). Follow-up and family study of anxious depression. *American Journal of Psychiatry, 148,* 1512–1517.

Coryell, W., Endicott, J., & Andreasen, N. C. (1998). Depression and panic attacks: The significance of overlap as reflected in follow-up and family study data. *American Journal of Psychiatry, 145,* 293–300.

Daley, S. E., Hammen, C., & Rao, U. (2000). Predictors of first onset and recurrence of major depression in young women during the 5 years following high school graduation. *Journal of Abnormal Psychology, 109,* 525–533.

Depression Guideline Panel. (1993). *Depression in primary care: Vol. 2. Treatment of major depression* (Clinical Practice Guideline No. 5). Rockville, MD: U.S. Department of Health and Human Services, Public Health Service, Agency for Health Care Policy and Research.

Fava, M., Rankin, M. A., Wright, E. C., Alpert, J. E., Nierenberg, A. A., Pava, J., et al. (2000). Anxiety disorders in major depression. *Comprehensive Psychiatry, 41,* 97–102.

Frank, E., Prien, R. F., Jarrett, R. B., Keller, M. B., Kupfer, D. J., Lavori, P. W., et al. (1991). Conceptualization and rationale for consensus definitions of terms in major depressive disorder: Remission, recovery, relapse, and recurrence. *Archives of General Psychiatry, 48,* 851–855.

Gilchrist, G., & Gunn, J. (2007). Observational studies of depression in primary care: What do we know? *BMC Family Practice, 8,* 1471–2296.

Hirschfeld, R. M., Russell, J. M., Delgado, P. L., Fawcett, J., Freidman, R. A., Harrison, W. M., et al. (1998). Predictors of response to acute treatment of chronic and double depression with sertraline or imipramine. *Journal of Clinical Psychiatry, 59,* 669–675.

Judd, L. L., Akiskal, H. S., & Zeller, P. J. (2000). Psychosocial disability during the long-term course of unipolar major depressive disorder. *Archives of General Psychiatry, 57,* 375–380.

Katz, M., & Klerman, G. L. (1979). Introduction: Overview of the Clinical Studies Program. *American Journal of Psychiatry, 136,* 49–51.

Keitner, G. I., Ryan, C. E., Miller, I. W., Kohn, R., & Epstein, N. B. (1991). Twelve month outcome of patients with major depression and comorbid psychiatric or medical illness (compound depression). *American Journal of Psychiatry, 148,* 345–350.

Keitner, G. I., Ryan, C. E., Miller, I. W., & Norman, W. H. (1992). Recovery and major depression: Factors associated with twelve-month outcome. *American Journal of Psychiatry, 149,* 93–99.

Keller, M. B., & Boland, R. J. (1998). Implications of failing to achieve successful long-term maintenance treatment of recurrent unipolar major depression. *Biological Psychiatry, 44,* 348–360.

Keller, M. B., Lavori, P. W., Endicott, J., Coryell, W., & Klerman, G. L. (1983). "Double depression": Two-year follow-up. *American Journal of Psychiatry, 140,* 689–694.

Keller, M. B., Lavori, P. W., Lewis, C. E., & Klerman, G. L. (1983). Predictors of relapse in major depressive disorder. *Journal of the American Medical Association, 250,* 3299–3304.

Keller, M. B., Lavori, P. W., Mueller, T. I., Endicott, J., Coryell, W., Hirschfield, R. M., et al. (1992). Time to recovery, chronicity, and levels of psychopathology in major depression: A 5-year prospective follow-up of 431 subjects. *Archives of General Psychiatry, 49,* 809–816.

Keller, M. B., & Shapiro, R. W. (1982). "Double depression": Superimposition of acute depressive episodes on chronic depressive disorders. *American Journal of Psychiatry, 139,* 438–442.

Keller, M. B., Shapiro, R., Lavori, P. W., & Wolfe, N. (1982). Recovery in major depressive disorder: Analysis with the life table and regression models. *Archives of General Psychiatry, 39,* 905–910.

Kendler, K. S., Gatz, M., Gardner, C. O., & Pedersen, N. L. (2006). A Swedish national twin study of lifetime major depression. *American Journal of Psychiatry, 163,* 109–114.

Kendler, K. S., Thornton, L. M., & Gardner, C. O. (2000). Stressful life events and previous episodes in the etiology of major depression in women: An evaluation of the "kindling" hypothesis. *American Journal of Psychiatry, 157,* 1243–1251.

Kerr, T. A., Roth, M., Schapira, K., & Gurney, C. (1972). The assessment and prediction of outcome in affective disorders. *British Journal of Psychiatry, 121,* 167–174.

Kessler, R. C., & Magee, W. J. (1994). Childhood family violence and adult recurrent depression. *Journal of Health and Social Behavior, 35,* 13–27.

Kessler, R. C., Nelson, C. B., McGonagle, K. A., Liu, J., Swartz, M., & Blazer, D. G. (1996). Comorbidity of DSM-III-R major depressive disorder in the general population: Results from the U.S. National Comorbidity Survey. *British Journal of Psychiatry, 168*(Suppl. 30), 17–30.

Klein, D. N., Shankman, S. A., & Rose, S. (2006). Ten-year prospective follow-up study of the naturalistic course of dysthymic disorder and double depression. *American Journal of Psychiatry, 163,* 872–880.

Koenig, H. G., Johnson, J. L., & Peterson, B. L. (2006). Major depression and physical illness trajectories in heart failure and pulmonary disease. *Journal of Nervous and Mental Disease, 194,* 909–916.

Kokkevi, A., & Stefanis, C. (1995). Drug abuse and psychiatric comorbidity. *Comprehensive Psychiatry, 36,* 329–337.

Lavori, P. W., Keller, M. B., Mueller, T. I., & Scheftner, W. (1994). Recurrence after recovery in unipolar major depressive disorder: An observational follow-up study of clinical predictors and somatic treatment as a mediating factor. *International Journal of Methods in Psychological Research, 4,* 211–229.

Lavretsky, H., Kitchen, C., Mintz, J., Kim, M. D., Estanol, L., & Kumar, A. (2002). Medical burden, cerebrovascular disease, and cognitive impairment in geriatric depression: Modeling the relationships with the CART analysis. *CNS Spectrums, 7,* 716–722.

Lavretsky, H., Lesser, I. M., Wohl, M., & Miller, B. L. (1998). Relationship of age, age at onset, and sex to depression in older adults. *American Journal of Geriatric Psychiatry, 6,* 248–256.

Lewinsohn, P. M., Allen, N. B., Seeley, J. R., & Gotlib, I. H. (1999). First onset versus recurrence of depression: Differential processes of psychosocial risk. *Journal of Abnormal Psychology, 108,* 483–489.

Limosin, F., Loze, J. Y., Zylberman-Bouhassira, M., Schmidt, M. E., Perrin, E., & Rouillon, F. (2004). The course of depressive illness in general practice. *Canadian Journal of Psychiatry, 49,* 119–123.

Maciejewski, P. K., Prigerson, H. G., & Mazure, C. M. (2001). Sex differences in event-related risk for major depression. *Psychological Medicine, 31,* 593–604.

MaGPIe Research Group. (2003). The nature and prevalence of psychological problems in New Zealand primary healthcare: A report on Mental Health and General Practice Investigation (MaGPIe). *New Zealand Medical Journal, 116,* U379.

McCullough, J. P., Klein, D. N., Borian, F. E., Howland, R. H., Riso, L. P., Keller, M. B., et al. (2003). Group comparisons of DSM-IV subtypes of chronic depression: Validity of the distinctions, part 2. *Journal of Abnormal Psychology, 112,* 614–622.

McCullough, J. P., McCune, K. J., Kaye, A. L., Braith, J. A., Friend, R., Roberts, W. C., et al. (1994). Comparison of a community dysthymia sample at screening with matched group of a nondepressed community controls. *Journal of Nervous and Mental Disease, 182,* 402–407.

Merikangas, K., & Gelernter, C. (1990). Comorbidity for alcoholism and depression. *Psychiatric Clinics of North America, 13,* 613–632.

Moffitt, T. E., Harrington, H., Caspi, A., Kim-Cohen, J., Goldberg, D., Gregory, A. M., et al. (2007). Depression and generalized anxiety disorder: Cumulative and sequential comorbidity in a birth cohort followed prospectively to age 32 years. *Archives of General Psychiatry, 64,* 651–660.

Monroe, S. M., & Harkness, K. L. (2005). Life stress, the "kindling" hypothesis, and the recurrence of depression: Considerations from a life stress perspective. *Psychological Review, 112,* 417–445.

Moos, R. H., & Cronkite, R. C. (1999). Symptom-based predictors of a 10-year chronic course of treated depression. *Journal of Nervous and Mental Disease, 187,* 360–368.

Morse, J. Q., Pilkonis, P. A., Houck, P. R., Frank, E., & Reynolds, C. F., III. (2005). Impact of cluster C personality disorders on outcomes of acute and maintenance treatment in late-life depression. *American Journal of Geriatric Psychiatry, 13,* 808–814.

Moses, T., Leuchter, A. F., Cook, I., & Abrams, M. (2006). Does the clinical course of depression determine improvement in symptoms and quality of life? *Journal of Nervous and Mental Disease, 194,* 241–248.

Mueller, T. I., Keller, M. B., Leon, A., Solomon, D. D., Shea, M. T., Coryell, W., et al. (1996). Recovery after five years of unremitting major depressive disorder. *Archives of General Psychiatry, 53,* 794–799.

Mueller, T. I., Kohn, R., Leventhal, N., Leon, A. C., Solomon, D., Coryell, W., et al. (2004). The course of depression in elderly patients. *American Journal of Geriatric Psychiatry, 12,* 22–29.

Mueller, T. I., Lavori, P. W., Keller, M. B., Swartz, A., Warshaw, M., Hasin, D., et al. (1994). Prognostic effect of the variable course of alcoholism on the 10-year course of depression. *American Journal of Psychiatry, 151,* 701–706.

NIMH Consensus Development Conference Statement. (1985). Mood disorders: Pharmacologic prevention of recurrences. *American Journal of Psychiatry, 142,* 469–476.

Ormel, J., Oldehinkel, A. J., & Brilman, E. I. (2001). The interplay and ecological continuity of neuroticism, difficulties, and life events in the etiology of major and subsyndromal, first and recurrent depressive episodes in later life. *American Journal of Psychiatry, 158,* 885–891.

Ormel, J., Oldehinkel, T., Brilman, E., & van den Brink, W. (1993). Outcome of depression and anxiety in primary care: A three-wave 3½-year study of psychopathology and disability. *Archives of General Psychiatry, 50,* 759–766.

Oslin, D. W., Katz, I. R., Edell, W. S., & Ten Have, T. R. (2000). Effects of alcohol consumption on the treatment of depression among elderly patients. *American Journal of Geriatric Psychiatry, 8,* 215–220.

Parker, G., Holmes, S., & Manicavasagar, V. (1986). Depression in general practice attenders: "Caseness," natural history and predictors of outcome. *Journal of Affective Disorders, 10,* 27–35.

Post, R. M. (2002). Do the epilepsies, pain syndromes, and affective disorders share common kindling-like mechanisms? *Epilepsy Research, 50,* 203–219.

Posternak, M. A., Solomon, D. A., & Leon, A. C. (2006). The naturalistic course of unipolar major depression in the absence of somatic therapy. *Journal of Nervous and Mental Disease, 194,* 324–329.

Rao, A. V., & Nammalvar, N. (1977). The course and outcome in depressive illness: A follow-up study of 122 cases in Madurai, India. *British Journal of Psychiatry, 130,* 392–396.

Rao, U., Hammen, C., & Daley, S. E. (1999). Continuity of depression during the transition to adulthood: A 5-year longitudinal study of young women. *Journal of the American Academy of Child and Adolescent Psychiatry, 38,* 908–915.

Regier, D. A., Farmer, M. E., Rae, D. S., Locke, B. Z., Keith, S. J., Judd, L. L., et al. (1990). Comorbidity of mental disorders with alcohol and other drug abuse: Results from the Epidemiologic Catchment Area (ECA) Study. *Journal of the American Medical Association, 264,* 2511–2518.

Reich, J. H., & Green, A. I. (1991). Effect of personality disorders on outcome of treatment. *Journal of Nervous and Mental Disease, 179,* 74–82.

Rounsaville, B. J., Prusoff, B. A., & Padian, N. (1980). Chronic mood disorders in depression outpatients: A prospective 16-month study of ambulatory patients. *Journal of Nervous and Mental Disease, 168,* 406–411.

Rybakowski, J. K., Nawacka, D., & Kiejna, A. J. (2004). One-year course of the first vs. multiple episodes of depression—Polish naturalistic study. *European Psychiatry, 19,* 258–263.

Rytsälä, H. J., Melartin, T. K., Leskelä, U. S., Lestelä-Mielonen, P. S., Sokero, T. P., & Isometsä, E. T. (2006). Determinants of functional disability and social adjustment in major depressive disorder: A prospective study. *Journal of Nervous and Mental Disease, 194,* 570–576.

Schmitz, N., Wang, J., Malla, A., & Lesage, A. (2007). Joint effect of depression and chronic conditions on disability: Results from a population-based study. *Psychosomatic Medicine, 69,* 332–338.

Schoevers, R. A., Deeg, D. J., van Tilburg, W., & Beekman, A. T. (2005). Depression and generalized anxiety disorder: Co-occurrence and longitudinal patterns in elderly patients. *American Journal of Geriatric Psychiatry, 13,* 31–39.

Shea, M. T. (1996). The role of personality in recurrent and chronic depression. *Current Opinion in Psychiatry, 9,* 117–120.

Simon, G. E., Fleck, M., Lucas, R., & Bushnell, D. M. (2004). Prevalence and predictors of depression treatment in an international primary care study. *American Journal of Psychiatry, 161,* 1626–1634.

Solomon, D. A., Keller, M. B., Leon, A. C., Mueller, T. I., Lavori, P. W., Shea, M. T., et al. (2000). Multiple recurrences of major depressive disorder. *American Journal of Psychiatry, 157,* 229–233.

Solomon, D. A., Keller, M. B., Leon, A. C., Mueller, T. I., Shea, M. T., Warshaw, M., et al. (1997). Recovery from major depression: A 10-year prospective follow-up across multiple episodes. *Archives of General Psychiatry, 54,* 1001–1006.

Steffens, D. C., & McQuoid, D. R. (2005). Impact of symptoms of generalized anxiety disorder on the course of late-life depression. *American Journal of Geriatric Psychiatry, 13,* 40–47.

Steffens, D. C., Snowden, M., Fan, M. Y., Hendrie, H., Katon, W. J., Unutzer, J., et al. (2006). Cognitive impairment and depression outcomes in the IMPACT study. *American Journal of Geriatric Psychiatry, 14,* 401–409.

Swendsen, J. D., & Merikangas, K. R. (2000). The comorbidity of depression and substance use disorders. *Clinical Psychology Review, 20,* 173–189.

Volkow, N. D. (2004). The reality of comorbidity: Depression and drug abuse. *Biological Psychiatry, 56,* 714–717.

Weissman, M. M., & Kasl, S. V. (1976). Help-seeking in depressed out-patients following maintenance therapy. *British Journal of Psychiatry, 129,* 252–260.

Wells, K. B., Stewart, A., Hays, R. D., Burnam, A., Rogers, W., Daniel, M., et al. (1989). The functioning and well-being of depressed patients—results of the Medical Outcomes Study. *Journal of the American Medical Association, 262,* 914–919.

Williamson, D. E., Birmaher, B., Axelson, D. A., Ryan, N. D., & Dahl, R. E. (2004). First episode of depression in children at low and high familial risk for depression. *Journal of the American Academy of Child and Adolescent Psychiatry, 43,* 291–297.

Woolfolk, R. L., Gara, M. A., & Ambrose, T. K. (1999). Self-complexity and the persistence of depression. *Journal of Nervous and Mental Disease, 187,* 393–399.

Zimmerman, M., Chelminski, I., & McDermut, W. (2002). Major depressive disorder and Axis I diagnostic comorbidity. *Journal of Clinical Psychiatry, 63,* 187–193.

CHAPTER 3

Assessment of Depression

Arthur M. Nezu, Christine Maguth Nezu,
Jill Friedman, *and* Minsun Lee

In this chapter, we provide an update of material presented in the first edition (Nezu, Nezu, McClure, & Zwick, 2002), as well as new information on more recently developed measures of depression. In a review of the history of measuring depression, Santor, Gregus, and Welch (2006) note that more than 280 measures of depressive severity have been developed since 1918. Simply to list all such measures is beyond the scope of this chapter. Consequently, we refer the reader to A. M. Nezu, Ronan, Meadows, and McClure (2000) for a review of over 90 measures of depression and depression-related constructs. In the first section of this chapter, we provide an overview of more than 20 depression measures, listed in alphabetical order and divided in two categories—clinician ratings and self-report inventories. Some measures were chosen based on their widespread usage (e.g., Beck Depression Inventory; Beck, Ward, Mendelson, Mock, & Erbaugh, 1961), whereas others were included as a function of their recent appearance in the literature (e.g., Cardiac Depression Scale; Hare & Davis, 1996). In addition, we include two measures that focus on the assessment of bipolar disorder—the Screening Assessment of Depression—Polarity (Solomon et al., 2006) and the Mood Disorder Questionnaire (Hirschfeld et al., 2000).

Because a plethora of depression measures do exist, we attempt in a subsequent section to answer the question: *What measures should clinicians/researchers use?* Because the answer depends to a large degree on several key concerns—the specific goals of the assessment, the amount of time one has to accomplish the evaluation, the amount of training necessary to validly administer the test, and what specific population one is evaluating—to name just a few—we offer a set of decision-making guidelines to aid in this selection process. We conclude with a section highlighting important future directions.

CLINICIAN RATINGS

Diagnostic Interview Schedule

The Diagnostic Interview Schedule (DIS-IV) is the sixth version of the DIS, initially developed in 1978 for use in the National Institute of Mental Health's (NIMH) Epidemiologic Catchment Area program (ECA; Robins, Helzer, Croughan, & Ratcliff, 1981). Since then, the DIS has been revised to be compatible with the current *Diagnostic and Statistical Manual of Mental Disorders*; thus, the DIS-IV is compatible with DSM-IV (American Psychiatric Association, 1994). The DIS-IV is a highly structured interview designed to allow laypersons to determine DSM diagnoses. It comprises 22 individual modules, most of which focus on specific diagnoses (e.g., generalized anxiety disorder) or groups of diagnoses (e.g., specific phobia, social phobia, agoraphobia). Questions are structured such that the interviewer can exit the module at various points as it becomes determined that the disorder in question is not present. All answers are coded according to explicit guidelines, with the coded answers entered into a computer to yield specific diagnoses. The DIS requires between 90 and 120 minutes to complete all modules. Note that extensive training of lay interviewers is required.

Because few measures cover the full range of DSM diagnoses, comparing the DIS to other measures has been difficult. Therefore, the validity of the DIS has been estimated in studies that compare DIS diagnoses with those obtained by trained professionals, such as psychiatrists. Unfortunately, results have been somewhat disappointing. For example, Anthony and colleagues (1985) found kappa values of agreement between lay-administered DIS diagnoses and those made by psychiatrists in a sample of 810 community residents to be relatively low (mean across diagnoses, 0.15).

Hamilton Rating Scale for Depression

The Hamilton Rating Scale for Depression (HAMD; Hamilton, 1960) was originally designed to evaluate the severity of depressive symptoms among patients previously diagnosed with a depressive disorder. It is historically the most widely used clinician rating of depression and is often viewed as the "gold standard." The HAMD contains 21 items, only 17 of which are typically scored. It takes approximately 10 minutes to complete this scale using information gleaned from a semistructured interview. To improve its reliability and to foster its use by lay interviewers, Williams (1988) developed a structured guide delineating specific questions to ask in order to validly complete the HAMD.

Despite its continued popularity, concerns have been raised regarding the reliability and validity of the HAMD. For example, based on an assessment of 70 studies published subsequent to a previous literature review (Hedlund & Vieweg, 1979), Bagby, Ryder, Schuller, and Marshall (2004) voiced serious concerns about the status of the HAMD as a "gold standard." They examined three major psychometric properties—reliability (internal, interrater, test–retest), item response, and validity (content, convergent, discriminant, factorial and predictive). In general, Bagby and colleagues found that internal, interrater, and retest reliabilities at the *scale* level were acceptable, but at the *item* level, interrater and retest reliabilities were inconsistent and questionable. Furthermore, they found low correlations between the HAMD and the Structured Clinical Interview for DSM-IV (SCID; First, Spitzer, Gibbon, & Williams, 1997) to be problematic. Important features of the DSM-IV definition of depression were not fully captured by the HAMD, and some symptoms were not assessed at all. Whereas convergent and discriminant validity coefficients were found to be adequate, the multidimensional nature of the HAMD was noted to lead to difficulties in interpreting the meaning of the total score. For example, Bagby and colleagues noted that certain items contribute more to the total score than do others. Particularly striking is the contrast between items addressing similar constructs, for example, psychomotor retardation versus agitation. Specifically, whereas the most severe form of the first symptom contributes 4 points to the total HAMD score, an equally severe manifestation of the second symptom contributes only 2 points. This occurs in the absence of any evidence to support such differential item weightings.

Bagby and colleagues (2004) further argued that because the HAMD was developed several decades ago, many symptoms of depression now thought to be important are not contained in this inventory. They concluded that the HAMD is conceptually and psychometrically flawed, and that a substantial revision or complete rejection of the HAMD should be considered. They claimed that any new instrument should measure the contemporary definition of depression and must be developed using item response theory.

As one might expect, this position was met with disagreement. For example, Corruble and Hardy (2005) argued that the HAMD was originally designed to measure depression severity and clinical changes in patients *already* diagnosed as being depressed. Thus, they suggested that Bagby and colleagues (2004) actually incorrectly extended the original aim of the scale by including studies carried out with both depressed and nondepressed patients. Corruble and Hardy (2005) also suggested that the HAMD should not be compared to DSM-IV criteria, because the two measures have different objectives (i.e., the HAMD assesses depression *severity* in depressed patients, whereas the DSM-IV defines a *diagnosis* of depression).

HAMD-7

Due in part to criticisms of the multidimensionality of the HAMD, researchers have developed shorter versions of the HAMD based on a unidimensional core group of depression symptoms. One such scale, the HAMD-7, includes the following items: depressed mood, guilt, suicide, work and interests, psychic anxiety, somatic anxiety, and general somatic symptoms. McIntyre, Kennedy, Bagby, and Bakish (2002) found estimates of reliability and validity to be comparable among mental health patients across this shortened version and the full 17-item HAMD. The cutoff score ≤ 3 for the HAMD-7 representing full remission was found to be comparable to that determined by the HAMD-17 (≤ 7). Moreover, the HAMD-7 demonstrated high rates of sensitivity (.95), specificity (.84), positive predictive power (.94), and negative predictive power (.86).

GRID-HAMD

The GRID-HAMD (Kalali et al., 2002) was developed by the Depression Rating Scale Standardization Team (DRSST), formed in 1999 to address concerns regarding the lack of standardization in administering and scoring the HAMD. The DRSST comprises researchers from academia, the pharmaceutical industry, clinical practice, and government, and is sponsored by the International Society for CNS Drug Development. This group presented its recommendations at the 2001 National Institute of Mental Health (NIMH)–sponsored New Clinical Drug Evaluation Unit (NCDEU) conference, which advocated a new approach to administering and scoring the HAMD. Changes included a GRID structure that operationalized the intensity and frequency of each item while allowing each to be rated simultaneously. Structured interview prompts and scoring guidelines were also provided. The

DRSST suggested that standardizing the administration and scoring of the HAMD would improve the current scale and lay the groundwork for developing a new measure, with the hope that validation studies would be conducted in the future. The GRID-HAMD is currently available at *www.iscdd.org*.

Depression Interview and Structured Hamilton

The Depression Interview and Structured Hamilton (DISH; Freedland et al., 2002) is a semistructured interview developed specifically for the Enhancing Recovery in Coronary Heart Disease (ENRICHD; ENRICHD Investigators, 2000) study, a multicenter clinical trial of treatment for depression and/or low social support for patients who have had a myocardial infarction. The purpose of the DISH is to (1) screen medical patients for depression; (2) diagnose major depressive disorder (MDD), dysthymia, and minor depression according to DSM-IV criteria; (3) assess the depressive severity with the 17-item HAMD using Williams's (1988) structured interview guide; and (4) document the history and course of a patient's depression.

An initial validity study found that a SCID diagnosis made by either a clinical social worker or clinical psychologist agreed with a DISH diagnosis (made by a trained nurse or lay interviewer) on 88% of the interviews. In the actual ENRICHD trial, clinicians agreed with 93% of research nurses' DISH diagnoses. Based on such initial findings, a National Heart, Lung, and Blood Institute (NHLBI) Working Group regarding the assessment and treatment of patients with cardiovascular disease recommends the use of the DISH for "diagnostic ascertainment" with regard to clinical trials (Davidson et al., 2006).

Schedule for Affective Disorders and Schizophrenia

The Schedule for Affective Disorders and Schizophrenia (SADS; Endicott & Spitzer, 1978) is a clinician-administered interview protocol designed to aid the process of diagnosis and to assess the severity of psychiatric symptoms as specified by Research Diagnostic Criteria (RDC; Spitzer, Endicott, & Robins, 1978). Several versions of the SADS exist—some to measure change in psychiatric status, a lifetime version, and versions modified for specific syndromes such as bipolar mood disorders. The current SADS version covers 24 major psychiatric disorders, as well as specific subtypes (e.g., recurrent MDD, endogenous MDD). The structured interview takes between 90 and 120 minutes to complete and requires interviewers that are trained mental health professionals.

Recently, Rogers (2001) summarized 21 investigations that assessed the interrater and test–retest reliability of the SADS. He found that most studies produced high interrater reliability estimates (e.g., most were associated with median kappa values greater than .85). Test–retest reliability for the SADS was also strong but slightly lower (intraclass coefficients were generally greater than .70). With regard to the reliability of diagnoses made through SADS interviews, Spitzer and colleagues (1978) reported a kappa value of .90 regarding the diagnosis of MDD, and .81 for minor depressive disorder.

Because the SADS is a well-validated and established Axis I interview protocol, it has frequently been used to validate other psychological measures. The SADS was also validated for the full spectrum of adult populations, from young adult to geriatric populations. It has been translated into several languages and has been widely used in clinical research. Consequently, it has a substantial body of empirical data to support its utility. It seems, however, that an effort to make the SADS compatible with more recent versions of the DSM has not yet been made, thus limiting its current applicability.

Structured Clinical Interview for DSM-IV Axis I Disorders

The Structured Clinical Interview for DSM-IV Axis I Disorders (SCID; First et al., 1997) provides a standardized clinical interview to determine DSM-IV (American Psychiatric Association, 1994) diagnoses and differential diagnoses. Six scores are derived for mood episodes, psychotic symptoms, psychotic disorders, mood disorders, substance use disorders, anxiety, and other disorders. Whereas this instrument is structured to match specific DSM-IV diagnostic criteria, it utilizes the skills of trained clinicians by allowing them to probe, restate questions, challenge respondents, and ask for clarification. Administration of the entire SCID ranges from 45 to 90 minutes. In certain cases, however, it is possible to administer specific modules, such as the mood disorder module, if time is a factor.

The SCID was first published in 1983 and has evolved along with the revisions of the DSM-III, DSM-III-R, DSM-IV, and DSM-IV-TR. The psychometric properties of the most current version of the SCID have not yet been published and are commonly estimated based on the previous version. The validity of this instrument can be evaluated in terms of how well it reflects the DSM-IV (American Psychiatric Association, 1994) diagnostic criteria and measures the constructs they purport to represent. Segal, Hersen, and Van Hasselt (1994) provided a review of studies reported until 1994, suggesting that the SCID demonstrates adequate reliability.

There are two versions of the SCID: (1) Structured Clinical Interview for DSM-IV Axis I Disorders—Clinician Version (SCID-CV; First et al., 1997); and (2) Structured Clinical Interview for DSM-IV Axis I Disorders—Research Version (SCID-RV; First, Gibbon, Spitzer, & Williams, 1996). The SCID-RV is longer than the SCID-CV, because it contains more disorders, subtypes, severity, and course specifiers. As research has expanded to include participants who may have limited resources (e.g., persons with lower income levels, concomitant medical illnesses), the SCID has been conducted over the telephone to overcome transportation or mobility problems. However, one study found that participants were more likely to receive a lifetime diagnosis of MDD after an in-person interview than after a telephone interview (Cacciola, Alterman, Rutherford, McKay, & May, 1999). The SCID has also been administered and evaluated in studies screening for depression in medically ill populations, including individuals with chronic pulmonary disease (Koenig, 2006) and primary care patients (Vuorilehto, Melartin, & Isometsä, 2006).

Screening Assessment of Depression—Polarity

Because patients with bipolar disorder are frequently misdiagnosed with MDD (Hirschfeld, Lewis, & Vornik, 2003), researchers have recently attempted to develop evidenced-based assessment procedures to differentiate between these diagnostic entities. The Screening Assessment of Depression—Polarity (SAD-P; Solomon et al., 2006) was developed within the NIMH Collaborative Program on the Psychobiology of Depression Longitudinal Study, which followed individuals with a variety of mood disorders for a median length of 16 years. In essence, the SAD-P is a rating scale of three items administered by clinicians with respect to patients who currently are experiencing a major depressive episode. The first item pertains to the number of prior episodes of major depression (where 0 = *No prior episodes* and 1 = *One or more prior episodes*), whereas the second focuses on family (i.e., first-degree relative) history of depression or mania (where 0 = *Negative history* and 1 = *Positive history*). The third and final item addresses the presence of delusions (e.g., persecutory, grandiose) during the current depressive episode (where 0 = *No delusions* and 1 = *One or more delusions present*). A total score of 2 and greater suggest that the individual's current depressive episode may be part of bipolar illness, and that a more in-depth assessment is warranted. Data from the NIMH Collaborative Program indicated that the SAD-P has adequate psychometric properties in distinguishing unipolar from bipolar disorder. Specifically, over-all sensitivity in accurately identifying patients with bipolar disorder was found to be .82; .72 in the bipolar I cross-validation sample, and .58 in the bipolar II cross-validation sample.

SELF-REPORT MEASURES

Beck Depression Inventory

The Beck Depression Inventory (BDI; Beck et al., 1961) is one of the most widely used self-report measures of depressive symptomatology across a variety of patient and nonpatient populations. The original BDI was developed as a clinician rating scale and published by Beck and colleagues in 1961, revised as a self-report instrument in 1971, and revised (BDI-II) to make its symptom content more reflective of the diagnostic criteria contained in DSM-IV (Beck, Steer, & Brown, 1996). Although it still comprises 21 items, in contrast to its predecessor, the BDI-II contains four new symptoms—agitation, worthlessness, concentration difficulty, and loss of energy—and now inquires about sleep and appetite *increases*, compared to only decreases. In addition, respondents are requested to use the past 2 weeks as the time frame during which such symptoms may have occurred, which is compatible with DSM-IV.

The BDI-II has demonstrated strong psychometric properties. For example, when the BDI-II was administered to individuals with psychiatric diagnoses and to other populations, such as college students, the results yielded high internal consistency coefficients (α = .92 and .93, respectively) and test–retest reliability (r = .93) (Beck et al., 1996). The factor structure of the BDI-II has been found to comprise two components—cognitive symptoms (e.g., pessimism, guilt, suicidal thoughts) and somatic–affective symptoms (e.g., sadness, loss of pleasure, crying, agitation). Comparisons between the BDI and the BDI-II suggest that the BDI-II is a stronger instrument in terms of its factor structure (Dozios, Ahnberg, & Dobson, 1998). The BDI-II has also been validated in a primary care setting (Arnau, Meagher, Norris, & Bramson, 2001), as well as in a sample of Southern, rural African American women (Gary & Yarandi, 2004).

BDI for Primary Care

The BDI for Primary Care (BDI-PC; Beck, Guth, Steer, & Ball, 1997) is a seven-item screening instrument developed to be a primary care modification of the BDI-II. To avoid confounding the symptoms of a medical condition that may be due to biological, medical, or substance abuse disorders, the somatic and behavioral symptoms of depression were not included. Thus, the BDI-PC minimizes the possibility of yielding spuriously high estimates of depression for patients with medical problems by focusing on psychological/cognitive symptoms, such as sadness, pessimism, past failure, loss of pleasure, self-dislike, self-criticalness, and suicidal thoughts or wishes. These seven items were chosen because they loaded saliently ($\geq$ .35) on the cognitive dimension of BDI-II scores.

BDI—Fast Screen

The BDI—Fast Screen (BDI-FS; Beck, Steer, & Brown, 2000), the most recent version of the BDI-PC, is an abbreviated self-report inventory designed to screen medical patients for depression rapidly using DSM-IV criteria (American Psychiatric Association, 1994). This measure primarily comprises the cognitive items of depression (e.g., statements that assess pessimism, self-dislike, previous failure, self-criticalness), which are included because they are considered to reflect the archetypal mood state of depression, independent of medical illness features. Items assessing sadness and loss of interest or pleasure in activities are also included. The last item on the BDI-FS assesses suicidal thoughts, which is regarded as an indicator of suicidal risk (Beck, Steer, & Brown, 2000). The BDI-FS has been found to be a psychometrically sound depression screening measure in a variety of medical populations, including patients with sickle-cell disease (Jenerette, Funk, & Murdaugh, 2005) and individuals diagnosed with multiple sclerosis (Benedict, Fishman, McClellan, Bakshi, & Weinstock-Guttman, 2003).

Cardiac Depression Scale

Research has increasingly documented the high prevalence and incidence of MDD among various cardiac patient populations (Nezu, Nezu, & Jain, 2005). As such, cardiac researchers have sought to develop measures of depression specifically validated on cardiac patient samples. The Cardiac Depression Scale (CDS) represents such a measure and was originally developed and validated in Australia (Hare & Davis, 1996). It comprises 26 items representing symptoms specific to depressed cardiac patients and uses a 7-point Likert-type scale. A brief, visual analog version of the scale was recently developed for rapid or repeated assessments (Di Benedetto, Lindner, Hare, & Kent, 2005). High internal consistency ($\alpha = .90$) and test–retest reliability ($r = .86$) estimates have been reported for the CDS. An initial factor analysis revealed the following seven factors: Sleep, Anhedonia, Uncertainty, Mood, Cognition, Hopelessness, and Inactivity.

According to its authors, the CDS has advantages over other depression scales used in medical populations. For example, it was developed and validated specifically for cardiac patients, whereas other measures were developed and validated in psychiatric populations. Thus, the CDS can be more sensitive in detecting the type of depression specific to cardiac patients, which is often characterized as subclinical or "reactive" (Di Benedetto et al., 2005). In addition, the CDS is posited as being psychometrically advantageous over the BDI, a commonly used scale in the cardiac literature. Compared with the BDI, which typically produces a positively skewed distribution, CDS scores have a normal distribution, enabling the CDS to differentiate scores in the lower range (Hare & Davis, 1996). The CDS also has an advantage over the Hospital Anxiety and Depression Scale (HADS; Zigmond & Snaith, 1983), another commonly used scale for medical populations, in that it includes items of somatic symptoms relevant to cardiac patients. Because the HADS omits somatic symptoms of depression and focuses on anhedonia, CDS developers claim that it loses important information, because somatic symptoms such as fatigue and reduced concentration are significant symptoms that some researchers believe to be related more to emotional distress (i.e., depression) than to the cardiac symptoms themselves (Lespérance & Frasure-Smith, 2000).

Center for Epidemiologic Studies Depression Scale

The Center for Epidemiologic Studies developed a 20-item, self-report, symptom rating scale to assess depressive symptomatology in the general population (Radloff, 1977). The Center for Epidemiologic Studies Depression Scale (CES-D) has been used as a tool for epidemiological studies of depression, screening for treatment studies, and measuring change over time in symptom severity. Scale items were originally chosen from previously developed scales (e.g., BDI) to represent the major symptoms of clinical depression. The instrument was designed to be brief, and takes less than 10 minutes to complete.

Based on a principal components analysis of data from general population samples, four major factors have been identified—Depressed Affect, Positive Affect, Somatic and Retarded Activity, and an Interpersonal factor (Radloff, 1977). The CES-D has also been found to be a reliable and valid measure of depression in samples of cancer patients (Hann, Winter, & Jacobsen, 1999) and individuals diagnosed with multiple sclerosis (Verdier-Talilefer, Gourlet, Fuhrer, & Alperovitch, 2001).

The CES-D has been used in many countries and has also been adapted for use in computer-assisted and telephone interviews. Studies have indicated that the psychometric properties of the computerized version are equivalent to those of the paper-and-pencil format (Ogles, France, Lunnen, Bell, & Goldfarb, 1998). Using the CES-D for voice recognition, computer-assisted interviews has been advantageous for overcoming language barriers and disabilities, and educating underserved populations (Muñoz, McQuaid, Gonzalez, Dimas, & Rosales, 1999).

CES-D—Revised

This 10-item version was derived from the original CES-D to correspond more closely with DSM-IV criteria for depression (Irwin, Artin, & Oxman, 1999). It was also revised to accommodate to the needs of elderly respondents, who may find the response format confusing, the questions emotionally stressful, and the time to complete it burdensome. Another stated purpose for this revision is to retain the advantageous qualities of a measure that has been valuable to community-based researchers, while increasing its generalizability to current psychiatric understanding. The CES-D—Revised (CES-D-R) has demonstrated high internal consistency ($\alpha = .87$; Turvey, Wallace, & Herzog, 1999), as well as good specificity (81–93%) and sensitivity (79–100%) when using a ≥ 4 cutoff score (Irwin et al., 1999).

Depression in the Medically Ill–18 and Depression in the Medically Ill–10

The Depression in the Medically Ill–18 and –10 (DMI-18 and DMI-10, respectively; Parker, Hilton, Bains, & Hadzi-Pavlovic, 2002) scales were specifically designed to measure depression in medically ill patients. To avoid confounding by symptoms of medical illness, both scales comprise solely cognitive-based items, whereas somatic items (e.g., sleep disturbance, appetite disturbance) are specifically excluded. Both versions exclude items regarding suicidal ideation and intent. The scale developers view the assessment of suicide as appropriate only in the context of face-to-face interaction, not as part of a self-report.

With regard to psychometric properties, Parker and colleagues (2002) estimated internal consistency for both the DMI-18 and DMI-10 to be high (.93 and .89, respectively). The DMI-18 was further found to be strongly correlated with both the BDI-PC and the HADS, as was the DMI-10. Using a ≥ 9 cutoff score for the DMI-10 yielded sensitivity estimates ranging between 93.5 and 100.0%. Specificity estimates ranged between 65.7 and 69.8%. A DMI-18 cutoff point ≥ 20 yielded sensitivity estimates ranging from 91.7 to 95.0% and specificity estimates between 68.1 and 72.4%. The sound psychometric properties of these scales have also been obtained in a variety of patient populations, including medically ill patients visiting general practitioners (Parker, Hilton, Hadzi-Pavlovic, & Irvine, 2003), psychiatric outpatients (Parker & Gladstone, 2004), and cardiac patients (Hilton et al., 2006).

Harvard Department of Psychiatry/National Depression Screening Day

The Harvard Department of Psychiatry/National Depression Screening Day (HANDS), a 10-item self-report questionnaire, was developed specifically to be used in the National Depression Screening Day (NDSD) in the United States (Baer et al., 2000). It is intended to be a brief, easy-to-score scale that provides guidelines for possible referral for mental health services. Items were derived from other psychometrically sound depression inventories, such as the BDI and Zung's Self-Rating Depression Scale (SDS; Zung, 1965), using item response theory. HANDS developers were careful to test its properties with participants reflecting the group that might participate in the NDSD. A cutoff score of 9 or higher (range of 0–30) yielded a sensitivity of 95% regarding individuals who met criteria for a DSM-IV diagnosis of MDD as produced via structured clinical interviews. This measure is also characterized by strong reliability properties (e.g., internal consistency is .87).

The HANDS has also been used to assess depression in both psychiatric and medical patient populations. For example, in examining the prevalence of cognitive and physical side effects of antidepressant medication, Fava and colleagues (2006) used the HANDS to define the treatment response/remission rates (i.e., scores < 9) and to assess the severity of residual depressive symptoms among patients diagnosed with MDD according to DSM-IV criteria. In addition, Wexler and colleagues (2006) used the HANDS to measure depression severity in patients with type 2 diabetes to investigate factors that affect the quality of life of primary care patients.

Hospital Anxiety and Depression Scale

The Hospital Anxiety and Depression Scale (HADS) was initially developed by Zigmond and Snaith (1983) to identify caseness of anxiety and depressive disorders among medical, nonpsychiatric patients. Fourteen items are equally distributed into two scales—Anxiety and Depression. All items are associated with a 4-point scale (0–3), producing a range on each scale of 0–21. To prevent overlap and inflated associations with somatic disorders, all symptoms of either anxiety or depression also relating to physical disorders (e.g., dizziness, headaches, insomnia, fatigue) were excluded. In a review of over 200 studies that used the HADS, Herrmann (1997) concluded that this clinically meaningful screening tool is also sensitive to changes related to the natural course of depression, as well as to responses due to both psychological and pharmacological interventions. More recently, Bjelland, Dahl, Haug, and Neckelmann (2002) reviewed an additional 747 studies published since the 1997 review to assess validity of the HADS. In general, this review indicated that factor-analytic studies revealed that the two-factor solution (i.e., Anxiety and Depression) was valid, that the Cronbach's alpha for the depression scale ranged between .67 and .90 (M = 0.82), and that a score of 8 and above on the depression scale yielded a sensitivity and specificity of .80. Overall, these authors concluded that the HADS performed effectively in identifying depression caseness across somatic, psychiatric, primary care, and nonpatient populations.

Inventory of Depressive Symptomatology

The Inventory of Depressive Symptomatology (IDS) was originally developed by Rush and colleagues (1986) to improve upon existing measures of depression by (1) providing equivalent weightings for each symptom item; (2) delineating clearly stated anchors; (3) including all DSM-IV criteria required to diagnose MDD; and (4) providing matched clinician and patient ratings. The original scales included 28 items in both versions and intended specifically to capture the following dimensions: vegetative symptoms, cognitive changes, mood disturbance, and anxiety symptoms. It was later increased to 30 items per version to include all DSM-IV atypical symptom features (Rush, Gullion, Basco, Jarrett, & Trivedi, 1996). Overall, the IDS was designed to provide a reliable method of measuring symptom severity and symptom change. Comparison of the psychometric properties of the 28- and 30-item versions led to the conclusion that the 30-item inventory was superior. Cronbach's alpha was found to range between .92 and .94 among a sample of depressed outpatients (Rush et al., 1996), to correlate highly with the HAMD, and to be sensitive to changes in symptom severity as a function of antidepressant medication.

Quick IDS

More recently, the IDS was revised to yield a shortened version, the 16-item Quick IDS (QIDS; Rush, Carmody, & Reimitz, 2000). Only those items that specifically addressed DSM-IV diagnostic symptom criteria were included in this version. The nine addressed DSM-IV domains include sad mood, concentration, self-criticism, suicidal ideation, interest, fatigue, sleep disturbance, appetite problems, and psychomotor agitation/retardation. An evaluation of the psychometric properties of the QIDS in a sample of patients with chronic depression yielded estimates of high internal consistency ($\alpha = .86$) and strong associations with the HAMD (Rush et al., 2003). Additional evaluations among patients in the Sequenced Treatment Alternatives to Relieve Depression (STAR*D; Rush et al., 2006) trial and among outpatients diagnosed with either MDD or bipolar disorder (Trivedi et al., 2004) further support the clinical utility and sensitivity of both the IDS and the QIDS.

Mood Disorder Questionnaire

The Mood Disorder Questionnaire (MDQ; Hirschfeld et al., 2000) is a self-report inventory developed to help screen for individuals who potentially experience bipolar spectrum disorder. It includes 13 yes–no items derived from both DSM-IV criteria and clinical experience. These items address whether several of any reported manic or hypomanic symptoms or behaviors (e.g., elevated energy levels, elevated interest in sex) were experienced during the same period of time. In addition, the respondent is asked to indicate the severity of impairment of such symptoms on a 4-point scale. Miller, Klugman, Berv, Rosenquist, and Ghaemi (2004) evaluated the sensitivity and specificity of the MDQ in a group of 37 patients with bipolar spectrum disorder and 36 patients with unipolar depression. Results indicated that the overall sensitivity was .58, but higher in patients with bipolar I disorder (.69) compared to those with bipolar II disorder (.30). A recent factor analysis of the MDQ identified a two-factor structure—an Elevated Mood Overactivity factor and an Irritable Behavior factor (Mangelli, Benazzi, & Fava, 2005). Due to the recency of this instrument, more extensive psychometric evaluations have not yet taken place.

Patient Health Questionnaire Depression Scale

The Primary Care Evaluation of Mental Disorders (PRIME-MD; Spitzer et al., 1994) is a clinician-administered instrument developed to assist primary care physicians when making criteria-based diagnoses of five common types of DSM-IV disorders, including depression.

The Patient Health Questionnaire (PHQ; Spitzer, Kroenke, & Williams, 1999) is the self-report version of the PRIME-MD developed to reduce clinician time required to evaluate a patient's responses. The Patient Health Questionnaire Depression Scale (PHQ-9; Kroenke, Spitzer, & Williams, 2001), the 9-item depression module from the full PHQ, asks patients to select the frequency of depressive symptoms they experienced in the past 2 weeks. It generally takes less than 10 minutes to complete. PHQ-9 items come directly from the nine signs and symptoms of major depression delineated in DSM-IV. Major depression is diagnosed if five or more of these nine criteria have been present at least *more than half the days* during the past 2 weeks and if one of the symptoms is depressed mood or anhedonia. One of the nine symptom criteria ("Thoughts that you would be better off dead or of hurting yourself in some way") counts, if present at all, regardless of duration.

PHQ-9 scores range from 0 to 27. Cutoff points of 5, 10, 15, and 20 represent the thresholds for *Mild*, *Moderate*, *Moderately severe*, and *Severe* depression, respectively. For a single screening cutpoint, a PHQ-9 score of 10 or greater was initially recommended (Kroenke et al., 2001). Internal consistency (Cronbach's α ranging from .86 to .89) and test–retest reliability (intraclass correlations ranging from .81 to .96) of the PHQ-9 have been found to be adequate (Kroenke et al., 2001). In addition, the PHQ has been validly applied to various medical populations, such as patients undergoing dialysis (Watnick, Wang, Demadura, & Ganzini, 2005) and individuals with traumatic brain injury (Fann et al., 2005).

In addition, the PHQ-9 has been validated and translated into many languages, including Spanish (Diez-Quevedo, Rangil, Sanchez-Planell, Kroenke, & Spitzer, 2001), German (Löwe, Grafe, et al., 2004), and Nigerian (Adewuya, Ola, & Afolabi, 2006). Moreover, Huang, Chung, Kroenke, Delucchi, and Spitzer (2006) found that the PHQ-9 measures a common construct of depression across diverse population samples (i.e., black, Chinese American, Latino, non-Hispanic white patient groups).

The PHQ-2 (Kroenke, Spitzer, & Williams, 2003) was developed as a two-item version of the PHQ-9 to address the need for briefer measures in busy clinical settings. This version inquires only about depressed mood and anhedonia. Kroenke and colleagues (2003) evaluated the criterion validity of the PHQ-2 with reference to the structured interview conducted by independent mental health professionals. They reported that the PHQ-2 was able to detect MDD with a sensitivity of 83% and a specificity of 92%, using an optimal cutoff score of 3.

Zung Self-Rating Depression Scale

The SDS (Zung, 1965) is among the most popular self-rating depression scales. This 20-item questionnaire was developed to assess quickly the cognitive, behavioral, and affective symptoms of depression. The psychometric properties of the SDS have been examined in a number of different cultures, including Dutch, Finnish, and Japanese populations. One study of 85 depressed and 28 nondepressed patients in a Dutch day clinic (de Jonghe & Baneke, 1989) found the internal consistency to be .82 and the split-half reliability to be .79. Factor analyses of the SDS have also been conducted. In general, although three factors tend to emerge from these analyses, they have been interpreted differently. For example, Sakamoto, Kijima, Tomoda, and Kambara (1998) assigned the following labels to the factors that emerged from their principal components analysis: cognitive, affective, and somatic symptoms. The analysis based on a sample of 2,187 Japanese college students resulted in a goodness-of-fit index (GFI) of .94. It was further supported by a confirmatory factor analysis in a sample of 597 Japanese undergraduates (GFI = .92). On the other hand, Kivela and Pahkala (1987) labeled the three factors differently that emerged from a principal components factor analysis with varimax rotation: depressed mood, loss of self-esteem, and irritability and agitation. This study was conducted in Finland with a sample of 290 depressed adults age 60 and older. It is possible that age or culturally related factors contributed to differences among these factors.

DECISION-MAKING GUIDELINES
FOR SELECTING DEPRESSION MEASURES

Given the plethora of psychometrically sound measures of depression, the question naturally arises: *Which one do I choose?* Moreover, because each depressed individual's difficulties are unique and no "textbook" strategy is readily apparent (Nezu & Nezu, 1993), effective decision-making guidelines are required (C. M. Nezu, Nezu, & Foster, 2000). As such, we recommend that the following questions should be considered when choosing assessment tools:

1. What are the goals of assessment?
2. Who is to be assessed?
3. What is the value of a given measure?
4. Who is the source of the information?

What Are the Goals of Assessment?

With regard to assessing depression, a variety of objectives can be identified, including (1) screening, (2) diagnosis and classification, (3) description of problem areas and symptoms, (4) case formulation and clinical hypothesis testing, (5) treatment planning, (6) prediction of behavior, and (7) outcome evaluation.

Screening

In clinical settings, screening provides a timely indication of whether further assessment is warranted. For research purposes, it is often helpful to determine whether a given individual might meet initial inclusion criteria. To be useful, scores from screening instruments should be highly correlated with scores provided by a more comprehensive assessment regarding the presence or absence of the disorder being assessed (i.e., adequate criterion-related validity). Cutoff scores are often required when screening instruments are used, along with information about the types of errors one may make when using such cutoffs. *Sensitivity* refers to the ability of a measure to identify accurately persons who have a given characteristic in question based on a given cutoff score, for example, the proportion of people with major depression who are correctly identified as such by their score on a given measure. *Specificity*, on the other hand, refers to the degree to which a measure accurately identifies individuals who do *not* have the characteristic being measured, for example, the proportion of people who in reality do not have a diagnosis of MDD, and who are correctly identified as *not* depressed by their score on a given depression measure. Measures originally identified as screening protocols include the HANDS, the PHQ, and the HADS.

Diagnosis and Classification

Accurate diagnostic classification serves two important purposes: (1) It provides for a common clinical language, and (2) it offers specific "content area" or index terms by which to search the scientific literature for accurate, reliable, and valid evaluation and treatment procedures (Nezu & Nezu, 1989). For research purposes, such classifications provide important demarcations among clinical samples, thus improving the validity and replicability of findings across studies. Instruments designed specifically for formulating diagnoses warrant particular scrutiny for their content validity; that is, a diagnostic instrument should contain content that clearly corresponds to the criteria required for diagnosis by a formal diagnostic system, such as the DSM-IV-TR (American Psychiatric Association, 2000). The content should exclude extraneous material and weigh symptoms as required by the classification system. Furthermore, the diagnosis that the instrument points to should be reliable over time and, when clinical judgment is involved, should demonstrate good interrater agreement when the system is implemented by independent evaluators assessing the same individual. Such a measure should also lead to an accurate differential diagnosis; that is, it should correctly denote not only the diagnosis for which a person qualifies but also diagnoses for which he or she does *not* qualify, especially when there is symptom overlap across diagnoses. Examples of such assessment procedures described earlier include the DIS, the DISH, the SAD-P, the SADS, and the SCID.

Description of Symptoms and Symptom Severity

Many assessment tools measure various dimensions of depression, such as the topography, range, severity, and/or frequency of symptoms. Such measures often provide specific idiographic information for persons within a specific diagnostic group (e.g., sleep difficulties, suicidal ideation, difficulties in concentration). Severity of depressive symptomatology is the most frequent assessment goal in both clinical and research settings given that such evaluations are important for treatment success. To usefully provide such information, measures of symptom severity especially need to be documented to be reliable over time. Most of the measures previously described, such as the BDI, the CDS, the CES-D, and the PHQ-9, assess depressive severity.

Clinical Hypothesis Testing

To develop a valid case formulation for a given individual, it is important to understand the etiology, function, and maintaining factors of that person's presenting problems (Nezu, Nezu, & Lombardo, 2004). Consequently, assessment focuses on identifying hypothesized *mechanisms of action*. Such variables, often referred to as *instrumental outcome variables*, can involve cognitive, emotional, behavioral, social, or biomedical factors that are theoretically or empirically connected to the symptoms or complaints for which an individual is seeking to achieve a given treatment objective or *ultimate outcome goal* (e.g., to decrease depression). From a research perspective, instrumental outcomes can be thought of as *independent variables*, whereas ultimate outcomes can be viewed as *dependent variables*. Clinically, changes in instrumental outcomes (e.g., poor problem-solving ability, as measured by the Social Problem-Solving Inventory—Revised; D'Zurilla, Nezu, & Maydeu-Olivares, 2002) are hypothesized to lead to changes in ultimate outcomes (e.g., problem-solving therapy lead to decreases in depressive symptoms, as posited by Nezu & Nezu, in press).

Treatment Planning

Assessing instrumental outcome variables can help therapists to develop treatment plans for depression (Nezu, Nezu, & Cos, 2007). For example, a clinician following a cognitive model of depression might first test for the presence of cognitive distortions using, for example, the Dysfunctional Attitude Scale (Weissman & Beck, 1978). The therapist is measuring not only depression (i.e., the referral complaint or ultimate reason for seeking treatment) but also a cognitive mediational style that is hypothesized to serve as an important causal factor of depression (an instrumental outcome). Therefore, the clinician would be able to determine whether, in fact, a cognitive model of depression is applicable to *this* patient. If so, then a cognitive restructuring approach may be recommended. If not, such an intervention might be inappropriate and potentially ineffective. In general, measures of instrumental outcomes can be useful for evaluating the idiographic importance of various mechanisms of action that are nomothetically linked to the clinical phenomena of interest. Measurement of both types of variables also underscores the importance of outcomes assessment in both clinical and research settings (Nezu, 1996). To usefully predict which treatments are likely to work and which are not, a measure ideally should provide some evidence that its use leads to more effective or efficient treatment than would occur in its absence.

Prediction of Behavior

Assessment is also important for behavioral prediction in academic, research, and clinical settings. Particularly relevant to clinical situations is the prediction of behavior that carries a high risk of danger to self or others. Relevant to depression, one example involves assessing the likelihood of suicidal risk (e.g., the Suicidal Ideation Questionnaire; Reynolds, 1987). In this case, previous studies of predictive validity are important, so that the clinician can determine how well the assessment tool actually predicts the outcome for which it was intended, as well as the nature and range of prediction errors that occur.

Treatment Outcome

Assessment protocols can also help to monitor therapeutic progress and to evaluate the efficacy of treatment. As such, the content of the measure should specifically address the behaviors targeted by the treatment plan. It is important that the measure be stable in the absence of conditions that produce change (i.e., that it demonstrate acceptable test–retest reliability in the absence of treatment or changes in the individual's circumstances). The measure should also be sufficiently sensitive to detect change. Investigations of whether changes in scores on the measure following treatment correlate significantly with changes in scores on other measures of the same construct provide further evidence of treatment sensitivity, as well as convergent validity. With respect to depression, measures that assess symptom severity, such as the BDI, often serve as instruments that provide information about the effects of treatment (e.g., a decrease in symptom severity).

Whom Are We Assessing?

People with depression represent a heterogeneous group. Therefore, in addition to determining an assessment plan based on particular goals for a given individual, it is important to use measures developed specifically for that particular subgroup of "depressed" people.

Age Differences

One patient variable of consequence is age. For example, adult measures of depression would be potentially inappropriate for children not only due to language differences but also with regard to the potential divarications in the overall constellation of symptoms and their behavioral expression. As such, a variety of depression measures have been developed specifically for children and adolescents, such as the Children's Depression Inventory (CDI; Kovacs, 1992) and the Reynolds Child Depression Inventory (Reynolds, 1989). Measures have also been developed specifically for older persons. A popular measure is the Geriatric Depression Scale (Yesavage et al., 1983), a self-report questionnaire geared for adults age 65 years and older. The Depression Rating Scale (Cohen-Mansfield & Marx, 1988) was developed to assess both depression and social functioning, specifically among older adult nursing home residents.

Concomitant Diagnoses

Another potential individual-difference variable is the presence of additional psychiatric or medical diagnoses. In certain cases, these concomitant problems can limit the validity of depression measures that do not take these disorders into account. One example is the Calgary Depression Scale for Schizophrenia (Addington, Addington, & Maticka-Tyndale, 1993), a clinician-rated protocol developed in response to the observation that other assessment instruments for depression did not accurately represent depressive symptoms or syndromes in persons with schizophrenia. In the Medical-Based Emotional Distress Scale (Overholser, Schubert, Foliart, & Frost, 1993), developed to provide a more valid assessment of distress, including dysphoria, the results are posited as not being biased by physical symptoms of the co-occurring medical disorder. Other, previously described examples of measures developed specifically or validated to assess depression in various medical populations include the BDI-FS, CDS, DMI-18, HADS, and PHQ-9.

Another relevant patient sample involves individuals with mental retardation. Although the prevalence of psychopathology in such individuals is significantly greater than among persons with normal intellectual functioning (C. M. Nezu, Nezu, & Gill-Weiss, 1992), the availability of psychometrically sound instruments to assess such problems is very limited. One such example is the Psychopathology Inventory for Mentally Retarded Adults (PIMRA; Matson, 1988), which includes eight clinical scales, one of which is an Affective Disorders scale. This interview-based instrument was developed and normed specifically on adult populations with mental retardation.

Cultural Differences

Of particular importance regarding interindividual differences is the potential influence of ethnic and cultural backgrounds. It is not enough to ensure that a self-report measure has been competently back-translated into another language (e.g., Spanish); it is critical also to demonstrate that it actually addresses constructs that have meaning within the given culture. Research has shown that whereas some similarities are evident in the expression of depression across various cultures, differences do exist (Kaiser, Katz, & Shaw, 1998). Such differences (e.g., headaches and "nerves" in Latino and Mediterranean cultures, fatigue and "imbalance" among Asian cultures, and "problems of the heart" in Middle Eastern countries, according to DSM-IV-TR; American Psychiatric Association, 2000) may be a function of varying values among cultures, or the manner in which Western society interprets these values. Cultures also vary in the manner in which they judge the seriousness or appropriateness of dysphoria (Parker, Gladstone, & Chee, 2001).

The importance of considering cultural background when conducting a differential diagnosis is emphasized in DSM-IV-TR (American Psychiatric Association, 2000). It is recommended that, in addition to the five standard diagnostic axes, the clinician consider five additional categories when working with multicultural environments: (1) cultural identity of the individual (e.g., the person's self-identified cultural group, his or her degree of acculturation, as well as his or her current involvement in the host culture); (2) cultural explanations of the individual's disorder (e.g., the causal attributions and significance of the "condition" that is promulgated by the individual's culture); (3) cultural factors related to one's psychosocial environment and levels of functioning (e.g., the availability of social support and the cultural interpretation of social stressors); (4) cultural elements of the relationship between the person and the clinician (e.g., the differences in both culture and social status between the clinician and the patient); and (5) overall assessment for diagnosis and care (e.g., the cultural factors that might impact upon the patient's diagnosis and treatment).

Using a cognitive-behavioral perspective, Tanaka-Matsumi, Seiden, and Lam (1996) suggest a similar approach when conducting a "culturally informed functional analysis." Specifically, they suggest eight concrete steps: (1) Assess cultural identity and degree of acculturation; (2) assess and evaluate clients' presenting problems with reference to their cultural norms; (3) evaluate clients' causal attributions regarding their problems; (4) conduct a functional analysis; (5) compare one's case formulation with a patient's belief system; (6) negotiate treatment objectives and methods with the patient; (7) discuss with the patient the need for data collection to assess treatment progress; and (8) discuss treatment duration, course, and expected outcome with the client.

Various measures of depression, initially developed in Western cultures, have been demonstrated to be applicable across a variety of cultures and have been translated into numerous languages, such as the BDI, the PHQ-9, and the Zung SDS. An example of a measure of depression specifically developed for a non-Western culture is the Vietnamese Depression Scale (VDS; Kinzie et al., 1982), which was developed in conjunction with Vietnamese mental health professionals; cultural group norms were considered at every stage of its development. Another example, the Chinese Depressive Symptom Scale (Lin, 1989), was specifically developed on the basis of research with community residents of Tianjin, China.

What Is the Value of a Given Measure?

We define the *value* of a measure as the joint function of (1) the probability that a given measure will provide the appropriate type of information for a given goal and (2) the cost–benefit ratio regarding practical concerns. The first aspect focuses on the strength of the psychometric properties of a measure, especially in relation to the specific goal at hand. As noted in the previous section on assessment goals, certain psychometric properties were identified as being particularly important relative to a given objective, for example, the need for a measure of depressive symptom severity to be reliable over time.

A cost–benefit analysis of various practical concerns should address the following issues: (1) the amount of time required by both the patient and the assessor; (2) potential risks or dangers associated with a given assessment procedure; (3) potential ethical violations associated with a given measure; (4) the effects of a given procedure on involved others (e.g., family members); (5) short- versus long-term benefits or liabilities related to a given assessment procedure; and (6) the incremental utility of the measure (e.g., how much unique information the measure offers).

One additional issue to be considered regarding practical issues is the cognitive complexity (e.g., length and number of individual items, readability, linguistic problems) of a particular measure. Shumway, Sentell, Unick, and Bamberg (2004) assessed the cognitive complexity of 15 self-administered depression measures and found considerable variability among them. With regard to measures described in this chapter, the BDI was found to be one of the most complex, whereas the Zung SDS and the HANDS were among the least complex. Consequently, when one is concerned about the ability of a given patient or research participant to understand and respond accurately to a given depression measure, because of limited educational background, levels of cognitive complexity need to be taken into account.

Who Is the Source of the Information?

Depression measures can be divided into two categories based on the source of the information—self-report and clinician-rated measures. Each method has its advantages and disadvantages. For example, whereas self-report questionnaires are relatively brief and require less time to complete than do clinician-rated measures, they are more vulnerable to respondent bias (e.g., patients may be less than truthful or wish to present themselves in a particularly "good or bad light"). Clinician-rated measures are likely to produce more reliable results than self-report inventories but often require special training in the structured interviews that may accompany such procedures. All else being equal, a combination of both procedures likely yields the most valid and comprehensive picture of a given patient. It is important, however, that the reader consider all the questions posed in this decision-making guide when choosing among the various measures of depression.

CONCLUSIONS AND FUTURE DIRECTIONS

We began this chapter by noting that close to 300 measures of depression have been developed during the past century. Most are not currently in active use, which suggests that new measures may be unnecessary. We firmly believe, however, that despite the plethora of current measures, it is important that researchers and clinicians continue to develop new measures and to engage in major revisions of existing instruments. We argue this point to address (1) the changing definition of depression (i.e., changes in diagnostic criteria) and the need to have measures that are consistent with contemporary thinking; (2) the changing nature of how depression is experienced and expressed by various subcultures of individuals who will be acculturated during the next several decades into mainstream Western society in varying degrees; (3) the improved understanding of how depression is expressed concomitantly with other mental health (e.g., anxiety disorders, bipolar disorder) and medical or physical health (e.g., cardiovascular disease, cancer, diabetes) diagnoses; and (4) the need to have psychometrically sound but user-friendly (e.g., brief, physically accessible, cognitively understandable) measures to accommodate a variety of patient needs. The final paragraphs of this chapter include what we consider to be important areas of future research and conceptual focus regarding the assessment of depression, including (1) definitional issues, (2) diversity issues, (3) advances in technology, and (4) conceptualization of depression as a public health issue.

Definitional Issues

As we noted earlier in describing the various measures of depression, new inventories have been developed or existing measures have been revised to be more consistent and current relative to changes in the definition of depression over the past decades (i.e., changes in DSM diagnostic criteria). Measures of depression must continue to be current, especially in light of controversies regarding the appropriateness of the "gold standard" status that certain measures currently enjoy as a function of tradition rather than of validity (e.g., the HAMD). The construction of the GRID-HAMD and future efforts of the DRSST to improve the HAMD are excellent examples of such efforts. In addition, not only do older measures need to be revised, but also basic research on the psychometric properties of such revisions must continue.

A related issue involves differences in what various researchers believe constitutes "core symptoms" of depression. For example, some measures were specifically developed to assess all nine DSM-IV diagnostic criteria dimensions (e.g., IDS, QID), whereas others were constructed to exclude deliberately certain criteria, such as suicidal ideation (e.g., DMI-10). Because it is unlikely that any single study will be administered to compare simultaneously the psychometric properties of a large number of measures, it will be difficult to ascertain which assessment tool is more reliable and valid across different populations and testing settings. One major divarication that currently appears unresolved is the definition of depression as it is experienced by samples of medical patients. As we noted earlier, several measures of depression were developed specifically for such individuals, with the notion of deliberately excluding somatic symptoms, such as fatigue and sleep disturbances (e.g., BDI-FS, BDI-PC, DMI-10, DMI-18, HADS); other measures, however, were not (e.g., CDS, PHQ, PHQ-9). In fact, the CDS, which was developed specifically for patients with cardiovascular disease, contains items addressing somatic symptoms, such as fatigue, with the notion that fatigue in depressed heart patients is related more to mood disturbance than to the cardiovascular problems. Interestingly, the NHLBI Working Group recommended that the first edition of the BDI be used as the measure of choice for both epidemiological and treatment outcome research due to its widespread usage and extensive database, with the caveat that the BDI-II, in the future, may accumulate additional psychometric properties to support its use (Davidson et al., 2006). It is important to note, however, that if cardiac researchers follow this recommendation, assuming that several measures of depression are not likely to be administered in the same study, the goal of collecting additional evidence for other inventories that do not have the history of the BDI, even the BDI-II, appears limited. Given that fatigue is a highly prevalent symptom of various cardiovascular disorders, particularly of heart failure, it is critical that research in the future focus on establishing a more valid definition of depression in medical patient populations, such as individuals with heart disease, to obtain a more comprehensive understanding of the experience and impact of this mood disorder.

Diversity Issues

As mentioned earlier in this chapter, the phenomenology and expression of depression can vary across differing ethnically based cultures (Kaiser et al., 1998), thus calling into question the validity of measures originally developed with samples of white, middle-class adults. In addition, because of their minority status, various ethnically diverse populations in the United States may have had limited access to traditional mental health services, thus creating further obstacles to this validation process. For example, Latinos represent a U.S. population that is frequently underserved. One study found that only 11% of Mexican Americans who met diagnostic criteria for major depression had sought mental health services (Muñoz et al., 1999). Spanish-speaking patients may experience a language barrier that inhibits them from seeking services. In general, we need to understand better how depression is conceptualized in both its experience and expression across different cultures, then develop psychometrically sound measures that better assess depression among such ethnically diverse populations. As immigrant populations increase in the United States, so does acculturation, making this endeavor particularly difficult. For example, Lin (1989) noted that whereas a review of the literature continues to support the hypothesis that Chinese individuals tend to deny depression or to express it somatically, rather than psychologically, Western influences in China have actually modified this behavioral pattern. Thus, what may currently be relevant and valid measures of depression among various cultures may become outdated in the near future.

Future research should also focus on improving the assessment of depression among (1) individuals residing in rural areas, (2) those who have lower economic status and literacy rates, (3) older adults, and (4) disabled people. Increasing the number of valid and reliable assessment modalities for such populations can lead to two important outcomes: (1) The degree and amount of treatment interventions aimed at reducing depression for these groups will expand; and (2) the accuracy of the estimate of the incidence and prevalence of depression in the general population will also be improved.

Advances in Technology

After considering the varied populations in need of future research and some of the obstacles faced by clinicians, it is not surprising that recent research efforts have attempted to reduce these barriers by expanding beyond traditional paper-and-pencil or interview techniques. Computerized voice recognition programs have the capability to evaluate depression among non-English-speaking persons, disabled patients, low-literacy populations, and geriatric samples (González et al., 2000). In addition, they can record and chart a patient's weekly assessment, increase the public's awareness of depression, improve the detection and treatment of depression in the general population, as well as objectify assessments and be cost- and time-efficient (Ogles et al., 1998).

Nevertheless, such technologically advanced protocols are not without problems. For example, it has been suggested that state anxiety can increase as a result of the computerized testing situation and potentially confound results (Merten & Ruch, 1996). Furthermore, computerized screening poses a dilemma in the treatment of patients who are suicidal or who have acute crises (Ogles et al., 1998). In addition, Cacciola and colleagues (1999) found that participants are more likely to receive a lifetime diagnosis of MDD when they are administered an in-person SCID rather than a telephone-based SCID. Therefore, substantial research is needed both to improve upon this technology and to identify, and subsequently resolve, important ethical dilemmas.

Depression as a Public Health Issue

The 2000 report on mental health by the Surgeon General of the United States (National Institute of Mental Health, 2000) underscored the need to view mental health as a public health issue. In addition, researchers have called for a greater synthesis between psychological and public health research to develop broad-based community interventions for depression (Nezu, Nezu, Trunzo, & McClure, 1998). In this context, assessment procedures need to be developed that examine the impact of depression has on public health, and the efficacy and effectiveness of community-based interventions. The HANDS (Baer et al., 2000) is one of the first measures to move in this direction by focusing on screening the general public for clinically significant depression by promoting a National Depression Screening Day. The effort to better equip primary care personnel to screen depression (e.g., PHQ-2) is another example of our improved ability to detect depression in large samples. Future research should continue to focus on the validity of using depression measures for public health purposes, the social and financial impact of depression on the community, and the likelihood of accessing and/or maintaining effective treatment as a result of public health assessment, prevention, and intervention.

REFERENCES

Addington, D., Addington, J., & Maticka-Tyndale, E. (1993). Rating depression in schizophrenia: A comparison of a self-report and an observer report scale. *Journal of Nervous and Mental Disease*, *181*, 561–565.

Adewuya, A. O., Ola, B. A., & Afolabi, O. O. (2006). Validity of the Patient Health Questionnaire (PHQ-9) as a screening tool for depression amongst Nigerian university students. *Journal of Affective Disorders*, *96*, 89–93.

American Psychiatric Association. (1994). *Diagnostic and statistical manual of mental disorders* (4th ed.). Washington, DC: Author.

American Psychiatric Association. (2000). *Diagnostic and statistical manual of mental disorders* (4th ed., text rev.). Washington, DC: Author.

Anthony, J. C., Folstein, M., Romanoski, A. J., Von Korff, M. R., Nestadt, G. R., Chahal, R., et al. (1985). Comparison of the lay Diagnostic Interview Schedule and a standardized psychiatric diagnosis: Experience in eastern Baltimore. *Archives of General Psychiatry*, *42*, 667–675.

Arnau, R. C., Meagher, M. W., Norris, M. P., & Bramson, R. (2001). Psychometric evaluation of the Beck Depression Inventory–II with primary care medical patients. *Health Psychology*, *20*, 112–119.

Baer, L., Jacobs, D. G., Meszler-Reizes, J., Blais, M., Fava, M., Kessler, R., et al. (2000). Development of a brief screening instrument: The HANDS. *Psychotherapy and Psychosomatics*, *69*, 35–41.

Bagby, R. M., Ryder, A. G., Schuller, D. R., & Marshall, M. B. (2004). The Hamilton Depression Rating Scale: Has the gold standard become a lead weight? *American Journal of Psychiatry*, *161*, 2163–2177.

Beck, A. T., Guth, D., Steer, R. A., & Ball, R. A. (1997). Screening for major depression disorders in medical inpatients with the Beck Depression Inventory for Primary Care. *Behaviour Research, and Therapy*, *35*, 785–791.

Beck, A. T., Steer, R. A., & Brown, G. K. (1996). *Manual for the BDI-II.* San Antonio, TX: Psychological Corporation.

Beck, A. T., Steer, R. A., & Brown, G. K. (2000). *Manual for the Beck Depression Inventory—Fast Screen for medical patients.* San Antonio, TX: Psychological Corporation.

Beck, A. T., Ward, C. H., Mendelson, M., Mock, J., & Erbaugh, J. (1961). An inventory for measuring depression. *Archives of General Psychiatry*, *4*, 561–571.

Benedict, R. H. B., Fishman, I., McClellan, M. M., Bakshi, R., & Weinstock-Guttman, B. (2003). Validity of the Beck Depression Inventory—Fast Screen in multiple sclerosis. *Multiple Sclerosis*, *9*, 393–396.

Bjelland, I., Dahl, A. A., Haug, T. T., & Neckelmann, D. (2002). The validity of the Hospital Anxiety and Depression Scale: An updated review. *Journal of Psychosomatic Research*, *52*, 69–77.

Cacciola, J. S., Alterman, A. I., Rutherford, M. J., McKay, J. R., & May, D. J. (1999). Comparability of telephone and in-person structured clinical interview for DSM-III-R (SCID) diagnoses. *Assessment*, *6*, 235–242.

Cohen-Mansfield, J., & Marz, M. S. (1988). Relationship between depression and agitation in nursing home residents. *Comprehensive Gerontology B: Behavioral, Social, and Applied Sciences*, *2*, 141–146.

Corruble, E., & Hardy, P. (2005). Why the Hamilton Depression Rating Scale endures. *American Journal of Psychiatry*, *162*, 2394.

Davidson, K. W., Kupfer, D. J., Bigger, J. T., Califf, R. M., Carney, R. M., Coyne, J. C., et al. (2006). Assessment and treatment of depression in patients with cardiovascular disease: National Heart, Lung, and Blood Institute Working Group Report. *Annals of Behavioral Medicine*, *32*, 121–126.

de Jonghe, J. F., & Baneke, J. J. (1989). The Zung Self-Rating Depression Scale: A replication study on reliability, validity and prediction. *Psychological Reports*, *64*, 833–834.

Di Benedetto, M., Lindner, H., Hare, D. L., & Kent, S. (2005). A Cardiac Depression Visual Analogue Scale for the brief and rapid assessment of depression following acute coronary syndromes. *Journal of Psychosomatic Research*, *59*, 223–229.

Diez-Quevedo, C., Rangil, T., Sanchez-Planell, L., Kroenke, K., & Spitzer, R. L. (2001). Validation and utility of the Patient Health Questionnaire in diagnosing mental disorders in 1003 general hospital Spanish inpatients. *Psychosomatic Medicine*, *63*, 679–686.

Dozois, D. J. A., Ahnberg, J. L., & Dobson, K. S. (1998). A psychometric evaluation of the Beck Depression Inventory–II. *Psychological Assessment*, *10*, 83–89.

D'Zurilla, T. J., Nezu, A. M., & Maydeu-Olivares, A. (2002). *Social Problem-Solving Inventory—Revised (SPSI-R): Technical manual*. North Tonawanda, NY: Multi-Health Systems.

Endicott, J., & Spitzer, R. L. (1978). A diagnostic interview: The Schedule for Affective Disorders and Schizophrenia. *Archives of General Psychiatry*, *35*, 837–844.

ENRICHD Investigators. (2000). Enhancing Recovery in Coronary Heart Disease Patients (ENRICHD): Study design and methods. *American Heart Journal*, *139*, 1–9.

Fava, M., Graves, L. M., Benazzi, F., Scalia, M. J., Iosifescu, D. V., Alpert, J. E., et al. (2006). A cross-sectional study of the prevalence of cognitive and physical symptoms during long-term antidepressant treatment. *Journal of Clinical Psychiatry*, *67*, 1754–1759.

Fann, J. R., Bombardier, C. H., Dikmen, S., Esselman, P., Warms, C. A., Pelzer, E., et al. (2005). Validity of the Patient Health Questionnaire–9 in assessing depression following traumatic brain injury. *Journal of Head Trauma and Rehabilitation*, *20*, 501–511.

First, M. B., Gibbon, M., Spitzer, R. L., & Williams, J. B. (1996). *Structured Clinical Interview for DSM-IV Axis I Disorders—Non-Patient Edition* (SCID-I/NP, Version 2.0). New York: Biometrics Research Department, New York State Psychiatric Institute.

First, M. B., Spitzer, R. L., Gibbon, M., & Williams, J. B. (1997). *User's guide for the Structure Clinical Interview for DSM-IV Axis I Disorders*. Washington, DC: American Psychiatric Press.

Freedland, K. E., Skala, J. A., Carney, R. M., Raczynski, J. M., Taylor, C. B., Mendes de Leon, C. F., et al. (2002). The Depression Interview and Structured Hamilton (DISH): Rationale, development, characteristics, and clinical validity. *Psychosomatic Medicine*, *64*, 897–905.

Gary, F. A., & Yarandi, H. N. (2004). Depression among southern rural African American women: A factor analysis of the Beck Depression Inventory–II. *Nursing Research*, *53*, 251–259.

González, G. M., Winfrey, J., Sertic, M., Salcedo, J., Parker, C., & Mendoza, S. (2000). A bilingual telephone-enabled speech recognition application for screening depression symptoms. *Professional Psychology: Research and Practice*, *31*, 398–403.

Hann, D., Winter, K., & Jacobsen, P. (1999). Measurement of depressive symptoms in cancer patients: Evaluation of the Center for Epidemiological Studies—Depression Studies Depression Scale (CES-D). *Journal of Psychosomatic Research*, *46*, 437–443.

Hamilton, M. (1960). Development of a rating scale for depression. *Journal of Neurology, Neurosurgery, and Psychiatry*, *23*, 56–62.

Hare, D. L., & Davis, C. R. (1996). Cardiac Depression Scale: Validation of a new depression scale for cardiac patients. *Journal of Psychosomatic Research*, *40*, 379–386.

Hedlund, J. L., & Vieweg, B. W. (1979). The Hamilton Rating Scale for Depression: A comprehensive review. *Journal of Operational Psychiatry*, *10*, 149–165.

Herrmann, C. (1997). International experiences with the Hospital Anxiety and Depression Scale—a review of validation data and clinical results. *Journal of Psychosomatic Research*, *42*, 17–41.

Hilton, T. M., Parker, G., McDonald, S., Heruc, G. A., Olley, A., Brotchie, H., et al. (2006). A validation study of two brief measures of depression in the cardiac population: The DMI-10 and DMI-18. *Psychosomatics*, *47*, 129–135.

Hirschfeld, R. M., Lewis, L., & Vornik, L. A. (2003). Perceptions and impact of bipolar disorder: How far have we really come: Results of the National Depressive and Manic–Depressive Association 2000 survey of individuals with bipolar disorder. *Journal of Clinical Psychiatry, 64*, 161–174.

Hirschfeld, R. M. A., Williams, J. B. W., Spitzer, R. L., Calabrese, J. R., Flynn, L., Keck, P. E., Jr., et al. (2000). Development and validation of a screening instrument for bipolar spectrum disorder: The Mood Disorder Questionnaire. *American Journal of Psychiatry, 157*, 1873–1875.

Huang, F. Y., Chung, H., Kroenke, K., Delucchi, K. L., & Spitzer, R. L. (2006). Using the Patient Health Questionnaire–9 to measure depression among racially and ethnically diverse primary care patients. *Journal of General Internal Medicine, 21*, 547–552.

Irwin, M., Artin, K., & Oxman, M. N. (1999). Screening for depression in the older adult. *Archives of Internal Medicine, 159*, 1701–1704.

Jenerette, C., Funk, M., & Murdaugh, C. (2005). Sickle cell disease: A stigmatizing condition that may lead to depression. *Issues in Mental Health Nursing, 26*, 1081–1101.

Kaiser, A. S., Katz, R., & Shaw, B. F. (1998). Cultural issues in the management of depression. In S. S. Kazarian & D. E. Evans (Eds.), *Cultural clinical psychology: Theory, research, and practice* (pp. 177–214). New York: Oxford University Press.

Kalali, A., Bech, P., Williams, J., Kobak, K., Lipsitz, J., Engelhardt, N., et al. (2002). The new GRID-HAM-D—results from field trials. *European Neuropsychopharmacology, 12*(S3), 239.

Kinzie, J. D., Manson, S. M., Vino, T. D., Tolan, N. T., Anh, B., & Pho, T. N. (1982). Development and validation of a Vietnamese language rating scale. *American Journal of Psychiatry, 139*, 1276–1281.

Kivela, S., & Pahkala, K. (1987). Factor structure of the Zung Self-Rating Depression Scale among a depressed elderly population. *International Journal of Psychology, 22*, 289–300.

Koenig, H. G. (2006). Predictors of depression outcomes in medical inpatients with chronic pulmonary disease. *American Journal of Geriatric Psychiatry, 14*, 939–948.

Kovacs, M. (1992). *Children's Depression Inventory manual*. North Tonawanda, NY: Multi-Health Systems.

Kroenke, K., Spitzer, R. L., & Williams, J. B. W. (2001). The PHQ-9: Validity of a brief depression severity measure. *Journal of General Internal Medicine, 16*, 606–613.

Kroenke, K., Spitzer, R. L., & Williams, J. B. (2003). The Patient Health Questionnaire–2: Validity of a two-item depression screener. *Medical Care, 41*, 1284–1292.

Lespérance, F., & Frasure-Smith, N. (2000). Depression in patients with cardiac disease: A practical review. *Journal of Psychosomatic Research, 48*, 379–391.

Lin, N. (1989). Measuring depressive symptomatology in China. *Journal of Nervous and Mental Disease, 177*, 121–131.

Löwe, B., Gräfe, K., Zipfel, S., Witte, S., Loerch, B., & Herzog, W. (2004). Diagnosing ICD-10 depressive episodes: Superior criterion validity of the Patient Health Questionnaire. *Psychotherapy and Psychosomatics, 73*, 386–390.

Mangelli, L., Benazzi, F., & Fava, G. A. (2005). Assessing the community prevalence of bipolar spectrum symptoms by the Mood Disorder Questionnaire. *Psychotherapy and Psychosomatics, 74*, 120–122.

Matson, J. L. (1988). *The PIMRA manual*. New Orleans, LA: International Diagnostic Systems.

McIntyre, R. S., Kennedy, S., Bagby, R. M., & Bakish, D. (2002). Assessing full remission. *Journal of Psychiatry and Neuroscience, 27*, 235–239.

Merten, T., & Ruch, W. (1996). A comparison of computerized and conventional administration of the German versions of the Eysenck Personality Questionnaire and the Carroll Rating Scale for Depression. *Personality and Individual Differences, 20*, 281–291.

Miller, C. J., Klugman, J., Berv, D. A., Rosenquist, K. J., & Ghaemi, S. N. (2004). Sensitivity and specificity of the Mood Disorder Questionnaire for detecting bipolar disorder. *Journal of Affective Disorders, 81*, 167–171.

Muñoz, R. F., McQuaid, J. R., Gonzalez, G. M., Dimas, J., & Rosales, V. A. (1999). Depression screening in a women's clinic using automated Spanish and English language voice recognition. *Journal of Consulting and Clinical Psychology, 67*, 502–510.

National Institute of Mental Health. (2000). *Mental health: A report of the Surgeon General* (DSL 2000-0134-P). Washington, DC: U.S. Government Printing Office.

Nezu, A. M. (1996). What are we doing to our patients and should we care if anyone else knows? *Clinical Psychology: Science and Practice, 3*, 160–163.

Nezu, A. M., & Nezu, C. M. (Eds.). (1989). *Clinical decision making in behavior therapy: A problem-solving perspective*. Champaign, IL: Research Press.

Nezu, A. M., & Nezu, C. M. (1993). Identifying and selecting target problems for clinical interventions: A problem-solving model. *Psychological Assessment, 5*, 254–263.

Nezu, A. M., & Nezu, C. M. (in press). Problem solving as a risk factor for depression. In K. S. Dobson & D. Dozois (Eds.), *Risk factors for depression*. New York: Elsevier Science.

Nezu, A. M., Nezu, C. M., & Cos, T. A. (2007). Case formulation for the behavioral and cognitive therapies: A problem-solving perspective. In T. D. Eells (Ed.), *Handbook of psychotherapy case formulation* (2nd ed., pp. 349–378). New York: Guilford Press.

Nezu, A. M., Nezu, C. M., & Jain, D. (2005). *The emotional wellness way to cardiac health: How letting go of depression, anxiety, and anger can heal your heart*. Oakland, CA: New Harbinger.

Nezu, A. M., Nezu, C. M., & Lombardo, E. R. (2004). *Cognitive-behavioral case formulation and treatment design: A problem-solving approach*. New York: Springer.

Nezu, A. M., Nezu, C. M., McClure, K. S., & Zwick, M. L. (2002). Assessment of depression. In I. H. Gotlib & C. L. Hammen (Eds.), *Handbook of depression* (pp. 61–85). New York: Guilford Press.

Nezu, A. M., Nezu, C. M., Trunzo, J. J., & McClure, K. S. (1998). Treatment maintenance for unipolar depression: Relevant issues, literature review, and recommendations for research and clinical practice. *Clinical Psychology: Science and Practice, 5*, 496–512.

Nezu, A. M., Ronan, G. F., Meadows, E. A., & McClure, K. S. (2000). *Practitioner's guide to empirically based measures of depression*. New York: Kluwer Academic/Plenum Press.

Nezu, C. M., Nezu, A. M., & Foster, S. L. (2000). A 10-step guide to selecting assessment measures in clinical and research settings. In A. M. Nezu, G. F. Ronan, E. A. Meadows, & K. S. McClure (Eds.), *Practitioner's guide to empirically based measures of depression* (pp. 17–24). New York: Kluwer Academic/Plenum Press.

Nezu, C. M., Nezu, A. M., & Gill-Weiss, M. J. (1992). *Psychopathology of persons with mental retardation: Clinical guidelines for assessment and treatment*. Champaign, IL: Research Press.

Ogles, B. M., France, C. R., Lunnen, K. M., Bell, M. T., & Goldfarb, M. (1998). Computerized depression screening and awareness. *Community Mental Health Journal, 34*, 27–38.

Overholser, J. C., Schubert, D. S. P., Foliart, R., & Frost, F. (1993). Assessment of emotional distress following a spinal cord injury. *Rehabilitation Psychology, 38*, 187–198.

Parker G., & Gladstone, G. (2004). Capacity of the DMI-10 depression in the medically ill screening measure to detect depression "caseness" in psychiatric out-patients. *Psychiatry Research, 127*, 283–287.

Parker, G., Gladstone, G., & Chee, K. T. (2001). Depression in the planet's largest ethnic group: The Chinese. *American Journal of Psychiatry, 158*, 857–864.

Parker, G., Hilton, T., Bains, J., & Hadzi-Pavlovic, D. (2002). Cognitive-based measures screening for depression in the medically ill: The DMI-10 and DMI-18. *Acta Psychiatrica Scandinavica, 105*, 419–426.

Parker, G., Hilton, T., Hadzi-Pavlovic, D., & Irvine, P. (2003). Clinical and personality correlates of a new measure of depression: A general practice study. *Australian and New Zealand Journal of Psychiatry, 37*, 104–109.

Radloff, L. S. (1977). The CES-D Scale: A self-report depression scale for research in the general population. *Applied Psychological Measurement, 1*, 385–401.

Reynolds, W. M. (1987). *Suicide Ideation Questionnaire: Professional manual*. Odessa, FL: Psychological Assessment Resources.

Reynolds, W. M. (1989). *Reynolds Child Depression Scale: Professional manual*. Odessa, FL: Psychological Assessment Resources.

Robins, L. N., Helzer, J. E., Croughan, J. L., & Ratcliff, K. S. (1981). National Institute of Mental Health Diagnostic Interview Schedule: Its history, characteristics, and validity. *Archives of General Psychiatry, 38*, 381–389.

Rogers, R. (2001). Schedule of Affective Disorders and Schizophrenia (SADS). In R. Rogers, *Handbook of diagnostic and structured interviewing* (pp. 84–102). New York: Guilford Press.

Rush, A. J., Bernstein, I. H., Trivedi, M. H., Carmody, T. J., Wisniewski, S., Mundt, J. C., et al. (2006). An evaluation of the Quick Inventory of Depressive Symptomatology and the Hamilton Rating Scale for Depression: A sequenced treatment alternatives to relieve depression trial report. *Biological Psychiatry*, 59, 493–501.

Rush, A. J., Carmody, T., & Reimitz, P. E. (2000). The Inventory of Depressive Symptomatology (IDS): Clinician (IDS-C) and Self-Report (IDS-SR) ratings of depressive symptoms. *International Journal of Methods in Psychiatric Research*, 9, 45–59.

Rush, A. J., Giles, D. E., Schlesser, M. A., Fulton, C. L., Weissenburger, J., & Burns, C. (1986). The Inventory for Depressive Symptomatology (IDS): Preliminary findings. *Psychiatry Research*, 18, 65–87.

Rush, A. J., Gullion, C. M., Basco, M. R., Jarrett, R. B., & Trivedi, M. H. (1996). The Inventory of Depressive Symptomatology (IDS): Psychometric properties. *Psychological Medicine*, 26, 477–486.

Rush, A. J., Trivedi, M. H., Ibrahim, H. M., Carmody, T. J., Arnow, B., Klein, D. N., et al. (2003). The 16-item Quick Inventory of Depressive Symptomatology (QIDS), Clinician Rating (QIDS-C), and Self-Report (QIDS-SR): A psychometric evaluation in patients with chronic major depression. *Biological Psychiatry*, 54, 573–583.

Sakamoto, S., Kijima, N., Tomoda, A., & Kambara, M. (1998). Factor structures of the Zung Self-Rating Depression Scale (SDS) for undergraduates. *Journal of Clinical Psychology*, 54, 477–487.

Santor, D. A., Gregus, M., & Welch, A. (2006). Eight decades of measurement in depression. *Measurement*, 4, 135–155.

Segal, D. L., Hersen, M., & Van Hasselt, V. B. (1994). Reliability of the Structured Clinical Interview for DSM-III-R: Evaluative review. *Comprehensive Psychiatry*, 35, 316–327.

Shumway, M., Sentell, T., Unick, G., & Bamberg, W. (2004). Cognitive complexity of self-administered depression measures. *Journal of Affective Disorders*, 83, 191–198.

Solomon, D. A., Leon, A. C., Maser, J. D., Truman, C. J., Coryell, W., Endicott, J., et al. (2006). Distinguishing bipolar major depression from unipolar major depression with the Screening Assessment of Depression—Polarity (SAD-P). *Journal of Clinical Psychiatry*, 67, 434–442.

Spitzer, R. L., Endicott, J., & Robins, E. (1978). Research Diagnostic Criteria. *Archives of General Psychiatry*, 35, 773–782.

Spitzer, R. L., Kroenke, K., & Williams, J. B. (1999). Patient Health Questionnaire Study Group: Validity and utility of a self-report version of PRIME-MD: The PHQ Primary Care Study. *Journal of the American Medical Association*, 282, 1737–1744.

Spitzer, R. L., Williams, J. B., Kroenke, K., Linzer, M., deGruy, F. V., Hahn, S. R., et al. (1994). Utility of a new procedure for diagnosing mental disorders in primary care: The PRIME-MD 1000 study. *Journal of the American Medical Association*, 272, 1749–1756.

Tanaka-Matsumi, J., Seiden, D. Y., & Lam, K. N. (1996). The Culturally Informed Functional Assessment (CIFA) interview: A strategy for cross-cultural behavioral practice. *Cognitive and Behavioral Practice*, 3, 215–234.

Trivedi, M. H., Rush, A. J., Ibrahim, H. M., Carmody, T. J., Biggs, M. M., Suppes, T., et al. (2004). The Inventory of Depressive Symptomatology, Clinician Rating (IDS-C) and Self-Report (IDS-SR), and the Quick Inventory of Depressive Symptomatology, Clinician Rating (QIDS-C), and Self-Report (QIDS-SR) in public sector patients with mood disorders: A psychometric evaluation. *Psychological Medicine*, 34, 73–82.

Turvey, C. L., Wallace, R. B., & Herzog, R. (1999). A revised CES-D measure of depressive symptoms and DSM-based measure of major depressive episode in the elderly. *International Journal of Psychogeriatrics*, 11, 139–148.

Verdier-Talilefer, M. H., Gourlet, V., Fuhrer, R., & Alperovitch, A. (2001). Psychometric properties of the Center for Epidemiologic Studies—Depression Scale in multiple sclerosis. *Neuroepidemiology*, 20, 262–267.

Vuorilehto, M., Melartin, T., & Isometsa, E. (2006). Depressive disorders in primary care: Recurrent, chronic, and co-morbid. *Psychological Medicine*, 35, 673–682.

Watnick, S., Wang, P. L., Demadura, T., & Ganzini, L. (2005). Validation of 2 depression screening tools in dialysis patients. *American Journal of Kidney Diseases*, 46, 919–924.

Weissman, A., & Beck, A. T. (1978, November). *Development and validation of the Dysfunctional Attitude Scale.* Paper presented at the annual meeting of the Association for Advancement of Behavior Therapy, Chicago.

Wexler, D. J., Grant, R. W., Wittenberg, E., Bosch, J. L., Cagliero, E., & Delahanty, L. (2006). Correlates of health-related quality of life in type 2 diabetes. *Diabetologia, 49,* 1489–1497.

Williams, J. B. W. (1988). A structured interview guide for the Hamilton Depression Rating Scale. *Archives of General Psychiatry, 45,* 742–747.

Yesavage, J. A., Brink, T. L., Rose, T. L., Lum, O., Huang, V., Adey, M., et al. (1983). Development and validation of a geriatric depression screening scale: A preliminary report. *Journal of Psychiatric Research, 17,* 37–49.

Zigmond, A. S., & Snaith, R. P. (1983). The Hospital Anxiety and Depression Scale. *Acta Psychiatrica Scandinavica, 67,* 361–370.

Zung, W. W. K. (1965). A self-rating depression scale. *Archives of General Psychiatry, 12,* 63–70.

CHAPTER 4

Methodological Issues in the Study of Depression

Rick E. Ingram *and* Greg J. Siegle

The appearance of the second edition of this *Handbook* underscores the enormous interest in understanding depression. Whether from a research or a clinical practice perspective, knowledge of depression is arguably necessary for all mental health professionals and students. It is simply not possible to comprehend depression meaningfully in the absence of methodologically sound research. Thus, our purpose in this chapter is to examine relevant issues and strategies for conducting research on depression. No single chapter, or even a book devoted to methodology, can examine all of the basic methodological issues that must guide the conduct of scientific research (issues such as random selection and internal and external validity). Nor can a single chapter articulate all of the important details to consider in every study of depression. Moreover, each area of depression research has specific methodological issues and challenges that cannot be covered in a single chapter. In this chapter, therefore, we focus on several major issues that are broadly important for research efforts on depression. We assume that sound general methodological techniques are well understood by researchers; consequently, we do not comment on these unless they are particularly germane to a topic of depression research.

DEFINING THE CONSTRUCT FOR RESEARCH: WHAT IS DEPRESSION?

It is imperative that investigators begin with a clear definition of the type of depression in which they are interested. There is arguably no more important factor in depression research than to define who is depressed and by what criteria. Thus, we examine both some conceptual and operational definitions of depression that researchers may wish to consider.

Depression as a Theoretical Construct

Depression has historically been conceived of as encompassing states that range from emotional distress to despondency to melancholia. Major depressive disorder (MDD) is currently conceptualized as a group of related symptoms, some of which are seen as criteria for the disorder (e.g., sad mood) and others of which are not (e.g., being discouraged about the future). Moreover, according to DSM-IV-TR (American Psychiatric Association, 2000), a certain number, but not a certain constellation, of symptoms must be present for a diagnosis. Consequently, very different conditions can receive the same diagnostic label of depression. The fact that some symptoms are recognized for a disorder, whereas others are not, underscores the idea that what is defined as *depression* is constructed from a group of symptoms that the scientific community has collectively termed to be depression. Thus, depression is a construct that is part of a broader class of psychological ideas. Should the scientific community decide that depression comprises a different group of symptoms (e.g., that suicidal ideation rather than sad mood is the defining feature of depression), the nature of depression itself would change, the characteristics of people diagnosed with depression would be different, and epidemiological data on the prevalence of depression would be transformed. Thus, how we define a construct such as depression is by a consensus of the scientific community.

Depression as a Clinical Syndrome

DSM-IV-TR is widely recognized as the classification system that defines depression for research and clinical purposes. DSM-IV-TR employs a categorical approach to psychological disorders; disorders are viewed as discrete entities that occur independently of other discrete disorders, although these other discrete disorders can also occur and give rise to comorbidity. Thus, depression is one of many distinct categories of disorders.

The manner in which depression is characterized in sources such as DSM-IV-TR has important implications for not only how depression is conceptualized by researchers (both implicitly and explicitly), but also how it is measured. For example, DSM-IV-TR requires the selection of research participants who meet certain inclusion criteria and do not meet certain exclusion criteria. Therefore, the categorical inclusion and exclusion diagnostic criteria established in DSM-IV-TR provide one way for researchers to define MDD operationally.

It is important to note that dimensional assumptions, which suggest that mild and severe depression are different ends of the same continuum, can be contrasted to the categorical assumptions inherent in DSM-IV-TR. For the study of MDD, differing assumptions do not necessarily affect the nature of the research. For example, an investigator who assumes that depression is continuous can still study depression by selecting participants on the basis of meeting DSM-IV-TR criteria for depression.

On the other hand, if an investigator assumes a dimensional view of depression, in which subclinical depressive states can be used as proxies to understand clinically significant depression, this assumption can have a dramatic impact on the nature of participant samples, on obtained results, and on the conclusions that are drawn. A number of researchers have questioned the advisability of attempting to understand clinical depression using such subclinical samples (Kendall & Flannery-Schroeder, 1995; Tennen, Hall, & Affleck, 1995), with some suggesting that doing so runs the risk of not only trivializing depression research but also diminishing the contributions of psychology in the eyes of science in general and of psychiatry in particular (Coyne, 1994). Several researchers have offered methodological suggestions for dealing with some of these issues (Ingram & Hamilton, 1999; Kendall, Hollon, Beck, Hammen, & Ingram, 1987).

Can the research with subclinical states, accompanied by the assumption of continuity, generalize to MDD? There seems to be a growing body of evidence, if not a consensus, that depression has at least some, if not many, dimensional qualities (Ruscio & Ruscio, 2000). Does this, then, suggest that it is wise to attempt to understand clinically significant depression by studying subclinical depression? Probably not. There are several reasons for this conclusion. First, the research addressing this issue, although suggestive, is not yet definitive. We may yet see evidence suggesting that the underlying structure of these states has qualitative differences. Second, questions of continuity focus on addressing depressive syndromes of differing severity, but, as we note later in this chapter, symptom-focused methodologies are in many cases a better alternative to this approach. Third, even if depression does fall on a continuum, some correlates may be so small in magnitude at the low end that they escape detection. To give a very simple illustration, an investigator interested in how depression is related to interpersonal disturbance might very well find little interpersonal disturbance when studying mild depressive states. However, given the widespread recognition that clinically significant depression is accompanied by problematic interpersonal functioning (Joiner & Coyne, 1999), generalization of such a subclinical finding to severe depression would be inappropriate and misleading. Fourth, and in a somewhat related fashion, even if many of the features of depression are dimensional, they may potentiate categorical processes at the severe end of the spectrum. Consider an example of sleep disturbances, which are common in depression (Hamilton, Luxton, & Karlson, in press). Suppose that sleep disturbances are themselves dimensional, so that mild sleep disturbances are observed in mild depression and serious sleep disturbances are observed in severe depression. However, if serious, but not mild, sleep disturbances disrupt biological regulation, then this may also cause qualitatively different problems in MDD that are absent in subclinical depression. Thus, studying sleep in subclinically depressed participants to understand the implications of sleep disturbances in clinical depression would be misguided, even if the research demonstrated that sleep disturbances do vary on a continuum.

So a decision to try to understand the features of MDD requires the selection of research participants who meet specified criteria for MDD. As we have noted, although it is theoretically possible to use other criteria, these criteria, for all practical purposes, will be those specified in DSM-IV-TR. Similarly, *dysthymia* is defined in DSM-IV-TR as the presence of at least two depressive symptoms lasting for at least 2 years. As with MDD, investigators interested in this construct are obligated to provide a clear operational definition of the construct for research purposes and, if they do not rely on DSM-IV-TR criteria, need to make a case for how the measure they use maps onto this construct. Bipolar disorder, along with its division into bipolar I (characterized by the presence of a manic episode) and bipolar II (the presence of a hypomanic episode), requires similar attention to both conceptual and operational clarity.

Depression as a Subclinical Syndrome

There are several reasons why an investigator might choose to study subclinical or minor depression. For example, subclinical depression may represent a risk factor for MDD, and may be conceptualized as one way to study risk. Another reason is that such mild states often represent more than just ordinary unhappiness, sad mood, or simply having a bad mood day (Gotlib, Lewinsohn, & Seeley, 1995). Indeed, it is possible for these states to be accompanied by at least some clear depressive symptoms (mild to moderate levels of motivational and cognitive deficits, vegetative signs, disruptions in interpersonal relationships, etc.). The symptoms of mild depression, though less serious than their clinical counterparts, may also interfere with significant aspects of individuals' lives. Thus, the emotionally problematic, disruptive, and common nature of mild or subclinical depressive states would appear to justify their study.

It is important to note that there is some confusion surrounding the concept and terminology of subclinical depression. Most broadly, *subclinical depression* tends be operationalized as any state in which depressive symptoms are present, but not in either sufficient number or severity to qualify as MDD, or in which symptoms have not been assessed in a manner that would warrant the determination of a diagnosis of MDD (e.g., through the use of self-report questionnaires). Procedures defining depression this way are so broad that they obscure important conceptual and methodological issues; therefore, they are not particularly useful. We briefly discuss several concepts that seem to fall under the label of *subclinical depression*, each of which has received some research attention and has some unique methodological issues to which attention should be directed.

Subclinical Depression Defined by DSM-IV-TR

DSM-IV includes *minor depressive disorder* as a proposal for a new category of psychological problem and specifies that this disorder is identical to MDD, with the exception that one must experience at least two but fewer than five depressive symptoms, and that less impairment be present. Such a condition clearly seems to fall under the rubric of subclinical depression, although it rarely appears as such in the research literature. Nevertheless, an investigator who wishes to study this type of depression has an available conceptual and operational definition of the disorder in DSM-IV-TR.

Subclinical Depression Defined by Elevated Scores on Depression Questionnaires

By far the most common approach to studying subclinical depression is to select individuals (almost always college students) on the basis of scores elevated above some cutoff on a depression questionnaire. In the vast majority of these cases the questionnaire used is the Beck Depression Inventory (BDI; Beck, 1967) and, although we confine our comments to subclinical depression defined by the BDI, our comments generally apply to other questionnaire procedures as well.

Aside from the considerable reliability and validity data that have accrued on the BDI (Beck, Steer, & Garbin, 1988), an important feature of this measure is the specification of cutoff points. For the BDI-IA (Beck, Rush, Shaw, & Emery, 1979) the cutoff for mild depressive states is a score of 10, whereas for the BDI-II, it is 14. The availability of cutoff points raises two related questions concerning how subclinical depression is operationalized. First does adherence to cutoff points capture the essential features of the subclinically depressed state, and second, is this minimum cutoff adequate for defining a sufficiently depressed subclinical sample?

Assuming that investigators of subclinical depression are interested in studying individuals who, even at a mild level, are experiencing one of the two cardinal features of depression, either sad mood or a loss of interest, is a cutoff score of 10 or 14 sufficient for determining that these essential features are present? Several investigators have expressed skepticism. For example, Tennen and colleagues (1995) have argued that such scores may be obtained even though the essential features of sad mood or loss of interest may not be endorsed by many respondents. A related consideration is the intensity of the endorsed critical symptoms. For instance, to count as endorsing a critical symptom, does one only need to check "I feel sad" on the BDI rather than the other available options, such as "I am so sad or unhappy that I can't stand it"? Clearly, on a measure with scores that can range as high as 63, a score of 10 or 14 may be obtained by individuals who are not experiencing cardinal symptoms with much intensity. Fortunately, the solution for this problem is relatively straightforward: selecting only participants who, depending on the investigator's interest, endorse either or both of the essential diagnostic features of depression. Investigators interested in more problematic subclinical states may want to require not only the endorsement of these items but also that they be endorsed at the higher levels available on the BDI.

Just as establishing minimum cutoffs is critical for studies of subclinical depression, so too is establishing upper cutoffs. Studies of "subclinical" depression that take all comers above a specified minimum cutoff will recruit some research participants who are clinically depressed. Such a study mixes subclinical depression and MDD in the same sample, which may yield misleading results, if assumptions of continuity turn out to be incorrect. Thus, researchers interested in subclinical depression would be well advised to, at minimum, set an upper cutoff, and would be even better advised to use a measure such as the Structured Clinical Interview for DSM-IV (SCID) to rule out MDD in sample participants.

Assessing Depressive Symptoms

There are a variety of reasons for investigators to study symptomatology in depression. Rather than studying a syndrome defined by either clinical or subclinical depression, an investigator may wish to examine the relation between the degree or severity of depressive symptoms and some other construct. Or investigators may wish to examine the relations among a few select symptoms, or even between one symptom and another construct, or a constellation of symptoms that cluster together (e.g., vegetative symptoms) and some other variable. For example, investigators may wish to understand specific mechanisms of depression they believe to be independent of other aspects of depression, in which case, the most appropriate strategy may be to examine individuals without the entire depressive syndrome. Several strategies exist for such studies, with at least one strategy that is both common and inappropriate. We note this strategy first.

Assessing Calculus Interests among Preschoolers: Studying Symptoms in Unselected Samples

One strategy to assess the association between depression and variables of some theoretical interest is to examine the correlation between these variables in an unselected sample. Studies employing this strategy are based on assumptions that both depression and its association with some other variable are continuous, relatively normally distributed, meaningful at both the high and low ends of the symptom spectrum, and that the associations between these variables are linear.

How reasonable are such assumptions? Not very. To note one reason why, the majority of subjects in any given sample will have very few depressive symptoms. Thus, studies that adopt this correlational strategy are assessing the relation between depression and some other variable in a sample in which little depression is present. Such a strategy is akin to studying interest in learning calculus among preschoolers. Because preschoolers have no such interest, correlations between scores on a questionnaire measuring this interest (undoubtedly randomly distributed) and some other measure would be meaningless, as is research that attempts to study the relation between a construct and depressive symptoms in a relatively nondepressed sample.

There are several appropriate ways to examine relations involving depressive symptomatology. One approach is to study only individuals who score above some cutoff point, that is, individuals who are experiencing depressive symptoms. A sample that comprises research participants who score above 13 on the BDI-II is more appropriate for answering questions about relations between degree of symptomatology and other variables. Indeed, it has been demonstrated that results can vary in important ways depending on whether associations are examined in the entire sample or in those who exceed the cutoff for a depressed subsample (Ingram & Hamilton, 1999).

Another strategy is to ensure that the full range of depressive symptoms is represented in the sample. For example, the researcher interested in this type of question could adopt a stratified sampling approach. This would involve selecting equal numbers of participants falling within equal intervals on the depression measure (e.g., on the BDI, selecting the same number of participants who score a 0, 1, 2, etc., up to some cutoff). Such a strategy creates an artificial sample, but it does so in a way that allows investigators to examine the genuine correlations between depressive symptoms, even at the very low end, and other variables.

Symptom Profile Research Strategies and Subtype Strategies

SYMPTOM PROFILES

Although there is general agreement that depression is phenotypically diverse, numerous studies rely on assessing individuals who evidence some constellation of depressive symptoms (i.e., a syndrome-based approach is used to define and then study depression). Several investigators, however, have pointed out the limitations of the syndrome-based approach (Costello, 1992; Ingram, Miranda, & Segal, 1998; Kendall & Brady, 1995; Persons, 1986). These limitations stem from the fact that this approach implicitly assumes that individuals with the same syndrome are equivalent in all or most important psychological ways—an assumption that is clearly not correct. For example, Kendall and Brady (1995) note that the symptoms of psychological disorders are so diverse that two people could be diagnosed with the same disorder but actually have very few symptoms in common. In the specific case of depression, only five of the nine criteria detailed in DSM-IV-TR are necessary for a diagnosis; thus, it is possible that two depressed individuals could have only one common symptom, and even the nature and experience of that one symptom could vary. Indeed, except for a diagnosis of depression, these two individuals could have virtually nothing in common, including the variables that caused the disorder and that determine its course. Moreover, relying solely on the concept of a syndrome to study a problem such as depression may miss important information (Persons, 1986). Thus, a sample of "depressed" individuals, selected only because they have enough symptoms to qualify as depressed, represents a phenotypically heterogeneous group.

It seems likely that different causal processes give rise to various symptom patterns that are clustered under the label of *depression*. Few would dispute at least some causal heterogeneity, yet few empirical data are available to help sort out the parameters of the different causal pathways that are both possible and potentially numerous. Indeed, although the possible subtypes of depression may not be endless, they are potentially so diverse that they may functionally defy conceptual classification and empirical scrutiny. Nevertheless, to disregard conceptually the possibility of different subtypes, or to acquiesce methodologically to the complexity of possible causal heterogeneity by ignoring the implications of lumping together various subtypes in research studies, likely hinders efforts to understand the nature of depression. Given this state of affairs, at least two broad sets of assumptions can guide methodological decision making: conceptual proposals for various subtypes, and a more empirically derived approach focused on examination of different subsets of symptoms.

Depending on the precise conceptual questions posed by investigators, a symptom-based conceptualization may be a viable alternative to the pure syndrome-based approach. Rather than group all individuals together because they have met some threshold of depressive symptoms, a symptom profile approach targets specific symptoms that are considered important. For example, negative affect is a variable that is critical to the definition of depression, and it is also thought to play a significant role in determining psychological and social functioning of depressed people. Investigators who are interested in negative affect might choose to study this variable in the context of a depressive state, yet it is important to realize that depressed (clinical, subclinical, dysthymia), anxious (general anxiety states, as well as more specific anxious states such as phobia and obsessive–compulsive problems), and physically ill (acute and chronically ill) people all experience negative affect. If negative affect is studied only in the context of a depressive syndrome, then important aspects of this phenomenon may be missed. Alternatively, a focus on negative affect rather than on the syndrome of depression allows for the study of individuals who share this state and are similar in important respects.

Using symptom clusters, or even one symptom, to select research participants does not rule out obtaining other information from participants. For instance, if a specific measure of negative affect is used, a depression syndrome can still be assessed. Indeed, in the case of a variable such as negative affect, this procedure allows investigators to determine whether a depressive syndrome (or other syndromes), or some pattern of depressive (or other) symptoms, contributes to explaining variance over and above that associated with negative affect. Hence, a specific focus on negative affect allows investigators to determine the correlates and possible causes of a process that may be fundamental to many types of psychopathology, and also to examine how this variable is associated with other symptoms and behaviors. Negative affect is, of course, merely an example. Investigators may decide to focus on other target symptoms or on clusters of similar symptoms.

It may therefore be worthwhile for researchers to consider examining depressive symptom profiles or clusters rather than (or perhaps in addition to) the aggregation of symptoms represented by classifying people as depressed. Of course, if researchers are interested in a depression construct characterized by the experience of a variety of symptoms (and are uninterested in specific subtypes), then the syndrome approach is warranted. Clearly, though, the symptom profile approach encompasses a high degree of flexibility and potentially addresses a number of questions that are simply not possible when participants are only selected for high versus low scores on a depression self-report measure, or when they exceed some clinical threshold of depressive symptoms. It also allows researchers to allow more precise conceptual questions.

SUBTYPES

Virtually all investigators operate from a theoretical framework that specifies at least some idea about causal processes. Unless they propose that all cases meeting the criteria for depression are caused by the same factors, it is possible conceptually to stipulate different subtypes, then proceed to test subtypes based on the predictions derived from a given model. These predictions presumably involve proposals about the symptoms and features that should follow from the proposed causal process, along with prevention and treatment implications. Thus, it should be possible to identify empirically those individuals who exhibit the proposed subtype, then to determine whether they become depressed when the "right" circumstances occur as specified by the particular subtype model (e.g., certain life events).

Abramson and Alloy (1990) have laid out similar logic in methodologies to test their proposals for a negative cognition subtype of depression. Inasmuch as some of the symptoms that typify certain subtypes may occur in various types of depression, they argue that studies may not do justice to possible subtypes if they lump all research participants together on the basis of exceeding a symptom threshold; in essence, this obscures the ability to find the possible causal pathways occurring in only a subset of the larger sample. They followed this logic to test their proposed negative cognition subtype of depression (Alloy & Abramson, 1999). They selected college students who were not depressed but who evidenced the kind of negative thinking patterns and attributional tendencies specified by the model, and followed them over the course of several years, assessing their likelihood of becoming depressed, as well as symptom patterns and features that should follow from their causal model. In a different application of this type of reasoning, Drevets (1999) developed a biological model of a novel subtype, *familial pure depression* (depression with no family history of alcoholism, antisocial personality, or mania), and subsequently selected for neuroimaging assessment individuals who were depressed and had relevant family histories to test his theory. We mention these particular proposals to illustrate that rather than lumping all individuals into studies based on a pure symptom approach, investigators can specify the types of causal processes that underlie their model, select individuals for whom the model seems to apply (i.e., the particular depression subtype), then assess the kinds of clinical symptoms and features that should follow from the model.

METHODOLOGICAL ISSUES AND CHALLENGES RELATED TO THE STUDY OF DEPRESSION

Having now presented some of the issues involved in defining depression operationally, we turn to a consideration of methodological issues for the purposes of adequately studying one of these depressive states (or patterns of symptoms). In particular, we examine some common problems in depression research and suggest possible solutions to these difficulties.

Third Variables: Broad and Specific Perspectives

Both broad and more specific ways to consider third-variable confounding can be considered; either or both are applicable depending on the particular questions being asked. The broader perspective focuses on the idea of "nuisance variables" (Meehl, 1978) and is a concern not only in depression studies but also in all studies that examine individual-difference variables (Campbell & Stanley, 1966). This represents a problem for research regardless of whether the focus is on MDD, subclinical depression, or symptom profiles. The more specific area of concern for depression is reflected in comorbidity, presenting more of an issue for studies of MDD than for research on subclinical depression or symptom-driven approaches. It is well known that depression is correlated with other emotionally dysfunctional states (Smith & Rhodewalt, 1991), thus making it difficult to know whether results are largely a function of depression alone, of some correlated state, or of a combination of depression and other states (Ingram, 1989).

In a similar fashion, consideration of physical comorbidities has become increasingly important in recent years. For example, mortality associated with post–myocardial infarction (MI) is greatly increased in the presence of depression; the extent to which post-MI depression represents a unique subtype is unclear. Moreover, physical and mental comorbidities may interact. For instance, nearly all post-MI depressed patients have significant anxiety (Denollet, Strik, Lousberg, & Honig, 2006). Another reason to consider physical comorbidities is that physical conditions and their associated treatments may induce depressions that are different in character from most naturally occurring depressions: Steroid- and cytokine-induced depressions, postpartum depressions, and lesion and psychoactive drug-induced depressions also have unique characteristics, highlighting the potential utility of attending to these features in more general studies of depression.

In theory, solutions to the presence of nuisance variables are relatively straightforward. For example, a researcher interested in depression could assess possibly correlated nuisance variables, such as anxiety, then statistically control for them in subsequent results. A second method also involves assessing the nuisance variable, then selecting only research participants who endorse depressive symptoms but do not endorse more than an average number of anxiety symptoms. However, even when investigators adhere to exclusion criteria that rule out comorbid diagnoses or problems, a subclinical comorbid state may still exist, as might the existence of other unassessed problems.

Depending on the theoretical context that guides the work, covariation is not necessarily a problem and may in fact lead to a more precise description of the causes and correlates of depression, as well as other symptom patterns. Natural covariation in and of itself, however, is not a sufficient justification for research practices that simply fail to distinguish between depressed states and other conditions. For example, Tennen and colleagues (1995) noted a growing body of research that has demonstrated important distinctions in the correlates of depression and anxiety despite their high correlation (Ingram, 1989; Kendall & Watson, 1989). Failing to produce a precise definition of the affective condition or conditions in which an investigator is interested, these differences belie the idea that not distinguishing empirically between these states is appropriate.

Solutions to the problem of third (and fourth, fifth, etc.) variables tend to fall into the broad categories of statistical control (if the third variable can be adequately measured) or exclusionary criteria (if a third variable can be identified). However, there is no "one size fits all" solution to nuisance-variable issues. How to deal with these confounds is ultimately up to the investigator. The investigator who is interested in assessing "pure" depression will make different decisions than will the one who is interested in depression as it naturally occurs.

Interacting Comorbidity

Comorbid states may interact with depression, for example, by making depression particularly severe or changing the nature of depression in the presence of the comorbid condition. In this context, attempts to decouple naturally co-occurring affective states may create an artificial condition. Hence, this situation would represent not simple nuisance covariation, but a condition in need of more subtle decomposition, for the comorbidity is part and parcel of the depressed state. For instance, the nature of the association between depression and anxiety is still a matter of debate. Whereas some investigators maintain that depression and anxiety lie on a continuum, others contend that depression and anxiety represent orthogonal dimensions, for which particular combinations (e.g., mixed anxiety–depression) represent a qualitatively different disorder than having just one condition (e.g., Angst & Merikangas, 1998; Barlow & Campbell, 2000). This consideration is particularly important, because over half of depressed adults report significant anxiety (Fawcett & Howard, 1983). Because comorbid patients take longer to recover than do "purely" depressed people (Angst, 1997), this distinction is particularly important. For understanding the individual with mixed depression–anxiety, the same considerations are applied as those used to understand a person with bipolar disorder, which is seen as a condition separate from unipolar depression (see Johnson, Cuellar, & Miller, Chapter 7, this volume).

Regardless of whether comorbidity is conceptualized as a nuisance variable to be controlled or as an important part of depression, investigators would be well advised to be aware of the issues of third variables and to develop a plan for dealing with them. In virtually all cases investigators would be wise to attempt to assess systematically those states that are known or suspected to be associated with depression. What they do with this assessment is then a function of the particular question being addressed.

Stability Considerations

Issues concerning depression stability have important methodological implications. Arguably the most significant effect of depressive states is that they endure over some period of time. Thus, we would be wise to focus our research efforts on those states that evidence this stability. This is especially important in studies of subclinical depression, because the milder nature of these states suggests that they will be less stable than MDD or (by definition) dysthymia. Thus, the meaningfulness of research on subclinical depression is enhanced by showing that the depressed state being studied endures over some period of time rather than remitting quickly. Although more stable, even MDD is not immune from stability issues.

Stability considerations bring with them some important methodological requirements. Most research on depression is pragmatically a two-step process, the first of which involves measuring the presence of depressive symptoms on one occasion, then conducting the research on a second occasion with individuals who meet the initial criteria for depression. For example, scores on depression measures can change, sometimes dramatically, over even relatively short periods of time. Thus, a group of individuals initially selected for high levels of depression may include a substantial number of people who no longer fall into a depressed range when experimental testing commences. Functionally, such research is testing hypotheses in a "depressed" sample in which not everyone is depressed. The best-case scenario in such a situation is that error variance increases, rendering detection of differences more difficult. A worst-case scenario is that such a procedure may produce misleading or erroneous results.

MDD represents a potentially different set of stability issues. Because of the severity and typical course of a state such as MDD, in most cases one can assume that these individuals will continue to meet criteria for depression at the time of experimental testing (although it is still wise to verify this). If an investigator is only interested in whether such criteria are met, then little further work is required. Beyond simply meeting criteria, however, the severity of depression (e.g., the number and intensity of symptoms) can vary, sometimes substantially, over the course of days or weeks. Such variability is commonly assessed in treatment studies (e.g., Jarrett, Vittengl, Doyle, & Clark, 2007), but this is less frequently the case in nontreatment studies. In addition, the pattern of symptoms may change over time. Beyond continuing to meet criteria, researchers' conclusions should take into account the symptom patterns and intensities at the time of experimental testing rather than those present at the time of selection into the study.

So researchers are well advised to establish the stability of the depressive state in which they are interested. Kendall and colleagues (1987) and Tennen and colleagues (1995) have argued for the use of multiple-gating procedures in which researchers establish appropriate depression scores or criteria at selection, readminister the depression measure at testing, then analyze data from only those individuals who score in the specified range, or who meet criteria, on both occasions. This helps to ensure that (1) this phenomenon has been stable over some period of time; (2) that participants are actually depressed at the time of testing and, depending on what is assessed; and that (3) patterns of depressive symptoms are consistent.

Depression across the Lifespan: Developmental Considerations

The extent to which depression in adults and children represents the same disorder is the subject of debate (e.g., Kaufman, Martin, King, & Charney, 2001). Current DSM criteria for child and adult depression are similar. Yet diagnosis in children is often more difficult, because children may have trouble reporting symptoms and may experience different patterns of symptoms. Thus, clinicians often rely on observations, such as tearfulness or academic problems, to make an early-onset diagnosis (Ryan, 2001). Symptom measures also suggest that at early ages, depression and other disorders, such as anxiety and attention-deficit/hyperactivity disorder (ADHD), may overlap considerably (Angold, Costello, & Erkanli, 1999). Also, biological measures associated with depression may not generalize to children (Kaufman et al., 2001). For example, event-related brain potentials suggest that depressed adults display greater brain responses to errors than do healthy adults (Tucker, Luu, Frishkoff, Quiring, & Poulsen, 2003). The event-related potential is late to develop and is not easily detectable in children (Ladouceur, Dahl, & Carter, 2007). Similarly, hypofrontality is a key biological measure in adult depression Siegle, Thompson, Carter, Steinhauer, & Thase, 2007). Because the prefrontal cortex is still developing through adolescence (Giedd, 2004), it is unclear what effect hypofrontality would have in the developing brain.

These issues become more complicated when we consider developmental factors. In subsequent sections, we discuss issues pertaining to research with children, but we note here that any discussion of children must be in reference to their particular age. Studies examining depression in a sample that ranges from age 4 to 14 years will, at best, evidence enormous variance; there is little in common between a 4-year-old and a 14-year-old, except that they are both children. Even the definition of childhood is unclear. Whereas some federal entities (e.g., the Draft Board) recognize childhood as ending at age 18, others, such as the National Institute of Mental Health (NIMH), make the distinction at age 21. Studies of childhood depression variables need to consider carefully the pros and cons of various age cutoff points for samples.

Choices of cutoff points in depression in older adults are less developmental in nature but still important; for example, at what point does a person become old and no longer eligible for studies of midlife depression? The distinction is important, because even though older adult depression shares many qualities with midlife depression, its unique aspects have led to the consideration that there may be distinct subtypes of older adult depression (see Blazer & Hybels, Chapter 21, this volume). In particular, a *depression executive syndrome* has been identified, in which prefrontally mediated executive control is specifically impaired (Alexopoulos, Kiosses, Klimstra, Kalayam, & Bruce, 2002). This diagnosis has clear biological correlates, probable differential etiology, and implications for differential treatment response (Alexopoulos et al., 2000). Thus, considering age-dependent factors in defining depression will be increasingly important, as will considering the effects of those factors on the onset and course of depression.

Cultural Factors

Race and Culture

The complexity of cultural considerations makes the difficult, age-related concerns we have just discussed seem straightforward and simple. In the past, culture was commonly seen, at least implicitly, as synonymous with race; indeed, in some cases (e.g., NIMH guidelines) it still is. Although race is a well-established biological construct (Bonham, Warshauer-Baker, & Collins, 2005), political considerations have created a controversy over its existence and meaning that, misguided or not, may prove to be a benefit to the extent that it forces research to focus on shared cultural experiences as important variables (see Chentsova-Dutton & Tsai, Chapter 16, this volume).

Unfortunately, there are no reliable guidelines beyond the identification of race for identifying culture. Federally funded research is required to attempt to recruit underrepresented groups, and to estimate before funding the numbers of participants defined by racial identification. American Psychological Association journals (e.g., *Journal of Consulting and Clinical Psychology*) strongly encourage investigators to report the racial composition of their samples. Ideally, in both of these instances, analyses could compare responses for different groups, although sufficient data are rarely available for doing so.

To the extent that culture represents a shared set of beliefs, experiences, and attitudes, it accounts for some portion of variance that will be important to explain. Yet it is also important to note that this may represent a relatively small portion of variance. Given the lack of measures of culture (and little consensus on definitions of culture), racial identification, however flawed, will likely remain the most common way to address culture for the time being.

Gender

Assuming that men and women have different shared experiences, gender may also be considered a cultural variable and has the advantage of being easily identified. Gender clearly plays a role in the epidemiology of depression, with women diagnosed with depression at twice the rate of men (Goodwin, Jacobi, Bittner, & Wittchen, 2006; Nolen-Hoeksema & Hilt, Chapter 17, this volume). Two types of questions are generated by consideration of gender in depression research. First, men and women (either depressed or at risk) may respond differently to research procedures. Although some investigators treat gender as a nuisance variable they need to control, doing so obscures potentially important differences in the processes linked to depression. Investigators may not know why men and women respond differently, but such knowledge might have significant implications.

Beyond reporting whether men and women respond differently, another issue concerns the more specific exploration of the nature of gender differences themselves. If the first question is "Do they differ?", the second question is "Why do they differ?" Although some investigators have spent considerable energy examining these questions, they are in the minority among depression researchers. Indeed, other than specific theories of gender differences (e.g., Nolen-Hoeksema, 2006), major theories of depression tend to be silent about gender differences. Likewise, among the thousands of published studies investigating various processes in depression, only a small minority has sought to understand the nature of these differences. Epidemiological data show that these differences are an important and ripe area for future research.

ISSUES IN UNDERSTANDING CAUSALITY

Understanding causal issues is important, if not essential, for many research efforts. Yet, what is *causality*? The simplest view refers to the onset of depression, the transition from a relatively normal state into a state of psychological disorder. However, because depression can develop over time, is not static after its onset, and recurs in many cases, a causal cycle may be a better formulation of this idea.

The Causal Cycle of Depression

Vulnerability

One cause of depression involves the idea of vulnerability to the disorder. Definitions of vulnerability vary, but Ingram and colleagues (1998) and Ingram and Price (2000) suggest several core features that characterize most accounts of vulnerability to depression.[1] A core feature is that vulnerability is a trait as opposed to a kind of state that characterizes the actual appearance of the depression. Depending on the level of analysis used, vulnerability can be seen as residing in genetic factors, biological substrates, or psychological variables. In addition, vulnerability is usually conceptualized as a latent endogenous process that is reactive to the effects of stress. Vulnerability is synonymous with the diathesis in the diathesis–stress approach that is common among current models of depression.

Onset

Following vulnerability, onset of the disorder is the next stage of the causal sequence. Onset is perhaps the most easily conceptualized aspect of causality, because it tends to be treated as synonymous with causality. However, *onset* is more precisely defined as the appearance of depressive symptoms. If the type of MDD specified by DSM-IV-TR is of interest, then *onset* is defined as the appearance of at least five out of nine symptoms, one of which comprises sad mood or loss of pleasure, and all of which persist for at least 2 weeks.

Course or Maintenance of Depression

Another aspect of the causal sequence is maintenance of the depressed state. By virtually all estimates, depression is a persistent disorder with symptoms lasting many months (sometimes even with effective treatment), and years in some cases (e.g., dysthymia; see Boland & Keller, Chapter 2, this volume). There is some consensus among investigators that untreated depression lasts between 6 months and a year, although the disorder may last up to 2 years in more severe cases (Keller, Shapiro, Lavori, & Wolfe, 1982). In fact, symptoms that endure for an extended period of time are most likely linked to the disruption and personal turmoil that accompany depression. Thus, the factors involved in the perpetuation of depression can be considered to be causal.

Response, Remission, and Recovery

Rush and colleagues (2006) recommend that *response* be defined as a clinically significant reduction in symptoms. Although descriptions of clinical significance have typically been described as a 50% reduction in symptoms (Frank et al., 1991), Rush and colleagues suggest that rather than use a universal definition, investigators should determine response rates in reference to specific patient characteristics. For example, they argue that rather than a 50% symptom reduction for all patients, a 25% reduction is a reasonable criterion for cases of treatment-resistant depression. In relation to response, *remission* is defined as the complete, or near complete, disappearance of all criterion symptoms, accompanied by the assumption that variables underlying the disorder may still be present. This is particularly the case when some symptoms, although diminished beyond clinical significance, are still present. On the other hand, *recovery* suggests the disappearance of symptoms criteria *and* the underlying processes. Rush and colleagues suggest that *remission* be defined as the lack of sufficient symptoms for a period of at least 3 consecutive weeks, and that *recovery* be defined as the lack of sufficient symptoms for a 4-month period.

Treatment Effects

The current "gold standard" in treatment research is the randomized controlled design in which participants are assigned to a treatment or to a placebo–waiting-list–alternative treatment condition. Other, more complex designs involving selective applications of adjunctive treatments, or algorithmic interventions (e.g., starting with a single treatment, then augmenting or switching between or among treatments) are also gaining popularity. These designs can increase our understanding of the extent to which specific treatments affect specific mechanisms of disorder.

Arguably, the power of treatment designs lies in the nature of assessments before, during, and after treatment. Assessment of symptoms alone results in the ability to understand the time course of recovery. Additional assessment of cognitive, social, and biological mechanisms can provide insights on the mechanisms of recovery. The more often the investigator performs such assessments, the more likely that he or she can begin to make claims regarding mediation and moderation of recovery by assessed factors (Kraemer, Stice, Kazdin, Offord, & Kupfer, 2001).

For example, treatments such as antidepressant medications are designed to affect brain mechanisms proximally associated with symptoms, presumably leaving trait-vulnerability mechanisms in place (Hollon, Thase, & Markowitz, 2002). Assessment of biological mechanisms before, during, and after antidepressant treatment could help us understand the extent to which medications are associated with change in underlying biological vulnerabilities. In contrast, cognitive therapy focuses on changing underlying vulnerabilities and is associated with reduction of future risk for depression (Hollon, Stewart, & Strunk, 2006). Designs contrasting such intervention, along with pre- and postassessments, could allow examination of differential mechanisms of change and their effects on underlying vulnerability factors across interventions.

Yet inferring that specific aspects of a treatment are directly associated with remission or recovery is difficult, in that multiple, nonspecific factors may also contribute to symptom change. For example, momentary symptom reduction due to antidepressants may lead to lifestyle changes that promote continued risk reduction. Comparison with placebo treatments can help us understand the extent to which specific aspects of recovery are uniquely associated with treatment mechanisms. Possibly adjunctive application of interventions that specifically target circumscribed mechanisms (e.g., Siegle, Ghinassi, & Thase, 2007) may be particularly revealing in this regard, because they can suggest which aspects of depression are dependent on specific brain mechanisms. Prospective interventions, such as those employed with vulnerable youth who are not yet depressed, may also be revealing, providing evidence of whether, if specific vulnerability mechanisms are addressed, depression will develop. Assessments of specific changes in brain and behavioral functioning associated with symptom reduction (e.g., as afforded by neuroimaging, information processing, and ecological momentary assessments) can also aid in this regard.

Vulnerability to Recurrence and Relapse

Vulnerability occurs at both the beginning and the end of the causal chain. Although cases of depression can and do occur when no obvious vulnerability is present, once depression has subsided, persons at risk are vulnerable to future episodes (barring the introduction of some intervening factor). This is the essence of one core feature of vulnerability: Vulnerability is a trait. This continuing vulnerability underscores the general fact that depression for many people is a recurrent disorder (Goodwin et al., 2006), as well as the more specific ideas of recurrence and relapse. Depressive relapse signifies the return of the index episode and implies the continuation of the initial episode, whereas recurrence suggests the onset of a new episode following recovery from the index episode (Frank et al., 1991; Rush et al., 2006).

Necessary, Sufficient, and Contributory Causality

An important factor in assessing causal models of depression concerns distinctions among necessary, sufficient, and contributory causal variables. *Necessary causal factors* are those that *must* occur for symptoms to develop (Abramson, Alloy, & Metalsky, 1988); if variables are necessary, then symptoms cannot occur in the absence of these variables. *Sufficient variables* are those whose presence ensures symptom onset. *Contributory causal factors* are those whose presence enhances the probability that symptoms will occur, but that in themselves are neither necessary nor sufficient.

As should be evident from this discussion, causality is a complex concept. What methodological insights can we glean from a consideration of the conceptual issues revolving around the idea of causality? We examine several issues below, especially those most relevant to the study of vulnerability to depression.

METHODOLOGICAL ISSUES IN THE STUDY OF VULNERABILITY TO DEPRESSION

Understanding vulnerability is arguably the most important aspect of contemporary depression research (Ingram et al., 1998; Ingram & Price, 2000). There are many reasons for this, but chief among them is that vulnerability research speaks most directly to issues of causality. Understanding what makes people vulnerable to depression not only provides important clues about why people become (or stay) depressed but also has significant implications for prevention and treatment. Many contemporary studies of depression have implications for understanding vulnerability, and vulnerability is the stated primary concern in an increasing number of studies. The methodological considerations that guide vulnerability research are becoming increasingly germane to depression researchers. We are not able to cover all of these issues, but we highlight several methodological concerns that are particularly critical for researchers to consider if they intend to examine vulnerability.

Differentiating Distal from Proximal Vulnerability Factors

Vulnerability factors can be either distal or proximal. Proximal factors precede depression relatively shortly before its onset. Distal factors, on the other hand, are less temporally close to the appearance of depression but nevertheless contribute to vulnerability. This distinction is important not only for conceptual reasons but also because it necessitates different methodological requirements for vulnerability research. Just as distal and proximal vulnerability must be distinguished to appreciate the full range of vulnerability, so too must the research designs that are appropriate to study these processes. Therefore, we examine these designs here (a more detailed examination is available in Ingram et al., 1998).

Methodological Strategies and Issues in the Study of Proximal Vulnerability

In this section we examine several designs used to assess proximal vulnerability, including (1) cross-sectional designs, (2) remission designs, and (3) priming designs.

Cross-Sectional Designs

Although cross-sectional designs have generated an enormous amount of data, their ability to uncover vulnerability, at least vulnerability to the onset of depression, is limited, because cross-sectional studies are explicitly correlational in nature. Consequently, they do not permit differentiation among causal variables, consequential variables, or third-variable causality (Garber & Hollon, 1991). Temporal antecedence must be demonstrated to infer onset; the features must precede the onset of the disorder if they are to be considered a cause of the disorder (Garber & Hollon, 1991), and correlational studies do not allow for such an assessment. An exception to this limitation is that cross-sectional designs may be used to investigate causality for features that are believed to be constant throughout the lifespan and depression (e.g., family history, genetic factors, or aspects of brain morphology), because these factors existed before the onset of the depression.

Remission Designs

The remission approach assesses individuals who were once, but are no longer, depressed. This strategy assumes that remitted individuals, by virtue of their previous depression, possess some characteristics that place them at risk for depression. For obvious reasons, it is inappropriate for participants in remission studies to be currently experiencing depression or any other psychopathological condition. Pertaining to vulnerability, the intent of most remission studies is to examine the functioning of vulnerable individuals, without the confound of current symptoms, and the stability of potentially causative factors, with the assumption that these factors should be stable and, if stable, should be empirically detectable.

The remission approach provides information about vulnerability factors that are both stable *and* accessible after remission. However, a remission design is a poor methodological choice to test the postulates of a model in which there is theoretical reason to believe that vulnerability factors may be stable but not easily accessible (Ingram et al., 1998). Such assumptions are made by diathesis–stress models, in which the diathesis is only accessed under stress. To test such a theory appropriately, studies must model the complexity of diathesis–stress models (Hollon, 1992); therefore, investigators must either simulate the stress activation of vulnerability factors in the lab or find a way to assess such activating features naturalistically.

Priming Designs

Priming designs follow the logic of the diathesis–stress idea and may in many cases be considered a subset of remission designs, because they expose remitted depressed individuals to an experimental stimulus, then examine subsequent reactions. By incorporated triggering agents into empirical evaluations, such procedures model the relations among variables that are specified by diathesis–stress theories. In this vein, several investigators emphasized that the empirical search for markers of depression is methodologically predicated on the need to understand how various systems respond when challenged, regardless of which system is of interest to the investigator (Scher, Ingram, & Segal, 2005). Indeed, Hollon (1992) noted the remarkable similarity between the biological dysregulation models that dominate psychiatric research and the assumptions of psychologically based priming studies. A strong argument for the construct validity of priming designs is that they closely model the actual complexities of diathesis–stress assumptions that are fundamental to contemporary depression models. Thus, priming designs enable the study of key variables when symptoms are not currently present, allowing researchers to make a distinction between processes that are symptomatic of depression and those that may precede it, therefore constituting vulnerability.

Methodological Strategies and Issues in the Study of Distal Vulnerability

High-Risk Research: The Offspring Design

Studying the offspring of individuals diagnosed with a disorder is a well-known research approach with empirical roots in the first investigations of vulnerability to schizophrenia (e.g., Mednick & Schulsinger, 1968). A crucial assumption of this strategy is that the offspring of depressed parents should possess characteristics that make them more likely than the offspring of nondepressed parents to develop depression. Moreover, beyond assessing risk factors for the development of a specific disorder, offspring designs provide a wealth of additional data, such as whether those offspring who do not emerge with the disorder are at risk for some other manner of psychological distress or, alternatively, whether there are factors that protect high-risk children from psychological problems.

A number of considerations are essential to the conduct of well-executed offspring designs. Some of these represent variations on basic research principles, whereas others are unique to this kind of approach to vulnerability. Hammen (1991) has examined a number of these considerations in her excellent work on the social context of risk in children of depressed mothers. We summarize these here.

DIAGNOSTIC AND DEMOGRAPHIC STATUS OF PARENTS AND THEIR CHILDREN

It is critical for investigators who assess the offspring of depressed parents to describe explicitly how they define and measure depression, and to rule out possible comorbidity, if the design calls for assessing relatively "pure" depression. A number of variables beyond depression are also important to assess in high-risk offspring designs, such as whether one or both parent(s) meet criteria for various types of depression (Hammen, 1991). In a similar fashion, demographic characteristics, such as parents' socioeconomic status (SES), age, education level, and ethnicity, are also important to assess for their possible impact on the development of vulnerability. Of course, the same clarity and precision needed to assess parents adequately in offspring studies are required to assess children in these studies.

MEDIATING PROCESSES IN BOTH PARENTS AND CHILDREN

Although demographic and diagnostic statuses are important, such data by themselves do not tell us much about the actual processes of vulnerability; that is, these data are informative about risk factors but not about risk mechanisms (Goodman & Gotlib, 1999). This is true even if a particular theory specifies that offspring are at increased risk for depression for a given set of reasons. For example, some theories predict that the children of depressed parents are more likely to develop depression because of the genetic transmission of vulnerability. However, even though it is well documented that the children of depressed parents are more likely to experience depression (Garber & Flynn, 2000; Goodman & Gotlib, 1999), this does not tell us what the genetic mechanism is, or even whether it is a genetic mechanism at all rather than some other variable. Thus, the finding that the children of depressed parents are more likely to become depressed does not itself support or validate a particular theory; additional strategies are necessary to examine potential mediating factors within the context of offspring designs.

High-Risk Paradigm: Parental Designs

If offspring designs suggest that it is informative to study the offspring of depressed parents, the reverse is also true; it is also important to study the parents of depressed offspring, or of offspring who are thought to be at risk for depression. For example, such designs allow investigators to examine what parental characteristics may be related to offspring depression or risk for depression. Of course, the same methodological considerations that apply to offspring designs also apply to these designs (careful consideration of the descriptive characteristics of the sample, etc.). In contrast to high-risk designs defined by depressed parents, such methodologies can address a number of additional issues, such as determining whether the parental characteristics differ between depressed and nondepressed child samples, whether the interactions between children and their parents are different across samples, and so forth.

Longitudinal Designs

Longitudinal designs comprise a group of strategies that assess cohorts at different points in time, with the goal of determining which variables predict the subsequent occurrence of depressive symptoms. The length of longitudinal designs can vary considerably, ranging from hours to days to months to years (e.g., for a longitudinal study spanning almost 20 years, see Zuroff, Koestner, & Powers, 1994). Likewise, assessment intervals also may vary considerably. Variables, such as length and timing of assessment, are determined by the theoretical context for the research and the corresponding empirical questions of interest to the researcher. Pragmatic factors, such as the resources available for the research, may also play a role in determining the type, length, and timing of assessments.[2] Several types of longitudinal designs may be used to study distal vulnerability factors.

Prospective longitudinal designs seek to identify variables thought to be linked to risk in individuals who are not yet depressed. Prior to the onset of depression, participants are assessed, then followed over some period of time. *Catch-up designs* using previously collected data, typically for another purpose, examine whether these data can predict current depression. *Cross-sequential designs* represent a combination of longitudinal and cross-sectional research (Vasta, Haith, & Miller, 1992). As in cross-sectional designs, different groups or cohorts are compared with one another, but, as in longitudinal designs, these different cohorts are also followed over time. For example, groups of 2-year-olds might be assessed along with groups of 4- and 6-year-olds, and followed over time. Such designs provide a potent method for tracking changes in possible risk processes, determining whether some of these changes are associated with later depression, and assessing whether variables that become prominent at certain times in the developmental process are related to vulnerability and depression.

Retrospective designs seek to understand the influence of vulnerability factors through recall of information relevant to vulnerability. For example, research participants might be asked to recall earlier events from childhood or adolescence that the investigator hypothesizes are related to vulnerability. Retrospective designs can also be supplemented by experimental conditions to examine different aspects of presumed vulnerability. Although they potentially provide a wealth of information, these designs are also vulnerable to criticisms that retrospective reports are likely to be unreliable and invalid. Based on an extensive review of research, Brewin, Andrews, and Gotlib (1993) classified several concerns over memory reliability, but argued that data generally do not substantiate these concerns. Nevertheless, they also suggested that retrospective reports are unlikely ever to be completely free of possible problems, and suggested supplementing retrospective reports with information from other informants, or examining independent records obtained by other sources.

CONCLUSIONS AND A CAUTIONARY NOTE ON DEMONSTRATING CAUSALITY

Problems in demonstrating causality afflict all of the methodological designs we have examined, even longitudinal research. Recall that such designs are uniquely equipped to demonstrate temporal antecedence. Yet it is also important to note that temporal antecedence is necessary, but not sufficient, to show causality. As a prerequisite to showing that a variable is causal, data must demonstrate that the variable in question predicts depressive symptomatology (e.g., Segal et al., 2006). Satisfying this prerequisite, however, is not enough; showing that a variable predicts the occurrence of depression is an important step, but in and of itself it does not establish a cause and effect. For example, even if a longitudinal design shows that certain responses predict subsequent depression, other processes that are correlated with the variables in question may serve as the actual causative factors for depression. As such, third-variable causality is extremely difficult to rule out.

To further illustrate this, consider the example of treatment studies within the context of the longitudinal design. Even though treatment targeted at a specific process may yield improvement in depression and change the process that it targeted, this does not prove that the targeted variable was the process responsible for the improvement (or responsible for the depression to begin with) (Garratt, Ingram, Rand, & Sawalani, 2007). There are any number of reasons why treatment may work, some of which may have little to do with the processes targeted by treatment. Thus, the problem of demonstrating causality applies to virtually all research designs, regardless of their theoretical framework. We can move closer to understanding causality in depression through well-conducted designs that adequately address the various issues that we and others (see Kazdin, 2003) have discussed, but proving causality is a goal that is likely to elude the field for some time to come.

The methodological cautions and suggestions presented in this chapter lead naturally to a number of potential future directions that are likely to yield useful insights into the nature of depression. We began with a discussion of lay notions of depression as an amalgam of many theoretical constructs. If different factors operate in the onset of different types of depression, then it will be increasingly important to understand their identification and differentiation. New techniques for distinguishing truly categorical subtypes of depression (e.g., taxonometric techniques capable of detecting noncontinuous distinctions within populations; Meehl, 1995), along with recognition of more continuously varying aspects of depression in formal diagnostic systems, could facilitate such investigations.

We end this chapter with a point that we have noted a number of times throughout this chapter, but that nevertheless warrants repeated emphasis. The appropriateness of many of the strategies and tactics that we and others have discussed relative to depression research depends on the precise conceptual questions and hypotheses proposed. Some tactics may be perfectly appropriate for one type of question concerning depression and grossly inappropriate for another. Far too infrequently, however, do investigators elaborate the specific conceptual question in which they are interested, with precise reference to a given depressed population. As we have noted, for example, we think there are legitimate reasons to study subclinical depression, but the field would be well-served if investigators always stated exactly why the questions they address relative to this particular group are important. Similarly, investigators interested in a "pure" major depressive state that is not associated with the conditions that typically co-occur with clinical depression would serve the field well by explicitly addressing why only this sample is of interest. Overall, precise conceptual and empirical questions will guide a more precise choice of research procedures and samples that ultimately increase our understanding of depression (Ingram & Hamilton, 1999).

In a general sense, we believe that the field has labored implicitly for too long under a uniformity myth, wherein depression is a single phenomenon that can always, or virtually always, be investigated with a few straightforward research strategies. This uniformity myth is giving way to a much more complex understanding of depression, and with it, the need to employ complex research strategies. Depression research was simpler when the field adhered implicitly to this uniformity myth, but more sophisticated strategies are beginning to reveal important aspects of the processes that underlie depression in ways that earlier and simpler studies could not. To continue this progress, we must appreciate the complexity of the specific phenomena that characterize what we broadly call *depression*; state very clearly our theoretical questions, with precise reference to the depression type and phenomena to which they are to be applied; then select a research strategy that matches the type of depression we want to understand. We must confront both the complexity of depression and the methodological strategies that can be used to investigate it, then make the best choices possible.

Certainly, some researchers may yearn for a return to an earlier time when depression research was simply a matter of comparing depressed and nondepressed groups, as assessed by a questionnaire. In the version of this chapter that appeared in the first edition of this *Handbook* (Ingram & Siegle, 2002) we made reference to a television commercial that at the time attempted to entice people to buy the new Oldsmobile by noting that it was "not your father's Oldsmobile." That commercial, thankfully, has disappeared, but the analogy still applies. Contemporary research on depression is no longer our father's Oldsmobile. That car was cheaper and easy to service but not all that reliable. New cars are more expensive to buy and to operate, and much more complicated and difficult to service. Yet the ride is better, more reliable, and we are more assured of getting to our ultimate destination. It is time to trade up.

NOTES

1. It is important to note that even though vulnerability is sometimes conceptualized as a trait, vulnerability is not necessarily permanent or unalterable (although psychological vulnerability is stable and relatively resistant to change). Corrective experiences can occur that may attenuate the vulnerability or, alternatively, certain experiences may increase vulnerability factors. It is further important to note that whereas vulnerability focuses on mechanisms, *risk* refers to any variable that is correlated with a higher likelihood of becoming depressed (e.g., being a woman). Although conceptually separate, it is noteworthy that risk and vulnerability are not empirically unrelated; vulnerability and risk can interact to produce and maintain disorders such as depression. Thus, the person who is "at risk" because he or she lives in a particularly stressful environment will see this risk realized in disorder if he or she also possesses the vulnerability mechanisms. This is, of course, the essence of the diathesis–stress approach that characterizes numerous models of depression.
2. Although longitudinal designs can be applied to the study of either proximal or distal factors, we examine them only in the context of distal research.

REFERENCES

Abramson, L. Y., & Alloy, L. B. (1990). Search for the "negative cognition" subtype of depression. In D. C. McCann & N. Endler (Eds.), *Depression: New directions in theory, research, and practice* (pp. 77–109). Toronto: Wall & Thompson.

Abramson, L. Y., Alloy, L. B., & Metalsky, G. I. (1988). The cognitive diathesis–stress theories of depression: Toward an adequate evaluation of the theories' validities. In L. B. Alloy (Ed.), *Cognitive processes in depression* (pp. 3–30). New York: Guilford Press.

Alexopoulos, G. S., Kiosses, D. N., Klimstra, S., Kalayam, B., & Bruce, M. L. (2002). Clinical presentation of the "depression–executive dysfunction syndrome" of late life. *American Journal of Geriatric Psychiatry, 10,* 98–106.

Alexopoulos, G. S., Meyers, B. S., Young, R. C., Kalayam, B., Kakuma, T., & Gabrielle, M. (2000). Executive dysfunction and long-term outcomes of geriatric depression. *Archives of General Psychiatry, 57,* 285–290.

Alloy, L. B., & Abramson, L. Y. (1999). The Temple–Wisconsin Cognitive Vulnerability to Depression Project: Conceptual background, design, and methods. *Journal of Cognitive Psychotherapy, 13,* 227–262.

American Psychiatric Association. (2000). *Diagnostic and statistical manual of mental disorders* (4th ed., text rev.). Washington, DC: Author.

Angold, A., Costello, J. E., & Erkanli, A. (1999). Comorbidity. *Journal of Child Psychology and Psychiatry, 40,* 57–87

Angst, J. (1997). Depression and anxiety: Implications for nosology, course, and treatment. *Journal of Clinical Psychiatry, 58,* 3–5.

Angst, J., & Merikangas, K. R. (1998). Mixed anxiety depression. *Psychiatria Hungarica, 3,* 263–268.

Barlow, D. H., & Campbell, L. A. (2000). Mixed anxiety–depression and its implications for models of mood and anxiety disorders. *Comprehensive Psychiatry, 41,* 55–60.

Beck, A. T. (1967). *Depression: Causes and treatment.* Philadelphia: University of Pennsylvania Press.

Beck, A. T., Rush, A. J., Shaw, B. F., & Emery, G. (1979). *Cognitive therapy of depression.* New York: Guilford Press.

Beck, A. T., Steer, R. A., & Garbin, M. G. (1988). Psychometric properties of the Beck Depression Inventory: Twenty-five years of evaluation. *Clinical Psychology Review*, *8*, 77–100.

Bonham, V. L., Warshauer-Baker, E., & Collins, F. S. (2005). Race and ethnicity in the genome era: The complexity of the constructs. *American Psychologist*, *60*, 9–15.

Brewin, C. R., Andrews, B., & Gotlib, I. (1993). Psychopathology and early experience: A reappraisal of retrospective reports. *Psychological Bulletin*, *113*, 82–98.

Campbell, D. T., & Stanley, J. C. (1966). *Experimental and quasi-experimental designs for research*. Chicago: Rand McNally.

Costello, C. G. (1992). Conceptual problems in current research in cognitive vulnerability to psychopathology. *Cognitive Therapy and Research*, *16*, 379–390.

Coyne, J. C. (1994). Self-reported distress: Analog or ersatz depression? *Psychological Bulletin*, *116*, 29–45.

Denollet, J., Strik, J. J., Lousberg, R., & Honig, A. (2006). Recognizing increased risk of depressive comorbidity after myocardial infarction: Looking for 4 symptoms of anxiety-depression. *Psychotherapy and Psychosomatics*, *75*, 346–352.

Drevets, W. C. (1999). Emerging neuroscience approaches to understanding cognition and psychopathology: Positron-emission tomography imaging. In C. R. Cloninger (Ed.), *Personality and psychopathology* (pp. 369–408). Washington, DC: American Psychiatric Association.

Fawcett, J., & Howard, M. (1983). Anxiety syndromes and their relationship to depressive illness. *Journal of Clinical Psychiatry*, *444*, 8–11.

Frank, E., Prien, R. F., Jarret, R. B., Keller, M. B., Kupfer, D. J., Lavori, P. W., et al. (1991). Conceptualization and rationale for consensus definitions of terms in major depressive disorder: Remission, recovery, relapse, and recurrence. *Archives of General Psychiatry*, *48*, 851–855.

Garber, J., & Flynn, C. (2001). Vulnerability to depression in children and adolescence. In R. E. Ingram & J. M. Price (Eds.), *Vulnerability to psychopathology: Risk across the lifespan* (pp. 175–225). New York: Guilford Press.

Garber, J., & Hollon, S. D. (1991). What can specificity designs say about causality in psychopathology research? *Psychological Bulletin*, *110*, 129–136.

Garratt, G., Ingram, R. E., Rand, K. L., & Sawalani, G. (2007). Cognitive processes in cognitive therapy: Evaluation of the mechanisms of change in the treatment of depression. *Clinical Psychology: Science and Practice*, *14*, 224–239.

Giedd, J. N. (2004). Structural magnetic resonance imaging of the adolescent brain. *Annals of the New York Academy of Science*, *1021*, 77–85.

Goodman, S. H., & Gotlib, I. H. (1999). Risk for psychopathology in the children of depressed mothers: A developmental model for understanding mechanisms of transmission. *Psychological Review*, *106*, 458–490.

Goodwin, R. D., Jacobi, F., Bittner, A., & Wittchen, H. (2006). Epidemiology of depression. In D. J. Stein, D. J. Kupfer, & A. F. Schatzberg (Eds.), *Textbook of mood disorders* (pp. 33–54). Washington, DC: American Psychiatric Publishing.

Gotlib, I. H., Lewinsohn, P. M., & Seeley, J. R. (1995). Symptoms versus a diagnosis of depression: Differences in psychosocial functioning. *Journal of Consulting and Clinical Psychology*, *63*, 90–100.

Hamilton, N. A., Luxton, D., & Karlson, C. (in press). Sleep and depression. In R. E. Ingram (Ed.), *International encyclopedia of depression*. New York: Springer.

Hammen, C. (1991). *Depression runs in families: The social context of risk and resilience in children of depressed mothers*. New York: Springer-Verlag.

Hollon, S. D. (1992). Cognitive models of depression from a psychobiological perspective. *Psychological Inquiry*, *3*, 250–253.

Hollon, S. D., Stewart, M., & Strunk, D. (2006). Enduring effects for cognitive behavior therapy in the treatment of depression and anxiety. *Annual Review of Psychology*, *57*, 285–315.

Hollon, S. D., Thase, M., & Markowitz, J. (2002). Treatment and prevention of depression. *Psychological Science in the Public Interest*, *3*, 39–77.

Ingram, R. E. (1989). Affective confounds in social-cognitive research. *Journal of Personality and Social Psychology*, *57*, 715–722.

Ingram, R. E., & Hamilton, N. A. (1999). Evaluating precision in the social psychological assessment of depression: Methodological considerations, issues, and recommendations. *Journal of Social and Clinical Psychology, 18,* 160–180.

Ingram, R. E., Miranda, J., & Segal, Z. V. (1998). *Cognitive vulnerability to depression.* New York: Guilford Press.

Ingram, R. E., & Price, J. M. (2000). The role of vulnerability in understanding psychopathology. In R. E. Ingram & J. M. Price (Eds.), *Vulnerability to psychopathology: Risk across the lifespan* (pp. 3–19). New York: Guilford Press.

Ingram, R. E., & Siegle, G. J. (2002). Methodological issues in depression research: Not your father's Oldsmobile. In I. Gotlib & C. Hammen (Eds.), *Handbook of depression* (3rd ed., pp. 86–114). New York: Guilford Press.

Jarrett, R. B., Vittengl, J. R., Doyle, K., & Clark, L. A. (2007). Changes in cognitive content during and following cognitive therapy for recurrent depression: Substantial and enduring but not predictive of change in depressive symptoms. *Journal of Consulting and Clinical Psychology, 75,* 432–446.

Joiner, T., & Coyne, J. C. (1999). *The interactional nature of depression: Advances in interpersonal approaches.* Washington, DC: American Psychological Association.

Kaufman, J., Martin, A., King, R., & Charney, D. (2001). Are child-, adolescent-, and adult-onset depression one and the same disorder? *Biological Psychiatry, 49,* 980–1001.

Kazdin, A. E. (2003). *Methodological issues and strategies in clinical research* (3rd ed.). Washington, DC: American Psychological Association.

Keller, M. B., Shapiro, R. W., Lavori, P. W., & Wolfe, N. (1982). Relapse in RDC major depressive disorders: Analysis with the life table. *Archives of General Psychiatry, 39,* 911–915.

Kendall, P. C., & Brady, E. U. (1995). Comorbidity in the anxiety disorders of childhood: Implications for validity and clinical significance. In K. D. Craig & K. S. Dobson (Eds.), *Anxiety and depression in adults and children* (pp. 3–35). Thousand Oaks, CA: Sage.

Kendall, P. C., & Flannery-Schroeder, E. C. (1995). Rigor, but not rigor mortis, in depression research. *Journal of Personality and Social Psychology, 68,* 892–894.

Kendall, P. C., Hollon, S. D., Beck, A. T., Hammen, C. L., & Ingram, R. E. (1987). Issues and recommendations regarding use of the Beck Depression Inventory. *Cognitive Therapy and Research, 11,* 289–299.

Kendall, P. C., & Watson, D. (Eds.). (1989). *Anxiety and depression: Distinctive and overlapping features.* San Diego, CA: Academic Press.

Kraemer, H. C., Stice, E., Kazdin, A., Offord, D., & Kupfer, D. (2001). How do risk factors work together? Mediators, moderators, and independent, overlapping, and proxy risk factors. *American Journal of Psychiatry, 158,* 848–856.

Ladouceur, C. D., Dahl, R. E., & Carter, C. S. (2007). The development of action monitoring through adolescence into adulthood: ERP and source localization. *Developmental Science, 10,* 874–891.

Mednick, S. A., & Schulsinger, F. (1968). Some premorbid characteristics related to breakdown in children of with schizophrenic mothers. In D. Rosenthal & S. S. Kety (Eds.), *Transmission of schizophrenia* (pp. 267–291). Oxford, UK: Pergamon.

Meehl, P. E. (1978). Theoretical risks and tabular asterisks: Sir Karl, Sir Ronald, and the slow progress of soft psychology. *Journal of Consulting and Clinical Psychology, 46,* 806–834.

Meehl, P. E. (1995). Bootstrap taxometrics: Solving the classification problem in psychopathology. *American Psychologist, 50,* 266–275.

Nolen-Hoeksema, S. (2006). The etiology of gender differences in depression. In C. Mazure, C. M. Keita, & G. Puryear (Eds.), *Understanding depression in women: Applying empirical research to practice and policy* (pp. 9–43). Washington, DC: American Psychological Association.

Persons, J. B. (1986). The advantages of studying psychological phenomena rather than psychiatric diagnoses. *American Psychologist, 41,* 1252–1260.

Ruscio, J., & Ruscio, A. (2000). Informing the continuity controversy: A taxometric analysis of depression. *Journal of Abnormal Psychology, 109,* 473–487.

Rush, A. J., Kraemer, H. C., Sackeim, H. A., Fava, M., Trivedi, M. H., Frank, E., et al. (2006). Report by the ACNP Task Force on Response and Remission in Major Depressive Disorder. *Neuropsychopharmacology, 31,* 1841–1853.

Ryan, D. (2001). Diagnosing pediatric depression. *Biological Psychiatry, 49,* 1050–1054.

Scher, C. D., Ingram, R. E., & Segal, Z. V. (2005). Cognitive reactivity and vulnerability: Empirical evaluation of construct activation and cognitive diathesis in unipolar depression. *Clinical Psychology Review, 25,* 487–510.

Segal, Z. V., Kennedy, M. D., Gemar, M., Hood, K., Pedersen, R., & Buis, T. (2006). Cognitive reactivity to sad mood provocation and the prediction of depressive relapse. *Archives of General Psychiatry, 63,* 749–755.

Siegle, G. J., Ghinassi, F., & Thase, M. E. (2007). Neurobehavioral therapies in the 21st century: Summary of an emerging field and an extended example of Cognitive Control Training for depression. *Cognitive Therapy and Research, 31,* 235–262.

Siegle, G. J., Thompson, W., Carter, C. S., Steinhauer, S. R., & Thase, M. E. (2007). Increased amygdala and decreased dorsolateral prefrontal BOLD responses in unipolar depression: Related and independent features. *Biological Psychiatry, 61,* 198–209.

Smith, T. W., & Rhodewalt, F. (1991). Methodological challenges at the social/clinical interface. In C. R. Snyder & D. R. Forsyth (Eds.), *Handbook of social and clinical psychology: The health perspective* (pp. 739–756). New York: Pergamon Press.

Tennen, H., Hall, J. A., & Affleck, G. (1995). Depression research methodologies in the *Journal of Personality and Social Psychology*: A review and critique. *Journal of Personality and Social Psychology, 68,* 870–884.

Tucker, D. M., Luu, P., Frishkoff, G., Quiring, J., & Poulsen, C. (2003). Frontolimbic response to negative feedback in clinical depression. *Journal of Abnormal Psychology, 112*(4), 667–678.

Vasta, R., Haith, M. M., & Miller, S. A. (1992). *Child psychology: The modern science.* New York: Wiley.

Zuroff, D. C., Koestner, R., & Powers, T. A. (1994). Self-criticism at age 12: Longitudinal study of adjustment. *Cognitive Therapy and Research, 18,* 267–386.

CHAPTER 5

Personality and Mood Disorders

Daniel N. Klein, C. Emily Durbin, *and* Stewart A. Shankman

The hypothesis that there is an association between personality and depression can be traced to antiquity, when Hippocrates, and later Galen, argued that particular "humors" were responsible for specific personality types and forms of psychopathology. In this chapter, we discuss a number of models that have been proposed to explain the association between personality and depression, comment on some important conceptual and methodological issues in this area, and selectively review the empirical literature on the relation between personality and the mood disorders. Because of space limitations, we do not consider a number of constructs that may be included within the domain of personality, such as perfectionism, self-esteem, cognitive styles, coping styles, and rumination.

Personality has traditionally been conceptualized as having two components: *temperament*, or early-emerging individual differences that derive, at least in part, from biological influences; and *character*, which is the product of socialization. The distinctions among personality, temperament, and character have been increasingly questioned in recent years, however, and the terms *personality* and *temperament* are now often used interchangeably (Caspi & Shiner, 2006).

The literature on personality and mood disorders has developed along several distinct lines: (1) early clinical psychiatrists' descriptions of affective temperaments; (2) research on the structure and neurobiology of personality; (3) psychoanalytic and cognitive-behavioral theory and observations; (4) developmental psychologists' work on temperament; and (5) clinical research on comorbidity between personality disorders and mood disorders. Because most of this work has focused on major depressive disorder (MDD) rather than on bipolar disorder, we emphasize MDD in this chapter.

MODELS OF PERSONALITY AND DEPRESSION

Various models of the relation between personality and mood disorders have been proposed. They include (1) personality and mood disorders having common causes; (2) personality as a precursor of mood disorders; (3) personality predisposing to the development of mood disorders; (4) personality having pathoplastic effects on mood disorders; (5) personality features as state-dependent concomitants of mood disorder episodes; and (6) personality features as complications (or scars) of mood disorders. The distinctions between some of these models can be problematic. Moreover, other models, as well as combinations of these models, are plausible. However, these six models provide a useful conceptual framework for approaching the issue.

The common cause model views personality and mood disorders as arising from the same, or at least an overlapping, set of etiological processes. The precursor model views personality as an early manifestation or *formes frustes* of mood disorder. Both models view personality and mood disorders as being caused by the same set of etiological factors. The precursor model differs from the common cause model, however, in that it assumes that the personality features are phenomenologically similar to the mood disorder and precede it temporally.

The predisposition model is similar to the precursor model, in that personality features are assumed to precede the onset of mood disorder. In the precursor model, however, personality and mood disorder derive from the same set of etiological processes. In contrast, in the predisposition model, personality is determined by a different set of processes than those that lead to mood disorders, and personality subsequently has a direct causal impact on psychopathology by increasing the risk of developing a mood disorder. In addition, the predisposition model does not assume that personality features and mood disorder symptoms are phenomenologically similar.

The pathoplasticity model is similar to the predisposition model, in that personality is viewed as influencing mood disorders. Rather than contributing to the onset of mood disorder, however, personality influences the expression of the disorder after onset. This influence can include the severity or pattern of symptomatology, response to treatment, and the course of the mood disorder.

The final two models reverse the direction of temporal sequencing. In the concomitants (or state-dependent) model, assessments of personality are colored, or distorted, by the individual's mood state. This model implies that personality returns to its baseline form after recovery from the episode. In contrast, the complications (or scar) model holds that mood disorder has an enduring effect on personality, such that changes in personality persist after recovery.

METHODOLOGICAL ISSUES

A number of methodological issues must be considered in evaluating the relation between personality and mood disorders, including (1) study design, (2) heterogeneity of mood disorders, and (3) assessment of personality.

Study Design

A number of research designs may be useful in studying the relation between personality and the mood disorders. Multivariate twin studies, prospective longitudinal studies of persons prior to the onset of mood disorders, and studies of populations at increased risk for mood disorders may be used to test the common cause, precursor, and predisposition models. Twin studies demonstrating that the same genes predispose individuals to both personality and mood disorders would support both the common cause and precursor models. Prospective longitudinal studies of persons with no prior history of mood disorder, showing that particular personality traits predict the onset of mood disorders, would support both the precursor and predisposition models. Studies demonstrating personality differences between persons at high and low risk for developing mood disorders may provide additional, albeit less direct, evidence for the precursor and predisposition models. Whereas no single design can distinguish among all three models, a combination of designs can do so. Finding substantial common genetic variance in twin studies but no evidence of developmental sequencing in longitudinal studies would support the common cause model; substantial common genetic variance and developmental sequencing would support the precursor model (particularly if the trait were also phenomenologically similar to the mood disorder); and developmental sequencing, but little common genetic variance, would support the predisposition model.

The concomitants model can be tested in cross-sectional studies comparing persons who have recovered from episodes of mood disorder and healthy controls or, even better, in longitudinal studies assessing individuals when they are having an episode and again after they have recovered. The presence of personality abnormalities in remission would suggest that they are trait markers rather than concomitants of mood episodes. The complications (or scar) hypothesis can be evaluated by assessing persons before and after a mood disorder episode. Personality abnormalities that are not evident before the episode but appear after would suggest that "scarring" has occurred. Finally, the pathoplasticity model can be evaluated in cross-sectional and longitudinal studies of persons with mood disorders by examining the associations among temperament traits and clinical features, course, and treatment response. It is difficult to rule out the possibility, however, that the personality trait is a marker for a more severe, chronic, or etiologically distinct subgroup rather than having a causal influence on the expression of the disorder.

Heterogeneity

The mood disorders are clinically, and probably etiologically, heterogeneous. Hence, it is likely that the role of personality factors differs in different forms of mood disorder. The current nosology of mood disorders is based on clinical features and is probably a poor approximation of etiological distinctions. Nonetheless, it is important to consider whether the role of personality varies as a function of the specific form of mood disorder (e.g., bipolar disorder, MDD, dysthymic disorder); the subtype of mood disorder (e.g., psychotic, melancholic, atypical); and key clinical characteristics, such as age of onset, recurrence, chronicity, and symptom severity. In addition, given the substantial comorbidity between mood disorders and other Axis I conditions, it is also important to consider whether an apparent association between personality and mood disorders may actually be due to an association between personality and a co-occurring nonmood, Axis I disorder. Finally, finding associations between personality and specific subtypes and clinical characteristics raises the question of whether the differences reflect heterogeneity or pathoplasticity. Whereas the former implies that there are etiological differences between the subgroups, the latter suggests that although personality influences symptom presentation and/or course, the primary etiological process is the same.

Assessment

Personality traits and disorders may be assessed with a variety of methods, including self-report inventories, semistructured interviews, informants' reports, observation in naturalistic settings, and laboratory tasks. The use of multiple methods is important, because the assessment of personality can be complicated by current state, limited insight, response styles, and the difficulty of distinguishing personality traits from the effects of stable environmental contexts. It is important to note, however, that studies using different methods or instruments can produce different findings even when examining the same construct. While there is moderate-to-good agreement between self-reports and informants' reports of most personality traits, the level of concordance between interviews with participants and informants, and between self-report inventories and diagnostic interviews, is poor for personality disorders (Zimmerman, 1994). Similarly, there is often poor agreement between parents' reports and observational measures of temperament in children (Rothbart & Bates, 2006). Finally, some assessment approaches may have greater validity than others in detecting associations between personality and mood disorders (e.g., self-report inventories may be more susceptible than semistructured interviews to mood-state biases).

Another issue concerns the overlap between some personality constructs and mood disorder symptoms. For example, many items on neuroticism scales are similar to depressive symptoms (Ormel, Rosmalen, & Famer, 2004). This can inflate associations between measures of personality and mood disorders. Moreover, even when personality is assessed in participants who do not currently have a mood disorder, it raises the possibility that associations between personality and previous or subsequent mood disorders are due to subthreshold or residual symptomatology.

AFFECTIVE TEMPERAMENTS

The classical European descriptive psychopathologists observed that many patients with major mood disorders, as well as their relatives, had premorbid personalities that appeared to be attenuated versions of their affective illnesses. For example, Kraepelin (1921) described four patterns of personality that he considered to be the "fundamental states" underlying manic–depressive illness: depressive, manic, irritable, and cyclothymic temperament. Two variants of these types, cyclothymic disorder and dysthymic disorder, are included as mood disorder diagnoses in DSM-IV. However, they are defined as more severe, symptomatic conditions than the affective temperaments described by Kraepelin.

Much of the research in this area has focused on depressive personality, in part due to its inclusion in the DSM-IV Appendix. A central question has been whether depressive personality can be distinguished from dysthymic disorder. In this context, studies indicate that although there is moderate overlap between the two constructs, a substantial number of individuals who meet criteria for one of these conditions do not meet criteria for the other (e.g., Klein & Bessaha, in press). Individuals with depressive personality have an increased rate of mood disorders in their relatives, even when participants with a history of mood disorder are excluded. In addition, relatives of patients with MDD, particularly those with MDD superimposed on dysthymic disorder (double depression), have increased levels of depressive personality traits. Finally, young adults with depressive personality and no comorbid Axis I and II disorders are at increased risk for developing dysthymic disorder but not MDD (Klein & Bessaha, in press).

Although common cause, precursor, and predisposition models are difficult to distinguish, the phenomenological similarity, familial coaggregation, and temporal relation between depressive personality and Axis I depressive disorders (particularly chronic depression) are consistent with a precursor conceptualization. There is also support for pathoplasticity, because depressive personality is associated with a poorer course of MDD and dysthymia (Klein & Bessaha, in press).

There are a growing number of studies of hypomanic personality (or hyperthymic temperament) and the other affective personality types. Unlike the research on depressive personality, which has generally involved diagnostic interviews, most research on the other affective temperaments has involved self-report inventories. This work indicates that relatives of patients with bipolar disorder have elevated levels of hyperthymic temperament (Kesebir et al., 2005), and that hypomanic personality traits predict the development of bipolar disorder (Kwapil et al., 2000). Surprisingly, however, several researchers report that healthy controls exhibit higher levels of hyperthymic temperament than do patients with current and past mood disorders and their relatives (e.g., Evans et al., 2005), highlighting the difficulty of distinguishing hypomanic personality from the upper end of normal-range extraversion.

Although the work on affective temperaments is important in identifying precursors of mood disorders and delineating a spectrum of mood disorder phenotypes, it is unlikely that these types actually reflect basic temperamental processes that originate in early childhood. Instead, the complex cognitive and interpersonal characteristics included in these temperament types are likely to be intermediate outcomes that reflect the interaction of basic temperament processes that become elaborated across development in conjunction with early socialization and the environment.

PERSONALITY DIMENSIONS

The affective temperaments are generally conceptualized in a categorical framework. In contrast, the two lines of work we discuss in this section conceptualize personality in dimensional terms. The first line of research includes the major structural models of personality, such as the five-factor model, and Gray's (1994) and Cloninger, Svrakic, and Przybeck's (1993) psychobiological models. Although most of this research is rooted in personality psychology, in some cases (e.g., Gray, 1994) it was originally derived from neurobiological models of animal behavior. The second line of research developed from psychoanalytic (Blatt, 1974) and cognitive (Beck, 1983) theories, and focuses on two groups of related traits: dependency/sociotropy and obsessionality/self-criticism/autonomy.

Neuroticism and Extraversion

Most models of personality structure conceptualize personality as being organized hierarchically, with three to five "superfactors" at the highest level, each divisible into a number of narrower traits or *facets*. The two personality superfactors included in all major structural models of personality are *neuroticism* (N; or *negative emotionality* [NE]) and extraversion (E; or *positive emotionality* [PE]). N/NE reflects sensitivity to negative stimuli, resulting in a range of negative moods, including sadness, fear, anxiety, guilt, and anger. E/PE includes positive affect (joy, enthusiasm), energy, affiliation, dominance and, in some conceptualizations, venturesomeness.

E/PE and N/NE, the two most widely studied personality dimensions in the mood disorders, are closely related to the affective temperament types discussed in the previous section. For example, Watson and Clark (1995) proposed that the melancholic (or depressive) temperament represents the combination of low PE and high NE. Indeed, depressive personality is associated with elevated N/NE and diminished E/PE (Klein & Bessaha, in press).

Individuals with MDD report higher levels of N/NE and lower levels E/PE than do controls and normative samples. These differences are not specific to MDD, because most forms of psychopathology are associated with elevated N/NE (Clark, 2005). Low PE is more specific to depression, although it is also evident in other conditions, such as schizophrenia, anorexia nervosa, and social phobia. This apparent lack of specificity may indicate that broad temperament dimensions underlie a variety of forms of psychopathology and contribute to the high rates of comorbidity between psychiatric disorders (Clark, 2005).

Studies of personality and psychopathology can be complicated by the influence of participants' mood states on reports of their personalities (the concomitants model). For example, many studies have found that individuals with MDD report higher levels of N/NE when they are depressed than when they are not depressed (e.g., Hirschfeld, Klerman, Clayton, Keller, McDonald-Scott, et al., 1983; Kendler, Neale, Kessler, Heath, & Eaves, 1993; Ormel, Oldehinklel, & Vollebergh, 2004). Thus, the association between depression and N/NE may be inflated when personality is assessed during a MDD episode. In contrast, the evidence for mood state effects on E/PE is weaker and less consistent (e.g., De Fruyt, Van Leeuwen, Bagby, Rolland, & Rouillon, 2006; Kendler et al., 1993).

To avoid the potentially confounding effects of mood state, a number of studies have compared persons with a history of depression when they are *euthymic*, or significantly improved, to nondepressed controls or population norms. These studies indicate that formerly depressed individuals report diminished levels of E/PE, but data for N/NE are less consistent (e.g., Hirschfeld, Klerman, Clayton, & Keller, 1983). The conflicting results for N/NE may be due to a number of factors, including: (1) insufficiently stringent criteria for recovery, thereby possibly confounding personality and residual symptoms; (2) use of normative data collected by other investigators, which may introduce demographic and sociocultural differences between the formerly depressed and comparison samples; and (3) selection effects. As N is associated with a poorer course, samples of remitted depressives may include a disproportionate number with low N.

The presence of personality abnormalities in the remitted state is consistent with the complications, common cause, precursor, and predisposition models; consequently, more sophisticated designs are required to provide more specific tests of these models. Several studies have tested the complications (or *scar*) hypothesis by comparing personality measures in depressed individuals before and after an MDD episode. Most of these studies have not observed increases in N, or decreases in E, after a MDD episode (Kendler et al., 1993; Ormel, Oldehinkel, et al., 2004; Shea et al., 1996). Moreover, "scarring" does not appear to be related to the number or duration of episodes (Ormel, Oldehinkel, et al., 2004).

A number of studies have tested the precursor and predisposition models by examining personality traits in the never-depressed relatives of patients with MDD. Most of these studies have failed to find differences between the never-depressed relatives of probands with mood disorders and controls on N and E (e.g., Hecht, van Calker, Berger, & von Zerssen, 1998; Ouimette, Klein, & Pepper, 1996). However, personality traits may not play the same role in risk for depression among familial and nonfamilial forms of depression. In addition, there may be selection biases in samples using relatives who are partly through the risk period for mood disorder, given that individuals with personality vulnerabilities may already have developed the disorder and are excluded from the analyses.

A more direct approach to testing the precursor and predisposition models is to conduct prospective studies of personality in never-depressed participants to determine whether personality characteristics predict the subsequent onset of MDD. Several studies using large community samples have reported that higher levels of N/NE predict the onset of first life-time MDD episodes (de Graaf, Bijl, Ravelli, Smit, & Vollebergh, 2002; Kendler et al., 1993; Kendler, Gatz, Gardner, & Pedersen, 2006; Ormel, Oldehinkel, et al., 2004). In addition, several studies using measures of other traits that overlap with N/NE or its facets have reported similar findings (Clayton, Ernst, & Angst, 1994; Hirschfeld et al., 1989; Rorsman, Grasbeck, Hagnell, Isberg, & Otterbeck, 1993).

Although there is some evidence that E/PE predicts the first onset of MDD (Kendler et al., 2006; Rorsman et al., 1993), it is much weaker, and several studies have failed to find an association (Hirschfeld et al., 1989; Kendler et al., 1993). However, Verkerk, Denollet, Van Heck, Van Son, and Pop (2005) recently reported that pregnant women with both high N and low E had an increased risk for a first lifetime onset of depressive disorders during the year after childbirth.

As we discussed earlier, to distinguish among the common cause, precursor, and predisposition models, it is necessary to consider the findings from a variety of research designs. When this is done, the weight of the evidence appears to support the precursor model, at least with respect to N. Thus, in two large twin samples, Kendler and colleagues (1993, 2006) reported significant associations between the liabilities to N and MDD, which were largely due to shared genetic risk factors. These data are more consistent with the common cause and precursor models than with the predisposition model, because the former posit that personality and depression share the same etiological influences, whereas the predisposition model presumes that the determinants of personality differ from those of depression. At the same time, the evidence reviewed here suggests that elevated levels of N precede the onset of MDD, supporting the precursor and predisposition models over the common cause model. Finally, the phenomenological similarity between N and MDD favors the precursor model over the common cause and predisposition models. Thus, when the full set of designs needed to tease these models apart is considered, the precursor model is the most consistent with the full range of evidence: N is phenomenologically similar to depressive symptoms; N and MDD share substantial genetic variance; and elevated levels of N precede the onset of MDD.

For both the precursor and predisposition models, a full understanding of the personality–mood disorder pathway requires identifying the factors and processes that lead from trait to disorder. Stressful life events appear to play an important role in the escalation to (in the precursor model), or precipitation of (in the predisposition model), mood disorder episodes. Thus, several studies have reported that individuals with high levels of N are more likely than persons with lower levels of N to experience an MDD episode following a stressful life event (e.g., Kendler, Kuhn, & Prescott, 2004).

N/NE and E/PE may also have a pathoplastic influence on the expression and course of depression after the onset of the disorder. For example, many studies have reported that N predicts a poorer course and response to treatment (e.g., Duggan, Lee, & Murray, 1990). Instead of personality having pathoplastic effects on the expression and course of depression, however, these associations could reflect diagnostic heterogeneity, with personality dysfunction serving as a marker for a more severe or etiologically distinct group. Indeed, there is evidence that the nonmelancholic subtype is characterized by more vulnerable personality styles than is melancholia (Boyce et al., 1990), and that chronic depressions are associated with higher N and lower E than is nonchronic MDD (Klein, in press).

Watson and Clark (1995) hypothesize that depression is characterized by high NE *and* low PE, raising the possibility that the combination of the two traits is particularly important in depressive disorders. Few studies, however, have examined the joint (or interactive) effects of these dimensions. Verkerk and colleagues (2005) found that the combination of high N and low E predicted the onset of depressive disorder, but they did not formally test the interaction of these dimensions. However, in a sample of college students, Gershuny and Sher (1998) found that N and E interacted to predict scores on a dimensional measure of depression 3 years later, such that N predicted depression only among participants who were low in E.

In conclusion, N/NE, is the most widely studied personality trait in depression. It appears to be influenced by clinical state (the concomitants model), to share genetic variance with depression (common cause and precursor models), to predict the subsequent onset of depression (precursor and predisposition models), and to influence the course of depression (pathoplasticity model). However, it does not appear to be changed by experience of depressive episodes (complications model). The role played by E/PE in depression is less clear. It is not influenced by clinical state or changed by the experience of depressive episodes. E appears to be abnormally low even during remission, suggesting that it may share causal determinants with depression, or serve as a precursor or predisposing factor. However, the genetic overlap between E and MDD is low (Kendler et al., 2006), and the evidence that E predicts the onset of MDD in prospective longitudinal studies is weak. Finally, data on the effects of E on the presentation and course of depression are limited and inconsistent.

The majority of studies have examined N/NE and E/PE at the superfactor level. It is possible, however, that only particular facets play a role in the development of MDD. Hence, it is important that future studies examine whether the common variance of subtraits reflected in the superfactors is associated with depression, or whether the unique variance of distinct facets, such as approach/reward sensitivity in E/PE, accounts for most of the association with depression. Given that many self-report measures of N/NE include items with content that is highly similar to symptoms of mood disorders (Ormel, Rosmalen, et al., 2004), it is also important to test the extent to which N/NE–depression associations are driven by facets and measures with overlapping content, or whether they extend to facets that are further from sad mood states. In addition, in parsing the domains of N/NE and E/PE, it will be important to use interview, informant, observational, and laboratory-based methods to complement traditional self-report inventories.

Behavioral Activation and Inhibition Systems

Gray's (1994) influential theory proposes that there are several neurobehavioral systems that underlie behavior, including the *behavioral activation system* (BAS), which responds to signals of reward, and the *behavioral inhibition system* (BIS), which is sensitive to cues for punishment. Similar to E/PE and N/NE, it has been hypothesized that depression is associated with reduced BAS and/or heightened BIS sensitivity. Several recent studies have examined self-report measures of BAS and BIS sensitivity in MDD. Consistent with Gray's model, compared to healthy controls, currently depressed patients report lower levels of BAS and higher levels of BIS, and patients with a past history of MDD report lower levels of BAS (Pinto-Meza et al., 2006). In addition, low BAS is associated with a poorer course of MDD (e.g., Kasch, Rottenberg, Arnow, & Gotlib, 2002), suggesting that it may have a pathoplastic effect on depression.

Cloninger's Model

Cloninger and colleagues (1993) have proposed a model of personality that comprises four temperament and three character dimensions. The temperament dimensions include *novelty seeking* (an appetitive/approach system that responds to signals of novelty and potential reward), *harm avoidance* (an inhibition/avoidance system that responds to aversive stimuli), *reward dependence* (a behavior maintenance system that is responsive to signals of social approval and attachment), and *persistence*. The character dimensions are *self-directedness* (responsible, goal-directed), *cooperativeness* (helpful, empathic vs. hostile, alienated), and *self-transcendence* (imaginative, unconventional). Although the dimensions in Cloninger's model are only modestly correlated with those of the Big Five and Gray's model, harm avoidance is conceptually and empirically associated with BIS, and novelty seeking and persistence are associated with BAS. Similarly, harm avoidance is correlated positively with N/NE and negatively with E/PE; self-directedness is negatively correlated with N/NE, and novelty seeking and persistence are associated with E/PE (e.g., DeFruyt, Van De Wiele, & Van Heeringen, 2000).

Most of these dimensions are influenced by the respondent's mood state (e.g., Farmer et al., 2003). However, a number of studies have reported that even after remission, patients with MDD report higher levels of harm avoidance and lower levels of self-directedness than do healthy controls (e.g., Smith, Duffy, Stewart, Muir, & Blackwood, 2005). Increased harm avoidance and lower self-directedness are also characteristic of most anxiety disorders, however, indicating that these effects are not specific to MDD, and suggesting that comorbid anxiety disorders may contribute to the associations between these trait dimensions and depressive disorders (Öngür, Farabaugh, Iosifescu, Perils, & Fava, 2005).

Few studies have explicitly tested the common cause, precursor, predisposition, and complications hypotheses for Cloninger's model. Farmer and colleagues (2003) found that never-depressed siblings of patients with MDD reported significantly greater harm avoidance and less self-directedness than did never-depressed sibs of healthy controls. In addition, Cloninger, Svrakic, and Przybeck (2006) recently reported that, in a large community sample, high harm avoidance and persistence, and low self-directness predicted an increase in self-reported depressive symptoms 12 months later. Finally, consistent with the pathoplasticity model, a number of studies have reported that low harm avoidance and self-directness are associated with a poor response to treatment (e.g., Mulder, Joyce, Frampton, Luty, & Sullivan, 2006).

In summary, consistent associations between high harm avoidance and low self-directedness, and the depressive disorders have been reported. This is consistent with the findings we reviewed earlier, indicating that depression is associated with increased sensitivity to punishment and a disposition to experience negative affect. Attempts to elucidate the nature of the relationship between Cloninger's traits and depressive disorders have been more limited; however, there is support for the concomitants, precursor and/or predisposition, and pathoplasticity models.

Dependency/Sociotropy and Obsessionality/Self-Criticism/Autonomy

A separate line of research on personality and depression has developed from the psychoanalytic and cognitive-behavioral traditions. Psychoanalysts have long emphasized the role of dependent and obsessional traits in the development of mood disorders. Subsequently, psychoanalytic and cognitive theorists proposed similar, personality-based theories of MDD (Beck, 1983; Blatt, 1974).

Blatt (1974) distinguished between *anaclitic* (or dependent) and *introjective* (or self-critical) forms of depression, with the former characterized by interpersonal concerns involving care and approval, and the latter by concerns of self-definition and self-worth. Beck (1983) proposed a similar distinction between *sociotropic* depressives, who have an intense need for close relationships, and *autonomous* depressives, who have a high need for independence and achievement. For both theorists, these traits are hypothesized to predispose individuals to depression in the face of "matching" life events (interpersonal loss for dependent/sociotropic individuals, and threats to autonomy and achievement for self-critical/autonomous individuals). In addition, both theorists posit that dependent/sociotropic individuals and self-critical/autonomous individuals exhibit different patterns of symptomatology when depressed; whereas the former are characterized by helplessness, tearfulness, and mood reactivity, the latter are characterized by guilt, feelings of worthlessness, anhedonia, social withdrawal, and lack of reactivity.

Patients with MDD generally report higher levels of dependency/sociotropy than do healthy controls (e.g., Enns & Cox, 1997), although they may not differ from patients with other forms of psychopathology, such as anxiety disorders (e.g., Bagby et al., 1992). Consistent with the concomitants model, depressed persons' sociotropy scores decline after recovery; however, there is less evidence for state effects on dependency, and the findings vary according to the measure used (e.g., Hirschfeld, Klerman, Clayton, Keller, McDonald-Scott, et al., 1983; Zuroff, Mongrain, & Santor, 2004). Data addressing the common cause, precursor, and predisposition models are limited. The majority of studies have reported that recovered depressives exhibit higher levels of dependency and sociotropy than do healthy controls (e.g., Hirschfeld, Klerman, Clayton, & Keller, 1983; Zuroff et al., 2004). However, most family studies have reported that the never-depressed relatives of patients with MDD do not differ from the relatives of healthy controls relative to dependency and sociotropy (e.g., Ouimette et al., 1996). Prospective longitudinal studies of never-depressed participants have found that dependency predicts first lifetime MDD episodes in middle-age and older adults (Hirschfeld et al., 1989; Rohde, Lewinsohn, & Seeley, 1990), but not in adolescents and young adults (Hirschfeld et al., 1989; Rohde, Lewinsohn, & Seeley, 1994). Finally, a number of studies that have tested the personality–life events congruence (or *matching*) hypothesis, although not for first-onset cases, have produced inconsistent findings (Zuroff et al., 2004). The limited data addressing the complications model indicate that dependent traits may increase after MDD episodes in adolescents (Rohde et al., 1994), but not in adults (Rohde et al., 1990; Shea et al., 1996). Finally, a number of studies have addressed the pathoplasticity model. Most of these studies have examined whether dependent/sociotropic traits are associated with the distinctive profile of depressive symptoms posited by Blatt (1974) and Beck (1983). Although these findings have been inconsistent (e.g., Robins, Bagby, Rector, Lynch, & Kennedy, 1997), there is evidence that dependent and sociotropic traits are associated with a poorer course of MDD (e.g., Lewinsohn, Rohde, Seeley, Klein, & Gotlib, 2000).

Similar to the findings for dependency and sociotropy, depressed individuals tend to exhibit higher levels of self-criticism and autonomy than do nondepressed controls (e.g., Enns & Cox, 1997). Self-criticism has a significant state component, because scores decrease after remission; however, autonomy does not appear to be influenced by clinical state (Zuroff et al., 2004). Again, data on the common cause, precursor, and predisposition models are sparse. Even after recovery, formerly depressed individuals tend to exhibit higher levels of self-criticism and autonomy than do healthy controls (Zuroff et al., 2004). However, the healthy relatives of patients with MDD and controls do not differ on self-criticism and autonomy (e.g., Ouimette et al., 1996). Unfortunately, there are no prospective, longitudinal studies examining whether self-criticism and autonomy predict the onset of MDD. Moreover, as noted earlier, the evidence for the personality–life events congruence hypothesis is mixed (Zuroff et al., 2004). To our knowledge, there are no data addressing the complications model. Finally, as noted earlier, studies testing whether self-criticism and autonomy are associated with the distinctive symptom profiles described by Blatt (1974) and Beck (1983) have yielded inconsistent results. However, these traits appear to be associated with a poorer course and response to treatment (e.g., Mongrain & Blackburn, 2005).

In contrast to dependency, sociotropy, self-criticism, and autonomy, the results of comparisons between depressed and nondepressed individuals on levels of obsessionality have yielded inconsistent results (Enns & Cox, 1997). Obsessionality does not appear to be influenced by clinical state (Hirschfeld, Klerman, Clayton, Keller, McDonald-Scott, et al., 1983). Both the results of comparisons between individuals who have recovered from depression and healthy controls (e.g., Hirschfeld, Klerman, Clayton, & Keller, 1983), and studies of the relatives of depressed and healthy probands (e.g., Hecht et al., 1998) have yielded inconsistent results, and prospective studies indicate that obsessionality does not predict the subsequent onset of MDD (Hirschfeld et al., 1989). Finally, there is no evidence of "scar" effects (Shea et al., 1996), and obsessionality does not influence the long-term course of depression (Duggan et al., 1990).

In conclusion, the nature of dependency, sociotropy, self-criticism, autonomy, and obsessionality relations with depressive disorders remains uncertain. One reason for the inconsistent findings may be that most of these constructs are multidimensional, and some subscales have stronger associations with depression than do others (e.g., Zuroff et al., 2004). Nonetheless, there is growing evidence that dependency/sociotropy and self-criticism/autonomy are associated with interpersonal difficulties, increased life stress, and maladaptive cognitive and coping styles that could potentially serve as mediators in a pathway(s) between personality and depression (Zuroff et al., 2004).

Personality in Bipolar Disorder

The role of personality in bipolar disorder is unclear. Although a number of researchers have reported that remitted patients with bipolar disorder have higher levels of E/PE than do remitted patients with MDD (e.g., Bagby et al., 1996), they do not differ from never-ill controls or population norms (e.g., Hecht et al., 1998). In addition, N/NE comparisons of patients with bipolar disorder both to patients with MDD and to healthy controls have yielded mixed results (e.g., Bagby et al., 1996; Hecht et al., 1998). Findings of researchers using Cloninger's system have been more consistent. Several studies have found that remitted patients with bipolar disorder report greater harm avoidance and less reward dependence, self-directness, and cooperativeness than do nonpatient controls (e.g., Engström, Brändström, Sigvardsson, Cloninger, & Nylander, 2004).

Part of the reason for the inconsistent findings for E/PE and N/NE may be the heterogeneity of bipolar disorder. For example, few studies have distinguished between bipolar I and bipolar II disorders. Thus, it is noteworthy that Akiskal and colleagues (2006) found that patients with bipolar I disorder were similar to healthy controls in terms of personality, whereas patients with bipolar II disorder were characterized by higher levels of both E- and N-like traits.

In the one prospective study examining precursors/predispositions to bipolar disorder, Clayton and colleagues (1994) reported that the premorbid personalities of young men who later developed bipolar disorder did not differ from those who remained well on a broad range of personality measures. In addition, several studies found that never-depressed relatives of bipolar patients did not differ from relatives of normal controls on N and E (e.g., Hecht, Genzwürker, Helle, & van Calker, 2005). Finally, there is some evidence that personality has a pathoplastic influence on the course of bipolar disorder, with higher levels of NE being associated with greater depression, and higher levels of PE being associated with greater mania/hypomania (e.g., Hecht et al., 1998).

CHILD TEMPERAMENT

Much of the work on personality and depression has conceptualized personality in temperamental terms, that is, as early emerging individual differences in the affective components of personality. Because most of the literature has focused on adults, however, it has been difficult to test the critical assumption that these temperamental vulnerabilities are indeed evident in early childhood. Research that is grounded in the child temperament literature in developmental psychology can help to identify the actual manifestations of temperamental vulnerabilities to mood disorders in young children, trace their development and continuity across the lifespan, and examine whether their influence is mediated via cognitive and interpersonal processes that have previously been implicated in the pathogenesis of mood disorders (Klein, Dougherty, Laptook, & Olino, in press).

Most major models of child temperament include the superordinate traits of PE and NE, which correspond fairly closely to E/PE and N/NE in adult models of personality (Caspi & Shiner, 2006; Rothbart & Bates, 2006). A third temperament trait that has also received attention with regard to risk for mood disorders in the developmental literature is *behavioral inhibition* (BI), which refers to wariness/fear, diminished activity, and a lack of approach in novel situations (Kagan, Reznick, & Snidman, 1987). BI, a complex combination of aspects of both PE (low approach) and NE (fear and anxiety proneness), does not have a direct analogue in most models of adult personality. Cross-sectional and longitudinal studies of child clinical and nonclinical samples using self-report measures have replicated the findings from the adult literature that low PE and high NE are associated with depression (e.g., Lonigan, Phillips, & Hooe, 2003). Observational studies of the children of depressed mothers also indicate that these traits may be associated with risk for depression. For instance, Durbin, Klein, Hayden, Buckley, and Moerk (2005) reported that preschoolers of mothers with a history of mood disorder exhibited low PE in structured, emotion-eliciting laboratory tasks; effects were particularly pronounced among offspring of mothers with chronic or recurrent depression. These children also exhibited elevated levels of NE; however, this was evident only in contexts in which the NE was nonnormative (e.g., tasks eliciting positive affect in most children). Furthermore, low PE in preschoolers predicted depressotypic cognitions (helplessness in a structured laboratory task, and failure to recall previously endorsed, positive self-descriptors in a delayed recall task) at age 7 (Hayden, Klein, Durbin, & Olino, 2006).

BI may be related to risk for both mood and anxiety disorders. For example, Rosenbaum and colleagues (2000) assessed BI using laboratory measures in 2- to 6-year-old children of parents with a history of MDD episodes and/or panic disorder, and parents with no history of mood or anxiety disorders. The children of patients with both MDD episodes and panic disorder exhibited significantly greater BI than did children of parents with no history of mood or anxiety disorder. Children of parents with MDD episodes alone had an intermediate level of BI that did not differ significantly from that of children of parents with both MDD episodes and panic disorder, parents with panic disorder alone, and parents with no history of mood or anxiety disorders. To the extent that there is a link between BI and risk for MDD, it is not clear whether it is driven by the low PE (low approach) or high NE (anxiety) elements of BI.

Hirshfeld-Becker and colleagues (2006) recently reported on secondary analyses of this sample to determine whether the small subgroup of offspring of parents with a history of both MDD and manic/hypomanic episodes were characterized by the opposite of BI, behavioral disinhibition. Indeed, although the offspring of bipolar and nonbipolar parents did not differ on BI, the former group exhibited a significantly higher rate of behavioral disinhibition. Behavioral disinhibition is not specific to bipolar disorder, however, because it is also evident in children with externalizing disorders.

Finally, there is some direct evidence that personality traits assessed in childhood predict the development of mood disorders in adults. Caspi, Moffitt, Newman, and Silva (1996) reported that children rated as socially reticent, inhibited, and easily upset at age 3 had elevated rates of depressive (but not anxiety or substance use) disorders at age 21. Similarly, van Os, Jones, Lewis, Wadsworth, and Murray (1997) found that physicians' ratings of children's behavioral apathy at ages 6, 7, and 11 were predictive of both adolescent mood disorder and chronic depression in middle adulthood.

COMORBIDITY BETWEEN MOOD AND PERSONALITY DISORDERS

Since the introduction of Axis II into DSM-III in 1980, there has been considerable interest in the relation between personality disorders (PDs) and Axis I disorders, with comorbidity between PDs and mood disorders receiving particular attention. Because self-report measures appear to overestimate the prevalence of personality disorders (Zimmerman, 1994), we focus in this section on studies using semistructured diagnostic interviews.

Reported rates of PDs in patients with MDD have varied, with most studies falling within the range of 50–85% for inpatients and 20–50% for outpatients (e.g., Corruble, Ginestet, & Guelfi, 1996). Knowledgeable informants also report high rates of PDs in patients with mood disorders (e.g., Pepper et al., 1995). In most studies, Cluster C (dependent, avoidant, and obsessive–compulsive) PDs are the most common Axis II conditions in MDD, and Cluster A (paranoid, schizoid, schizotypal) PDs are the least common. Contrary to clinical lore, the rate of PDs appears to be similar in melancholic and nonmelancholic MDD; however PDs are more common in early-onset than in late-onset depression (e.g., Garyfallos et al., 1999). Dysthymic disorder appears to be associated with an even higher rate of PDs than does MDD (e.g., Garyfallos et al., 1999; Pepper et al., 1995). Cluster B (antisocial, borderline, histrionic, narcissistic) and Cluster C PDs are particularly common.

Given the difficulty of assessing PDs when patients are in an acute manic state, the most valid prevalence rates in bipolar disorder come from euthymic samples. Studies using semistructured diagnostic interviews in euthymic patients with bipolar disorder have generally found that about one-third to one-half of patients exhibit PDs (e.g., George, Miklowitz, Richards, Simoneau, & Taylor, 2003). The most common PDs in bipolar disorder are from Cluster B and Cluster C. Compared to patients with MDD, patients with bipolar disorder have higher rates of narcissistic PD and lower rates of Cluster C disorders (Mantere et al., 2006).

In light of these high comorbidity rates, it is important to try to understand the nature of the relation between mood disorders and PDs. Determining the reasons for comorbidity is a challenging task (for an extended discussion, see Klein & Riso, 1993). However, a number of the conceptual models we discussed earlier with respect to personality and mood disorders have also been used in conceptualizing the comorbidity between mood disorders and

PDs. In particular, investigators have been interested in determining whether comorbidity between mood disorders and PDs reflects shared etiological factors (the common causes model); whether personality disorders predict or play a causal role in the development or maintenance of mood disorders (similar, although not identical, to the precursor and predisposition models); whether mood disorders play a causal role in the development or maintenance of PDs (again similar, but not identical, to the complications model); whether the assessment of PDs is influenced by the individual's mood state (the concomitants model); and whether PDs influence the presentation, treatment, or course of mood disorders (the pathoplasticity model). In addition, similar to the earlier discussion regarding the relation between N/NE and MDD, rates of comorbidity may also be inflated by overlapping content in diagnostic criteria (e.g., the criteria for borderline personality disorder and MDD both include dysphoric affect and suicidal behavior), although, in fact, removal of overlapping criteria does not substantially reduce comorbidity.

A number of studies have reported data for many PDs that are relevant to the concomitants and pathoplasticity models. The assessment of PDs is significantly influenced by clinical state, with patients reporting more PD traits during an episode than after recovery (Zimmerman, 1994). This effect may be reduced, although probably not eliminated, by careful interviewing and use of informant reports. There is also considerable support for the pathoplasticity model, because many (although not all) studies have reported that comorbid PDs are associated with earlier onset, longer and more frequent episodes, and poorer response to treatment (e.g., Grilo et al., 2005; Mulder et al., 2006). Fewer studies, however, have attempted to explore other models of the association between mood disorders and PDs.

The one Axis II condition whose relation to the mood disorders has received the greatest consideration is borderline personality disorder (BPD). Most of this work has explored whether BPD and MDD have shared or overlapping etiologies by comparing BPD and MDD on biological correlates, family history, and treatment response. In addition, several studies have examined the relations between BPD and MDD symptoms over time. Although these studies do not directly address the precursor, predisposition, and complications models, they are relevant in that they attempt to determine the direction of influences between BPD and MDD.

There appears to be overlap between BPD and MDD on biological abnormalities and familial aggregation of mood disorders and PDs, suggesting the possibility of shared etiological factors. Shortened rapid eye movement (REM) latencies are common in MDD and also evident in never-depressed patients with BPD (e.g., De la Fuente, Bobes, Vizuete, & Mendlewicz, 2001). In addition, there is an elevated rate of mood disorders in relatives of never-depressed patients with BPD (e.g., Riso, Klein, Anderson, & Ouimette, 2000). In contrast, MDD and BPD differ with respect to response to antidepressant medication. Antidepressants can be helpful in managing some aspects of BPD; however, many of the core features of the disorder tend not to respond to pharmacotherapy (Soloff, 2000). This suggests that there may also be etiological and pathophysiological features that are unique to each disorder.

Two studies have used longitudinal designs to investigate the direction of the effects between depressive symptoms and BPD traits. Klein and Schwartz (2002) compared a series of models of the longitudinal relations between depressive symptoms and BPD traits over a 5-year follow-up. The best-fitting model included a common factor that affected both disorders and unique influences on depression and BPD traits. A model in which BPD traits influenced depressive symptoms over time also provided an adequate, although not quite as good, fit. In contrast, the model positing that depressive symptoms influence subsequent BPD traits did not fit the data. Similarly, when Gunderson and colleagues (2004) examined the relation between depressive symptoms and BPD traits over 3 years, they found that BPD traits predicted changes in depressive symptoms, but depression did not predict changes in BPD traits. However, they did not examine a model in which a common factor influenced both depressive symptoms and BPD features over time.

There has also been considerable interest in the relation between bipolar disorder and BPD. Because affective instability is characteristic of both conditions, some researchers have conceptualized BPD as a "dysphoric facet" of bipolar conditions such as bipolar II disorder and cyclothymic disorder (Smith, Muir, & Blackwood, 2004). There is little evidence, however, for familial coaggregation between bipolar disorder and BPD, and longitudinal studies have found that only a small proportion of persons with BPD later develop bipolar disorder, suggesting that the causal processes underlying these two disorders are fairly distinct (Gunderson et al., 2006).

Although the evidence is not conclusive, available data suggest that the mood disorders and BPD are distinct conditions with some shared etiological influences. At the same time, BPD may influence the course of depression. An important area for future research is to identify the common causal factors and processes, with leading candidates including genes, early childhood maltreatment, and serotonergic dysregulation (Klein & Schwartz, 2002). In addition, it may be useful to disaggregate the BPD construct and examine the nature of the associations between mood disorders and selected facets of BPD, such as affective dysregulation. Finally, it is likely that the reasons for comorbidity with mood disorders differ for different PDs and dimensions of personality dysfunction. Hence, there is a need for research to elucidate the mechanisms and processes responsible for the covariation between mood disorders and other forms of Axis II psychopathology.

CONCLUSIONS AND FUTURE DIRECTIONS

The topic of the relation between PDs and mood disorders has produced a sprawling literature, with many gaps and inconsistent findings. Nonetheless, it is possible to draw a number of tentative conclusions. First, reports of many traits (e.g., N/NE, harm avoidance, dependency) are influenced by clinical state, although some traits (e.g., E/PE, obsessionality, autonomy) appear to be independent of mood state. Further work is needed to determine whether mood state biases can be reduced by using interviews rather than self-report inventories. Second, there appear to be common causes/shared etiological factors between some personality traits and PDs, such as N and BPD, and mood disorders. Third, there is substantial support for the view that depressive personality is closely related etiologically to, and may be a precursor of, Axis I depressive disorders, particularly more chronic forms such as dysthymic disorder and double depression. More work is needed, however, that examines other affective temperament types, such as cyclothymic temperament. Fourth, there is mounting evidence that N/NE is a precursor of MDD, although the overlap between items used to assess N/NE and depressive symptomatology is an important potential confound. In addition, the possibility that low E/PE and dependency may also play roles as precursors or predisposing factors should continue to be investigated. Fifth, although further data addressing the complications model are needed, it appears unlikely that mood disorders produce enduring changes in personality. Sixth, many personality traits and disorders appear to have pathoplastic effects on the course of mood disorders, and may also influence treatment response. Greater attention needs to be paid, however, to the possible confound of heterogeneity. Finally, although the issue of diagnostic specificity has not been investigated for all of the personality types and dimensions reviewed here, available evidence suggests that most of the personality features associated with mood disorders are also evident in other forms of psychopathology, particularly anxiety disorders. This may reflect the phenomenon of *multifinality*, in which variables that occur early in the causal chain can lead to multiple outcomes, presumably due to the effects of subsequent moderators. On the other hand, it is also conceivable that some of the Axis I disorders that are currently viewed as distinct are actually variants of a single disorder, and that personality–Axis I relationships may provide important information for revising our classification system (Clark, 2005).

To make further progress in elucidating the relation between PDs and mood disorders, future studies should be guided by five broad considerations: (1) examining personality and temperament constructs at a greater level of specificity; (2) going beyond the traditional self-report inventory assessment methodology; (3) considering the heterogeneity of mood disorders; (4) conducting prospective longitudinal studies that begin prior to the period of risk for mood disorders; and (5) identifying moderators and mediators of the personality–mood disorders relation.

First, the literatures on affective temperament types, personality trait dimensions, and child temperament appear to be converging on the potential role of NE and PE as precursors or predisposing factors in the mood disorders. Much of this work, however, has been conducted at the superfactor level. It is important to determine whether a more specific level of analysis will yield more powerful effects and increase the specificity of associations between personality constructs and particular forms of psychopathology. This will require finer-grained analyses that parse the key components of the personality–temperament superfactors. For example, within E/PE, it is critical to distinguish between positive affect, appetitive/approach behavior, sociability, dominance, and venturesomeness. In addition, it is important to explore combinations of traits (e.g., high NE and low PE) and to break trait-relevant behaviors down into more specific parameters (e.g., frequency, intensity, duration, reactivity, and appropriateness to situational context of emotional experience and expression).

Second, self-report inventories may not be capable of the fine-grained analyses necessary to make these distinctions. Thus, it is important to develop semistructured interviews for personality traits that can reduce the effects of mood state biases and response styles, and make subtle distinctions between related constructs. It is also important to explore the utility of supplementing self-report data with informants' reports. Finally, it is noteworthy that the studies reporting prospective associations between childhood personality and adult mood disorders employed observational measures of personality (Caspi et al., 1996; van Os et al., 1997). This highlights the value of developing and refining observational measures of affect and behavior in naturalistic and in laboratory settings.

Third, the role of personality–temperament may vary for different forms of mood disorder. Personality appears to play an especially important role in early-onset, chronic, and recurrent depressive conditions (e.g., Duggan et al., 1990; Garyfallos et al., 1999; van Os et al., 1997). Examining the relations between personality–temperament and broad diagnostic categories such as MDD may obscure important associations with particular forms of depression; hence, future studies need to give greater consideration to the heterogeneity of mood disorders.

Fourth, there is a critical need for prospective, longitudinal studies. Unfortunately, most existing studies have examined adolescents or adults. In recent years, it has become evident that many cases of mood disorder have already developed by late childhood/early adolescence. Therefore, to test the precursor and predisposition models, and to trace the development and impact of potential personality–temperamental vulnerabilities, it is necessary to conduct longitudinal studies that start in early childhood to obtain a sufficient number of first-onset cases and avoid selection biases caused by excluding participants who already have a history of mood disorder at initial assessment.

Finally, if personality is a precursor of, or predisposes, individuals to the development of mood disorders, it is critical to identify the moderating factors and mediating processes involved in these pathways. Some evidence suggests that moderators may include gender, early adversity, and life stress, and mediators may include interpersonal deficits, depressotypic cognitions, maladaptive coping, and behavioral and neurobiological stress reactivity (Klein et al., in press). There is a need for more systematic research examining multiple moderators and mediators in a longitudinal framework.

REFERENCES

Akiskal, H. S., Kilzieh, N., Maser, J. D., Clayton, P. J., Schettler, P. J., Shea, M. T., et al. (2006). The distinct temperament profiles of bipolar I, bipolar II, and MDD patients. *Journal of Affective Disorders, 92,* 19–33.

Bagby, R. M., Cox, B. J., Schuller, D. R., Levitt, A. J., Swinson, R. P., & Joffe, R. T. (1992). Diagnostic specificity of the dependent and self-critical personality dimensions in major depression. *Journal of Affective Disorders, 26,* 59–64.

Bagby, R. M., Young, L. T., Schuller, D. R., Bindseil, K. D., Cooke, R. G., Dickens, S. E., et al. (1996). Bipolar disorder, unipolar depression and the five-factor model of personality. *Journal of Affective Disorders, 41,* 25–32.

Beck, A. T. (1983). Cognitive therapy of depression: New approaches. In P. Clayton & J. Barrett (Eds.), *Treatment of depression: Old and new approaches* (pp. 265–290). New York: Raven Press.

Blatt, S. J. (1974). Levels of object representation in anaclitic and introjective depression. *Psychoanalytic Study of the Child, 29,* 107–157.

Boyce, P., Parker, G., Hickie, I., Wilhelm, K., Brodaty, H., & Mitchell, P. (1990). Personality differences between patients with remitted melancholic and nonmelancholic depression. *American Journal of Psychiatry, 147,* 1476–1483.

Caspi, A., Moffitt, T. E., Newman, D. L., & Silva, P. A. (1996). Behavioral observations at age 3 years predict adult psychiatric disorders. *Archives of General Psychiatry, 53,* 1033–1039.

Caspi, A., & Shiner, R. L. (2006). Personality development. In W. Damon, R. Lerner, & N. Eisenberg (Eds.), *Handbook of child psychology: Vol. 3. Social, emotional, and personality development* (6th ed., pp. 300–365). New York: Wiley.

Clark, L. A. (2005). Temperament as a unifying basis for personality and psychopathology. *Journal of Abnormal Psychology, 114,* 505–521.

Clayton, P. J., Ernst, C., & Angst, J. (1994). Premorbid personality traits of men who develop unipolar or bipolar disorders. *European Archives of Psychiatry and Clinical Neuroscience, 243,* 340–346.

Cloninger, C. R., Svrakic, D. M., & Przybeck, T. R. (1993). A psychobiological model of temperament and character. *Archives of General Psychiatry, 50,* 975–990.

Cloninger, C. R., Svrakic, D. M., & Przybeck, T. R. (2006). Can personality predict future depression: A twelve-month follow-up of 631 subjects. *Journal of Affective Disorders, 92,* 35–44.

Corruble, E., Ginestet, D., & Guelfi, J. D. (1996). Comorbidity of personality disorders and unipolar major depression: A review. *Journal of Affective Disorders, 37,* 157–170.

DeFruyt, F., Van De Wiele, L., & Van Heeringen, C. (2000). Cloninger's psychobiological model of temperament and character and the five-factor model of personality. *Personality and Individual Differences, 29,* 441–452.

De Fruyt, F., Van Leeuwen, K., Bagby, R. M., Rolland, J.-P., & Rouillon, F. (2006). Assessing and inter-preting personality change and continuity in patients treated for major depression. *Psychological Assessment, 18*, 71–80.

de Graaf, R., Bijl, R. V., Ravelli, A., Smit, F., & Vollebergh, W. A. (2002). Predictors of first incidence of DSM-III-R psychiatric disorders in the general population: Findings from the Netherlands Mental Health Survey and Incidence Study. *Acta Psychiatrica Scandinavica, 106*, 303–313.

De la Fuente, J. M., Bobes, J., Vizuete, C., & Mendlewicz, J. (2001). Sleep-EEG in borderline patients without concomitant major depression: A comparison with major depressives and normal control subjects. *Psychiatry Research, 105*, 87–95.

Duggan, C. F., Lee, A. S., & Murray, R. M. (1990). Does personality predict long-term outcome in de-pression? *British Journal of Psychiatry, 157*, 19–24.

Durbin, C. E., Klein, D. N., Hayden, E. P., Buckley, M. E., & Moerk, K. C. (2005). Temperamental emo-tionality in preschoolers and parental mood disorders. *Journal of Abnormal Psychology, 114*, 28–37.

Engström, C., Brändström, S., Sigvardsson, S., Cloninger, R., & Nylander, P.-O. (2004). Bipolar disorder: I. Temperament and character. *Journal of Affective Disorders, 82*, 131–134.

Enns, M. W., & Cox, P. J. (1997). Personality dimensions and depression: Review and commentary. *Ca-nadian Journal of Psychiatry, 42*, 274–284.

Evans, L., Akiskal, H. S., Keck, P. E., Jr., McElroy, S., Sadovnick, A. D., Remick, R. A., et al. (2005). Familiality of temperament in bipolar disorder: Support for a genetic spectrum. *Journal of Affective Disorders, 85*, 153–168.

Farmer, A., Mahmood, A., Redman, K., Harris, T., Sadler, S., & McGuffin, P. (2003). A sib-pair study of the temperament and character scales in major depression. *Archives of General Psychiatry, 60*, 490–496.

Garyfallos, G., Adamopoulou, A., Karastergiou, A., Voikli, M., Sotiropoulou, A., Donias, S., et al. (1999). Personality disorders in dysthymia and major depression. *Acta Psychiatrica Scandinavica, 99*, 332–340.

George, E. L., Miklowitz, D. J., Richards, J. A., Simoneau, T. L., & Taylor, D. O. (2003). The comorbidity of bipolar disorders and Axis II personality disorders: Comorbidity and clinical correlates. *Bipolar Disorders, 5*, 115–122.

Gershuny, B. S., & Sher, K. J. (1998). The relation between personality and anxiety: Findings from a 3-year prospective study. *Journal of Abnormal Psychology, 107*, 252–262.

Gray, J. A. (1994). Framework for a taxonomy of psychiatric disorder. In S. H. M. van Goozen & N. E. Van de Poll (Eds.), *Emotions: Essays on emotion theory* (pp. 29–59). Hillsdale, NJ: Erlbaum.

Grilo, C. M., Sanislow, C. A., Shea, M. T., Skodol, A. E., Stout, R. L., Gunderson, J. G., et al. (2005). Two-year prospective naturalistic study of remission from major depressive disorder as a function of personality disorder comorbidity. *Journal of Consulting and Clinical Psychology, 73*, 78–85.

Gunderson, J. G., Morey, L. C., Stout, R. L., Skodol, A. E., Shea, M. T., McGlashan, T. H., et al. (2004). Major depression disorder and borderline personality disorder revisited: Longitudinal interactions. *Journal of Clinical Psychiatry, 65*, 1049–1056.

Gunderson, J. G., Weinberg, I., Daversa, M. T., Kueppenbender, K. D., Zanarini, M. D., Shea, T. M., et al. (2006). Descriptive and longitudinal observations on the relationship of borderline personality dis-order and bipolar disorder. *American Journal of Psychiatry, 163*, 1173–1178.

Hayden, E. P., Klein, D. N., Durbin, C. E., & Olino, T. M. (2006). Low positive emotionality at age three predicts depressotypic cognitions in seven-year old children. *Development and Psychopathology, 18*, 409–423.

Hecht, H., Genzwürker, S., Helle, M., & van Calker, D. (2005). Social functioning and personality of subjects at familial risk for affective disorder. *Journal of Affective Disorders, 84*, 33–42.

Hecht, H., van Calker, D., Berger, M., & von Zerssen, D. (1998). Personality in patients with affective disorders and their relatives. *Journal of Affective Disorders, 51*, 33–43.

Hirschfeld, R. M. A., Klerman, G. L., Clayton, P. J., & Keller, M. B. (1983). Personality and depression: Empirical findings. *Archives of General Psychiatry, 40*, 993–998.

Hirschfeld, R. M. A., Klerman, G. L., Clayton, P. J., Keller, M. B., McDonald-Scott, P., & Larkin, B. H. (1983). Assessing personality: Effects of the depressive state on trait measurement. *American Jour-nal of Psychiatry, 140*, 695–699.

Hirschfeld, R. M. A., Klerman, G. L., Lavori, P., Keller, M. B., Griffith, P., & Coryell, W. (1989). Premorbid personality assessments of first onset of major depression. *Archives of General Psychiatry*, *46*, 345–350.

Hirshfeld-Becker, D. R., Biederman, J., Henin, A., Faraone, S. V., Cayton, G. A., & Rosenbaum, J. F. (2006). Laboratory-observed behavioral disinhibition in the young offspring of parents with bipolar disorder: A high-risk pilot study. *American Journal of Psychiatry*, *163*, 265–271.

Kagan, J., Reznick, J. S., & Snidman, N. (1987). The physiology and psychology of behavioral inhibition in children. *Child Development*, *55*, 1459–1473.

Kasch, K. L., Rottenberg, J., Arnow, B. A., & Gotlib, I. H. (2002). Behavioral activation and inhibition systems and the severity and course of depression. *Journal of Abnormal Psychology*, *111*, 589–597.

Kendler, K. S., Gatz, M., Gardner, C. O., & Pedersen, N. L. (2006). Personality and major depression. *Archives of General Psychiatry*, *63*, 1113–1120.

Kendler, K. S., Kuhn, J., & Prescott, C. A. (2004). The interrelationship of neuroticism, sex, and stressful life events in the prediction of episodes of major depression. *American Journal of Psychiatry*, *161*, 631–636.

Kendler, K. S., Neale, M. C., Kessler, R. C., Heath, A. C., & Eaves, L. J. (1993). A longitudinal twin study of personality and major depression in women. *Archives of General Psychiatry*, *50*, 853–862.

Kesebir, S., Vahip, S., Akdeniz, F., Yüncü, Z., Alkan, M., & Akiskal, H. (2005). Affective temperaments as measured by TEMPS-A in patients with bipolar I disorder and their first-degree relatives: A controlled study. *Journal of Affective Disorders*, *85*, 127–133.

Klein, D. N. (in press). Dysthymia and chronic depression. In W. E. Craighead, D. J. Miklowitz, & L. W. Craighead (Eds.), *Psychopathology: History, theory, and diagnosis*. Hoboken, NJ: Wiley.

Klein, D. N., & Bessaha, M. L. (in press). Depressive personality disorder. In T. Millon, P. H. Blaney, & R. D. Davis (Eds.), *Oxford textbook of psychopathology* (2nd ed.). New York: Oxford University Press.

Klein, D. N., Dougherty, L. R., Laptook, R. S., & Olino, T. M. (in press). Temperament and risk for mood disorders in adolescents. In N. Allen & L. Sheeber (Eds.), *Adolescent emotional development and the emergence of depressive disorders*. Cambridge, UK: Cambridge University Press.

Klein, D. N., & Riso, L. P. (1993). Psychiatric diagnoses: Problems of boundaries and co-occurrences. In C. G. Costello (Ed.), *Basic issues in psychopathology* (pp. 19–66). New York: Guilford Press.

Klein, D. N., & Schwartz, J. E. (2002). The relation between depressive symptoms and borderline personality disorder features over time in dysthymic disorder. *Journal of Personality Disorders*, *16*, 523–535.

Kraepelin, É. (1921). *Manic-depressive insanity and paranoia*. Edinburgh, UK: Livingstone.

Kwapil, T. R., Miller, M. B., Zinser, M. C., Chapman, L. J., Chapman, J., & Eckblad, M. (2000). A longitudinal study of high scorers on the Hypomanic Personality Scale. *Journal of Abnormal Psychology*, *109*, 222–226.

Lewinsohn, P. M., Rohde, P., Seeley, J. R., Klein, D. N., & Gotlib, I. H. (2000). The natural course of adolescent major depressive disorder: II. Predictors of depression recurrence in young adults. *American Journal of Psychiatry*, *157*, 1584–1591.

Lonigan, C. J., Phillips, B. M., & Hooe, E. S. (2003). Relations of positive and negative affectivity to anxiety and depression in children: Evidence from a latent-variable longitudinal study. *Journal of Consulting and Clinical Psychology*, *71*, 465–481.

Mantere, O., Melartin, T. K., Suominen, K., Rytsälä, H. J., Valtonen, H. M., Arvilommi, P., et al. (2006). Differences in Axis I and Axis II comorbidity between bipolar I and II disorders and major depressive disorder. *Journal of Clinical Psychiatry*, *67*, 584–593.

Mongrain, M., & Blackburn, S. (2005). Cognitive vulnerability, lifetime risk, and the recurrence of major depression in graduate students. *Cognitive Therapy and Research*, *29*, 747–768.

Mulder, R. T., Joyce, P. R., Frampton, C. M. A., Luty, S. E., & Sullivan, P. F. (2006). Six months of treatment for depression: Outcome and predictors of the course of illness. *American Journal of Psychiatry*, *163*, 95–100.

Öngür, D., Farabaugh, A., Iosifescu, D. V., Perils, R., & Fava, M. (2005). Tridimensional Personality Questionnaire factors in major depressive disorder: Relationship to anxiety disorder comorbidity and age of onset. *Psychotherapy and Psychosomatics*, *74*, 173–178.

Ormel, J., Oldehinkel, A. J., & Vollebergh, W. (2004). Vulnerability before, during, and after a major depressive episode. *Archives of General Psychiatry, 61,* 990–996.

Ormel, J., Rosmalen, A., & Farmer, A. (2004). Neuroticism: A non-informative marker of vulnerability to psychopathology. *Social Psychiatry and Psychiatric Epidemiology, 39,* 906–912.

Ouimette, P. C., Klein, D. N., & Pepper, C. M. (1996). Personality traits in the first degree relatives of outpatients with depressive disorders. *Journal of Affective Disorders, 39,* 43–53.

Pepper, C. M., Klein, D. N., Anderson, R. L., Riso, L. P., Ouimette, P. C., & Lizardi, H. (1995). DSM-III-R Axis II comorbidity in dysthymia and major depression. *American Journal of Psychiatry, 152,* 239–247.

Pinto-Meza, A., Caseras, X., Soler, J., Puigdemont, D., Pérez, V., & Torrubia, R. (2006). Behavioral inhibition and behavioral activation systems in current and recovered major depression participants. *Personality and Individual Differences, 40,* 215–226.

Riso, L. P., Klein, D. N., Anderson, R. L., & Ouimette, P. C. (2000). A family study of outpatients with borderline personality disorder and no history of mood disorder. *Journal of Personality Disorders, 14,* 208–217.

Robins, C. J., Bagby, R. M., Rector, N. A., Lynch, T. R., & Kennedy, S. H. (1997). Sociotropy, autonomy, and patterns of symptoms in patients with major depression: A comparison of dimensional and categorical approaches. *Cognitive Therapy and Research, 21,* 285–300.

Rohde, P., Lewinsohn, P. M., & Seeley, J. R. (1990). Are people changed by the experience of having an episode of depression?: A further test of the scar hypothesis. *Journal of Abnormal Psychology, 99,* 264–271.

Rohde, P., Lewinsohn, P. M., & Seeley, J. R. (1994). Are adolescents changed by an episode of major depression? *Journal of the American Academy of Child and Adolescent Psychiatry, 33,* 1289–1298.

Rorsman, B., Grasbeck, A., Hagnell, O., Isberg, P.-E., & Otterbeck, L. (1993). Premorbid personality traits and psychometric background factors in depression: The Lundby Study 1957–1972. *Neuropsychobiology, 27,* 72–79.

Rosenbaum, J. F., Biederman, J., Hirshfeld-Becker, D. R., Kagan, J., Snidman, N., Friedman, D., et al. (2000). A controlled study of behavioral inhibition in children of parents with panic disorder and depression. *American Journal of Psychiatry, 157,* 2002–2010.

Rothbart, M. K., & Bates, J. E. (2006). Temperament. In N. Eisenberg, W. Damon, & R. M. Lerner (Eds.), *Handbook of child psychology: Vol. 3. Social, emotional, and personality development* (6th ed., pp. 99–166). Hoboken, NJ: Wiley.

Shea, M. T., Leon, A. C., Mueller, T. I., Solomon, D. A., Warshaw, M. G., & Keller, M. B. (1996). Does major depression result in lasting personality change? *American Journal of Psychiatry, 153,* 1404–1410.

Smith, D. J., Duffy, L., Stewart, M. E., Muir, W. J., & Blackwood, D. H. R. (2005). High harm avoidance and low self-directedness in euthymic young adults with recurrent, early-onset depression. *Journal of Affective Disorders, 87,* 83–89.

Smith, D. J., Muir, W. J., & Blackwood, D. H. R. (2004). Is borderline personality disorder part of the bipolar spectrum? *Harvard Review of Psychiatry, 12,* 133–139.

Soloff, P. H. (2000). Psychopharmacology of borderline personality disorder. *Psychiatric Clinics of North America, 23,* 169–192.

van Os, J., Jones, P., Lewis, G., Wadsworth, M., & Murray, R. (1997). Developmental precursors of affective illness in a general population birth cohort. *Archives of General Psychiatry, 54,* 625–631.

Verkerk, G. J. M., Denollet, J., Van Heck, G. L., Van Son, M. J. M., & Pop, V. J. M. (2005). Personality factors as determinants of depression in postpartum women: A prospective 1-year follow-up study. *Psychosomatic Medicine, 67,* 632–637.

Watson, D., & Clark, L. A. (1995). Depression and the melancholic temperament. *European Journal of Personality, 9,* 351–366.

Zimmerman, M. (1994). Diagnosing personality disorders: A review of issues and research models. *Archives of General Psychiatry, 51,* 225–245.

Zuroff, D. C., Mongrain, M., & Santor, D. A. (2004). Conceptualizing and measuring personality vulnerability to depression: Comment on Coyne and Whiffen (1995). *Psychological Bulletin, 130,* 489–511.

CHAPTER 6

Depression and Medical Illness

Kenneth E. Freedland *and* Robert M. Carney

In the past, the relationship between depression and medical illness generated relatively little interest outside of medical psychology and consultation–liaison psychiatry, now known as the psychiatric subspeciality of psychosomatic medicine. It has since become one of the most active areas of research in behavioral medicine and health psychology. Because depression is one of the most common conditions in primary care, it has also gained attention in the internal medicine and health services research literatures. This chapter examines the relationship between depression and medical illness, controversies and challenges in the assessment and treatment of depression in medically ill patients, and some directions for future research.

RELATIONSHIPS BETWEEN DEPRESSION AND MEDICAL ILLNESS

Comorbidity

The probability that two conditions co-occur by chance is equal to the product of their prevalence rates (Kraemer, 1995). For example, if 5% of a population has depression and 7% has diabetes, these two conditions would be expected to co-occur by chance alone in less than 1% of the population ($.05 \times .07 = .0035$). If they co-occur substantially more often, then there are probably reasons other than chance for their comorbidity.

Many studies have found comorbidity rates between depression and medical conditions that greatly exceed chance. Such findings should be interpreted with caution. In epidemiological surveys, medical conditions are usually ascertained by self-report. Depression is associated with high rates of medically unexplained symptoms (Katon, Sullivan, & Walker, 2001). Thus, reliance on self-reported health status may inflate medical comorbidity estimates in depressed populations.

Some studies have found high comorbidity between depression and medical conditions in hospitalized patients (e.g., Freedland et al., 2003). Access to objective medical records reduces or eliminates reliance on self-reported health status and is a key advantage of this type of research. However, these studies are vulnerable to Berkson's bias (Berkson, 1946). If the combination of two conditions (disorders A and B) increases the risk of hospitalization, the prevalence of disorder B will necessarily be higher in patients with than in those without disorder A. The combination of depression and chronic medical illness can increase the risk of hospitalization, thereby setting the stage for Berkson's bias. For example, depression predicts nonadherence to medical treatment regimens (DiMatteo, Lepper, & Croghan, 2000), and nonadherent patients may be more likely to require hospitalization than are adherent but otherwise comparable patients.

However, the "bias" in Berkson's bias pertains to overestimation of comorbidity in the population at large, or in outpatients, from studies of hospitalized patients. Berkson's bias does not invalidate estimates of the comorbidity of depression and medical illness among hospitalized patients; it simply gives us one more reason to avoid overgeneralizing them.

Another reason for caution is that the "meaningful" proportion of comorbidity is not self-evident. For example, if 25% of patients admitted to a hospital had diabetes, and 25% had major depression, 5% would be expected to have both conditions by chance. If 20% were found to have both conditions, would this mean that they co-occur by chance in 5% of the cases and for some more interesting reason (e.g., shared etiology) in 15%? Not necessarily. Although 5% of the cases *could* have occurred by chance, this does not mean that 5% *did* occur by chance. Even if chance expectation did carry that implication, there would not be any obvious way to discern which of the co-occurrences were meaningful and which were merely coincidental.

A similar question arises with regard to depression as a risk factor for medical morbidity and mortality. For example, depression increases the risk of mortality after acute myocardial infarction (MI; Frasure-Smith, Lespérance, & Talajic, 1993), but the risk is much less than 100%. Apparently, some depressed patients are at high risk, and others are not (Carney & Freedland, 2007). The high- and low-risk subsets might differ in many different ways, but a fundamental possibility is that the association between major depression and acute MI may be coincidental in some cases and consequential in others.

Medical Illness as a Predictor of Depression

Medical illness is often listed as a risk factor for depression (e.g., Dubovsky, Davis, & Dubovsky, 2003), but this is based on few truly prospective studies of the lifetime incidence of depression. Such studies are difficult to conduct, because chronic medical conditions seldom emerge until middle or old age, whereas the incidence of depression increases sharply in adolescence and rises in an approximately linear manner thereafter. Furthermore, the age at onset has declined over successive birth cohorts (Kessler et al., 2003). Thus, the lifetime onset of major depression not only precedes the onset of any major chronic medical illnesses in most cases but also it often does so by several decades.

In the Health and Retirement Study (Polsky et al., 2005), 8,387 adults ages 51–61 years were recruited in 1992 and followed biennially from 1994 through 2000. At each survey wave, the participants were assessed for depression and asked whether a physician had told them, during the 2 years since the previous interview, that they had any specific medical conditions. The timing of new diagnoses of specific medical conditions, such as hypertension, was determined by identifying the follow-up interval in which the condition was first reported.

Overall, 5.5% of participants reported depression within the first 2 years. The rates were no higher for subjects with a new diagnosis of heart disease or diabetes (5.5%), and they were actually a little lower for those with newly diagnosed hypertension (3.5%) or arthritis (4.4%). In contrast, the rates were 9.1% within 2 years after a stroke, 12.7% after the diagnosis of chronic lung disease, and 13.1% after the diagnosis of cancer. When adjusted hazard ratios were examined for each 2-year period within each medical condition, a more complicated picture emerged. The hazard of depression after a diagnosis of cancer or lung disease was quite high initially but decreased in succeeding years. In contrast, the adjusted hazard of depression was relatively low in the first 2 years after the diagnosis of arthritis or heart disease, but it subsequently increased.

This suggests that there is no simple answer to the question of whether newly diagnosed medical conditions increase the risk for depression. The answer depends on the medical condition, and on when it was diagnosed. It also raises the possibility that diverse medical conditions may increase the risk of depression for different reasons. For example, the high risk of depression in cancer patients might be due in part to the use of agents such as interferon alpha (Musselman et al., 2001). These agents are not used to treat most of the other medical conditions that carry a high risk of depression. Other potentially influential factors vary within and between medical conditions as well (e.g., how painful, disabling, or disfiguring the condition is; its prognostic implications; and the financial, social, and other burdens it imposes on the patient). So, for example, malignant melanoma and chronic obstructive pulmonary disease might increase the risk of depression not only for some of the same reasons but also for different reasons.

Chronic medical illness predicts depression in older individuals, but its relationship to first-ever episodes of major depression in the elderly is complicated by the possible involvement of central nervous system (CNS) abnormalities. Subtle CNS abnormalities may be involved in "vascular depression" (Krishnan, Hays, & Blazer, 1997). More profound CNS abnormalities may also be involved. Major depressive syndrome is common after the onset of cognitive impairment in patients with Alzheimer's disease and, in the majority of cases, there is no known premorbid history of major depression (Zubenko et al., 2003). Depression, even in adolescence or young adulthood, is also a risk factor for Alzheimer's disease (Green et al., 2003; Ownby, Crocco, Acevedo, John, & Lowenstein, 2006).

These complexities aside, a number of prospective studies have shown that chronic medical illness is a risk factor for depression, especially in older adults. The Alameda County Study evaluated community residents age 50 years or older. Poor health was one of the strongest independent predictors of depression (Roberts, Kaplan, Shema, & Strawbridge, 1997). The Canadian National Population Health Survey (NPHS), a national probability sample of over 17,000 Canadian residents, identified predictors of major depression. Respondents with chronic medical conditions had about twice the risk of developing a new major depressive episode. Painful conditions, including migraine headaches and back pain, were among the strongest predictors (Patten, 2001). In the Medical Outcomes Study (MOS), physical health status and depression data were obtained at three assessment points over 4 years. Poor physical health predicted subsequent depression and vice versa. However, the former relationship was more robust than the latter (Hays, Marshall, Wang, & Sherbourne, 1994).

A recent review of 20 prospective studies indicated that medical illness and poor health status were often identified as risk factors for depression among elderly community residents, but neither was an *independent* risk factor in a quantitative meta-analysis. In contrast, bereavement, sleep disturbances, disability, prior depression, and female gender were independent risk factors (Cole & Dendukuri, 2003). These findings, along with those of the NPHS, suggest that pain and physical disability, which are often, but not always, associated with an identifiable chronic illness, may be more important risk factors than is medical illness per se.

There is ample evidence from cross-sectional studies that depression is more prevalent among medically ill than among physically healthy individuals. A Canadian study of over 2,500 households documented major depressive episodes within the past year. Medical conditions were identified by self-report. Individuals with chronic medical conditions had a higher prevalence of major depression than those with no medical illnesses. This held after adjustment for age, sex, social support, and stressful life events (Gagnon & Patten, 2002).

The Canadian Community Health Survey (CCHS) randomly sampled over 115,000 subjects from the general population and administered structured interviews to assess major depression and chronic medical illnesses. Unlike the Gagnon and Patten (2002) study, the CCHS sample included individuals as young as 18 years old. After adjustment for age and sex, chronic fatigue syndrome (CFS) and fibromyalgia were the conditions most strongly associated with major depression. Weaker associations were found for diabetes, heart disease, gastrointestinal disorders, and other medical conditions that tend to be less painful or fatiguing than CFS or fibromyalgia (Patten et al., 2005). This raises further questions about whether medical illness per se contributes to depression after pain and disability have been taken into account.

Nevertheless, it is often simply assumed that medical illness causes depression. This may be due in part to the logical fallacy *post hoc, ergo propter hoc.* A patient has a heart attack, undergoes further evaluation, and is found to be depressed. The depression is assumed, with little or no evidence, to have been *caused* by the heart attack, simply because the depression was discovered after the medical condition. Causality seems plausible because heart attacks are aversive, stressful, "depressing" experiences. However, many patients who are depressed after a serious medical event were depressed before the event; many have histories of depression that began years or even decades before any physical health problems; and many other patients who have the same kind of medical event do not become depressed. For example, the 20% prevalence of major depression after acute MI implies that about 80% of patients do *not* have major depression. Some of them have minor or subsyndromal depression, but if MIs literally caused major depression in the same sense that they can cause heart failure, then even more patients would probably have major depression. It also suggests that MIs may precipitate depression only under certain circumstances or in patients with certain characteristics.

Medical Illness as a Cause of Depression

There may be circumstances in which medical illness actually does cause depression instead of merely predicting it. However, the etiology of depression is poorly understood. A central innovation of DSM-III (American Psychiatric Association, 1980) was that it removed etiological considerations, wherever possible, from psychiatric nosology and replaced them with descriptive criteria. This improved the reliability of psychiatric diagnosis and eliminated much of the etiological guesswork that had previously dominated it. Although this represents a major breakthrough, it breaks down when applied to psychiatric comorbidity in medical illness. Consideration of the possible etiological role of medical illness is necessary when it co-occurs with depression. There is reason to doubt that conditions such as heart disease play a causal role in the development of depression, but this does not rule out the possibility. Furthermore, certain medical conditions, such as hypothyroidism, definitely cause depressive symptoms and possibly full, syndromal depression as well (Gold, Pottash, & Extein, 1981; Kolakowska & Swigar, 1977).

DSM-IV-TR (American Psychiatric Association, 2000) provides stringent criteria for etiological judgments. Major depression is not to be classified as a mental disorder due to a general medical condition unless its symptoms are *due solely to the direct, physiological effects* of a medical condition. It is difficult to prove that symptoms are due entirely to direct, physiological effects of medical illness, and not at all due to depression. Symptoms can be multiply determined (simultaneously produced by two or more disorders; e.g., depression and a medical illness). Furthermore, medical conditions can contribute to depressive symptoms via indirect pathways. For example, patients with heart failure might have insomnia because of difficulty breathing at night, a noisy hospital environment, worries about health, and/or depression. The insomnia may be only partially due to the direct physiological effects of heart failure. It might also be due to other factors, so it cannot be attributed solely to the medical condition and discounted as a symptom of depression. DSM-IV asserts that the benefit of the doubt should be given to the psychiatric disorder. It also implies that depression should not be classified as being due to a medical condition, even if it can be explained entirely by the patient's inability to cope with it, because that is not a direct physiological effect of the illness.

The same logic applies to questions about whether depression is due to a medication. For example, dysphoric mood is a common side effect of beta-blockers. It is sometimes assumed that if a depressed patient is taking a beta-blocker, the depression must be *due* to the medication. However, there is no association between beta-blockade and clinical depression (Bright & Everitt, 1992; Carney et al., 1987; van Melle et al., 2006). There is stronger evidence for attributing depression to certain other agents, such as interferon-alpha, but even so, it is difficult to prove that a patient's depression is due *solely* to their direct, physiological effects. If interferon-alpha is being used to treat malignant melanoma, for example, the depression might also be due in part to the distressing psychological effects of cancer. In some cases, it may be possible for the treating physician to evaluate the role of direct physiological effects of a medication by adjusting the dosage, switching agents, or discontinuing treatment. This might show that the medication is wholly responsible for a syndrome that merely resembles depression. However, most major depressive episodes in medical patients are true cases of depression, not medication side effects.

The phenomenology of depression may also offer clues as to the role of direct, physiological effects of medical illnesses and medications. In a clinical trial (Capuron et al., 2002), 40 patients with malignant melanoma who were about to start interferon-alpha treatment were randomly assigned to either paroxetine or placebo. They were assessed at regular intervals for depression, anxiety, and neurotoxic side effects. Anorexia, fatigue, and pain emerged within the first 2 weeks of interferon-alpha treatment in a many cases, but dysphoric mood, anxiety, and cognitive impairment did not appear until later in treatment, and primarily in the subset of patients who met full DSM-IV criteria for major depression. Furthermore, the latter symptoms were more responsive to treatment with paroxetine than were the fatigue, anorexia, and pain. This did not establish that symptoms such as fatigue were due *solely* to interferon-alpha. It did suggest, however, that whereas interferon-alpha may have been the predominant cause of these symptoms, it did not account for the full syndrome of major depression. It is tempting to exclude symptoms such as fatigue when diagnosing depression in such circumstances, but the DSM-IV rule favors their inclusion.

The MOS (Wells et al., 1989) provided further evidence that depression is not merely epiphenomenal in medical patients. The MOS assessed depression in 11,242 outpatients. Patients who had either depressive symptoms or a depressive disorder had worse functional impairment, worse perceived health, and more physical pain than patients with no chronic conditions. The level of functional impairment uniquely attributable to depression was comparable to or worse than that associated with eight different medical conditions, such as arthritis and diabetes. Depression and these medical conditions had additive effects on functional impairment (e.g., impairment was roughly twice as severe in patients with comorbid diabetes and depression as in patients with diabetes alone). This is inconsistent with the view that depression is nothing more than an "understandable," inconsequential reaction to medical illness.

Depression as a Predictor of the Onset of Medical Illness

The Western Electric Study was one of the first to find that depression in a relatively healthy cohort predicts the incidence of medical illness later in life. Depression was assessed in over 2,000 middle-aged male employees. It predicted the incidence of cancer during over 10 years of follow-up, and cancer mortality over 20 years (Persky, Kempthorne-Rawson, & Shekelle, 1987). In the Stirling County Study, depression and anxiety disorders among 1,003 adults predicted somatic disorders in 618 survivors over a 16-year follow-up and vice versa (Murphy et al., 1992).

The Framingham Heart Study recently produced two reports about depression as a risk factor for medical illness. Depression was measured by the Center for Epidemiologic Studies Depression Scale (CES-D) in 3,634 participants in the original and offspring cohorts. Over a 6-year follow-up, 83 participants had cardiac events and 133 participants died. A CES-D score ≥ 16 did not predict cardiac events, but it did predict all-cause mortality. The risk of death was 33% higher in the second than in the first CES-D tertile, and 88% higher in the third (Wulsin et al., 2005). The second report (Salaycik et al., 2007) included 4,120 participants with up to 8 years of follow-up data. In those younger than 65 years, depression increased risk of stroke fourfold. It did not predict stroke in older adult participants.

Other recent studies have shown that depression is an independent predictor of various medical conditions. For example, the Healthy Women Study, a prospective cohort study initiated in 1983, showed that depression at baseline was an independent predictor of the onset of the metabolic syndrome over an average of 15 years of follow-up (Raikkonen, Matthews, & Kuller, 2007).

Depression as a Risk Factor for Morbidity and Mortality in Medical Illness

There has been more research on depression as a risk factor for morbidity and mortality in patients with established medical illness than for the onset of illness. Numerous studies have examined depression's role in heart disease, cancer, and other major medical illnesses. Although depression has been established as an independent risk factor for further morbidity and mortality in certain medical conditions, there is considerable uncertainty as to whether it is a *causal* risk factor in any of them. Several formidable hurdles confront researchers in this area. First, observational studies are often plagued by questions about residual confounding (Fewell, Davey Smith, & Sterne, 2007). Rigorous studies adjust for multiple potential confounders (e.g., Ang, Choi, Kroenke, & Wolfe, 2005), but one can never be certain that researchers accounted for other important confounders. For example, subclinical risk factors (e.g., undiagnosed diabetes) may be missed. Measurement error can contribute to residual confounding, and it can be difficult to obtain "gold standard" data on medical confounders. For example, left ventricular ejection fraction (LVEF) is a key indicator of the severity of heart disease, but it is not an error-free measure, and it is unobtainable in some cases.

Because this type of research is expensive, many studies have small samples, and small samples severely constrain the number of confounders that can be included in statistical models (Babyak, 2004). Paradoxically, it is more difficult to obtain "gold standard" medical measures in large studies than in small ones. In a large epidemiological study, for example, the severity of heart disease might be measured by a few simple questions, such as "Have you ever had a heart attack?" In a smaller study, it might be possible to obtain more rigorous measures, such as cardiac troponin levels and LVEF, but the sample might not be large enough to adjust for other potentially important covariables. Thus, both large and small observational studies are vulnerable to questions about residual confounding, but often for different reasons.

Complex mechanisms link depression to disease outcomes. How does depression increase the risk of mortality after an MI, for example? Many possibilities, including both behavioral (e.g., poor adherence to medical treatment) and physiological (e.g., cardiovascular autonomic dysregulation) factors are being studied (Skala, Freedland, & Carney, 2006). There may be multiple links in the mechanistic chain, and the mechanisms may interact in complex ways. If the mechanisms can ever be mapped out in exquisite detail, the causal role (if any) of depression in disease outcomes will be clear. That, however, may require another generation or two of research.

Finally, clinical trials are widely regarded as the crucible of risk factor research. Failure to demonstrate that treatment modifies the effect of a risk factor on a disease outcome raises doubts about whether the risk factor is causal rather than merely a risk marker. However, there are more ways for a trial to fail than to succeed. For example, the Enhancing Recovery in Coronary Heart Disease (ENRICHD) clinical trial tested the hypothesis that treating depression and low perceived social support after an acute MI reduces the risk of recurrent MI and death. Not only did the intervention have no effect on the primary medical outcome, but it also had only modest effects on depression and social support (Berkman et al., 2003). Thus, ENRICHD did not provide a very strong test of the hypothesis. It is not unique in this regard. For example, it took numerous clinical trials to establish that hypercholesterolemia could be modified in ways that have favorable effects on cardiovascular outcomes (Baigent et al., 2005; Thavendiranathan, Bagai, Brookhart, & Choudhry, 2006). A key difference, though, is that whereas hundreds of millions of dollars have been spent studying the effects of cholesterol-lowering agents on cardiovascular outcomes in hundreds of thousands of patients, ENRICHD (a study of only 2,481 patients) is one of a very small number of trials that have investigated whether treating depression improves medical outcomes. More trials will have to be conducted before definitive conclusions can be reached.

Biobehavioral Mechanisms Linking Depression to Medical Illness

Depression increases the risk of various forms of medical morbidity and mortality, but how it does so is unclear. Candidate mechanisms are factors that are affected by depression and that contribute to the pathogenesis or progression of disease. Some factors are candidates in multiple diseases (Mykletun et al., 2007). Others are more specific. For example, procoagulant factors might help to explain why depression predicts major adverse cardiovascular events (Serebruany et al., 2003), but not why it predicts mortality in women with AIDS (Cook et al., 2004).

Several physiological correlates of depression have dominated the search for mechanisms. Depression is associated with altered autonomic tone (Veith et al., 1994), and autonomic dysregulation has been studied extensively as a mechanism linking depression to adverse cardiovascular outcomes (e.g., Carney et al., 1999, 2001; Carney, Freedland, & Veith, 2005; Gehi, Mangano, Pipkin, Browner, & Whooley, 2005). Elevated circulating levels of inflammatory mediators such as interleukin-6 (IL-6), C-reactive protein (CRP), and tumor necrosis factor-alpha (TNF-α) have been found in depressed but otherwise healthy individuals (Danner, Kasl, Abramson, & Vaccarino, 2003; Miller, Stetler, Carney, Freedland, & Banks, 2002). Some of the same factors have been implicated in the progression of coronary disease (Libby, Ridker, & Maseri, 2002). Consequently, a number of studies have examined, with mixed results, whether inflammatory cytokines can help to explain the relationship between depression and cardiovascular disease (Frasure-Smith et al., 2007; Lespérance, Frasure-Smith, Theroux, & Irwin, 2004; Miller, Freedland, & Carney, 2005; Miller, Freedland, Duntley, & Carney, 2005; Ranjit et al., 2007; Schins et al., 2005). Similarly, depression is associated with insulin resistance (Winokur, Maislin, Phillips, & Amsterdam, 1988). This has inspired numerous studies of the roles of insulin resistance and glucose dysregulation in the associations among depression, diabetes, and metabolic syndrome (Gans, 2006; Heiskanen et al., 2006; Herva, Rasanen, et al., 2006; Kinder, Carthenon, Palaniappan, King, & Fortmann, 2004; Lustman, Anderson, et al., 2000; McCaffery, Niaura, Todaro, Swan, & Carmelli, 2003; Raikkonen et al., 2007; Vogelzangs et al., 2007). Research on physiological mechanisms has also fueled efforts to identify their genetic substrates (de Geus, 2006; McCaffery et al., 2006; Otte, McCaffery, Ali, & Whooley, 2007).

Some of the behavioral effects of depression have also been identified as candidate mechanisms. Nonadherence is a prominent example. Depression triples the risk of nonadherence to a wide variety of medical treatments (DiMatteo et al., 2000), and it may help to explain why depressed patients have worse medical outcomes (Carney, Freedland, Eisen, Rich, & Jaffe, 1995; Gehi, Haas, Pipkin, & Whooley, 2005).

ASSESSMENT OF DEPRESSION IN MEDICALLY ILL PATIENTS

Diagnosis of Depressive Disorders

Most arguments about whether to exclude ambiguous features when diagnosing depressive disorders in medical patients focus on somatic symptoms, such as insomnia, fatigue, or decreased appetite. However, medical illnesses and medications can also produce other, depression-like symptoms, such as poor concentration, dysphoric mood, or anhedonia. Furthermore, cognitive and affective symptoms can be just as difficult to evaluate as somatic symptoms. For example, how does one determine whether a hospitalized patient with a serious medical illness has lost interest or pleasure in his or her usual activities? The patient is obviously in no position to engage in usual activities, whatever they might be. Under such circumstances, it is difficult even to determine whether anhedonia is present, much less to judge its etiology.

Several different diagnostic rules have been proposed for ambiguous symptoms in medical patients. The *inclusive* rule counts them, regardless of whether they might be better explained by a general medical condition. The *exclusive* rule disallows them, even if they might be due to depression. The *etiological* rule counts them except if there is evidence that they are due to medical illness. The *substitutive* rule replaces them with others, such as hopelessness, that are not part of the standard criteria for major depression. Several variants and combinations of these rules have also been proposed (Cohen-Cole & Stoudemire, 1987).

DSM-IV is etiological, but with a stringent threshold for attributing symptoms to medical illness. It is more inclusive, at least in principle, than the inconsistent and vaguely etiological approach that is sometimes employed in practice. In that approach, symptoms may be disallowed if they *might* be due to a medical illness, if they are *mostly* due to illness, and/or if they are due to indirect or psychological effects of illness. This approach is not in accord with the DSM-IV rule.

The choice of a diagnostic rule is consequential. In a large study of medical inpatients, the prevalence of major depression ranged from 10 to 21%, depending on the diagnostic rule. The inclusive rule was the most sensitive and reliable, and an *exclusive etiological* rule had the highest specificity for severe, persistent depression. The DSM-IV rule yielded a prevalence of major depression (17%) that was intermediate between the most inclusive and the most restrictive rules (Koenig, George, Peterson, & Pieper, 1997). In a recent study of cancer patients, the exclusive rule yielded the strongest association between major depression and a serotonin-related biomarker (Uchitomi et al., 2001). In general, though, ambiguous symptoms are valid indicators of depression in medical patients (Simon & Von Korff, 2006). Usually, the best approach is to adhere to the DSM-IV rule.

Measurement of Depression Symptoms

More has been written about exclusion of somatic symptoms from continuous measures of depression than from diagnostic interviews. This is reflected in the multiplicity of measures used to study depression in medical patients. For example, the Beck Depression Inventory (BDI—Beck, Steer, & Brown, 1996; Beck, Ward, Mendelson, Mock, & Erbaugh, 1961) is one of the most widely used measures of depression in studies of medical patients, and it includes somatic symptoms. The Hospital Anxiety and Depression Scale (HADS; Zigmond & Snaith, 1983) is also frequently used, particularly in Europe. One of the reasons for its popularity is that it *excludes* somatic symptoms.

The role of somatic symptoms in depression measurement has been studied in a variety of ways. For example, Lustman, Freedland, Carney, Hong, and Clouse (1992) compared the BDI symptom profiles of three groups of patients: diabetic patients with major depression, nondepressed diabetic patients, and depressed but otherwise healthy psychiatric patients. Twelve out of 13 cognitive BDI symptoms, and five out of eight somatic symptoms, did not differ in prevalence or severity between the two depressed groups. The nondepressed group differed significantly in prevalence and severity from both depressed groups on every symptom except for weight loss. This suggests that depression has a similar presentation in diabetic and psychiatric patients, and it supports the inclusion of somatic symptoms when measuring depression in diabetic patients.

Lustman, Clouse, Griffith, Carney, and Freedland (1997) subsequently administered the BDI and the Diagnostic Interview Schedule (DIS; Robins, Helzer, Croughan, & Ratcliff, 1981) to 172 diabetic outpatients classified as having major depression or no depressive disorder. The Cognitive subscale was slightly more accurate vis-à-vis the DIS than was the Somatic subscale, but the BDI Total Score outperformed both subscales. Even if the cognitive items are more specific than the somatic items, it is still better to retain the somatic items and administer the entire BDI when studying patients with diabetes.

A second approach compares the screening performance of scales that include or exclude somatic symptoms. In a recent review, Thombs and colleagues (2007) reported that the BDI and the HADS were the most frequently used measures with post-MI patients. The HADS is slightly more sensitive and less specific than the BDI for major depression. Neither one is unequivocally superior to the other. An earlier study (Strik, Honig, Lousberg, & Denollet, 2001) reached similar conclusions.

Another way is to consider whether scales such as the BDI predict medical outcomes primarily because the somatic items are predictive. If so, this might suggest that the somatic items reflect medical illness rather than depression, and that more severe medical illness, rather than depression, increases the risk of adverse outcomes. Most studies contradict this view. When differences are found, the cognitive symptoms are often better predictors than the somatic symptoms (e.g., Barefoot et al., 2000; Irvine et al., 1999). These would be improbable findings if the somatic items were determined primarily by medical illness and negligibly by depression.

Thus, the evidence that somatic items should be excluded from measures of depression in medical patients is far from conclusive. In addition, there are disadvantages to removing them: information of potential clinical value is lost, criterion symptoms of major depression are not assessed, and modified rather than standard versions of instruments such as the BDI are required. On balance, the advantages of retaining the somatic items outweigh the disadvantages.

TREATMENT OF DEPRESSION IN MEDICAL PATIENTS

Medical comorbidity affects treatment responsiveness in major depression (Bogner et al., 2005; Iosifescu et al., 2003, 2005), but medical illness is an exclusion criterion in most clinical trials of treatments for depression (Keitner, Posternak, & Ryan, 2003). It is risky to generalize from these trials to the treatment of depression in medical patients, yet there have been few depression trials for patients with specific medical comorbidities. More trials are needed, both to test safety and efficacy and to determine whether standard treatments have to be modified for medical patients.

For example, behavioral activation is a key component of cognitive-behavioral therapy (CBT) for depression (Dimidjian et al., 2006). It is also used to treat depression in ambulatory medical patients (ENRICHD Investigators, 2001). However, it may carry a risk of triggering serious adverse events (SAEs) in vulnerable medical patients. A behavioral activation plan that includes getting back out on the golf course would be innocuous for a depressed but otherwise healthy individual, but potentially dangerous for a medical patient who cannot tolerate physical exertion. This does not mean that behavioral activation cannot be used with medical patients. It means that the patient's physician should be consulted, that medical contraindications must be taken into account, and that the invention must be modified accordingly (Skala, Freedland, & Carney, 2005).

Two safety issues constrain antidepressant options for medical patients. First, there are medical contraindications for some antidepressants; for example, tricyclics can cause tachycardia and orthostatic hypotension, and they are risky for patients with conduction disorders and arrhythmias (Roose & Miyazaki, 2005). Second, antidepressants can interact with other medications. For example, selective serotonin reuptake inhibitors (SSRIs) are generally safe for patients with coronary heart disease (CHD; Roose & Miyazaki, 2005), but they can interact in harmful ways with drugs that are metabolized by the same cytochrome P450 liver enzymes (Nemeroff, Preskorn, & Devane, 2007).

Psychotherapy can also have adverse interactions with medical illnesses and treatments. In Lustman, Griffith, Freedland, Kissel, and Clouse's (1998) trial of CBT for depression in diabetes, the intervention group received CBT plus supportive diabetes education, and the control group received only supportive diabetes education. The CBT group had better depression outcomes, and better glycemic control at follow-up, but diabetes complications and poor adherence to glucose self-monitoring predicted worse depression outcomes in CBT (Lustman, Freedland, Griffith, & Clouse, 1998). Conversely, glucose self-monitoring decreased during the treatment phase in the CBT than the control arm (Lustman, Griffith, et al., 1998).

An adverse interaction was also observed in the Canadian Cardiac Randomized Evaluation of Antidepressant and Psychotherapy Efficacy (CREATE) trial (Lespérance et al., 2007). Patients with CHD and major depression were double-randomized to 12 weeks of interpersonal therapy (IPT) plus clinical management (CM) or to CM only, and to 12 weeks of citalopram or pill placebo treatment. Citalopram was superior to placebo for depression, but IPT plus CM was not superior to CM alone. To the contrary, CM alone produced slightly more improvement, especially in patients with low social support or substantial functional impairment.

These studies do not suggest that psychotherapy is harmful or contraindicated for medical patients. They show that patients have finite time and capacity for treatment and self-care. Time and energy spent on CBT or IPT is unavailable for disease self-management and medical care, and vice versa. This should be taken into account in treatment planning and monitoring, especially with patients who have limited social, physical, or financial resources.

Depression trials are conducted for two reasons in medical patient populations. One reason is to evaluate treatment safety and/or efficacy. These studies are similar to standard psychiatric and psychological trials, except that they are conducted in medical patient populations. For example, the Sertraline Antidepressant Randomized Heart Attack Trial (SADHART; Glassman et al., 2002) tested the safety and efficacy of sertraline for major depression in patients hospitalized for an acute coronary syndrome. The primary safety outcome was change in LVEF; secondary safety outcomes included other cardiovascular parameters and major adverse cardiovascular events. There was no between-group difference in Hamilton Rating Scale for Depression (HAMD) scores in the overall sample, but sertraline was superior in the subgroup with severe, recurrent depression. There was no evidence that sertraline is unsafe. Instead, there was a trend toward better cardiovascular outcomes in the sertraline arm than in the placebo arm.

The other reason is to determine whether treatment of depression (or a particular kind of treatment) can improve medical outcomes. ENRICHD is an example of this type of trial. Patients hospitalized for an acute MI were randomly assigned to usual care or to CBT augmented by sertraline when indicated. The primary medical endpoint was recurrent MI or death. There was no between-group difference on this endpoint (Berkman et al., 2003), perhaps because the intervention had only weak effects on depression and social support. A subgroup analysis revealed a lower risk of late mortality in patients whose depression improved during the intervention compared to those whose depression persisted or worsened (Carney et al., 2004).

These two types of studies differ not only in their aims but also in their size and design. Trials such as ENRICHD require much larger samples and different control conditions than do trials like SADHART. Despite their differences, they are interdependent. Without safe and highly efficacious interventions, depression treatment cannot possibly improve medical outcomes. Without the hope of improved medical outcomes, there would be less interest in developing safe and highly efficacious interventions. Of course, depression is a serious disorder in its own right, and it has multiple adverse effects besides increasing the risk of medical morbidity and mortality. Thus, increased treatment efficacy for comorbid depression in medical illness is an important objective, even if the goal of better medical outcomes remains elusive (Carney & Freedland, 2007).

Another type of intervention research aims to improve the quality and effectiveness of depression treatment in primary care settings. Some studies include patients with a broad range of medical conditions. For example, the Improving Mood: Promoting Access to Collaborative Treatment (IMPACT; Unutzer et al., 2002) study randomized 1,801 patients from 18 primary care clinics in five states. Intervention patients had a depression care manager and an interventionist who provided education, care management, problem-solving therapy, and consultation with physicians. The intervention group had better depression and functional outcomes, higher quality of life, and higher treatment satisfaction. Other primary care studies focus on depression in patients with specific medical conditions. The Pathways Study (Katon et al., 2004), an example of this type of trial, involved 329 patients with diabetes from nine primary care clinics. The intervention was similar to the one developed for IMPACT, and it produced similar benefits.

DEPRESSION IN RELATION TO SPECIFIC MEDICAL CONDITIONS

Obesity

Pediatric depression predicts adult obesity in both genders, but especially in women (Franko, Striegel-Moore, Thompson, Schreiber, & Daniels, 2005; Pine, Goldstein, Wolk, & Weissman, 2001; Richardson et al., 2003), and pediatric obesity may also predict depression in adult women (Herva, Laitinen, et al., 2006). There is an association between lifetime history of major depression and obesity in both genders, particularly in women with severe obesity (Dong, Sanchez, & Price, 2004; McIntyre, Konarski, Wilkins, Soczynska, & Kennedy, 2006; Simon et al., 2006). Positive associations have also been found between current depression and obesity (Hach, Ruhl, Klotsche, Klose, & Jacobi, 2006; Heo, Pietrobelli, Fontaine, Sirey, & Faith, 2006; Herva, Laitinen, et al., 2006; Johnston, Johnson, McLeod, & Johnston, 2004; Lahiri, Rettig-Ewen, Bohm, & Laufs, 2007; Onyike, Crum, Lee, Lyketsos, & Eaton, 2003; Scott et al., 2008).

Depression and obesity are unlikely companions in that loss of appetite and weight loss are common symptoms of major depression. However, hyperphagia and weight gain are symptoms of atypical major depression, and the atypical subtype is more common than its name implies. In the National Comorbidity Survey (NCS), 36% of participants with major depression had atypical depression, based on the presence of hypersomnia and hyperphagia. In a substudy of 1,500 participants with major depression in the Sequenced Treatment Alternatives to Relieve Depression (STAR*D) trial, 18% had atypical features (Novick et al., 2005). The STAR*D criteria included hypersomnia, hyperphagia, and several other features. Thus, between one-fifth and one-third of patients with major depression have the atypical subtype. Whether this explains the association between depression and obesity remains to be investigated.

Metabolic Syndrome

Several cardiac risk factors that were once thought to be essentially independent are now known to co-occur in the metabolic syndrome. National Cholesterol Education Program (NCEP) criteria for the metabolic syndrome require at least three of the following: (1) abdominal obesity, (2) hypertriglyceridemia, (3) low high-density lipoprotein (HDL) cholesterol, (4) hypertension, and (5) high fasting glucose. The overall prevalence of the metabolic syndrome in the United States is 22%, but it ranges from 7% among individuals in their 20s to 43% among those in the 60s (Ford, Giles, & Dietz, 2002). This syndrome increases the risk of type 2 diabetes (Hanley et al., 2005; Macchia et al., 2006) and cardiovascular disease (Gami et al., 2007).

Several different kinds of studies have produced evidence of a relationship between depression and the metabolic syndrome. A large, population-based health survey found that women with a history of major depression were twice as likely as other women to have the metabolic syndrome (Kinder et al., 2004). A recent longitudinal study found that severe depressive symptoms predicted incident metabolic syndrome in middle-aged women (Raikkonen et al., 2007). An analysis of male twin-pairs from the National Heart, Blood, and Lung Institute (NHLBI) Twin Study found an association between depressive symptoms and the metabolic syndrome, attributable to nongenetic (environmental) factors (McCaffery et al., 2003). There is also evidence that this relationship may be mediated by unhealthy behaviors, including poor diet, smoking, and physical inactivity (Bonnet et al., 2005), and moderated by hypercortisolemia (Vogelzangs et al., 2007).

Diabetes Mellitus

There is a voluminous literature on depression in relation to type 2 diabetes. Depression predicts incident diabetes (Carnethon, Kinder, Fair, Stafford, & Fortmann, 2003; Everson-Rose et al., 2004), and a recent meta-analytic review concluded that depressed adults have a 37% increased risk of developing type 2 diabetes (Knol et al., 2006). Depression is also highly comorbid with type 2 diabetes. Depressive disorders are approximately twice as common in diabetic as in otherwise comparable nondiabetic patients. Among patients with diabetes, depression is approximately twice as common in women as in men (Ali, Stone, Peters, Davies, & Khunti, 2006; Anderson, Freedland, Clouse, & Lustman, 2001). Although the prevalence of clinical depression is lower in type 1 than in type 2 diabetes, it is approximately four times higher in patients with type 1 diabetes than in controls (Barnard, Skinner, & Peveler, 2006).

Depression has adverse medical implications for patients with diabetes. It is associated with poor glycemic control (Lustman, Anderson, et al., 2000) and predicts diabetes complications, including retinopathy, nephropathy, neuropathy, macrovascular disorders, and sexual dysfunction (de Groot, Anderson, Freedland, Clouse, & Lustman, 2001). It may also accelerate the onset of coronary disease (Clouse et al., 2003).

Fortunately, randomized clinical trials have shown that depression in patients with diabetes can be treated with CBT (Lustman, Griffith, et al., 1998) or with carefully chosen antidepressants (Lustman, Freedland, et al., 2000). A recent maintenance-phase trial also showed that sertraline can help to prevent recurrence of major depression after successful treatment (Lustman et al., 2006). Furthermore, the IMPACT (Williams et al., 2004) and Pathways (Kinder et al., 2006; Simon et al., 2007) trials demonstrated the effectiveness, particularly for patients with multiple diabetes complications, of collaborative depression treatment in primary care settings. Treatment of depression per se does not improve diabetes self-care (Lin et al., 2006; Lustman, Griffith, et al., 1998), yet it does improve glycemic control (Lustman, Freedland, Griffith, & Clouse, 2000; Lustman, Griffith, et al., 1998; Lustman et al., 2006). It is not entirely clear whether this is due to biological changes associated with depression remission or to the direct effects of therapy (Lustman & Clouse, 2002).

Sleep Apnea

Patients with obstructive sleep apnea–hypopnea syndrome (OSAHS) have frequent episodes of breathing cessation during sleep, frequent arousals, and excessive daytime sleepiness. OSAHS is especially common in obese individuals and in older men, and it increases the risks of metabolic syndrome, hypertension, and cardiovascular events (Patil, Schneider, Schwartz, & Smith, 2007). A Veterans Administration (VA) health care database study found that 22% of patients with OSAHS also had a depressive disorder (Sharafkhaneh, Giray, Richardson, Young, & Hirshkowitz, 2005). Major depression is associated with longer obstructive episodes in men and women with OSAHS, and more frequent episodes in men (Carney et al., 2006). Depression is also associated with more severe fatigue and worse subjective sleep quality in patients with OSAHS (Bardwell, Ancoli-Israel, & Dimsdale, 2007; Bardwell, Moore, Ancoli-Israel, & Dimsdale, 2003; Wells, Day, Carney, Freedland, & Duntley, 2004; Wells, Freedland, Carney, Duntley, & Stepanski, 2007).

Coronary Heart Disease

Depression has been studied much more extensively in relation to CHD than to any other illness. Meta-analytic reviews estimate that depression confers a relative risk of 1.64 for incident coronary disease (Wulsin & Singal, 2003), and that it approximately doubles the odds of mortality after an acute MI (Barth, Schumacher, & Herrmann-Lingen, 2004; van Melle et al., 2004). A more comprehensive meta-analysis (Nicholson, Kuper, & Hemingway, 2006) recently produced similar findings. In the World Mental Health surveys of populations in 17 countries, the presence of heart disease doubled the odds of major depression (Ormel et al., 2007). In the 52-nation INTERHEART study, depression was significantly more common among 11,119 subjects with MI than among 13,648 controls (24 vs. 18%; odds ratio, 1.55) (Rosengren et al., 2004). Converging evidence that depression accelerates the clinical expression of coronary disease, and that it increases the risks of further morbidity and mortality in established CHD, has inspired numerous studies of the underlying biobehavioral mechanisms (Skala et al., 2006).

Several large, multicenter clinical trials have recently shown that we have a lot to learn about how to treat depression in patients with CHD. The disappointing primary results of the SADHART (Glassman et al., 2002) and ENRICHD (Berkman et al., 2003) studies were discussed previously. In the Myocardial INfarction and Depression—Intervention Trial (MIND-IT), the latest disappointment, 331 patients who met the ICD-10 criteria for a current depressive episode between 3 and 12 months after an acute MI were randomly assigned, in a complex design, to an "intervention" arm or to usual care. There were no significant between-group differences in depression or in cardiac event rates (van Melle et al., 2007).

Secondary analyses of these trials have revealed that severe, recurrent, treatment-resistant major depression may have worse prognostic implications than other forms of depression for post-MI patients. In ENRICHD, patients with these characteristics were at approximately three times higher risk than treatment responders of late mortality (Carney et al., 2004). Similar findings were recently published by the MIND-IT investigators (de Jonge et al., 2007). Neither study identified any strong baseline predictors of treatment response. This suggests that future trials should incorporate procedures for rapid identification and remediation of nonresponse.

Heart Failure

The prevalence of chronic heart failure is increasing as the population ages, and interest in the role of depression in heart failure is rising accordingly. Depression increases the risk for heart failure in certain high-risk groups, including elderly women (Williams et al., 2002), and in patients with isolated systolic hypertension (Abramson, Berger, Krumholz, & Vaccarino, 2001) or a recent acute MI (Powell et al., 2005). The overall prevalence of depression is approximately 17–20% in patients with chronic heart failure, but it is considerably higher in younger and more debilitated patients (Freedland et al., 1991, 2003). Depression increases the risks of hospitalization and mortality in patients with heart failure (Freedland et al., 1991; Jiang et al., 2001, 2007; Sherwood et al., 2007; Williams et al., 2002). Treatment research in this area is still at an early stage (Gottlieb et al., 2007; Lespérance et al., 2003).

Cerebrovascular Accident

Stroke has one of the most complex and interesting relationships to depression of any medical condition, primarily because of the etiological questions it raises. Major depression affects approximately 19% of patients hospitalized for stroke, and 23% of outpatients (Robinson, 2003). An early study suggested that the risk of early poststroke depression depended on the location of the brain lesion; patients with left anterior strokes were particularly vulnerable (Starkstein, Robinson, Berthier, & Price, 1988). This was confirmed in a study that also suggested that later-onset depression may be associated more strongly with poststroke disability than with lesion location (Parikh, Lipsey, Robinson, & Price, 1988). Subsequent studies cast doubt on the early findings (Carson et al., 2000; Morris et al., 1996). In a recent effort to clarify this phenomenon, a significant inverse correlation between the severity of depression and the distance of the lesion from the frontal pole in patients with left-hemisphere strokes was found (Narushima, Kosier, & Robinson, 2003). Researchers have also begun to consider whether proinflammatory cytokines may help to explain this relationship (Spalletta et al., 2006).

Treatment research has yielded some promising findings for depressed stroke patients. One of the earliest placebo-controlled trials demonstrated that nortriptyline was efficacious for poststroke depression (Lipsey, Robinson, Pearlson, Rao, & Price, 1984). Nortriptyline is superior to fluoxetine for short-term depression outcomes (Robinson et al., 2000), but fluoxetine may produce better long-term results (Chemerinski, Robinson, Arndt, & Kosier, 2001). There is also evidence suggesting that these agents may improve other outcomes, including executive functions (Narushima, Paradiso, Moser, Jorge, & Robinson, 2007), activities of daily living (Chemerinski et al., 2001), irritability (Chan, Campayo, Moser, Arndt, & Robinson, 2006), and mortality (Jorge, Robinson, Arndt, & Starkstein, 2003). However, most of the existing studies are relatively small; larger trials are needed.

Cancer

Cancer is one of the most controversial areas in behavioral medicine, particularly regarding whether depression or other psychological factors increase the risk of developing cancer, and whether psychotherapy improves chances of cancer survival. Despite some positive findings, there is slim evidence for either possibility (Bergelt et al., 2005; Coyne, Stefanek, & Palmer, 2007; Eysenck, 1993; Hahn & Petitti, 1988; Spiegel & Giese-Davis, 2003; Zonderman, Costa, & McCrae, 1989). Recent reports have also shown that antidepressants are overprescribed to cancer patients (Coyne, Palmer, & Shapiro, 2004; Coyne, Palmer, Shapiro, Thompson, & DeMichele, 2004), and question the efficacy of psychotherapy for their distress and depression (Andrykowski & Manne, 2006; Coyne, Lepore, & Palmer, 2006; Manne & Andrykowski, 2006).

On the other hand, there is growing evidence that depression is associated with shorter survival times in cancer patients (Brown, Levy, Rosberger, & Edgar, 2003; Faller, Bulzebruck, Drings, & Lang, 1999; Faller & Schmidt, 2004; Persky et al., 1987; Prieto et al., 2005; Stommel, Given, & Given, 2002; Watson, Haviland, Greer, Davidson, & Bliss, 1999). Depression has other adverse implications in cancer as well. It may exacerbate cancer-related pain (Spiegel, Sands, & Koopman, 1994) and functional impairment (Hegel et al., 2006), interfere with acceptance of chemotherapy (Colleoni et al., 2000), and increase the desire for hastened death among terminally ill cancer patients (Breitbart et al., 2000). Taken together, these findings underscore the need to develop more efficacious treatments for depression in cancer, and to ensure that the patients who receive them are also the ones who need them.

HIV/AIDS

Depression is prevalent among individuals (and especially women) with AIDS (Ciesla & Roberts, 2001; Morrison et al., 2002), but there is uncertainty regarding the relationship between the course of HIV/AIDS and the course of depression. A large cohort study found that depressive symptoms remained stable in HIV-seropositive individuals until about a year before AIDS diagnosis, at which time symptom severity increased. It then reached a plateau about 6 months before AIDS developed (Lyketsos et al., 1996). More stable patterns have also been found (Rabkin et al., 1997).

Depression is associated with HIV risk behaviors such as needle sharing, although the direction of this relationship is unclear (Hutton, Lyketsos, Zenilman, Thompson, & Erbelding, 2004; Stein, Solomon, Herman, Anderson, & Miller, 2003). There is also growing evidence that depression may accelerate the progression of HIV/AIDS and increase the risk of mortality (Cook et al., 2004; Cruess et al., 2005; Evans et al., 2002; Ickovics et al., 2001; Leserman et al., 1997). Antidepressant treatment of depression is challenging in HIV/ AIDS patients due to side effects, polypharmacy, and attrition, but there is at least limited evidence for the efficacy of fluoxetine and paroxetine in these patients (Elliott et al., 1998; Rabkin, Wagner, & Rabkin, 1999). Psychotherapy (Markowitz et al., 1998) and dehydro-epiandrosterone (DHEA) (Rabkin, McElhiney, Rabkin, McGrath, & Ferrando, 2006) have also shown promise. Little is known about whether treatment of depression can alter the course of HIV/AIDS, but the possibility deserves further investigation.

FUTURE DIRECTIONS

There is great interest in depression as a risk factor for the development of medical illness, and for impairment, morbidity, and mortality after the onset of conditions such as obesity, diabetes, heart disease, stroke, cancer, and HIV/AIDS. However, research lags far behind in some of these conditions compared to others. The literature on depression in cancer, for example, is much smaller than those for heart disease and diabetes. Depression may be more difficult to study in some diseases than in others; nevertheless, more work is needed in these areas.

Sparseness of data about *exposure* to depression is a pervasive problem. We know, for example, that patients who are depressed after an acute MI are at higher risk of death within the next 3 years (e.g., Carney et al., 2003). It is not clear, though, that episodes of depression around the time of an acute MI have anything directly to do with the deaths that occur 1 or 2 years later. It is possible that depression also has to be present *at the time* of a recurrent MI to increase its lethality. Perhaps depression at the time of the index MI is simply a harbinger of subsequent depressive episodes, some of which just happen to coincide with periods of cardiovascular vulnerability. To address such questions, it is necessary to collect depression data at frequent intervals over lengthy follow-ups. That such data are difficult to obtain helps to explain why we need to know much more about the timing of exposure, as well as *cumulative* exposure, to depression in relation to medical illness and medical outcomes.

Complete delineation of the *biobehavioral mechanisms* linking depression to medical illness is one of the most daunting challenges. Certain candidate mechanisms, such as autonomic dysregulation, inflammatory processes, physical inactivity, and poor adherence to medical treatment regimens, may underlie the relationships between depression and a number of different medical illnesses. Others may play a more exclusive role. For example, glucose dysregulation may help to account for the effects of depression on diabetes (Lustman, Anderson, et al., 2000), but not for its ability to predict cancer mortality after stem cell transplantation (Prieto et al., 2005). Less is known about some candidate mechanisms than about others. We have only just begun, for example, to investigate the genetic substrates of the relationship between depression and CHD (de Geus, 2006; McCaffery et al., 2006). Finally, we know little about the interrelationships among these mechanistic variables. Most studies have examined individual mechanisms, or classes of mechanisms. For example, the associations among autonomic dysregulation, inflammatory processes, and procoagulant processes in depressed patients with CHD have been studied only recently (Carney et al., 2007). The ultimate goal of work in this area is to develop comprehensive causal models of the relationship of depression to specific disease outcomes. We are at a very early stage in that work.

Most studies focus on the role of depression in specific, chronic medical conditions, but these conditions may not occur in isolation. A study of over 60,000 general practice patients (van den Akker, Buntinx, Metsemakers, Roos, & Knottnerus, 1998) showed that 30% of patients have two or more chronic medical conditions. The rate increases with age, such that 78% of patients age 80 years and older have at least two chronic conditions. Rigorous studies of depression as a risk factor for specific medical outcomes take medical comorbidity into account by adjusting either for specific comorbidities (e.g., Grunau, Sheps, Goldner, & Ratner, 2006) or for a comorbidity index, such as the Cumulative Illness Rating Scale (Linn, Linn, & Gurel, 1968) or the Charlson Comorbidity Index (Charlson, Pompei, Ales, & MacKenzie, 1987). These are useful approaches, but they oversimplify the associations among illnesses. Although it has not yet penetrated very far into psychiatric research, the concept of *multimorbidity* is well known in chronic disease epidemiology. Multimorbidity coefficients have distinct advantages over traditional methods (Batstra, Bos, & Neeleman, 2002). With very few exceptions, they have not yet been utilized in studies of the relationship between depression and medical illness (Fortin et al., 2006). The next generation of research in this area should incorporate state-of-the-art multimorbidity methods.

Last, but not least, there is a critical shortage of clinical trial data. Large, rigorous trials are needed to develop more efficacious treatments and to determine whether treating depression can improve medical outcomes (Carney & Freedland, 2007; Davidson et al., 2006; Freedland, Miller, & Sheps, 2006; Kaufmann, 2003; Sheps, Freedland, Golden, & McMahon, 2003). The clinical importance of a risk factor such as depression depends to a considerable extent on whether it is modifiable, and whether modifying it improves medical outcomes. We need to learn much more about how to treat this risk factor.

REFERENCES

Abramson, J., Berger, A., Krumholz, H. M., & Vaccarino, V. (2001). Depression and risk of heart failure among older persons with isolated systolic hypertension. *Archives of Internal Medicine, 161,* 1725–1730.

Ali, S., Stone, M. A., Peters, J. L., Davies, M. J., & Khunti, K. (2006). The prevalence of co-morbid depression in adults with type 2 diabetes: A systematic review and meta-analysis. *Diabetic Medicine, 23,* 1165–1173.

American Psychiatric Association. (1980). *Diagnostic and statistical manual of mental disorders* (3rd ed.) Washington, DC: Author.

American Psychiatric Association. (2000). *Diagnostic and statistical manual of mental disorders* (4th ed., text rev.). Washington, DC: Author.

Anderson, R. J., Freedland, K. E., Clouse, R. E., & Lustman, P. J. (2001). The prevalence of comorbid depression in adults with diabetes: A meta-analysis. *Diabetes Care, 24,* 1069–1078.

Andrykowski, M. A., & Manne, S. L. (2006). Are psychological interventions effective and accepted by cancer patients?: I. Standards and levels of evidence. *Annals of Behavioral Medicine, 32,* 93–97.

Ang, D. C., Choi, H., Kroenke, K., & Wolfe, F. (2005). Comorbid depression is an independent risk factor for mortality in patients with rheumatoid arthritis. *Journal of Rheumatology, 32,* 1013–1019.

Babyak, M. A. (2004). What you see may not be what you get: A brief, nontechnical introduction to overfitting in regression-type models. *Psychosomatic Medicine, 66,* 411–421.

Baigent, C., Keech, A., Kearney, P. M., Blackwell, L., Buck, G., Pollicino, C., et al. (2005). Efficacy and safety of cholesterol-lowering treatment: Prospective meta-analysis of data from 90,056 participants in 14 randomised trials of statins. *Lancet, 366,* 1267–1278.

Bardwell, W. A., Ancoli-Israel, S., & Dimsdale, J. E. (2007). Comparison of the effects of depressive symptoms and apnea severity on fatigue in patients with obstructive sleep apnea: A replication study. *Journal of Affective Disorders, 97,* 181–186.

Bardwell, W. A., Moore, P., Ancoli-Israel, S., & Dimsdale, J. E. (2003). Fatigue in obstructive sleep apnea: Driven by depressive symptoms instead of apnea severity? *American Journal of Psychiatry, 160,* 350–355.

Barefoot, J. C., Brummett, B. H., Helms, M. J., Mark, D. B., Siegler, I. C., & Williams, R. B. (2000). Depressive symptoms and survival of patients with coronary artery disease. *Psychosomatic Medicine, 62,* 790–795.

Barnard, K. D., Skinner, T. C., & Peveler, R. (2006). The prevalence of co-morbid depression in adults with type 1 diabetes: Systematic literature review. *Diabetic Medicine, 23,* 445–448.

Barth, J., Schumacher, M., & Herrmann-Lingen, C. (2004). Depression as a risk factor for mortality in patients with coronary heart disease: A meta-analysis. *Psychosomatic Medicine, 66,* 802–813.

Batstra, L., Bos, E. H., & Neeleman, J. (2002). Quantifying psychiatric comorbidity—lessons from chronic disease epidemiology. *Social Psychiatry and Psychiatric Epidemiology, 37,* 105–111.

Beck, A. T., Steer, R. A., & Brown, G. K. (1996). *Manual for the Beck Depression Inventory–II.* San Antonio, TX: Psychological Corporation.

Beck, A. T., Ward, C. H., Mendelson, M., Mock, J. E., & Erbaugh, J. K. (1961). An inventory for measuring depression. *Archives of General Psychiatry, 4,* 561–571.

Bergelt, C., Christensen, J., Prescott, E., Gronbaek, M., Koch, U., & Johansen, C. (2005). Vital exhaustion and risk for cancer: A prospective cohort study on the association between depressive feelings, fatigue, and risk of cancer. *Cancer, 104,* 1288–1295.

Berkman, L. F., Blumenthal, J., Burg, M., Carney, R. M., Catellier, D., Cowan, M. J., et al. (2003). Effects of treating depression and low perceived social support on clinical events after myocardial infarction: The Enhancing Recovery in Coronary Heart Disease Patients (ENRICHD) randomized trial. *Journal of the American Medical Association, 289,* 3106–3116.

Berkson, J. (1946). Limitations of the application of fourfold table analysis to hospital data. *Biometrics Bulletin, 2,* 47–53.

Bogner, H. R., Cary, M. S., Bruce, M. L., Reynolds, C. F., III, Mulsant, B., Ten Have T., et al. (2005). The role of medical comorbidity in outcome of major depression in primary care: The PROSPECT study. *American Journal of Geriatric Psychiatry, 13,* 861–868.

Bonnet, F., Irving, K., Terra, J. L., Nony, P., Berthezene, F., & Moulin, P. (2005). Depressive symptoms are associated with unhealthy lifestyles in hypertensive patients with the metabolic syndrome. *Journal of Hypertension, 23,* 611–617.

Breitbart, W., Rosenfeld, B., Pessin, H., Kaim, M., Funesti-Esch, J., Galietta, M., et al. (2000). Depression, hopelessness, and desire for hastened death in terminally ill patients with cancer. *Journal of the American Medical Association, 284,* 2907–2911.

Bright, R. A., & Everitt, D. E. (1992). Beta-blockers and depression: Evidence against an association. *Journal of the American Medical Association, 267,* 1783–1787.

Brown, K. W., Levy, A. R., Rosberger, Z., & Edgar, L. (2003). Psychological distress and cancer survival: A follow-up 10 years after diagnosis. *Psychosomatic Medicine, 65,* 636–643.

Capuron, L., Gumnick, J. F., Musselman, D. L., Lawson, D. H., Reemsnyder, A., Nemeroff, C. B., et al. (2002). Neurobehavioral effects of interferon-alpha in cancer patients: Phenomenology and paroxetine responsiveness of symptom dimensions. *Neuropsychopharmacology, 26,* 643–652.

Carnethon, M. R., Kinder, L. S., Fair, J. M., Stafford, R. S., & Fortmann, S. P. (2003). Symptoms of depression as a risk factor for incident diabetes: Findings from the National Health and Nutrition Examination Epidemiologic Follow-Up Study, 1971–1992. *American Journal of Epidemiology, 158,* 416–423.

Carney, R. M., Blumenthal, J. A., Catellier, D., Freedland, K. E., Berkman, L. F., Watkins, L. L., et al. (2003). Depression as a risk factor for mortality after acute myocardial infarction. *American Journal of Cardiology, 92,* 1277–1281.

Carney, R. M., Blumenthal, J. A., Freedland, K. E., Youngblood, M., Veith, R. C., Burg, M. M., et al. (2004). Depression and late mortality after myocardial infarction in the Enhancing Recovery in Coronary Heart Disease (ENRICHD) study. *Psychosomatic Medicine, 66,* 466–474.

Carney, R. M., Blumenthal, J. A., Stein, P. K., Watkins, L., Catellier, D., Berkman, L. F., et al. (2001). Depression, heart rate variability, and acute myocardial infarction. *Circulation, 104,* 2024–2028.

Carney, R. M., & Freedland, K. E. (2007). Does treating depression improve survival after acute coronary syndrome?: Invited commentary on . . . effects of antidepressant treatment following myocardial infarction. *British Journal of Psychiatry, 190,* 467–468.

Carney, R. M., Freedland, K. E., Eisen, S. A., Rich, M. W., & Jaffe, A. S. (1995). Major depression and medication adherence in elderly patients with coronary artery disease. *Health Psychology, 14,* 88–90.

Carney, R. M., Freedland, K. E., Stein, P. K., Miller, G. E., Steinmeyer, B., Rich, M. W., et al. (2007). Heart rate variability and markers of inflammation and coagulation in depressed patients with coronary heart disease. *Journal of Psychosomatic Research, 62,* 463–467.

Carney, R. M., Freedland, K. E., & Veith, R. C. (2005). Depression, the autonomic nervous system, and coronary heart disease. *Psychosomatic Medicine, 67*(Suppl. 1), S29–S33.

Carney, R. M., Freedland, K. E., Veith, R. C., Cryer, P. E., Skala, J. A., Lynch, T., et al. (1999). Major depression, heart rate, and plasma norepinephrine in patients with coronary heart disease. *Biological Psychiatry, 45,* 458–463.

Carney, R. M., Howells, W. B., Freedland, K. E., Duntley, S. P., Stein, P. K., Rich, M. W., et al. (2006). Depression and obstructive sleep apnea in patients with coronary heart disease. *Psychosomatic Medicine, 68,* 443–448.

Carney, R. M., Rich, M. W., teVelde, A., Saini, J., Clark, K., & Freedland, K. E. (1987). Prevalence of major depressive disorder in patients receiving beta-blocker therapy versus other medications. *American Journal of Medicine, 83*, 223–226.

Carson, A. J., MacHale, S., Allen, K., Lawrie, S. M., Dennis, M., House, A., et al. (2000). Depression after stroke and lesion location: A systematic review. *Lancet, 356*, 122–126.

Chan, K. L., Campayo, A., Moser, D. J., Arndt, S., & Robinson, R. G. (2006). Aggressive behavior in patients with stroke: Association with psychopathology and results of antidepressant treatment on aggression. *Archives of Physical Medicine and Rehabilitation, 87*, 793–798.

Charlson, M. E., Pompei, P., Ales, K. L., & MacKenzie, C. R. (1987). A new method of classifying prognostic comorbidity in longitudinal studies: Development and validation. *Journal of Chronic Diseases, 40*, 373–383.

Chemerinski, E., Robinson, R. G., Arndt, S., & Kosier, J. T. (2001). The effect of remission of poststroke depression on activities of daily living in a double-blind randomized treatment study. *Journal of Nervous and Mental Disease, 189*, 421–425.

Ciesla, J. A., & Roberts, J. E. (2001). Meta-analysis of the relationship between HIV infection and risk for depressive disorders. *American Journal of Psychiatry, 158*, 725–730.

Clouse, R. E., Lustman, P. J., Freedland, K. E., Griffith, L. S., McGill, J. B., & Carney, R. M. (2003). Depression and coronary heart disease in women with diabetes. *Psychosomatic Medicine, 65*, 376–383.

Cohen-Cole, S. A., & Stoudemire, A. (1987). Major depression and physical illness: Special considerations in diagnosis and biologic treatment. *Psychiatric Clinics of North America, 10*, 1–17.

Cole, M. G., & Dendukuri, N. (2003). Risk factors for depression among elderly community subjects: A systematic review and meta-analysis. *American Journal of Psychiatry, 160*, 1147–1156.

Colleoni, M., Mandala, M., Peruzzotti, G., Robertson, C., Bredart, A., & Goldhirsch, A. (2000). Depression and degree of acceptance of adjuvant cytotoxic drugs. *Lancet, 356*, 1326–1327.

Cook, J. A., Grey, D., Burke, J., Cohen, M. H., Gurtman, A. C., Richardson, J. L., et al. (2004). Depressive symptoms and AIDS-related mortality among a multisite cohort of HIV-positive women. *American Journal of Public Health, 94*, 1133–1140.

Coyne, J. C., Lepore, S. J., & Palmer, S. C. (2006). Efficacy of psychosocial interventions in cancer care: Evidence is weaker than it first looks. *Annals of Behavioral Medicine, 32*, 104–110.

Coyne, J. C., Palmer, S. C., & Shapiro, P. J. (2004). Prescribing antidepressants to advanced cancer patients with mild depressive symptoms is not justified. *Journal of Clinical Oncology, 22*, 205–206.

Coyne, J. C., Palmer, S. C., Shapiro, P. J., Thompson, R., & DeMichele, A. (2004). Distress, psychiatric morbidity, and prescriptions for psychotropic medication in a breast cancer waiting room sample. *General Hospital Psychiatry, 26*, 121–128.

Coyne, J. C., Stefanek, M., & Palmer, S. C. (2007). Psychotherapy and survival in cancer: The conflict between hope and evidence. *Psychological Bulletin, 133*, 367–394.

Cruess, D. G., Douglas, S. D., Petitto, J. M., Ten Have, T., Gettes, D., Dube, B., et al. (2005). Association of resolution of major depression with increased natural killer cell activity among HIV-seropositive women. *American Journal of Psychiatry, 162*, 2125–2130.

Danner, M., Kasl, S. V., Abramson, J. L., & Vaccarino, V. (2003). Association between depression and elevated C-reactive protein. *Psychosomatic Medicine, 65*, 347–356.

Davidson, K. W., Kupfer, D. J., Bigger, J. T., Califf, R. M., Carney, R. M., Coyne, J. C., et al. (2006). Assessment and treatment of depression in patients with cardiovascular disease: National Heart, Lung, and Blood Institute Working Group Report. *Psychosomatic Medicine, 68*, 645–650.

de Geus, E. J. (2006). Genetic pleiotropy in depression and coronary artery disease. *Psychosomatic Medicine, 68*, 185–186.

de Groot, M., Anderson, R., Freedland, K. E., Clouse, R. E., & Lustman, P. J. (2001). Association of depression and diabetes complications: A meta-analysis. *Psychosomatic Medicine, 63*, 619–630.

de Jonge, P., Honig, A., van Melle, J. P., Schene, A. H., Kuyper, A. M., Tulner, D., et al. (2007). Nonresponse to treatment for depression following myocardial infarction: Association with subsequent cardiac events. *American Journal of Psychiatry, 164*, 1371–1378.

DiMatteo, M. R., Lepper, H. S., & Croghan, T. W. (2000). Depression is a risk factor for noncompliance with medical treatment: Meta-analysis of the effects of anxiety and depression on patient adherence. *Archives of Internal Medicine, 160*, 2101–2107.

Dimidjian, S., Hollon, S. D., Dobson, K. S., Schmaling, K. B., Kohlenberg, R. J., Addis, M. E., et al. (2006). Randomized trial of behavioral activation, cognitive therapy, and antidepressant medication in the acute treatment of adults with major depression. *Journal of Consulting and Clinical Psychology, 74,* 658–670.

Dong, C., Sanchez, L. E., & Price, R. A. (2004). Relationship of obesity to depression: A family-based study. *International Journal of Obesity and Related Metabolic Disorders, 28,* 790–795.

Dubovsky, S. L., Davis, R., & Dubovsky, A. N. (2003). Mood disorders. In R. E. Hales & S. C. Yudofsky (Eds.), *The American Psychiatric Publishing textbook of clinical psychiatry* (4th ed., pp. 439–542). Washington, DC: American Psychiatric Publishing.

Elliott, A. J., Uldall, K. K., Bergam, K., Russo, J., Claypoole, K., & Roy-Byrne, P. P. (1998). Randomized, placebo-controlled trial of paroxetine versus imipramine in depressed HIV-positive outpatients. *American Journal of Psychiatry, 155,* 367–372.

ENRICHD Investigators. (2001). Enhancing Recovery in Coronary Heart Disease (ENRICHD) study intervention: Rationale and design. *Psychosomatic Medicine, 63,* 747–755.

Evans, D. L., Ten Have, T. R., Douglas, S. D., Gettes, D. R., Morrison, M., Chiappini, M. S., et al. (2002). Association of depression with viral load, CD8 T lymphocytes, and natural killer cells in women with HIV infection. *American Journal of Psychiatry, 159,* 1752–1759.

Everson-Rose, S. A., Meyer, P. M., Powell, L. H., Pandey, D., Torrens, J. I., Kravitz, H. M., et al. (2004). Depressive symptoms, insulin resistance, and risk of diabetes in women at midlife. *Diabetes Care, 27,* 2856–2862.

Eysenck, H. J. (1993). Prediction of cancer and coronary heart disease mortality by means of a personality inventory: Results of a 15-year follow-up study. *Psychological Reports, 72,* 499–516.

Faller, H., Bulzebruck, H., Drings, P., & Lang, H. (1999). Coping, distress, and survival among patients with lung cancer. *Archives of General Psychiatry, 56,* 756–762.

Faller, H., & Schmidt, M. (2004). Prognostic value of depressive coping and depression in survival of lung cancer patients. *Psycho-Oncology, 13,* 359–363.

Fewell, Z., Davey Smith, G., & Sterne, J. A. (2007). The impact of residual and unmeasured confounding in epidemiologic studies: A simulation study. *American Journal of Epidemiology, 166,* 646–655.

Ford, E. S., Giles, W. H., & Dietz, W. H. (2002). Prevalence of the metabolic syndrome among U.S. adults: Findings from the third National Health and Nutrition Examination Survey. *Journal of the American Medical Association, 287,* 356–359.

Fortin, M., Bravo, G., Hudon, C., Lapointe, L., Dubois, M. F., & Almirall, J. (2006). Psychological distress and multimorbidity in primary care. *Annals of Family Medicine, 4,* 417–422.

Franko, D. L., Striegel-Moore, R. H., Thompson, D., Schreiber, G. B., & Daniels, S. R. (2005). Does adolescent depression predict obesity in black and white young adult women? *Psychological Medicine, 35,* 1505–1513.

Frasure-Smith, N., Lespérance, F., Irwin, M. R., Sauve, C., Lespérance, J., & Theroux, P. (2007). Depression, C-reactive protein and two-year major adverse cardiac events in men after acute coronary syndromes. *Biological Psychiatry, 62,* 302–308.

Frasure-Smith, N., Lespérance, F., & Talajic, M. (1993). Depression following myocardial infarction: Impact on 6-month survival. *Journal of the American Medical Association, 270,* 1819–1825.

Freedland, K. E., Carney, R. M., Rich, M. W., Caracciolo, A., Krotenberg, J. A., Smith, L. J., et al. (1991). Depression in elderly patients with congestive heart failure. *Journal of Geriatric Psychiatry, 24,* 59–71.

Freedland, K. E., Miller, G. E., & Sheps, D. S. (2006). The great debate, revisited. *Psychosomatic Medicine, 68,* 179–184.

Freedland, K. E., Rich, M. W., Skala, J. A., Carney, R. M., Davila-Roman, V. G., & Jaffe, A. S. (2003). Prevalence of depression in hospitalized patients with congestive heart failure. *Psychosomatic Medicine, 65,* 119–128.

Gagnon, L. M., & Patten, S. B. (2002). Major depression and its association with long-term medical conditions. *Canadian Journal of Psychiatry, 47,* 149–152.

Gami, A. S., Witt, B. J., Howard, D. E., Erwin, P. J., Gami, L. A., Somers, V. K., et al. (2007). Metabolic syndrome and risk of incident cardiovascular events and death: A systematic review and meta-analysis of longitudinal studies. *Journal of the American College of Cardiology, 49,* 403–414.

Gans, R. O. (2006). The metabolic syndrome, depression, and cardiovascular disease: Interrelated conditions that share pathophysiologic mechanisms. *Medical Clinics of North America, 90,* 573–591.

Gehi, A., Haas, D., Pipkin, S., & Whooley, M. A. (2005). Depression and medication adherence in outpatients with coronary heart disease: Findings from the Heart and Soul Study. *Archives of Internal Medicine, 165,* 2508–2513.

Gehi, A., Mangano, D., Pipkin, S., Browner, W. S., & Whooley, M. A. (2005). Depression and heart rate variability in patients with stable coronary heart disease: Findings from the Heart and Soul Study. *Archives of General Psychiatry, 62,* 661–666.

Glassman, A. H., O'Connor, C. M., Califf, R. M., Swedberg, K., Schwartz, P., Bigger, J. T., Jr., et al. (2002). Sertraline treatment of major depression in patients with acute MI or unstable angina. *Journal of the American Medical Association, 288,* 701–709.

Gold, M. S., Pottash, A. L., & Extein, I. (1981). Hypothyroidism and depression: Evidence from complete thyroid function evaluation. *Journal of the American Medical Association, 245,* 1919–1922.

Gottlieb, S. S., Kop, W. J., Thomas, S. A., Katzen, S., Vesely, M. R., Greenberg, N., et al. (2007). A double-blind placebo-controlled pilot study of controlled-release paroxetine on depression and quality of life in chronic heart failure. *American Heart Journal, 153,* 868–873.

Green, R. C., Cupples, L. A., Kurz, A., Auerbach, S., Go, R., Sadovnick, D., et al. (2003). Depression as a risk factor for Alzheimer disease: The MIRAGE Study. *Archives of Neurology, 60,* 753–759.

Grunau, G. L., Sheps, S., Goldner, E. M., & Ratner, P. A. (2006). Specific comorbidity risk adjustment was a better predictor of 5-year acute myocardial infarction mortality than general methods. *Journal of Clinical Epidemiology, 59,* 274–280.

Hach, I., Ruhl, U. E., Klotsche, J., Klose, M., & Jacobi, F. (2006). Associations between waist circumference and depressive disorders. *Journal of Affective Disorders, 92,* 305–308.

Hahn, R. C., & Petitti, D. B. (1988). Minnesota Multiphasic Personality Inventory–rated depression and the incidence of breast cancer. *Cancer, 61,* 845–848.

Hanley, A. J., Karter, A. J., Williams, K., Festa, A., D'Agostino, R. B., Jr., Wagenknecht, L. E., et al. (2005). Prediction of type 2 diabetes mellitus with alternative definitions of the metabolic syndrome: The Insulin Resistance Atherosclerosis Study. *Circulation, 112,* 3713–3721.

Hays, R. D., Marshall, G. N., Wang, E. Y., & Sherbourne, C. D. (1994). Four-year cross-lagged associations between physical and mental health in the Medical Outcomes Study. *Journal of Consulting and Clinical Psychology, 62,* 441–449.

Hegel, M. T., Moore, C. P., Collins, E. D., Kearing, S., Gillock, K. L., Riggs, R. L., et al. (2006). Distress, psychiatric syndromes, and impairment of function in women with newly diagnosed breast cancer. *Cancer, 107,* 2924–2931.

Heiskanen, T. H., Niskanen, L. K., Hintikka, J. J., Koivumaa-Honkanen, H. T., Honkalampi, K. M., Haatainen, K. M., et al. (2006). Metabolic syndrome and depression: A cross-sectional analysis. *Journal of Clinical Psychiatry, 67,* 1422–1427.

Heo, M., Pietrobelli, A., Fontaine, K. R., Sirey, J. A., & Faith, M. S. (2006). Depressive mood and obesity in US adults: Comparison and moderation by sex, age, and race. *International Journal of Obesity (London), 30,* 513–519.

Herva, A., Laitinen, J., Miettunen, J., Veijola, J., Karvonen, J. T., Laksy, K., et al. (2006). Obesity and depression: Results from the longitudinal Northern Finland 1966 Birth Cohort Study. *International Journal of Obesity (London), 30,* 520–527.

Herva, A., Rasanen, P., Miettunen, J., Timonen, M., Laksy, K., Veijola, J., et al. (2006). Co-occurrence of metabolic syndrome with depression and anxiety in young adults: The Northern Finland 1966 Birth Cohort Study. *Psychosomatic Medicine, 68,* 213–216.

Hutton, H. E., Lyketsos, C. G., Zenilman, J. M., Thompson, R. E., & Erbelding, E. J. (2004). Depression and HIV risk behaviors among patients in a sexually transmitted disease clinic. *American Journal of Psychiatry, 161,* 912–914.

Ickovics, J. R., Hamburger, M. E., Vlahov, D., Schoenbaum, E. E., Schuman, P., Boland, R. J., et al. (2001). Mortality, CD4 cell count decline, and depressive symptoms among HIV-seropositive women: Longitudinal analysis from the HIV Epidemiology Research Study. *Journal of the American Medical Association, 285,* 1466–1474.

Iosifescu, D. V., Clementi-Craven, N., Fraguas, R., Papakostas, G. I., Petersen, T., Alpert, J. E., et al. (2005). Cardiovascular risk factors may moderate pharmacological treatment effects in major depressive disorder. *Psychosomatic Medicine, 67,* 703–706.

Iosifescu, D. V., Nierenberg, A. A., Alpert, J. E., Smith, M., Bitran, S., Dording, C., et al. (2003). The impact of medical comorbidity on acute treatment in major depressive disorder. *American Journal of Psychiatry, 160,* 2122–2127.

Irvine, J., Basinski, A., Baker, B., Jandciu, S., Paquette, M., Cairns, J., et al. (1999). Depression and risk of sudden cardiac death after acute myocardial infarction: Testing for the confounding effects of fatigue. *Psychosomatic Medicine, 61,* 729–737.

Jiang, W., Alexander, J., Christopher, E., Kuchibhatla, M., Gaulden, L. H., Cuffe, M. S., et al. (2001). Relationship of depression to increased risk of mortality and rehospitalization in patients with congestive heart failure. *Archives of Internal Medicine, 161,* 1849–1856.

Jiang, W., Kuchibhatla, M., Clary, G. L., Cuffe, M. S., Christopher, E. J., Alexander, J. D., et al. (2007). Relationship between depressive symptoms and long-term mortality in patients with heart failure. *American Heart Journal, 154,* 102–108.

Johnston, E., Johnson, S., McLeod, P., & Johnston, M. (2004). The relation of body mass index to depressive symptoms. *Canaian Journal of Public Health, 95,* 179–183.

Jorge, R. E., Robinson, R. G., Arndt, S., & Starkstein, S. (2003). Mortality and poststroke depression: A placebo-controlled trial of antidepressants. *American Journal of Psychiatry, 160,* 1823–1829.

Katon, W., Sullivan, M., & Walker, E. (2001). Medical symptoms without identified pathology: Relationship to psychiatric disorders, childhood and adult trauma, and personality traits. *Annals of Internal Medicine, 134,* 917–925.

Katon, W. J., Von, K. M., Lin, E. H., Simon, G., Ludman, E., Russo, J., et al. (2004). The Pathways Study: A randomized trial of collaborative care in patients with diabetes and depression. *Archives of General Psychiatry, 61,* 1042–1049.

Kaufmann, P. G. (2003). Depression in cardiovascular disease: Can the risk be reduced? *Biological Psychiatry, 54,* 187–190.

Keitner, G. I., Posternak, M. A., & Ryan, C. E. (2003). How many subjects with major depressive disorder meet eligibility requirements of an antidepressant efficacy trial? *Journal of Clinical Psychiatry, 64,* 1091–1093.

Kessler, R. C., Berglund, P., Demler, O., Jin, R., Koretz, D., Merikangas, K. R., et al. (2003). The epidemiology of major depressive disorder: Results from the National Comorbidity Survey Replication (NCS-R). *Journal of the American Medical Association, 289,* 3095–3105.

Kinder, L. S., Carnethon, M. R., Palaniappan, L. P., King, A. C., & Fortmann, S. P. (2004). Depression and the metabolic syndrome in young adults: Findings from the Third National Health and Nutrition Examination Survey. *Psychosomatic Medicine, 66,* 316–322.

Kinder, L. S., Katon, W. J., Ludman, E., Russo, J., Simon, G., Lin, E. H., et al. (2006). Improving depression care in patients with diabetes and multiple complications. *Journal of General Internal Medicine, 21,* 1036–1041.

Knol, M. J., Twisk, J. W., Beekman, A. T., Heine, R. J., Snoek, F. J., & Pouwer, F. (2006). Depression as a risk factor for the onset of type 2 diabetes mellitus: A meta-analysis. *Diabetologia, 49,* 837–845.

Koenig, H. G., George, L. K., Peterson, B. L., & Pieper, C. F. (1997). Depression in medically ill hospitalized older adults: Prevalence, characteristics, and course of symptoms according to six diagnostic schemes. *American Journal of Psychiatry, 154,* 1376–1383.

Kolakowska, T., & Swigar, M. E. (1977). Thyroid function in depression and alcohol abuse: A retrospective study. *Archives of General Psychiatry, 34,* 984–988.

Kraemer, H. C. (1995). Statistical issues in assessing comorbidity. *Statistics in Medicine, 14,* 721–733.

Krishnan, K. R., Hays, J. C., & Blazer, D. G. (1997). MRI-defined vascular depression. *American Journal of Psychiatry, 154,* 497–501.

Lahiri, K., Rettig-Ewen, V., Bohm, M., & Laufs, U. (2007). Perceived psychosocial stress and cardiovascular risk factors in obese and non-obese patients. *Clinical Research on Cardiology, 96,* 365–374.

Leserman, J., Petitto, J. M., Perkins, D. O., Folds, J. D., Golden, R. N., & Evans, D. L. (1997). Severe stress, depressive symptoms, and changes in lymphocyte subsets in human immunodeficiency virus-infected men: A 2-year follow-up study. *Archives of General Psychiatry, 54,* 279–285.

Lespérance, F., Frasure-Smith, N., Koszycki, D., Laliberte, M. A., van Zyl, L. T., Baker, B., et al. (2007). Effects of citalopram and interpersonal psychotherapy on depression in patients with coronary artery disease: The Canadian Cardiac Randomized Evaluation of Antidepressant and Psychotherapy Efficacy (CREATE) trial. *Journal of the American Medical Association, 297*, 367–379.

Lespérance, F., Frasure-Smith, N., Laliberte, M. A., White, M., Lafontaine, S., Calderone, A., et al. (2003). An open-label study of nefazodone treatment of major depression in patients with congestive heart failure. *Canadian Journal of Psychiatry, 48*, 695–701.

Lespérance, F., Frasure-Smith, N., Theroux, P., & Irwin, M. (2004). The association between major depression and levels of soluble intercellular adhesion molecule 1, interleukin-6, and C-reactive protein in patients with recent acute coronary syndromes. *American Journal of Psychiatry, 161*, 271–277.

Libby, P., Ridker, P. M., & Maseri, A. (2002). Inflammation and atherosclerosis. *Circulation, 105*, 1135–1143.

Lin, E. H., Katon, W., Rutter, C., Simon, G. E., Ludman, E. J., Von, K. M., et al. (2006). Effects of enhanced depression treatment on diabetes self-care. *Annals of Family Medicine, 4*, 46–53.

Linn, B. S., Linn, M. W., & Gurel, L. (1968). Cumulative illness rating scale. *Journal of the American Geriatrics Society, 16*, 622–626.

Lipsey, J. R., Robinson, R. G., Pearlson, G. D., Rao, K., & Price, T. R. (1984). Nortriptyline treatment of post-stroke depression: A double-blind study. *Lancet, 1*, 297–300.

Lustman, P. J., Anderson, R. J., Freedland, K. E., de Groot, M., Carney, R. M., & Clouse, R. E. (2000). Depression and poor glycemic control: A meta-analytic review of the literature. *Diabetes Care, 23*, 934–942.

Lustman, P. J., & Clouse, R. E. (2002). Treatment of depression in diabetes: Impact on mood and medical outcome. *Journal of Psychosomatic Research, 53*, 917–924.

Lustman, P. J., Clouse, R. E., Griffith, L. S., Carney, R. M., & Freedland, K. E. (1997). Screening for depression in diabetes using the Beck Depression Inventory. *Psychosomatic Medicine, 59*, 24–31.

Lustman, P. J., Clouse, R. E., Nix, B. D., Freedland, K. E., Rubin, E. H., McGill, J. B., et al. (2006). Sertraline for prevention of depression recurrence in diabetes mellitus: A randomized, double-blind, placebo-controlled trial. *Archives of General Psychiatry, 63*, 521–529.

Lustman, P. J., Freedland, K. E., Carney, R. M., Hong, B. A., & Clouse, R. E. (1992). Similarity of depression in diabetic and psychiatric patients. *Psychosomatic Medicine, 54*, 602–611.

Lustman, P. J., Freedland, K. E., Griffith, L. S., & Clouse, R. E. (1998). Predicting response to cognitive behavior therapy of depression in type 2 diabetes. *General Hospital Psychiatry, 20*, 302–306.

Lustman, P. J., Freedland, K. E., Griffith, L. S., & Clouse, R. E. (2000). Fluoxetine for depression in diabetes: A randomized double-blind placebo-controlled trial. *Diabetes Care, 23*, 618–623.

Lustman, P. J., Griffith, L. S., Freedland, K. E., Kissel, S. S., & Clouse, R. E. (1998). Cognitive behavior therapy for depression in type 2 diabetes mellitus: A randomized, controlled trial. *Annals of Internal Medicine, 129*, 613–621.

Lyketsos, C. G., Hoover, D. R., Guccione, M., Dew, M. A., Wesch, J. E., Bing, E. G., et al. (1996). Changes in depressive symptoms as AIDS develops: The Multicenter AIDS Cohort Study. *American Journal of Psychiatry, 153*, 1430–1437.

Macchia, A., Levantesi, G., Borrelli, G., Franzosi, M. G., Maggioni, A. P., Marfisi, R., et al. (2006). A clinically practicable diagnostic score for metabolic syndrome improves its predictivity of diabetes mellitus: The Gruppo Italiano per lo Studio della Sopravvivenza nell'Infarto Miocardico (GISSI)-Prevenzione Scoring. *American Heart Journal, 151*, 754.

Manne, S. L., & Andrykowski, M. A. (2006). Are psychological interventions effective and accepted by cancer patients?: II. Using empirically supported therapy guidelines to decide. *Annals of Behavioral Medicine, 32*, 98–103.

Markowitz, J. C., Kocsis, J. H., Fishman, B., Spielman, L. A., Jacobsberg, L. B., Frances, A. J., et al. (1998). Treatment of depressive symptoms in human immunodeficiency virus–positive patients. *Archives of General Psychiatry, 55*, 452–457.

McCaffery, J. M., Frasure-Smith, N., Dube, M. P., Theroux, P., Rouleau, G. A., Duan, Q., et al. (2006). Common genetic vulnerability to depressive symptoms and coronary artery disease: A review and development of candidate genes related to inflammation and serotonin. *Psychosomatic Medicine, 68*, 187–200.

McCaffery, J. M., Niaura, R., Todaro, J. F., Swan, G. E., & Carmelli, D. (2003). Depressive symptoms and metabolic risk in adult male twins enrolled in the National Heart, Lung, and Blood Institute twin study. *Psychosomatic Medicine, 65,* 490–497.

McIntyre, R. S., Konarski, J. Z., Wilkins, K., Soczynska, J. K., & Kennedy, S. H. (2006). Obesity in bipolar disorder and major depressive disorder: Results from a national community health survey on mental health and well-being. *Canadian Journal of Psychiatry, 51,* 274–280.

Miller, G. E., Freedland, K. E., & Carney, R. M. (2005). Depressive symptoms and the regulation of proinflammatory cytokine expression in patients with coronary heart disease. *Journal of Psychosomatic Research, 59,* 231–236.

Miller, G. E., Freedland, K. E., Duntley, S., & Carney, R. M. (2005). Relation of depressive symptoms to C-reactive protein and pathogen burden (cytomegalovirus, herpes simplex virus, Epstein–Barr virus) in patients with earlier acute coronary syndromes. *American Journal of Cardiology, 95,* 317–321.

Miller, G. E., Stetler, C. A., Carney, R. M., Freedland, K. E., & Banks, W. A. (2002). Clinical depression and inflammatory risk markers for coronary heart disease. *American Journal of Cardiology, 90,* 1279–1283.

Morris, P. L., Robinson, R. G., de Carvalho, M. L., Albert, P., Wells, J. C., Samuels, J. F., et al. (1996). Lesion characteristics and depressed mood in the Stroke Data Bank Study. *Journal of Neuropsychiatry and Clinical Neurosciences, 8,* 153–159.

Morrison, M. F., Petitto, J. M., Ten Have, T., Gettes, D. R., Chiappini, M. S., Weber, A. L., et al. (2002). Depressive and anxiety disorders in women with HIV infection. *American Journal of Psychiatry, 159,* 789–796.

Murphy, J. M., Monson, R. R., Olivier, D. C., Zahner, G. E., Sobol, A. M., & Leighton, A. H. (1992). Relations over time between psychiatric and somatic disorders: The Stirling County Study. *American Journal of Epidemiology, 136,* 95–105.

Musselman, D. L., Lawson, D. H., Gumnick, J. F., Manatunga, A. K., Penna, S., Goodkin, R. S., et al. (2001). Paroxetine for the prevention of depression induced by high-dose interferon alfa. *New England Journal of Medicine, 344,* 961–966.

Mykletun, A., Bjerkeset, O., Dewey, M., Prince, M., Overland, S., & Stewart, R. (2007). Anxiety, depression, and cause-specific mortality: The HUNT study. *Psychosomatic Medicine, 69,* 323–331.

Narushima, K., Kosier, J. T., & Robinson, R. G. (2003). A reappraisal of poststroke depression, intra- and inter-hemispheric lesion location using meta-analysis. *Journal of Neuropsychiatry and Clinical Neurosciences, 15,* 422–430.

Narushima, K., Paradiso, S., Moser, D. J., Jorge, R., & Robinson, R. G. (2007). Effect of antidepressant therapy on executive function after stroke. *British Journal of Psychiatry, 190,* 260–265.

Nemeroff, C. B., Preskorn, S. H., & Devane, C. L. (2007). Antidepressant drug–drug interactions: Clinical relevance and risk management. *CNS Spectrums, 12,* 1–13.

Nicholson, A., Kuper, H., & Hemingway, H. (2006). Depression as an aetiologic and prognostic factor in coronary heart disease: A meta-analysis of 6,362 events among 146,538 participants in 54 observational studies. *European Heart Journal, 27,* 2763–2774.

Novick, J. S., Stewart, J. W., Wisniewski, S. R., Cook, I. A., Manev, R., Nierenberg, A. A., et al. (2005). Clinical and demographic features of atypical depression in outpatients with major depressive disorder: Preliminary findings from STAR*D. *Journal of Clinical Psychiatry, 66,* 1002–1011.

Onyike, C. U., Crum, R. M., Lee, H. B., Lyketsos, C. G., & Eaton, W. W. (2003). Is obesity associated with major depression?: Results from the Third National Health and Nutrition Examination Survey. *American Journal of Epidemiology, 158,* 1139–1147.

Ormel, J., Von, K. M., Burger, H., Scott, K., Demyttenaere, K., Huang, Y. Q., et al. (2007). Mental disorders among persons with heart disease: Results from World Mental Health surveys. *General Hospital Psychiatry, 29,* 325–334.

Otte, C., McCaffery, J., Ali, S., & Whooley, M. A. (2007). Association of a serotonin transporter polymorphism (5-HTTLPR) with depression, perceived stress, and norepinephrine in patients with coronary disease: The Heart and Soul Study. *American Journal of Psychiatry, 164,* 1379–1384.

Ownby, R. L., Crocco, E., Acevedo, A., John, V., & Loewenstein, D. (2006). Depression and risk for Alzheimer disease: Systematic review, meta-analysis, and metaregression analysis. *Archives of General Psychiatry, 63*, 530–538.

Parikh, R. M., Lipsey, J. R., Robinson, R. G., & Price, T. R. (1988). A two year longitudinal study of poststroke mood disorders: Prognostic factors related to one and two year outcome. *International Journal of Psychiatry in Medicine, 18*, 45–56.

Patil, S. P., Schneider, H., Schwartz, A. R., & Smith, P. L. (2007). Adult obstructive sleep apnea: Pathophysiology and diagnosis. *Chest, 132*, 325–337.

Patten, S. B. (2001). Long-term medical conditions and major depression in a Canadian population study at Waves 1 and 2. *Journal of Affective Disorders, 63*, 35–41.

Patten, S. B., Beck, C. A., Kassam, A., Williams, J. V., Barbui, C., & Metz, L. M. (2005). Long-term medical conditions and major depression: Strength of association for specific conditions in the general population. *Canadian Journal of Psychiatry, 50*, 195–202.

Persky, V. W., Kempthorne-Rawson, J., & Shekelle, R. B. (1987). Personality and risk of cancer: 20-year follow-up of the Western Electric Study. *Psychosomatic Medicine, 49*, 435–449.

Pine, D. S., Goldstein, R. B., Wolk, S., & Weissman, M. M. (2001). The association between childhood depression and adulthood body mass index. *Pediatrics, 107*, 1049–1056.

Polsky, D., Doshi, J. A., Marcus, S., Oslin, D., Rothbard, A., Thomas, N., et al. (2005). Long-term risk for depressive symptoms after a medical diagnosis. *Archives of Internal Medicine, 165*, 1260–1266.

Powell, L. H., Catellier, D., Freedland, K. E., Burg, M. M., Woods, S. L., Bittner, V., et al. (2005). Depression and heart failure in patients with a new myocardial infarction. *American Heart Journal, 149*, 851–855.

Prieto, J. M., Atala, J., Blanch, J., Carreras, E., Rovira, M., Cirera, E., et al. (2005). Role of depression as a predictor of mortality among cancer patients after stem-cell transplantation. *Journal of Clinical Oncology, 23*, 6063–6071.

Rabkin, J. G., Goetz, R. R., Remien, R. H., Williams, J. B., Todak, G., & Gorman, J. M. (1997). Stability of mood despite HIV illness progression in a group of homosexual men. *American Journal of Psychiatry, 154*, 231–238.

Rabkin, J. G., McElhiney, M. C., Rabkin, R., McGrath, P. J., & Ferrando, S. J. (2006). Placebo-controlled trial of dehydroepiandrosterone (DHEA) for treatment of nonmajor depression in patients with HIV/AIDS. *American Journal of Psychiatry, 163*, 59–66.

Rabkin, J. G., Wagner, G. J., & Rabkin, R. (1999). Fluoxetine treatment for depression in patients with HIV and AIDS: A randomized, placebo-controlled trial. *American Journal of Psychiatry, 156*, 101–107.

Raikkonen, K., Matthews, K. A., & Kuller, L. H. (2007). Depressive symptoms and stressful life events predict metabolic syndrome among middle-aged women: A comparison of World Health Organization, Adult Treatment Panel III, and International Diabetes Foundation definitions. *Diabetes Care, 30*, 872–877.

Ranjit, N., Diez-Roux, A. V., Shea, S., Cushman, M., Seeman, T., Jackson, S. A., et al. (2007). Psychosocial factors and inflammation in the multi-ethnic study of atherosclerosis. *Archives of Internal Medicine, 167*, 174–181.

Richardson, L. P., Davis, R., Poulton, R., McCauley, E., Moffitt, T. E., Caspi, A., et al. (2003). A longitudinal evaluation of adolescent depression and adult obesity. *Archives of Pediatrics and Adolescent Medicine, 157*, 739–745.

Roberts, R. E., Kaplan, G. A., Shema, S. J., & Strawbridge, W. J. (1997). Does growing old increase the risk for depression? *American Journal of Psychiatry, 154*, 1384–1390.

Robins, L. N., Helzer, J. E., Croughan, J., & Ratcliff, K. S. (1981). National Institute of Mental Health Diagnostic Interview Schedule: Its history, characteristics, and validity. *Archives of General Psychiatry, 38*, 381–389.

Robinson, R. G. (2003). Poststroke depression: Prevalence, diagnosis, treatment, and disease progression. *Biological Psychiatry, 54*, 376–387.

Robinson, R. G., Schultz, S. K., Castillo, C., Kopel, T., Kosier, J. T., Newman, R. M., et al. (2000). Nortriptyline versus fluoxetine in the treatment of depression and in short-term recovery after stroke: A placebo-controlled, double-blind study. *American Journal of Psychiatry, 157*, 351–359.

Roose, S. P., & Miyazaki, M. (2005). Pharmacologic treatment of depression in patients with heart disease. *Psychosomatic Medicine, 67*(Suppl. 1), S54–S57.

Rosengren, A., Hawken, S., Ounpuu, S., Sliwa, K., Zubaid, M., Almahmeed, W. A., et al. (2004). Association of psychosocial risk factors with risk of acute myocardial infarction in 11,119 cases and 13,648 controls from 52 countries (the INTERHEART study): Case–control study. *Lancet, 364,* 953–962.

Salaycik, K. J., Kelly-Hayes, M., Beiser, A., Nguyen, A. H., Brady, S. M., Kase, C. S., et al. (2007). Depressive symptoms and risk of stroke: The Framingham Study. *Stroke, 38,* 16–21.

Schins, A., Tulner, D., Lousberg, R., Kenis, G., Delanghe, J., Crijns, H. J., et al. (2005). Inflammatory markers in depressed post-myocardial infarction patients. *Journal of Psychiatric Research, 39,* 137–144.

Scott, K. M., Bruffaerts, R., Simon, G. E., Alonso, J., Angermeyer, M., de Girolamo, G., et al. (2008). Obesity and mental disorders in the general population: Results from the World Mental Health surveys. *International Journal of Obesity (London), 32,* 192–200.

Serebruany, V. L., Glassman, A. H., Malinin, A. I., Nemeroff, C. B., Musselman, D. L., van Zyl, L. T., et al. (2003). Platelet/endothelial biomarkers in depressed patients treated with the selective serotonin reuptake inhibitor sertraline after acute coronary events: The Sertraline Antidepressant Heart Attack Randomized Trial (SADHART) Platelet Substudy. *Circulation, 108,* 939–944.

Sharafkhaneh, A., Giray, N., Richardson, P., Young, T., & Hirshkowitz, M. (2005). Association of psychiatric disorders and sleep apnea in a large cohort. *Sleep, 28,* 1405–1411.

Sheps, D. S., Freedland, K. E., Golden, R. N., & McMahon, R. P. (2003). ENRICHD and SADHART: Implications for future biobehavioral intervention efforts. *Psychosomatic Medicine, 65,* 1–2.

Sherwood, A., Blumenthal, J. A., Trivedi, R., Johnson, K. S., O'Connor, C. M., Adams, K. F., Jr., et al. (2007). Relationship of depression to death or hospitalization in patients with heart failure. *Archives of Internal Medicine, 167,* 367–373.

Simon, G. E., Katon, W. J., Lin, E. H., Rutter, C., Manning, W. G., Von, K. M., et al. (2007). Cost-effectiveness of systematic depression treatment among people with diabetes mellitus. *Archives of General Psychiatry, 64,* 65–72.

Simon, G. E., & Von Korff, M. (2006). Medical co-morbidity and validity of DSM-IV depression criteria. *Psychological Medicine, 36,* 27–36.

Simon, G. E., Von Korff, M., Saunders, K., Miglioretti, D. L., Crane, P. K., Van Belle, G., et al. (2006). Association between obesity and psychiatric disorders in the U.S. adult population. *Archives of General Psychiatry, 63,* 824–830.

Skala, J. A., Freedland, K. E., & Carney, R. M. (2005). *Heart disease.* Toronto: Hogrefe & Huber.

Skala, J. A., Freedland, K. E., & Carney, R. M. (2006). Coronary heart disease and depression: A review of recent mechanistic research. *Canadian Journal of Psychiatry, 51,* 738–745.

Spalletta, G., Bossu, P., Ciaramella, A., Bria, P., Caltagirone, C., & Robinson, R. G. (2006). The etiology of poststroke depression: A review of the literature and a new hypothesis involving inflammatory cytokines. *Molecular Psychiatry, 11,* 984–991.

Spiegel, D., & Giese-Davis, J. (2003). Depression and cancer: Mechanisms and disease progression. *Biological Psychiatry, 54,* 269–282.

Spiegel, D., Sands, S., & Koopman, C. (1994). Pain and depression in patients with cancer. *Cancer, 74,* 2570–2578.

Starkstein, S. E., Robinson, R. G., Berthier, M. L., & Price, T. R. (1988). Depressive disorders following posterior circulation as compared with middle cerebral artery infarcts. *Brain, 111*(2), 375–387.

Stein, M. D., Solomon, D. A., Herman, D. S., Anderson, B. J., & Miller, I. (2003). Depression severity and drug injection HIV risk behaviors. *American Journal of Psychiatry, 160,* 1659–1662.

Stommel, M., Given, B. A., & Given, C. W. (2002). Depression and functional status as predictors of death among cancer patients. *Cancer, 94,* 2719–2727.

Strik, J. J., Honig, A., Lousberg, R., & Denollet, J. (2001). Sensitivity and specificity of observer and self-report questionnaires in major and minor depression following myocardial infarction. *Psychosomatics, 42,* 423–428.

Thavendiranathan, P., Bagai, A., Brookhart, M. A., & Choudhry, N. K. (2006). Primary prevention of cardiovascular diseases with statin therapy: A meta-analysis of randomized controlled trials. *Archives of Internal Medicine, 166,* 2307–2313.

Thombs, B. D., Magyar-Russell, G., Bass, E. B., Stewart, K. J., Tsilidis, K. K., Bush, D. E., et al. (2007). Performance characteristics of depression screening instruments in survivors of acute myocardial infarction: Review of the evidence. *Psychosomatics, 48,* 185–194.

Uchitomi, Y., Kugaya, A., Akechi, T., Nakano, T., Wenner, M., Okamura, H., et al. (2001). Three sets of diagnostic criteria for major depression and correlations with serotonin-induced platelet calcium mobilization in cancer patients. *Psychopharmacology (Berlin), 153,* 244–248.

Unutzer, J., Katon, W., Callahan, C. M., Williams, J. W., Jr., Hunkeler, E., Harpole, L., et al. (2002). Collaborative care management of late-life depression in the primary care setting: A randomized controlled trial. *Journal of the American Medical Association, 288,* 2836–2845.

van den Akker, M., Buntinx, F., Metsemakers, J. F., Roos, S., & Knottnerus, J. A. (1998). Multimorbidity in general practice: Prevalence, incidence, and determinants of co-occurring chronic and recurrent diseases. *Journal of Clinical Epidemiology, 51,* 367–375.

van Melle, J. P., de Jonge, P., Honig, A., Schene, A. H., Kuyper, A. M., Crijns, H. J., et al. (2007). Effects of antidepressant treatment following myocardial infarction. *British Journal of Psychiatry, 190,* 460–466.

van Melle, J. P., de Jonge, P., Spijkerman, T. A., Tijssen, J. G., Ormel, J., van Veldhuisen, D. J., et al. (2004). Prognostic association of depression following myocardial infarction with mortality and cardiovascular events: A meta-analysis. *Psychosomatic Medicine, 66,* 814–822.

van Melle, J. P., Verbeek, D. E., van den Berg, M. P., Ormel, J., van der Linde, M. R., & de Jonge, P. (2006). Beta-blockers and depression after myocardial infarction: A multicenter prospective study. *Journal of the American College of Cardiology, 48,* 2209–2214.

Veith, R. C., Lewis, N., Linares, O. A., Barnes, R. F., Raskind, M. A., Villacres, E. C., et al. (1994). Sympathetic nervous system activity in major depression: Basal and desipramine-induced alterations in plasma norepinephrine kinetics. *Archives of General Psychiatry, 51,* 411–422.

Vogelzangs, N., Suthers, K., Ferrucci, L., Simonsick, E. M., Ble, A., Schrager, M., et al. (2007). Hypercortisolemic depression is associated with the metabolic syndrome in late-life. *Psychoneuroendocrinology, 32,* 151–159.

Watson, M., Haviland, J. S., Greer, S., Davidson, J., & Bliss, J. M. (1999). Influence of psychological response on survival in breast cancer: A population-based cohort study. *Lancet, 354,* 1331–1336.

Wells, K. B., Stewart, A., Hays, R. D., Burnam, M. A., Rogers, W., Daniels, M., et al. (1989). The functioning and well-being of depressed patients: Results from the Medical Outcomes Study. *Journal of the American Medical Association, 262,* 914–919.

Wells, R. D., Day, R. C., Carney, R. M., Freedland, K. E., & Duntley, S. P. (2004). Depression predicts self-reported sleep quality in patients with obstructive sleep apnea. *Psychosomatic Medicine, 66,* 692–697.

Wells, R. D., Freedland, K. E., Carney, R. M., Duntley, S. P., & Stepanski, E. J. (2007). Adherence, reports of benefits, and depression among patients treated with continuous positive airway pressure. *Psychosomatic Medicine, 69,* 449–454.

Williams, J. W., Jr., Katon, W., Lin, E. H., Noel, P. H., Worchel, J., Cornell, J., et al. (2004). The effectiveness of depression care management on diabetes-related outcomes in older patients. *Annals of Internal Medicine, 140,* 1015–1024.

Williams, S. A., Kasl, S. V., Heiat, A., Abramson, J. L., Krumholz, H. M., & Vaccarino, V. (2002). Depression and risk of heart failure among the elderly: A prospective community-based study. *Psychosomatic Medicine, 64,* 6–12.

Winokur, A., Maislin, G., Phillips, J. L., & Amsterdam, J. D. (1988). Insulin resistance after oral glucose tolerance testing in patients with major depression. *American Journal of Psychiatry, 145,* 325–330.

Wulsin, L. R., Evans, J. C., Vasan, R. S., Murabito, J. M., Kelly-Hayes, M., & Benjamin, E. J. (2005). Depressive symptoms, coronary heart disease, and overall mortality in the Framingham Heart Study. *Psychosomatic Medicine, 67,* 697–702.

Wulsin, L. R., & Singal, B. M. (2003). Do depressive symptoms increase the risk for the onset of coronary disease?: A systematic quantitative review. *Psychosomatic Medicine, 65,* 201–210.

Zigmond, A. S., & Snaith, R. P. (1983). The hospital Anxiety and Depression Scale. *Acta Psychiatrica Scandinavica, 67,* 361–370.

Zonderman, A. B., Costa, P. T., Jr., & McCrae, R. R. (1989). Depression as a risk for cancer morbidity and mortality in a nationally representative sample. *Journal of the American Medical Association, 262,* 1191–1195.

Zubenko, G. S., Zubenko, W. N., McPherson, S., Spoor, E., Marin, D. B., Farlow, M. R., et al. (2003). A collaborative study of the emergence and clinical features of the major depressive syndrome of Alzheimer's disease. *American Journal of Psychiatry, 160,* 857–866.

CHAPTER 7

Bipolar and Unipolar Depression

A Comparison of Clinical Phenomenology, Biological Vulnerability, and Psychosocial Predictors

Sheri L. Johnson, Amy K. Cuellar, *and* Christopher Miller

Although clinical lore and the very name of the disorder suggest that bipolar disorder necessarily involves depression, this is not the case. Rather, the diagnosis of bipolar I disorder is based on a single lifetime manic or mixed episode and does not require an episode of depression (American Psychiatric Association, 1994). In nontreatment samples, as many as 20–33% of individuals with bipolar disorder report no lifetime episode of major depression (cf. Karkowski & Kendler, 1997; Kessler, Rubinow, Holmes, Abelson, & Zhao, 1997). Despite the evidence that many people with mania report no history of major depressive episodes, some of these cases may be diagnosed inaccurately or might develop depression over time. Indeed, in one 20-year follow-up study of those initially diagnosed with unipolar mania, 20 of 27 people did develop depressive episodes (Solomon et al., 2003). Nonetheless, even with this extensive follow-up, some people continued to display unipolar mania. Moreover, analyses of epidemiological data suggest that the absence of depression is not related to the duration of illness (Kessler et al., 1997). Rather, it appears that some people with bipolar disorder do not experience depressive episodes.

Even among the people with bipolar disorder who do experience depressive episodes, there is dramatic variability in the expression of depression. For some, though, depressive symptoms can be quite chronic and severe. In a naturalistic National Institute of Mental Health study of 146 patients with bipolar I disorder, followed for an average of 12.8 years, subsyndromal symptoms of depression or dysthymia were present for almost 25% of the time, and major depressive episodes were present for 9% of weeks (Judd et al., 2002). Depressive symptoms can also cause serious impairment and are more likely than manic symptoms to trigger help seeking (Calabrese, Hirschfeld, Frye, & Reed, 2004). Understanding the nature of bipolar depression, then, is important.

Because depression occurs in both bipolar and unipolar mood disorders, an obvious question is whether these depressions are similar or different. This chapter presents research on clinical features, neurobiology, and psychosocial triggers for depressive episodes. Throughout, we focus on whether unipolar and bipolar depressions share similar mechanisms in the genesis of episodes.

In considering these questions, we note that many studies of bipolar disorder fail to differentiate between mania and depression. Because the predictors of depression and mania within bipolar disorder may differ (Johnson, Winters, & Meyer, 2006), we focus only on studies that have disentangled depression and mania.

Most of the studies covered have focused on bipolar I disorder. DSM-IV includes criteria for other forms of disorder, including bipolar II disorder, defined on the basis of *hypomania* (a milder form of mania), as well as *cyclothymia*, defined on the basis of recurrent mood changes (both upward and downward) that do not meet full criteria for manic or depressive episodes. Although it is believed that bipolar II disorder and cyclothymia are more common than bipolar I disorder (Merikangas et al., 2007), they have been less of a research focus. Perhaps most importantly, the interrater reliability of the most commonly used diagnostic instruments is poor for hypomania and milder symptoms of mania (Johnson, Eisner, & Miller, 2008). Hence, unless noted otherwise, we focus on bipolar I disorder.

COURSE OF THE DISORDER

In this section, we examine studies that have compared bipolar and unipolar depression on different course parameters, such as age of onset, duration, episode frequency, and severity (see Table 7.1 for included studies and their methods). To ensure comparability of studies, we set certain minimal criteria for inclusion in the review. The decision to include a particular study was based on (1) whether the investigators compared bipolar and unipolar depression directly rather than comparing the disorders without regard to episode polarity, (2) a focus on bipolar I disorder rather than bipolar spectrum disorders, (3) adequate sample size (at least 70 participants) for statistical power, and (4) use of a semistructured diagnostic interview. Before beginning, it is worth noting that two designs have been common within these studies. Most studies have compared the previous course of disorder among people with current major depressive disorder and those with bipolar depression. Beyond these retrospective studies, a growing number of researchers have recruited persons during episodes of major depressive disorder, then followed participants longitudinally, typically using the Longitudinal Interval Follow-Up Examination (LIFE) interview to determine whether course parameters predict who develops a first episode of mania.

In reviewing studies of the course of disorder that met our criteria, one of the most consistent findings is that age of onset is earlier in bipolar depression than in unipolar depression. Earlier age of onset has been reported in retrospective reports of currently diagnosed bipolar disorder and major depressive disorder (Endicott et al., 1985; Winokur, Coryell, Endicott, & Akiskal, 1993; Wozniak et al., 2004). Prospective studies also have consistently identified earlier age of onset of major depressive episodes as a key risk factor for a switch to bipolar disorder (Akiskal et al., 1983; Geller, Zimerman, Williams, Bolhofner, & Craney, 2001; Othmer et al., 2007).

Beyond age of depression onset, researchers have focused on comparing the duration of depressive episodes between bipolar and unipolar disorder. In general, current research appears to support a view of the duration of bipolar depression as shorter than that of unipolar

TABLE 7.1. Comparisons of Course of Depression between Bipolar Disorder and Major Depressive Disorder

Author (year)	n	Sample
		Retrospective/current designs
Chengappa et al. (2003)	1,218	Stanley Center Bipolar Registry
Goel et al. (2002)	165	Parents with seasonal affective disorder
Endicott et al. (1985)	226	Inpatients and outpatients
Perlis et al. (2006)	1,551	Nonpsychotic outpatients
Serretti et al. (2002)	1,832	Inpatient
Smith et al. (2005)	87	Outpatient university students
Wozniak et al. (2004)	280	Childhood depression with comorbid ADHD
		Prospective designs
Akiskal et al. (1995)	559	NIMH Collaborative Study participants (79.7% inpatient, unipolar depression)
Akiskal et al. (1983)	203	Outpatients with unipolar depression
Coryell et al. (1987)	372	Inpatients and outpatients with primary major depressive disorder
Coryell et al. (1989)	559	Inpatients and outpatients
Furukawa et al. (2000)	116	Inpatients and outpatients
Geller et al. (2001)	100	Prepubertally depressed children
Winokur, Coryell, et al. (1993)	320	Inpatients

major depression in three (Akiskal et al., 1983; Coryell et al., 1989; Furukawa et al., 2000) out of four studies (for an exception, see Coryell, Andreasen, Endicott, & Keller, 1987).

Do unipolar and bipolar depression episodes differ in severity? Two retrospective studies have suggested greater severity of depression in bipolar disorder compared to unipolar disorder (Goel, Terman, & Terman, 2002; Wozniak et al., 2004). Congruently, one prospective study found that more severe depressive episodes predicted greater likelihood of a manic onset (Akiskal et al., 1995). Nevertheless, one study of undergraduate students found no significant difference in severity between bipolar disorder and major depressive disorder (Smith, Harrison, Muir, & Blackwood, 2005). One might assume, however, that undergraduate samples do not provide a representative sample of bipolar disorder in the community. To date, then, the three strongest of four studies suggest that bipolar disorder is related to more severe depressive episodes.

Finally, it is less clear whether bipolar and unipolar depression differ on number of depressive episodes. Two studies have examined whether people who have more depressive episodes are likely to develop manic episodes. The findings of one prospective study with 320 persons suggested that number of previous episodes did not predict manic onset (Winokur, Coryell, Keller, Endicott, & Akiskal, 1993), whereas findings of a study of 1,551 persons suggested that people with more depressive episodes are at increased risk of developing mania (Perlis, Brown, Baker, & Nierenberg, 2006). Hence, it is not clear at this point whether more frequent episodes indicate risk for mania.

In summary, across cross-sectional and longitudinal research, bipolar disorder appears to be differentiated from unipolar depression by a younger age of depressive onset, shorter depressive episodes, and more severe depressive episodes. Findings on the frequency of depressive episodes are not consistent. Some of the cross-study inconsistencies in findings might reflect methodological issues. For example, differences between bipolar and unipolar disorder might be so small as to require substantial sample sizes. As noted earlier, differences in the frequency of depressive episodes were documented only in a study of over 1,500 persons.

Beyond sample size, other methodological issues are pervasive in the literature comparing the course of bipolar and unipolar disorder. Many studies have failed to attend to confounds, such as medication regimens. In addition, developmental cohort differences might account for discrepant findings. For example, prepubertal onset of bipolar disorder was found to be significantly more common in a cohort born after 1940 compared to one born before 1940 (Chengappa et al., 2003). Although the best available cross-sectional and longitudinal research suggests that bipolar disorder is characterized by course parameters such as early age of onset, shorter duration of episodes, and greater severity, these methodological limitations make our conclusions tentative. More definitive studies are needed to address these limitations in the literature.

SYMPTOMATOLOGY

Early research and clinical lore on symptom profiles suggested that major depressive disorder is characterized by more classic vegetative features and affective symptoms, whereas bipolar depression involves more atypical vegetative features (for a review, see Depue & Monroe, 1978). Since that time, substantial research has been conducted on symptom patterns. In Table 7.2, we categorized these studies by the type of study design (cross-sectional or prospective). We used the same criteria described in the previous section to determine inclusion in the literature review.

We begin by describing one symptom for which differences are consistently observed—psychosis. In many studies, psychosis has been found to be more common among patients with bipolar depression than among those with major depressive disorder (Endicott et al., 1985; Guze, Woodruff, & Clayton, 1975; Parker, Roy, Wilhelm, Mitchell, & Hadzi-Pavlovic, 2000), with only one study finding no significant differences (Breslau & Meltzer, 1998). Intriguingly, psychosis during major depressive episodes also has been found consistently to predict a switch into bipolar disorder (Akiskal et al., 1983; Coryell et al., 1995; Goldberg, Harrow, & Whiteside, 2001; Othmer et al., 2007; Solomon et al., 2006).

Bipolar depression appears to be characterized by greater psychomotor retardation, with the exception of findings in one study; that is, in comparisons with major depressive disorder, bipolar depression was characterized as having significantly more psychomotor retardation in two cross-sectional studies (Parker et al., 2000; Serretti, Mandelli, Lattuada, Cusin, & Smeraldi, 2002) as well as in a prospective study of switches from major depressive disorder to bipolar disorder (Akiskal et al., 1983). Nevertheless, in contrast to the previously mentioned results, one study found significantly less psychomotor retardation in bipolar depression (Goel et al., 2002).

A set of studies has found that differences in a particular cognitive or emotional symptom differentiate between major depressive disorder from bipolar depression, but in each case, only one available study met our methodological criteria. For example, bipolar depression is characterized by significantly more pessimism (Perlis et al., 2006), guilt (Parker et al., 2000), anger attacks (Perlis et al., 2004), and suicidal ideation (Perlis et al., 2006), but less reactive mood (Parker et al., 2000), sadness (Perlis et al., 2006), and anxiety (Perlis et al.,

TABLE 7.2. Studies of Symptomatology in Major Depressive Disorder and Bipolar Disorder Depressive Episodes

Author (year)	*n*	Sample	Symptom measures
Retrospective/current designs			
Guze, Woodruff, & Clayton (1975)	253	Inpatient with primary or secondary affective disorder	Structured interview
Serretti et al. (2002)	1,832	Inpatient with depression	SCID, SADS, OPCRIT, HAMD
Breslau & Meltzer (1988)	111	Voluntary admission inpatients with psychotic depression	PSE, psychiatric and family history schedule, and HAMD or SADS-C
Goel, Terman, & Terman (2002)	165	Patients with seasonal affective disorder	SCID, HAMD, SIGH-SAD, HIGH-R
Parker et al. (2000)	987	Inpatient and outpatient bipolar disorder and unipolar depression	DSM-III–defined, 18 items measuring symptoms of melancholia
Perlis et al. (2006)	1,551	Nonpsychotic outpatients	SCID or MINI for diagnosis, CGI, HAMD, MADRS
Perlis et al. (2004)	79	Outpatients in a mood disorder clinic	SCID, Symptom Questionnaire, and CGI for current depression; Anger Attacks Questionnaire
Endicott et al. (1985)	292	Inpatient recurrent unipolar depression, bipolar I disorder, and bipolar II disorder	SADS, observation, chart review, informants
Prospective studies of manic onset			
Coryell et al. (1995)	605 depression, 96 mania	Inpatients and outpatients with major depressive disorder, schizoaffective disorder, or bipolar disorder	SADS, LIFE
Akiskal et al. (1983)	203	Outpatients with depression and no history of mania	Semistructured interview
Goldberg, Harrow, & Whiteside (2001)	74	Inpatients hospitalized for unipolar depression	SADS, Schizophrenia State Inventory
Solomon et al. (2006)	429	NIMH Collaborative Depression Study participants (79.7% inpatient)	SADS; LIFE for first 2 years of follow-up, LIFE-II for years 2–5, SLICE for years 6+

Note. CGI, Clinical Global Impression Severity scale; HAMD, Hamilton Rating Scale for Depression; HIGH-R, Hypomania Interview Guide—Retospective Assessment Version; LIFE, Longitudinal Interval Follow-Up Examination; MADRS, Montgomery–Asberg Depression Rating Scale; MINI, Mini-International Neuropsychiatric Interview; OPCRIT, Operational Criteria for Psychotic Illness Checklist; PSE, Present State Examination; SADS, Schedule for Affective Disorders and Schizophrenia; SCID, Structured Clinical Interview for DSM-IV; SIGH-SAD, Structured Interview Guide for the Hamilton Depression Rating Scale—Seasonal Affective Disorder Version; SLICE, Streamlined Longitudinal Interval Continuation Evaluation.

2006). Without replication, it remains possible that such findings are spurious due to the multiple tests conducted within such research.

In terms of vegetative symptoms, bipolar depression has been related more to appetite loss than has major depressive disorder (Parker et al., 2000). One study found less insomnia (Perlis et al., 2006) in bipolar depression compared to major depressive disorder, although another study found no significant difference (Parker et al., 2000). In another prospective study, switches from major depressive disorder to bipolar disorder were predicted by greater hypersomnia (Akiskal et al., 1983). As with cognitive and emotional symptoms, findings for appetite and sleep symptoms remain unreplicated within studies that met our design criteria.

In summary, psychosis appears to be more common in bipolar than in unipolar depression. In addition, three out of four findings suggest that psychomotor retardation is more common in bipolar than in unipolar depression.

Strong conclusions are difficult to make about other symptomatology differences between bipolar disorder and major depressive disorder. Findings for emotion, sleep, and appetite have not been replicated in carefully designed studies. Two major factors might help to explain why so many symptoms differentiate groups in only one study. First, studies have included varied symptom measures, some of which have quite poor coverage of certain symptoms, such as atypical vegetative symptoms. Perhaps the most important concern is that most studies of symptomatology have conducted many statistical tests without correcting alpha levels; type I errors may yield artificially elevated reports of group differences that could help explain some of the inconsistent findings across studies.

Beyond the paucity of high-quality studies on many symptoms, it is important to note other limitations in the available studies. On the whole, these studies are characterized by little attention to confounds, such as demographic characteristics (e.g., age, gender), the severity of depression (for an exception, see Perlis et al., 2006), or the complicated medication regimens within bipolar disorder. Available studies also fail to control for subthreshold symptoms of mania or anxiety, which could account for some of the differences seen (e.g., anger, anxiety, or insomnia).

Despite these limitations, some differences between bipolar disorder and major depressive disorder emerge consistently. There appears to be both cross-sectional and prospective evidence that bipolar depression is characterized by more psychosis and psychomotor retardation than is unipolar depression.

BIOLOGICAL VULNERABILITY

Although a comprehensive review of biological vulnerability is beyond the scope of this chapter (for a review, see Goodwin & Jamison, 2007), this overview highlights current biological models of depression. Genetic influences play an important role in the etiology of bipolar disorder, with heritability estimates as high as .85 (McGuffin et al., 2003). Early studies examined the familial associations between bipolar disorder (defined as mania with and without depression) and major depressive disorder. Relatives of major depressive disorder probands do not appear to be at elevated risk for mania (Winokur & Tsuang, 1996). In contrast, relatives of bipolar disorder probands are at higher risk of major depressive disorder than are relatives of non-affectively-disordered probands (Karkowski & Kendler, 1997; Plomin, DeFries, McClearn, & Rutter, 1997).

Surprisingly, though, few studies have differentiated family history patterns among persons with bipolar disorder with and without depression. Those that have distinguished bipolar probands by depression history find that family rates of depression are elevated among probands with a personal history of depression, but not among probands with no personal history of depression (Angst, Gerber-Werder, Zuberbühler, & Gamma, 2004; Perris, 1984).

Although family history studies provide important information, twin studies are preferable for disentangling whether the patterns observed are attributable to genetic or environmental influences. One twin study found that the heritabilities for depression and mania were correlated, but the correlation was low enough that these vulnerabilities should be considered as distinct (McGuffin et al., 2003). One way in which genetic vulnerability for a mood disorder may manifest itself is in neurobiology. This provides important evidence that one might want to consider neurobiological and neuroimaging findings that distinguish between risk for mania and depression. Unfortunately, few studies have done this. Here, we focus on studies that have at least examined the neurobiological correlates of bipolar depressive episodes.

Indeed, neuroimaging studies suggest that the same brain regions are involved during the depressive episodes of unipolar and bipolar disorders. Both unipolar and bipolar depression appear related to increased activation of the amygdala (a region involved in early responses to emotionally salient and novel stimuli). This evidence of increased amygdala activity (Abercrombie et al., 1998; Drevets, 1998) is particularly robust when participants are viewing faces with sad or threatening facial expressions (Sheline et al., 2001; Yurgelun-Todd et al., 2000). The hyperactivity of the amygdala appears to be coupled with diminished responsiveness during depressive episodes of regions involved in emotion regulation, such as the dorsal anterior cingulate and the prefrontal cortex (Stoll, Renshaw, Yurgelun-Todd, & Cohen, 2001). In summary, imaging studies of bipolar depression suggest parallels between bipolar depression and major depressive disorder, particularly in studies of neural responses to emotion-relevant stimuli.

Beyond neuroanatomical correlates, substantial research has focused on neurotransmitter irregularities associated with affective disturbances. We focus here on deficits in the functioning of dopamine, serotonin, and norepinephrine, which have been a dominant focus of research. Although these systems are believed to increase risk in interaction with other neurobiological variables, research comparing bipolar disorder and major depressive disorder has rarely examined more sophisticated models of membrane function, second messenger systems, and receptor sensitivity.

Much of the historical research on neurotransmitters has focused on the levels of neurotransmitters, ideally measured within the cerebrospinal fluid (CSF). Generally, studies of CSF metabolites show remarkable consistency in the patterns evidenced among patients with bipolar disorder and major depressive disorder. Both bipolar disorder and major depressive disorder are associated with low CSF levels of the serotonin metabolite 5-hydroxyindoleacetic acid (5-HIAA) compared to levels among healthy controls (e.g., Bowers, Heninger, & Gerbode, 1969; Sjostrom & Roos, 1973). Many findings suggest that bipolar disorder and major depressive disorder are associated with comparable CSF levels of the dopamine metabolite homovanillic acid (Goodwin & Jamison, 2007). In a review of over 80 studies on neurobiological and neurotransmitter studies of major depressive disorder and bipolar disorder depressive episodes, Yatham and colleagues (2000) reported that any differences observed between the disorders have failed to replicate.

Although findings on neurotransmitter metabolites have dominated the historical literature, more recent research has shifted to studies of how well a given neurotransmitter system functions; that is, beyond levels of a neurotransmitter, key components of the system include the density and sensitivity of receptors, as well as mechanisms involved in the reuptake and metabolism of neurotransmitters. New technologies allow for more sophisticated tests of the function of neurotransmitter systems, by providing a "challenge" to the system by changing levels of a given neurotransmitter and measuring neurological, behavioral, affective, or cognitive responses. These studies have tended to focus on dopamine and serotonin.

In one paradigm, a dopamine agonist is administered, and then growth hormone is measured as an index of the sensitivity to dopamine. These studies have yielded no group differences in comparisons of persons with major depressive disorder, bipolar depression, and healthy control groups (Jimerson et al., 1984; McPherson, Walsh, & Silverstone, 2003).

Beyond the small number of studies of dopamine agonists, sleep deprivation paradigms provide one window into studying dopamine function. It has been suggested that increases in dopamine functioning may mediate sleep deprivation effects (Ebert & Berger, 1998), such that sleep deprivation may provide another form of challenge to the dopamine system. Experimentally induced sleep deprivation appears to produce temporary symptom relief for both bipolar depression (Barbini et al., 1998) and major depressive disorder (Wu & Bunney, 1991). Direct comparisons of responses to sleep deprivation among persons with bipolar disorder and major depressive disorder do suggest some differences in the ability to regulate in response to this challenge. Barbini and colleagues (1998) found that repeated sleep deprivation over a 7-night period produced greater abatement in depressive symptoms in people with bipolar disorder compared to those with major depressive disorder; that is, bipolar disorder, compared to major depressive disorder, may be related to increased reactivity to sleep deprivation.

Several pharmacological challenges for studying serotonin system sensitivity have been well-validated within major depressive disorder. As reviewed by Sobczak, Riedel, Booij, Het Rot, and Deutz (2002), four studies suggest that people with unipolar and bipolar depression demonstrate similarly blunted hormonal responses to *d*-fenfluramine (which triggers the release of serotonin and inhibits reuptake) or tryptophan (a precursor to serotonin). More recently, Sher and colleagues (2003) found that people with bipolar depression, as well as those with major depressive disorder, demonstrate a blunted shift in prolactin after *d*-fenfluramine administration compared to healthy control participants. Unaffected family members of persons with bipolar disorder demonstrate atypical cognitive (Sobczak, Riedel, et al., 2002) and mood responses (Quintin et al., 2001) to serotonin challenges, suggesting that deficits in serotonin functioning are not secondary to medication effects or scars of previous episodes.

In summary, bipolar disorder and major depressive disorder appear to share many neurobiological features. Both types of depressive episodes appear related to deficits in brain regions involved in emotional reactivity and regulation. Several lines of evidence suggest deficits in the functioning of the serotonin and dopamine systems for both bipolar depression and major depressive disorder. Despite neurobiological similarities between bipolar disorder and major depressive disorder, some differences have been found. Perhaps most importantly, even though people with bipolar depression and those with major depressive disorder demonstrate mood shifts with sleep deprivation, these effects are stronger in bipolar disorder than they are in major depressive disorder, suggesting that there might be greater dopamine dysregulation in bipolar disorder.

PSYCHOSOCIAL ANTECEDENTS TO DEPRESSION

The psychosocial antecedents to major depressive disorder have been well documented. Among socioenvironmental variables, robust evidence has emerged for negative life events and expressed emotion as predictors of major depressive disorder (Brown & Harris, 1978; Butzlaff & Hooley, 1998). Personality traits have also received considerable attention (Klein, Durbin, & Shankman, Chapter 5, this volume). Cognitive styles have been studied extensively (see Joormann, Chapter 13, this volume). In the next sections, we describe studies examining whether these same variables predict bipolar depression. First, though, we review methodological issues that must be addressed to study antecedents of bipolar depression.

Methodological Issues

Studies in this field vary in the use of cross-sectional versus prospective designs. Most researchers are well aware that cross-sectional studies fail to distinguish between the precursors and the consequences of symptoms. An ideal prospective study would administer psychosocial measures before the onset of manic or depressive symptoms. Given the low prevalence of bipolar disorder, however, this is rarely accomplished (but see Hillegers et al., 2004). A more practical design would involve administering psychosocial measures to euthymic bipolar disorder I patients and following them to see if psychosocial characteristics predict the severity of depressive symptoms over time. Within prospective studies, the choice of an appropriate outcome variable is complicated. Many prospective studies in this field have focused on occurrence of episodes. Categorizing an episode as manic or depressive, however, may obscure recognition of symptoms from the opposite pole (mixed states); that is, depressive symptoms are common during manic and hypomanic episodes. Sato, Bottlender, Kleindienst, and Möller (2002) conducted cluster analyses of symptoms present during a manic episode. Although one group of individuals appeared to have pure manic episodes, 68 of the 576 participants with mania experienced significant depressive symptoms. Minor depressive symptoms appear to be even more common. Indeed, in one study, most (hypo)manic episodes involved depressive symptoms (Bauer, Simon, Ludman, & Unutzer, 2005). In short, categorizing an episode as "manic" or "depressed" may obscure important variance. Depressive symptoms may influence the severity and duration of manic episodes. Given this, studies that estimate changes in depressive and manic symptom severity separately are more informative for this chapter than are studies of episodes. Relatively few studies have met this criterion.

Studies that have addressed psychosocial factors and bipolar depression can be categorized into cross-sectional (or retrospective) studies and prospective studies. In either group, almost no studies have compared unipolar and bipolar depression directly.

Socioenvironmental Predictors

Although many studies have focused on life events in bipolar disorder, few studies are prospective, and few have evaluated whether events are dependent on or caused by a person's illness (for a review, see Johnson & Fingerhut, 2006). Several retrospective life event studies have examined rates of severe, independent life events occurring before depression episodes of bipolar disorder (Hunt, Bruce-Jones, & Silverstone, 1992; Perris, 1984). A study by Malkoff-Schwartz and colleagues (2000) deserves particular mention, because it used a rigorous interview design to rule out confounds in the assessment of life events (e.g., stressors caused by symptomatic behavior). As with the other research, the findings of this study suggest that severe, independent, negative life events were equally common before episodes of bipolar depression and major depressive disorder.

Isometsä, Heikinen, Henriksson, Aro, and Lonnquist (1995) compared the prevalence of life events preceding completed suicides of individuals with bipolar disorder and major depressive disorder. Next of kin completed the Recent Life Change Survey regarding stressors experienced by deceased persons before their death. Negative life events appeared to be equally common precipitants to suicide, in that 64% of individuals with bipolar disorder and 66% of those with unipolar disorder had experienced at least one negative life event shortly before their death.

Beyond these retrospective studies, several studies have examined whether negative life events prospectively predict the course of bipolar depression. In three prospective studies (Cohen, Hammen, Henry, & Daley, 2004; Johnson, Winett, Meyer, Greenhouse, & Miller, 1999; Johnson et al., 2008), life events and social support predicted depression, but neither predicted mania. Johnson and colleagues (in press) replicated the finding that severe negative life events predict increases in bipolar depression, but not in mania. Hammen (1995) found comparable rates of negative life events before episodes of bipolar depression and major depressive disorder.

Among 38 adolescents with bipolar disorder, depressive symptoms over time were highly correlated with the level of chronic stress in family and interpersonal relationships (Kim, Miklowitz, Biuckians, & Mullen, 2007).

One study is particularly intriguing because it examined the role of life events in predicting the onset of mood disorders among 140 offspring of parents with bipolar disorder. Hillegers and colleagues (2004) used the adolescent version of the Life Events and Difficulties Schedule to examine the influence of life events among 140 offspring of 86 parents with BPD. At 5-year follow-up, 34 of the children had developed depressive disorders and 4 had developed bipolar spectrum disorders, according to the SADS for School-Aged Children. The onset of these mood disorders was clearly related to the cumulative number of severe negative life events over a 5-year period: Each severe life event increased risk of future onset by approximately 10%. Findings, however, were limited by the 5-year period covered by interviews. Indeed, analyses of the data suggested that participants forgot about 11% of severe events per year, such that about half of the events from 5 years before would have been forgotten. In subsequent analyses, the authors addressed this difficulty with recall by examining links between severe life events and episodes (either new onsets or recurrences) of mood disorders that occurred within 14 months of interview (Wals et al., 2005). As with previous analyses, life events were clearly tied to mood disorders, and particularly to depression. Hence, negative life events appear to be important in understanding first episodes of depression among those at risk for bipolar disorder.

Beyond life events, *expressed emotion* (EE), defined as either overinvolvement, hostility or criticism by family members toward the patient, is a robust predictor of major depressive disorder (Butzlaff & Hooley, 1998). EE predicted more severe depressive symptoms of bipolar disorder in two studies (Kim & Miklowitz, 2004; Yan, Hammen, Cohen, Daley, & Henry, 2004).

People with major depressive disorder and bipolar depression appear to experience comparable rates of independent negative life events before episode onsets or suicides. In summary, the social environment appears to be important for understanding the course of bipolar depression. Negative life events often precede increases in depressive symptoms. As with major depressive disorder, episodes of bipolar depression appear to be related to low social support and high EE. This body of evidence suggests strong overlap between the environmental triggers of unipolar and bipolar depression.

Personality Traits

Personality traits have been a focus in bipolar disorder research for the better part of 100 years; early psychodynamic theory hypothesized higher achievement-striving levels in this population. Compared to people with major depressive disorder, euthymic individuals with bipolar disorder appear to experience comparably elevated levels of neuroticism (Goodwin & Jamison, 2007). Not surprisingly given the nature of mania, people with bipolar disorder also appear to report heightened positive affect and extraversion compared to people with major depressive disorder (Goodwin & Jamison, 2007). Neuroticism and positive affect scores within bipolar disorder, though, appear correlated with the relative severity of depression and mania, respectively (Hecht, van Calker, Berger, & von Zerssen, 1998; Murray, Goldstone, & Cunningham, 2007). These cross-sectional studies of personality, however, have been criticized for failing to attend to the effects of illness on personality measures (cf. Hirschfeld et al., 1983).

Relatively few studies have examined how personality predicts depression in people with bipolar disorder. Neuroticism predicted increases in bipolar disorder depressive symptoms (but not manic symptoms) over time in one study of 39 people (Lozano & Johnson, 2001), congruent with the literature on major depressive disorder (Gunderson, Triebwasser, Phillips, & Sullivan, 1999).

In addition to traditional personality dimensions, such as neuroticism, recent research has focused on what might be conceptualized as *subaffective syndromes*: characteristics that bridge the gap between personality and mild, but long-term, affective traits. These studies have focused on the correlates of mania within bipolar disorder rather than the correlates of depression. Therefore, this literature appears to be answering the question: "If someone has a depressive episode, which personality factors predict whether he or she will have a manic episode?" Mood lability and cyclothymia, characteristics that include a tendency toward positive moods, have been found to predict the development of first manic episodes (Akiskal et al., 1995; Egeland, Hostetter, Pauls, & Sussex, 2000; Regeer et al., 2006). These findings, then, suggest that mania onset is predicted by traits that are similar to, though of lesser severity than, full-blown manic symptoms.

The literature we have reviewed has attempted to address the question of predicting mania in persons with depression. So far, however, few studies have addressed the related question: "If someone has a manic episode, which personality factors predict whether he or she will have a depressive episode?" Initial findings suggest that depressive temperament is related more to depressive episodes than to manic episodes among those with euthymic bipolar disorder (Gandotra & Paul, 2004; Henry et al., 1999). However, we could not identify any prospective studies of depressive temperament.

In summary, research suggests that neuroticism predicts depressive symptoms within both bipolar disorder and major depressive disorder. In regard to temperament research, there is a need for prospective designs. Also of concern is that many temperament studies have focused on bipolar spectrum disorders (including bipolar I disorder, bipolar II disorder, and even bipolar disorder not otherwise specified). The low reliability of diagnoses for the milder forms of bipolar disorder, as well as subtle differences in diagnostic criteria used in different studies, makes generalizing across studies difficult.

Cognitive Styles

Many aspects of cognition have been studied in mood disorders, from neuropsychological deficits to self-reported thought content to information-processing parameters. Neuropsychological research suggests that bipolar disorder appears to be related to deficits in executive functioning (Martinez-Arán et al., 2004). Verbal memory deficits have been found to correlate with the number of previous depressive episodes for both major depressive disorder and bipolar depression (Fossati et al., 2004). Here, though, we focus on negative cognitive styles.

Comparable to major depressive disorder, bipolar disorder is associated with a range of negative cognitive styles during depression, including elevated scores on the Attributional Style Questionnaire (ASQ), the Automatic Thoughts Questionnaire (ATQ), and the Dysfunctional Attitudes Scale (DAS), as well as measures of rumination and low self-esteem (for a review, see Cuellar, Johnson, & Winters, 2005; see also Jones, Sellwood, & McGovern, 2005). People with bipolar depression appear similar to those with major depressive disorder in that their reaction times are slowed when they are asked to ignore negative words on the Stroop Color-Naming Task (Lyon, Startup, & Bentall, 1999). A larger question, posed in research on both unipolar depression and bipolar disorder is whether these cognitive characteristics can be documented outside of a depressive episode, or whether they merely reflect the influence of current mood state on thought content and processes.

Many of the negative cognitive facets documented during bipolar depression diminish with recovery. During remission, individuals with bipolar disorder and major depressive disorder have been shown to obtain scores within the normal range on the DAS (Tracy, Bauwens, Martin, Pardoen, & Mendlowicz, 1992) and the ATQ (Hollon, Kendall, & Lumry, 1986), and to report self–ideal discrepancies, self-esteem levels, and attributions for negative events that are comparable to those of healthy controls (Bentall, Kinderman, & Mason, 2005; Bentall & Thompson, 1990; Daskalopoulou et al., 2002; Lyon et al., 1999; Scott, Stanton, Garland, & Ferrier, 2000; Scott & Pope, 2003; Tracy et al., 1992; Wolf & Mueller-Oerlinghausen, 2002). Persons with remitted bipolar disorder also performed comparably to healthy controls on an affective go/no-go task, designed to measure the ability to inhibit responses to negative and positively valenced words (Rubinsztein, Michael, Paykel, & Sahakian, 2000). In some studies of remitted individuals, persons with bipolar disorder make less stable attributions for negative events and report higher self-esteem than do persons with major depressive disorder (Ashworth, Blackburn, & McPherson, 1985; Tracy et al., 1992; Winters & Neale, 1985).

In contrast, other studies suggest that during remission, individuals with bipolar disorder evidence overly negative cognitive styles. For example, Scott and colleagues (2000) found that a euthymic bipolar disorder group demonstrated elevated scores on sociotropy and perfectionism compared to a healthy control group, even after they controlled for subsyndromal symptom levels. In two studies (Mansell & Lam, 2004; Scott et al., 2000), people with remitted bipolar disorder displayed a tendency to have overly general autobiographical memories of negative events (e.g., collapsing across several incidents of a failure or a success), consistent with similar findings in unipolar depression (Mackinger, Pachinger, Leibetseder, & Fartacek, 2000).

In summary, evidence is mixed about whether negative cognitive styles can be documented after remission among persons with bipolar disorder. These cross-study discrepancies may be related to two issues: heterogeneity in depression within bipolar disorder and insensitivity of some cognitive measures. We briefly discuss these two issues.

Heterogeneity in Depression

As we noted at the outset, not all people with bipolar disorder experience depression. Several studies have suggested that negative cognitive styles might be elevated only among those bipolar participants with a history of depression (Alloy, Reilly-Harrington, Fresco, Whitehouse, & Zechmeister, 1999) or current depressive symptoms (Eisner, Johnson, & Carver, 2008; Thomas & Bentall, 2002). Although few studies have considered the issue in bipolar disorder, findings in the depression literature suggest that even mildly negative affective states might be important to consider as well (Ingram, Bernet, & McLaughlin, 1994).

Differences across Measures in Sensitivity to Negative Cognition within Bipolar Disorder

Psychodynamic authors described the "manic defense" in the early part of the 20th century (e.g., Abraham, 1911/1927). This construct has continued to receive attention, because several authors have suggested that defensiveness among people with bipolar disorder may interfere with the assessment of negative cognitive styles. In an early study, Winters and Neale (1985) noted that people with bipolar disorder appear similar to healthy controls on overt measures of self-esteem. However, on a task described as more subtle, the Pragmatic Inference Task (PIT), people with remitted bipolar disorder obtain scores reflecting self-blaming attributions for failure that were comparable to those of people with remitted major depressive disorder. In addition, although PIT and self-esteem scores were correlated for individuals with major depressive disorder and those with no disorder, these scores were not correlated among individuals with bipolar disorder. In short, during remission, people with bipolar disorder appear to describe themselves more positively than do those with major depressive disorder on some, but not all, measures. Across measures, there is greater inconsistency in the self-descriptions of persons with bipolar disorder.

Given these findings, Bentall and his colleagues (2005) recommended that bipolar disorder cognition should be measured with more subtle cognitive tasks, such as the PIT and an Emotion Stroop Task, rather than the Rosenberg Self-Esteem Scale or the ASQ. Consistent with this idea, the Bentall team found that people with mania were slower when asked to ignore depressive words on an Emotion Stroop Task even when other cognitive measures did not demonstrate negative biases (Lyon et al., 1999). At this early stage of research, then, some measures appear more sensitive to a negative cognitive style than others, particularly during remission.

Summary of Cross-Sectional Cognitive Studies

During depression, people with bipolar disorder and major depressive disorder manifest strikingly parallel cognitive styles. Much of the research suggests that cognitive styles are relatively state-dependent in bipolar disorder, in that many negative cognitive style parameters observed during depression are less demonstrable with recovery. It will be important for future research to attend carefully to heterogeneity in depression and issues related to defensiveness, to get a better picture of the role of cognitive styles in bipolar disorder.

Cognitive Styles and Low Self-Esteem as Predictors of Depression

Despite ambiguity on whether remitted bipolar disorder is consistently correlated with negative cognitive styles, several studies suggest that, when present, negative cognitive styles predict a poorer course of symptoms within bipolar disorder. For example, Scott and Pope (2003) found a trend in which negative self-esteem predicted relapse (either manic or depressive) among patients with bipolar disorder. We found that low self-esteem and negative cognitive styles predicted greater increases over time in depression but not mania (Johnson et al., 1999; Johnson & Fingerhut, 2004). Hence, early data suggest that negative cognitive styles and low self-esteem, when present, may help to predict bipolar depression, although it remains unclear whether the effect sizes for such variables are similar for bipolar and unipolar depression.

PSYCHOSOCIAL TREATMENT

Given the concordance between the risk factors for bipolar disorder and major depressive disorder, one might expect that effective treatment strategies for major depressive disorder would help to alleviate bipolar depression. To date, three of the most carefully researched psychotherapies for bipolar disorder—family therapy, cognitive therapy, and interpersonal psychotherapy—appear to relieve bipolar depression more than they relieve mania (Frank et al., 2000; Lam, Hayward, Watkins, Wright, & Sham, 2005; Miklowitz et al., 2000). Given evidence for the effectiveness of these approaches for major depressive disorder (DeRubeis & Crits-Cristoph, 1998), bipolar depression might be similar to major depressive disorder in terms of responsiveness to specific psychotherapies.

FUTURE DIRECTIONS

Bipolar depression and major depressive disorder appear to share remarkable overlap in symptoms and neurobiology. Moreover, many of the variables that contribute to the course of major depressive disorder also appear to contribute to the course of bipolar depression; that is, negative life events, low social support, EE, neuroticism, negative cognitive styles, and low self-esteem may each help to predict depression within bipolar disorder. Given the applicability of psychosocial models of major depressive disorder to bipolar depression, it is not surprising that psychosocial treatments with strong effects on major depressive disorder have fared well in addressing bipolar depression.

In this chapter we have emphasized comparisons between unipolar and bipolar depression. Obviously, any comprehensive model of bipolar disorder must consider mania. In this regard, it is of interest that many of the psychosocial variables that predict unipolar and bipolar depression appear less important in the prediction of mania (Johnson et al., 1999, in press; Miklowitz et al., 2000). Although a consideration of mania is beyond the scope of this chapter, the interested reader is referred to articles that focus on unique biological (Chiaroni et al., 2000), temperament (Johnson, 2005), and life event (Johnson et al., in press; Malkoff-Schwartz et al., 2000) predictors of mania.

Setting aside the prediction of mania, are the depressive episodes in bipolar disorder and unipolar disorder entirely similar? Clinical intuition and preliminary data suggest a unique aspect of the pathology of bipolar disorder that is important in considering depression. Bipolar disorder appears to be characterized by marked extremes and fluctuations. We described earlier the evidence for a set of characteristics that differentiate people with mania from those with unipolar depressive disorder. These characteristics include earlier age of onset, shorter duration of episodes, more severe episodes, more symptoms of psychosis and psychomotor retardation, as well as interepisode mood lability and cyclothymia. Not only do these characteristics appear to differentiate between groups within cross-sectional studies, but they also predict development of the first manic episode. Bipolar disorder also appears related to more extreme reactivity to sleep deprivation compared to major depressive disorder. Depue, Krauss, and Spoont (1987) have emphasized dysregulation as a core component of the neurobiology of bipolar disorder, and people with bipolar spectrum disorders appear to have greater difficulties in mood and cortisol regulation following challenges than do controls (Depue et al., 1987). The theme of dysregulation, then, appears to emerge across studies on the neurobiology, course, and symptom patterns of bipolar disorder. Although Hollon (1992) has noted the importance of dysregulation in major depressive disorder, we note that bipolar disorder appears to be related even more to dysregulation than does major depressive disorder. Therefore, one might expect more dramatic responses to psychosocial or biological challenges in persons with bipolar disorder compared to those with major depressive disorder. Unfortunately, studies of this type are rare.

We join others (Joffe, Young, & MacQueen, 1999; Schweitzer, Maguire, & Ng, 2005) in calling for recognition that research and clinical work would be furthered by differentiating between mania and depression. Our model suggests three testable tenets: (1) Bipolar depression and major depressive disorder are predicted by comparable psychosocial variables; (2) mania and depression are predicted by separate psychosocial variables within bipolar disorder; and (3) bipolar disorder (including both depressive and manic poles) is characterized by more dysregulation than is major depressive disorder. Evidence for each tenet is quite limited, however, and each needs more careful longitudinal and integrative research.

As researchers begin to conduct such studies, we hope that this review has highlighted several key methodological issues in sample definition, measurement, and study design. For example, future research must consider confounds, such as the duration of illness, number of episodes, and medication profiles.

In summary, there is evidence to suggest that drawing from the literature on major depressive disorder will foster greater understanding of the depressive symptoms of bipolar disorder. We hope that others will be encouraged to consider the intriguing comparisons between unipolar depression and bipolar depression. We believe that such investigations will yield new insights into etiological models and treatment strategies.

REFERENCES

Abercrombie, H. C., Schaefer, S. M., Larson, C. L., Oakes, T. R., Lindgren, K. A., & Holden, J. E. (1998). Metabolic rate in the right amygdala predicts negative affect in depressed patients. *NeuroReport, 9,* 3301–3307.

Abraham, K. (1927). Notes on the psychoanalytic investigations and treatment of manic–depressive insanity and allied conditions. In E. Jones (Ed.), *Selected papers of Karl Abraham* (pp. 418–480). London: Hogarth Press. (Original work published 1911)

Akiskal, H. S., Maser, J. D., Zeller, P. J., Endicott, J., Coryell, W., Keller, M., et al. (1995). Switching from "unipolar" to bipolar II: An 11-year prospective study of clinical and temperamental predictors of 559 patients. *Archives of General Psychiatry, 52,* 114–123.

Akiskal, H. S., Walker, P., Puzantian, V. R., King, D., Rosenthal, T. L., & Dranon, M. (1983). Bipolar outcome in the course of depressive illness: Phenomenologic, familial, and pharmacologic predictors. *Journal of Affective Disorders, 5,* 115–128.

Alloy, L. B., Reilly-Harrington, N., Fresco, D. M., Whitehouse, W. G., & Zechmeister, J. S. (1999). Cognitive styles and life events in subsyndromal unipolar and bipolar disorders: Stability and prospective prediction of depressive and hypomanic mood swings. *Journal of Cognitive Psychotherapy, 13,* 21–40.

American Psychiatric Association. (1994). *Diagnostic and statistical manual of mental disorders* (4th ed.). Washington, DC: Author.

Angst, J., Gerber-Werder, R., Zuberbühler, H. U., & Gamma, A. (2004). Is bipolar disorder heterogeneous? *European Archives of Psychiatry and Clinical Neuroscience, 254,* 82–91.

Ashworth, C. M., Blackburn, I. M., & McPherson, F. M. (1985). The performance of depressed and manic patients on some repertory grid measures: A cross-sectional study. *British Journal of Medical Psychology, 55*, 247–255.

Barbini, B., Colombo, C., Benedetti, F., Campori, E., Bellodi, L., & Smeraldi, E. (1998). The unipolar–bipolar dichotomy and the response to sleep deprivation. *Psychiatry Research, 79*, 43–50.

Bauer, M. S., Simon, G. E., Ludman, E., & Unutzer, J. (2005). "Bipolarity" in bipolar disorder: Distribution of manic and depressive symptoms in a treated population. *British Journal of Psychiatry, 187*, 87–88.

Bentall, R. P., Kinderman, P., & Mason, K. (2005). Self discrepancies in bipolar disorder: Comparisons of manic, depressed, remitted and normal patients. *British Journal of Clinical Psychology, 44*, 457–473.

Bentall, R. P., & Thompson, M. (1990). Emotional stroop performance and the manic defense. *British Journal of Clinical Psychology, 29*, 235–237.

Bowers, M. B., Henninger, J. G. R., & Gerbode, G. (1969). Cerebrospinal fluid 5-hydroxy-indoleacetic acid and homovanillic acid in psychiatric patients. *Journal of Neuropharmacology, 8*, 255–262.

Breslau, N., & Meltzer, H. Y. (1988). Validity of subtyping psychotic depression: Examination of phenomenology and demographic characteristics. *American Journal of Psychiatry, 145*, 35–40.

Brown, G. W., & Harris, T. O. (1978). *Social origins of depression: A study of psychiatric disorder in women.* New York: Free Press.

Butzlaff, R. L., & Hooley, J. M. (1998). Expressed emotion and psychiatric relapse: A meta-analysis. *Archives of General Psychiatry, 55*, 547–552.

Calabrese, J., Hirschfeld, R. M. A., Frye, M. A., & Reed, M. L. (2004). Impact of depressive symptoms compared to manic symptoms in the community: Results of a U.S. community-based sample. *Journal of Clinical Psychiatry, 65*, 1499–1504.

Chengappa, K. N. R., Kupfer, D. J., Frank, E., Houck, P. R., Grochocinski, V. J., Cluss, P. A., et al. (2003). Relationship of birth cohort and early age of onset of illness in a bipolar disorder case of registry. *American Journal of Psychiatry, 160*, 1636–1642.

Chiaroni, P., Azorin, J. M., Dassa, D., Henry, J. M., Giudicelli, S., Malthiery, Y., et al. (2000). Possible involvement of the dopamine D3 receptor locus in subtypes of bipolar affective disorder. *Psychiatric Genetics, 10*, 43–49.

Cohen, A. N., Hammen, C., Henry, R. M., & Daley, S. E. (2004). Effects of stress and social support on recurrence in bipolar disorder. *Journal of Affective Disorders, 82*, 143–147.

Coryell, W., Andreasen, N. C., Endicott, J., & Keller, M. (1987). The significance of past mania or hypomania in the course and outcome of major depression. *American Journal of Psychiatry, 144*, 309–315.

Coryell, W., Endicott, J., Maser, J. D., Keller, M. B., Leon, A. C., & Akiskal, H. (1995). Long-term stability of polarity distinctions in the affective disorders. *American Journal of Psychiatry, 152*, 385–390.

Coryell, W., Keller, M., Endicott, J., Andreasen, N., Clayton, P., & Hirschfeld, R. (1989). Bipolar II illness: Course and outcome over a five-year period. *Psychological Medicine, 19*, 129–141.

Cuellar, A. K., Johnson, S. L., & Winters, R. (2005). Distinctions between bipolar and unipolar depression. *Clinical Psychological Review, 25*, 307–339.

Daskalopoulou, E. G., Dikeos, D. G., Papadimitriou, G. N., Souery, D., Blairy, S., Massat, I., et al. (2002). Self-esteem, social adjustment and suicidality in affective disorders. *European Psychiatry, 17*, 265–271.

Depue, R. A., Krauss, S. P., & Spoont, M. R. (1987). A two-dimensional threshold model of seasonal bipolar affective disorder. In D. Magnuson & A. Ohman (Eds.), *Psychopathology: An interactional perspective* (pp. 95–123). San Diego, CA: Academic Press.

Depue, R. A., & Monroe, S. M. (1978). The unipolar-bipolar distinction in the depressive disorders. *Psychological Bulletin, 85*, 1001–1029.

DeRubeis, R. J., & Crits-Christoph, P. (1998). Empirically supported individual and group psychological treatments for adult mental disorders. *Journal of Consulting and Clinical Psychology, 66*, 37–52.

Drevets, W. C. (1998). Functional neuroimaging studies of depression: The anatomy of melancholia. *Annual Review of Medicine, 49*, 341–361.

Ebert, D., & Berger, M. (1998). Neurobiological similarities in antidepressant sleep deprivation and psychostimulant use: A psychostimulant theory of antidepressant sleep deprivation. *Psychopharmacology, 140*, 1–10.

Egeland, J. A., Hostetter, A. M., Pauls, D. L., & Sussex, J. N. (2000). Prodromal symptoms before onset of manic–depressive disorder suggested by first hospital admission histories. *Journal of the American Academy of Child and Adolescent Psychiatry, 39*, 1245–1252.

Eisner, L., Johnson, S. L., & Carver, C. S. (2008). Cognitive responses to failure and success relate uniquely to bipolar disorder depression versus mania. *Journal of Abnormal Psychology, 117*, 154–163.

Endicott, J., Nee, J., Andreasen, N., Clayton, P., Keller, M., & Coryell, W. (1985). Bipolar II: Combine or keep separate? *Journal of Affective Disorders, 8*, 17–28.

Fossati, P., Harvey, P. O., Le Bastard, G., Ergis, A. M., Jouvent, R., & Allilaire, J. F. (2004). Verbal memory performance of patients with a first depressive episode and patients with unipolar and bipolar recurrent depression. *Journal of Psychiatric Research, 38*, 137–144.

Frank, E., Kupfer, D. J., Gibbons, R., Houck, P., Kostelnik, B., & Mallinger, A. (2000). *Interpersonal and social rhythm therapy prevents depressive symptoms in patients with bipolar I disorder.* In D. Miklowitz (Chair), Is the course of manic–depressive illness influenced by psychosocial factors?: Lessons from observational and treatment studies. Symposium conducted at the 15th annual meeting of the Society for Research on Psychopathology, Boulder, CO.

Furukawa, T. A., Konno, W., Morinobu, S., Harai, H., Kitamura, T., & Takahashi, K. (2000). Course and outcome of depressive episodes: Comparison between bipolar, unipolar and subthreshold depression. *Psychiatry Research, 96*, 211–220.

Gandotra, S., & Paul, S. E. (2004). Affective temperaments and polarity in bipolar I disorder: Relationship and predictive value. *Hong Kong Journal of Psychiatry, 14*, 15–23.

Geller, B., Zimerman, B., Williams, M., Bolhofner, K., & Craney, J. L. (2001). Bipolar disorder at prospective follow-up of adults who had prepubertal major depressive disorder. *American Journal of Psychiatry, 158*, 125–127.

Goel, N., Terman, M., & Terman, J. S. (2002). Depressive symptomatology differentiates subgroups of patients with seasonal affective disorder. *Depression and Anxiety, 15*, 34–41.

Goldberg, J. F., Harrow, M., & Whiteside, J. E. (2001). Risk for bipolar illness in patients initially hospitalized for unipolar depression. *American Journal of Psychiatry, 158*, 1265–1270.

Goodwin, F. K., & Jamison, K. R. (2007). *Manic–depressive illness.* Oxford, UK: Oxford University Press.

Gunderson, J. G., Triebwasser, J., Phillips, K. A., & Sullivan, C. N. (1999). Personality and vulnerability to affective disorders. In R. C. Cloninger (Ed.), *Personality and psychopathology* (pp. 3–32). Washington, DC: American Psychiatric Press.

Guze, S. B., Woodruff, R. A., & Clayton, P. J. (1975). The significance of psychotic affective disorders. *Archives of General Psychiatry, 32*, 1147–1150.

Hammen, C. L. (1995). Stress and the course of unipolar and bipolar disorders. In C. M. Mazure (Ed.), *Does stress cause psychiatric illness?* (pp. 87–110). Washington, DC: American Psychiatric Association.

Hecht, H., van Calker, D., Berger, M., & von Zerssen, D. (1998). Personality in patients with affective disorders and their relatives. *Journal of Affective Disorders, 51*, 33–43.

Henry, C., Lacoste, J., Bellivier, F., Verdoux, H., Bourgeois, M. L., & Leboyer, M. (1999). Temperament in bipolar illness: Impact on prognosis. *Journal of Affective Disorders, 56*, 103–108.

Hillegers, M. H., Burger, H., Wals, M., Reichart, C. G., Verhulst, F. C., Nolen, W. A., et al. (2004). Impact of stressful life events, familial loading and their interaction on the onset of mood disorders. *British Journal of Psychiatry, 185*, 97–101.

Hirschfeld, R. M. A., Klerman, G. L., Clayton, P. J., Keller, M. B., Mcdonald-Scott, P., & Larkin, B. H. (1983). Assessing personality: Effects of the depressive state on trait measurement. *American Journal of Psychiatry, 140*, 695–699.

Hollon, S. D. (1992). Cognitive models of depression from a psychobiological perspective. *Psychological Inquiry, 3*, 250–253.

Hollon, S. D., Kendall, P. C., & Lumry, A. (1986). Specificity of depressotypic cognitions in clinical depression. *Journal of Abnormal Psychology, 95,* 52–59.

Hunt, N., Bruce-Jones, W. D., & Silverstone, T. (1992). Life events and relapse in bipolar affective disorder. *Journal of Affective Disorders, 25,* 13–20.

Ingram, R. E., Bernet, C. Z., & McLaughlin, S. C. (1994). Attentional allocation processes in individuals at risk for depression. *Cognitive Therapy and Research, 18,* 317–332.

Isometsä, E., Heikinen, M., Henriksson, M., Aro, H., & Lonnquist, J. (1995). Recent life events and completed suicide in bipolar affective disorder: A comparison with major depressive suicides. *Journal of Affective Disorders, 33,* 99–106.

Jimerson, D. C., Cutler, N. R., Post, R. M., Rey, A., Gold, P. W., Brown, G. M., et al. (1984). Neuroendocrine responses to apomorphine in depressed patients and healthy control subjects. *Psychiatry Research, 13,* 1–12.

Joffe, R. T., Young, L. T., & MacQueen, G. M. (1999). A two-illness model of bipolar disorder. *Bipolar Disorders, 1,* 25–30.

Johnson, S. L. (2005). Mania and dysregulation in goal pursuit. *Clinical Psychology Review, 25,* 241–262.

Johnson, S. L., Cuellar, A., Ruggero, C., Perlman, C., Goodnick, P., White, R., et al. (2008). Life events as predictors of mania and depression in bipolar I disorder. *Journal of Abnormal Psychology, 117,* 268–277.

Johnson, S. L., Eisner, L. R., & Miller, C. (2008). Bipolar disorder. In J. Hunsley & E. J. Mash (Eds.), *Guide to assessments that work* (pp. 121–137). New York: Oxford University Press.

Johnson, S. L., & Fingerhut, R. (2004). Negative cognitions predict the course of bipolar depression, not mania. *Journal of Cognitive Psychotherapy, 18,* 149–162.

Johnson, S. L., & Fingerhut, R. (2006). Life events as predictors of relapse, depression, and mania in bipolar disorder. In S. Jones & R. Bentall (Eds.), *The psychology of bipolar disorder: New developments and research strategies* (pp. 47–72). Oxford, UK: Oxford University Press.

Johnson, S. L., Winett, C., Meyer, B., Greenhouse, W., & Miller, I. (1999). Social support and the course of bipolar disorder. *Journal of Abnormal Psychology, 108,* 558–566.

Johnson, S. L., Winters, R., & Meyer, B. (2006). A polarity-specific model of bipolar disorder. In T. Joiner, J. Brown, & J. Kistner (Eds.), *The interpersonal, cognitive, and social nature of depression* (pp. 153–171). Washington, DC: American Psychological Association.

Jones, S. H., Sellwood, W., & McGovern, J. (2005). Psychological therapies for bipolar disorder: The role of model-driven approaches to therapy integration. *Bipolar Disorders, 7,* 22–32.

Judd, L. L., Akiskal, H. S., Schettler, P. J., Endicott, J., Maser, J., Solomon, D. J., et al. (2002). The long-term natural history of the weekly symptomatic status of bipolar I disorder. *Archives of General Psychiatry, 59,* 530–545.

Karkowski, L. M., & Kendler, K. S. (1997). An examination of the genetic relationship between bipolar and unipolar illness in an epidemiological sample. *Psychiatric Genetics, 7,* 159–163.

Kessler, R. C., Rubinow, D. R., Holmes, C., Abelson, J. M., & Zhao, S. (1997). The epidemiology of DSM-III-R bipolar I disorder in a general population survey. *Psychological Medicine, 27,* 1079–1089.

Kim, E. Y., & Miklowitz, D. J. (2004). Expressed emotion as a predictor of outcome among bipolar patients undergoing family therapy. *Journal of Affective Disorders, 82,* 343–52.

Kim, E. Y., Miklowitz, D. J., Biuckians, A., & Mullen, K. (2007). *Life stress and the course of early-onset bipolar disorder.* Manuscript under review.

Lam, D. H., Hayward, P., Watkins, E. R., Wright, K., & Sham, P. (2005). Relapse prevention in patients with bipolar disorder: Cognitive therapy outcome after 2 years. *American Journal of Psychiatry, 162,* 324–329.

Lozano, B., & Johnson, S. L. (2001). Personality traits on the NEO-V as predictors of depression and mania. *Journal of Affective Disorders, 63,* 103–111.

Lyon, H. M., Startup, M., & Bentall, R. P. (1999). Social cognition and the manic defense: Attributions, selective attention, and self-schema in bipolar affective disorder. *Journal of Abnormal Psychology, 108,* 273–282.

Mackinger, H. F., Pachinger, M. M., Leibetseder, M. M., & Fartacek, R. R. (2000). Autobiographical memories in women remitted from major depression. *Journal of Abnormal Psychology, 109,* 331–334.

Maier, W., Minges, J., Lichtermann, D., Franke, P., & Gansicke, M. (1995). Personality patterns in subjects at risk for affective disorders. *Psychopathology, 28*, 59–72.

Malkoff-Schwartz, S., Frank, E., Anderson, B., Hlastala, S. A., Luther, J. F., Sherrill, J. T., et al. (2000). Social rhythm disruption and stressful life events in the onset of bipolar and unipolar episodes. *Psychological Medicine, 30*, 1005–1016.

Mansell, W., & Lam, D. (2004). A preliminary study of autobiographical memory in remitted bipolar and unipolar depression and the role of imagery in the specificity of memory. *Memory, 12*, 437–446.

Martinez-Arán, A., Vieta, E., Colom, F., Torrent, C., Sánchez-Moreno, J., Reinares, M., et al. (2004). Cognitive impairment in euthymic bipolar patients: Implications for clinical and functional outcome. *Bipolar Disorders, 6*, 224–232.

McGuffin, P., Rijsdijk, F., Andrew, M., Sham, P., Katz, R., & Cardno, A. (2003). The heritability of bipolar affective disorder and the genetic relationship to unipolar depression. *Archives of General Psychiatry, 6*, 497–502.

McPherson, H., Walsh, A., & Silverstone, T. (2003). Growth hormone and prolactin response to apomorphine in bipolar and unipolar depression. *Journal of Affective Disorders, 76*, 121–125.

Merikangas, K. R., Akiskal, H. S., Angst, J., Greenberg, P. E., Hirschfeld, R. M. A., Petukhova, M., et al. (2007). Lifetime and 12-month prevalence of bipolar spectrum disorder in the National Comorbidity Replication Survey. *Archives of General Psychiatry, 64*, 543–552.

Miklowitz, D. J., Simoneau, T. L., George, E. L., Richards, J. A., Kalbag, A., & Sachs-Ericsson, N. (2000). Family-focused treatment of bipolar disorder: 1-year effects of a psychoeducational program in conjunction with pharmacotherapy. *Biological Psychiatry, 48*, 582–592.

Murray, G., Goldstone, E., & Cunningham, E. (2007). Personality and the predisposition(s) to bipolar disorder: Heuristic benefits of a two-dimensional model. *Bipolar Disorders, 9*, 453–461.

Othmer, E., DeSouza, C. M., Penick, E. C., Nickel, E. J., Hunter, E. E., Othmer, S. C., et al. (2007). Indicators of mania in depressed outpatients: A retrospective analysis of data from the Kansas 1500 study. *Journal of Clinical Psychiatry, 68*, 47–51.

Parker, G., Roy, K., Wilhelm, K., Mitchell, P., & Hadzi-Pavlovic, D. (2000). The nature of bipolar depression: Implications for the definition melancholia. *Journal of Affective Disorders, 59*, 217–224.

Perlis, R. H., Brown, E., Baker, R. W., & Nierenberg, A. A. (2006). Clinical features of bipolar depression versus major depressive disorder in large multicenter trials. *American Journal of Psychiatry, 163*, 225–231.

Perlis, R. H., Smoller, J. W., Fava, M., Rosenbaum, J. F., Nierenberg, A. A., & Sachs, G. S. (2004). The prevalence and clinical correlates of anger attacks during depressive episodes in bipolar disorder. *Journal of Affective Disorders, 79*, 291–295.

Perris, H. (1984). Life events and depression: Part 2. Results in diagnostic subgroups and in relation to the recurrence of depression. *Journal of Affective Disorders, 7*, 25–36.

Plomin, R., DeFries, J. C., McClearn, G. E., & Rutter, M. (1997). *Behavioral genetics* (3rd ed.). New York: Freeman.

Quintin, P., Benkelfat, C., Launay, J. M., Arnulf, I., Pointereau-Bellenger, A., Barbault, S., et al. (2001). Clinical and neurochemical effect of acute tryptophan depletion in unaffected relatives of patients with bipolar affective disorder. *Biological Psychiatry, 50*, 184–190.

Regeer, E. J., Krabbendam, L., De-Graaf, R., Ten-Have, M., Nolen, W. A., & Van Os, J. (2006). A prospective study of the transition rates of subthreshold (hypo)mania and depression in the general population. *Psychological Medicine, 36*, 619–627.

Rubinsztein, J. S., Michael, A., Paykel, E. S., & Sahakian, B. J. (2000). Cognitive impairment in remission in bipolar affective disorder. *Psychological Medicine, 30*, 1025–1036.

Sato, T., Bottlender, R., Kleindienst, N., & Möller, H. J. (2002). Syndromes and phenomenological subtypes underlying acute mania: A factor analytic study of 576 manic patients. *American Journal of Psychiatry, 159*, 968–974.

Schweitzer, I., Maguire, K., & Ng, C. H. (2005). Should bipolar disorder be viewed as manic disorder?: Implications for bipolar depression. *Bipolar Disorders, 7*, 418–423.

Scott, J., & Pope, M. (2003). Cognitive styles in individuals with bipolar disorder. *Psychological Medicine, 33*, 1081–1088.

Scott, J., Stanton, B., Garland, A., & Ferrier, I. N. (2000). Cognitive vulnerability in patients with bipolar disorder. *Psychological Medicine, 30,* 467–472.

Serretti, A., Mandelli, L., Lattuada, E., Cusin, C., & Smeraldi, E. (2002). Clinical and demographic features of mood disorder subtypes. *Psychiatry Research, 112,* 195–210.

Sheline, Y. I., Barch, D. M., Donnelly, J. M., Ollinger, J. M., Snyder, A. Z., & Mintun, M. A. (2001). Increased amygdala response to masked emotional faces in depressed subjects resolves with antidepressant treatment: An fMRI study. *Biological Psychiatry, 50,* 651–658.

Sher, L., Oquendo, M. A., Li, S., Ellis, S., Brodsky, B. S., Malone, K. M., et al. (2003). Prolactin response to fenfluramine administration in patients with unipolar and bipolar depression and healthy controls. *Psychoneuroendocrinology, 28,* 559–573.

Sjostrom, R., & Roos, B. E. (1973). 5-Hydroxyindolacetic acid and homovanillic acid in cerebrospinal fluid in manic–depressive psychosis. *European Journal of Clinical Pharmacology, 4,* 170–176.

Smith, D. J., Harrison, N., Muir, W., & Blackwood, D. H. R. (2005). The high prevalence of bipolar spectrum disorders in young adults with recurrent depression: Toward an innovative diagnostic framework. *Journal of Affective Disorders, 84,* 167–178.

Sobczak, S., Honig, A., van Duinen, M. A., & Riedel, W. J. (2002). Serotonergic dysregulation in bipolar disorders: A literature review of serotonergic challenge studies. *Bipolar Disorders, 4,* 347–356.

Sobczak, S., Riedel, W. J., Booij, I., Het Rot, A. M., & Deutz, N. E. P. (2002). Cognition following acute tryptophan depletion: Difference between first-degree relatives of bipolar disorder patients and matched healthy control volunteers. *Psychological Medicine, 32,* 503–512.

Solomon, D. A., Leon, A. C., Endicott, J., Coryell, W. H., Mueller, T. I., Posternak, M. A., et al. (2003). Unipolar mania over the course of a 20-year follow-up study. *American Journal of Psychiatry, 160,* 2049–2051.

Solomon, D. A., Leon, A. C., Maser, J. D., Truman, C. J., Coryell, W., Endicott, J., et al. (2006). Distinguishing bipolar major depression from unipolar major depression with the Screening Assessment of Depression—Polarity (SAD-P). *Journal of Clinical Psychiatry, 67,* 434–442.

Stoll, A. L., Renshaw, P. F., Yurgelun-Todd, D. A., & Cohen, B. M. (2000). Neuroimaging in bipolar disorder: What have we learned? *Biological Psychiatry, 48,* 505–517.

Thomas, J., & Bentall, R. P. (2002). Hypomanic traits and response styles to depression. *British Journal of Clinical Psychology, 41,* 309–313.

Tracy, A., Bauwens, F., Martin, F., Pardoen, D., & Mendlowicz, J. (1992). Attributional style and depression: A controlled comparison of remitted unipolar and bipolar patients. *British Journal of Clinical Psychology, 31,* 83–84.

Wals, M., Hillegers, M. H. J., Reichart, C. G., Verhulst, F. C., Nolen, W. A., & Ormel, J. (2005). Stressful life events and onset of mood disorders in children of bipolar parents during 14-month follow-up. *Journal of Affective Disorders, 87,* 253–263.

Winokur, G., Coryell, W., Endicott, J., & Akiskal, H. (1993). Further distinctions between manic–depressive illness (bipolar disorder) and primary depressive disorder (unipolar depression). *American Journal of Psychiatry, 150,* 1176–1181.

Winokur, G., Coryell, W., Keller, M., Endicott, J., & Akiskal, H. (1993). A prospective follow-up of patients with bipolar and primary unipolar affective disorder. *Archives of General Psychiatry, 50,* 457–465.

Winokur, G., & Tsuang, M. T. (1996). *The natural history of mania, depression, and schizophrenia.* Washington, DC: American Psychiatric Press.

Winters, K. C., & Neale, J. (1985). Mania and low self-esteem. *Journal of Abnormal Psychology, 94,* 282–290.

Wolf, T., & Mueller-Oerlinghausen, B. (2002). The influence of successful prophylactic drug treatment on cognitive dysfunction in bipolar disorders. *Bipolar Disorders, 4,* 263–270.

Wozniak, K., Spencer, T., Biederman, J., Kwon, A., Monuteaux, M., & Rettew, J. (2004). The clinical characteristics of unipolar vs. bipolar major depression in ADHD youth. *Journal of Affective Disorders, 82,* 59–69.

Wu, J., & Bunney, W. E. (1991). The biological basis of an antidepressant response to sleep deprivation and relapse: Review and hypothesis. *American Journal of Psychiatry, 147,* 14–21.

Yan, L. J., Hammen, C., Cohen, A. N., Daley, S. E., & Henry, R. M. (2004). Expressed emotion versus relationship quality variables in the prediction of recurrence in bipolar patients. *Journal of Affective Disorders, 83,* 199–206.

Yatham, L. N., Liddle, P. F., Shiah, I., Scarrow, G., Lam, R. W., Adam, M. J., et al. (2000). Brain serotonin$_2$ receptors in major depression: A positron emission tomography study. *Archives of General Psychiatry, 57,* 850–858.

Yurgelun-Todd, D. A., Gruber, S. A., Kanayama, G., Killgore, W. D., Baird, A. A., & Young, A. D. (2000). fMRI during affect discrimination in bipolar affective disorder. *Bipolar Disorders, 2,* 237–248.

PART II

VULNERABILITY, RISK, AND MODELS OF DEPRESSION

Many approaches have been taken by theorists in attempts to understand the origins of depression. Whereas some of these theories involve genetics and biological functioning, other approaches focus on personal characteristics of individuals who are believed to be vulnerable to depressive episodes, and on aspects of the social environments that are hypothesized to increase risk for depression. The eight chapters in this section describe approaches and models developed to explain vulnerability and risk for unipolar depression. Levinson describes (Chapter 8) the genetic foundations of depression and discusses results of studies that have examined the heritability of this disorder. Continuing with a focus on biological factors in depression Thase (Chapter 9) and by Davidson, Pizzagalli, and Nitschke (Chapter 10) describe biological aspects of depressive disorders. Whereas Thase focuses on the role of neurotransmitters in the onset and maintenance of depression, Davidson and colleagues describe neuroanatomical structures and the neural circuitry that has recently been implicated in this disorder. Goodman and Brand (Chapter 11) also discuss biological aspects of vulnerability to depression, but broaden the focus to include psychosocial factors early in life that appear to increase risk for depression. Hammen (Chapter 12) reviews the growing literature that documents the adverse effects of parental depression on children's functioning, focusing on methodological issues in this research, and on mechanisms and mediators of the effects of parental depression. Joormann (Chapter 13) describes the large body of research examining cognitive models of vulnerability to depression and recent work using paradigms adapted from experimental cognitive psychology to assess information processing in depression. Joiner and Timmons (Chapter 14) describe aspects of the interpersonal context of depression, and Monroe, Slavich, and Georgiades (Chapter 15) complement this chapter by adopting a diathesis–stress perspective in examining the social environment of depressed individuals.

CHAPTER 8

Genetics of Major Depression

Douglas F. Levinson

Increasingly powerful molecular-genetics methodologies are being applied to the search for specific genetic sequence variations that increase one's risk of developing complex disorders and traits—*complex* meaning that they are influenced by multiple genetic and nongenetic factors rather than by a single dominant or recessive gene. Major depressive disorder (MDD) and depression-related personality traits are among the most common targets of this research. The purpose of this chapter is to introduce the reader to the epidemiological data that motivate current research strategies and to the methodologies employed, then to review genetic association and linkage studies of depression and related traits. The chapter closes with a discussion of future directions in research on the genetics of depression.

On a *clinical* level, the conceptualization of *phenotypes* (definitions of measurable, heritable categories and dimensions) for genetic studies rests on four lines of research. The most important of these is the series of *family and twin studies* that established modern psychiatric diagnostic criteria based on specific signs, symptoms, and longitudinal course (Research Diagnostic Criteria [RDC] in 1975, *Diagnostic and Statistical Manual of Mental Disorders* [DSM-III] in 1979, and *International Classification of Diseases* [ICD-10] in 1990). These categories were validated primarily by demonstration of elevated risks in relatives and in twins (i.e., in *monozygotic*, or identical, twins more than in *dizygotic* twins) of *probands* (index cases) from the same category and were at least partially independent of other categories in terms of familial risks. These criteria dramatically influenced depression research: They separated unipolar depression from bipolar disorder; defined MDD as a combination of affective, cognitive, and physiological features; and replaced previous definitions of *neurotic* and *reactive* depression, which confused the clinician's causal theory with objective signs and symptoms. This approach, while imperfect, reflects dramatic advances in knowledge.

Operationalized diagnostic categories have received support from studies of evolving *pharmacological* treatments. MDD criteria have proven to be reasonably predictive of response to antidepressant drugs or electroconvulsive therapy; lithium, a remarkably effective acute and preventive treatment for mania, was much less effective for acute depression and not at all effective for schizophrenia. Although the pharmacological evidence generally supported the separation of bipolar disorder from unipolar depression, as well as from schizophrenia, it is important to note that no drug is specific to a diagnosis; consequently, diagnoses remain imperfect predictors of drug response.

Personality research consistently identifies a higher-order factor related to a general tendency toward experiencing more negative (dysphoric, anxious, phobic) emotional responses. As measured by Eysenck's (1967) *neuroticism* scales, this trait has a heritability of 40–50%, is reasonably stable across adult life, and is a significant predictor of future onset of MDD, with an approximately 55% overlap of the genetic risk factors for MDD and for neuroticism (reviewed in Fanous & Kendler, 2004). These common genetic factors seem to extend to generalized anxiety disorder, less strongly to panic disorder and social phobia, but not to obsessive–compulsive disorder or simple phobias (Hettema, Prescott, Myers, Neale, & Kendler, 2005; Mineka, Watson, & Clark, 1998). Thus, some genetic studies target neuroticism scores or combined measures of depressive and anxiety symptoms.

The risk of major depression during adulthood has also been shown to be increased by traumatic childhood experiences such as physical and sexual abuse, emotional neglect, family disorganization, and parental loss (Kendler, Kuhn, & Prescott, 2004). A major issue for future genetic research is to determine whether and how these experiences interact with genes in influencing risk. For example, do certain combinations of genotypes have their greatest effect on risk in people who have experienced trauma? It is becoming more common for investigators to measure these nongenetic factors directly (and sometimes prospectively) in large-scale twin studies, so that the effects of genes, environment, and *gene–environment interactions* can be estimated, and in genetic association studies, in which interactions with specific genotypes can be analyzed. Unless environmental factors are measured, standard twin heritability estimates attribute to genes the portion of the variance that is actually due to an interaction of genes with shared environment (whether physiological or psychological) (Heath et al., 2002). Thus, it is likely that as more powerful technologies are applied to large samples in which environmental variables have also been measured, it will be possible to achieve a more complex understanding of gene–environment interactions.

Four major *molecular*-genetics methodologies are now being applied to the study of major depression: genomewide linkage and association, candidate gene association, and large-scale resequencing.

A *linkage* study requires assays of hundreds or thousands of DNA markers in families with combinations of two or more ill relatives whose relationships to each other permit statistical analysis of whether a particular DNA sequence variant (*allele*) has been inherited by ill individuals more frequently than would be expected by chance. Or, for a continuous trait such as neuroticism, one can test all available relatives or pairs drawn from the same or opposite extremes of the distribution. Depending on the size of the genetic effect and of the sample, linkage analysis can identify the approximate locations of susceptibility genes (e.g., pointing to regions of 50–200 genes). Further studies of specific genes can then be undertaken. Starting in the late 1980s, there have been multiple linkage studies of disorders with high heritability estimates (80% or greater), such as schizophrenia and bipolar disorder. Investigators avoided MDD, with its lower heritability (40–70%, see below) and presumed high etiological heterogeneity. Gradually, clinical methods were developed for recruiting and assessing larger numbers of families, and advances in molecular, statistical, and computational technologies made larger studies feasible. Thus, several large linkage studies of MDD and related traits have now been carried out.

The selection of a *candidate gene* requires either linkage evidence or an etiological hypothesis (e.g., antidepressants alter monoamine neurotransmission; therefore, genes involved in these systems might influence risk of depression). Most MDD candidate gene studies have considered a small number of *functional polymorphisms* (DNA sequence variations that alter protein chemistry or gene expression levels) in key genes in monoaminergic pathways. More recently, it has become possible to study genes more comprehensively. The HapMap Project (International HapMap Consortium, 2003) has catalogued many of the common sequence variants in the genome—those found on more than 5% of chromosomes. Because nearby single nucleotide polymorphisms (SNPs) are often correlated (i.e., the variant present at one location predicts the nearby variant), most common variation in a gene can be assayed with a subset of known SNPs (*tag SNPs*) (Gabriel et al., 2002). Despite the promise of this methodology, however, few studies of depression have been carried out using comprehensive tag SNP sets for candidate genes or for chromosomal candidate regions in large clinical samples.

Genomewide association (GWA) studies of MDD and related traits are currently being conducted. The HapMap project was based on the *common disease–common variant* hypothesis (Lander, 1996): Because most of the DNA sequence variation in any one human genome is "old" (i.e., most surviving mutations occurred hundreds of thousands or millions of years ago) and relatively common (i.e., 5% or more of chromosomes carry the evolutionarily more recent variant), it is likely that some, rather than most, of the more common complex human diseases are influenced by common variants. There are now genotyping technologies that can screen thousands of subjects (cases vs. controls, or constellations of family members) using 500,000–1,000,000 SNPs, providing information (directly or by correlation) about most of the common SNPs in the genome. Highly significant genetic associations have already been discovered with these methods for such diseases as type II diabetes (Frayling, 2007), Crohn's disease (Mathew, 2008) and cancer (Savage & Greene, 2007). These assays also detect deletions and duplications of short or long stretches of DNA (*copy number variants* [CNVs]), which are common in the genome and are believed to contribute to disease risks in some cases (McCarroll & Altshuler, 2007).

A related and complementary hypothesis suggests that rare genetic variants are likely to influence common diseases (i.e., there could be many different rare sequence variations that alter the function of a gene or a pathway of interacting genes). *Resequencing* (determining the sequence of an individual's DNA) of each gene in many people would be required to determine whether rare variants are more common in ill individuals. New technologies are making large-scale resequencing studies possible for the first time, and resequencing of entire genomes might be cost-effective in the future.

GENETIC EPIDEMIOLOGY OF MDD

MDD is a common disorder: The lifetime prevalence is at least 10%, with the risk in females twice that in males (Moldin, Reich, & Rice, 1991; see Kessler & Wang, Chapter 1, this volume). Twin studies suggest that genes account for 40–50% of the susceptibility to MDD in the population (reviewed in Sullivan, Neale, & Kendler, 2000), although heritability might be higher in clinically identified probands (e.g., McGuffin, Katz, Watkins, & Rutherford, 1996). In fact, heritability was estimated to be as high as 70% when subjects were interviewed twice, then diagnosed with MDD, if during either interview they recalled an episode at some point during their life (Kendler, Neale, Kessler, Heath, & Eaves, 1993). Adoption studies also support the operation of genetic factors (Sullivan et al., 2000). Studies of MDD in families have been inconclusive about how it is inherited, but multiple genes likely interact to increase an individual's susceptibility (Moldin et al., 1991). As noted above, part of the genetic effect on depression risk is probably due to specific gene–environment interactions.

The power of a genetic study to detect a specific, risk-altering locus depends in part on how much that locus increases the risk of the disease in the population (Risch, 1987). This is commonly measured as relative risk (RR), the risk of the disease in first-degree relatives of ill probands divided by the risk in the general population (which should be estimated from control families using the same clinical methodology). The overall RR for MDD is 2–3 (Sullivan et al., 2000), probably resulting from the interaction of several or many genes, so that each contributes a small increase in risk. This seems generally to be the case for common, genetically complex disorders: Successful association studies are detecting specific sequence variants that increase risk by perhaps 15–30%. It is generally assumed that genetic studies should target phenotypes that predict the largest possible total RR, in the hope that this also maximizes the RR attributable to any single factor.

Three characteristics of MDD probands have generally been shown to predict a larger increase in risk to their relatives: recurrent episodes (see Sullivan et al., 2000); earlier age at onset (AO) (reviewed in Levinson et al., 2003); and severity, as indexed by the number of MDD criteria endorsed by each subject (Kendler, Gatz, Gardner, & Pedersen, 2007). Whereas there has been a consensus in the field that recurrence is a strong predictor of familial risk, investigators' assessments of the predictive effect of AO have differed. According to my reading of the literature, RR is not substantially above 1 for the relatives of probands with AO after the age of 40, and it rises significantly as the proband's AO drops from the 30s to the 20s, to the teens, and particularly to the pre-pubertal period (although there also appears to be a subset of individuals with onset of depression during adolescence, without recurrence in adulthood, so this conclusion appears more applicable to those with at least one adult episode). It is important to note, however, that the combined effects of AO and recurrence have generally not been studied in large, population-based samples. Recently, Kendler and colleagues (2007) reported that in a sample of almost 14,000 adult twin pairs from the Swedish National Twin Registry, AO, recurrence, and number of endorsed criteria each modestly predicted increased familial risk, but RR was not computed directly. Other data suggest that the RR of MDD with both recurrence *and* early onset (MDD-RE) could be as high as 4–5 (Levinson et al., 2003), which makes this an attractive phenotype for genetic studies (see the later discussion of linkage studies); not all investigators, however, select on these variables.

Unipolar and bipolar (BP) mood disorders may share at least some genetic determinants, given the increased risk of MDD in the relatives of probands with bipolar disorder. On the other hand, relatives of MDD probands are not at increased risk of *bipolar I disorder* (BP-I) (episodes meeting full manic criteria, including functional role impairment; Maier et al., 1993). Given that MDD is much more common than BP, it seems likely that much of the genetic susceptibility to MDD is independent of that of BP. Research evidence fails to support the anecdotal clinical observation that patients with BP have different symptom patterns (e.g., excessive rather than reduced sleep and appetite) (Blacker, Lavori, Faraone, & Tsuang, 1993). Some early studies suggested that there could be a genetic relation between MDD and bipolar II disorder (BP-II) (recurrent major depression plus mild, brief manic episodes without gross impairment; Endicott et al., 1985; Gershon et al., 1982), but the issue has not been addressed adequately by well-controlled family studies. It remains for future findings in molecular genetics to clarify the extent to which common versus distinct genetic factors underlie MDD, BP-I, and BP-II.

Another unexplained finding is that in several large, well-designed family studies, a higher lifetime risk of MDD has been observed in first-degree relatives of probands with schizophrenia than in relatives of control probands (Gershon et al., 1982; Maier et al., 1993). Maier and colleagues (1993) found that this result could not be explained by confounding factors such as assortative mating, an atypical symptom profile in these relatives, or emergence of MDD after the onset of schizophrenia in the proband (a likely stressor for relatives). Relatives of probands with MDD are not at increased risk of schizophrenia, although there is some evidence for familial cosegregation of schizophrenia and MDD with psychotic features.

ASSOCIATION STUDIES OF CANDIDATE GENES

Monoaminergic Candidate Genes

Most candidate gene studies of depression and related traits have focused on functional polymorphisms in a small set of genes involved in monoaminergic neurotransmission. Most of these genes are involved in the synthesis, degradation, or neurotransmission of serotonin (5-hydroxytryptamine, 5-HT). The single most widely studied gene (*SLC6A4*, also known as *5-HTT*) encodes the serotonin transporter, which affects the "reuptake" of serotonin back into the presynaptic (releasing) cell. This site is blocked by many antidepressant drugs, including the serotonin-specific reuptake inhibitor (SSRI) class, thus increasing the amount of serotonin that remains in the synaptic space during the first several weeks of antidepressant treatment, before other mechanisms produce a new homeostasis (Goodnick & Goldstein, 1998). Other genes relevant to monoaminergic systems that have been studied include those encoding the 5-HT_{2A} receptor (5HTR2A), *tyrosine hydroxylase* (*TH*, an enzyme necessary for dopamine synthesis), *tryptophan hydroxylase* (*TPH1* and *TPH2* isoforms, enzymes involved in serotonin synthesis, with *TPH2* active in brain), catechol-*o*-methyltransferase (COMT, an enzyme that degrades dopamine) and the dopamine (D_4) receptor (DRD4).

5-HTTLPR, Depression, and Stress

The single most-studied variant is 5-HTTLPR (5-HT-linked promoter region), a 44-base pair (bp) insertion–deletion polymorphism in *SLC6A4*. Almost all studies have analyzed counts or genotypes for the two alleles (variants) defined by the presence (long, or L allele) or absence (short, or S allele) of the insertion sequence. S alleles produce fewer transporter molecules that bind less serotonin, and this should decrease reuptake capacity (Lesch et al., 1996). Many antidepressants (including SSRIs) block this same reuptake site, and these drugs have diverse effects on mood, anxiety, cognition, and behavior. Thus, it is reasonable to predict that this DNA variant will have some significant effects on mood and behavior.

However, most studies have not considered other variants in *SLC6A4* that have substantial effects on gene expression or function, other than an intronic variable number of tandem repeats (VNTR) polymorphism described at the same time as 5-HTTLPR and also affecting expression. More recently, an adenine/guanine (A/G) SNP (rs25531) was described (Hu et al., 2006; Nakamura, Ueno, Sano, & Tanabe, 2000) that is apparently within the 5-HTTLPR L allele sequence. The L_G allele variant is found on approximately 10% of chromosomes in European populations (24% in African Americans) and shows reduced activity similar to that of the S allele. Martin, Cleak, Willis-Owen, Flint, and Shifman (2007) identified 55 SNPs in or near the gene and measured expression levels of the gene transcript in lymphocytes from subjects with different genotypes at combinations of these SNPs and of 5-HTTLPR. Two SNPs (rs2020933 and rs16965628) were highly correlated with each other and predicted expression levels more strongly than did 5-HTTLPR. It is important to note, however, that only around 10% of individuals carry one of these SNPs, whereas a majority carry the 5-HTTLPR S allele. Martin and colleagues could not confirm reduced expression in L_G carriers, although the sample size for this comparison was small. It is not clear how the results of 5-HTTLPR association studies will be altered when genotypes at rs25531 and rs2020933/rs16965628 are incorporated into more analyses. Furthermore, neither Shioe and colleagues (2003) nor Parsey and colleagues (2006) could demonstrate an effect of biallelic or triallelic 5-HTTLPR genotype (respectively) on serotonin binding in the brain.

Meta-analyses have failed to detect an association between L/S alleles or genotypes and MDD diagnosis (Table 8.1). Meta-analyses have reported an association of S alleles or S/S genotypes with neuroticism, but two analyses supported association only for neuroticism as measured by the NEO Personality Inventory, and not for the related but not identical dimension of harm avoidance (Schinka, Busch, & Robichaux-Keene, 2004; Sen, Burmeister, & Ghosh, 2004), whereas a third analysis was positive only for harm avoidance (Munafo, Clark, & Flint, 2005). More recently, Willis-Owen, Turri, and colleagues (2005) were unable to detect any association between neuroticism scores and either 5-HTTLPR or rs2020933 in a large sample of subjects drawn from the extremes of the neuroticism distribution in over 80,000 subjects from a population sample; and Middeldorp and colleagues (2007) found no association of 5-HTTLPR with neuroticism or other measures of depression or anxiety in families with over 1,200 offspring from a twin registry. These reports cast doubt on the hypothesis that there is any very substantial association between 5-HTTLPR and trait measures of proneness to anxiety and depression. Several meta-analyses have suggested an association between S alleles and suicidal behavior, although most of the evidence for this association came from subjects with alcoholism rather than from mood disorder subjects (reviewed in Levinson, 2005).

A more provocative and influential set of findings has emerged from studies testing the hypothesis that there is a significant interaction among 5-HTTLPR alleles or genotypes, depression, and stress (gene–environment interaction). In 847 subjects whose development was followed from ages 3 to 26, Caspi and colleagues (2003) reported that the number of stressful life events between ages 21 and 25 predicted a subsequent major depressive episode (or increase in depressive symptoms), and that individuals with more S alleles were more likely to experience depression after stress ($p < .05$ for scores, $p = .056$ for MDD diagnosis). S alleles also were reported to predict the probability of depression in people with higher ratings of childhood maltreatment between ages 3 and 11. Consistent with the meta-analyses described earlier, depression diagnosis was not predicted by genotype alone. Thus, the study supported an effect of 5-HTTLPR genotype on stress reactivity rather than directly on depression (a point that seems to be missed in most media and some academic reports).

Many studies now support this hypothesis. There are some negative studies, and there is some inconsistency in results: is the relevant genetic factor the number of S (or low activity) alleles, or the S/S or low/low genotype, and are S or S/S individuals most different in their response to a single stress or low-stress event (Cervilla et al., 2007; Kendler, Kuhn, Vittum, Prescott, & Riley, 2005), or do they show enhanced response as the number of stressors or the severity of stress increases? But the number of studies supporting some kind of mediation of stress response by this polymorphism suggests that there is a real effect. Positive findings include increased onsets of depressive episodes after stressful events in S carriers

TABLE 8.1. Meta-Analyses of Mood Disorder Genetic Association Studies

Polymorphism	Disorder	Ref	Studies	Cases/cont	Effect	OR	CI	p	Het	Pub bias	Comments
HTR2A T102C	MDD c-c	a	7	768/959	Alleles	0.96	0.84–1.11	NS	NS	NS	
SLC6A4											
5-HTTLPR	MDD c-c	b	14	1,961/3,402	S	1.05	0.96–1.14	NS	+	NS	No effect of ethnicity
	MDD c-c	c	10	910/2,017	S; each GT				+		Europeans: S/S OR = 1.16 (p < .05), dependent on one study; NS due to multiple tests
Neuroticism/Harm avoid		d,e	23	5,629	NEO+TPQ			.087	+	NS	T-scores (mean 50, SD 10)
					NEO only (10)			.000016			
Neuroticism (NEO)		f	11	2,231*				NS			Also NS for GT, dom or rec
Harm avoid (TPQ)			13	2,598*	SS vs. SL+LL			.0021			Also p = .0082 for SS vs. LL
Intron 2 VNTR	MDD c-c	b	9	1,817/653	Length (contin)	0.99	0.92–1.06	NS	NS	NS	
		c	11	706/2,242	9,10,12 rpts			NS	NS	NS	Each allele NS for Asian, Eur separately
TH tetranucleotide repeat	MDD	g	3	204/359	Alleles 2,3,4,5			NS	NS		
DRD4 48 bp rpt	MDD c-c	h	12	318/814	2-rpt allele	1.73	1.29–2.32	<.003	+		Corrected for multiple testing

Note. All studies used random- and/or fixed-effects meta-analysis methods. Ref, reference; cont, controls; OR, odds ratio; CI, 95% confidence interval; contin, allele length analyzed as continuous variable; c-c, case–control studies only; Eur, European; GT, genotype; rpt, repeat; Harm avoid, harm avoidance; Het, test for heterogeneity among studies; NS, not statistically significant; NEO, NEO Personality Inventory; TPQ, Tridimensional Personality Questionnaire; S, short alleles; SL, short/long genotype; LL, long/long genotype.

References: *a*—Anguelova, Benkelfat, and Turecki (2003); *b*—Lasky-Su, Faraone, Glatt, and Tsuang (2005); *c*—Lotrich and Pollock (2004); *d*—data shown are from Sen, Burmeister, and Ghosh (2004); *e*—similar conclusions reached by Schinka, Busch, and Robichaux-Keene (2004), details not shown; *f*—Munafo, Clark, and Flint (2005); *g*—Furlong et al. (1999); *h*—López-León et al. (2005).

*Analysis included only general population samples (no patient samples), and excluded studies with deviation from Hardy–Weinberg equilibrium.

(Kim et al., 2007; Zalsman et al., 2006) or with S/S genotypes (Cervilla et al., 2007; Jacobs et al., 2006; Kendler et al., 2005; Wilhelm et al., 2006); S alleles or S/S genotypes predicting increased depression in members of alcoholism families who reported unemployment, relationship problems, or poor health (Dick et al., 2007); higher depression scores in maltreated children, if they lacked social supports (Kaufman et al., 2004); increased adrenocorticotropic hormone (ACTH) response to separation in female (but not male) rhesus monkeys with previous adversity (Barr et al., 2004); increased history of adult suicide attempts in psychiatric inpatients with histories of childhood sexual and physical abuse (Gibb, McGeary, Beevers, & Miller, 2006); and increased depression, perceived stress, and excreted norepinephrine in patients with chronic coronary disease (Otte, McCaffery, Ali, & Whooley, 2007).

There are also reports, however, that raise questions about these findings. Gillespie, Whitfield, Williams, Heath, and Martin (2004) reported that in 1,206 twins, stress predicted MDD, but with no interaction with 5-HTTLPR genotype. Jacobs and colleagues (2006) suggested that this might be due to the older age of this sample. Chorbov and colleagues (2007) reported increased depression following stress in young adult twins with *high* activity genotypes (L_A/L_A, L_A/S, L_A/L_G). In a small study, Taylor and colleagues (2006) reported that the S/S genotype was associated with *more* depression in individuals who reported early adversity, but S/S individuals without early adversity were *less* likely to develop depression—a puzzling finding. In a careful prospective study, Jacobs and colleagues reported that whereas S/S genotype predicted increased depression after stress, this effect was related to the presence of neuroticism, a finding that is not supported by other, large, recent studies of neuroticism, as described earlier.

If this effect is real, then what is its mechanism? Several imaging findings support the possible neurobiological relevance of carrying S alleles. Hariri and colleagues (2005) have reported increased amygdala activation (measured by functional magnetic resonance imaging [fMRI]) in response to aversive stimuli in S allele carriers. Dannlowski and colleagues (2007) supported this finding for polymorphisms in 5-HTT and 5-HT1A (a step toward testing hypotheses that extend beyond 5-HTTLPR). Hickie and colleagues (2007) reported smaller caudate (but not amygdala or hippocampal) volumes in S carriers with major depression. But neurochemically, the effect seems paradoxical: Short alleles are less active, which should have an effect similar to that of antidepressant drug treatment, which typically reduces the risk of depressive episodes, with or without stress. Hariri and colleagues suggested an explanation based on downstream postsynaptic effects, and Gotlib, Joorman, Minor, and Hallmayer (2008) reported that adolescent girls with S/S genotypes showed increased cortisol responses to laboratory stress. The exact mechanism of this apparent set of gene–environment interactions remains unclear.

Other Monoaminergic Candidate Genes

TPH is an attractive candidate gene, because it is a key enzyme in the synthesis of serotonin; thus, genetically induced changes in enzyme activity could plausibly influence mood. In response to reports of association between SNPs in the *TPH* (*TPH1*) gene and suicidal behavior, several meta-analyses had reported a lack of overall association (see Levinson, 2005). Whereas the most recent meta-analyses claimed to support an association, it is likely that the number of tests performed on the data would overwhelm any positive finding (see Li & He, 2006, for a recent analysis and a review of previous studies). More recently, Zill, Baghai, and colleagues (2004) reported that the *TPH2* isoform is predominant in the brain, and that MDD is associated with one of 10 *TPH2* SNPs and with SNP haplotypes in 300 patients with MDD compared to 265 controls. Association of the same SNP was observed in 263 suicide completers compared to controls (Zill, Buttner, et al., 2004). The finding was a "protective" effect associated with intronic (noncoding) SNPs (lower frequency of associated variants in cases). There have been both positive and negative studies, as reviewed recently by López de Lara and colleagues (2007), who reported evidence in favor of the association, and Mann and colleagues (2008), who reported negative data and also reviewed mixed evidence regarding possible association of *TPH2* with bipolar disorder. No meta-analysis is available, because different SNPs were genotyped in different studies. Zhang and colleagues (2005) reported a loss-of-function polymorphism in *TPH2*, which they found in only a small subset of MDD cases and not in controls, but three collaborative studies totaling thousands of cases and controls were unable to find this polymorphism in any subject (Glatt et al., 2005; Van Den Bogaert et al., 2005; Zhou et al., 2005).

The other serotonin-related gene that has been studied frequently is *5HTR2A*, the gene encoding the serotonin 2A receptor. A meta-analysis of seven studies failed to support association of the T102C functional polymorphism in this gene to MDD (Anguelova, Benkelfat, & Turecki, 2003). Li, Duan, and He (2006) reported that in studies of suicidal ideation and suicide attempts, meta-analysis produced no significant evidence for association with the functional T102C polymorphism in the 25 included studies, but there was some support for association of the A-1483G promoter polymorphism, although in only seven studies, and only for one genotypic split but a test of allele frequencies. López León and colleagues (2005) have also reported support for association of MDD with the 2-repeat allele of the 48-bp variable repeat site in *DRD4* (encoding the D_4 receptor) in a meta-analysis of 12 studies, but the analysis included only 318 MDD cases. There are many other genes in which polymorphisms have been studied by one or several groups, but with no recent meta-analyses to assess the evidence across studies. The interested reader is also referred to the growing literature on monoamine-related gene polymorphisms and antidepressant responsiveness (reviewed by Perlis, 2007), which is beyond the scope of this review.

Other Candidate Gene Findings

An intriguing hypothesis about the etiology of major depression is that neurotoxic effects (possibly related to excessive corticotropin activity and/or to inflammatory effects of cytokines) damage or kill hippocampal cells, which in turn mediates many depressive symptoms, with deficient function of neuroprotective peptides possibly constituting one of the genetic predispositions, and with antidepressants enhancing these neuroprotective effects (Manji, Drevets, & Charney, 2001). *Brain-derived neurotrophic factor* (BDNF) is one such neuroprotective protein. There were initial reports of reduced serum BDNF in MDD (Karege et al., 2002) and of an association between polymorphisms in BDNF and BP (Neves-Pereira et al., 2002; Sklar et al., 2002). There was also a report of association between the *Val66Met* polymorphism and neuroticism (Sen et al., 2003), although a large subsequent study produced negative results (Willis-Owen, Fullerton, et al., 2005). Subsequent studies of BDNF in mood disorders have produced inconsistent results (reviewed by Levinson, 2006). Surtees and colleagues (2007) reported more recently that *Val66Met* did not predict mood status in a community sample of 7,389 individuals, of whom 1,214 reported a positive lifetime history of MDD. Similar results were observed in a community sample of 568 individuals (Grünblatt et al., 2006). No meta-analysis is available for MDD.

Angiotensin-converting enzyme (ACE) was proposed as a candidate gene for MDD for two reasons. Angiotension influences blood pressure via the hypothalamic–pituitary axis, which is known to be dysregulated in patients with MDD; thus, it could influence depression-related processes as well. Also, an association between MDD and a functional insertion–deletion polymorphism in *ACE* was reported in a small sample (Arinami et al., 1996). A recent meta-analysis did not support association for this polymorphism (López-León et al., 2006). A recent study of a more comprehensive set of common SNPs in *ACE* did provide some support for association to a SNP in the gene promoter region, which also appeared to be weakly associated with increased cortisol response to corticotropin-releasing hormone (CRH) (Baghai et al., 2006). In this analysis, a deviation from expected genotype distributions was observed in controls, which was found to be due not to genotyping error but was attributed to the exclusion of individuals with depression from the control group. This finding will require replication.

There is some evidence supporting an association between MDD and the *methylenetetrahydrofolate reductase encoding (MTHFR)* gene, an enzyme involved in the degradation of homocysteine, although meta-analysis fails to support a significant association (Zintzaras, 2006). The gene is of interest, because increases in homocysteine are thought to predispose to vascular inflammation and heart disease, which may in turn be associated with depression (see Freedland & Carney, Chapter 6, this volume). The *P2RX7* gene, which was reported to be associated with BP in a study of the genetically isolated population of Lac St. Jean, Québec (Barden et al., 2006), has also been reported to be weakly associated with MDD in a German case–control sample (Lucae et al., 2006). Hashimoto and colleagues (2006) reported a weak association between MDD and a functional polymorphism in *DISC1* (*dysbindin-1*), a gene that has reportedly been associated with schizophrenia. Svenningsson and colleagues (2006) suggested that the *p11* gene, which encodes a member of the S100 protein family, should be considered a candidate gene for MDD based on compelling evidence that it is involved with serotonergic transmission, interacts with 5-HT_{1B} receptors, is underexpressed in a mouse model of depression and in postmortem brain tissue from MDD patients, and is overexpressed after administration of antidepressants or electroconvulsive therapy. But no evidence for association was observed in a resequencing and tag SNP study of a sample of 640 MDD cases versus 650 controls (Verma et al., 2007). Finally, in a region of chromosome 12, where Abkevich and colleagues (2003) reported strong evidence for genetic linkage of MDD in males, Harlan and colleagues (2006) referred to evidence (apparently as yet unpublished) for *APAF1* (encoding *apoptosis protease activating factor 1*) as an MDD candidate gene in these families based on resequencing, and demonstrated that the putatively implicated mutation increases apoptotic activity, an interesting potential mechanism. Evaluation of the finding awaits publication of the association evidence.

GENETIC LINKAGE STUDIES

Table 8.2 summarizes the samples and phenotype definitions of genomewide linkage studies of MDD and of depression-related traits. Most of the MDD scans attempted to select families based on features that predict higher relative risk. Zubenko and colleagues (2003), for example, selected MDD probands with recurrence, as well as AO before age 25, then analyzed data using narrower or broader criteria for relatives. Holmans and colleagues (2007) selected probands with recurrent MDD with AO before age 31 and relatives with AO before age 41, and McGuffin and colleagues (2005) selected probands and siblings with recurrent

TABLE 8.2. Linkage Studies of Major Depression and Neuroticism-Related Personality Traits

First author (year)	Families	Cases	Phenotype(s)
MDD			
Zubenko et al. (2003)	81	NA	MDD-RE, MDD-R, "major" mood disorders, "all" mood disorders, "depressive spectrum" disorders"; sex and "2q linkage" as covariates
Utah study[a]			
Abkevich (2003)	110	1,107	MDD or BP-I or BP-II
Camp (2005)	87 (19–112)[b]	75–718[b]	MDD-RE; MDD-RE or anxiety disorder; MDD-RE plus anxiety disorder; secondary analysis divided by sex
Holmans (2007)	656	1,748	MDD-RE
McGuffin (2005)	412	891	MDD-R
Personality		*n* (genotyped)	
Cloninger (1998)	105	987	Harm avoidance (in alcoholism pedigrees)
Fullerton (2003)	561	1,122	Neuroticism; extreme concordant–discordant pairs drawn from a population sample of 88,141
Nash (2004)	283	757	Composite index of anxiety and depression; neuroticism; extreme concordant–discordant pairs drawn from a population sample of 6,387 sibships)
Neale (2005)	129	343	Neuroticism (families ascertained for nicotine dependence)
Kuo (2007)	486	1,022	Neuroticism (families ascertained for alcohol dependence)

Note. Shown are the sample characteristics and phenotype definitions in linkage genome scans of major depression and of neuroticism and related personality traits. MDD-RE, recurrent, early-onset MDD (onset before age 25 in Zubenko et al.; before age 31 in Holmans et al. [before 41 for cases other than probands] and in Camp et al.); MDD-R, recurrent MDD (Fullerton et al. studied pairs in which each sib was in the top or bottom 2.5th percentile of scores; Nash et al. selected the 10% "most informative" pairs); NA, not available.

[a]Abkevich et al. and Camp et al. drew their pedigrees from the same Utah sample. Abkevich et al. considered all MDD cases plus BP-I and BP-II as affected, and selected families with four or more such cases. Camp et al. considered MDD-RE cases (and/or, in alternative analyses, all DSM-IV anxiety disorders) as affected, excluded BP cases, and selected families with three or more MDD-RE cases.

[b]Eighty-seven large families were studied. *p*-values were corrected for multiple testing: For each of three diagnostic models, pedigrees were split for analysis by limiting the genealogies to 3, 4, 5, or 6 generations. The *n* of "independent" families and of "affected" cases varied with diagnostic model and genealogical rule.

MDD (and the average AO turned out to be similar to that in the Holmans et al. [2007] studies). Two of the reports (Abkevich et al., 2003; Camp et al., 2005) were based on the same sample of families recruited in Utah. The families were identified on the basis of an MDD proband and multiple relatives with MDD, but because these were large families in which distant relatives could often be recruited, relatives with BP-I and BP-II disorders were often identified and were included in the sample. Abkevich and colleagues (2003) analyzed linkage in males and females separately, including all MDD and BP cases. Camp and colleagues (2005) then reanalyzed the data after excluding BP relatives, defining MDD-RE in terms of recurrence and onset before age 31, and considering three alternative phenotypes (MDD-RE; MDD-RE *or* any anxiety disorder; MDD-RE *plus* any anxiety disorder). Note that they grouped all anxiety disorders together, regardless of the weight of evidence for genetic relatedness to depressive disorders. Nevertheless, most of the anxiety diagnoses were categories (panic disorder, agoraphobia, social phobia) that have shown such a relation (Hettema et al., 2005; Mineka et al., 1998).

All of the trait-based linkage–genomewide linkage studies carried out quantitative analyses of linkage of DNA markers to factor scores derived from personality questionnaires. Two studies (Fullerton et al., 2003; Nash et al., 2004) that used the strategy of selecting extremely concordant and extremely discordant sib pairs recruited from large population-based samples elegantly demonstrated the potential efficiency and power of trait-based designs. Neale, Sullivan, and Kendler (2005) and Kuo and colleagues (2007) analyzed neuroticism scores in samples of families recruited for nicotine and alcohol dependence studies, respectively. Cloninger and colleagues (1998) analyzed scores for the harm avoidance factor of the Tridimensional Personality Questionnaire (TPQ), which is related, but not identical, to neuroticism.

Three studies (Abkevich et al., 2003; Holmans et al., 2007; Zubenko et al., 2003) have reported evidence for linkage that achieved genomewide statistical significance (i.e., after correction for multiple testing), and one study (Fullerton et al., 2003) reported several significant linkages to neuroticism. Abkevich and colleagues (2003) reported significant linkage in males, but not in females, in a region of chromosome 12q. Camp and colleagues (2005) failed to find significant linkage in this region when they analyzed the same data but included only MDD-RE cases. Levinson and colleagues (2007) reported significant linkage on chromosome 15q after genotyping SNP markers across the region. Zubenko and colleagues (2003) reported multiple significant linkage results, but I question whether correction for multiple testing was handled correctly in this report, as discussed elsewhere (Levinson, 2006).

Findings that have received some support in more than one study are listed in Table 8.3. In the absence of meta-analytic data to compare results across studies, chromosomal regions are listed if two or more studies reported "positive" results based on rank (the top 10 findings in each study regardless of *p* value) or logarithm of the odds (LOD) scores > 2 without covariates (a typical threshold for "suggestive linkage" (Lander & Kruglyak, 1995). Each study produced additional findings that, although not yet strongly supported by other studies, could represent true evidence for weak genetic effects; the reader is referred to the original papers for details. Several investigators are planning to complete a formal combined linkage analysis once the McGuffin and colleagues (2005) results are available for the full 1,000 affected sib pairs in their study (the published report is for the first half of the sample).

The data in Table 8.3 suggest that some degree of convergence of linkage evidence across studies might emerge and, if so, these chromosomal regions will deserve close attention as fine-grained association and resequencing studies proceed. Power is a fundamental problem here. Linkage power analyses suggested that reliable detection of a genetic locus that contributed a 25–30% increase in risk to siblings of affected probands would require samples of 900–1,000 affected sibling pairs (ASPs; Levinson et al., 2003). We have only one linkage study of MDD so far with a sample of more than 900 ASPs (Holmans et al., 2007; Levinson et al., 2007), plus one study of neuroticism (Fullerton et al., 2003), which despite a smaller sample probably had similar power, because its strategy was to study a quantitative

TABLE 8.3. Depression and Neuroticism Linkage Findings with Support in More Than One Genome Scan

Chromosome	Region (centiMorgans)	Best linkage evidence	Supportive evidence (logarithm of the odds [LOD] or ordinal rank)
1	126–137	Neuroticism[a]: 2nd	Neuroticism[b]: 2nd
3	105	MDD-RE/Anx, MDD-RE[c]: 1st	Neuroticism[b]: 4th
4	151–176	Neuroticism[a]: 3rd	MDDRE/Anx[c]: LOD > 2 (females)
6	31–47	Neuroticism[d]): 1st	
8	8–26	Harm avoidance[f]: 1st	Neuroticism[a]: 7th; 1st in males MDD-RE[e]: 4th; 2nd in M-M pairs
11	85–99	Neuroticism[a]: 6th	MDD-RE[g]: LOD > 2
12	100–105	MD+BP[h]: 1st in males)	Neuroticism[a]: 1st; 1st in females
MDD-R[i]: 4th Neuroticism[j]: 3rd			
15	105–125	MDD-RE[e]: 1st	MDD-RE[c]): 1st in males
18	75–88	MDD-RE/Anx[c]): 2nd	MDD-RE[c]): 5th
Mood Dis[g]: LOD > 2 (also harm avoidance[f], 3rd)			

Note. Results are described in most cases in terms of relative strength of evidence for linkage; that is, best linkage result in the primary scan analysis = "1st," etc. (if no specific subtype listed) or for a phenotype or subset (if listed), or LOD score (without covariates) > 2 (see text). MDD-RE, recurrent early-onset MDD (onset <31 in c, e; <25 in f); MDD-R, recurrent MDD; MDD-RE/ Anx, the LOD score was maximized over three diagnostic models (MDD-RE alone, MDD-RE or any anxiety disorder, MDD-RE plus any anxiety disorder); MD+BP, analysis of families with multiple MDD probands, with BP (bipolar disorder) relatives included as affected), same sample as c; Mood Dis, any mood disorder (broad diagnosis); M-M, male–male affected pairs.

References: a—Fullerton et al. (2003); b—Neale et al. (2005); c—Camp et al. (2005); d—Nash et al. (2004); e—Holmans et al. (2007); f—Cloninger et al. (1998); g—Zubenko et al. (2003); h—Abkevich et al. (2003); i—McGuffin et al. (2007); j—Kuo et al. (2007).

trait in extremely discordant sibling pairs. Thus, we cannot determine for sure whether there is a locus that would produce replicable results in multiple samples this large. (See our later discussion of the difference between the contribution of a locus to increased sibling risk and the increased risk to individuals conferred by an allele or genotype.)

The strongest finding that emerges from a large set of statistical tests tends to reflect the "winner's curse"; that is, the effect was detected because it happened to appear large in this sample. If, for example, linkage is actually present at that locus in some, but not most, families, the number of families with evidence for linkage vary stochastically from study to study (and this variance is greater in sets of small samples, each with inadequate power); one will initially detect linkage when a study happens to recruit a higher proportion of such families than are present in the entire population. Then, as evidence accumulates from more studies, the large effect fails to replicate, and the real effect ultimately proves to be substantially smaller (Goring, Terwilliger, & Blangero, 2001).

The Holmans and colleagues (2007), Abkevich and colleagues (2003), and Fullerton and colleagues (2003) studies were relatively large and used appropriate statistical criteria for genomewide linkage, so it is more likely that their findings are real (i.e., in the absence of linkage, such a large effect would rarely be observed). However, the actual genetic effects in these regions are probably more modest than these original reports have suggested. Note also that linkage to the chromosome 12q region (Abkevich et al., 2003) has been more frequently reported for BP (see discussion in Barden et al., 2006). Given that evidence for this locus disappeared when Camp and colleagues (2005) removed the bipolar relatives from the analysis, it is possible that a linkage in the region is more closely related to BP, or that it is somehow related to the genetic overlap between these two disorders. As noted earlier, a possible candidate gene in this region has been discussed (Harlan et al., 2006), but the actual evidence for association of MDD to this gene has not yet been published.

Are linkage studies relevant to future research? One of the motivations for the HapMap Project and the development of genomewide SNP chip assays was the realization that association studies are more powerful than linkage studies (Risch & Merikangas, 1996). One way to understand this is to think about the parameters that predict the power of each type of study. For a linkage study of a categorical trait, power is related in part to the locus-specific RR to siblings of ill individuals (λ_{sibs}; i.e., if a *specific* locus accounts for a 30% increase in the disease risk of ill probands' siblings, averaged across all families in the population, then λ_{sibs} is 1.3). A particular locus could have a small effect in all families or a larger effect in a proportion of families. A large study (1,000 ASPs) can detect linkage reliably if the locus-specific λ_{sibs} is 1.3 or slightly less (a 25–30% increase in risk), with a rapid drop in power below 1.25 (Levinson et al., 2003). For an association study, the relevant parameter is allelic or genotypic relative risk (the increased risk to a carrier of that variant), depending on type of inheritance model. A study of 2,000 ill cases and 2,000 control subjects can often detect a more common variant, with a RR of 1.3–1.6. But to construct a model that predicts a λ_{sibs} of 1.3, one must typically assume an allelic or genotypic RR in the range of 3 to 10, because no plausible model of a complex disease can assume that every proband carries any single risk allele, and a sibling has only a 50% chance of inheriting the same specific allele as the proband. So, if one can assay the actual risk variant, or a highly correlated one nearby, association methods are much more powerful, and the GWA approach makes this possible for the more common variants in the genome.

Linkage studies do provide valuable information, however. A linkage signal can be detected if sequence variation at one or more locations in a region accounts for a substantial increase in disease risk, even if there are a large number of very rare variants in different families. Current large-scale association methods would fail in the case of multiple rare variants, or if the risk variant and any nearby correlated variants were not represented on the genotyping array. Thus, a linkage signal that emerges from a large study or meta-analysis tells us that association signals in the region should be taken particularly seriously, and it has been suggested that linkage evidence should be used formally to up-weight statistical evidence for association based on linkage evidence (Roeder, Bacanu, Wasserman, & Devlin, 2006). If no associations are initially observed, the region will deserve further study as more powerful assays (including resequencing) are developed.

FUTURE DIRECTIONS:
GENOMEWIDE ASSOCIATION AND BEYOND

The next major step in depression genetics research will be a set of GWA studies using chip-based arrays of common SNPs. At the very least, GWA studies of between 1,000 and 2,000 cases versus control groups are likely to be reported during 2008 by six research groups, led by Dr. Patrick Sullivan of University of North Carolina and collaborators in the Netherlands (as part of the Genetic Association Information Network program, see *www.fnih.org*), Dr. Steve Hamilton and collaborators from the Sequenced Treatment Alternatives to Relieve Depression (STAR*D) study, Dr. Markus Nöthen (University of Bonn) and colleagues in Germany, two pharmaceutical industry research groups (Glaxo and Pfizer), and Levinson and colleagues in the Genetics of Recurrent Early-Onset Depression (GenRED) collaboration. A seventh project, led by Dr. Peter McGuffin at the Institute of Psychiatry in London, carried out a GWA analysis using pooled genotyping (genotyping pools of large numbers of DNA specimens, each several times, to estimate case and control frequencies), and is now carrying out a study with individual genotyping. A meta-analysis (combined analysis) of individually genotyped GWA studies is also being planned.

These data will provide an important initial test of the ability of the current generation of high-throughput genotyping chips (the Affymetrix, Illumina, and Perlegen platforms) to detect associations between MDD and common SNPs or CNVs of around 10,000 base pairs or longer. The best possible outcome would be that combined data from these and other, future studies will clearly support association to SNPs that alter the functioning of genes that ultimately prove to be relevant to the etiology of depression—perhaps genes whose relevance was previously unsuspected, providing new theories of etiology and targets for drug therapy. If no clearcut associations emerged, then one could conclude that either no single variant had a sufficient genetic effect to be detected in the total sample, or one or more such variants were not adequately assayed by the current chips. Given that the combined sample size will be around 10,000 cases, it is quite possible that there will not be adequate power to detect the effects of loci with allelic relative risk (ARR) or genotype relative risk (GRR) in the range of 1.1–1.2. We know even less about what to expect from studies that are able to assay CNVs, a field that is really just beginning with the development of the latest chip assays.

Technologies for *resequencing* (determining the sequence of) individual subjects are also undergoing rapid development. New methods typically involve cutting the target DNA sequences into small pieces, analyzing the sequences in parallel and redundantly by novel, rapid methods, then "assembling" the entire sequence from the short segments using computer software techniques. A brief review with relevant references and links is found in Mardis (2008). It has been a widely publicized goal of the field to achieve the "thousand dollar genome" (i.e., to be able to resequence the entire genome of an individual for that sum), but the power and accuracy of these methods in the short term are just beginning to be tested adequately. It is widely believed, however, that as these methods evolve further, they will permit the more routine application of *deep resequencing*—the determination of the DNA sequence of target genes (or of elements in these genes; e.g., exons) in large numbers of subjects. Evolutionary models of disease genetics suggest that both common and rare DNA sequence variants could play important roles in the etiology of common, complex disorders, sometimes in the same genes (Botstein & Risch, 2003; Pritchard, 2001). Although current GWA methods provide reasonable assays of common SNPs and of CNVs, large-scale resequencing studies will eventually be needed to test the hypothesis that, within some susceptibility genes, there are many different, very rare variants (each found in very few people in a population, or in only one person), each of which can increase disease risk. Early successes in this area have come in the study of lipid disorders, for which resequencing studies of hundreds of individuals (e.g., Cohen et al., 2006) have demonstrated an excess of rare coding SNPs in people with very high versus very low values for lipid measurements relevant to heart disease. The size of resequencing studies (sample size, as well as amount of sequence studied) will increase rapidly over the next few years.

Progress is also likely in areas of bioinformatics related to the cataloguing of interacting networks or "pathways" of genes and proteins (e.g., Moriya, Itoh, Okuda, Yoshizawa, & Kanehisa, 2007). Greater understanding of these interactions is likely to lead to better approaches in the analysis of genetic data. Currently, for example, association data are typically analyzed one or two variants at a time, at great cost in terms of statistical power to detect genetic effects. As the pathways likely to be relevant to depression become clearer, it will be possible to test a smaller number of hypotheses that combine evidence across all genes in a pathway, thereby increasing power. For example, emerging data might begin to support interacting effects predicted by recent theories of depression (as discussed earlier), involving neurotrophic and neurotoxic processes, inflammation, and regulation of cortisol secretion by the hypothalamic–pituitary axis. Or, GWA or other studies could implicate novel pathways, suggesting an entirely new set of candidate genes and a new set of research strategies relevant to those particular genes and pathways.

Now that it is feasible to study large numbers of genetic variants in many subjects, it should also be a priority of the field to find more cost-effective ways to measure putative "endophenotypes" in large samples (i.e., biological phenomena that could lie closer to the site of action of depression-related genetic variation) (Hasler, Drevets, Manji, & Charney, 2004), so that large-scale gene mapping studies could be undertaken for these phenotypes. These variables might include cortisol hypersecretion (Ehlert, Gaab, & Heinrichs, 2001), dysregulation of sleep (Riemann, Berger, & Voderholzer, 2001), and structural changes in the hippocampus and subgenual prefrontal cortex (Botteron, Raichle, Drevets, Heath, & Todd, 2002; Drevets, 2001; see Davidson, Pizzagalli, & Nitschke, Chapter 10, this volume). Some of these variables have been studied in small samples of relatives of subjects with MDD (Giles, Biggs, Rush, & Roffwarg, 1988; Modell et al., 1998; Sitaram, Dubé, Keshavan, Davies, & Reynal, 1987), but much larger studies will be needed to select which variables are the best candidates for gene mapping. Similarly, the merger of large-scale genotyping and resequencing methods and large-scale population-based studies of environmental variables should make it possible to test gene–environment hypotheses more systematically rather than one polymorphism at a time.

In conclusion, we currently know little about the genetic underpinnings of susceptibility to depression and related traits. There is no clear association of MDD with DNA sequence variants in genes in monoaminergic pathways. Genetic linkage studies have demonstrated some convergent findings, but formal meta-analyses have not yet been carried out. There is a promising set of studies of the interaction among a functional insertion–deletion variant in the serotonin transporter gene, stress, and onset of major depressive symptoms and episodes. Although this variant does not appear to contribute substantially to lifetime risk of MDD, these studies have created an interesting model for approaching the important question of gene–environment interactions. Meanwhile, the era of GWA studies is upon us, and multiple studies of MDD will appear during 2008. Studies of common SNPs (GWA methods), rare SNPs (deep resequencing methods) and CNVs are likely to identify some of the genes that contribute to depression susceptibility, leading to new, testable theories about the relevant biological mechanisms and their possible interactions with environmental factors.

REFERENCES

Abkevich, V., Camp, N. J., Hensel, C. H., Neff, C. D., Russell, D. L., Hughes, D. C., et al. (2003). Predisposition locus for major depression at chromosome 12q22-12q23.2. *American Journal of Human Genetics*, 73, 1271–1281.

Anguelova, M., Benkelfat, C., & Turecki, G. (2003). A systematic review of association studies investigating genes coding for serotonin receptors and the serotonin transporter: I. Affective disorders. *Molecular Psychiatry, 8,* 574–591.

Arinami, T., Li, L., Mitsushio, H., Itokawa, M., Hamaguchi, H., & Toru, M. (1996). An insertion/deletion polymorphism in the angiotensin converting enzyme gene is associated with both brain substances P contents and affective disorders. *Biological Psychiatry, 40,* 1122–1127.

Baghai, T. C., Binder, E. B., Schule, C., Salyakina, D., Eser, D., Lucae, S., et al. (2006). Polymorphisms in the angiotensin-converting enzyme gene are associated with unipolar depression, ACE activity and hypercortisolism. *Molecular Psychiatry, 11,* 1003–1015.

Barden, N., Harvey, M., Gagné, B., Shink, E., Tremblay, M., Raymond, C., et al. (2006). Analysis of single nucleotide polymorphisms in genes in the chromosome 12Q24.31 region points to *P2RX7* as a susceptibility gene to bipolar affective disorder. *American Journal of Medical Genetics B, 141*(4), 374–382.

Barr, C. S., Newman, T. K., Schwandt, M., Shannon, C., Dvoskin, R. L., Lindell, S. G., et al. (2004). Sexual dichotomy of an interaction between early adversity and the serotonin transporter gene promoter variant in rhesus macaques. *Proceedings of the National Academy of Sciences USA, 101,* 12358–12363.

Blacker, D., Lavori, P. W., Faraone, S. V., & Tsuang, M. T. (1993). Unipolar relatives in bipolar pedigrees: A search for indicators of underlying bipolarity. *American Journal of Medical Genetics B, 48*(4), 192–199.

Botstein, D., & Risch, N. (2003), Discovering genotypes underlying human phenotypes: Past successes for Mendelian disease, future approaches for complex disease. *Nature Genetics, 33*(Suppl.), 228–237.

Botteron, K. N., Raichle, M. E., Drevets, W. C., Heath, A. C., & Todd, R. D. (2002). Volumetric reduction in left subgenual prefrontal cortex in early onset depression. *Biological Psychiatry, 51,* 342–344.

Camp, N. J., Lowry, M. R., Richards, R. L., Plenk, A. M., Carter, C., Hensel, C. H., et al. (2005). Genome-wide linkage analyses of extended Utah pedigrees identifies loci that influence recurrent, early-onset major depression and anxiety disorders. *American Journal of Medical Genetics B, 135,* 85–93.

Caspi, A., Sugden, K., Moffitt, T. E., Taylor, A., Craig, I. W., Harrington, H., et al. (2003). Influence of life stress on depression: Moderation by a polymorphism in the *5-HTT* gene. *Science, 301,* 386–389.

Cervilla, J. A., Molina, E., Rivera, M., Torres-González, F., Bellón, J. A., Moreno, B., et al. (2007). The risk for depression conferred by stressful life events is modified by variation at the serotonin transporter 5HTTLPR genotype: Evidence from the Spanish PREDICT-Gene cohort. *Molecular Psychiatry, 12*(8), 748–755.

Chorbov, V. M., Lobos, E. A., Todorov, A. A., Heath, A. C., Botteron, K. N., & Todd, R. D. (2007). Relationship of 5-HTTLPR genotypes and depression risk in the presence of trauma in a female twin sample. *American Journal of Medical Genetics B, 144*(6), 830–833.

Cloninger, C. R., Van Eerdewegh, P., Goate, A., Edenberg, H. J., Blangero, J., Hesselbrock, V., et al. (1998). Anxiety proneness linked to epistatic loci in genome scan of human personality traits. *American Journal of Medical Genetics, 81,* 313–317.

Cohen, J. C., Pertsemlidis, A., Fahmi, S., Esmail, S., Vega, G. L., Grundy, S. M., et al. (2006). Multiple rare variants in NPC1L1 associated with reduced sterol absorption and plasma low-density lipoprotein levels. *Proceedings of the National Academy of Sciences USA, 103*(6), 1810–1815.

Dannlowski, U., Ohrmann, P., Bauer, J., Kugel, H., Baune, B. T., Hohoff, C., et al. (2007). Serotonergic genes modulate amygdala activity in major depression. *Genes, Brain, and Behavior, 7,* 672–676.

Dick, D. M., Plunkett, J., Hamlin, D., Nurnberger, J., Jr., Kuperman, S., Schuckit, M., et al. (2007). Association analyses of the serotonin transporter gene with lifetime depression and alcohol dependence in the Collaborative Study on the Genetics of Alcoholism (COGA) sample. *Psychiatric Genetics, 17*(1), 35–38.

Drevets, W. C. (2001). Neuroimaging and neuropathological studies of depression, implications for the cognitive-emotional features of mood disorders. *Current Opinion in Neurobiology, 11,* 240–249.

Ehlert, U., Gaab, J., & Heinrichs, M. (2001). Psychoneuroendocrinological contributions to the etiology of depression, posttraumatic stress disorder, and stress-related disorders: The role of the hypothalamus–pituitary–adrenal axis. *Biological Psychology, 57,* 141–152.

Endicott, J., Nee, J., Andreasen, N., Clayton, P., Keller, M., & Coryell, W. (1985). Bipolar II: Combine or keep separate. *Journal of Affective Disorders, 8,* 17–28.

Eysenck, H. J. (1967). *The biological basis of personality.* Springfield, IL: Thomas.

Fanous, A. H., & Kendler, K. S. (2004). The genetic relationship of personality to major depression and schizophrenia. *Neurotoxicity Research, 6*(1), 43–50.

Frayling, T. M. (2007). Genome-wide association studies provide new insights into type 2 diabetes aetiology. *Nature Reviews: Genetics, 8*(9), 657–662.

Fullerton, J., Cubin, M., Tiwari, H., Wang, C., Bomhra, A., Davidson, S., et al. (2003). Linkage analysis of extremely discordant and concordant sibling pairs identifies quantitative-trait loci that influence variation in the human personality trait neuroticism. *American Journal of Human Genetics, 72*(4), 879–890.

Furlong, R. A., Rubinsztein, J. S., Ho, L., Walsh, C., Coleman, T. A., Muir, W. J., et al. (1999). Analysis and meta-analysis of two polymorphisms within the tyrosine hydroxylase gene in bipolar and unipolar affective disorders. *American Journal of Medical Genetics B, 88,* 88–94.

Gabriel, S. B., Schaffner, S. F., Nguyen, H., Moore, J. M., Roy, J., Blumenstiel, B., et al. (2002). The structure of haplotype blocks in the human genome. *Science, 296,* 2225–2229.

Gershon, E. S., Hamovit, J., Guroff, J. J., Dibble, E., Leckman, J. F., Sceery, W., et al. (1982). A family study of schizoaffective, bipolar I, bipolar II, unipolar, and normal control probands. *Archives of General Psychiatry, 39,* 1157–1167.

Gibb, B. E., McGeary, J. E., Beevers, C. G., & Miller, I. W. (2006). Serotonin transporter (5-HTTLPR) genotype, childhood abuse, and suicide attempts in adult psychiatric inpatients. *Suicide and Life-Threatening Behavior, 36*(6), 687–693.

Giles, D. E., Biggs, M. M., Rush, A. J., & Roffwarg, H. P. (1988). Risk factors in families of unipolar depression: I. Psychiatric illness and reduced REM latency. *Journal of Affective Disorders, 14,* 51–59.

Gillespie, N. A., Whitfield, J. B., Williams, B., Heath, A. C., & Martin, N. G. (2005). The relationship between stressful life events, the serotonin transporter (5-HTTLPR) genotype and major depression. *Psychological Medicine, 35,* 101–111.

Glatt, C. E., Carlson, E., Taylor, T. R., Risch, N., Reus, V. I., & Schaefer, C. A. (2005). Response to Zhang et al. (2005): Loss-of-function mutation in tryptophan hydroxylase-2 identified in unipolar major depression, *Neuron 45,* 11–16. *Neuron, 48*(5), 704–705.

Goodnick, P. J., & Goldstein, B. J. (1998). Selective serotonin reuptake inhibitors in affective disorders: I. Basic pharmacology. *Journal of Psychopharmacology, 12*(3, Suppl. B), S5–S20.

Goring, H. H., Terwilliger, J. D., & Blangero, J. (2001). Large upward bias in estimation of locus-specific effects from genomewide scans. *American Journal of Medical Genetics B, 69,* 1357–1369.

Gotlib, I. H., Joormann, J., Minor, K. L., & Hallmayer J. (2008). HPA axis reactivity: A mechanism underlying the associations among 5-HTTLPR, stress, and depression. *Biological Psychiatry, 63,* 847–851.

Grünblatt, E., Hupp, E., Bambula, M., Zehetmayer, S., Jungwirth, S., Tragl, K. H., et al. (2006). Association study of BDNF and CNTF polymorphism to depression in non-demented subjects of the "VITA" study. *Journal of Affective Disorders, 96*(1–2), 111–116.

Hariri, A. R., Drabant, E. M., Munoz, K. E., Kolachana, B. S., Mattay, V. S., Egan, M. F., et al. (2005). A susceptibility gene for affective disorders and the response of the human amygdala. *Archives of General Psychiatry, 62,* 146–152.

Harlan, J., Chen, Y., Gubbins, E., Mueller, R., Roch, J. M., Walter, K., et al. (2006). Variants in Apaf-1 segregating with major depression promote apoptosome function. *Molecular Psychiatry, 11*(1), 76–85.

Hashimoto, R., Numakawa, T., Ohnishi, T., Kumamaru, E., Yagasaki, Y., Ishimoto, T., et al. (2006). Impact of the DISC1 *Ser704Cys* polymorphism on risk for major depression, brain morphology and ERK signaling. *Human Molecular Genetics, 15,* 3024–3033.

Hasler, G., Drevets, W. C., Manji, H. K., & Charney, D. S. (2004). Discovering endophenotypes for major depression. *Neuropsychopharmacology, 29,* 1765–1781.

Heath, A. C., Todorov, A. A., Nelson, E. C., Madden, P. A., Bucholz, K. K., & Martin, N. G. (2002). Gene–environment interaction effects on behavioral variation and risk of complex disorders: The example of alcoholism and other psychiatric disorders. *Twin Research, 5*(1), 30–37.

Hettema, J. M., Prescott, C. A., Myers, J. M., Neale, M. C., & Kendler, K. S. (2005). The structure of genetic and environmental risk factors for anxiety disorders in men and women. *Archives of General Psychiatry, 62*(2), 182–189.

Hickie, I. B., Naismith, S. L., Ward, P. B., Scott, E. M., Mitchell, P. B., Schofield, P. R., et al. (2007). Serotonin transporter gene status predicts caudate nucleus but not amygdala or hippocampal volumes in older persons with major depression. *Journal of Affective Disorders, 98*(1–2), 137–142.

Holmans, P., Weissman, M. M., Zubenko, G. S., Scheftner, W. A., Crowe, R. R., Depaulo, J. R., Jr., et al. (2007). Genetics of Recurrent Early-Onset Major Depression (GenRED): Final genome scan report. *American Journal of Psychiatry, 164*(2), 248–258.

Hu, X. Z., Lipsky, R. H., Zhu, G., Akhtar, L. A., Taubman, J., Greenberg, B. D., et al. (2006). Serotonin transporter promoter gain-of-function genotypes are linked to obsessive–compulsive disorder. *American Journal of Human Genetics, 78*(5), 815–826.

International HapMap Consortium. (2003). The International HapMap Project. *Nature, 426,* 789–796.

Jacobs, N., Kenis, G., Peeters, F., Derom, C., Vlietinck, R., & van Os, J. (2006). Stress-related negative affectivity and genetically altered serotonin transporter function: Evidence of synergism in shaping risk of depression. *Archives of General Psychiatry, 63*(9), 989–996.

Karege, F., Perret, G., Bondolfi, G., Schwald, M., Bertschy, G., & Aubry, J. M. (2002). Decreased serum brain-derived neurotrophic factor levels in major depressed patients. *Psychiatry Research, 109,* 143–148.

Kaufman, J., Yang, B. Z., Douglas-Palumberi, H., Houshyar, S., Lipschitz, D., Krystal, J. H., et al. (2004). Social supports and serotonin transporter gene moderate depression in maltreated children. *Proceedings of the National Academy of Sciences USA, 101,* 17316–17321.

Kendler, K. S., Gatz, M., Gardner, C. O., & Pedersen, N. L. (2007). Clinical indices of familial depression in the Swedish Twin Registry. *Acta Psychiatrica Scandinavica, 115*(3), 214–220.

Kendler, K. S., Kuhn, J. W., & Prescott, C. A. (2004). Childhood sexual abuse, stressful life events and risk for major depression in women. *Psychological Medicine, 34,* 1475–1482.

Kendler, K. S., Kuhn, J. W., Vittum, J., Prescott, C. A., & Riley, B. (2005). The interaction of stressful life events and a serotonin transporter polymorphism in the prediction of episodes of major depression: A replication. *Archives of General Psychiatry, 62,* 529–535.

Kendler, K. S., Neale, M. C., Kessler, R. C., Heath, A. C., & Eaves, L. J. (1993). The lifetime history of major depression in women: Reliability of diagnosis and heritability. *Archives of General Psychiatry, 50,* 863–870.

Kim, J. M., Stewart, R., Kim, S. W., Yang, S. J., Shin, I. S., Kim, Y. H., et al. (2007). Interactions between life stressors and susceptibility genes (5-HTTLPR and BDNF) on depression in Korean elders. *Biological Psychiatry, 62*(5), 423–428.

Kuo, P. H., Neale, M. C., Riley, B. P., Patterson, D. G., Walsh, D., Prescott, C. A., et al. (2007). A genome-wide linkage analysis for the personality trait neuroticism in the Irish affected sib-pair study of alcohol dependence. *American Journal of Medical Genetics B, 144*(4), 463–468.

Lander, E., & Kruglyak, L. (1995). Genetic dissection of complex traits: Guidelines for interpreting and reporting linkage results. *Nature Genetics, 11*(3), 241–247.

Lander, E. S. (1996). The new genomics: Global views of biology. *Science, 274,* 536–539.

Lasky-Su, J. A., Faraone, S. V., Glatt, S. J., & Tsuang, M. T. (2005). Meta-analysis of the association between two polymorphisms in the serotonin transporter gene and affective disorders. *American Journal of Medical Genetics, 133,* 110–115.

Lesch, K. P., Bengel, D., Heils, A., Sabol, S. Z., Greenberg, B. D., Petri, S., et al. (1996). Association of anxiety-related traits with a polymorphism in the serotonin transporter gene regulatory region. *Science, 274,* 1527–1531.

Levinson, D. F. (2005). Meta-analysis in psychiatric genetics. *Current Psychiatry Reports, 7,* 143–151.

Levinson, D. F. (2006). The genetics of depression: A review. *Biological Psychiatry, 60*(2), 84–92.

Levinson, D. F., Evgrafov, O. V., Knowles, J. A., Potash, J. B., Weissman, M. M., Scheftner, W. A., et al. (2007). Genetics of recurrent early-onset major depression (GenRED): Significant linkage on chromosome 15q25-q26 after fine mapping with single nucleotide polymorphism markers. *American Journal of Psychiatry, 164*(2), 259–264.

Levinson, D. F., Zubenko, G. S., Crowe, R. R., DePaulo, J. R., Scheftner, W. S., Weissman, M. M., et al. (2003). Genetics of Recurrent Early-Onset Depression (GenRED): Design and preliminary clinical characteristics of a repository sample for genetic linkage studies. *American Journal of Medical Genetics B, 119,* 118–130.

Li, D., Duan, Y., & He, L. (2006). Association study of serotonin 2A receptor (5-HT2A) gene with schizophrenia and suicidal behavior using systematic meta-analysis. *Biochemical and Biophysical Research Communications, 340*(3), 1006–1015.

Li, D., & He, L. (2006). Further clarification of the contribution of the tryptophan hydroxylase (TPH) gene to suicidal behavior using systematic allelic and genotypic meta-analyses. *Human Genetics, 119*(3), 233–240.

López de Lara, C., Brezo, J., Rouleau, G., Lesage, A., Dumont, M., Alda, M., et al. (2007). Effect of tryptophan hydroxylase-2 gene variants on suicide risk in major depression. *Biological Psychiatry, 62*(1), 72–80.

López-León, S., Croes, E. A., Sayed-Tabatabaei, F. A., Claes, S., Van Broeckhoven, C., & van Duijn, C. M. (2005). The dopamine D4 receptor gene 48-base-pair-repeat polymorphism and mood disorders: A meta-analysis. *Biological Psychiatry, 57*(9), 999–1003.

Lotrich, F. E., & Pollock, B. G. (2004). Meta-analysis of serotonin transporter polymorphisms and affective disorders. *Psychiatric Genetics, 14,* 121–129.

Lucae, S., Salyakina, D., Barden, N., Harvey, M., Gagné, B., Labbé, M., et al. (2006). *P2RX7,* a gene coding for a purinergic ligand-gated ion channel, is associated with major depressive disorder. *Human Molecular Genetics, 15,* 2438–2445.

Maier, W., Lichtermann, D., Minges, J., Hallmayer, J., Heun, R., Benkert, O., et al. (1993). Continuity and discontinuity of affective disorders and schizophrenia: Results of a controlled family study. *Archives of General Psychiatry, 50,* 871–883.

Manji, H. K., Drevets, W. C., & Charney, D. S. (2001). The cellular neurobiology of depression. *Nature Medicine, 7,* 541–547.

Mann, J. J., Currier, D., Murphy, L., Huang, Y. Y., Galfalvy, H., Brent, D., et al. (2008). No association between a TPH2 promoter polymorphism and mood disorders or monoamine turnover. *Journal of Affective Disorders, 106*(1-2), 117–121.

Mardis, E. R. (2008). The impact of next-generation sequencing technology on genetics. *Trends in Genetics, 24*(3), 133–141.

Martin, J., Cleak, J., Willis-Owen, S. A., Flint, J., & Shifman, S. (2007). Mapping regulatory variants for the serotonin transporter gene based on allelic expression imbalance. *Molecular Psychiatry, 12*(5), 421–422.

Mathew, C. G. (2008). New links to the pathogenesis of Crohn disease provided by genome-wide association scans. *Nature Reviews: Genetics, 9*(1), 9–14.

McCarroll, S. A., & Altshuler, D. M. (2007). Copy-number variation and association studies of human disease. *Nature Genetics, 39*(Suppl. 7), S37–S42.

McGuffin, P., Katz, R., Watkins, S., & Rutherford, J. (1996). A hospital-based twin register study of the heritability of DSM-IV unipolar depression. *Archives of General Psychiatry, 53,* 129–136.

McGuffin, P., Knight, J., Breen, G., Brewster, S., Boyd, P. R., Craddock, N., et al. (2005). Whole genome linkage scan of recurrent depressive disorder from the depression network study. *Human Molecular Genetics, 14*(22), 3337–3345.

Middeldorp, C. M., de Geus, E. J., Beem, A. L., Lakenberg, N., Hottenga, J. J., Slagboom, P. E., et al. (2007). Family based association analyses between the serotonin transporter gene polymorphism (5-HTTLPR) and neuroticism, anxiety and depression. *Behavior Genetics, 37*(2), 294–301.

Mineka, S., Watson, D., & Clark, L. A. (1998). Comorbidity of anxiety and unipolar mood disorders. *Annual Review of Psychology, 49,* 377–412.

Modell, S., Lauer, C. J., Schreiber, W., Huber, J., Krieg, J. C., & Holsboer, F. (1998). Hormonal response pattern in the combined DEX-CRH test is stable over time in subjects at high familial risk for affective disorders. *Neuropsychopharmacology, 18,* 253–262.

Moldin, S. O., Reich, T., & Rice, J. P. (1991). Current perspectives on the genetics of unipolar depression. *Behavior Genetics, 21,* 211–242.

Moriya, Y., Itoh, M., Okuda, S., Yoshizawa, A. C., & Kanehisa, M. (2007). KAAS, an automatic genome annotation and pathway reconstruction server. *Nucleic Acids Research, 35,* W182–W185.

Munafo, M. R., Clark, T., & Flint, J. (2005). Does measurement instrument moderate the association between the serotonin transporter gene and anxiety-related personality traits?: A meta-analysis. *Molecular Psychiatry, 10,* 415–419.

Nakamura, M., Ueno, S., Sano, A., & Tanabe, H. (2000). The human serotonin transporter gene linked polymorphism (5-HTTLPR) shows 10 novel allelic variants. *Molecular Psychiatry, 5,* 32–38.

Nash, M. W., Huezo-Diaz, P., Williamson, R. J., Sterne, A., Purcell, S., Hoda, F., et al. (2004). Genome-wide linkage analysis of a composite index of neuroticism and mood-related scales in extreme selected sibships. *Human Molecular Genetics, 13,* 2173–2182.

Neale, B. M., Sullivan, P. F., & Kendler, K. S. (2005). A genome scan of neuroticism in nicotine dependent smokers. *American Journal of Medical Genetics B, 132,* 65–69.

Neves-Pereira, M., Mundo, E., Muglia, P., King, N., Macciardi, F., & Kennedy, J. L. (2002). The brain-derived neurotrophic factor gene confers susceptibility to bipolar disorder: Evidence from a family-based association study. *American Journal of Human Genetics, 71,* 651–655.

Otte, C., McCaffery, J., Ali, S., & Whooley, M. A. (2007). Association of a serotonin transporter polymorphism (5-HTTLPR) with depression perceived stress, and norepinephrine in patients with coronary disease: The Heart and Soul Study. *American Journal of Psychiatry, 164*(9), 1379–1384.

Parsey, R. V., Hastings, R. S., Oquendo, M. A., Hu, X., Goldman, D., Huang, Y. Y., et al. (2006). Effect of a triallelic functional polymorphism of the serotonin-transporter-linked promoter region on expression of serotonin transporter in the human brain. *American Journal of Psychiatry, 163*(1), 48–51.

Perlis, R. H. (2007). Pharmacogenetic studies of antidepressant response: How far from the clinic? *Psychiatric Clinics of North America, 30*(1), 125–138.

Pritchard, J. K. (2001). Are rare variants responsible for susceptibility to complex diseases? *American Journal of Human Genetics, 69,* 124–137.

Riemann, D., Berger, M., & Voderholzer, U. (2001). Sleep and depression—results from psychobiological studies: An overview. *Biological Psychology, 57,* 67–103.

Risch, N. (1987). Assessing the role of HLA-linked and unlinked determinants of disease. *American Journal of Human Genetics, 40,* 1–14.

Risch, N., & Merikangas, K. (1996). The future of genetic studies of complex human diseases. *Science, 273,* 1516–1517.

Savage, S. A., & Greene, M. H. (2007). The evidence for prostate cancer risk loci at 8q24 grows stronger. *Journal of the National Cancer Institute, 99,* 1499–1501.

Schinka, J. A., Busch, R. M., & Robichaux-Keene, N. (2004). A meta-analysis of the association between the serotonin transporter gene polymorphism (5-HTTLPR) and trait anxiety. *Molecular Psychiatry, 9,* 197–202.

Sen, S., Burmeister, M., & Ghosh, D. (2004). Meta-analysis of the association between a serotonin transporter promoter polymorphism (5-HTTLPR) and anxiety-related personality traits. *American Journal of Medical Genetics B, 127,* 85–89.

Sen, S., Nesse, R. M., Stoltenberg, S. F., Li, S., Gleiberman, L., Chakravarti, A., et al. (2003). A BDNF coding variant is associated with the NEO personality inventory domain neuroticism: A risk factor for depression. *Neuropsychopharmacology, 28*(2), 397–401.

Shioe, K., Ichimiya, T., Suhara, T., Takano, A., Sudo, Y., Yasuno, F., et al. (2003). No association between genotype of the promoter region of serotonin transporter gene and serotonin transporter binding in human brain measured by PET. *Synapse, 48*(4), 184–188.

Sitaram, N., Dubé, S., Keshavan, M., Davies, A., & Reynal, P. (1987). The association of supersensitive cholinergic REM-induction and affective illness within pedigrees. *Journal of Psychiatric Research, 21,* 487–497.

Sklar, P., Gabriel, S. B., McInnis, M. G., Bennett, P., Lim, Y. M., Tsan, G., et al. (2002). Family-based association study of 76 candidate genes in bipolar disorder: BDNF is a potential risk locus. *Molecular Psychiatry, 7,* 579–593.

Sullivan, P. F., Neale, M. C., & Kendler, K. S. (2000). Genetic epidemiology of major depression: Review and meta-analysis. *American Journal of Psychiatry, 157,* 1552–1562.

Surtees, P. G., Wainwright, N. W., Willis-Owen, S. A., Sandhu, M. S., Luben, R., Day, N. E., et al. (2007). No association between the BDNF Val66Met polymorphism and mood status in a non-clinical community sample of 7,389 older adults. *Journal of Psychiatric Research, 41*(5), 404–409.

Svenningsson, P., Chergui, K., Rachleff, I., Flajolet, M., Zhang, X., El Yacoubi, M., et al. (2006). Alterations in 5-HT1B receptor function by *p11* in depression-like states. *Science, 311,* 77–80.

Taylor, S. E., Way, B. M., Welch, W. T., Hilmert, C. J., Lehman, B. J., & Eisenberger, N. I. (2006). Early family environment, current adversity, the serotonin transporter promoter polymorphism, and depressive symptomatology. *Biological Psychiatry, 60*(7), 671–676.

Van Den Bogaert, A., De Zutter, S., Heyrman, L., Mendlewicz, J., Adolfsson, R., Van Broeckhoven, C., et al. (2005). Response to Zhang et al. (2005): Loss-of-function mutation in tryptophan hydroxylase-2 identified in unipolar major depression, *Neuron 45,* 11–16. *Neuron, 48*(5), 704.

Verma, R., Cutler, D. J., Holmans, P., Knowles, J. A., Crowe, R. R., Scheftner, W. A., et al. (2007). Investigating the role of *p11* (S100A10) sequence variation in susceptibility to major depression. *American Journal of Medical Genetics B, 144*(8), 1079–1082.

Wilhelm, K., Mitchell, P. B., Niven, H., Finch, A., Wedgwood, L., Scimone, A., et al. (2006). Life events, first depression onset and the serotonin transporter gene. *British Journal of Psychiatry, 188,* 210–215.

Willis-Owen, S. A., Fullerton, J., Surtees, P. G., Wainwright, N. W., Miller, S., & Flint, J. (2005). The *Val66Met* coding variant of the brain-derived neurotrophic factor (BDNF) gene does not contribute toward variation in the personality trait neuroticism. *Biological Psychiatry, 58*(9), 738–742.

Willis-Owen, S. A., Turri, M. G., Munafò, M. R., Surtees, P. G., Wainwright, N. W., Brixey, R. D., et al. (2005). The serotonin transporter length polymorphism, neuroticism, and depression: A comprehensive assessment of association. *Biological Psychiatry, 58*(6), 451–456.

Zalsman, G., Huang, Y. Y., Oquendo, M. A., Burke, A. K., Hu, X. Z., Brent, D. A., et al. (2006). Association of a triallelic serotonin transporter gene promoter region (5-HTTLPR) polymorphism with stressful life events and severity of depression. *American Journal of Psychiatry, 163*(9), 1588–1593.

Zhang, X., Gainetdinov, R. R., Beaulieu, J. M., Sotnikova, T. D., Burch, L. H., Williams, R. B., et al. (2005). Loss-of-function mutation in tryptophan hydroxylase-2 identified in unipolar major depression. *Neuron, 45,* 11–16.

Zhou, Z., Peters, E. J., Hamilton, S. P., McMahon, F., Thomas, C., McGrath, P. J., et al. (2005). Response to Zhang et al. (2005): Loss-of-function mutation in tryptophan hydroxylase-2 identified in unipolar major depression, *Neuron 45,* 11–16. *Neuron, 48*(5), 702–703.

Zill, P., Baghai, T. C., Zwanzger, P., Schule, C., Eser, D., Rupprecht, R., et al. (2004). SNP and haplotype analysis of a novel tryptophan hydroxylase isoform (*TPH2*) gene provide evidence for association with major depression. *Molecular Psychiatry, 9,* 1030–1036.

Zill, P., Buttner, A., Eisenmenger, W., Moller, H. J., Bondy, B., & Ackenheil, M. (2004). Single nucleotide polymorphism and haplotype analysis of a novel tryptophan hydroxylase isoform (*TPH2*) gene in suicide victims. *Biological Psychiatry, 56,* 581–586.

Zintzaras, E. (2006). C677T and A1298C methylenetetrahydrofolate reductase gene polymorphisms in schizophrenia, bipolar disorder and depression: A meta-analysis of genetic association studies. *Psychiatric Genetics, 16*(3), 105–115.

Zubenko, G. S., Maher, B., Hughes, H. B. III, Zubenko, W. N., Stiffler, J. S., Kaplan, B. B., et al. (2003). Genome-wide linkage survey for genetic loci that influence the development of depressive disorders in families with recurrent, early-onset, major depression. *American Journal of Medical Genetics B, 123*(1), 1–18.

CHAPTER 9

Neurobiological Aspects of Depression

Michael E. Thase

Since antiquity, there have been speculations about the biological basis of depression. To take but one example, the term *melancholia*, which is currently used to describe one of the most severe forms of depression, reflects the ancient Greek theory that mood disorders were caused by an imbalance of black bile (Jackson, 1986). Only during the past 50 years, however, has the methodology been available to study directly alterations in brain function associated with depression. What has emerged from this half-century of research has been an iterative and evolving process, answering some questions and opening new and more sophisticated lines of inquiry. One certainty is that the heterogeneous conditions grouped together under the construct of *clinical depression* are biopsychosocial disorders that—much more often than not—have multifactorial causality.

My colleagues and I reviewed evidence pertaining to neurobiological disturbances associated with depression in the previous volume of this *Handbook*, including a wide range of neurochemical, neuroendocrine, neurophysiological, and neuroanatomical parameters (Thase, Jindal, & Howland, 2002). Over the past two decades, various hypotheses have been advanced, tested, and either rejected or modified as research paradigms have evolved and knowledge about the function of the central nervous system (CNS) in health, in disease, and in response to various states of duress has grown. A number of new hypotheses also have been advanced. Some research tools, such as measurement of catecholamine metabolites in urine, blood, and cerebrospinal fluid (CSF) or electrophysiological recordings of neuronal activity, that were *de rigueur* in the 1970s and 1980s are now seldom used; others that were not technologically feasible, such as functional magnetic resonance imaging (fMRI), positron emission tomography (PET) imaging of receptor binding, and fast through-put genotyping, are now commonplace.

Perhaps the most notable advances have come from research on the intracellular processes that link receptors, second messengers, and various transcription factors to the up- or down-regulation of gene activity. Elsewhere in this volume, the current status of research on the genetics (Levinson, Chapter 8, this volume) and studies using brain imaging techniques to examine normal and pathological processes that accompany emotional expression (Davidson, Pizzagalli, & Nitschke, Chapter 10, this volume) is reviewed in detail. In this chapter, research using other neurobiological paradigms is emphasized, with a particular focus on developments that have taken place since our last comprehensive review of this literature (Thase et al., 2002). The overarching conceptual framework of this review centers on two basic tenets: (1) Clinical forms of depression comprise a related yet heterogeneous group of syndromes associated with disturbances of the brain systems that regulate the normal processes of mood, cognition, and appetitive behavior; and (2) most—if not all—forms of depression involve dysfunctional adaptations of the brain systems that regulate adaptations to stress.

BACKGROUND

Research on the neurobiology of depression began in earnest in the late 1950s, when converging lines of evidence pointed to the possibility of dysfunction of CNS systems subserved by the monoamine neurotransmitters, particularly the catecholamine norepinephrine (NE) and the indoleamine serotonin (also known as 5-hydroxytryptamine, or 5-HT). Early studies indicated that these neurotransmitters are important regulators of bodily functions that are commonly disturbed in depression, including sleep, appetite, libido, and psychomotor tone; by the mid-1960s, there was strong evidence that both types of medication used to treat depression, tricyclic antidepressants (TCAs) and monoamine oxidase inhibitors (MAOIs), directly affect NE and/or 5-HT neurons.

Because the TCAs and MAOIs immediately increased the amount of monoamine activity at neuronal synapses, researchers initially thought that depression was caused by a deficit of 5-HT or NE activity, and presumed that mania was caused by increased NE activity, perhaps in the context of a deficit of counterbalancing 5-HT activity (Bunney & Davis, 1965; Glassman, 1969; Schildkraut, 1965). Although the role of a third monoamine neurotransmitter, dopamine (DA), was generally thought to be more relevant to psychosis and to the activity of the phenothiazine-type medications used to treat schizophrenia, some theorists also emphasized the putative role of DA in symptoms such as fatigue, anhedonia, and psychomotor retardation (Korf & van Praag, 1971). Research over the next two decades failed to support the most simplistic models (e.g., deficit states corrected by medications that "restored" neuronal monoaminergic activity), but it confirmed that the therapeutic effects of antidepressants were initiated by actions on 5-HT and/or NE neurons, and investigators documented disturbed monoaminergic function in subgroups of individuals with mood disorders (e.g., see Duman, Heninger, & Nestler, 1997; Maes & Meltzer, 1995; Nemeroff, 1998; Schatzberg & Schildkraut, 1995; Willner, 1995).

Three findings from the first generation of research on the neurobiology of depression have ongoing relevance. First, although depression is no longer thought to be caused by deficits of NE or 5-HT, it is true that subgroups of patients with depression have either low urinary levels of the NE metabolite 3-methoxy-4-hydroxyphenylglycol (MHPG) (Ressler & Nemeroff, 1999; Schatzberg & Schildkraut, 1995) or low CSF levels of the serotonin metabolite 5-hydroxyindoleacetic acid (5-HIAA) (Maes & Meltzer, 1995). These findings have ongoing import, because the former abnormality is associated with psychomotor retardation (and, possibly, with preferential response to antidepressants that strongly affect noradrenergic neurotransmission; Schatzberg & Schildkraut, 1995), whereas low CSF 5-HIAA has been associated with increased risk of suicide, potentially lethal suicide attempts, and other violent, life-threatening behaviors (Maes & Meltzer, 1995; Mann, Brent, & Arango, 2001), although not with preferential response to medications that powerfully affect 5-HT neurons (Maes & Meltzer, 1995). Low CSF 5-HIAA levels subsequently have been shown to be at least partly under heritable control and, across primate species, appear to be a trait-like phenomenon associated with various types of aggressivity and impulsivity (Mann et al., 2001).

A second enduring and well-replicated finding concerns the hypersecretion of the glucocorticoid hormone *cortisol*, the primary effector of stress responses of humans. Cortisol is synthesized in the adrenal cortex and released into the systemic circulation in response to a cascade of *neuropeptides* (i.e., small chains of amino acids that act as neurotransmitters). The stress response cascade is initiated by corticotropin-releasing factor (CRF; also known as corticotropin-releasing hormone, or CRH), which is released in the cerebral cortex and hypothalamus in response to perceived stress. Recent research has established a link between a polymorphism of the gene coding for the CRF receptor and risk of depression (Liu et al., 2006). CRF in turn triggers the release of adrenocorticotropic hormone (ACTH), which is secreted by specialized neuroendocrine cells in the anterior pituitary gland and travels via systemic circulation to stimulate cortisol release from the adrenal glands. Plasma cortisol levels (i.e., the end product of the hypothalamic–pituitary–adrenocortical [HPA] axis in humans) normally follow a well-regulated diurnal rhythm: highest in the morning and lowest in the late evening. Intracellular actions of cortisol are mediated by intracellular glucocorticoid receptors, the expression of which are under genetic control (van Rossum et al., 2006) and can be up- or down-regulated by a number of factors that are relevant to depression (Neigh & Nemeroff, 2006).

A significant minority of individuals with depression show elevated cortisol levels throughout the day and blunting of the normal circadian secretory rhythm. Given the importance of glucocorticoids in systemic responses to a variety of acute stresses, including infection, hypothermia, and traumatic injury, elevated plasma cortisol levels are associated with measurably increased concentrations in virtually all body fluids, including urine, saliva, and CSF (Holsboer, 1995; Swaab, Bao, & Lucassen, 2005). In addition to elevated cortisol concentrations, increased HPA activity can be detected by several challenge paradigms, such as the dexamethasone (DEX) suppression test (DST) and the combined DST/CRH test (Holsboer, 2001). In studies of depression, various indicators of hypercortisolism are linked to older age and increased syndromal symptom severity, including psychosis and suicidal ideation, as well as a lower response to placebo and nonspecific therapeutic interventions (Thase et al., 2002).

A history of severe maltreatment or trauma during critical developmental periods can have lasting effects on regulation of the HPA axis (Heim, Mletzko, Purselle, Musselman, & Nemeroff, 2008; Newport, Heim, Bonsall, Miller, & Nemeroff, 2004). In some individuals with a history of neglect or maltreatment during childhood, including those who have never developed depression, there is blunting of the axis, with reduced cortisol secretion in response to experimentally contrived stresses, such as a public speaking task (Carpenter et al., 2007). Blunted HPA response to stress is also seen in individuals with posttraumatic stress disorder (PTSD) and chronic fatigue syndrome (Bremner, 2006). Those with a history of early trauma and depression, by contrast, are more likely to show an exaggerated HPA response to stress and a state-dependent increase in plasma cortisol (Bremner, 2006; Holsboer, 2001).

The third set of pivotal findings emanate from various experimental paradigms that measure the activity of localized neuronal circuits within the brain, including several subregions of the prefrontal cortex and the core structures that comprise the limbic system (Thase et al., 2002). Before it was possible to visualize subtle changes in regional cerebral activity in the living human, researchers obtained evidence of depression-related alterations in neuronal activity using all-night electroencephalographic (EEG) recordings during sleep (see Thase, 2006, for a comprehensive review). Such polysomnographic (PSG) recordings revealed a decrease of "deeper" slow-wave sleep (SWS) and an intensification in the amount and intensity of rapid eye movement (REM) sleep, and provided objective documentation of the difficulties that people with depression experience falling asleep and remaining asleep. Although neither of these alterations is pathognomonic to depression, the combination was shown to be relatively specific and of direct pathophysiological relevance. Because waking EEGs generally did not reveal characteristic alterations in depression, sleep appeared to unmask a characteristic alteration in the electrical activity of nuclei in the brain under the control of 5-HT and NE (Thase, Frank, & Kupfer, 1985). The PSG abnormalities associated with depression were somewhat more prevalent than was hypercortisolemia, but were nevertheless also age-dependent and more commonly observed among people with more severe, recurrent depressions (Thase et al., 2002).

More recently, studies of alterations of neuronal circuitry in depression have utilized neuroimaging strategies, including PET and fMRI scans, to measure both the structural integrity and functional activity (i.e., metabolic activity and regional blood flow at rest and in response to experimental challenges) (Drevets, 2000; Mayberg, 2003). Results of these studies, reviewed later in this chapter, have underscored the heterogeneity of depression and yielded evidence of several prototypical abnormalities, including increased activity of the amygdala, decreased activity of the dorsolateral prefrontal cortex (DLPFC), and reduced hippocampal volume (see also Davidson et al., Chapter 10, this volume).

ABNORMALITIES OF MONOAMINERGIC SYSTEMS

Noradrenergic Systems

Almost all of the NE cell bodies in the brain are located in a single nucleus, the locus ceruleus (LC), which is located in the rostral brainstem. Noradrenergic neurons project from the LC to the thalamus, hypothalamus, limbic system, basal ganglia, and cerebral cortex (see Figure 9.1) (Kandel, Schwartz, & Jessell, 1991; Kingsley, 2000). Such diffuse ascending projections reflect the role of NE in initiating and maintaining arousal in the brainstem, limbic system, and cerebral cortex, and as a modulator of other neural systems. Noradrenergic projections to the amygdala and hippocampus have been implicated in behavioral sensitization to stress (Ferry, Roozendaal, & McGaugh, 1999), and stimulation of noradrenergic fibers in the medial forebrain bundle enhances attention and increases levels of goal-directed or reward-seeking behavior (Aston-Jones, Rajkowski, & Cohen, 1999).

Noradrenergic neurotransmission plays an essential role in the experience of stress. Perception of novel or threatening stimuli is relayed from the cerebral cortex to the LC via the thalamus and hypothalamus, and from the periphery via the nucleus prepositus hypoglossi. These inputs can provoke an almost immediate increase in NE activity. Thus, cognitive processes affecting perception can amplify or dampen NE cellular responses to internal or external stimuli. In addition, activation from fibers projecting from the nucleus paragiganto-cellularis (probably using a small, excitatory neurotransmitter, e.g., glutamate), and release of CRH can "turn on" the LC (Nestler, Alreja, & Aghajanian, 1999). The peripheral component of stress response to stress is transmitted from the LC via the sympathoadrenal pathway to the endochromafin cells in the medulla of the adrenal glands, which in turn release

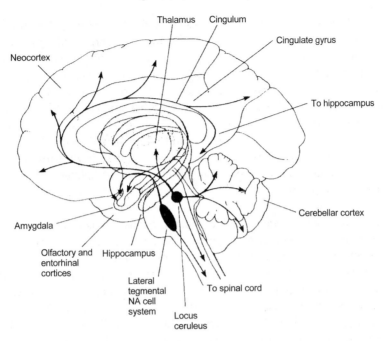

FIGURE 9.1. A lateral view of the brain demonstrates the course of the major noradrenergic pathways emanating from the locus ceruleus and from the lateral brainstem tegmentum. From Kandel, Schwartz, and Jessell (1991). Copyright 1991 by Appleton & Lange. Reprinted by permission.

NE into systemic circulation. Thus, the principal effectors of peripheral stress response, NE and cortisol, are released from glands that are located only a few centimeters apart, deep in the abdomen. The peripherally arousing effects of the sympathoadrenal response are largely mediated by cells expressing the α_1 and ß-type of NE receptors.

The activity of NE neurons is regulated in part by the autoinhibitory effects of α_2 receptors. Neuronal release of NE almost immediately begins to decrease the sensitivity of LC neurons to repeated firing. α_2 receptors also are located on serotoninergic cell bodies, and stimulation of these *heteroceptors* activates nearby (colocalized) inhibitory 5-HT neurons. A sustained increase in LC firing (i.e., a normal response to persistent stress) also causes the number of α_1 and ß-receptors to decrease, a process known as *down-regulation* or *desensitization*. Together, these four actions (i.e., α_2 autoinhibition, α_1 and ß-receptor down-regulation, and activation of adjacent inhibitory 5-HT neurons) constitute a homeostatic counterregulatory force that dampens an excessive response to a transient threat. If, however, the stress is sustained or unresolvable, intracellular stores of NE may become depleted when demand begins to exceed synthetic capacity. When this occurs, there is diminished inhibitory α_2 and 5-HT input to the LC. Thus, homeostasis of NE neurotransmission may become dysregulated, resulting in increased firing of the LC but inefficient signal transduction. Over time, the net effect is that ascending central NE neurotransmission decreases (which probably causes reduced urinary excretion of MHPG in depressed patients with psychomotor retardation), although the output of the adrenal medulla may remain high (which may explain the observation of high levels of NE and its metabolites in some severely depressed patients).

The consequences of sustained stress on NE systems in animal studies include decreased exploratory and consummatory behavior, as illustrated in studies using the learned helplessness paradigm (Maier & Seligman, 1976; Maier & Watkins, 2005). Learned helplessness should not be thought of as strictly analogous to human depression: Cognitive constructs such as entrapment, powerlessness, hopelessness, and guilt distinguish depression in humans from the behavioral states experienced by rodents and dogs in learned helplessness experiments (Gilbert, 1992). Nevertheless, the changes in NE activity observed in learned helplessness experiments do parallel those associated with other animal models of depression and are associated with other neurobiological correlates of depression, including elevated glucocorticoid activity, reduced 5-HT activity, and alterations in gene transcription factors (Berton et al., 2007; Maier & Watkins, 2005; Weiss & Kilts, 1998). Moreover, recognition of the mediators of individual differences in development of helplessness—both inherited and acquired—has opened new avenues for research (Berton et al., 2007; Krishnan et al., 2007).

Despite the continued relevance of NE neurotransmission as a reliable target for medications that exert antidepressant effects, studies in the 1990s indicated that it is unlikely that dysfunction of NE systems has a primary role in the etiology of depression (Anand et al., 2000; Ressler & Nemeroff, 1999). Nevertheless, several polymorphisms associated with either synthesis of NE or its signal transduction may be associated with excessive responses to stress, which may in turn increase the risk of depression during vulnerable periods (Jabbi et al., 2007; Shelton, 2007). Altered NE response to stress may likewise play a role as a modulator of other implicated factors in depression, including both pathological processes, such as the proinflammatory cytokines (Szelényi & Vizi, 2007), and processes that promote neuronal resilience, such as those mediated by brain-derived neurotropic factor (Chen, Nguyen, Pike, & Russo-Neustadt, 2007).

The therapeutic relevance of NE is supported by several converging lines of evidence. First, antidepressants that selectively block neuronal reuptake of NE have overall clinical efficacy that is roughly comparable to that of the selective serotonin reuptake inhibitors (SSRIs) (Nutt et al., 2007; Papakostas, Nelson, Kasper, & Möller, 2007). Second, the specific additive therapeutic effect of enhancing NE is also suggested by the modest yet reproducible advantage of the so-called *dual-reuptake inhibitors* (i.e., medications that inhibit reuptake of both 5-HT and NE) versus SSRIs in meta-analyses of controlled clinical trials (Nemeroff et al., 2008; Papakostas, Thase, Fava, Nelson, & Shelton, 2007; Thase et al., 2007). Third, studies of the physiological effects of selective NE reuptake inhibitors (NRIs) have documented normalization of a variety of functional disturbances associated with depression, including pineal secretion of melatonin and blood pressure responses to changes in posture (Golden, Markey, Risby, Cowdry, & Potter, 1988; Ressler & Nemeroff, 1999). Fourth, inhibition of the synthetic enzyme tyrosine hydroxylase via administration of α-methylparatyrosine, an analogue of the NE precursor tyrosine, rapidly reverses the effects of NRIs but not of SSRIs (Delgado, 2004). Together, these data indicate that NE plays an important neuromodulatory role in the activity of antidepressant medications.

Serotoninergic Systems

Most of the serotonin (5-HT) in the brain is synthesized in clusters of cell bodies known as the dorsal raphé nuclei, located in the pons. From the dorsal brainstem, these 5-HT neurons project to the cerebral cortex, hypothalamus, thalamus, basal ganglia, septum, and hippocampus (see Figure 9.2) (Kandel et al., 1991; Kingsley, 2000). Serotonin pathways are largely colocalized with NE pathways and generally have tonic and inhibitory effects that counterbalance NE activity. For example, much evidence indicates that 5-HT input to the

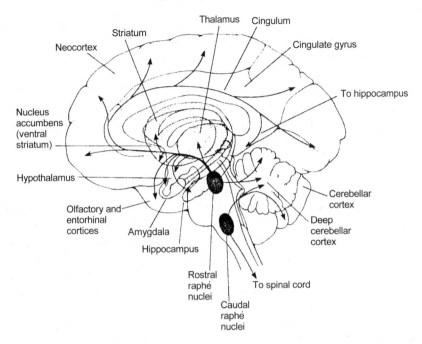

FIGURE 9.2. A lateral view of the brain demonstrates the course of the major serotoninergic pathways. Although the raphé nuclei form a fairly continuous collection of cell groups throughout the brainstem, they are graphically illustrated here as two groups, one rostral and one caudal. From Kandel, Schwartz, and Jessell (1991). Copyright 1991 by Appleton & Lange. Reprinted by permission.

thalamus is an important facilitator of appetite (Kingsley, 2000). Serotoninergic neurons projecting to the suprachiasmatic nucleus (SCN) of the anterior hypothalamus help to regulate circadian rhythms (e.g., sleep–wake cycles, body temperature, and HPA axis function) (Bunney & Bunney, 2000; Duncan, 1996). An intact 5-HT system also is needed to modulate the 90-minute infraradian cycle of alternating periods of REM and non-REM sleep (Duncan, 1996).

There are at least 15 types of serotonin receptors in the mammalian brain, each of which is under genetic control. Two of these receptors, $5\text{-}HT_{1A}$ and $5\text{-}HT_{2A}$, have been of greatest relevance to the pathophysiology of depression and/or the mechanism of antidepressant action (Mann et al., 2001), although research on some of the more recently identified receptors, such as the $5\text{-}HT_4$ and $5\text{-}HT_7$, is in its infancy. All 5-HT neurons express membrane-bound transporters (5-HTT), which permit the uptake of 5-HT from the synaptic cleft. The activity of many antidepressants is initiated by blocking this transporter, including, of course, the most widely used antidepressants in contemporary clinical practice, the SSRIs. As I discuss later in this chapter, identification of a functional polymorphism in the promoter region of the gene that codes for the 5-HTT has opened multiple new lines of research and helps to explain individual differences in response to stress and antidepressant medications.

An intact basal or tonic level of 5-HT neurotransmission is necessary for both affiliative social behaviors (Insel & Winslow, 1998) and the expression of goal-directed motor and consummatory behaviors primarily mediated by NE and DA. In experimental paradigms, defeat reliably lowers basal 5-HT tone across essentially all vertebrates studied and, in the wild, primates with lower levels of tonic 5-HT neurotransmission (as measured by CSF 5-HIAA levels) are more impulsive, aggressive, and generally have lower rankings on social dominance hierarchies than do animals with higher basal levels of 5-HT "tone" (Higley, Mehlman, Higley, et al., 1996; Higley, Mehlman, Poland, et al., 1996). Conversely, a rise in social dominance is accompanied by an increase in CSF 5-HIAA (Mehlman et al., 1995), and treatment with SSRIs decreases impulsive aggression (Fairbanks, Melega, Jorgensen, Kaplan, & McGuire, 2001). There is ample documentation of parallel associations in humans and low 5-HIAA is associated with suicide and other violent behaviors (Mann et al., 2001).

The tonic level of 5-HT neurotransmission in primates is relatively stable, with a slight seasonal variation (i.e., higher levels in the summer than in the fall) (Zajicek et al., 2000). Central serotoninergic tone is partly under genetic control (Higley, Mehlman, Poland, et al., 1996), with heritability at least partly determined by a polymorphism in the promoter region of the gene that codes for 5-HT-T. In primates, animals manifesting at least one copy of the short (S) allele, which is less functional (i.e., less transporter is synthesized, resulting in reduced uptake capability), show greater behavioral dysfunction and more exaggerated responses to stress than do animals who have two copies of the more common long (L) form of the allele (Barr et al., 2003, 2004; Shannon et al., 2005).

Humans show a similar polymorphism of 5-HTT, with the recent identification of a third variant (a less functional variant of the L form) (Firk & Markus, 2007; Levinson, 2006). Studies of the association of these polymorphisms and vulnerability to depression have yielded relatively consistent evidence of gene × environment interactions. A relation among the S allele of the serotonin transporter, stress, and increased risk of depression and suicidal ideation was first reported by Caspi and colleagues (2003) and subsequently widely (albeit not universally) replicated (e.g., see Jacobs et al., 2006; Kendler, Kuhn, Vittum, Prescott, & Riley, 2005). Importantly, individuals with one or two copies of the S allele are not at increased risk of depression per se, but are at increased risk of depression when exposed to life stress (Firk & Markus, 2007; Levinson, 2006). Such heightened vulnerability to stress is apparent at several levels, including increased limbic blood flow (Hariri et al., 2002) or cortisol secretion (Gotlib, Joorman, Minor, & Hallmayer, 2007) in response to experimentally induced threat, elevated levels of trait-like neuroticism (Jacobs et al., 2006) or dysfunctional attitudes (Hayden et al., 2008), and use of less active coping strategies (Wilhelm et al., 2007). That this inherited vulnerability is typically manifest early in life is indirectly reflected by the results of Baune and colleagues (in press), who found that the melancholic form of depression—which typically has a later age of onset—is disproportionately associated with L alleles for the serotonin transporter. Although results of individual studies are not fully consistent, a recent meta-analysis of 15 studies found a significant association between the S allele and a lower likelihood of response or remission (Serretti, Kato, De Ronchi, & Kinoshita, 2007; see also Levinson, Chapter 8, this volume).

Reduced numbers of 5-HT uptake transporters also have been demonstrated in blood platelets (Maes & Meltzer, 1995) in the brains of depressed individuals who committed suicide (Lin & Tsai, 2004; Mann et al., 2001), and by *in vivo* receptor imaging in depressed patients (Parsey et al., 2006). This reduction in 5-HTT capacity appears to be linked directly to inheritance of the S allele of 5-HTT (Li & He, 2007; Wasserman et al., 2007).

Available evidence from studies using receptor imaging techniques suggests that dysfunction of 5-HT$_{1A}$ receptors is clearly implicated in depression (Drevets et al., 2007). Although this abnormality could be an artifact of exposure to antidepressant medication, it has recently been demonstrated in a study of treatment-naive individuals (Hirvonen et al.,

2007). Down-regulation of 5-HT$_{1A}$ receptors is a consequence of exposure to chronic stress, however, which—in the absence of a heritable risk factor—is the most likely explanation (López et al., 1999; Maier & Watkins, 2005). Nevertheless, an allelic variation of the 5-HT$_{1A}$ receptor has recently been reported to be associated with risk of depression during interferon therapy (Kraus et al., 2007), so the potential contribution of a heritable vulnerability cannot be discounted.

The integrity of 5-HT neurotransmission also can be transiently compromised by dietary manipulation, specifically, by eliminating the precursor tryptophan (one of the essential amino acids) from the food source. Complete disruption of 5-HT synthesis has little immediate impact on mood in studies of healthy individuals, but it does impact more subtle aspects of cognitive–affective processing, such as enhanced anticipation of punishment (Cools, Robinson, & Sahakian, in press) and reduction of the normal attentional bias to positive emotionally valenced stimuli (Roiser et al., in press). In studies of depressed people, a brief period of tryptophan depletion does not worsen untreated depression, but it does significantly increases depressive symptoms in some unmedicated people with remitted depressive episodes (e.g., see Neumeister et al., 2006). Neumeister and colleagues (2006) also found that response to tryptophan depletion differs significantly between remitted depressed individuals and controls as a function of genetic vulnerability. Within the group of remitted depressed people, tryptophan depletion had stronger effects in individuals with at least one copy of the L allele of the 5-HTT, whereas within normal controls, only those who had two copies of the S polymorphism showed an increase in depressive symptoms.

Among patients treated for depression, tryptophan depletion can reverse acute response overnight in about 50 to 60% of people treated with SSRI antidepressants (Delgado, 2004; Delgado et al., 1991; Moore et al., 2000). Tryptophan depletion does not reverse response to placebo (Delgado, 2004). The lack of effect of tryptophan depletion on the improvement of patients treated with NRIs (Delgado, 2004), repetitive transcranial magnetic stimulation (O'Reardon et al., 2006), and cognitive therapy (O'Reardon et al., 2004) also points to the specificity of this mechanism.

Dopaminergic Systems

There are four principal DA pathways in the brain (see Figure 9.3) (Kandel et al., 1991; Kingsley, 2000). The tuberoinfundibular system projects from cell bodies in the hypothalamus to the pituitary and inhibits secretion of the hormone prolactin. The nigrostriatral system, which helps to regulate psychomotor activity, originates from cell bodies in the substantia nigra and projects to the basal ganglia. The mesolimbic pathway begins with cell bodies located in the ventral tegmentum and projects to the nucleus accumbens, amygdala, hippocampus, medial dorsal nucleus of the thalamus, and cingulate gyrus. The mesolimbic DA pathway modulates emotional expression and goal-directed or consummatory behavior. Because down-regulation of this pathway invariably accompanies learned helplessness and social defeat identifying individual differences in susceptibility has important implications for research on depression (Krishnan et al., 2007). The mesocortical DA pathway, which projects from the ventral tegmentum orbitofrontal and prefrontal cerebral cortex, subserves motivation, initiation of goal-directed tasks, and "executive" cognitive processes. Decreased DA activity has obvious implications in the motoric, hedonic, and cognitive symptoms of depression (Nestler & Carlezon, 2006; Willner, 1995). Recently, an allelic variation in the gene coding for the enzyme catechol-O-methyl transferase (COMT)—the *Val158Met* polymorphism—was found to be associated with significant differences in the experience of pos-

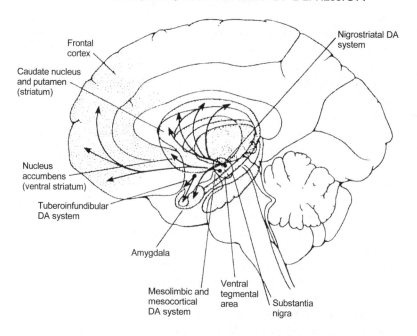

FIGURE 9.3. A lateral view of the brain demonstrates the course of the four major dopaminergic tracts. From Kandel, Schwartz, and Jessell (1991). Copyright 1991 by Appleton & Lange. Reprinted by permission.

itive affect in daily life, with individuals with one or two Met alleles experiencing significantly greater positive responses to pleasant events than those with the Val alleles (Wichers et al., in press). DA activity is also potentiated by stimulation of nicotine receptors (a subtype of receptors for acetylcholine), which may help to explain the high prevalence of tobacco consumption among depressed people (Glassman, 1993; see Freedland & Carney, Chapter 6, this volume). A selective increase in DA activity in mesocortical regions, perhaps induced by elevated cortisol levels, also may be implicated in development of hallucinations and delusions, which characterize about 10% of the most severely depressed patients (Schatzberg & Rothschild, 1992).

As with the other monoamines, chronic stress reduces DA levels and results in behavioral changes suggestive of depression (Nestler & Carlezon, 2006; Willner, 1995). For example, in an animal model of depression, chronic mild stress reduces the reinforcing effects of low concentrations of sucrose solution. Dopaminergic neurotransmission also is partly dependent on the integrity of 5-HT systems (Dremencov et al., 2004; Sasaki-Adams & Kelley, 2001), providing another example of how dysfunction in one system can provoke secondary changes in the others. Although none of the currently available antidepressants can truly be considered strongly dopaminergic, the MAOIs and perhaps bupropion and sertraline have some dopaminergic activity, and animal studies utilizing a variety of antidepressants have found that they can reverse or prevent the DA dysfunction caused by chronic stress (Cuadra, Zurito, Gioino, & Molina, 2001; Dremencov et al., 2004; Nestler & Carlezon, 2006; Willner, 1997). Among the various DA receptors that have been identified, the D_2 receptor appears to be most relevant to antidepressant activity (Gershon, Vishne, & Grunhaus, 2007). Active efforts continue to develop "triple reuptake" inhibitors, although such efforts have been difficult because of toxicity and the likelihood that a strongly dopaminergic drug would prove to be habit forming and have abuse potential.

STRESS, MONOAMINES, AND THE HPA AXIS

The foregoing discussion has emphasized the changes in monoamine function that are linked to depression, particularly in relation to the neurobiological consequences of sustained, unresolvable stress. In this section, the role of the HPA axis is considered in more detail.

Elevated HPA activity is the hallmark of mammalian stress responses, and the regulation of the axis is partly under the control of phasic NE (activating) and tonic 5-HT (inhibitory) neurotransmission. This axis has four levels of organization and modulation. In relevant areas of the cerebral cortex, the threat and contextual significance of the stressor are perceived, and the signal is relayed to the HPA. With respect to the role of the higher brain regions in HPA regulation, neurons containing the neuropeptides CRH and arginine vasopressin are diffusely located throughout the cerebral cortex, with particularly high concentrations within the thalamus, amygdala, and other components of the limbic system. Studies measuring CRH synthesis demonstrate that these brain regions "light up" immediately following exposure to stress (Holsboer, 1995; Swaab et al., 2005). Furthermore, because CRH activates the LC, which in turn further stimulates the thalamus, hypothalamus, and amygdala, sustained stress can provoke a *reverberating circuit*, or a positive feedback loop. Activating inputs from neurons are transmitted to the hypothalamus, where CRH also is released and travels systemically to the adjacent pituitary. Specialized cells in the anterior pituitary respond to CRH via release of ACTH, which travels via the bloodstream to the cortex of the adrenal glands, where glucocorticoids are released and, if the stressor is sustained, synthesis is increased. The impact of CRH stimulation is increased by simultaneous release of arginine vasopressin, which in turn is intensified during chronic stress (Swaab et al., 2005).

The cellular effects of glucocorticoids are triggered by intracellular glucocorticoid receptors (GRs), which migrate between the cell membrane and cell nuclei (Holsboer, 2000; Swaab et al., 2005). Thus, cortisol can rapidly modulate changes in the activity of a number of genes. Cortisol is the principal glucocorticoid hormone of humans. Once cortisol release is stimulated by ACTH, it is released into the circulation and exerts a large number of physiological actions on various end organs, including anti-inflammatory effects on immune function and insulin–antagonist effects on glucose and lipid metabolism. Overall, these acute changes promote short-term survival in response to overwhelming or life-threatening circumstances. Such benefits are time-limited, however, and negative compensatory (allostatic) changes begin to accumulate if cortisol levels remain elevated for prolonged periods (McEwen, 2000). Such allostatic changes include increased risks of hypertension, obesity, heart disease, osteoporosis, and autoimmune diseases, all of which appear to be increased in people with mood disorders (Evans et al., 2005).

The HPA axis, like the NE and 5-HT components of stress response, is regulated by a redundant, multilevel system of inhibitory control. This type of negative feedback inhibition occurs at all levels of the axis, including the hippocampus, hypothalamus, pituitary, and adrenal cortex. As acute stresses pass or resolve, the elevated plasma cortisol levels of healthy humans normalize within a matter of minutes or hours.

Sustained hypercortisolism thus can result from increased CRH drive (from the hypothalamus or cerebral cortex), increased secretion of ACTH (e.g., by a pituitary tumor), unrestrained noradrenergic stimulation from the LC, and/or the failure of one or more mechanisms of feedback inhibition (Holsboer, 1995; Swaab et al., 2005). There is evidence that sustained hypercortisolism can impair the integrity of HPA feedback inhibition (Bremner,

1999; Sapolsky, 1996). Exposure to various forms of stress early in life has been shown to compromise the regulation of HPA activity for a lifetime (Bremner, 1999; Coplan et al., 2001). In animal models of early trauma, even brief periods of maternal separation can result in longstanding changes in stress responses (Coplan et al., 2001, 2006). Fortunately, this effect can be partly mitigated by competent maternal behavior (Macri & Würbel, 2006). Stress in later life appears to accelerate the slow decline in the integrity of HPA axis regulation that normally accompanies aging. This age-dependent change has been shown to result, in part, from death of cells containing GRs in the hippocampus (Sapolsky, 1996), coupled with a decline in neurogenesis (i.e., the process of generation of new neurons) (Bremner, 2006). Hypercortisolism may suppress neurogenesis by decreasing neuronal synthesis of brain-derived neurotropic factor (BDNF) and is thought to play a role in the reductions in the volume of several areas of the cortex associated with depression (Bremner, 2006). Importantly, treatments that effectively reduce hypercortisolism have also been shown to at least partly reverse hippocampal volume reduction in other conditions, including PTSD (Bremner, 1999) and Cushing's disease (Starkman et al., 1999). However, because reduced hippocampal volume has been shown to be partly heritable in free-ranging primates (Lyons, Yang, Sawyer-Glover, Moseley, & Schatzberg, 2001) and has been documented in patients experiencing their first lifetime depressive episode (Frodl et al., 2002), this may be a risk factor, as well as a consequence, for hypercortisolism. Consistent with this view, primates with smaller hippocampal volumes were shown to have increased cortisol responses to experimentally induced stress (Lyons, Parker, Zeitzer, Buckmaster, & Schatzberg, 2007).

Like stress itself, hypercortisolism is not unique to depression. A significant minority of people with acute schizophrenia, mania, PTSD, and other distressing mental disorders manifest one or more signs of hypercortisolism. Across mental disorders, intensity of dysphoric arousal increases the likelihood of hypercortisolism (Thase & Howland, 1995). Abnormalities of HPA regulation also commonly occur in advanced Alzheimer's disease, presumably due to acceleration of hippocampal cell death (Swaab et al., 2005). Nevertheless, dysregulation of HPA activity plays an important role in the pathophysiology of depression and may ultimately prove to be a target for novel therapeutics of severe depressive disorders (Holsboer, 2000; Nemeroff, 1998; see Gitlin, Chapter 24, this volume).

ANTIDEPRESSANTS, MONOAMINE RECEPTORS, AND INTRACELLULAR MECHANISMS

Although it was known by the mid-1960s that TCAs and MAOIs enhance NE and 5-HT neurotransmission, several puzzling discrepancies indicated that the mechanisms underlying antidepressant response were not due simply to monoamine agonist effects. For example, although increased NE or 5-HT levels were available in the synaptic cleft within hours of administration of NE or 5-HT reuptake inhibitors, antidepressant responses took weeks to emerge (Duman, Heninger, & Nestler, 1997; Shelton, 2007). By contrast, some NE agonists, as exemplified by cocaine, were shown to have rapid mood-elevating properties but no sustained antidepressant effects. The MAOIs, which increase synaptic monoamine levels by inhibiting intracellular degradation of NE, 5-HT, and DA, similarly were associated with a time course of antidepressant effects that typically lagged at least several weeks behind the biochemical effects. Subsequently, other compounds that did not have clear-cut monoamine agonist effects, such as mianserin, also were identified to be effective antidepressants.

It is now clear that the synaptic effects of antidepressant medications initiate a sequence or cascade of effects that culminate within the nuclei of serotoninergic and noradrenergic neurons, modulating the activity of specific genes (Duman, Schlesinger, Kodama, Russell, & Duman, 2007; Shelton, 2007; Warner-Schmidt & Duman, 2006). Thus, the interplay resulting from effects on monoamine reuptake transporters and changes in the "signal" of cellular electrical activity is transduced into a series of intracellular reactions of second- and third-messengers that activate or inhibit the activity of selected genes. The pathway of action of antidepressant medication initiates an effect at 5-HT or NE receptors, whether by diffusely increasing the availability of monoamines at the synapse (i.e., the MAOIs), selectively blockading reuptake of serotonin (SSRIs), norepinephrine (NRIs; e.g., desipramine or reboxetine) or both (the SNRIs venlafaxine and duloxetine) selectively at specific receptor subtypes (e.g., the 5-HT_2 blocking antidepressants trazodone, nefazodone, mianserin, and mirtazapine). Receptor binding activates membrane-bound guanine nucleotide-binding (G) proteins and enzymes such as phospholipase C (PLC), protein kinase C, and adenylate cyclase (AC) (Shelton, 2007). These enzymes catalyze the formation of the so-called "second messengers" (which actually are at least the third step in the sequence), such as cyclic adenomonophosphate (cAMP) and diacylglycerol. The second messengers, in turn, activate intracellular enzymes, protein kinases A and C (PKA and PKC, respectively), which phosphorylate the gene transcription factor CREB (cAMP response element binding protein). CREB appears to be the first common step shared by antidepressants that selectively modulate NE or 5-HT neurotransmission (Shelton, 2007).

Phosphorylated CREB regulates the activity of a number of genes related to stress responses, including the genes that code for CRH, GRs, BDNF, and TRKB, which is the intracellular receptor for BDNF (Duman et al., 2007; Shelton, 2007). As noted earlier, BDNF is receiving increased attention, because it has been shown to reverse or inhibit stress-induced apoptosis, it is necessary for neurogenesis, and it plays a key role in neuroplasticity (Pittenger & Duman, 2008; Warner-Schmidt & Duman, 2006). BDNF levels are significantly decreased by a variety of stressors and increased by a variety of antidepressant interventions (Martinowich & Lu, 2008; Pittenger & Duman, 2008). Importantly, whereas BDNF promotes stress resilience in brain regions such as the hippocampus, it reduces appetitive and exploratory behavior in mesolimbic regions and plays an important role in mediating behavioral responses to social defeat (Berton et al., 2006; Krishnan et al., 2007). Levels of BDNF have been shown to be reduced in the plasma of depressed people (Aydemir et al., 2006; Huang, Lee & Liu, 2009). This abnormality appears to be reversed by effective antidepressant treatment (Aydemir et al., 2006; Huang et al., 2007; Martinowich & Lu, 2008; Yoshimura et al., 2007).

OTHER NEUROTRANSMITTER DISTURBANCES

Neuron fibers containing acetylcholine (ACH) are distributed diffusely throughout the cerebral cortex and interact extensively with monoamine and glucocorticoid systems (Kingsley, 2000). At the most general level, ACH neurons have alerting or activating acute effects on brain systems, as reflected by increased release of ACTH and cortisol, increased nocturnal awakenings, and increased firing of LC neurons (Janowsky & Overstreet, 1995). The two principal subtypes of ACH receptors are called *nicotinic* and *muscarinic* receptors. Although muscarinic receptors have received the most attention, the interaction between DA and nicotinic neurotransmission also is significant (Glassman, 1993; Stolerman & Reavill, 1989).

It has long been known that drugs with agonist and antagonist effects on ACH have opposing effects on depressive symptoms (Janowsky & Overstreet, 1995). Behavioral changes following administration of an ACH agonist include lethargy, anergia, and psychomotor retardation in normal subjects and, among patients, exacerbation of depression, as well as weak and transient antimanic effects (Janowsky & Overstreet, 1995).

There is evidence from studies of animals and humans that heightened muscarinic ACH receptor sensitivity can induce some of the neurobiological changes associated with depression (Janowsky & Overstreet, 1995). For example, a mice strain bred to be supersensitive to cholinergic effects develops learned helplessness quickly when exposed to inescapable stress (Overstreet, 1993). Similarly, some remitted patients with recurrent mood disorders, as well as their never-ill first-degree relatives, manifest a trait-like supersensitivity to cholinergic agonists (Sitaram, Dubé, Keshavan, Davies, & Reynal, 1987). Elevated choline levels in depression likewise have been detected by *in vivo* studies utilizing magnetic resonance spectroscopy, particularly in basal ganglia regions (Yildiz-Yesiloglu & Ankerst, 2006). A specific gene accounting for such heightened activity has not yet been confirmed, although a polymorphism of the type 2 muscarinic receptor has been implicated (Wang et al., 2004). A state of cholinergic supersensitivity also can be induced by attenuating adrenergic activity (Schittecatte et al., 1992). Interest in the therapeutic potential of cholinergic antagonists has recently been reactivated by the work of Furey and Drevets (2006), who found that intravenous doses of scopalomine bromide have robust and relatively sustained antidepressant effects.

Gamma-aminobutyric acid (GABA) has inhibitory effects on NE and DA pathways. GABA receptors are densely localized in the thalamus and ascending mesocortical and mesolimbic systems (Kingsley, 2000; Paul, 1995). GABA is released in a calcium (Ca^{+2})-dependent fashion from interneurons in the cortex, brainstem, and spinal cord, and dampens the activity of excitatory neural circuits. Through this mechanism, inhibitory GABA-ergic neurons help to mediate the expression of the behaviors associated with learned helplessness (Berton et al., 2007). There are two principal subtypes of GABA receptors, referred to as A and B (Paul, 1995). Benzodiazepines and barbiturates attach to $GABA_A$ receptors, which serve to "gate" the control of membrane chloride (Cl^-) ion channels. This results in localized hyperpolarization of neurons, which decreases their responsivity to excitatory neurotransmitters. $GABA_B$ receptors are indirectly coupled to membrane potassium (K^+) channels via a G-protein and have uncertain clinical relevance (Kingsley, 2000; Paul, 1995).

Chronic stress can reduce or deplete GABA levels in these regions of the brain, perhaps reflecting, yet again, an example of an excessive demand outstripping the capacity for synthesis (Weiss & Kilts, 1998). Reduction of GABA levels in people with depressive disorders has been observed in plasma and CSF specimens (Petty, 1995), in postmortem tissues of individuals who completed suicide (Rajkowska et al., 2007; Sequeria et al., 2007), and in studies using proton magnetic resonance spectroscopy *in vivo* (Hasler et al., 2007). Reductions of cortical volume in regions of the prefrontal cortex and hippocampus, at least in part, appear to be the result of reductions in GABA-ergic interneurons in the surrounding glia (Rajkowska et al., 2007). Although sustained normalization of GABA function has not yet been demonstrated in longitudinal studies of clinical populations, some evidence does suggest normal GABA function among recently remitted individuals (Hasler et al., 2005).

The excitatory amino acid glutamate is one of the most widely distributed neurotransmitters in the CNS (Kingsley, 2000). There are two broad types of glutamate receptors: the α-amino-3-hydroxy-5-methylisoxazole-4-propionic acid (AMPA) receptor and the N-methyl-D-aspartate (NMDA) receptor. AMPA receptors are ionotropic (i.e., cation channels) transmembrane receptors that mediate fast synaptic transmission in the brain. AMPA receptors (AMPARs) are essential for development of long-term potentiation (LTP) of neurons, one of the best-studied forms of neuroplasticity. AMPARs comprise four types of glutamate subunits, designated as Glu_{R1}, Glu_{R2}, Glu_{R3}, and Glu_{R4}, which combine to form tetramers. Most AMPARs are either homotetramers (i.e., four units of Glu_{R1} or Glu_{R4}) or symmetric combinations of two units of Glu_{R2} and a second dimer that comprises Glu_{R1}, Glu_{R3}, or Glu_{R4}; each subunit has a binding site for glutamate. The ion channel opens when at least two sites are occupied. Most AMPARs in the brain include Glu_{R2} subunits, which are impermeable to calcium, hence helping to guard against neurotoxicity.

The NMDA receptor is an ionotropic receptor for glutamate (and, to a lesser extent, aspartate); activation of these receptors opens nonselective ion channels that allow sodium and calcium influx and potassium efflux. It is the calcium influx that results in the critical role that NMDA receptors play in both synaptic plasticity and neurotoxicity. NMDA receptors comprise heterodimers formed by NR_1 and NR_2 subunits; multiple receptor isoforms are characterized by distinct patterns of distribution within the brain and unique functional properties. Each receptor has three regions, which constitute the extracellular, membrane, and intracellular domains. The extracellular domain includes NR_1 subunits that bind to glycine and NR_2 subunits that bind to glutamate. The membrane domain includes the channel pores, which are highly permeable to calcium and are subject to a voltage-dependent magnesium block. The intracellular domain contain residues that are modifiable by protein kinases and protein phosphatases.

The potential relevance of drugs that activate AMPARs or block NMDA receptors to a range of CNS disorders is increasingly recognized (Bleakman, Alt, & Witkin, 2007; Palucha & Pilc, 2005; Pittenger, Sanacora, & Krystal, 2007). Importantly, intracellular accumulation of glutamate has neurotoxic effects, particularly for glial cells (Rajkowska & Miguel-Hidalgo, 2007), and neurons and glial cells in the hippocampus and amygdala have high concentrations of NMDA receptors (Mathew et al., 2001; Rajkowska & Miguel-Hidalgo, 2007). With respect to antidepressant effects, the recent findings of Zarate and colleagues (2006) are of considerable interest: They confirmed that infusions of the NMDA antagonist ketamine have rapid, robust, and relatively sustained therapeutic effects in a small, but well-controlled, study of patients with refractory depressive disorders. Although both the mode of administration (intravenous) and the propensity for psychomimetic effects necessarily delimit the therapeutic utility of ketamine per se, extensive research directed at identifying other compounds without these drawbacks is ongoing in a number of laboratories.

ABNORMALITIES OF HORMONAL REGULATORY SYSTEMS

HPA Axis Dysregulation

As briefly noted earlier, increased secretion of plasma cortisol is one of the best documented biological correlates of depression. Beyond simply measuring cortisol concentrations in various body fluids at one point in time, more detailed investigations have collected integrated measures of HPA axis activity across a number of hours or cortisol responses to various provocative challenges, including the much-maligned DST or the more refined combined DST/CRH infusion test.

That hypercortisolemia in depression is heavily severity-dependent is readily apparent in differences in prevalence: Whereas only 20–40% of depressed outpatients show elevated cortisol concentrations in plasma or urine specimens, up to 60–80% of depressed inpatients manifest increased cortisol concentrations. Consistent with this observation, hypercortisolemia is at least twice as likely in studies of patients with melancholic (i.e., endogenous) or psychotic forms of depression as in studies of individuals with less severe forms of major depressive disorder (Holsboer, 1995; Thase & Howland, 1995).

Hypercortisolism has several therapeutic implications. Patients with increased HPA activity appear to be less responsive to placebo (Ribeiro, Tandon, Grunhaus, & Greden, 1993) or psychotherapy (Thase et al., 1996) than are individuals with more normal HPA activity, and persistent hypercortisolemia—despite apparently effective antidepressant therapy—is associated with an increased risk of subsequent relapse (Holsboer, 1995; Ribeiro et al., 1993). Development of safer, more selective CRH antagonists was once considered by some to be the area of greatest therapeutic promise (Holsboer, 2000; Nemeroff, 1998), although slow progress in this area has somewhat dampened enthusiasm.

Thyroid Axis Dysregulation

Thyroid gland dysfunction has long been known to be associated with increased risk for depression (Fountoulakis et al., 2006; Thase et al., 1985). In addition to *hypothyroidism* (a clinical diagnosis based on low basal levels of thyroid hormone and characteristic symptoms, e.g., fatigue, weight gain, cold intolerance, and dry skin), there are less clear-cut cases of "subclinical" hypothyroidism in which basal thyroid hormone levels are still within normal limits but there is evidence of diminished response to the hypothalamic (thyrotropin-releasing hormone; TRH) or pituitary (thyroid-stimulating hormone; TSH) neuropeptides that drive the thyroid axis (Fountoulakis et al., 2006; Thase et al., 1985). It is important to note, however, that relatively few people seeking treatment for depression have frank hypothyroidism, and only a small percentage may be considered to have subclinical hypothyroidism (Fountoulakis et al., 2006; Thase et al., 1985). Normal thyroid function is nevertheless essential for the integrity of CNS processes such as energy metabolism (Bauer et al., 2003) and neurogenesis (Montero-Pedrazuela et al., 2006); moreover, there is evidence that even subtle reductions in the activity of the thyroid axis may be associated with reduced responsiveness to antidepressants or greater risk of relapse (Cole et al., 2002; Joffe & Marriott, 2000). Because of these characteristics, augmentation of an ineffective antidepressant medication with thyroid hormone is a reasonably well-tolerated strategy that benefits a minority of patients with treatment-resistant depression (Nierenberg et al., 2006) and may actually speed antidepressant response in treatment-naive, depressed patients (Cooper-Kazaz et al., 2007).

A significant minority of depressed patients with otherwise normal basal thyroid hormone levels—up to 40% in studies of depressed inpatients—manifest a blunted TSH response to a test dose of TRH (Mason, Garbutt, & Prange, 1995). This altered response, which paradoxically would normally be suggestive of hyperthyroidism, does not rapidly reverse with effective treatment and is predictive of increased risk of relapse (Kirkegaard & Faber, 1998). Within the context of normal basal levels of thyroid hormones, a blunted TSH response to TRH is indicative of down-regulation of thyrotropin responsiveness as a consequence of increased extrahypothalamic "drive" on the thyroid axis (Holsboer, 1995). Like the increased drive on the HPA axis, this appears to be part of the brain's homeostatic response to sustained dysphoric activation.

Growth Hormone and Somatostatin

Growth hormone (GH) is secreted by cells in the anterior pituitary in response to the hypothalamic neuropeptide growth hormone–releasing factor (GHRF), as well as noradrenergic stimulation via α_2 receptor stimulation of NE (Holsboer, 1995). GH secretion is principally inhibited by the neuropeptides somatostatin and CRH. Significant concentrations of somatostatin are found in the amygdala, hippocampus, nucleus accumbens, prefrontal cortex, and LC (Plotsky, Owens, & Nemeroff, 1995). In addition to its inhibitory effects on GH release, somatostatin dampens the effects of other activating neuropeptides, including CRH. GH secretion normally follows a 24-hour circadian rhythm, with highest levels between 2300 and 0200 hours. Thus, the nocturnal rise in GH secretion is normally synchronized with the first few hours of sleep, especially during the first non-REM sleep period, in concert with the greatest amount of deep, slow-wave sleep (SWS; Steiger, 2007). The most consistent alteration of GH associated with depression is blunted release in response to a variety of agents with noradrenergic agonist effects, including various antidepressants and the selective α_2 agonist clonidine (Holsboer, 1995; Thase & Howland, 1995). Blunted GH release has been documented in childhood-onset depression (Dahl et al., 2000) and appears to be both trait-like (Coplan et al., 2000) and most pronounced among depressed people with diminished SWS (Steiger, 2007).

Prolactin

Prolactin, which is involved in regulation of reproductive functions, such as nursing and menstruation, is released from the pituitary in response to stimulation of 5-HT_{1A} receptors and inhibited by stimulation of D_2 receptors (Kingsley, 2000). Although most studies of basal prolactin secretion have not detected abnormalities in depressed patients, blunted prolactin response to various 5-HT agonists has been found in some, but not all, studies (Maes & Meltzer, 1995; Mann et al., 2001). Of note, blunted prolactin responsivity is less likely to be found in studies of premenopausal women, which suggests that higher levels of circulating estrogen have a facilitative effect on 5-HT_{1A} neurotransmission (Parry & Haynes, 2000). Elevated prolactin levels, on the other hand, may be a consequence of therapy with most of the older antipsychotic medications, as well as several of the newer generation of antipsychotics, such as risperidone.

ALTERATIONS OF SLEEP NEUROPHYSIOLOGY

The neurochemical processes mediating sleep are fairly well characterized (Steiger, 2007). The propensity to sleep follows a circadian rhythm marked by a nocturnal rise in the pineal hormone melatonin and by low levels of ACTH and cortisol. Melatonin is released from the pineal gland following the onset of darkness in response to ß-adrenergic stimulation. The sleep–wake circadian rhythm is "paced" by the suprachiasmatic nucleus of the hypothalamus. There is also a 90-minute infradian cycle oscillating between REM and non-REM sleep; this cycle is normally suppressed during wakefulness. The desynchronization of EEG rhythms following sleep onset partly reflects decreased activity of the LC and increased inhibitory activity of GABA-ergic and 5-HT neurons; the latter effect appears to be mediated by 5-HT_2 receptors (Horne, 1992; Steiger, 2007). Beyond facilitating sleep onset, 5-HT neurons tonically inhibit the onset of REM sleep; this effect appears to be mediated by 5-HT_{1A} receptors. Near the end of each 90-minute REM–non-REM cycle, 5-HT neurons cease firing, which "releases" the pontine cholinergic neurons that initiate REMs. The depth of sleep also is facilitated by certain neuropeptides, including ghrelin, galanin, and neuropeptide Y, and disrupted by others, including CRH and somatostatin (Steiger, 2007).

As noted earlier, a significant proportion of people with depression manifest reduced SWS and an early onset of the first period of REM (also referred to as *reduced REM latency*; Benca, Obermeyer, Thisted, & Gillin, 1992; Thase, 2006). Reduced REM latency and decreased SWS are significantly correlated, in large part because 30 to 40 minutes of SWS during the first non-REM sleep period normally inhibits the onset of the first REM period. SWS propensity is partly under genetic control, and consistent with trait-like behavior, reduced SWS often persists following clinical recovery (Kupfer & Ehlers, 1989; Thase, Fasiczka, Berman, Simons, & Reynolds, 1998). Although both of these changes in sleep electrophysiology are observed with aging, depression appears to accelerate this process by a decade or more (Thase, 2006). The findings are more evident among men and postmenopausal women than among premenopausal women, perhaps reflecting the "sparing" effects of estrogen on deep sleep (Thase, 2006).

Compared to age-matched healthy controls, people with depression also experience an increase in nocturnal awakenings and a decrease in total sleep time. Whereas reduced SWS appears to be state-independent, sleep continuity disturbances associated with depression are to some extent correlated with symptom severity. Unlike normal aging, depression is also associated with an increase in the frequency and amplitude of REM sleep (Thase, 2006). Such changes in the phasic activity of REM sleep, which are quantified as measures of REM intensity or density, are greatest during the first several REM periods. Increased *phasic* REM sleep typically co-occurs with other state-dependent biological abnormalities, including hypercortisolemia (Kupfer & Ehlers, 1989; Thase & Howland, 1995). Increased phasic REM sleep is more pronounced in recurrent depression than in a single lifetime episode—both during depressive episodes (Thase et al., 1995) and following remission (Jindal et al., 2002)—and is one component of a profile of sleep disturbances associated with poorer response to psychotherapy (Thase et al., 1996, 1997). Although linked to severity and at least partly reversible with effective treatment, increased indices of phasic REM sleep also appear to identify people at high risk for depressive disorder (Modell, Ising, Holsboer, & Lauer, 2005).

Antidepressants have variable effects on measures of sleep efficiency that are largely linked to secondary properties, such as antihistaminergic effects (Sharpley & Cowen, 1995; Thase, 2006). Potent monoamine oxidase reuptake inhibitors that are not sedating tend to be relatively sleep-neutral, with some tendency for increased nocturnal awakenings to be slightly offset by improvements in subject complaints of insomnia (Thase, 2006). Drugs that block 5-HT_{2C} receptors, including mirtazapine and agomelatine, may have an advantage over SSRIs and SNRIs in terms of improvements in sleep efficiency (Thase, 2006; Zupancic & Guilleminault, 2006), although there is no evidence to indicate a stronger overall antidepressant effect.

Most antidepressants, including the SSRIs, SNRIs, TCAs, and MAOIs, rapidly delay the onset of REM sleep and suppress phasic REM sleep (Sharpley & Cowen, 1995; Thase, 2006). Pharmacological REM suppression is mediated by stimulation of 5-HT_{1A} receptors, as well as by less well-characterized effects of NE neurotransmission. Because nonpharmacological deprivation of REM sleep (implemented by EEG-monitored awakenings) also was shown to have at least transient antidepressant effects, for a time researchers postulated that REM suppression was a necessary action of antidepressant therapies (e.g., Thase & Kupfer, 1987). However, REM suppression is only weakly correlated with antidepressant efficacy (Thase & Kupfer, 1987) and neither a number of novel antidepressant medications, including bupropion (Nofzinger et al., 1995), nefazodone (Rush et al., 1998), and agomelatine (Zupancic & Guilleminault, 2006), nor psychosocial interventions, such as cognitive therapy (Thase et al., 1998), significantly suppress REM sleep. Together, these findings indicate that REM suppression is neither a necessary nor sufficient element of antidepressant therapy.

DEPRESSION AND CIRCADIAN RHYTHMS

Sleep disturbances, increased cortisol secretion, blunted nocturnal GH secretion, and elevated nocturnal body temperature all reflect abnormalities of circadian biological rhythms, with severe depression possibly representing an abnormal phase advancement of circadian rhythms (Wirz-Justice, 1995). Researchers also noted that depressed people have disruptions of the social zeitgebers ("time givers" such as mealtimes, periods of companionship, and exercise) that help to entrain circadian rhythms (Ehlers, Frank, & Kupfer, 1988). A review of later studies of depression suggested that the alterations in associated circadian rhythms were better viewed as a disorganization of functions than as a phase advance (Thase et al., 2002). Thus, the state of dysphoric activation that characterized more severe depressions—whether mediated by increased CRH and cortisol levels or decreased inhibitory neurotransmission from 5-HT or GABA pathways—may simply "overpower" the more subtle regulation of circadian rhythms. There is, however, evidence of a circadian phase delay in the subset of patients that experiences recurrent winter depression (Lewy et al., 2007) that is responsive to manipulations of the photoperiod via bright white, morning light or dawn stimulation (Avery et al., 2001; Lewy et al., 2007).

IMMUNOLOGICAL DISTURBANCES

Depressive disorders are associated with several immunological abnormalities, including decreased lymphocyte proliferation in response to mitogens and other forms of impaired cellular immunity (Irwin & Miller, 2007; Petito, Repetto, & Hartemink, 2001; Raison, Capuron, & Miller, 2006). These lymphocytes and macrophages produce proinflammatory peptides, such as C-reactive protein (CRP), and cytokines, such the interleukins (ILs), which in turn interact with neuromodulators, such as BDNF and CRH (Irwin & Miller, 2007; Petito et al., 2001; Raison et al., 2006). Although depression is not invariably associated with alterations in immune response, the number of studies reporting positive associations is too great to discount, and this relationship is at least likely to contribute to the increased risk of inflammatory diseases, including arthritis, allergy, and atherosclerosis, associated with depression (Glassman & Miller, 2007). Studies of the behavioral and neurochemical effects associated with interferon are illustrative (Felger et al., 2007; Lotrich, Rabinovitz, Gironda, & Pollock, 2007; Wichers et al., 2007). Of note, the risk of depression during interferon therapy may be linked to an allelic variation in the gene for the 5-HT_{1A} receptor (Kraus et al., 2007) and is attenuated by pretreatment with antidepressants (Raison et al., 2007).

CEREBRAL METABOLIC STUDIES IN DEPRESSIVE DISORDERS

The activity of neuronal circuitry may be visualized in the living brain via PET or fMRI scans. In studies utilizing PET to measure cerebral glucose utilization (because glucose is the primary source of energy for neurons, it is an excellent marker of neuronal activity), experimentally provoked dysphoria has been shown to increase cerebral blood flow (CBF) to the thalamus, medial prefrontal cortex, and amygdala in healthy individuals (Mayberg, 2003), with deactivation of the DLPFC observed in some studies (see Freed & Mann, 2007). The most widely replicated PET finding associated with clinical depression is reduced glucose utilization in the anterior cortical structures, including DLPFC (Drevets, 2000; Mayberg, 2003). Reductions in DLPFC activity have also been documented in studies using fMRI (Harvey et al., 2005; Siegle, Thompson, Carter, Steinhauser, & Thase, 2007). Because this relative hypofrontality has been observed in unipolar, bipolar, and secondary depressions (Baxter et al., 1989), it appears to reflect a common final pathway for diverse depressive states. Frontal hypometabolism has been shown to be reversible following switches from depression into mania in bipolar depression (Ketter et al., 1994), as well as in response to both psychotherapy and pharmacotherapy (Brody et al., 2001; Goldapple et al., 2004; Martin, Martin, Rai, Richardson, & Royall, 2001).

In addition to a global reduction of anterior cerebral metabolism, increased glucose metabolism has been observed in several limbic regions, most prominently in the amydala (Drevets, 2000). The strongest evidence of limbic hypermetabolism is found in studies of patients with a family history of severe, recurrent depression, hypercortisolemia, or PSG abnormalities (Drevets, 2000; Nofzinger et al., 2000). Among this high-risk group, limbic hypermetabolism is suppressed by effective pharmacotherapy, but appears to reemerge when patients are restudied off medication (Drevets, 2000) or following 5-HT depletion (Bremner et al., 1997; Neumeister et al., 2006). As initially reported by Hariri and colleagues (2002) in healthy control subjects manifesting the "at-risk" S allele of the 5-HTT, amygdalar hypermetabolism appears to be the emotional "amplifier" that helps to distort the signal of relatively minor stressors in vulnerable people. Interestingly, abnormalities of prefrontal and limbic systems appear to be unrelated (i.e., having one does not increase the likelihood of manifesting the other), at least in mildly to moderately depressed patients (Siegle et al., 2007); thus, they may represent distinctly different targets for intervention (Siegle, Carter, & Thase, 2006). There is some evidence that that cognitive-behavioral therapy and antidepressant medication result in different patterns of changes in CBF, with psychotherapy showing a greater impact on anterior cortical structures, and medication having a greater effect on subcortical structures, including the amygdala (Goldapple et al., 2004; Kennedy et al., 2007).

SUMMARY

Major depressive disorder is a heterogeneous clinical entity; not surprisingly, therefore, it has been associated with a wide range of neurobiological disturbances. The characteristics that have been shown to be at least partly state-dependent—including elevated peripheral levels of NE metabolites, increased phasic REM sleep, poor sleep maintenance, hypercortisolism, impaired cellular immunity, decreased DLPFC activity, and increased activity in the amygdala and related paralimbic regions—tend to coaggregate among more severely symptomatic patients, particularly older patients who have experienced recurrent depressive episodes; this constellation partly maps onto the classic clinical prototype of endogenous depression or melancholia.

The trait-like neurobiological characteristics of depression—including low 5-HIAA, decreased SWS, reduced REM latency, blunted nocturnal growth hormone response, increased responsivity to stress, and possibly reduced hippocampal volume—are associated with an early age of onset and a more chronic illness course, as well as greater heritability. In people manifesting these traits, symptom expression early in the course of the illness may be shaped by the developmental trajectory of functional inhibitory response systems (i.e., 5-HT and GABA), resulting in symptoms that are atypical of melancholia, such as overeating and oversleeping. Given that estrogen enhances these inhibitory responses, it is not surprising that reverse-neurovegetative features are most common among depressed premenopausal women.

Nevertheless, it is also true that responses to stress, aging, and neurobiological sequelae of recurrent depression are almost inextricably interwoven, and many individuals experience a shift in the predominant symptoms and response to treatment over time. During youth and young adult life, the onset of the first depressive episode is almost invariably associated with significant stress (Kendler, Karkowski, & Prescott, 1999); this relation is strongest in individuals with a history of increased genetic risk (Caspi et al., 2003; Kendler et al., 2005). This association unravels in midlife for individuals with a history of recurrent depressive episodes (Kendler, Thornton, & Gardner, 2001), however, in concert with the increasing prevalence of state-dependent neurobiological abnormalities. Relevant later-life diseases of the brain that impair brain function—including cerebrovascular disease and Alzheimer's disease—subsequently heighten vulnerability to depression, even among those with low heritable risk.

FUTURE DIRECTIONS

Although many aspects of the neurobiology of depression remain only partly understood—and some findings that appear quite promising in 2008 are likely to be false leads—there has been tremendous progress in the 6 years since publication of the first edition of this *Handbook*. The major developments include further clarification of the associations between both stress responses and antidepressant actions to intracellular processes, including those relevant to a large number of heritable factors that may be associated with individual differences in the vulnerability to, clinical characteristics of, and therapeutic responses in depression. Using messenger RNA as an indicator of gene activity, it is now possible to determine which genes are "turned on" or "turned off" by particular stressors or interventions. To the extent that gene products can be measured reliably in plasma or CSF or be "tagged" with radionucleotides that permit visualization of gene activity in the living brain, these techniques are increasingly relevant in clinical research. Even when *in vivo* measurement is not possible, research applications using relevant animal models of depression and postmortem brain tissue are providing important new data.

Following completion of mapping the human genome, it has become possible to study the relations among various polymorphisms for gene products relevant to neurotransmission (i.e., genes that code for proteins involved in the metabolism and signal transduction of monoamines, excitatory amino acids, and glucocorticoids) and familial risk for mood disorders. The explosion of research that followed recognition of the link between the less functional S allele of the serotonin transporter and increased response to stress in terms of limbic activation (Hariri et al., 2002) and risk of depression (Caspi et al., 2003) is illustrative of but one of many possible links to vulnerability. Research targeting heritable resilience factors (i.e., gene products that are shown to reduce the impact of other risk factors) holds comparable promise (Southwick, Vythilingam, & Charney, 2005). Not only will the next decade of research help to clarify further the complex biopsychosocial pathways of illness transmission, but it may also lead to identification of potential new mechanisms for intervention. The ultimate goal of such research will be development of treatments that have enduring or truly curative effects.

Finally, changes in relevant regions of the brain in response to various pharmacological or psychological mood induction paradigms, and in response to various information-processing tasks, have now been extensively studied. These studies reveal both similarities and differences between people suffering from depression and the sadness or distress experienced by healthy controls. Consistent with other lines of evidence, the overall pattern of these results supports a continuum of model of psychopathology, spanning the range across "normal" dysphoria, grief, and minor depression, and the mild, moderate, and most severe forms of major depressive episodes. Dysphoric affect is associated with activation of the amygdala and related limbic structures, with a progressive reduction of the DLPFC that is associated with increasing syndromal severity. The next generation of research will focus on the reversibility of structural changes associated with depression, such as increased amygdalar volume and decreased hippocampal size, as well as on development of more efficient and powerful interventions that directly target these abnormalities. Until such strategies are available, early recognition of depression, vigorous treatment leading to complete remission of symptoms, and subsequent prophylaxis to minimize the risk of relapse or recurrence represent the best means available to mental health professionals to lessen the functional and neurobiological consequences of this ubiquitous illness.

REFERENCES

Anand, A., Charney, D. S., Oren, D. A., Berman, R. M., Hu, X. S., Cappiello, A., et al. (2000). Attenuation of the neuropsychiatric effects of ketamine with lamotrigine: Support for hyperglutamatergic effects of N-methyl-D-aspartate receptor antagonists. *Archives of General Psychiatry, 57,* 270–276.

Aston-Jones, G., Rajkowski, J., & Cohen, J. (1999). Role of locus coeruleus in attention and behavioral flexibility. *Biological Psychiatry, 46,* 1309–1320.

Avery, D. H., Eder, D. N., Bolte, M. A., Hellekson, C. J., Dunner, D. L., Vitiello, M. V., et al. (2001). Dawn stimulation and bright light in the treatment of SAD: A controlled study. *Biological Psychiatry, 50,* 205–216.

Aydemir, C., Yalcin, E. S., Aksaray, S., Kisa, C., Yildirim, S. G., Uzbay, T., et al. (2006). Brain-derived neurotrophic factor (BDNF) changes in the serum of depressed women. *Progress in Neuro-Psychopharmacology and Biological Psychiatry, 30,* 1256–1260.

Barr, C. S., Newman, T. K., Becker, M. L., Parker, C. C., Champoux, M., Lesch, K. P., et al. (2003). The utility of the non-human primate: Model for studying gene by environment interactions in behavioral research. *Genes, Brain, and Behavior, 2,* 336–340.

Barr, C. S., Newman, T. K., Shannon, C., Parker, C., Dvoskin, R. L., Becker, M. L., et al. (2004). Rearing condition and rh5-HTTLPR interact to influence limbic–hypothalamic–pituitary–adrenal axis response to stress in infant macaques. *Biological Psychiatry, 55,* 733–738.

Bauer, M., London, E. D., Silverman, D. H., Rasgon, N., Kirchheiner, J., & Whybrow, P. C. (2003). Thyroid, brain and mood modulation in affective disorder: Insights from molecular research and functional brain imaging. *Pharmacopsychiatry, 36*(Suppl. 3), S215–S221.

Baune, B. T., Hohoff, C., Mortensen, J., Deckert, V., Arolt, V., & Domschke, K. (in press). Serotonin transporter polymorphism (5-HTTLPR) association with melancholic depression: A female specific effect? *Depression and Anxiety.*

Baxter, L. R., Schwartz, J. M., Phelps, M. E., Mazziotta, J. C., Guze, B. H., Selin, C. E., et al. (1989). Reduction of prefrontal cortex glucose metabolism common to three types of depression. *Archives of General Psychiatry, 46,* 243–250.

Benca, R. M., Obermeyer, W. H., Thisted, R. A., & Gillin, J. C. (1992). Sleep and psychiatric disorders: A meta-analysis. *Archives of General Psychiatry, 4,* 651–668.

Berton, O., Covington, H. E., III, Ebner, K., Tsankova, N. M., Carle, T. L., Ulery, P., et al. (2007). Induction of deltaFosB in the periaqueductal gray by stress promotes active coping responses. *Neuron*, 55, 289–300.

Berton, O., McClung, C. A., Dileone, R. J., Krishnan, V., Renthal, W., Russo, S. J., et al. (2006). Essential role of BDNF in the mesolimbic dopamine pathway in social defeat stress. *Science*, 311, 864–868.

Bleakman, D., Alt, A., & Witkin, J. M. (2007). AMPA receptors in the therapeutic management of depression. *Current Drug Targets: CNS and Neurological Disorders*, 6, 117–126.

Bremner, J. D. (1999). Does stress damage the brain? *Biological Psychiatry*, 45, 797–805.

Bremner, J. D. (2006). Traumatic stress: Effects on the brain. *Dialogues in Clinical Neuroscience*, 8(4), 445–461.

Bremner, J. D., Innis, R. B., Salomon, R. M., Staib, L. H., Ng, C. K., Miller, H. L., et al. (1997). Positron emission tomography measurement of cerebral metabolic correlates of tryptophan depletion-induced depressive relapse. *Archives of General Psychiatry*, 54, 364–374.

Brody, A. L., Saxena, S., Stoessel, P., Gillies, L. A., Fairbanks, L. A., Alborzian, S., et al. (2001). Regional brain metabolic changes in patients with major depression treated with either paroxetine or interpersonal therapy: Preliminary findings. *Archives of General Psychiatry*, 58, 631–640.

Bunney, W. E., & Bunney, B. G. (2000). Molecular clock genes in man and lower animals: Possible implications for circadian abnormalities in depression. *Neurospychopharmacology*, 22, 335–345.

Bunney, W. E., Jr., & Davis, J. M. (1965). Norepinephrine and depressive reactions: A review. *Archives of General Psychiatry*, 13, 483–494.

Carpenter, L. L., Carvalho, J. P., Tyrka, A. R., Wier, L. M., Mello, A. F., Mello, M. F., et al. (2007). Decreased adrenocorticotropic hormone and cortisol responses to stress in healthy adults reporting significant childhood maltreatment. *Biological Psychiatry*, 62, 1080–1087.

Caspi, A., Sugden, K., Moffitt, T. E., Taylor, A., Craig, I. W., Harrington, H., et al. (2003). Influence of life stress on depression: Moderation by a polymorphism in the 5-HTT gene. *Science*, 301, 386–389.

Chen, M. J., Nguyen, T. V., Pike, C. J., & Russo-Neustadt, A. A. (2007). Norepinephrine induces BDNF and activates the PI-3K and MAPK cascades in embryonic hippocampal neurons. *Cellular Signalling*, 19, 114–128.

Cole, D. P., Thase, M. E., Mallinger, A. G., Soares, J. C., Luther, J. F., Kupfer, D. J., et al. (2002). Lower pretreatment thyroid function predicts a slower treatment response in bipolar depression. *American Journal of Psychiatry*, 159, 116–121.

Cools, R., Robinson, O. J., & Sahakian, B. (in press). Acute tryptophan depletion in healthy volunteers enhances punishment prediction but does not affect reward prediction. *Neuropsychopharmacology*.

Cooper-Kazaz, R., Apter, J. T., Cohen, R., Karagichev, L., Muhammed-Moussa, S., Grupper, D., et al. (2007). Combined treatment with sertraline and liothyronine in major depression: A randomized, double-blind, placebo-controlled trial. *Archives of General Psychiatry*, 64(6), 679–688.

Coplan, J. D., Smith, E. L., Altemus, M., Mathew, S. J., Perera, T., Kral, J. G., et al. (2006). Maternal–infant response to variable foraging demand in nonhuman primates: Effects of timing of stressor on cerebrospinal fluid corticotropin-releasing factor and circulating glucocorticoid concentrations. *Annals of the New York Academy of Sciences*, 1071, 525–533.

Coplan, J. D., Smith, E. L. P., Altemus, M., Scharf, B. A., Owens, M. J., Nemeroff, C. B., et al. (2001). Variable foraging demand rearing: Sustained elevations in cisternal cerebrospinal fluid corticotropin-releasing factor concentrations in adult primates. *Biological Psychiatry*, 50, 200–204.

Coplan, J. D., Wolk, S. I., Goetz, R. R., Ryan, N. D., Dahl, R. E., Mann, J. J., et al. (2000). Nocturnal growth hormone secretion studies in adolescents with or without major depression re-examined: Integration of adult clinical follow-up data. *Biological Psychiatry*, 47, 594–604.

Cuadra, G., Zurita, A., Gioino, G., & Molina, V. (2001). Influence of different antidepressant drugs on the effect of chronic variable stress on restraint-induced dopamine release in frontal cortex. *Neuropsychopharmacology*, 25(3), 384–394.

Dahl, R. E., Birmaher, B., Williamson, D. E., Dorn, L., Perel, J., Kaufman, J., et al. (2000). Low growth hormone response to growth hormone-releasing hormone in child depression. *Biological Psychiatry*, 48, 981–988.

Delgado, P. L. (2004). How antidepressants help depression: Mechanisms of action and clinical response. *Journal of Clinical Psychiatry*, 65(Suppl. 4), 25–30.

Delgado, P. L., Price, L. H., Miller, H. L., Salomon, R. M., Licinio, J., Krystal, J. H., et al. (1991). Rapid serotonin depletion as a provocative challenge test for patients with major depression: Relevance to antidepressant action and the neurobiology of depression. *Psychopharmacology Bulletin, 27*, 321–330.

Dremencov, E., Gispan-Herman, I., Rosenstein, M., Mendelman, A., Overstreet, D. H., Zohar, J., et al. (2004). The serotonin–dopamine interaction is critical for fast-onset action of antidepressant treatment: *In vivo* studies in an animal model of depression. *Progress in Neuropsychopharmacology and Biological Psychiatry, 28*, 141–147.

Drevets, W. C. (2000). Functional anatomical abnormalities in limbic and prefrontal cortical structures in major depression. *Progress in Brain Research, 126*, 413–431.

Drevets, W. C., Thase, M. E., Moses-Kolko, E. L., Price, J., Frank, E., Kupfer, D. J., et al. (2007). Serotonin-1A receptor imaging in recurrent depression: Replication and literature review. *Nuclear Medicine and Biology, 34*, 865–877.

Duman, C. H., Schlesinger, L., Kodama, M., Russell, D. S., & Duman, R. S. (2007). A role for MAP kinase signaling in behavioral models of depression and antidepressant treatment. *Biological Psychiatry, 61*, 661–670.

Duman, R. S., Heninger, G. R., & Nestler, E. J. (1997). A molecular and cellular theory of depression. *Archives of General Psychiatry, 54*, 597–606.

Duncan, W. C., Jr. (1996). Circadian rhythms and the pharmacology of affective illness. *Pharmacology Therapy, 71*, 253–312.

Ehlers, C. L., Frank, E., & Kupfer, D. J. (1988). Social zeitgebers and biological rhythms: A unified approach to understanding the etiology of depression. *Archives of General Psychiatry, 45*, 948–952.

Evans, D. L., Charney, D. S., Lewis, L., Golden, R. N., Gorman, J. M., Krishnan, K. R., et al. (2005). Mood disorders in the medically ill: Scientific review and recommendations. *Biological Psychiatry, 58*, 175–189.

Fairbanks, L. A., Melega, W. P., Jorgensen, M. J., Kaplan, J. R., & McGuire, M. T. (2001). Social impulsivity inversely associated with CSF 5-HIAA and fluoxetine exposure in vervet monkeys. *Neuropsychopharmacology, 24*(4), 370–378.

Felger, J. C., Alagbe, O., Hu, F., Mook, D., Freeman, A. A., Sanchez, M. M., et al. (2007). Effects of interferon-alpha on rhesus monkeys: A nonhuman primate model of cytokine-induced depression. *Biological Psychiatry, 62*, 1324–1333.

Ferry, B., Roozendaal, B., & McGaugh, J. L. (1999). Role of norepinephrine in mediating stress hormone regulation of long-term memory storage: A critical involvement of the amygdala. *Biological Psychiatry, 46*, 1140–1152.

Firk, C., & Markus, C. R. (2007). Review: Serotonin by stress interaction: A susceptibility factor for the development of depression? *Journal of Psychopharmacology, 21*, 538–544.

Fountoulakis, K. N., Kantartzis, S., Siamouli, M., Panagiotidis, P., Kaprinis, S., Iacovides, A., et al. (2006). Peripheral thyroid dysfunction in depression. *World Journal of Biological Psychiatry, 7*(3), 131–137.

Freed, P. J., & Mann, J. J. (2007). Sadness and loss: Toward a neurobiopsychosocial model. *American Journal of Psychiatry, 164*, 28–34.

Frodl, T., Meisenzahl, E. M., Zetzsche, T., Born, C., Groll, C., Jäger, M., et al. (2002). Hippocampal changes in patients with a first episode of major depression. *American Journal of Psychiatry, 159*, 1112–1118.

Furey, M. L., & Drevets, W. C. (2006). Antidepressant efficacy of the antimuscarinic drug scopolamine: A randomized, placebo-controlled clinical trial. *Archives of General Psychiatry, 63*, 1121–1129.

Gershon, A. A., Vishne, T., & Grunhaus, L. (2007). Dopamine D2-like receptors and the antidepressant response. *Biological Psychiatry, 61*, 145–153.

Gilbert, P. (1992). *Depression: The evolution of powerlessness*. Hove, UK: Erlbaum.

Glassman, A. (1969). Indoleamines and affective disorders. *Psychosomatic Medicine, 31*, 107–114.

Glassman, A. H. (1993). Cigarette smoking: Implications for psychiatric illness. *American Journal of Psychiatry, 150*, 546–553.

Glassman, A. H., & Miller, G. E. (2007). Where there is depression, there is inflammation . . . sometimes! *Biological Psychiatry, 62*, 280–281.

Goldapple, K., Segal, Z., Garson, C., Lau, M., Bieling, P., Kennedy, S., et al. (2004). Modulation of corti-cal–limbic pathways in major depression: Treatment-specific effects of cognitive behavior therapy. *Archives of General Psychiatry*, *61*, 34–41.

Golden, R. N., Markey, S. P., Risby, E. D., Cowdry, R. W., & Potter, W. Z. (1988). Antidepressants reduce whole-body norepinephrine turnover while enhancing 6-hydroxymelatonin output. *Archives of General Psychiatry*, *45*, 150–154.

Gotlib, I. H., Joormann, J., Minor, K. L., & Hallmayer, J. (2008). HPA axis reactivity: A mechanism un-derlying the associations among *5-HTTLPR*, stress, and depression. *Biological Psychiatry*, *63*(9), 847–851.

Hariri, A. R., Mattay, V. S., Tessitore, A., Kolachana, B., Fera, F., Goldman, D., et al. (2002). Serotonin transporter genetic variation and the response of the human amygdala. *Science*, *297*, 400–403.

Harvey, P. O., Fossati, P., Pochon, J. B., Levy, R., LeBastard, G., Lehéricy, S., et al. (2005). Cognitive con-trol and brain resources in major depression: An fMRI study using the n-back task. *NeuroImage*, *26*, 860–869.

Hasler, G., Neumeister, A., van der Veen, J. W., Tumonis, T., Bain, E. E., Shen, J., et al. (2005). Normal prefrontal gamma-aminobutyric acid levels in remitted depressed subjects determined by proton magnetic resonance spectroscopy. *Biological Psychiatry*, *58*, 969–973.

Hasler, G., van der Veen, J. W., Tumonis, T., Meyers, N., Shen, J., & Drevets, W. C. (2007). Reduced prefrontal glutamate/glutamine and gamma-aminobutyric acid levels in major depression deter-mined using proton magnetic resonance spectroscopy. *Archives of General Psychiatry*, *64*, 193–200.

Hayden, E. P., Dougherty, L. R., Maloney, B., Olino, T. M., Sheikh, H., Durbin, C. E., et al. (2008). Early-emerging cognitive vulnerability to depression and the serotonin transporter promoter region poly-morphism. *Journal of Affective Disorders*, *107*(1–3), 227–230.

Heim, C., Mletzko, T., Purselle, D., Musselman, D. L., & Nemeroff, C. B. (2008). The dexamethasone/corticotropin-releasing factor test in men with major depression: Role of childhood trauma. *Biolog-ical Psychiatry*, *63*(4), 398–405.

Higley, J. D., Mehlman, P. T., Higley, S. B., Fernald, B., Vickers, J., Lindell, S. G., et al. (1996). Exces-sive mortality in young free-ranging male nonhuman primates with low cerebrospinal fluid 5-hydroxyindoleacetic acid concentrations. *Archives of General Psychiatry*, *53*, 537–543.

Higley, J. D., Mehlman, P. T., Poland, R. E., Taub, D. M., Vickers, J., Suomi, S. J., et al. (1996). CSF testos-terone and 5-HIAA correlate with different types of aggressive behaviors. *Biological Psychiatry*, *40*, 1067–1082.

Hirvonen, J., Karlsson, H., Kajander, J., Lepola, A., Markkula, J., Rasi-Hakala, H., et al. (2007). De-creased brain serotonin 5-HT1A receptor availability in medication-naive patients with major de-pressive disorder: An *in-vivo* imaging study using PET and [carbonyl-C]WAY-100635. *Interna-tional Journal of Neuropsychopharmacology*, *31*, 1–12.

Holsboer, F. (1995). Neuroendocrinology of mood disorders. In F. E. Bloom & D. J. Kupfer (Eds.), *Psychopharmacology: The fourth generation of progress* (pp. 957–969). New York: Raven Press.

Holsboer, F. (2000). The corticosteroid receptor hypothesis of depression. *Neuropsychopharmacology*, *23*, 477–501.

Holsboer, F. (2001). Stress, hypercortisolism and corticosteroid receptors in depression: Implications for therapy. *Journal of Affective Disorders*, *62*, 77–91.

Horne, J. (1992). Human slow-wave sleep and the cerebral cortex. *Journal of Sleep Research*, *1*, 122–124.

Huang, T. L., Lee, C. T., & Liu, Y. L. (2008). Serum brain-derived neurotrophic factor levels in patients with major depression: Effects of antidepressants. *Journal of Psychiatric Research*, *42*(7), 521–525.

Insel, T. R., & Winslow, J. T. (1998). Serotonin and neuropeptides in affiliative behaviors. *Biological Psy-chiatry*, *44*, 207–219.

Irwin, M. R., & Miller, A. H. (2007). Depressive disorders and immunity: 20 years of progress and dis-covery. *Brain, Behavior, and Immunity*, *21*, 374–383.

Jabbi, M., Kema, I. P., van der Pompe, G., Te Meerman, G. J., Ormel, J., & den Boer, J. A. (2007). Catechol-O-methyltransferase polymorphism and susceptibility to major depressive disorder mod-ulates psychological stress response. *Psychiatric Genetics*, *17*, 183–193.

Jackson, S. W. (1986). *Melancholia and depression from Hippocratic times to modern times*. New Haven, CT: Yale University Press.

Jacobs, N., Kenis, G., Peeters, F., Derom, C., Vlietinck, R., & van Os, J. (2006). Stress-related negative affectivity and genetically altered serotonin transporter function: Evidence of synergism in shaping risk of depression. *Archives of General Psychiatry, 63*(9), 989–996.

Janowsky, D. S., & Overstreet, D. H. (1995). The role of acetylcholine mechanisms in mood disorders. In F. E. Bloom & D. J. Kupfer (Eds.), *Psychopharmacology: The fourth generation of progress* (pp. 945–956). New York: Raven Press.

Jindal, R. D., Thase, M. E., Fasiczka, A. L., Friedman, E. S., Buysse, D. J., Frank, E., et al. (2002). Electroencephalographic sleep profiles in single episode and recurrent unipolar forms of major depression: II. Comparison during remission. *Biological Psychiatry, 51*, 230–236.

Joffe, R. T., & Marriott, M. (2000). Thyroid hormone levels and recurrence of major depression. *American Journal of Psychiatry, 157*, 1689–1691.

Kandel, E. R., Schwartz, J. H., & Jessell, T. M. (1991). *Principles of neural science* (3rd ed.). New York: Elsevier.

Kendler, K. S., Karkowski, L. M., & Prescott, C. A. (1999). Causal relationship between stressful life events and the onset of major depression. *American Journal of Psychiatry, 156*, 837–841.

Kendler, K. S., Kuhn, J. W., Vittum, J., Prescott, C. A., & Riley, B. (2005). The interaction of stressful life events and a serotonin transporter polymorphism in the prediction of episodes of major depression: A replication. *Archives of General Psychiatry, 62*, 529–535.

Kendler, K. S., Thornton, L. M., & Gardner, C. O. (2001). Genetic risk, number of previous depressive episodes, and stressful life events in predicting onset of major depression. *American Journal of Psychiatry, 158*, 582–586.

Kennedy, S. H., Konarski, J. Z., Segal, Z. V., Lau, M. A., Bieling, P. J., McIntyre, R. S., et al. (2007). Differences in brain glucose metabolism between responders to CBT and venlafaxine in a 16-week randomized controlled trial. *American Journal of Psychiatry, 164*, 778–788.

Ketter, T. A., George, M. S., Ring, H. A., Pazzaglia, P., Marangell, L., Kimbrell, T. A., et al. (1994). Primary mood disorders: Structural and resting functional studies. *Psychiatric Annals, 24*, 637–642.

Kingsley, R. E. (2000). *Concise text of neuroscience, second edition*. Philadelphia: Lippincott/Williams & Wilkins.

Kirkegaard, C., & Faber, J. (1998). The role of thyroid hormones in depression. *European Journal of Endocrinology, 138*, 1–9.

Korf, J., & van Praag, H. M. (1971). Retarded depressions and the dopamine metabolism. *Psychopharmacologia, 19*, 199–203.

Kraus, M. R., Al-Taie, O., Schäfer, A., Pfersdorff, M., Lesch, K. P., & Scheurlen, M. (2007). Serotonin-1A receptor gene HTR1A variation predicts interferon-induced depression in chronic hepatitis C. *Gastroenterology, 132*, 1279–1286.

Krishnan, V., Han, M. H., Graham, D. L., Berton, O., Renthal, W., Russo, S. J., et al. (2007). Molecular adaptations underlying susceptibility and resistance to social defeat in brain reward regions. *Cell, 131*, 391–404.

Kupfer, D. J., & Ehlers, C. L. (1989). Two roads to rapid eye movement latency. *Archives of General Psychiatry, 46*, 945–948.

Levinson, D. F. (2006). The genetics of depression: A review. *Biological Psychiatry, 15*, 84–92.

Lewy, A. J., Rough, J. N., Songer, J. B., Mishra, N., Yuhas, K., & Emens, J. S. (2007). The phase shift hypothesis for the circadian component of winter depression. *Dialogues in Clinical Neuroscience, 9*, 291–300.

Li, D., & He, L. (2007). Meta-analysis supports association between serotonin transporter (5-HTT) and suicidal behavior. *Molecular Psychiatry, 12*, 47–54.

Lin, P. Y., & Tsai, G. (2004). Association between serotonin transporter gene promoter polymorphism and suicide: Results of a meta-analysis. *Biological Psychiatry, 55*, 1023–1030.

Liu, Z., Zhu, F., Wang, G., Xiao, Z., Wang, H., Tang, J., et al. (2006). Association of corticotropin-releasing hormone receptor1 gene SNP and haplotype with major depression. *Neuroscience Letters, 404*, 358–362.

López, J. F., Liberzon, I., Vázquez, D. M., Young, E. A., & Watson, S. J. (1999). Serotonin 1A receptor messenger RNA regulation in the hippocampus after acute stress. *Biological Psychiatry, 45,* 934–937.

Lotrich, F. E., Rabinovitz, M., Gironda, P., & Pollock, B. G. (2007). Depression following pegylated interferon-alpha: Characteristics and vulnerability. *Journal of Psychosomatic Research, 63,* 131–135.

Lyons, D. M., Parker, K. J., Zeitzer, J. M., Buckmaster, C. L., & Schatzberg, A. F. (2007). Preliminary evidence that hippocampal volumes in monkeys predict stress levels of adrenocorticotropic hormone. *Biological Psychiatry, 62,* 1171–1174.

Lyons, D. M., Yang, C., Sawyer-Glover, A. M., Moseley, M. E., & Schatzberg, A. F. (2001). Early life stress and inherited variation in monkey hippocampal volumes. *Archives of General Psychiatry, 58,* 1145–1151.

Macri, S., & Würbel, H. (2006). Developmental plasticity of HPA and fear responses in rats: A critical review of the maternal mediation hypothesis. *Hormones and Behavior, 50,* 667–680.

Maes, M., & Meltzer, H. Y. (1995). The serotonin hypothesis of major depression. In F. E. Bloom & D. J. Kupfer (Eds.), *Psychopharmacology: The fourth generation of progress* (pp. 933–944). New York: Raven Press.

Maier, S. F., & Seligman, M. E. P. (1976). Learned helplessness: Theory and evidence. *Journal of Experimental Psychology, 105,* 3–46.

Maier, S. F., & Watkins, L. R. (2005). Stressor controllability and learned helplessness: The roles of the dorsal raphe nucleus, serotonin, and corticotropin-releasing factor. *Neuroscience and Biobehavioral Reviews, 29,* 829–841.

Mann, J. J., Brent, D. A., & Arango, V. (2001). The neurobiology and genetics of suicide and attempted suicide: A focus on the serotonergic system. *Neurospychopharmacology, 24,* 467–477.

Martin, S. D., Martin, E., Rai, S. S., Richardson, M. A., & Royall, R. (2001). Brain blood flow changes in depressed patients treated with interpersonal psychotherapy or venlafaxine hydrochloride: Preliminary findings. *Archives of General Psychiatry, 58,* 641–648.

Martinowich, K., & Lu, B. (2008). Interaction between BDNF and serotonin: Role in mood disorders. *Neuropsychopharmacology, 33,* 73–83.

Mason, G. A., Garbutt, J. C., & Prange, A. J., Jr. (1995). Thyrotropin-releasing hormone: Focus on basic neurobiology. In F. E. Bloom & D. J. Kupfer (Eds.), *Psychopharmacology: The fourth generation of progress* (pp. 493–503). New York: Raven Press.

Mathew, S. J., Coplan, J. D., Smith, E. L. P., Schloepp, D. D., Rosenblum, L. A., & Gorman, J. M. (2001). Glutamate–hypothalamic–pituitary–adrenal axis interactions: Implications for mood and anxiety disorders. *CNS Spectrums, 6,* 555–564.

Mayberg, H. S. (2003). Positron emission tomography imaging in depression: A neural systems perspective. *Neuroimaging Clinics of North America, 13,* 805–815.

McEwen, B. S. (2000). Allostasis and allostatic load: Implications for neuropsychopharmacology. *Neuropsychopharmacology, 22,* 108–124.

Mehlman, P. T., Higley, J. D., Faucher, I., Lilly, A. A., Taub, D. M., Vickers, J., et al. (1995). Correlation of CSF 5-HIAA concentration with sociality and the timing of emigration in free-ranging primates. *American Journal of Psychiatry, 152,* 907–913.

Modell, S., Ising, M., Holsboer, F., & Lauer, C. J. (2005). The Munich Vulnerability Study on Affective Disorders: Premorbid polysomnographic profile of affected high-risk probands. *Biological Psychiatry, 58,* 694–699.

Montero-Pedrazuela, A., Venero, C., Lavado-Autric, R., Fernández-Lamo, I., García-Verdugo, J. M., Bernal, J., et al. (2006). Modulation of adult hippocampal neurogenesis by thyroid hormones: Implications in depressive-like behavior. *Molecular Psychiatry, 11,* 361–371.

Moore, P., Landolt, H.-P., Seifritz, E., Clark, C., Bhatti, T., Kelso, J., et al. (2000). Clinical and physiological consequences of rapid tryptophan depletion. *Neuropsychopharmacology, 23,* 601–622.

Neigh, G. N., & Nemeroff, C. B. (2006). Reduced glucocorticoid receptors: Consequence or cause of depression? *Trends in Endocrinology and Metabolism, 17,* 124–125.

Nemeroff, C. B. (1998). Psychopharmacology of affective disorders in the 21st century. *Biological Psychiatry, 44,* 517–525.

Nemeroff, C. B., Entsuah, R., Benattia, I., Demitrack, M., Sloan, D. M., & Thase, M. E. (2008). Comprehensive Analysis of Remission (COMPARE) with venlafaxine versus SSRIs. *Biological Psychiatry*, *63*(4), 424–434.

Nestler, E. J., Alreja, M., & Aghajanian, G. K. (1999). Molecular control of locus coeruleus neurotransmission. *Biological Psychiatry*, *46*, 1131–1139.

Nestler, E. J., & Carlezon, W. A., Jr. (2006). The mesolimbic dopamine reward circuit in depression. *Biological Psychiatry*, *59*, 1151–1159.

Neumeister, A., Hu, X. Z., Luckenbaugh, D. A., Schwarz, M., Nugent, A. C., Bonne, O., et al. (2006). Differential effects of 5-HTTLPR genotypes on the behavioral and neural responses to tryptophan depletion in patients with major depression and controls. *Archives of General Psychiatry*, *63*, 978–986.

Newport, D. J., Heim, C., Bonsall, R., Miller, A. H., & Nemeroff, C. B. (2004). Pituitary–adrenal responses to standard and low-dose dexamethasone suppression tests in adult survivors of child abuse. *Biological Psychiatry*, *55*, 10–20.

Nierenberg, A. A., Fava, M., Trivedi, M. H., Wisniewski, S. R., Thase, M. E., McGrath, P. J., et al. (2006). A comparison of lithium and T(3) augmentation following two failed medication treatments for depression: A STAR*D report. *American Journal of Psychiatry*, *163*, 1519–1530.

Nofzinger, E. A., Fasiczka, A., Berman, S., & Thase, M. E. (2000). Bupropion SR reduces periodic limb movements associated with arousals from sleep in depressed patients with periodic limb movement disorder. *Journal of Clinical Psychiatry*, *61*, 858–862.

Nofzinger, E. A., Reynolds, C. F., III, Thase, M. E., Frank, E., Jennings, J. R., Fasiczka, A. L., et al. (1995). REM sleep enhancement by bupropion in depressed men. *American Journal of Psychiatry*, *152*, 274–276.

Nutt, D., Demyttenaere, K., Janka, Z., Aarre, T., Bourin, M., Canonico, P. L., et al. (2007). The other face of depression, reduced positive affect: The role of catecholamines in causation and cure. *Journal of Psychopharmacology*, *21*, 461–471.

O'Reardon, J. P., Chopra, M. P., Bergan, A., Gallop, R., DeRubeis, R. J., & Crits-Christoph, P. (2004). Response to tryptophan depletion in major depression treated with either cognitive therapy or selective serotonin reuptake inhibitor antidepressants. *Biological Psychiatry*, *55*, 957–959.

O'Reardon, J. P., Cristancho, P., Pilania, P., Bapatla, K. B., Chuai, S., & Peshek, A. D. (2006). Patients with a major depressive episode responding to treatment with repetitive transcranial magnetic stimulation (rTMS) are resistant to the effects of rapid tryptophan depletion. *Depression and Anxiety*, *24*, 537–544.

Overstreet, D. H. (1993). The Flinders sensitive line rats: A genetic animal model of depression. *Neuroscience and Biobehavioral Reviews*, *17*, 51–68.

Palucha, A., & Pilc, A. (2005). The involvement of glutamate in the pathophysiology of depression. *Drug News and Perspectives*, *18*, 262–268.

Papakostas, G. I., Nelson, J. C., Kasper, S., & Möller, H. J. (2007). A meta-analysis of clinical trials comparing reboxetine, a norepinephrine reuptake inhibitor, with selective serotonin reuptake inhibitors for the treatment of major depressive disorder. *European Neuropsychopharmacology*.

Papakostas, G. I., Thase, M. E., Fava, M., Nelson, J. C., & Shelton, R. C. (2007). Are antidepressant drugs that combine serotonergic and noradrenergic mechanisms of action more effective than the selective serotonin reuptake inhibitors in treating major depressive disorder?: A meta-analysis of studies of newer agents. *Biological Psychiatry*, *62*, 1217–1227.

Parry, B. L., & Haynes, P. (2000). Mood disorders and the reproductive cycle. *Journal of Gender-Specific Medicine*, *3*, 53–58.

Parsey, R. V., Hastings, R. S., Oquendo, M. A., Huang, Y. Y., Simpson, N., Arcement, J., et al. (2006). Lower serotonin transporter binding potential in the human brain during major depressive episodes. *American Journal of Psychiatry*, *163*, 52–58.

Paul, S. M. (1995). GABA and glycine. In F. E. Bloom & D. J. Kupfer (Eds.), *Psychopharmacology: The fourth generation of progress* (pp. 87–94). New York: Raven Press.

Petito, J. M., Repetto, M. J., & Hartemink, D. A. (2001). Brain–immune interactions in neuropsychiatry: Highlights of the basic science and relevance to pathogenic factors and epiphenomena. *CNS Spectrums*, *6*, 383–391.

Petty, F. (1995). GABA and mood disorders: A brief review and hypothesis. *Journal of Affective Disorders, 34*, 275–281.

Pittenger, C., & Duman, R. S. (2008). Stress, depression, and neuroplasticity: A convergence of mechanisms. *Neuropsychopharmacology, 33*, 88–109.

Pittenger, C., Sanacora, G., & Krystal, J. H. (2007). The NMDA receptor as a therapeutic target in major depressive disorder. *Current Drug Targets: CNS and Neurological Disorders, 6*, 101–115.

Plotsky, P. M., Owens, M. J., & Nemeroff, C. B. (1995). Neuropeptide alterations in mood disorders. In F. E. Bloom & D. J. Kupfer (Eds.), *Psychopharmacology: The fourth generation of progress* (pp. 971–981). New York: Raven Press.

Raison, C. L., Capuron, L., & Miller, A. H. (2006). Cytokines sing the blues: Inflammation and the pathogenesis of depression. *Trends in Immunology, 27*, 24–31.

Raison, C. L., Woolwine, B. J., Demetrashvili, M. F., Borisov, A. S., Weinreib, R., Staab, J. P., et al. (2007). Paroxetine for prevention of depressive symptoms induced by interferon-alpha and ribavirin for hepatitis C. *Alimentary Pharmacology and Therapeutics, 25*, 1163–1174.

Rajkowska, G., & Miguel-Hidalgo, J. J. (2007). Gliogenesis and glial pathology in depression. *Current Drug Targets: CNS and Neurological Disorders, 6*, 219–233.

Rajkowska, G., O'Dwyer, G., Teleki, Z., Stockmeier, C. A., & Miguel-Hidalgo, J. J. (2007). GABAergic neurons immunoreactive for calcium binding proteins are reduced in the prefrontal cortex in major depression. *Neuropsychopharmacology, 32*, 471–482.

Ressler, K. J., & Nemeroff, C. B. (1999). Role of norepinephrine in the pathophysiology and treatment of mood disorders. *Biological Psychiatry, 46*, 1219–1233.

Ribeiro, S. C. M., Tandon, R., Grunhaus, L., & Greden, J. F. (1993). The DST as a predictor of outcome in depression: A meta-analysis. *American Journal of Psychiatry, 150*, 1618–1629.

Roiser, J. P., Levy, J., Fromm, S. J., Wang, H., Hasler, G., Sahakian, B. J., et al. (in press). The effect of acute tryptophan depletion on the neural correlates of emotional processing in healthy volunteers. *Neuropsychopharmacology.*

Rush, A. J., Armitage, R., Gillin, J. C., Yonkers, K. A., Winokur, A., Moldofsky, H., et al. (1998). Comparative effects of nefazodone and fluoxetine on sleep in outpatients with major depressive disorder. *Biological Psychiatry, 44*, 3–14.

Sapolsky, R. M. (1996). Why stress is bad for your brain. *Science, 273*, 749–750.

Sasaki-Adams, D. M., & Kelley, A. E. (2001). Serotonin–dopamine interactions in the control of conditioned reinforcement and motor behavior. *Neuropsychopharmacology, 25*, 440–452.

Schatzberg, A. F., & Rothschild, A. J. (1992). Psychotic (delusional) major depression: Should it be included as a distinct syndrome in DSM-IV? *American Journal of Psychiatry, 149*, 733–745.

Schatzberg, A. F., & Schildkraut, J. J. (1995). Recent studies on norepinephrine systems in mood disorders. In F. E. Bloom & D. J. Kupfer (Eds.), *Psychopharmacology: The fourth generation of progress* (pp. 911–920). New York: Raven Press.

Schildkraut, J. J. (1965). The catecholamine hypothesis of affective disorder: A review of supporting evidence. *American Journal of Psychiatry, 122*, 509–522.

Schittecatte, M., Charles, G., Machowski, R., Garcia-Valentin, J., Mendlewicz, J., & Wilmotte, J. (1992). Reduced clonidine rapid eye movement sleep suppression in patients with primary major affective illness. *Archives of General Psychiatry, 49*, 637–642.

Sequeira, A., Klempan, T., Canetti, L., French-Mullen, J., Benkelfat, C., Rouleau, G. A., et al. (2007). Patterns of gene expression in the limbic system of suicides with and without major depression. *Molecular Psychiatry, 12*, 640–655.

Serretti, A., Kato, M., De Ronchi, D., & Kinoshita, T. (2007). Meta-analysis of serotonin transporter gene promoter polymorphism (*5-HTTLPR*) association with selective serotonin reuptake inhibitor efficacy in depressed patients. *Molecular Psychiatry, 12*(3), 247–257.

Shannon, C., Schwandt, M. L., Champoux, M., Shoaf, S. E., Suomi, S. J., Linnoila, M., et al. (2005). Maternal absence and stability of individual differences in CSF 5-HIAA concentrations in rhesus monkey infants. *American Journal of Psychiatry, 162*, 1658–1664.

Sharpley, A., & Cowen, P. (1995). Effect of pharmacologic treatment on the sleep of depressed patients. *Biological Psychiatry, 37*, 85–98.

Shelton, R. C. (2007). The molecular neurobiology of depression. *Psychiatric Clinics of North America, 30*, 1–11.

Siegle, G. J., Carter, C. S., & Thase, M. E. (2006). Use of fMRI to predict recovery in cognitive behavior therapy for unipolar depression. *American Journal of Psychiatry, 163*(4), 735–738.

Siegle, G. J., Thompson, W., Carter, C. S., Steinhauer, S. R., & Thase, M. E. (2007). Increased amygdala and decreased dorsolateral prefrontal BOLD responses in unipolar depression: Related and independent features. *Biological Psychiatry, 61*, 198–209.

Sitaram, N., Dubé, S., Keshavan, M., Davies, M., & Reynal, P. (1987). The association of supersensitive cholinergic REM-induction and affective illness within pedigrees. *Biological Psychiatry, 21*, 487–497.

Southwick, S. M., Vythilingam, M., & Charney, D. S. (2005). The psychobiology of depression and resilience to stress: Implications for prevention and treatment. *Annual Review of Clinical Psychology, 1*, 255–291.

Starkman, M. N., Giordani, B., Gebarski, S. S., Berent, S., Schork, M. A., & Schteingart, D. E. (1999). Decrease in cortisol reverses human hippocampal atrophy following treatment of Cushing's disease. *Biological Psychiatry, 46*, 1595–1602.

Steiger, A. (2007). Neurochemical regulation of sleep. *Journal of Psychiatric Research, 41*, 537–552.

Stolerman, I. P., & Reavill, C. (1989). Primary cholinergic and indirect dopaminergic mediation of behavioural effects of nicotine. *Progress in Brain Research, 79*, 227–237.

Swaab, D. F., Bao, A. M., & Lucassen, P. J. (2005). The stress system in the human brain in depression and neurodegeneration. *Ageing Research Reviews, 4*, 141–194.

Szelényi, J., & Vizi, E. S. (2007). The catecholamine cytokine balance: Interaction between the brain and the immune system. *Annals of the New York Academy of Sciences, 1113*, 311–324.

Thase, M. E. (2006). Depression and sleep: Pathophysiology and treatment. *Dialogues in Clinical Neuroscience, 8*, 217–226.

Thase, M. E., Dubé, S., Bowler, K., Howland, R. H., Myers, J. E., Friedman, E., et al. (1996). Hypothalamic–pituitary–adrenocortical activity and response to cognitive behavior therapy in unmedicated, hospitalized depressed patients. *American Journal of Psychiatry, 153*, 886–891.

Thase, M. E., Fasiczka, A. L., Berman, S. R., Simons, A. D., & Reynolds, C. F., III. (1998). Electroencephalographic sleep profiles before and after cognitive behavior therapy of depression. *Archives of General Psychiatry, 55*, 138–144.

Thase, M. E., Frank, E., & Kupfer, D. J. (1985). Biological processes of major depression. In E. E. Beckham & W. R. Leber (Eds.), *Handbook of depression: Treatment, assessment, and research* (pp. 816–913). Homewood, IL: Dorsey Press.

Thase, M. E., Greenhouse, J. B., Frank, E., Reynolds, C. F., III, Pilkonis, P. A., Hurley, K., et al. (1997). Treatment of major depression with psychotherapy or psychotherapy–pharmacotherapy combinations. *Archives of General Psychiatry, 54*, 1009–1015.

Thase, M. E., & Howland, R. H. (1995). Biological processes in depression: Updated review and integration. In E. E. Beckham & W. R. Leber (Eds.), *Handbook of depression* (2nd ed., pp. 213–279). New York: Guilford Press.

Thase, M. E., Jindal, R., & Howland, R. H. (2002). Biological aspects of depression. In I. H. Gotlib & C. L. Hammen (Eds.), *Handbook of depression* (pp. 192–218). New York: Guilford Press.

Thase, M. E., & Kupfer, D. J. (1987). Current status of EEG sleep in the assessment and treatment of depression. In G. D. Burrows & J. S. Werry (Eds.), *Advances in human psychopharmacology* (Vol. 4, pp. 93–148). Greenwich, CT: JAI Press.

Thase, M. E., Kupfer, D. J., Buysse, D. J., Frank, E., Simons, A. D., McEachran, A. B., et al. (1995). Electroencephalographic sleep profiles in single-episode and recurrent unipolar forms of major depression: 1. Comparison during acute depressive states. *Biological Psychiatry, 38*, 506–515.

Thase, M. E., Pritchett, Y. L., Ossanna, M. J., Swindle, R. W., Xu, J., & Detke, M. J. (2007). Efficacy of duloxetine and selective serotonin reuptake inhibitors: Comparisons as assessed by remission rates in patients with major depressive disorder. *Journal of Clinical Psychopharmacology, 27*, 672–676.

van Rossum, E. F., Binder, E. B., Majer, M., Koper, J. W., Ising, M., Modell, S., et al. (2006). Polymorphisms of the glucocorticoid receptor gene and major depression. *Biological Psychiatry, 59*, 681–688.

Wang, J. C., Hinrichs, A. L., Stock, H., Budde, J., Allen, R., Bertelsen, S., et al. (2004). Evidence of common and specific genetic effects: association of the muscarinic acetylcholine receptor M2 (CHRM2) gene with alcohol dependence and major depressive syndrome. *Human Molecular Genetics*, *13*, 1903–1911.

Warner-Schmidt, J. L., & Duman, R. S. (2006). Hippocampal neurogenesis: Opposing effects of stress and antidepressant treatment. *Hippocampus*, *16*(3), 239–249.

Wasserman, D., Geijer, T., Sokolowski, M., Frisch, A., Michaelovsky, E., Weizman, A., et al. (2007). Association of the serotonin transporter promotor polymorphism with suicide attempters with a high medical damage. *European Neuropsychopharmacology*, *17*(3), 230–233.

Weiss, J. M., & Kilts, C. D. (1998). Animal models of depression and schizophrenia. In A. F. Schatzberg & C. B. Nemeroff (Eds.), *Textbook of psychopharmacology* (2nd ed., pp. 89–131). Washington, DC: American Psychiatric Press.

Wichers, M., Aguilera, M., Kenis, G., Krabbendam, L., Myin-Germeys, I., Jacobs, N., et al. (in press). The catechol-O-methyl transferase *Val(158)Met* polymorphism and experience of reward in the flow of daily life. *Neuropsychopharmacology*.

Wichers, M. C., Kenis, G., Koek, G. H., Robaeys, G., Nicolson, N. A., & Maes, M. (2007). Interferon-alpha-induced depressive symptoms are related to changes in the cytokine network but not to cortisol. *Journal of Psychosomatic Research*, *62*, 207–214.

Wilhelm, K., Siegel, J. E., Finch, A. W., Hadzi-Pavlovic, D., Mitchell, P. B., Parker, G., et al. (2007). The long and the short of it: Associations between 5-HTT genotypes and coping with stress. *Psychosomatic Medicine*, *69*, 614–620.

Willner, P. (1995). Dopaminergic mechanisms in depression and mania. In F. E. Bloom & D. J. Kupfer (Eds.), *Psychopharmacology: The fourth generation of progress* (pp. 921–931). New York: Raven Press.

Willner, P. (1997). The mesolimbic dopamine system as a target for rapid antidepressant action. *International Clinical Psychopharmacology*, *12*(Suppl. 3), S7–S14.

Wirz-Justice, A. (1995). Biological rhythms in mood disorders. In F. E. Bloom & D. J. Kupfer (Eds.), *Psychopharmacology: The fourth generation of progress* (pp. 999–1017). New York: Raven Press.

Yildiz-Yesiloglu, A., & Ankerst, D. P. (2006). Review of 1H magnetic resonance spectroscopy findings in major depressive disorder: A meta-analysis. *Psychiatry Research*, *147*, 1–25.

Yoshimura, R., Mitoma, M., Sugita, A., Hori, H., Okamoto, T., Umene, W., et al. (2007). Effects of paroxetine or milnacipran on serum brain-derived neurotrophic factor in depressed patients. *Progress in Neuro-Psychopharmacology and Biological Psychiatry*, *31*, 1034–1037.

Zajicek, K. B., Price, C. S., Shoaf, S. E., Mehlman, P. T., Suomi, S. J., Linnoila, M., et al. (2000). Seasonal variation in CSF 5-HIAA concentrations in male rhesus monkeys. *Neuropsychopharmacology*, *22*, 240–250.

Zarate, C. A., Jr., Singh, J. B., Carlson, P. J., Brutsche, N. E., Ameli, R., Luckenbaugh, D. A., et al. (2006). A randomized trial of an N-methyl-D-aspartate antagonist in treatment-resistant major depression. *Archives of General Psychiatry*, *63*, 856–864.

Zupancic, M., & Guilleminault, C. (2006). Agomelatine: A preliminary review of a new antidepressant. *CNS Drugs*, *20*(12), 981–992.

CHAPTER 10

Representation and Regulation of Emotion in Depression

Perspectives from Affective Neuroscience

Richard J. Davidson, Diego A. Pizzagalli, *and* Jack B. Nitschke

Affective neuroscience is the subdiscipline that examines the underlying neural bases of mood and emotion. The application of this body of theory and data to the understanding of affective disorders is helping to generate a new understanding of the brain circuitry underlying these disorders. Moreover, parsing the heterogeneity of these disorders on the basis of known circuits in the brain is providing a novel and potentially very fruitful approach to subtyping that does not rely on the descriptive nosology of psychiatric diagnosis, but is based on a more objective characterization of the specific affective deficits in patients with mood disorders. At a more general level, this approach is helping to bridge the chasm between the literatures that focus on normal emotion and on the disorders of emotion. Historically, because these research traditions have had little to do with one another, they have emerged independently. However, affective neuroscience has helped to integrate these approaches into a more unified project that focuses on understanding individual differences in affective style, their constituent components, and the neural bases (see, e.g., Davidson, 2000; Davidson, Jackson, & Kalin, 2000). This chapter is an update of our Chapter 9 in the first edition of this *Handbook* and emphasizes findings published in the past 3 years.

Affective neuroscience takes as its overall aims a similar project to that pursued by its cognate discipline, cognitive neuroscience, though it focuses instead on affective processes. The decomposition of cognitive processes into more elementary constituents that can then be studied in neural terms has been remarkably successful. We no longer query subjects about the contents of their cognitive processes, because many of the processes so central to important aspects of cognitive function are opaque to consciousness (see Joormann, Chapter 13, this volume). Instead, contemporary cognitive scientists and neuroscientists have developed laboratory tasks to interrogate subjects and reveal more elementary cognitive function.

These more elementary processes can then be examined using imaging methods in humans, lesion methods in animals, and the study of human patients with focal brain damage. Affective neuroscience uses the same strategy to approach emotion. Global constructs of emotion are giving way to more specific and elementary constituents that can be examined with objective laboratory measures. For example, Davidson's laboratory has been developing methods to probe the chronometry of affect using both neuroimaging and peripheral startle measures. These measures allow us to examine an anticipatory period prior to the delivery of an emotional stimulus, a recovery period following the delivery of an emotional stimulus, and other, related parameters that can be assessed objectively and that reveal systematic individual differences (see Davidson, 1998, 2000; Jackson et al., 2003). Though it is still tempting and often important to obtain measures of subjects' conscious experience of the contents of their emotional states and traits, these self-reports no longer comprise the sole source of information about emotion.

Because there are recent basic literature reviews on the circuitry underlying emotion and emotion regulation (e.g., Davidson & Irwin, 1999; Davidson, Jackson, & Kalin, 2000; Davidson, Putnam, & Larson, 2000; Davidson, Pizzagalli, Nitschke, & Putnam, 2002; Ochsner & Gross, 2005; Rolls, 1999), we do not review these data systematically in this chapter. We wish to underscore at the outset that one of crucial issues that plagues research in this area is the heterogeneity of depression (see Ingram & Siegle, Chapter 4, this volume). From an examination of the inconsistencies across studies, it is apparent that traditional methods for parsing heterogeneity based on descriptive phenomenology are not yielding clean separation of underlying neural circuitry. For example, the melancholic versus nonmelancholic distinction does not systematically reveal differences in neural correlates (see below). Recommendations for moving beyond phenomenology are provided throughout this chapter.

We have three broad goals:

1. To review the functional role of the prefrontal cortices, anterior cingulate, hippocampus, and amygdala in affect and emotion regulation (see Figure 10.1 for an illustration of these structures and their locations).
2. To review the functional and structural abnormalities that have been found in these regions relative to depression.
3. Based on the first and second goals (a) to advance hypotheses about symptom clusters that may arise as a consequence of dysfunctions in specific regions; and (b) to offer suggestions for different ways of parsing the heterogeneity of depression to reflect more directly the circuitry of emotion and emotion regulation in the brain.

THE EMOTIONAL CIRCUITRY OF THE BRAIN AND ITS DYSFUNCTION IN DEPRESSION

Prefrontal Cortex

The Role of the Prefrontal Cortex in Emotion and Emotion Regulation

Abnormalities in activation of prefrontal regions in depression have been reported more frequently than those for any other brain region, mostly in the direction of decreased bilateral or predominantly left-sided activation (Davidson, Abercrombie, Nitschke, & Putnam, 1999; George, Ketter, & Post, 1994). Miller and Cohen (2001) outlined a comprehensive theory of

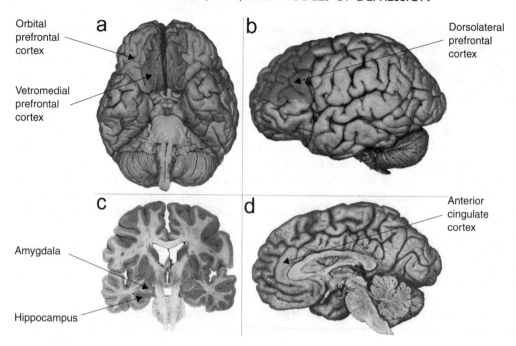

Orbital prefrontal cortex

Vetromedial prefrontal cortex

Dorsolateral prefrontal cortex

Anterior cingulate cortex

Amygdala

Hippocampus

FIGURE 10.1. Key brain regions involved in affect and mood disorders: (a) orbital prefrontal cortex and ventromedial prefrontal cortex; (b) dorsolateral prefrontal cortex; (c) hippocampus and amygdala; and (d) anterior cingulate cortex.

prefrontal function based on nonhuman primate anatomical and neurophysiological studies, human neuroimaging findings, and computational modeling. The core feature of their model holds that the prefrontal cortex (PFC) maintains the representation of goals and the means to achieve them. Particularly in situations that are ambiguous, the PFC sends bias signals to other areas of the brain to facilitate the expression of task-appropriate responses in the face of competition with potentially stronger alternatives. In the affective domain, we often confront situations in which the arousal of emotion is inconsistent with other goals that have already been instantiated. For example, the availability of an immediate reward offers a potent response alternative that may not be in the best service of the overall goals of the person. In such a case, the PFC is required to generate a bias signal to other brain regions that guide behavior toward the acquisition of a more adaptive goal, which, in this case, would entail delay of gratification. Affect-guided planning and anticipation that involves the experience of emotion associated with an anticipated choice is the hallmark of adaptive, emotion-based decision making that has repeatedly been found to become impaired in patients with lesions of ventromedial PFC (Damasio, 1994). The instantiation of affect-guided anticipation is most often accomplished in situations that are heavily laden with competition from potentially stronger alternatives. In such cases in particular, we would expect PFC activation to occur.

Our laboratory has contributed extensively to the literature on asymmetries in PFC function associated with approach- and withdrawal-related emotion and mood (e.g., Davidson & Irwin, 1999; Davidson, Jackson, & Kalin, 2000). In this context, we suggest that left-sided PFC regions are particularly involved in approach-related, appetitive goals. The instantiation of such goals, particularly in the face of strong alternative responses, requires left-sided PFC activation. In contrast, right-sided PFC regions are hypothesized to be particularly important in the maintenance of goals that require behavioral inhibition and withdrawal in situations that involve strong alternative response options to approach. The prototype of such a process has been captured in several neuroimaging studies that involve variants of a go/no-go task in which a dominant response set is established to respond quickly, except on those trials in which a cue to inhibit the response is presented. Several studies using event-related functional magnetic resonance imaging (fMRI) have found a lateralized focus of activation in the right lateral PFC (inferior frontal sulcus) to cues signaling response inhibition, presented in the context of other stimuli toward which a strong approach set was established (Garavan, Hester, Murphy, Fassbender, & Kelly, 2006; Garavan, Ross, & Stein, 1999; Konishi et al., 1999; see Dillon & Pizzagalli, 2007, for recent review).

Depressed individuals with hypoactivation in certain regions of the PFC may be deficient in instantiating goal-directed behavior and in overriding more automatic responses that may involve the perseveration of negative affect and dysfunctional attitudes. We would expect such deficits to be unmasked in situations in which decision making is ambiguous and the maintenance of goal-directed behavior is required in the face of potentially strong alternative responses. As we argue below, when strong alternative responses involve affect, which they often do, the ventromedial PFC is particularly implicated.

Results from recent neuroimaging and electrophysiological studies suggest that the orbital cortex, and the ventral frontal cortex in particular, is especially important for the representation of rewards and punishments, and that different sectors within this cortex may emphasize reward versus punishment (Kawasaki et al., 2001; O'Doherty, Kringelbach, Rolls, Hornak, & Andrews, 2001). More specifically, a left-sided medial region of the orbitofrontal cortex (OFC) appears particularly responsive to rewards, whereas a lateral right-sided region appears particularly responsive to punishments (O'Doherty et al., 2001). Differential behavioral responsivity to reward versus punishment has been found in two studies in our laboratory (Henriques & Davidson, 2000; Henriques, Glowacki, & Davidson, 1994). In particular, whereas normal individuals exhibited systematic modification of response bias to monetary reward, depressed patients failed to show such changes, but they did show response bias shifts in response to monetary punishment. Pizzagalli, Jahn, and O'Shea (2005) have more recently replicated and extended this finding, and demonstrated that individuals with elevated levels of depressive symptoms fail to show a response bias to reward. The precise neural correlates of individual differences in response bias to reward remain to be fully characterized.

PFC in Depression

Consistent with prior literature, recent reports have documented decreased activation in both dorsolateral and dorsomedial PFC, as well as the pregenual region of the anterior cingulate gyrus in depressed patients (see Drevets [1998] for a review of the early studies and Fitzgerald, Laird, Maller, & Daskalakis [2008] for a more recent review of this literature). The reduction in activation in this latter region, particularly on the left side, appears to be at least partially a function of a reduction in the volume of gray matter, as revealed by MRI-derived morphometric measures (Drevets et al., 1997). Consistent with the notion that the metabolic reduction found in this region is at least partially a function of the volume reduction, Drevets and colleagues (1997) have reported that remission of symptoms associated with successful treatment is not accompanied by a normalization of activation in this area.

This general decrease in dorsolateral PFC and in the pregenual region of the anterior cingulate cortex (ACC) tends to be accompanied by an increase in other regions of the PFC, particularly in the ventrolateral and orbital (lateral and medial) regions and also in the amygdala (Siegle, Thompson, Carter, Steinhauer, & Thase, 2007). Treatment studies have found that activation in dorsolateral PFC, particularly on the left side, increases following successful antidepressant treatment (Kennedy et al., 2001). Less consistent are findings for ventrolateral and orbital PFC regions: whereas some studies have found increases in these regions (Kennedy et al., 2001), others have reported decreases (e.g., Brody et al., 1999; Mayberg et al., 1999). In more recent work, investigators have developed behavioral paradigms hypothesized to differentiate more sensitively between depressed patients and controls. For example, we (Schaefer, Putnam, Benca, & Davidson, 2006) presented positive social stimuli in several different categories to depressed patients and controls on two occasions—the first prior to treatment when patients were in episode, and the second following approximately 22 weeks of treatment with venlaxafine. We found that at the initial testing occasion, when patients were in a depressive episode, there was hypoactivation in a circuit that included several regions of PFC, including medial, inferior, and superior frontal gyri. Similar results that also included a blunted ventral striatal response to positive stimuli have been reported by others (e.g., Epstein et al., 2006). Fu et al. (2007) reported a similar hypoactivated response to happy facial expressions.

As suggested earlier, recent reports of anatomical PFC differences between depressed patients and normal controls are of critical import to any claims made about functional differences between these two groups of individuals. Consistent with earlier work by Coffey and colleagues (1993), who found that depressed inpatients had 7% smaller frontal lobe volumes than those of nonpsychiatric controls, Drevets and colleagues (1997) reported that patients with unipolar and bipolar depression with a family history of mood disorders showed 48 and 39% reductions in subgenual PFC volume, respectively. In a postmortem study by the same group (Öngür, An, & Price, 1998), glial cell number was significantly reduced in subgenual PFC in both unipolar (24%) and bipolar patients (41%) with family history of major depressive disorder (MDD). No significant effects were observed for nonfamilial MDD or bipolar disorder (BD). Rajkowska (2000) has further examined alterations in neuronal and glial histopathology in postmortem brains of patients with mood disorders. She and her colleagues found that left prefrontal cortices (no other brain areas were examined) of subjects with MDD had decreases in cortical thickness, neuronal size, and neuronal and glial densities in upper cortical layers (II–IV) of left rostral OFC; decreases in neuronal size and glial densities in lower cortical layers (V–VI); and decreases in neuronal and glial size and density in supra- and infragranular layers. Of note, they found a 12–15% reduction of cortical thickness in the lateral OFC. Furthermore, they argued that the 22–37% reduction in density of large neurons and 6–27% increase of small neurons in the rostral OFC and dorsolateral PFC (DLPFC) may implicate cell atrophy rather than cell loss as the mechanism for the reduced cortical volume seen in depression. Similar results were observed in the left DLPFC of bipolar patients. These brains were characterized by a 16–22% reduction in neuronal density in Layer III, 17–30% reduction in pyramidal cell density in Layers III and V, and a 19% reduction in glial density in Sublayer IIIc. The fact that these anatomical differences in the brain of patients with mood disorders might account for some of the functional differences noted by Drevets and colleagues do not in itself provide any direct measures of causal influence. Longitudinal studies of patients at risk for mood disorders are needed to ascertain whether these structural differences are present prior to the onset of a depressive episode. Heritable factors can be examined by studying monozygotic twins discordant for mood disorders to ascertain whether the anatomical abnormalities are found in the affected twin only (see Levinson, Chapter 8, this volume).

The common observation in electroencephalographic (EEG) studies of an altered pattern of asymmetric activation in anterior scalp regions in the direction of reduced left relative to right activation in depressed or dysphoric individuals has also been replicated several times in recent years (Bell, Schwartz, Hardin, Baldwin, & Kline, 1998, Bruder et al., 1997; Debener et al., 2000; Gotlib, Ranganath, & Rosenfeld, 1998; Pauli, Wiedemann, & Nickola, 1999; but see Reid, Duke, & Allen [1998] for complications, Davidson [1998] for a rejoinder, and Davidson [2004] for a more recent review).

In an important extension of the work on electrophysiological asymmetries, Bruder and his colleagues (2001) examined whether brain electrical asymmetry measures acquired during a pretreatment period predicted response to selective serotonin reuptake inhibitor (SSRI) treatment. They found that, among women in particular, treatment responders had significantly less relative right-sided activation compared with the nonresponders, though this effect was present in both anterior and posterior scalp regions. Based on the role of right prefrontal regions in components of negative affect (Davidson, 2000) and right posterior regions in arousal and anxiety (Heller & Nitschke 1998), these findings imply that those subjects with global right-activation, who would be expected to have symptoms of negative affect and anxious arousal, are least likely to show improvements with SSRI treatment.

Anterior Cingulate Cortex

The Role of the Anterior Cingulate Cortex in Emotion and Emotion Regulation

Several theorists have proposed that the anterior cingulate cortex (ACC) acts as a bridge between attention and emotion (Bush, Luu, & Posner, 2000; Devinsky, Morrell, & Vogt, 1995; Ebert & Ebmeier, 1996; Mayberg et al., 1997; Vogt, Nimchinsky, Vogt, & Hof, 1995). In their review, Thayer and Lane (2000) described the ACC as "a point of integration for visceral, attentional, and affective information that is critical for self-regulation and adaptability" (p. 211). In light of its anatomical connections (see below), the ACC appears well equipped for assessing and responding to the behavioral significance of external stimuli. Critical roles of the ACC in selective attention (i.e., prioritizing incoming information), affect, and specific characteristic mammalian social behaviors have been described (Devinsky et al., 1995; Vogt, Finch, & Olson, 1992). However, to fully understand the role of the ACC in psychopathology, affective states, and emotional processing, it seems mandatory to recognize that the ACC is far from being a functionally homogeneous region, and at least two subdivisions can be discerned (Devinsky et al., 1995; Vogt et al., 1992, 1995). The first, referred to as the *affect subdivision*, encompasses rostral and ventral areas of the ACC (Brodmann's areas [BAs] 25, 32, 33, and rostral BA 24). The second, referred to as the *cognitive subdivision*, involves dorsal regions of the ACC (caudal BAs 24′ and 32′, cingulate motor area; see Bush et al., 2000). The affect subdivision possesses extensive connections with limbic and paralimbic regions, such as the amygdala, nucleus accumbens, OFC, periaqueductal gray, anterior insula, and autonomic brainstem motor nuclei, and is assumed to be involved in regulating visceral and autonomic responses to stressful behavioral and emotional events, emotional expression, and social behavior. Because of its strong connections with the lateral hypothalamus, the subgenual ACC (BA 25) is considered the most important autonomic region within the frontal region (Öngür et al., 1998).

Conversely, the cognitive subdivision is intimately connected with DLPFC (BA 46/9), posterior cingulate, parietal cortex (BA 7), supplementary motor area, and spinal cord, and plays an important role in response selection and processing of cognitively demanding information. In functional neuroimaging studies, some evidence points to a functional differentiation between ventral (affective) and dorsal (cognitive) ACC subdivisions (Bush et al., 1998, 2000; Whalen, Bush, et al., 1998) though other evidence, particularly from the pain literature, challenges this simple differentiation (Salomons, Johnstone, Backonja, & Davidson, 2004).

From a functional perspective, activation of the dorsal region of the ACC has been reported during interference between competing information sources (Pardo, Pardo, Janer, & Raichle, 1990), visual attention (Nobre et al., 1997), monitoring of cognitive (Carter et al., 2000; MacDonald, Cohen, Stenger, & Carter, 2000) and reward-related (Rogers et al., 1999) conflicts, task difficulty (Paus et al., 1997), and increased risk-associated outcome uncertainty (Critchley, Mathias, & Dolan, 2001), among other experimental manipulations. A common denominator among these experimental conditions is that they all required modulation of attention or executive functions and monitoring of competition (Bush et al., 2000). The role of the ACC in conflict monitoring has been especially emphasized by Cohen and colleagues (Carter, Botvinick, & Cohen, 1999; Carter et al., 2000; Miller & Cohen, 2001), who proposed that the ACC may serve an evaluative function, reflecting the degree of response conflict elicited by a given task. Conflict occurs when two or more possible task-related decisions compete or interfere with each other. According to the *competition monitoring hypothesis*, the cognitive subdivision of the ACC monitors conflicts or cross-talk between brain regions. If a signal of competition emerges, this output signals the need for controlled processing. The DLPFC (BA 9) is assumed to be critical for this form of controlled processing, in that it represents and maintains task demands necessary for such control, and inhibits (e.g., Garavan et al., 1999) or increases neural activity in brain regions implicated in the competition. Thus, dorsal ACC activation leading to a call for further processing by other brain regions may represent a mechanism for effortful control. From a functional perspective, activation of the ventral ACC has been reported during various emotional states and manipulations (for reviews, see Bush et al., 2000; Reiman, 1997). Collectively, recent findings suggest that the ventral ACC is critically involved in conscious experience of affect, and possibly of uncertainty, conflict, and expectancy violation arising from affectively and motivationally salient situations (see below).

In light of the many types of experimental manipulations that activate the ACC, is there a common denominator underlying activation of the rostral–ventral ACC in such disparate experimental conditions, such as pain, classical conditioning, transient mood, activation of primary drive states, Stroop task, and perceiving facial expressions, among others? A possible answer to this question is that the ventral subdivision of the ACC may be critical for assessing the presence of possible conflicts between the current functional state of the organism and incoming information with potentially relevant motivational and emotional consequences. This suggestion is based on the observation that the ventral subdivision of the ACC is involved in behaviors characterized by monitoring and evaluation of performance, internal states, and presence of reward or punishment, which often require change in behavior. Extant evidence suggests that ACC activation may be present when effortful emotional regulation is required in situations in which behavior is failing to achieve a desired outcome or when affect is elicited in contexts that are not normative, including most laboratory situations (Bush et al., 2000; Ochsner & Barrett, 2001). Relatedly, it is not surprising that the ACC is one of the most consistently activated regions in patients with different anxiety disorders, such as obsessive–compulsive disorder (OCD) (Breiter, Rauch, et al., 1996; Rauch,

Savage, Alpert, Fischman, & Jenike, 1997), simple phobia (Rauch et al., 1995), and posttraumatic stress disorder (PTSD) (Rauch et al., 1996; Shin et al., 1997), in which conflicts between response tendencies and environments are prominent. Interestingly, psychosurgical lesions of the ACC has been used as a treatment for mood and anxiety disorders (e.g., Baer et al., 1995; see Binder & Iskandar [2000] for a review), possibly because of a reduction of conflict monitoring and uncertainty that otherwise characterize these psychiatric conditions.

ACC in Depression

In major depression, decreased ACC activation relative to controls has been reported repeatedly. In single-photon emission computed tomography (SPECT) studies, decreased regional cerebral blood flow (rCBF) in the left (Curran, Tucker, Kutas, & Posner, 1993; Mayberg, Lewis, Regenold, & Wagner, 1994) or right (Ito et al., 1996) ACC has been found in medicated patients with unipolar depression compared to controls. Decreased ACC activation has been recently replicated with PET (Bench et al., 1992; Drevets et al., 1997; George et al., 1997; Kumar et al., 1993) and fMRI (Beauregard et al., 1998) techniques. Interestingly, the region of the ACC found to be hypoactive in major depression (dorsal ACC: dorsal region of BA 32; BAs 24' and 32') appears to be different from the region found to be hyperactive in eventual treatment responders (ventral and rostral ACC, including pregenual BAs 24 and 32). Whereas the state of being depressed is associated with reduced dorsal ACC activity (previously discussed), remission has been characterized by increased activity in the same region (Bench, Frackowiak, & Dolan, 1995; Buchsbaum et al., 1997; Mayberg et al., 1999). Based on the functional neuroimaging and animal literature reviewed earlier, it is conceivable to postulate that (1) hypoactivation in dorsal regions of the ACC (BAs 24' and 32') may be associated with impaired modulation of attention or executive functions and impaired monitoring of competition among various response options; (2) hypoactivation in ventral regions of the ACC (BAs 24 and 32) may be associated with blunted conscious experience of affect, hypoarousal, anhedonia, and reduced coping potential in situations characterized by uncertainty, conflict, and expectancy violation between the environment and one's affective state; and (3) hyperactivation in ventral regions of the ACC may be associated with increased attentional and behavioral responses to anxiety-provoking situations, especially in subjects with depression and comorbid anxiety. Such hyperactivation may cause attentional and affective stereotypies. Although future studies will be needed to test these assumptions more explicitly, recent findings are consistent with some of them. For example, in a fluorodeoxyglucose–positron emission tomography (FDG-PET) study, Brody and colleagues (2001) found that reduction of anxiety/somatization symptoms was associated with decreased activation in the ventral ACC. Conversely, improvement in psychomotor retardation symptoms was associated with increased activation in the dorsal ACC. In a combined EEG-PET study using source localization, we observed that melancholic depressed subjects showed evidence of hypoactivation in BA 25 compared to both nonmelancholic depressed and control subjects (Pizzagalli et al., 2004).

Several recent studies have examined differences between depressed and control subjects on cognitive and affective tasks hypothesized to be mediated by the ACC, along with either simultaneous recordings of ACC function or examination of baseline ACC function. In one of our studies, we administered the Eriksen flanker task to subjects whose levels of depressive symptoms differed (Pizzagalli, Peccoralo, Davidson, & Cohen, 2006). We found that subjects high in depressive symptoms showed significantly lower accuracy after incorrect versus correct trials. Moreover, using source localized high-density EEG recordings, we observed that these high depression subjects had significantly reduced baseline gamma activity (36–44 Hz) within the ventral but not the dorsal ACC. Extending these findings to a clinical sample, Holmes and Pizzagalli (2008) recently reported that unmedicated subjects with major depression were characterized by impaired performance in trials immediately following a mistake. Interestingly, subjects with depression showed hyperactivation in the rostral ACC 80 ms after committing an error. Moreover, unlike control subjects, patients failed to recruit DLPFC regions 472 ms after error commission. Based on these and related findings (e.g., Alexopoulos et al., 2007; Chiu & Deldin, 2007), Holmes and Pizzagalli concluded that behavioral impairments were associated with exaggerated automatic detection of unfavorable performance outcomes and inability to recruit cognitive control after error commission. In an important recent study using fMRI, Steele, Kumar, and Ebmeier (2007) investigated the response to feedback in patients with depression and healthy controls. They found that controls responded to negative feedback with an increase in reaction time and activation of the dorsal ACC. Patients with depression showed neither a change in reaction time following negative feedback nor an alteration of the signal in ACC. Knutson, Bhanji, Cooney, Atlas, and Gotlib (2007) examined the anticipation of monetary gain or loss in healthy controls and in patients with depression. They found accentuated activation of the ACC during anticipation of increasing gains, suggestive of increased conflict during the anticipation of gains.

As noted, early on Drevets and colleagues (1997) reported an anatomical difference in the pregenual region of the ACC, with depressed patients showing smaller gray matter volume in this region. Several more recent studies have also reported volume reductions in this and bordering areas of the ACC (Caetano et al., 2006; Coryell, Nopoulos, Drevets, Wilson, & Andreasen, 2005; Tang et al., 2007).

The interplay between the affective and cognitive subdivisions of the ACC is currently unknown. From a theoretical perspective, several authors have suggested that the affective subdivision of the ACC may integrate salient affective and cognitive information (e.g., that derived from environmental stimuli or task demands), and subsequently modulate attentional processes within the cognitive subdivision accordingly (Mayberg et al., 1997, 1999; Mega, Cummings, Salloway, & Malloy, 1997; Pizzagalli, Pascual-Marqui, et al., 2001). In agreement with this hypothesis, dorsal anterior and posterior cingulate pathways devoted to attentional processes and amygdalar pathways devoted to affective processing converge within BA 24 (Mega et al., 1997). These mechanisms may be especially important for understanding the repeatedly demonstrated finding that increased pretreatment activity in the rostral ACC is associated with eventual better treatment response (Chen et al., 2007; Ebert, Feistel, & Barocka, 1991; Mayberg et al., 1997; Pizzagalli, Pascual-Marqui, et al., 2001; Wu et al., 1992, 1999). In an influential article, Mayberg and colleagues (1997) reported that patients with unipolar depression who responded to treatment after 6 weeks showed higher pretreatment glucose metabolism in a rostral region of the ACC (BA 24a/b) compared to both nonresponders and nonpsychiatric comparison subjects. We (Pizzagalli, Pascual-Marqui, et al., 2001) replicated this finding with EEG source localization techniques and demonstrated that even among those patients who respond to treatment, the magnitude of treatment response was predicted by baseline levels of activation in the same region of the ACC as that identified by Mayberg and colleagues. In addition, we suggested that hyperactivation of the rostral ACC in depression might reflect an increased sensitivity to affective conflict, such that the disparity between one's current mood and the responses expected in a particular context activates this region of ACC, which in turn issues a call for further processing to help resolve the conflict. This call for further processing is hypothesized to aid the treatment response.

One of the major outputs from the ACC is a projection to PFC. This pathway may be the route through which the ACC issues a call to the PFC for further processing to address a conflict that has been detected. Thus, abnormalities in PFC function in depression may arise as a consequence of the failure of the normal signals from the ACC, may be intrinsic to the PFC, or both. Findings of disrupted functional connectivity within frontocingulate pathways during both resting (Pizzagalli, Oakes, & Davidson, 2003) and task-induced (Holmes & Pizzagalli, 2008) states in subjects with depression is consistent with the hypothesis that dysfunctional interaction between ACC and PFC regions might play an important role in the pathophysiology of depression. It is also possible, and even likely, that different subtypes of depression may involve primary dysfunction in one or another part of the circuitry that we review in this chapter. We address this issue in more detail at the end of the chapter; for now, it is important to underscore the possibility that there may exist a primary ACC-based depression subtype and a primary PFC-based depression subtype. These subtypes might not conform to the currently prevalent phenomenological and descriptive nosologies in the psychiatric literature.

Hippocampus

The Role of the Hippocampus in Emotion and Emotion Regulation

The hippocampus is critically involved in episodic, declarative, contextual, and spatial learning and memory (Fanselow, 2000; Squire & Knowlton, 2000). In addition, the hippocampus is also importantly involved in the regulation of adrenocorticotropic hormone (ACTH) secretion (Jacobson & Sapolsky, 1991). With respect to conditioning, rodent studies have convincingly shown that the hippocampus plays a key role in the formation, storage, and consolidation of contextual fear conditioning (for a review, see Fanselow, 2000), in part through its interaction with the amygdala (Maren & Hobin, 2007). In this form of hippocampal-dependent Pavlovian conditioning, fear (e.g., expressed in increased freezing) is acquired to places or contexts (e.g., a specific cage) previously associated with aversive events (e.g., shock). This fact has important implications for our understanding of the abnormalities in affective function that may arise as a consequence of hippocampal dysfunction.

In functional neuroimaging studies, hippocampal–parahippocampal activation has been reported during perception of several negatively valenced stimuli and/or the experience of negatively valenced affective states, such as trace conditioning (Büchel, Dolan, Armony, & Friston, 1999), perception of aversive complex stimuli (Lane, Fink, Chau, & Dolan, 1997), threat-related words (Isenberg et al., 1999), increasing music dissonance (Blood, Zatorre, Bermudez, & Evans, 1999), tinnitus-like aversive auditory stimulation (Mirz, Gjedde, Sodkilde-Jrgensen, & Pedersen, 2000), vocal expressions of fear (Phillips, Young, et al., 1998), aversive taste (Zald, Lee, Fluegel, & Pardo, 1998), anticipatory anxiety (Javanmard et al., 1999), procaine-induced affect (Ketter et al., 1996), and monetary penalties (Elliott & Dolan, 1999). However, it seems that valence is not the critical variable for evoking hippocampal activation. Indeed, hippocampal activation has been also reported during experimental manipulation of positive affect, such as reevoking pleasant affective autobiographical memories (Fink et al., 1996), increases in winning in a game-like task (Zalla et al., 2000), and perception of the loved person (Bartels & Zeki, 2000). Also, hippocampal activation has been found to be correlated with long-term recognition memory for pleasant films (Hamann, Ely, Grafton, & Kilts, 1999).

In reconciling these findings, we suggest that most of the experimental manipulations leading to hippocampal activation contain contextual cues (see Davidson, Jackson, & Kalin, 2000); that is, we assume that they involve the consolidation of a memory for an integrated representation of a context similar to that associated with the presented stimulus (Fanselow, 2000). This is clearly the case during not only Pavlovian and trace conditioning, for instance, but also presentation of both positively and negatively valenced visual, olfactory, and auditory cues that may induce reevocation and consolidation of contextual information associated with similar situation in the past (e.g., Nader, Schafe, & LeDoux, 2000). Although the mechanisms underlying contextual conditioning in humans are still unclear, it is possible that plasticity in functional connectivity between the hippocampus and regions crucially involved in decoding the behavioral significance of incoming information, such as the amygdala and the pulvinar, may critically contribute to contextual learning (Morris, Friston, & Dolan, 1997; Morris, Ohman, & Dolan, 1999), even when the information is presented below the level of conscious awareness (Morris et al., 1999). As reviewed by Davis and Whalen (2001), animal studies clearly suggest that the amygdala exerts a modulatory influence on hippocampal-dependent memory systems, possibly through direct projections from the basolateral nucleus of the amygdala. Consistent with this view, stimulation of the amygdala causes long-term potentiation (LTP) induction in the dentate gyrus of the hippocampus (Ikegaya, Abe, Saito, & Nishiyama, 1995). Conversely, lesions to (Ikegaya, Saito, & Abe, 1994) or local anesthetics within (Ikegaya, Saito, & Abe, 1995) the basolateral nucleus of the amygdala attenuate LTP in the dentate gyrus. Although drawing conclusions from these rodent studies to humans is speculative at this stage, it is intriguing that most of the human neuroimaging studies that report hippocampal activation during aversive affective manipulations have also found amygdalar activation (Büchel et al., 1999; Dougal, Phelps, & Davachi, 2007; Isenberg et al., 1999; Ketter et al., 1996; Mirz et al., 2000; Zald et al., 1998). Future neuroimaging studies should test directly the interplay between the hippocampus and the amygdala in these processes, and in fear-related learning and memory, especially in light of recent animal data suggesting an interplay between these regions in modulating extinction of conditioned fear (Corcoran & Maren, 2001).

Hippocampus in Depression

In their review, Davidson, Jackson, and Kalin (2000) noted that various form of psychopathology involving disorders of affect may be characterized as disorders in context-regulation of affect; that is, patients with mood and anxiety disorders often display normative affective responses, but in inappropriate contexts. Given the preclinical and functional neuroimaging literature reviewed earlier, one may hypothesize that patients showing inappropriate context regulation of affect may be characterized by hippocampal dysfunction. Consistent with this conjecture, recent morphometric studies using MRI indeed reported hippocampal atrophy in patients with major depression (Bremner et al., 2000; Colla et al., 2007; Lange & Irle, 2004; Maller, Daskalakis, & Fitzgerald, 2007; Mervaala et al., 2000; Neumeister et al., 2005; Shah, Ebmeier, Glabus, & Goodwin, 1998; Sheline, Sanghavi, Mintun, & Gado, 1999; Sheline, Wang, Gado, Csernansky, & Vannier, 1996; Steffens et al., 2000; von Gunten, Fox, Cipolotti, & Ron, 2000; but see Ashtari et al., 1999; Vakili et al., 2000), BD (Noga, Vladar, & Torrey, 2001), PTSD (Bremner et al., 1995; Bremner, Innis, et al., 1997; Stein, Koverola, Hanna, Torchia, & McClarty, 1997), and borderline personality disorder

(Driessen et al., 2000; for reviews, see Sapolsky, 2000; Sheline, 2000). Where hippocampal volume reductions in depression have been found, the magnitude of reduction ranges from 8 to 19%. Functional hippocampal abnormalities in major depression have been also reported at baseline by researchers using PET measures of glucose metabolism (e.g., Saxena et al., 2001). Whether hippocampal dysfunction precedes or follows onset of depressive symptomatology is still unknown.

In depression, inconsistencies across studies may be explained by several methodological considerations. First, as pointed out by Sheline (2000), studies reporting positive findings generally used MRI with higher spatial resolution (~0.5–2.0 mm) compared to those reporting negative findings (~3–10 mm). Second, it seems that age, severity of depression, and, most significantly, duration of recurrent depression may be important moderator variables. Indeed, researchers reporting negative findings either studied younger cohorts (e.g., Vakili et al., 2000: 38 ± 10 years vs. Sheline et al., 1996: 69 ± 10 years; von Gunten et al., 2000: 58 ± 9 years; Steffens et al., 2000: 72 ± 8 years) or less severe and less chronic cohorts (Ashtari et al., 1999 vs. Bremner et al., 2000; Shah et al., 1998; Sheline et al., 1996). In a study from our laboratory (Rusch, Abercrombie, Oakes, Schaefer, & Davidson, 2001), we also failed to find hippocampal atrophy in a relatively young subject sample (33.2 ± 9.5 years) with moderate depression severity. In a study of pediatric depression, Rosso and colleagues (2005) found no hippocampal volume difference between groups. Notably, in normal early adulthood (18–42 years), decreased bilateral hippocampal volume has been reported with increasing age in male, but not female, healthy subjects (Pruessner, Collins, Pruessner, & Evans, 2001). Finally, in females, initial evidence suggests that total lifetime duration of depression, rather than age, is associated with hippocampal atrophy (Sheline et al., 1999), inviting the possibility that hippocampal atrophy may be a symptom rather than a cause of depression. Other recent evidence suggests that the extent of hippocampal atrophy in depression may interact with specific genetic factors. For example, Frodl and colleagues (2007) found that both depressed patients and controls carrying the Met allele for brain-derived neutropic factor (BDNF) gene had significantly smaller hippocampal volumes than did comparison subjects homozygous for the Val-BDNF allele. In addition, Frodl and colleagues found that depressed patients as a group had significantly smaller hippocampal volumes than did controls. Taylor and colleagues (2005) observed a complex interaction between age of onset of depression and polymorphisms in the promoter region of the serotonin transporter gene on hippocampal volume. In the patients with early onset, those patients homozygous for the short allele (S/S genotype) had smaller hippocampal volumes than did comparison patients. In an important, recent study on monogygotic twins, de Geus and colleagues (2007) marshal evidence to show that volume reductions in the hippocampus are present only in the co-twin at risk for depression and anxiety compared to his or her identical co-twin. These findings convincingly demonstrate at least some important environmental etiology for the hippocampal volume reduction found in depression.

Structurally, the hippocampal changes may arise due to neuronal loss through chronic hypercortisolemia, glial cell loss, stress-induced reduction in neurotrophic factors, or stress-induced reduction in neurogenesis, but the precise mechanisms are not completely known (Sheline, 2000). In depression, the hypothesis of an association between sustained, stress-related elevations of cortisol and hippocampal damage has received considerable attention. This hypothesis is based on the observation that the pathophysiology of depression involves dysfunction in negative feedback of the hypothalamic–pituitary–adrenal (HPA) axis (see Pariante & Miller [2001] for a review), which results in increased levels of cortisol during depressive episodes (e.g., Carroll, Curtis, & Mendels, 1976). Higher levels of cortisol may in turn lead to neuronal damage in the hippocampus, because this region possesses high levels of glucocorticoid receptors (Reul & de Kloet, 1986), and glucocorticoids are neurotoxic (Sapolsky, Krey, & McEwen, 1986). Because the hippocampus is involved in negative-feedback control of cortisol (Jacobson & Sapolsky, 1991), hippocampal dysfunction may result in reduction of the inhibitory regulation of the HPA axis, which could then lead to hypercortisolemia. Consistent with this view, chronic exposure to increased glucocorticoid concentrations has been shown to lower the threshold for hippocampal neuronal degeneration in animals (Gold, Goodwin, & Chrousos, 1988; McEwen, 1998; Sapolsky, Uno, Rebert, & Finch, 1990) and humans (Lupien et al., 1998). At least in nonhuman primates, this association is qualified by the observation that chronically elevated cortisol concentrations in the absence of chronic "psychosocial" stress do not produce hippocampal neuronal loss (Leverenz et al., 1999). Conversely, naturalistic, chronic psychosocial stress has been shown to induce structural changes in hippocampal neurons of subordinate animals (Magarinos, McEwen, Flugge, & Fuchs, 1996). In depression, hippocampal volume loss has been shown to be associated with lifetime duration of depression (Sheline et al., 1999), consistent with the assumption that long-term exposure to high cortisol levels may lead to hippocampal atrophy. However, this conjecture has not been verified empirically in humans.

Although intriguing, these findings cannot inform us about the causality among hippocampal dysfunction, elevated levels of cortisol, and most importantly, inappropriate context regulation of affect in depression. In one of the few studies that examined associations between hippocampal volume and basal cortisol, Colla and colleagues (2007) found no relation between the variables. It may be that with a denser cortisol sampling protocol that includes assessment of dirurnal slope, such relations might be uncovered. Unfortunately, none of the structural neuroimaging studies of depression that investigated hippocampal volume were prospective and took into account cortisol data in an effort to unravel the causal link between cortisol output and hippocampal dysfunction.

The possibility of plasticity in the hippocampus deserves particular comment. Studies of rodents have shown hippocampal neurogenesis as a consequence of antidepressant pharmacological treatment (Chen, Rajkowska, Du, Seraji-Bosorgzad, & Manji, 2000; Malberg, Eisch, Nestler, & Duman, 2000), electroconvulsive shock (Madhav, Pei, Grahame-Smith, & Zetterstrom, 2000) and, most intriguingly, as a consequence of positive handling, learning, and exposure to an enriched environment (Kempermann, Kuhn, & Gage, 1997; for a review, see Gould, Tanapat, Rydel, & Hastings, 2000). In humans, neurogenesis in the adult human hippocampus has been also reported (Eriksson et al., 1998). Furthermore, in patients with Cushing's disease, who are characterized by very high levels of cortisol, increases in hippocampal volume were significantly associated with magnitude of cortisol decrease produced by microadrenomectomy (Starkman et al., 1999). As a corpus, these animal and human data clearly suggest that plasticity in the human hippocampus is possible (for reviews, see Duman, Malberg, Nakagawa, & D'Sa, 2000; Gould et al., 2000; Jacobs, Praag, & Gage, 2000), which suggests that structural and functional changes in the hippocampus of a depressed patient may be reversible. Indeed, recent formulations underscore the possible role of underlying hippocampal neurogenesis in some of the behavioral effects of antidepressant treatment (Sahay & Hen, 2007).

In summary, preclinical and clinical studies converge in suggesting an association between major depression and hippocampal dysfunction. Future studies should (1) assess whether hippocampal atrophy precedes or follows increased onset of depression; (2) assess the causal relation between hypercortisolemia and hippocampal volume reduction; (3) directly test a putative link between inappropriate, context-dependent affective responding and hippocampal atrophy; and (4) assess putative treatment-mediated plastic changes in the hippocampus.

Amygdala

The Role of the Amygdala in Emotion and Emotion Regulation

Although a link between amygdalar activity and negative affect has been a prevalent view in the literature, particularly when examined in response to exteroceptive aversive stimuli (e.g., LeDoux, 2000), recent findings from invasive animal studies, human lesion, and functional neuroimaging studies are converging on a broader view that regards the role of the amygdala in negative affect as a special case of its more general role in directing attention to affectively salient stimuli, and issuing a call for further processing of stimuli that have major significance for the individual. Extant evidence is consistent with the argument that the amygdala is critical for recruiting and coordinating cortical arousal and vigilant attention for optimizing sensory and perceptual processing of stimuli associated with underdetermined contingencies, such as novel, "surprising," or "ambiguous" stimuli (e.g., Davis & Whalen, 2001; Holland & Gallagher, 1999; Whalen, 1998). Most stimuli in this class may be conceptualized as having an aversive valence, because we tend to have a negativity bias in the face of uncertainty (Taylor, 1991).

The amygdala and the structures with which it is interconnected, particularly regions of the PFC, play a crucial role in the regulation of emotion (for a review, see Ochsner & Gross, 2005). Recently, Urry and colleagues (2006) demonstrated that voluntary regulation of emotion using cognitive reappraisal is associated with systematic changes in activation of the amygdala in normal subjects. Specifically, the down-regulation of emotion is associated with decreased activation in the amygdala compared with an attend control condition. In addition, in this study, we examined which brain regions were activated when the amygdala was down-regulated and found that the ventromedial prefrontal cortex (vmPFC) was strongly reciprocally related to the amygdala (correlations > .8). During the down-regulation of emotion, the vmPFC was activated. Moreover, in this study we demonstrated that those subjects with the greatest decrease in amygdala activation and the greatest increase in vmPFC activation during the down-regulation of emotion had the steepest slope of diurnal variation in basal cortisol. These individuals may be thought of as the good emotion regulators, and they especially showed low levels of evening cortisol (correlations in the range of .7).

The Role of the Amygdala in Depression

In major depression, structural and functional abnormalities in the amygdala have been reported. Relative to structure, several studies have reported an association between increased amygdalar volume and depression. This association has been found in depressed patients with bipolar disorders (Altshuler, Bartzokis, Grieder, Curran, & Mintz, 1998; Strakowski et al., 1999) as well as temporal lobe epilepsy (TLE; Tebartz van Elst, Woermann, Lemieux, & Trimble, 1999, 2000). Mervaala and colleagues (2000) observed significant asymmetry in amygdalar volumes (right smaller than left) in patients with MDD but not in controls. In patients with TLE and dysthymia, left amygdalar volume was positively correlated with depression severity, as assessed with the Beck Depression Inventory (BDI) (Tebartz van Elst et al., 1999). More recently, Munn and colleagues (2007) failed to find significant differences in amygdalar volume between depressed and control twin subjects. Zetzsche and colleagues

(2006) studied a sample of patients with borderline personality disorder, with and without major depression, and found that those with major depression had significantly larger amygdalar volumes than did those without major depression. Moreover, there was a significant association between severity of depressive symptoms and left amygdalar volume. Although these findings generally depict a relation between increased amygdalar volume and depression, it is important to stress that (1) the causal relations between the two entities are still unknown, and (2) some inconsistencies among studies are present. Indeed, some researchers reported either decreased bilateral volume in the amygdalar core nuclei (Sheline, Gado, & Price, 1998) or null findings (Ashtari et al., 1999; Coffey et al., 1993; Pantel et al., 1997). Although the reasons are still unclear, it is interesting to note that two null findings were found in studies of geriatric depression (Ashtari et al., 1999; Pantel et al., 1997).

Functionally, abnormal elevations of resting rCBF or glucose metabolism in the amygdala have been reported in depression during both wakefulness (Drevets et al., 1992) and sleep (Ho et al., 1996; Nofzinger et al., 1999). In an FDG-PET study, Ho and colleagues (1996) reported increased absolute cerebral glucose metabolic activity in several brain regions, particularly the amygdala (+44%), in 10 unmedicated men with unipolar depression during a non-REM sleep period. Furthermore, in his review, Drevets (2001) reports data from five consecutive studies in which increased rCBF or glucose metabolism has been consistently replicated in depressives with familial MDD or melancholic features. In a postmortem study, serotonin (5-HT_2) receptor density was significantly increased in the amygdalas of depressive patients who committed suicide (Hrdina, Demeter, Vu, Sotonyi, & Palkovits, 1993).

Abnormally increased amygdalar activation has also been reported in bipolar depression (Ketter et al., 2001) and in anxiety disorders, which often show high degree of comorbidity with depression (Birbaumer et al., 1998; Liberzon et al., 1999; Rauch et al., 1996, 2000; Schneider et al., 1999; Semple et al., 2000; Shin et al., 1997). Further establishing a link between depression and amygdalar activation, two studies have reported a positive correlation between amygdalar activation and depression severity or dispositional negative affect in patients with MDD (Abercrombie et al., 1998; Drevets et al., 1992). After pharmacologically induced remission from depression, amygdalar activation has been observed to decrease to normative values (Drevets, 2001). In familial pure depressive disease, however, increased (left) amygdalar activation persists during the remitted phases (Drevets et al., 1992), suggesting that, at least in some subtypes of depression, amygdalar dysfunction may be trait-like. Interestingly, patients with remitted MDD exhibiting symptom relapse as a consequence of serotonin depletion showed increased amygdalar activation prior to the depletion compared to those who did not relapse (Bremner, Randall, et al., 1997).

In one of the first fMRI studies using an activation paradigm, Yurgelun-Todd and colleagues (2000) reported higher left amygdalar activation for patients with BD than for controls in response to fearful faces. More recently, Fales and colleagues (2007) showed that a sample of 27 patients with major depression exhibited significantly greater activation in the amygdala in response to unattended fear-relevant stimuli compared with 24 healthy controls. Using a paradigm based on our prior studies of anticipatory anxiety (Nitschke, Sarinopoulos, Mackiewicz, Schaefer, & Davidson, 2006), Abler, Erk, Herwig, and Walter (2007) found that in response to a cue that predicted a negative picture, depressed patients showed greater activation in the extended amygdalar region compared with controls. They also found that depression severity was positively correlated with ventral amygdalar activation in response to negative pictures. Three recent studies focused on emotional memory found evidence of amygdalar differences in depression during encoding. Ramel and colleagues (2007) found that amygdalar activation during encoding predicted recall of nega-tive-valenced self-referent words in a subset of patients with remitted depression compared with never-depressed controls only in a condition that followed a sad mood induction, but not before the mood induction. In a sample of adolescents with major depression, Roberson-Nay and colleagues (2006) found that patients had greater left amygdalar activa-tion compared with healthy controls during successful versus unsuccessful encoding of faces. Finally, distinguishing among difference valences of stimuli, Hamilton and Gotlib (2008) found that depressed adults were characterized by greater right amygdalar activation than were nondepressed controls during the encoding of subsequently recalled negative, but not positive or neutral, stimuli.

To probe individual differences in connectivity between the amygala and the vmPFC, which we previously found to be inversely coupled in healthy controls (Urry et al., 2006), we compared patients with major depression to a new sample of healthy controls (John-stone, van Reekum, Urry, Kalin, & Davidson, 2007) on an emotion regulation task in the scanner. We replicated our previous finding of inverse coupling between the vmPFC and the amygdala in controls. Among depressed patients these brain regions were positively corre-lated. Moreover, measures of pupil dilation were obtained to index cognitive effort during emotion regulation. Although there was no main group effect on this measure, indicating that the patients and controls expended comparable effort to down-regulate their emotion, we did find a very different pattern of correlation between the pupil measures and brain ac-tivity. For the controls, the more effort they expended (as indexed by greater pupil dilation), the *less* the activation in emotion-related brain regions, such as the amygdala. However, for patients, this association was positive.

These latter findings suggest that one fundamental abnormality in depression may be associated with the regulation of negative affect. Despite what appear to be normal levels of effort and engagement, several of our findings suggest that such effort does not culminate in adaptive modulation of neural activity in emotion-processing regions. Our findings further suggest that there may be a subset of patients with depression who actually show exacerba-tions in symptoms during the voluntary regulation of negative affect. We believe that such strategies may be associated with rumination.

In light of the pivotal role of the amygdala in recruiting and coordinating vigilant be-havior toward stimuli with underdetermined contingencies, hyperactivation of the amygdala in major depression may bias initial evaluation of and response to incoming information. Although still a speculation, this mechanism may rely on norepinephrine, which is (1) often-times abnormally elevated in depression (e.g., Veith et al., 1994); (2) involved in amygdala-mediated emotional learning (Ferry, Roozendaal, & McGaugh, 1999); and (3) affected by glucocorticoid secretion, which is often elevated in MDD (e.g., Carroll et al., 1976). Thus, these findings may explain cognitive biases toward aversive or emotionally arousing infor-mation observed in depression.

Increased amygdalar activation in depression may also represent a possible biological substrate for anxiety, which often is comorbid with depression. In this respect, elevated lev-els of glucocortocoid hormones, which characterize at least some subgroups of patients with depression, may be especially relevant, because elevated glucocorticoid hormones have been shown to be associated with increased corticotropin-releasing hormone (CRH) in the amygdala. Increased CHR availability may increase anxiety, fear, and expectation of adver-sity (Schulkin, 1994).

Our findings on emotion regulation in depression raise the possibility that when abnor-mally high levels of amygdalar activation are observed in depression, they may reflect abnormalities in the modulation of amygdalar activity by regions of the PFC and, as such, re-flect problems in emotion regulation. Although some data support this conjecture, additional research is needed to determine whether these are state or trait abnormalities, and to deter-mine the specific profile of symptoms with which they may be associated.

SUMMARY AND FUTURE DIRECTIONS

In this chapter we have reviewed circuitry that underlies the representation and regulation of emotion. This circuitry exhibits different kinds of abnormalities in depression. Different ter-ritories of the PFC and ACC, the hippocampus, and the amygdala were considered. These structures are all interconnected in regionally specific ways and exhibit bidirectional feed-back. Abnormalities in the morphometry and functioning of each of these structures have been reported in depression. Because longitudinal studies that involve the measurement of brain structure and function in at-risk individuals have not yet been performed, we cannot specify at present which of the abnormalities may be primary in the sense of occurring first, and which may be secondary to dysfunctions initially occurring in another brain region. For example, PFC abnormalities may arise as a consequence of ACC abnormalities or be inde-pendent. In addition, a paucity of work has examined functional and/or structural connec-tivity among these regions. Some of the abnormalities in depression may arise as a conse-quence of impaired connectivity, either functional or structural, or both. Future research should include measures of both functional (e.g., Cordes et al., 2000) and structural connectiv-ity. The latter can be beautifully measured with diffusion tensor imaging (Le Bihan et al., 2001).

In the course of this review, we have drawn on the animal and human literature on ba-sic processes in emotion and emotion regulation to help interpret the abnormalities reported in depression and to highlight the kinds of studies that have not yet been performed but are important to conduct. The findings on the basic processes in animals and normal humans provide the foundation for a model of the major components in affect representation and regulation. The input to affect representation can be either a sensory stimulus or a memory. Most sensory stimuli are relayed through the thalamus and from there take a short route to the amygdala (LeDoux, 2000) and/or go up to cortex. From both association cortex and from subcortical regions, including the amygdala, information is relayed to different zones of the PFC. The PFC plays a crucial role in the representation of goals. In the presence of ambiguous situations, the PFC sends bias signals to other brain regions to facilitate the ex-pression of task-appropriate responses in the face of competition with potentially stronger alternatives. We have argued that, in the affective domain, the PFC implements affect-guided anticipatory processes. Left-sided PFC regions are particularly involved in approach-related appetitive goals, whereas right-sided PFC regions are involved in the maintenance of goals that require behavioral inhibition. Abnormalities in PFC function would be expected to compromise goal instantiation in patients with depression. Left-sided hypoactivation would result in deficits specifically in pregoal attainment forms of positive affect, whereas right-sided hyperactivation would result in excessive behavioral inhibition and anticipatory anxi-ety. Hypoactivation in regions of the PFC with which the amygdala is interconnected may result in a decrease in the regulatory influence on the amygdala and a prolonged time course of amygdalar activation in response to challenge. This might be expressed phenomenologi-cally as perseveration of negative affect and rumination.

The ACC is critically involved in conflict monitoring and is activated whenever an indi-vidual is confronted with a challenge that involves conflict among two or more response options. According to an influential theory of ACC function (Carter et al., 1999), the ACC monitors the conflicts or cross-talk among brain regions. When such conflict is detected, the ACC issues a call for further processing to the PFC, which then adjudicates among the various response options and guides behavior toward a goal. The ACC is very frequently activated in neuroimaging studies of human emotion (for a review, see Bush et al., 2000) in part because when emotion is elicited in the laboratory, it produces response conflict. There is the general expectation to behave in an unemotional fashion, because subjects are participating in a scientific experiment, yet there are the responses that are pulled by the emotional challenge, such as certain patterns of facial expression. This is commonly reported by subjects and is associated with ACC activation.

There is sometimes a conflict between an individual's mood state and the behavior that is expected of him or her in a particular social or role context. For example, dispositional mood state may predispose depressed individuals, to set few goals and engage in little intentional action, yet the demands of their environments may include expectations to behave and act in specific ways. In an individual with normal levels of ACC activation, the signal from ACC would call to other brain regions, the PFC being the most important, to resolve the conflict and to engage in appropriate goal-directed behavior. However, in an individual with abnormally low levels of ACC activation, the conflict between dispositional mood state and the expectations of context would not be effectively monitored; thus, the usual call for further processing would not be issued. The data on ACC function in depression most consistently reveal a pattern of decreased activation in certain regions of the ACC. Interestingly, as we noted earlier, those depressed patients with greater activation in the ventral ACC before antidepressant treatment are the ones most likely to show the largest treatment responses. In normal individuals, activation of the affective subdivision of the ACC may also be associated phenomonologically with the "will to change."

The hippocampus appears to play an important role in encoding context. Lesions to the hippocampus in animals impair context conditioning. In addition, this structure has a high density of glucocorticoid receptors, and elevated levels of cortisol in animal models have been found to produce hippocampal cell death. In humans, various stress-related disorders, including depression, have been found to be associated with hippocampal atrophy. Whether such hippocampal volume differences are a cause or a consequence of the depression cannot be determined from extant data. However, to the extent that hippocampal dysfunction is present, we would expect that such individuals would show abnormalities in the context-appropriate modulation of emotional behavior. This type of abnormality would be expressed as the display of normal emotion in inappropriate contexts. Thus, the persistence of sadness in situations that would ordinarily engender happiness could in part arise as a consequence of a hippocampus-dependent problem in the context modulation of emotional responses. We have shown such effects in rhesus monkeys (for a review, see Davidson, Jackson, & Kalin, 2000), though these effects have not yet been studied in depressed patients. The extensive connections between hippocampus and PFC would presumably provide the requisite anatomical substrate for conveying the contextual information to PFC to regulate emotional behavior in a context-appropriate fashion. The connections between hippocampus and PFC are another potential target of dysfunction in depression. It is possible that in a certain subtype of individual, contextual encoding is intact and PFC-implemented, goal-directed behavior is intact but context fails to guide and reprioritize goals adequately. In such cases, the functional and/or anatomical connectivity between hippocampus and PFC might be a prime candidate for dysfunction. As noted earlier, tools are now available to examine both types of connectivity with noninvasive measures.

The amygdala has long been viewed as a key site for both the perception of cues that signal threat and the production of behavioral and autonomic responses associated with aversive responding. As we noted earlier, current evidence suggests that the amygdala's role in negative affect may be a special case of its more general role in directing attention and resources to affectively salient stimuli, and issuing a call for further processing of stimuli that have potentially major significance for the individual. As with other parts of the circuit we have addressed, there are extensive connections between the amygdala and each of the other structures we have considered. The amygdala receives input from a wide range of cortical zones and has even more extensive projections back to cortex, which enables biasing of cortical processing as a function of the early evaluation of a stimulus as affectively salient. Also, like the other components of the circuit we have described, there are individual differences in amygdalar activation both at baseline (Schaefer et al., 2000) and in response to challenge (for a review, see Davidson & Irwin 1999). Moreover, as we noted earlier, it is likely that regions of the PFC play an important role in modulating activation in the amygdala, thus influencing the time course of amygdala-driven, negative affective responding (Johnstone et al., 2007; Urry et al., 2006). In light of the reported associations between individual differences in amygdalar activation and affect measures, it is likely that when it occurs, hyperactivation of the amygdala in depression is associated more with fear-like and anxiety components of the symptoms than with sad mood and anhedonia. In our own work, we have found that amygdalar activation predicts dispositional negative affect in depressed patients but is unrelated to variations in positive affect (Abercrombie et al., 1998). Excessive activation of the amygdala in depressed patients may also be associated with hypervigilance, particularly toward threat-related cues, which further exacerbates some of the symptoms of depression.

Several types of studies critically need to be performed in light of the extant evidence reviewed in this chapter. First, studies are needed that relate specific abnormalities in particular brain regions to objective laboratory tasks that are neurally inspired and designed to capture the particular kinds of processing hypothesized to be implemented in those brain regions. Relatively few studies of this kind have been conducted. Most studies on depressed patients that examine relations between individual differences in neural activity and behavioral phenomena almost always relate such neural variation to symptom measures that are either self-report or interview-based indices. In the future, it will be important to complement the phenomenological description with laboratory measures explicitly designed to highlight the processes implemented in different parts of the circuit we described.

Such future studies should include measures of both functional and structural connectivity to complement the activation measures. It is clear that interactions among the various components of the circuitry we describe are likely to play a crucial role in determining behavioral output. Moreover, it is possible that connectional abnormalities may exist in the absence of abnormalities in specific structures. This possibility underscores the real necessity of including measures of connectivity in future research.

As noted several times in this review, longitudinal studies of at-risk samples with the types of imaging measures featured in this review are crucial. We do not know whether any of the abnormalities we discussed, both of a structural and functional variety, precede the onset of the disorder, co-occur with the onset of the disorder, or follow after some time the expression of the disorder. It is likely that the timing of the abnormalities in relation to the clinical course of the disorder varies for different parts of the circuitry. The data we reviewed earlier showing a relation between the number of cumulative days depressed over the course of the lifetime and hippocampal volume suggest that this abnormality may follow the expression of the disorder and represent a consequence rather than a primary cause of the disorder. Before such a conclusion is accepted, however, it is important to conduct the requisite longitudinal studies to begin to disentangle these complex causal factors.

Finally, we regard the evidence presented in this review as offering strong support for the view that *depression* is a heterogeneous group of disorders. It is possible that depression spectrum disorders can be produced by abnormalities in many different parts of the circuitry reviewed. The specific subtype, symptom profile, and affective abnormalities should vary systematically with the location and nature of the abnormality. It is likely that some of the heterogeneity produced by deficits in particular components of the circuitry reviewed will not map precisely onto the diagnostic categories we have inherited from descriptive psychiatry. A major challenge for the future will be to build a more neurobiologically plausible scheme for parsing the heterogeneity of depression based on the location and nature of the abnormality in the circuitry featured in this review. We believe that this ambitious effort will lead to considerably more consistent findings at the biological level and also enable us to characterize more rigorously different endophenotypes that could then be exploited for genetic studies.

ACKNOWLEDGMENTS

The authors wish to thank Alexander J. Shackman and William Irwin for invaluable comments, and Andrew M. Hendrick, Kathryn A. Horras, Megan Zuelsdorff, and Susan Jensen for skilled and dedicated assistance in the preparation of the manuscript. Additional thanks to William Irwin for preparation of Figure 10.1. This work was supported by NIMH grants (Nos. MH40747, P50-MH52354, MH43454, and P50-MH61083) and by an NIMH Research Scientist Award (No. K05-MH00875) to Richard J. Davidson. Diego A. Pizzagalli was supported by NIMH (No. R01 MH68376) and NCCAM (No. R21 AT002974) grants. Jack B. Nitschke was supported by NIMH grants (Nos. R01-MH74847 and K08-MH63984) and a training grant (No. T32-MH18931).

REFERENCES

Abercrombie, H. C., Schaefer, S. M., Larson, C. L., Oakes, T. R., Holden, J. E., Perlman, S. B., et al. (1998). Metabolic rate in the right amygdala predicts negative affect in depressed patients. *NeuroReport*, 9, 3301–3307.

Abler, B., Erk, S., Herwig, U., & Walter, H. (2007). Anticipation of aversive stimuli activates extended amygdala in unipolar depression. *Journal of Psychiatric Research*, 41, 511–522.

Adamec, R., & Young, B. (2000). Neuroplasticity in specific limbic system circuits may mediate specific kindling induced changes in animal affect—implications for understanding anxiety associated with epilepsy. *Neuroscience and Biobehavioral Reviews*, 24, 705–723.

Adolphs, R., Cahill, L., Schul, R., & Babinsky, R. (1997). Impaired declariative memory for emotional material following bilateral amygdala damage in humans. *Learning and Memory*, 4, 291–300.

Adolphs, R., Damasio, H., Tranel, D., & Damasio, A. R. (1995). Fear and the human amygdala. *Journal of Neuroscience*, 15, 5879–5891.

Adolphs, R., Tranel, D., & Damasio, A. R. (1998). The human amygdala in social judgment. *Nature*, 393, 470–474.

Alexopoulos, G. S., Murphy, C. F., Gunning-Dixon, F. M., Kalayam, B., Katz, R., Kanellopoulos, D., et al. (2007). Event-related potentials in an emotional go/no-go task and remission of geriatric depression. *NeuroReport*, 18, 217–221.

Altshuler, L. L., Bartzokis, G., Grieder, T., Curran, J., & Mintz, J. (1998). Amygdala enlargement in bipolar disorder and hippocampal reduction in schizophrenia: An MRI study demonstrating neuroanatomic specificity. *Archives of General Psychiatry, 55*, 663–664.

Ashtari, M., Greenwald, B. S., Kramer-Ginsberg, E., Hu, J., Wu, H., Patel, M., et al. (1999). Hippocampal/amygdala volumes in geriatric depression. *Psychological Medicine, 29*, 629–638

Baer, L., Rauch, S. L., Ballantine, H. T. J., Martuza, R., Cosgrove, R., Cassem, E., et al. (1995). Cingulotomy for intractable obsessive–compulsive disorder: Prospective long-term follow-up of 18 patients. *Archives of General Psychiatry, 52*, 384–392.

Bartels, A., & Zeki, S. (2000). The neural basis of romantic love. *NeuroReport, 11*, 3829–3834.

Beauregard, M., Leroux, J. M., Bergman, S., Arzoumanian, Y., Beaudoin, G., Bourgouin, P., et al. (1998). The functional neuroanatomy of major depression: An fMRI study using an emotional activation paradigm. *NeuroReport, 9*, 3253–3258.

Bell, I. R., Schwartz, G. E., Hardin, E. E., Baldwin, C. M., & Kline, J. P. (1998). Differential resting quantitative electroencephalographic alpha patterns in women with environmental chemical intolerance, depressives, and normals. *Biological Psychiatry, 43*, 376–388.

Bench, C. J., Frackowiak, R. S., & Dolan, R. J. (1995). Changes in regional cerebral blood flow on recovery from depression. *Psychological Medicine, 25*, 247–251.

Bench, C. J., Friston, K. J., Brown, R. G., Scott, L. C., Frackowiak, S. J., & Dolan, R. J. (1992). The anatomy of melancholia: Focal abnormalities of cerebral blood flow in major depression. *Psychological Medicine, 22*, 607–615.

Binder, D. K., & Iskandar, B. J. (2000). Modern neurosurgery for psychiatric disorders. *Neurosurgery, 47*, 9–21.

Birbaumer, N., Grodd, W., Diedrich, O., Klose, U., Erb, E., Lotze, M., et al. (1998). fMRI reveals amygdala activation to human faces in social phobics. *NeuroReport, 9*, 1223–1226.

Blood, A. J., Zatorre, R. J., Bermudez, P., & Evans, A. C. (1999). Emotional responses to pleasant and unpleasant music correlate with activity in paralimbic brain regions. *Nature Neuroscience, 2*, 382–387.

Brannan, S., Liotti, M., Egan, G., Shade, R., Madden, L., Robillard, R., et al. (2001). Neuroimaging of cerebral activations and deactivations associated with hypercapnia and hunger for air. *Proceedings of the National Academy of Sciences USA, 98*, 2029–2034.

Breiter, H. C., Rauch, S. L., Kwong, K. K., Baker, J. R., Weisskoff, R. M., Kennedy, D. N., et al. (1996). Functional magnetic resonance imaging of symptom provocation in obsessive–compulsive disorder. *Archives of General Psychiatry, 53*, 595–606.

Bremner, J. D., Innis, R. B., Salomon, R. M., Staib, L. H., Ng, C. K., Miller, H. L., et al. (1997). Positron emission tomography measurement of cerebral metabolic correlates of tryptophan depletion-induced depressive relapse. *Archives of General Psychiatry, 54*, 364–374.

Bremner, J. D., Narayan, M., Anderson, E. R., Staib, L. H., Miller, H. L., & Charney, D. S. (2000). Hippocampal volume reduction in major depression. *American Journal of Psychiatry, 157*, 115–118.

Bremner, J. D., Randall, P., Scott, T. M., Bronen, R. A., Seibyl, J. P., Southwick, S. M., et al. (1995). MRI-based measurement of hippocampal volume in patients with combat-related posttraumatic stress disorder. *American Journal of Psychiatry, 152*, 972–981.

Bremner, J. D., Randall, P., Vermetten, E., Staib, L. H., Bronen, R. A., Mazure, C., et al. (1997). Magnetic resonance imaging-based measurement of hippocampal volume in posttraumatic stress disorder related to childhood physical and sexual abuse—a preliminary report. *Biological Psychiatry, 41*, 23–32.

Brody, A. L., Saxena, S., Mandelkern, M. A., Fairbanks, L. A., Ho, M. L., & Baxter, L. R., Jr. (2001). Brain metabolic changes associated with symptom factor improvement in major depressive disorder. *Biological Psychiatry, 50*(3), 171–178.

Brody, A. L., Saxena, S., Silverman, D. H., Alborzian, S., Fairbanks, L. A., Phelps, M. E., et al. (1999). Brain metabolic changes in major depressive disorder from pre- to post-treatment with paroxetine. *Psychiatry Research, 91*, 127–139.

Bruder, G. E., Stewart, J. W., Mercier, M. A., Agosti, V., Leite, P., Donovan, S., et al. (1997). Outcome of cognitive-behavioral therapy for depression: Relation to hemispheric dominance for verbal processing. *Journal of Abnormal Psychology, 106*, 138–144.

Bruder, G. E., Stewart, J. W., Tenke, C. E., McGrath, P. J., Leite, P., Bhattacharya, N., et al. (2001). Electroencephalographic and perceptual asymmetry differences between responders and non-responders to an SSRI antidepressant. *Biological Psychiatry, 49*, 416–425.

Büchel, C., Dolan, R., Armony, J. L., & Friston, K. J. (1999). Amygdala–hippocampal involvement in human aversive trace conditioning revealed through event-related functional magnetic resonance imaging. *Journal of Neuroscience, 19*, 10869–10876.

Buchsbaum, M. S., Wu, J., Siegel, B. V., Hackett, E., Trenary, M., Abel, L., et al. (1997). Effect of sertraline on regional metabolic rate in patients with affective disorder. *Biological Psychiatry, 41*, 15–22.

Bush, G., Luu, P., & Posner, M. I. (2000). Cognitive and emotional influences in anterior cingulate cortex. *Trends in Cognitive Sciences, 4*, 215–222.

Bush, G., Whalen, P. J., Rosen, B. R., Jenike, M. A., McInerney, S. C., & Rauch, S. L. (1998). The counting Stroop: An interference task specialized for functional neuroimaging–validation study with functional MRI. *Human Brain Mapping, 6*, 270–282.

Caetano, S. C., Kaur, S., Brambilla, P., Nicoletti, M., Hatch, J. P., Sassi, R. B., et al. (2006). Smaller cingulate volumes in unipolar depressed patients. *Biological Psychiatry, 59*(8), 702–706.

Carroll, B. J., Curtis, G. C., & Mendels, J. (1976). Cerebrospinal fluid and plasma free cortisol concentrations in depression. *Psychological Medicine, 6*, 235–244.

Carter, C. S., Botvinick, M. M., & Cohen, J. D. (1999). The contribution of the anterior cingulate cortex to executive processes in cognition. *Reviews in the Neurosciences, 10*, 49–57.

Carter, C. S., MacDonald, A. M., Botvinick, M., Ross, L. L., Stenger, V. A., Noll, D., et al. (2000). Parsing executive processes: Strategic vs. evaluative functions of the anterior cingulate cortex. *Proceedings of the National Academy of Sciences USA, 97*, 1944–1948.

Chen, C. H., Ridler, K., Suckling, J., Williams, S., Fu, C. H., Merio-Pich, E., et al. (2007). Brain imaging correlates of depressive symptom severity and predictors of symptom improvement after antidepressant treatment. *Biological Psychiatry, 62*(5), 407–414.

Chen, G., Rajkowska, G., Du, F., Seraji-Bozorgzad, N., & Manji, H. K. (2000). Enhancement of hippocampal neurogenesis by lithium. *Journal of Neurochemistry, 75*, 1729–1734.

Chiu, P., & Deldin, P. (2007). Neural evidence for enhanced error detection in major depressive disorder. *American Journal of Psychiatry, 164*, 608–616.

Coffey, C. E., Wilkinson, W. E., Weiner, R. D., Parashos, I. A., Djang, W. T., Webb, M. C., et al. (1993). Quantitative cerebral anatomy in depression: A controlled magnetic resonance imaging study. *Archives of General Psychiatry, 50*, 7–16.

Colla, M., Kronenberg, G., Deuschle, M., Meichel, K., Hagen, T., Bohrer, M., et al. (2007). Hippocampal volume reduction and HPA-system activity in major depression. *Journal of Psychiatric Research, 41*(7), 553–560.

Corcoran, K. A., & Maren, S. (2001). Hippocampal inactivation disrupts contextual retrieval of fear memory after extinction. *Journal of Neuroscience, 21*, 1720–1726.

Cordes, D., Haughton, V. M., Arfanakis, K., Wendt, G., Turski, P. A., Moritz, C. H., et al. (2000). Mapping functionally related regions of brain with functional connectivity MR imaging. *American Journal of Neuroradiology, 21*, 1636–1644.

Coryell, W., Nopoulos, P., Drevets, W., Wilson, T., & Andreasen, N. C. (2005). Subgenual prefrontal cortex volumes in major depressive disorder and schizophrenia: Diagnostic specificity and prognostic implications. *American Journal of Psychiatry, 162*(9), 1706–1712.

Critchley, H. D., Mathias, C. J., & Dolan, R. J. (2001). Neural activity in the human brain relating to uncertainty and arousal during anticipation. *Neuron, 29*, 537–545.

Curran, T., Tucker, D. M., Kutas, M., & Posner, M. I. (1993). Topography of the N400: Brain electrical activity reflecting semantic expectancy. *Electroencephalography and Clinical Neurophysiology, 88*, 188–209.

Damasio, A. R. (1994). *Descartes' error: Emotion, reason, and the human brain.* New York: Avon.

Davidson, R. J. (1998). Anterior electrophysiological asymmetries, emotion and depression: Conceptual and methodological conundrums. *Psychophysiology, 35*, 607–614.

Davidson, R. J. (2000). Affective style, psychopathology and resilience: Brain mechanisms and plasticity. *American Psychologist, 55*, 1193–1214.

Davidson, R. J. (2004). What does the prefrontal cortex "do" in affect?: Perspectives in frontal EEG asymmetry research. *Biological Psychology, 67*, 219–234.

Davidson, R. J., Abercrombie, H. C., Nitschke, J. B., & Putnam, K. M. (1999). Regional brain function, emotion and disorders of emotion. *Current Opinion in Neurobiology, 9*, 228–234.

Davidson, R. J., & Irwin, W. (1999). The functional neuroanatomy of emotion and affective style. *Trends in Cognitive Sciences, 3*, 11–21.

Davidson, R. J., Jackson, D. C., & Kalin, N. H. (2000). Emotion, plasticity, context and regulation. *Psychological Bulletin, 126*, 890–906.

Davidson, R. J., Pizzagalli, D., Nitschke, J. B., & Putnam, K. M. (2002). Depression: Perspectives from affective neuroscience. *Annual Review of Psychology, 53*, 545–574.

Davidson, R. J., Putnam, K. M., & Larson, C. L. (2000). Dysfunction in the neural circuitry of emotion regulation—a possible prelude to violence. *Science, 289*, 591–594.

Davis, M., & Whalen, P. J. (2001). The amygdala: Vigilance and emotion. *Molecular Psychiatry, 6*, 13–34.

Debener, S., Beauducel, A., Nessler, D., Brocke, B., Heilemann, H., & Kayser, J. (2000). Is resting anterior EEG alpha asymmetry a trait marker for depression?: Findings for healthy adults and clinically depressed patients. *Neuropsychobiology, 41*, 31–37.

de Geus, E. J., van't Ent, D., Wolfensberger, S. P., Heutink, P., Hoogendijk, W. J., Boomsma, D. I., et al. (2007). Intrapair differences in hippocampal volume in monozygotic twins discordant for the risk for anxiety and depression. *Biological Psychiatry, 61*(9), 1062–1071.

Devinsky, O., Morrell, M. J., & Vogt, B. A. (1995). Contributions of anterior cingulate cortex to behaviour. *Brain, 118*, 279–306.

Dillon, D. G., & Pizzagalli, D. A. (2007). Inhibition of action, thought, and emotion: A selective neurobiological review. *Applied and Preventive Psychology, 12*, 99–114.

Dougal, S., Phelps, E. A., & Davachi, L. (2007). The role of medial temporal lobe in item recognition and source recollection of emotional stimuli. *Cognitive, Affective and Behavioral Neuroscience, 7*(3), 233–242.

Drevets, W. C. (1998). Functional neuroimaging studies of depression: The anatomy of melancholia. *Annual Review of Medicine, 49*, 341–361.

Drevets, W. C. (2001). Neuroimaging and neuropathological studies of depression: Implications for the cognitive–emotional features of mood disorders. *Current Opinion in Neurobiology, 11*, 240–249.

Drevets, W. C., Price, J. L., Simpson, J. R. J., Todd, R. D., Reich, T., Vannier, M., et al. (1997). Subgenual prefrontal cortex abnormalities in mood disorders. *Nature, 386*, 824–827.

Drevets, W. C., Videen, T. O., Price, J. L., Preskorn, S. H., Carmichael, S. T., & Raichle, M. E. (1992). A functional anatomical study of unipolar depression. *Journal of Neuroscience, 12*, 3628–3641.

Driessen, M., Herrmann, J., Stahl, K., Zwaan, M., Meier, S., Hill, A., et al. (2000). Magnetic resonance imaging volumes of the hippocampus and the amygdala in women with borderline personality disorder and early traumatization. *Archives of General Psychiatry, 57*, 1115–1122.

Duman, R. S., Malberg, J., Nakagawa, S., & D'Sa, C. (2000). Neuronal plasticity and survival in mood disorders. *Biological Psychiatry, 48*, 732–739.

Ebert, D., & Ebmeier, K. P. (1996). The role of the cingulate gyrus in depression: From functional anatomy to neurochemistry. *Biological Psychiatry, 39*, 1044–1050.

Ebert, D., Feistel, H., & Barocka, A. (1991). Effects of sleep deprivation on the limbic system and the frontal lobes in affective disorders: A study with Tc-99m-HMPAO SPECT. *Psychiatry Research, 40*, 247–251.

Elliott, R., & Dolan, R. J. (1999). Differential neural responses during performance of matching and nonmatching to sample tasks at two delay intervals. *Journal of Neuroscience, 19*, 5066–5073.

Epstein, J., Pan, H., Kocsis, J. H., Yang, Y., Butler, T., Chusid, J., et al. (2006). Lack of ventral striatal response to positive stimuli in depressed versus normal subjects. *American Journal of Psychiatry, 163*(10), 1784–1790.

Eriksson, P. S., Perfilieva, E., Bjork-Eriksson, T., Alborn, A., Nordborg, C., Peterson, D. A., et al. (1998). Neurogenesis in the adult human hippocampus. *Nature Medicine, 4*, 1313–1317.

Fales, C. L., Barch, D. M., Rundle, M. M., Mintun, M. A., Snyder, A. Z., Cohen, J. D., et al. (2007). Altered emotional interference processing in affective and cognitive control brain circuitry in major depression. *Biological Psychiatry, 63*, 377–384.

Fanselow, M. S. (2000). Contextual fear, gestalt memories, and the hippocampus. *Behavioural Brain Research, 110*, 73–81.

Ferry, B., Roozendaal, B., & McGaugh, J. L. (1999). Role of norepinephrine in mediating stress hormone regulation of long-term memory storage: A critical involvement of the amygdala. *Biological Psychiatry, 46*, 1140–1152.

Fink, G. R., Markowitsch, H. J., Reinkemeier, M., Bruckbauer, T., Kessler, J., & Heiss, W. (1996). Cerebral representation of one's own past: Neural networks involved in autobiographical memory. *Journal of Neuroscience, 16*, 4275–4282.

Fitzgerald, P. B., Laird, A. R., Maller, J., & Daskalakis, Z. J. (2008). A meta-analytic study of changes in brain activation in depression. *Human Brain Mapping, 29*, 683–695.

Frodl, T., Schüle, C., Schmitt, G., Born, C., Baghai, T., Zill, P., et al. (2007). Association of the brain-deprived neurotrophic factor *Val66Met* polymorphism with reduced hippocampal volumes in major depression. *Archives of General Psychiatry, 64*(4), 410–416.

Fu, C. H., Williams, S. C., Brammer, M. J., Suckling, J., Kim, J., Cleare, A. J., et al. (2007). Neural responses to happy facial expression in major depression following antidepressant treatment. *American Journal of Psychiatry, 164*(4), 599–607.

Garavan, H., Hester, R., Murphy, K., Fassbender, C., & Kelly, C. (2006). Individual differences in the functional neuroanatomy of inhibitory control. *Brain Research, 1105*(1), 130–142.

Garavan, H., Ross, R. H., & Stein, E. A. (1999). Right hemispheric dominance of inhibitory control: An event-related functional MRI study. *Proceedings of the National Academy of Sciences USA, 96*, 8301–8306.

George, M. S., Ketter, T. A., Parekh, P. I., Rosinsky, N., Ring, H. A., Pazzaglia, P. J., et al. (1997). Blunted left cingulate activation in mood disorder subjects during a response interference task (the Stroop). *Journal of Neuropsychiatry and Clinical Neurosciences, 9*, 55–63.

George, M. S., Ketter, K. A., & Post, R. M. (1994). Prefrontal cortex dysfunction in clinical depression. *Depression, 2*, 59–72.

Gold, P. W., Goodwin, F. K., & Chrousos, G. P. (1988). Clinical and biochemical manifestations of depression: Relation to the neurobiology of stress. *New England Journal of Medicine, 314*, 348–353.

Gotlib, I. H., Ranganath, C., & Rosenfeld, J. P. (1998). Frontal EEG alpha asymmetry, depression, and cognitive functioning. *Cognition and Emotion, 12*, 449–478.

Gould, E., Tanapat, P., Rydel, T., & Hastings, N. (2000). Regulation of hippocampal neurogenesis in adulthood. *Biological Psychiatry, 48*, 715–720.

Hamann, S. B., Ely, T. D., Grafton, S. T., & Kilts, C. D. (1999). Amygdala activity related to enhanced memory for pleasant and aversive stimuli. *Nature Neuroscience, 2*, 289–293.

Hamilton, J. P., & Gotlib, I. H. (2008). Neural substrates of increased memory sensitivity for negative stimuli in major depression. *Biological Psychiatry, 63*, 1155–1162.

Heller, W., & Nitschke, J. B. (1998). The puzzle of regional brain activity in depression and anxiety: The importance of subtypes and comorbidity. *Cognition and Emotion, 12*, 421–447.

Henriques, J. B., & Davidson, R. J. (2000). Decreased responsiveness to reward in depression. *Cognition and Emotion, 15*, 711–724.

Henriques, J. B., Glowacki, J. M., & Davidson, R. J. (1994). Reward fails to alter response bias in depression. *Journal of Abnormal Psychology, 103*, 460–466.

Ho, A. P., Gillin, J. C., Buchsbaum, M. S., Wu, J. C., Abel, L., & Bunney, W. E., Jr. (1996). Brain glucose metabolism during non-rapid eye movement sleep in major depression: A positron emission tomography study. *Archives of General Psychiatry, 53*, 645–652.

Holland, P. C., & Gallagher, M. (1999). Amygdala circuitry in attentional and representational processes. *Trends in Cognitive Sciences, 3*, 65–73.

Holmes, A. J., & Pizzagalli, D. A. (2008). Spatio-temporal dynamics of error processing dysfunctions in major depressive disorder. *Archives of General Psychiatry, 65*, 179–188.

Hrdina, P. D., Demeter, E., Vu, T. B., Sotonyi, P., & Palkovits, M. (1993). 5-HT uptake sites and 5-HT$_2$ receptors in brain of antidepressant-free suicide victims/depressives: Increase in 5-HT$_2$ sites in cortex and amygdala. *Brain Research, 614*, 37–44.

Ikegaya, Y., Abe, K., Saito, H., & Nishiyama, N. (1995). Medial amygdala enhances synaptic transmission and synaptic plasticity in the dentate gyrus of rats *in vivo*. *Journal of Neurophysiology, 74,* 2201–2203.

Ikegaya, Y., Saito, H., & Abe, K. (1994). Attenuated hippocampal long-term potentiation in basolateral amygdala-lesioned rats. *Brain Research, 656,* 157–164.

Ikegaya, Y., Saito, H., & Abe, K. (1995). Requirement of basolateral amygdala neuron activity for the induction of long-term potentiation in the dentate gyrus *in vivo*. *Brain Research, 671,* 351–354.

Isenberg, N., Silbergswieg, D., Engelien, A., Emmerich, S., Malavade, K., Beattie, B., et al. (1999). Linguistic threat activates the human amygdala. *Proceedings of the National Academy of Sciences USA, 96,* 10456–10459.

Ito, H., Kawashima, R., Awata, S., Ono, S., Sato, K., Goto, R., et al. (1996). Hypoperfusion in the limbic system and prefrontal cortex in depression: SPECT with anatomic standardization technique. *Journal of Nuclear Medicine, 37,* 410–414.

Jackson, D. C., Mueller, C. J., Dolski, I., Dalton, K. M., Nitschke, J. B., Urry, H. L., et al. (2003). Now you feel it, now you don't: Frontal EEG asymmetry and individual differences in emotion regulation. *Psychological Science, 14,* 612–617.

Jacobs, B. L., Praag, H., & Gage, F. H. (2000). Adult brain neurogenesis and psychiatry: A novel theory of depression. *Molecular Psychiatry, 5,* 262–269.

Jacobson, L., & Sapolsky, R. M. (1991). The role of the hippocampus in feedback regulation of the hypothalamic–pituitary–adrenocortical axis. *Endocrine Reviews, 12,* 118–134.

Javanmard, M., Shlik, J., Kennedy, S. H., Vaccarino, F. J., Houle, S., & Bradwejn, J. (1999). Neuroanatomic correlates of CCK-4-induced panic attacks in healthy humans: A comparison of two time points. *Biological Psychiatry, 45,* 872–982.

Johnstone, T., van Reekum, C. M., Urry, H. L., Kalin, N. H., & Davidson, R. J. (2007). Failure to regulate: Counter-productive recruitment of top-down prefrontal–subcortical circuitry in major depression. *Journal of Neuroscience, 27,* 8877–8884.

Kawasaki, H., Adolphs, R., Kaufman, O., Damasio, H., Damasio, A. R., Granner, M., et al. (2001). Single-neuron responses to emotional visual stimuli recorded in human ventral prefrontal cortex. *Nature Neuroscience, 4,* 15–16.

Kempermann, G., Kuhn, H. G., & Gage, F. H. (1997). More hippocampal neurons in adult mice living in an enriched environment. *Nature, 386,* 493–495.

Kennedy, S. H., Evans, K. R., Kruger, S., Mayberg, H. S., Meyer, J. H., McCann, S., et al. (2001). Changes in regional brain glucose metabolism measured with positron emission tomography after paroxetine treatment of major depression. *American Journal of Psychiatry, 158,* 899–905.

Ketter, T. A., Andreason, P. J., George, M. S., Lee, C., Gill, D. S., Parekh, P. I., et al. (1996). Anterior paralimbic mediation of procaine-induced emotional and psychosensory experiences. *Archives of General Psychiatry, 53,* 59–69.

Ketter, T. A., Kimbrell, T. A., George, M. S., Dunn, R. T., Speer, A. M., Benson, B. E., et al. (2001). Effects of mood and subtype on cerebral glucose metabolism in treatment-resistant bipolar disorder. *Biological Psychiatry, 49,* 97–109.

Knutson, B., Bhanji, J. P., Cooney, R. E., Atlas, L. Y., & Gotlib, I. H. (2008). Neural responses to monetary incentives in major depression. *Biological Psychiatry, 63,* 686–692.

Konishi, S., Nakajima, K., Uchida, I., Kikyo, H., Kameyama, M., & Miyashita, Y. (1999). Common inhibitory mechanism in human inferior prefrontal cortex revealed by event-related functional MRI. *Brain, 122,* 981–991.

Kumar, A., Newberg, A., Alavi, A., Berlin, J., Smith, R., & Reivich, M. (1993). Regional glucose metabolism in late-life depression and Alzheimer disease: A preliminary positron emission tomography study. *Proceedings of the National Academy of Sciences USA, 90,* 7019–7023.

Lane, R. D., Fink, G. R., Chau, P. M., & Dolan, R. J. (1997). Neural activation during selective attention to subjective emotional responses. *NeuroReport, 8,* 3969–3972.

Lange, C., & Irle, E. (2004). Enlarged amygdala volume and reduced hippocampal volume in young women with major depression. *Psychological Medicine, 34*(6), 1059–1064.

Le Bihan, D., Mangin, J. F., Poupon, C., Clark, C. A., Pappata, S., Molko, N., et al. (2001). Diffusion tensor imaging: Concepts and applications. *Journal of Magnetic Resonance Imaging, 13,* 534–546.

LeDoux, J. E. (2000). Emotion circuits in the brain. *Annual Review of Neuroscience, 23,* 155–184.

Leverenz, J. B., Wilkinson, C. W., Wamble, M., Corbin, S., Grabber, J. E., Raskind, M. A., et al. (1999). Effect of chronic high-dose exogenous cortisol on hippocampal neuronal number in aged nonhuman primates. *Journal of Neuroscience, 19,* 2356–2361.

Liberzon, I., Taylor, S. F., Amdur, R., Jung, T. D., Chamberlain, K. R., Minoshima, S., et al. (1999). Brain activation in PTSD in response to trauma-related stimuli. *Biological Psychiatry, 45,* 817–826.

Lupien, S. J., de Leon, M., de Santi, S., Convit, A., Tarshish, C., Nair, N. P., et al. (1998). Cortisol levels during human aging predict hippocampal atrophy and memory deficits. *Nature Neuroscience, 1,* 69–73.

Nitschke, J. B., Sarinopoulos, I., Mackiewicz, K. L., Schaefer, H. S., & Davidson, R. J. (2006). Functional neuroanatomy of aversion and its anticipation. *NeuroImage, 29,* 106–116.

MacDonald, A. W., Cohen, J. D., Stenger, V. A., & Carter, C. S. (2000). Dissociating the role of the dorsolateral prefrontal and anterior cingulate cortex in cognitive control. *Science, 288,* 1835–1838.

Madhav, T. R., Pei, Q., Grahame-Smith, D. G., & Zetterstrom, T. S. (2000). Repeated electroconvulsive shock promotes the sprouting of serotonergic axons in the lesioned rat hippocampus. *Neuroscience, 97,* 677–683.

Magarinos, A. M., McEwen, B. S., Flugge, G., & Fuchs, E. (1996). Chronic psychosocial stress causes apical dendritic atrophy of hippocampal CA3 pyramidal neurons in subordinate tree shrews. *Journal of Neuroscience, 16,* 3534–3540.

Malberg, J. E., Eisch, A. J., Nestler, E. J., & Duman, R. S. (2000). Chronic antidepressant treatment increases neurogenesis in adult rat hippocampus. *Journal of Neuroscience, 20,* 9104–9110.

Maller, J. J., Daskalakis, Z. J., & Fitzgerald, P. B. (2007). Hippocampal volumetrics in depression: The importance of the posterior tail. *Hippocampus, 17*(11), 1023–1027.

Maren, S., & Hobin, J. A. (2007). Hippocampal regulation of context-dependent neuronal activity in the lateral amygdala. *Learning and Memory, 14*(4), 318–324.

Masserman, J. H., Levitt, M., McAvoy, T., Kling, A., & Pechtel, C. (1958). The amygdalae and behavior. *American Journal of Psychiatry, 115,* 14–17.

Mayberg, H. S. (1997). Limbic–cortical dysregulation: A proposed model of depression. *Journal of Neuropsychiatry and Clinical Neurosciences, 9,* 471–481.

Mayberg, H. S., Brannan, S. K., Mahurin, R. K., Jerabek, P. A., Brickman, J. S., Tekell, J. L., et al. (1997). Cingulate function in depression: A potential predictor of treatment response. *NeuroReport, 8,* 1057–1061.

Mayberg, H. S., Lewis, P. L., Regenold, W., & Wagner, H. N. (1994). Paralimbic hypoperfusion in unipolar depression. *Journal of Nuclear Medicine, 35,* 929–934.

Mayberg, H. S., Liotti, M., Brannan, S. K., McGinnis, S., Mahurin, R. K., Jerabek, P. A., et al. (1999). Reciprocal limbic–cortical function and negative mood: Converging PET findings in depression and normal sadness. *American Journal of Psychiatry, 156,* 675–682.

McEwen, B. S. (1998). Protective and damaging effects of stress mediators. *New England Journal of Medicine, 338,* 171–179.

Mega, M. S., Cummings, J. L., Salloway, S., & Malloy, P. (1997). The limbic system: An anatomic, phylogenetic, and clinical perspective. *Journal of Neuropsychiatry and Clinical Neurosciences, 9,* 315–330.

Mervaala, E., Fohr, J., Kononen, M., Valkonen-Korhonen, M., Vainio, P., Partanen, K., et al. (2000). Quantitative MRI of the hippocampus and amygdala in severe depression. *Psychological Medicine, 30,* 117–125.

Miller, E. K., & Cohen, J. D. (2001). An integrative theory of prefrontal cortex function. *Annual Review of Neuroscience, 24,* 167–202.

Mirz, F., Gjedde, A., Sodkilde-Jrgensen, H., & Pedersen, C. B. (2000). Functional brain imaging of tinnitus-like perception induced by aversive auditory stimuli. *NeuroReport, 11,* 633–637.

Morris, J. S., Friston, K. J., & Dolan, R. J. (1997). Neural responses to salient visual stimuli. *Proceedings of the Royal Society of London, 264,* 769–775.

Morris, J. S., Ohman, A., & Dolan, R. J. (1999). A subcortical pathway to the right amygdala mediating "unseen" fear. *Proceedings of the National Academy of Sciences USA, 96,* 1680–1685.

Munn, M. A., Alexopoulos, J., Nishino, T., Babb, C. M., Flake, L. A., Singer, T., et al. (2007). Amygdala volume analysis in female twins with major depression. *Biological Psychiatry, 62,* 415–422.

Nader, K., Schafe, G. E., & LeDoux, J. E. (2000). Fear memories require protein synthesis in the amygdala for reconsolidation after retrieval. *Nature, 406,* 722–726.

Neumeister, A., Wood, S., Bonne, O., Nugent, A. C., Luckenbaugh, D. A., Young, T., et al. (2005). Reduced hippocampal volume in unmedicated, remitted patients with major depression versus control subjects. *Biological Psychiatry, 57*(8), 935–937.

Nitschke, J. B., Sarinopoulos, I., Mackiewicz, K. L., Schaefer, H. S., & Davidson, R. J. (2006). Functional neuroanatomy of aversion and its anticipation. *NeuroImage, 29,* 106–116.

Nobre, A. C., Sebestyen, G. N., Gitelman, D. R., Mesulam, M. M., Frackowiak, R. S., & Frith, C. D. (1997). Functional localization of the system for visuospatial attention using positron emission tomography. *Brain, 120,* 515–533.

Nofzinger, E. A., Nichols, T. E., Meltzer, C. C., Price, J., Steppe, D. A., Miewald, J. M., et al. (1999). Changes in forebrain function from waking to REM sleep in depression: Preliminary analyses of [^{18}F]FDG PET studies. *Psychiatry Research, 91,* 59–78.

Noga, J. T., Vladar, K., & Torrey, E. F. (2001). A volumetric magnetic resonance imaging study of monozygotic twins discordant for bipolar disorder. *Psychiatry Research, 106,* 25–34.

Ochsner, K. N., & Barrett, L. F. (2001). A multiprocess perspective on the neuroscience of emotion. In T. J. Mayne & G. A. Bonanno (Eds.), *Emotions: Current issues and future directions* (pp. 38–81). New York: Guilford Press.

Ochsner, K. N., & Gross, J. J. (2005). The cognitive control of emotion. *Trends in Cognitive Sciences, 9*(5), 242–249.

O'Doherty, J., Kringelbach, M. L., Rolls, E. T., Hornak, J., & Andrews, C. (2001). Abstract reward and punishment representations in the human orbitofrontal cortex. *Nature Neuroscience, 4,* 95–102.

Öngür, D., An, X., & Price, J. L. (1998). Prefrontal cortical projections to the hypothalamus in macaque monkeys. *Journal of Comparative Neurology, 401,* 480–505.

Öngürm, D., Drevetsm, W. C., & Pricem, J. L. (1998). Glial reduction in the subgenual prefrontal cortex in mood disorders. *Proceedings of the National Academy of Sciences USA, 95,* 13290–13295.

Pantel, J., Schroder, J., Essig, M., Popp, D., Dech, H., Knopp, M. V., et al. (1997). Quantitative magnetic resonance imaging in geriatric depression and primary degenerative dementia. *Journal of Affective Disorders, 42,* 69–83.

Pardo, J. V., Pardo, P. J., Janer, K. W., & Raichle, M. E. (1990). The anterior cingulate cortex mediates processing selection in the Stroop attentional conflict paradigm. *Proceedings of the National Academy of Sciences USA, 87,* 256–259.

Pariante, C. M., & Miller, A. H. (2001). Glucocorticoid receptors in major depression: Relevance to pathophysiology and treatment. *Biological Psychiatry, 49,* 391–404.

Pauli, P., Wiedemann, G., & Nickola, M. (1999). Pain sensitivity, cerebral laterality, and negative affect. *Pain, 80,* 359–364.

Paus, T., Zatorre, R. J., Hofle, N., Caramanos, Z., Gotman, J., Petrides, M., et al. (1997). Time-related changes in neural systems underlying attention and arousal during the performance of an auditory vigilance task. *Journal of Cognitive Neurosciences, 9,* 392–408.

Phillips, M. L., Young, A. W., Scott, S. K., Calder, A. J., Andrew, C., Giampietro, V., et al. (1998). Neural responses to facial and vocal expressions of fear and disgust. *Proceedings of the Royal Society of London B: Biological Sciences, 265,* 1809–1817.

Pizzagalli, D. A., Jahn, A. L., & O'Shea, J. P. (2005). Toward an objective characterization of an anhedonic phenotype: A signal-detection approach. *Biological Psychiatry, 57*(4), 319–327.

Pizzagalli, D. A., Lehmann, D., Koenig, T., Regard, M., & Pascual-Marqui, R. D. (2000). Face-elicited ERPs and affective attitude: Brain electric microstate and tomography. *Clinical Neurophysiology, 111,* 521–531.

Pizzagalli, D. A., Oakes, T. R., & Davidson, R. J. (2003). Coupling of theta activity and glucose metabolism in the human rostral anterior cingulated cortex: An EEG/PET study of normal and depressed subjects. *Psychophysiology, 40,* 939–949.

Pizzagalli, D. A., Oakes, T. R., Fox, A. S., Chung, M. K., Larson, C. L., Abercrombie, H. C., et al. (2004). Functional but not structural subgenual prefrontal cortex abnormalities in melancholia. *Molecular Psychiatry, 9*, 393–405.

Pizzagalli, D. A., Pascual-Marqui, R. D., Nitschke, J. B., Oakes, T. R., Larson, C. L., Abercrombie, H. C., et al. (2001). Anterior cingulate activity as a predictor of degree of treatment response in major depression: Evidence from brain electrical tomography analysis. *American Journal of Psychiatry, 158*, 405–415.

Pizzagalli, D. A., Peccoralo, L. A., Davidson, R. J., & Cohen, J. D. (2006). Resting anterior cingulate activity and abnormal responses to errors in subjects with elevated depressive symptoms: A 128-channel EEG study. *Human Brain Mapping, 27*, 185–201.

Pruessner, J. C., Collins, D. L., Pruessner, M., & Evans, A. C. (2001). Age and gender predict volume decline in the anterior and posterior hippocampus in early adulthood. *Journal of Neuroscience, 21*, 194–200.

Rajkowska, G. (2000). Postmortem studies in mood disorders indicate altered numbers of neurons and glial cells. *Biological Psychiatry, 48*, 766–777.

Ramel, W., Goldin, P. R., Eyler, L. T., Brown, G. G., Gotlib, I. H., & McQuaid, J. R. (2007). Amygdala reactivity and mood-congruent memory in individuals at risk for depression. *Biological Psychiatry, 61*, 231–239.

Rauch, S. L., Savage, C. R., Alpert, N. M., Fischman, A. J., & Jenike, M. A. (1997). A study of three disorders using positron emission tomography and symptom provocation. *Biological Psychiatry, 42*, 446–452.

Rauch, S. L., Savage, C. R., Alpert, N. M., Miguel, E. C., Baer, L., Breiter, H. C., et al. (1995). A positron emission tomographic study of simple phobic symptom provocation. *Archives of General Psychiatry, 52*, 20–28.

Rauch, S. L., van der Kolk, B. A., Fisler, R. E., Alpert, N. M., Orr, S. P., Savage, C. R., et al. (1996). A symptom provocation study of posttraumatic stress disorder using positron emission tomography and script-driven imagery. *Archives of General Psychiatry, 53*, 380–387.

Rauch, S. L., Whalen, P. J., Shin, L. M., McInerney, S. C., Macklin, M. L., Lasko, N. B., et al. (2000). Exaggerated amygdala response to masked facial stimuli in posttraumatic stress disorder: A functional MRI study. *Biological Psychiatry, 47*, 769–776.

Reid, S. A., Duke, L. M., & Allen, J. J. B. (1998). Resting frontal electroencephalographic asymmetry in depression: What are the mediating factors? *Psychophysiology, 35*, 389–404.

Reiman, E. M. (1997). The application of positron emission tomography to the study of normal and pathologic emotions. *Journal of Clinical Psychiatry, 58*, 4–12.

Reul, J. M., & de Kloet, E. R. (1986). Anatomical resolution of two types of corticosterone receptor sites in rat brain with *in vitro* autoradiography and computerized image analysis. *Journal of Steroid Biochemistry and Molecular Biology, 24*(1), 269–272.

Roberson-Nay, R., McClure, E. B., Monk, C. S., Nelson, E. E., Guyer, A. E., Fromm, S. J., et al. (2006). Increased amygdale activity during successful memory encoding in adolescent major depressive disorder: An fMRI study. *Biological Psychiatry, 60*, 966–973.

Rogers, R. D., Owen, A. M., Middleton, H. C., Williams, E. J., Pickens, J., Sahakian, B. J., et al. (1999). Choosing between small, likely rewards and large, unlikely rewards activates inferior and orbital prefrontal cortex. *Journal of Neuroscience, 20*, 9029–9038.

Rolls, E. T. (1999). The functions of the orbitofrontal cortex. *Neurocase, 5*, 301–312.

Rosso, I. M., Cintron, C. M., Steingard, R. J., Renshaw, P. F., Young, A. D., & Yurgelun-Todd, D. A. (2005). Amygdala and hippocampus volumes in pediatric major depression. *Biological Psychiatry, 57*(1), 21–26.

Rusch, B. D., Abercrombie, H. C., Oakes, T. R., Schaefer, S. M., & Davidson, R. J. (2001). Hippocampal morphometry in depressed patients and control subjects: Relations to anxiety symptoms. *Biological Psychiatry, 50*, 960–964.

Sahay, A., & Hen, R. (2007). Adult hippocampal neurogenesis in depression. *Nature Neuroscience, 10*(9), 1110–1115.

Salomons, T. V., Johnstone, T., Backonja, M., & Davidson, R. J. (2004). Perceived controllability modulates the neural response to pain. *Journal of Neuroscience, 24,* 7199–7203.

Sapolsky, R. M. (2000). Glucocorticoids and hippocampal atrophy in neuropsychiatric disorders. *Archives of General Psychiatry, 57,* 925–935.

Sapolsky, R. M., Krey, L. C., & McEwan, B. S. (1986). The neuroendocrinology of stress and aging: The glucocorticoid cascade hypothesis. *Endocrine Reviews, 7,* 284–301.

Sapolsky, R. M., Uno, H., Rebert, C. S., & Finch, C. E. (1990). Hippocampal damage associated with prolonged glucocorticoid exposure in primates. *Journal of Neuroscience, 10,* 2897–2902.

Saxena, S., Brody, A. L., Ho, M. L., Alborzian, S., Ho, M. K., Maidment, K., et al. (2001). Cerebral metabolism in major depression and obsessive–compulsive disorder occurring separately and concurrently. *Biological Psychiatry, 50,* 159–170.

Schaefer, H. S., Putnam, K. M., Benca, R. M., & Davidson, R. J. (2006). Event-related fMRI measures of neural reactivity to positive social stimuli in pre- and post-treatment depression. *Biological Psychiatry, 60*(9), 974–986.

Schaefer, S. M., Abercrombie, H. C., Lindgren, K. A., Larson, C. L., Ward, R. T., Oakes, T. R., et al. (2000). Six-month test–retest reliability of MRI-defined PET measures of regional cerebral glucose metabolic rate in selected subcortical structures. *Human Brain Mapping, 10,* 1–9.

Schneider, F., Weiss, U., Kessler, C., Muller-Gartner, H. W., Posse, S., Salloum, J. B., et al. (1999). Subcortical correlates of differential classical conditioning of aversive emotional reactions in social phobia. *Biological Psychiatry, 45,* 863–871.

Schulkin, J. (1994). Melancholic depression and the hormones of adversity—a role for the amygdala. *Current Directions in Psychological Science, 3,* 41–44.

Semple, W. E., Goyer, P. F., McCormick, R., Donovan, B., Muzic, R. F. J., Rugle, L., et al. (2000). Higher brain blood flow at amygdala and lower frontal cortex blood flow in PTSD patients with comorbid cocaine and alcohol abuse compared with normals. *Psychiatry, 63,* 65–74.

Shah, P. J., Ebmeier, K. P., Glabus, M. F., & Goodwin, G. M. (1998). Cortical grey matter reductions associated with treatment-resistant chronic unipolar depression: Controlled magnetic resonance imaging study. *British Journal of Psychiatry, 172,* 527–532.

Sheline, Y. I. (2000). 3D MRI studies of neuroanatomic changes in unipolar major depression: The role of stress and medical comorbidity. *Biological Psychiatry, 48,* 791–800.

Sheline, Y. I., Gado, M. H., & Price, J. L. (1998). Amygdala core nuclei volumes are decreased in recurrent major depression. *NeuroReport, 9,* 2023–2028.

Sheline, Y. I., Sanghavi, M., Mintun, M. A., & Gado, M. H. (1999). Depression duration but not age predicts hippocampal volume loss in medically healthy women with recurrent major depression. *Journal of Neuroscience, 19,* 5034–5043.

Sheline, Y. I., Wang, P. W., Gado, M. H., Csernansky, J. G., & Vannier, M. W. (1996). Hippocampal atrophy in recurrent major depression. *Proceedings of the National Academy of Sciences USA, 93,* 3908–3913.

Shin, L. M., Kosslyn, S. M., McNally, R. J., Alpert, N. M., Thompson, W. L., Rauch, S. L., et al. (1997). Visual imagery and perception in posttraumatic stress disorder: A positron emission tomographic investigation. *Archives of General Psychiatry, 54,* 233–241.

Siegle, G. J., Thompson, W., Carter, C. S., Steinhauer, S. R., & Thase, M. E. (2007). Increased amygdala and decreased dorsolateral prefrontal BOLD responses in unipolar depression: Related and independent features. *Biological Psychiatry, 61*(2), 198–209.

Squire, L. R., & Knowlton, B. J. (2000). The medial temporal lobe, the hippocampus, and the memory systems of the brain. In M. S. Gazzaniga (Ed.), *The new cognitive neurosciences* (pp. 765–779). Cambridge, MA: MIT Press

Starkman, M. N., Giordani, B., Gebarski, S. S., Berent, S., Schork, M. A., & Schteingart, D. E. (1999). Decrease in cortisol reverses human hippocampal atrophy following treatment of Cushing's disease. *Biological Psychiatry, 46,* 1595–1602.

Steele, J. D., Kumar, P., & Ebmeier, K. P. (2007). Blunted response to feedback information in depressive illness. *Brain, 130,* 2367–2374.

Steffens, D. C., Byrum, C. E., McQuoid, D. R., Greenberg, D. L., Payne, M. E., Blitchington, T. F., et al. (2000). Hippocampal volume in geriatric depression. *Biological Psychiatry, 48*, 301–309.

Stein, M. B., Koverola, C., Hanna, C., Torchia, M. G., & McClarty, B. (1997). Hippocampal volume in women victimized by childhood sexual abuse. *Psychological Medicine, 27*, 951–959.

Strakowski, S. M., DelBello, M. P., Sax, K. W., Zimmerman, M. E., Shear, P. K., Hawkins, J. M., et al. (1999). Brain magnetic resonance imaging of structural abnormalities in bipolar disorder. *Archives of General Psychiatry, 56*, 254–260.

Tang, Y., Wang, F., Xie, G., Liu, J., Li, L., Su, L., et al. (2007). Reduced ventral anterior cingulated and amygdala volumes in medication-naive females with major depressive disorder: A voxel-based morphometric magnetic resonance imaging study. *Psychiatry Research, 156*(1), 83–86.

Taylor, S. E. (1991). Asymmetrical effects of positive and negative events: The mobilization–minimization hypothesis. *Psychological Bulletin, 110*, 67–85.

Taylor, W. D., Steffens, D. C., Payne, M. E., MacFall, J. R., Marchuk, D. A., Svenson, I. K., et al. (2005). Influence of serotonin transporter promoter region polymorphisms on hippocampal volumes in late-life depression. *Archives of General Psychiatry, 62*(5), 537–544.

Tebartz van Elst, L., Woermann, F. G., Lemieux, L., & Trimble, M. R. (1999). Amygdala enlargement in dysthymia: A volumetric study of patients with temporal lobe epilepsy. *Biological Psychiatry, 46*, 1614–1623.

Tebartz van Elst, L., Woermann, F., Lemieux, L., & Trimble, M. R. (2000). Increased amygdala volumes in female and depressed humans: A quantitative magnetic resonance imaging study. *Neuroscience Letters, 281*, 103–106.

Thayer, J. F., & Lane, R. D. (2000). A model of neurovisceral integration in emotion regulation and dysregulation. *Journal of Affective Disorders, 61*, 201–216.

Urry, H. L., van Reekum, C. M., Johnstone, T., Kalin, N. H., Thurow, M. E., Schaefer, H. S., et al. (2006). Amygdala and ventromedial prefrontal cortex are inversely coupled during regulation of negative affect and predict the diurnal pattern of cortisol secretion among older adults. *Journal of Neuroscience, 26*, 4415–4425.

Vakili, K., Pillay, S. S., Lafer, B., Fava, M., Renshaw, P. F., & Bonello-Cintron, C. M. (2000). Hippocampal volume in primary unipolar major depression: A magnetic resonance imaging study. *Biological Psychiatry, 47*, 1087–1090.

Veith, R. C., Lewis, N., Linares, O. A., Barnes, R. F., Raskind, M. A., Villacres, E. C., et al. (1994). Sympathetic nervous system activity in major depression: Basal and desipramine-induced alterations in plasma norepinephrine kinetics. *Archives of General Psychiatry, 51*, 411–422.

Vogt, B. A., Finch, D. M., & Olson, C. R. (1992). Functional heterogeneity in cingulate cortex: The anterior executive and posterior evaluative regions. *Cerebral Cortex, 2*, 435–443.

Vogt, B. A., Nimchinsky, E. A., Vogt, L. J., & Hof, P. R. (1995). Human cingulate cortex: surface features, flat maps, and cytoarchitecture. *Journal of Comparative Neurology, 359*, 490–506.

von Gunten, A., Fox, N. C., Cipolotti, L., & Ron, M. A. (2000). A volumetric study of hippocampus and amygdala in depressed patients with subjective memory problems. *Journal of Neuropsychiatry and Clinical Neurosciences, 12*, 493–498.

Whalen, P. J. (1998). Fear, vigilance, and ambiguity: Initial neuroimaging studies of the human amygdala. *Current Directions in Psychological Science, 7*, 177–188.

Whalen, P. J., Bush, G., McNally, R. J., Wilhelm, S., McInerney, S. C., Jenike, M. A., et al. (1998). The emotional Stroop paradigm: A functional magnetic resonance imaging probe of the anterior cingulate affective division. *Biological Psychiatry, 44*, 1219–1228.

Whalen, P. J., Rauch, S. L., Etcoff, N. L., McInerney, S. C., Lee, M. B., & Jenike, M. A. (1998). Masked presentations of emotional facial expressions modulate amygdala activity without explicit knowledge. *Journal of Neuroscience, 18*, 411–418.

Wu, J., Buschbaum, M. S., Gillin, J. C., Tang, C., Cadwell, S., Wiegland, M., et al. (1999). Prediction of antidepressant effects of sleep deprivation by metabolic rates in the ventral anterior cingulate and medical prefrontal cortex. *American Journal of Psychiatry, 156*, 1149–1158.

Wu, J. C., Gillin, J. C., Buchsbaum, M. S., Hershey, T., Johnson, J. C., & Bunney, W. E. (1992). Effect of sleep deprivation on brain metabolism of depressed patients. *American Journal of Psychiatry, 149,* 538–543.

Yurgelun-Todd, D. A., Gruber, S. A., Kanayama, G., Killgore, D. S., Baird, A. A., & Young, A. D. (2000). fMRI during affect discrimination in bipolar affective disorder. *Bipolar Disorders, 2,* 237–248.

Zald, D. H., Lee, J. T., Fluegel, K. W., & Pardo, J. V. (1998). Aversive gustatory stimulation activates limbic circuits in humans. *Brain, 121,* 1143–1154.

Zalla, T., Koechlin, E., Pietrini, P., Basso, G., Aquino, P., Sirigu, A., et al. (2000). Differential amygdala responses to winning and losing: A functional magnetic resonance imaging study in humans. *European Journal of Neuroscience, 12,* 1764–1770.

Zetzsche, T., Frodl, T., Preuss, U. W., Schmitt, G., Seifert, D., Leinsinger, G., et al. (2006). Amygdala volume and depressive symptoms in patients with borderline personality disorder. *Biological Psychiatry, 60,* 302–310.

CHAPTER 11

Depression and Early Adverse Experiences

Sherryl H. Goodman *and* Sarah R. Brand

For decades, researchers and clinicians seeking the keys to understanding depression have considered early adverse experiences as having potentially great etiological significance. Links have been drawn between depression, in both children and adults, and exposure to prenatal stress, inadequate parenting, abuse and neglect, early trauma, and loss of a parent. Exposure to these events, either acute or chronic, could potentially hold vital clues to etiological mechanisms and identification of groups at risk for the development of depression. Our purpose in this chapter is to examine knowledge about associations between early experiences and depression from a developmental psychopathology perspective. The advantages of this perspective include the opportunity to take into account both normal and abnormal processes, and alternative developmental pathways.

A developmental psychopathology perspective begins with a consideration of developmental processes. At a minimum, therefore, it is essential to know the timing of exposure to an adverse experience. Timing is important for at least two reasons. First, it is informative in terms of children's stage-salient needs at the time of exposure, which might be disrupted as a result of the adverse experiences. Second, consideration of timing allows one to take into account the potential advantage of developmental accomplishments that children might have achieved prior to any disruption associated with the adverse experiences. This chapter is organized around developmental course, beginning with prenatal experiences, then considering experiences during infancy and early childhood.

Furthermore, developmental psychopathology offers a wealth of constructs and models from many related disciplines that help us to understand the role of early experience in the emergence of depression. Thus, in this chapter we also consider several proposed conceptual models to explain the role of early experiences in the development of depression. Among those that we consider are biological systems (stress-related neurobiology, brain development, and psychophysiology), the attachment system, cognitive diathesis models, and emotional expression and regulation.

In addition, a developmental psychopathology perspective works toward models that integrate multiple transactional influences, and that consider the concepts of pathways, *multifinality* (the same risk factors being associated with different outcomes), and *equifinality* (the multiple pathways by which individuals may arrive at a particular outcome, in this case, depression) (Cicchetti & Rogosch, 1996). Therefore, these models are considered not only alone but also as parts of integrative models, including diathesis–stress, vulnerability, and transactional models. In the concluding sections of this chapter, we delineate some of the alternative developmental pathways. Finally, we suggest future directions for research.

EXPERIENCES DURING FETAL DEVELOPMENT: MATERNAL STRESS AND DEPRESSION

Studies of both animals and humans have revealed that mothers' stress during pregnancy contributes to risk for the development of a range of behavioral disturbances in their offspring, some of which might be associated with depression. Rhesus monkeys that are mildly stressed during pregnancy produce offspring with lower birthweight, poorer neuromotor maturation, delayed cognitive development, shorter attention span, more temperamental irritability, and less engagement in exploration of novel stimuli as infants (Schneider, Moore, & Kraemer, 2003). As juveniles, they demonstrate abnormal social behavior (less exploration and more clinging) and greater hypothalamic–pituitary–adrenal (HPA) activity (elevated cortisol) at baseline, and even more so in response to novelty. The effects are stronger if the mothers were stressed early rather than in middle to late pregnancy. Similarly, the offspring of rats that are stressed during pregnancy have lower birthweight, less vocalization during isolation in a novel environment, less exploration of novel environments, suppressed immune function, and persistent HPA axis hyperactivity (Kay, Tarcic, Poltyrev, & Weinstock, 1998; Williams, Hennessy, & Davis, 1998). Recent findings implicate the release of corticosterone (COR) during stress in the pregnant mothers, which interferes with fetal programming of HPA axis regulation, albeit in females more than in males (Zagron & Weinstock, 2006).

In humans, these early outcomes associated with fetal exposure to stress may contribute to the later development of depression in many ways. For example, dysregulated affect or behavior, if persistent, might leave children vulnerable to stress-induced depression. Similarly, tendencies toward behavioral inhibition, especially in response to novelty, might be associated with children failing to acquire adequate social relationships and competencies that protect against the later development of depression.

Inspired by the animal studies, researchers have also studied humans who were prenatally exposed to their mothers' adverse experiences. Among these results are the findings from the prospective Project Ice Storm, which showed that second-trimester exposure to the stressors associated with the storm predicted children's emotional and behavior problems at 3 to 4 years of age (King & Laplante, 2005; King, 2007). Others have extended the animal studies by examining levels of anxiety in pregnant women. These studies have particularly important implications for later development of depression in offspring given typically high associations between anxiety and depression both in pregnant (Goodman & Tully, in press) and in general samples (Clark, 1989). In one such prospective study, mothers' higher anxiety in early pregnancy and higher depression in later pregnancy predicted more infant sleep problems (O'Connor et al., 2007), whereas anxiety alone was associated with elevated levels of emotional problems in their children at 4 and 7 years of age (O'Connor, Heron, Golding, Beveridge, & Glover, 2002; O'Connor, Heron, Golding, & Glover, 2003). These findings remained significant even after researchers controlled for sociodemographic risk, obstetrical and antenatal risks, and postpartum levels of anxiety and depression. Other researchers focused on depression in pregnancy and found associations between depression in pregnancy and infants' lower scores on the Brazelton Neonatal Behavioral Assessment Scale (1984), specifically on subscales that measure orientation to face/voice stimulus and alertness (Hernandez-Reif, Field, Diego, & Ruddock, 2006), as well as excessive crying and fussiness at birth (Zuckerman, Bauchner, Parker, & Cabral, 1990). Although important in demonstrating a significant association between prenatal stress, anxiety, or depression and adverse outcome, this set of findings does not identify the primary mechanisms that account for these outcomes.

Researchers from several different theoretical perspectives have examined the fetal environment to identify possible mechanisms of abnormal fetal development that might be associated with maternal stress, anxiety, or depression, and that might place human infants at risk for the later development of depression. Among the aspects of fetal environment that have been considered are (1) neuroendocrine abnormalities, (2) reduced blood flow to the fetus, (3) altered fetal activity levels, (4) poor health behaviors, and (5) mothers' use of antidepressant medications.

Possible Mechanisms

Neuroendocrine Abnormalities

Because the fetus's first transactions with the mother occur at gestational day 13 or 14, when *in utero* blood flow is established, fetal exposure to the neuroendocrine correlates of the mother's stress or depression begins early and could potentially influence all aspects of fetal development. Knowledge of the neurobiology of depression leads to a concern for individuals who, as fetuses, might be exposed to corticotropin-releasing factor (CRF) hypersecretion. As reviewed by Graham, Heim, Goodman, Miller, and Nemeroff (1999), CRF is the prime regulator of the endocrine stress response. Evidence has been building for its role in coordinating the behavioral, immunological, and autonomic responses to stress. As such, the anticipated consequences for individuals exposed to CRF hypersecretion during fetal development include abnormal stress reactivity, abnormal behavioral and affective functioning, and abnormal electroencephalographic (EEG) patterns. Moreover, each of these aspects of functioning is known to be disrupted in adult depression (Davidson, Pizzagalli, & Nitschke, 2002). In children who had been exposed to CRF hypersecretion as fetuses, these indices of abnormal functioning may represent markers of risk for depression, especially the later emergence of stress-induced depression. Fetal exposure to high levels of cortisol could result in changes in HPA axis functioning that may not be reversible, and that are likely to be reflected in dysregulation of affect and behavior in infants. The latter are likely then to become part of a transactional system with the childrearing environment, which further contributes to risk for the development of depression.

Cortisol and corticotropin-releasing hormone (CRH) concentrations in plasma or urine are among the primary indices of HPA axis activity. Consequently, it has been important to know whether neuroendocrine correlates of stress or depression in pregnant women are circulated to the fetus. A few researchers have found that prenatal stress or depression is associated with the women's increased levels of plasma and urinary cortisol, ß-endorphins, CRH, catecholamines, epinephrine, and norepinephrine (Field et al., 2004; Handley, Dunn, Waldron, & Baker, 1980; Smith et al., 1990). Similarly, women's lower social support is associated with their levels of adrenocorticotropin-releasing factor (adrenocorticotropic hormone [ACTH]) (Wadhwa et al., 2002). Among these hormones, only cortisol has been found to cross the placenta to the fetus; at 20–36 weeks of pregnancy, maternal levels of cortisol accounted for 50% of the variance in the fetal levels of cortisol (Glover, 1999). Although evidence is still needed for associations between fluctuations in women's depression or stress/anxiety and their cortisol levels, researchers are beginning to identify associations between maternal cortisol levels and fetal and newborn functioning (for a review, see Field, Diego, & Hernandez-Reif, 2006).

Reduced Blood Flow to the Fetus

Another aspect of fetal development that might contribute to risk for the later development of depression involves the vascular system, specifically, reduced blood flow to the fetus. Glover and colleagues found maternal trait anxiety to be associated with impaired uterine blood flow in nonsmoking, healthy women in the third trimester of pregnancy (Teixeira, Fisk, & Glover, 1999). Reduced uterine blood flow was in turn associated with lower birthweight or prematurity of the babies. From birth these infants may be more difficult to care for, adding stress to an already anxious mother, and more likely to have an elevated stress response, both of which increase vulnerability to depression.

Altered Fetal Activity Levels

Researchers have consistently shown links between maternal stress and anxiety during pregnancy and altered fetal activity and heart rate (DiPietro, Irizarry, Costigan, & Gurewitsch, 2004). For example, fetuses of mothers with anxiety disorders had greater increases in heart rate after the mothers were exposed to a mild stressor compared to fetuses of mothers without anxiety disorders (Monk, Sloan, Myers, & Ellman, 2004). Fetal activity and heart rate have potential implications for emotional regulation later in life, as evidenced by fetal heart rate at 24 and 32 weeks of gestation predicting infant heart rate at 1 year (DiPietro et al., 2002).

Poor Health Behaviors

A fetus may be at risk for the later development of depression because of the pregnant mother's inadequate health care and engagement in risky behaviors that may endanger healthy fetal development. Depression during pregnancy has been associated with less frequent and less adequate prenatal care, more unhealthy eating and sleeping patterns, and more smoking, although the rates of smoking and drinking in pregnant women are relatively low (Marcus, Flynn, Blow, & Barry, 2003; Zuckerman, Amorao, Bauchner, & Cabral, 1989). Women with depression are also less likely to seek and to adhere to prenatal care (Kelly et al., 1999). Although these maternal behaviors have most often been associated with risk for externalizing disorders in the offspring (Milberger, Biederman, Faraone, Chen, & Jones, 1996), they may also contribute to the risk for depression through their association with other risk factors, such as inadequate parenting of the infant (Zuckerman & Bresnahan, 1991).

Mothers' Use of Antidepressant Medications

The subset of fetuses whose mothers are clinically depressed during pregnancy may also be exposed *in utero* to antidepressant medications. The two dominant medications prescribed for treatment of major depression, tricyclic antidepressants and fluoxetine, cross the placental barrier (Loughhead et al., 2006). Nonetheless, it is difficult to draw conclusions from studies of obstetrical and neonatal outcomes associated with antidepressant exposure. Many studies suffer from methodological shortcomings, such as having relied on self-report, retrospective data; outcome assessment not blinded to maternal status; and failing to control for relevant correlates, such as maternal tobacco use, comorbid psychiatric conditions, and severity of mental illness. Not surprisingly, findings with regard to rates of miscarriage, preterm delivery, and low birthweight have been mixed. Recent studies have accounted for maternal mental illness in assessments of infants in relation to fetal antidepressant exposure, and found lower birthweight and higher rates of neonatal symptoms (Oberlander et al., 2004) Further complicating efforts to understand risk associated with antidepressant exposure is an emergent understanding that individual differences may be explained by genetic polymorphisms influencing fetal medication exposure (Devane et al., 2006). Studies underway in our lab have the potential to contribute to the understanding of how and to what extent prenatal exposure to antidepressant medication contributes to risk for later development of depression.

Summary

In summary, adverse experiences during fetal development, including exposure to neuroendocrine abnormalities, reduced blood flow, the mother's poor health behaviors, and possibly the mother's use of antidepressant medications, may precipitate a set of events that contributed to the later emergence of depression in the offspring. Among the mechanisms that have been considered are an altered stress response system and a more difficult infant who stresses the mother–infant relationship. As we discuss later with regard to integrative models, each of these mechanisms is likely to involve hereditary factors in a complex manner and also to contribute to transactional processes, any number of which might result in depression.

EXPERIENCES DURING INFANCY AND EARLY CHILDHOOD

The predominant aspect of early life experiences of infants and young children associated with risk for depression is inadequate parenting, including the extreme of abuse. Inadequate parenting exposes children to maladaptive models of social skills and affective expression, stresses infants who experience inappropriate stimulation and inadequate arousal modulation, and, more broadly, interferes with healthy development to the extent that parents fail to provide for infants' and young children's stage-salient needs. Thus, infants and young children who experience inadequate parenting may develop problems such as emotion dysregulation, poorer interpersonal skills, and dysfunctional stress response, each of which may predispose children to the later development of depression.

As reviewed by Graham and colleagues (1999), evidence of elevated cortisol in response to physical stressors, such as physical illness or surgical procedures, in neonates suggests the capacity of humans to respond to stress very early in life. These findings underscore the importance of studies of stressors in infancy, in that high levels of stress hormones could potentially damage still-developing neurons, engendering vulnerability to future stressors (Essex, Klein, Cho, & Kalin, 2002; Hane & Fox, 2006).

Animal models have yielded helpful information on the effects of early life stressors in terms of both correlations with neurobiological alterations and behavioral consequences. Maternal separation in rats in the first few weeks of postnatal life has been reliably associated with both HPA axis alterations and behavioral changes that mimic adult depression (Kaffman & Meaney, 2007; Pihoker, Owens, Kuhn, Schanberg, & Nemeroff, 1993). Moreover, the alterations in HPA axis response to stress persist into adulthood in these early-stressed rats. In fact, the most recent studies suggest that an important mechanism of these alterations may be associated changes in maternal care when the pups are returned following separation. Studies of nonhuman primates separated from their mothers have produced similar findings (Byrne & Suomi, 1999). Thus, the animal studies provide strong support for a model of early loss, separation, or other alterations in maternal care disrupting the development of sensitive neurobiological systems, leaving the organism vulnerable to psychopathology.

Unresponsive or Neglectful Parenting

Both the mutual regulation model (Tronick & Gianino, 1986) and the psychobiological attunement model (Field, 1985) describe a mother who is inattentive and emotionally unresponsive, failing to respond to her infant's needs for help with behavioral or affective regulation and, ultimately, contributing to the infant's difficulty in developing arousal modulation. In both models, the infant becomes agitated in attempts to elicit responses from the mother, then withdraws and begins to show signs of depression. Findings consistent with these models come from studies of infants whose mothers were instructed to simulate depression, as well as studies of infants with depressed mothers.

When nondepressed mothers are instructed to respond to their infants' positive affect displays with a still face, infants respond with sober expressions and are found to avert their gaze from the mother (Adamson & Frick, 2003). Findings on infants' changes in physiology and behavior are consistent with the idea that infants experience the still-face procedure as stressful (Haley & Stansbury, 2003; Moore & Calkins, 2004).

In face-to-face interactions with their infants, depressed mothers have been observed to display less positive affect, more frequent expressions of sadness, and fewer expressions of interest than do well mothers (Pickens & Field, 1993). Infants with depressed mothers, in turn, engaged in more gaze and head aversion, consistent with the idea that the infants were using self-regulatory behaviors to minimize the negative affect associated with maternal unresponsiveness. Lyons-Ruth, Lyubchik, Wolfe, and Bronfman (2002) found that infants whose mothers related to them in a fearful and withdrawn manner, in contrast to intrusive mothers, as described in the next section, were more likely to develop disorganized–secure attachment styles, with signs of apprehension and dysphoria. Weinberg and Tronick (1996) found that boys were particularly vulnerable to a withdrawn maternal interaction style, which, they speculated, may be associated with boys' greater need for regulatory support. In a longitudinal study, Field (2002) found that infants of depressed mothers who had been withdrawn rather than intrusive (see the next section) showed less adaptive interactive behavior and lower Bayley Mental Scale scores. Thus, persistent exchanges with a sad and unresponsive caregiver disrupt infants' early affect development, failing to provide the help they need to learn to manage arousal, and socializing depression-like affective expressions. Moreover, from a social learning theory perspective (Bandura, 1986), infants and young children who experience low levels of contingent responsiveness to their initiatives may fail to learn healthy patterns of self-reward and adaptive attributional styles. The latter consideration is expanded in the later section, "Family Functioning."

Intrusive, Harsh, or Coercive Parenting

Inadequate parenting may also be characterized as intrusive, harsh, or coercive. Researchers have revealed that maternal depression is associated not only with a withdrawn, unresponsive pattern of interaction with infants but also a pattern of hostile–intrusive overstimulation. A subset of mothers has been observed to overstimulate, to be physically intrusive (e.g., poking and jabbing their infants), to interfere with infants' exploratory activities, and to show hostile and irritable affect (Cohn, Matias, Tronick, Lyons-Ruth, & Connell, 1986; Field, Healy, Goldstein, & Guthertz, 1990).

Maternal hostility and intrusiveness are associated with infant fussiness (Field et al., 1990) or avoidance (Cohn et al., 1986), especially in girls (Weinberg & Tronick, 1998). Each of these behavioral reactions, avoidance and fussiness, may contribute to risk for depression, especially in terms of the infant's contribution to parent–child transactional patterns of influence that unfold over time. Egeland, Pianta, and O'Brian (1993) suggest that intrusive or hostile mothers disrupt healthy psychological development by interfering with their infants' development of autonomous functioning.

Regardless of depression status, parents who engage in coercive and controlling parenting, particularly if it is a persistent quality of early parenting, might contribute to children's developing a sense of helplessness and a tendency to view themselves as having little control over outcomes (Racusin & Kaslow, 1991). Each of these sets of beliefs, and their associated behavior patterns, increases children's vulnerability to depression, as well as anxiety (Chorpita, 2001). Some support for these contentions comes from studies in which parents of clinically depressed or anxious children were found to use more coercion and were observed to be more controlling and less democratic compared to parents of nondepressed children (Dadds, Sanders, Morrison, & Rebgetz, 1992; McLeod, Wood, & Weisz, 2007).

Inconsistent Parenting

Some mothers, perhaps a distinct subgroup of depressed mothers, display inconsistencies in parenting their infants. Lyons-Ruth and colleagues (2002) theorized that these women's own ambivalence about attachment would lead them to engage in contradictory caregiving strategies with their infants. The infants may in turn develop disorganized–insecure attachment styles and hostile/punitive behavior. From a transactional perspective, it is important to follow groups of infants reared by mothers who engage in this behavior relative to other observed patterns of inadequate parenting to determine whether these patterns are associated with the development of different emotional or behavioral problems in the children.

Abuse

Physical or sexual abuse or neglect of a child by a parent represents the extreme of inadequate parenting and adverse early life experiences. Thus, it is no surprise that infants or toddlers who have been maltreated have high rates of disorganized attachment, negative views of themselves, and lower cortisol reactivity (Barnett, Ganiban, & Cicchetti, 1999; Hart, Gunnar, & Cicchetti, 1996). Infants and toddlers are the most frequently reported victims of physical abuse, which may reflect a tendency of individuals to be more likely to report suspected abuse of younger children, who are perceived as more vulnerable (Gelles, 1998). On the other hand, violence-prone parents may view infants' and toddlers' needs for protection from danger as justification for abuse.

Parents who abuse their children also may be depressed or may be abusing drugs or alcohol (Gelles, 1998). Other factors associated with abuse, such as high levels of stress in the family, social isolation, being single and young, being in an abusive partner relationship, and having low income, also contribute to the likelihood of an accumulation of early adverse experiences. Both Gelles (1998) and Belsky (1993) have developed models that describe the multiple adverse influences that converge in families in which parents abuse their children. Maternal depression and abuse may have independent effects on depression, and the combination may be associated with higher levels of depression in the children (Kinard, 1995).

Although the consequences of abuse in young children are wide ranging, of particular concern with regard to risk for depression are findings that the children are likely to have lower self-esteem, difficulty relating to peers, insecure attachment relationships, dysfunctional attributions, social-cognitive biases (being hypervigilant to cues of danger), neuroendocrine abnormalities, and, ultimately, depression (Jungmeen & Cicchetti, 2006). Children who experienced abuse in early life exhibit alterations in HPA axis activity; however, different alterations have been found based on the type of abuse (i.e., sexual, physical, emotional), showing that the effects of stress are variable and influenced by many factors (Nemeroff, 2004). For example, Heim and colleagues (2000) reported that a small group of adult women who had been sexually or physically abused as children showed persistent, hyperactive HPA axis responses to stress relative to women with no history of childhood abuse. This pattern was strongest among women who had been abused and also had a current major depression. A review of the child abuse and neglect literature also indicated that abuse is associated with overall volume loss in the hippocampus, corpus callosum, and prefrontal cortex, along with altered cortical symmetry in the frontal lobes and superior temporal gyrus (Kaufman & Charney, 2001). Each of these processes has been associated with later emergence of depression, even relative to children from neglectful homes.

Also important to consider is that the stressful context of the lives of many abuse victims likely contributes to the negative cascade of outcomes. Many of the correlates of child abuse are, in their own right, risk factors for depression. According to Crittenden (1998), many of the consequences of abuse can be attributed to the context of neglect and psychological maltreatment. In summary, abuse leaves children with behavioral, cognitive, emotional, and neuroendocrine vulnerabilities to depression.

Loss

The early experience of loss, particularly a parent's death and the associated grief, has long been considered a severe stressor that may place children at risk for depression. Recent studies, which included careful matching of risk and control samples, support links between the childhood experience of parental death and later depressive disorders (Cerel, Fristad, Verducci, Weller, & Weller, 2006; Schmiege, Khoo, Sandler, Ayers, & Wolchik, 2006). Researchers also continue to reveal how children's psychological responses vary as a function of the characteristics of the loss experience. Important variables include the extent to which the loss is associated with changes and ongoing disruptions in children's environment and routine; children's age and sex; and other family characteristics, such as depression, in the surviving parent and the availability of supportive others (Pfeffer, 1996).

Deprived Environments (Institutional Rearing)

For some children, loss of parents is followed by social, emotional, and intellectual deprivation. In particular, international conflicts have left orphaned many children, some of whom are raised in sparse, institutional orphanages; others are adopted either early or later in childhood. Several groups of researchers saw the opportunity to learn about what traditionally is called *maternal deprivation* by studying different groups of these children, most recently, in Romania. Overall, the strongest conclusion from these studies has been that whereas children who were adopted earlier (prior to 4 months of age) did not significantly differ from matched controls, children who were adopted later, especially those adopted after 2 years of age, showed attachment disorder behaviors, behavioral deficits, behavioral problems, and blunted circadian rhythm during day care at 3–4 years of age (Gunnar & van Dulmen, 2007; O'Connor, Rutter, & the English & Romanian Adoptees Study Team, 2000). Moreover, elevated cortisol levels were still evident 6–7 years later. Attachment disorder, particularly the disinhibited pattern, persisted into early adolescence (Rutter et al., 2007). In summary, consequences of the extremes of early deprivation might be overcome if children are adopted early; otherwise, children experience persistent adverse behavioral and neuroendocrine abnormalities that suggest vulnerability to stress-induced depression.

Family Functioning

In addition to the extreme family circumstances already described, a number of more common aspects of family functioning have also been hypothesized to be associated with the later emergence of depression. Abnormal family functioning may contribute to development of patterns of coping, beliefs, and interpersonal styles that leave children vulnerable to depression. One such pattern occurs when parents set overly stringent reward criteria, thus rewarding their children at low rates. According to social learning theory (Bandura, 1986), children of such parents may internalize those standards and contingencies for reinforcement (Cole & Rehm, 1986). These children may then engage in low rates of self-reward and high rates of self-criticism, attend selectively to negative feedback, and be more likely to blame themselves for negative outcomes and less likely to take credit for positive outcomes. Consistent with cognitive-behavioral models of depression, each of these processes has been associated with increased risk for depression.

Similarly, parents' level of emotional overinvolvement with their children may increase risk for depression. Emotional overinvolvement, along with criticism and hostility, is frequently studied in relation to the construct of *expressed emotion* (EE), which refers to the emotional aspects of family members' communication patterns (Hooley & Gotlib, 2000). In one study of children who became depressed, mothers of children with a gradual onset of depression were found to have high levels of emotional overinvolvement, in contrast to mothers of children with an acute onset of their depression episode (Hamilton, Asarnow, & Tompson, 1999). In a related study, young (ages 13 to 21 years old) mothers' depression symptom scale scores were associated with their judging their 3-month-old infants as being more "vulnerable" (Field et al., 1996). Furthermore, mothers' vulnerability scores explained associations between the mothers' depression scores and the infants' lower Bayley Scales of Infant Development motor and mental scores, and less exploratory play at 12 months of age. Other evidence suggests that mothers of inhibited 3- to 4-year-old children perceive their children as more vulnerable than do mothers of uninhibited children, and also interact with their children in ways that are less likely to validate their children's emotional experiences (Shamir-Essakow, Ungerer, Rapee, & Safier, 2004). The latter was particularly apparent in mothers of inhibited children who were insecurely attached. Further studies are needed to determine the mechanisms by which parents' emotional overinvolvement or perceptions of their child's vulnerability contribute to the development of depression in children, especially from a transactional perspective.

Another aspect of family functioning that might increase risk for depression involves interparental conflict. Several processes might be implicated in linking exposure to conflict and depression in children, particularly if the conflict is intense, aggressive, and unresolved and children are exposed repeatedly and at early ages (Davies & Cummings, 1994). Children may feel threatened and overwhelmed, have heightened emotional arousal (increased heart rate and elevated cortisol) and difficulty regulating their emotions (inability to suppress vagal tone), may develop depressotypic attributional styles, and may withdraw as a way of coping with their own level of distress (Davies & Cummings, 1994; Gottman & Katz, 2002; Grych & Fincham, 1990). Difficulty regulating emotions and focusing attention in stressful situations, along with these cognitive patterns, increase vulnerability to depression.

CONCEPTUAL MODELS TO EXPLAIN THE ROLE OF EARLY EXPERIENCES

Biological Systems

Neuroendocrine: Stress Hormones

The HPA system coordinates behavioral, immunological, endocrinological, and autonomic responses to stress (Arborelius, Owens, Plotsky, & Nemeroff, 1999). In adults, dysregulation of the HPA system is related to major depression and posttraumatic stress disorder (PTSD). Cortisol is the primary steroid hormone produced by the HPA system in humans in response to stress. By the age of 3 months, human infants have adult-equivalent levels of cortisol and are capable of responding to stress.

Brief elevations of cortisol levels are considered to be adaptive. Individuals may experience enhanced ability, both physiologically and behaviorally, to manage the stressor. In contrast, prolonged hyperactivity of the HPA axis, with persistently elevated cortisol levels, has been associated with negative effects on physiological and behavioral systems. In rats, chronic early life stress has been shown to result in dysregulation of the HPA system and in attenuated emotionality in adulthood. Early rearing conditions can permanently alter the CRF systems by altering the receptor types in certain areas of the brain (Plotsky et al., 2005). Early life stress is also likely to predispose children to at least transient, if not permanent, alterations in the CRF system, interfering with their ability to respond adaptively to later stressors (Gunnar & Vazquez, 2001). Findings previously described in this chapter regarding abused and institutionally reared children are consistent with this model, as are findings on associations between high maternal stress exposure (especially maternal depression) beginning in infancy and preschoolers' higher cortisol levels and higher levels of behavior problems (Essex et al., 2002). Overall, neuroendocrine abnormalities resulting from early exposure to stress hold promise for elucidating some of the mechanisms for the emergence of depression in association with early life stress.

Nervous System: Cardiac Vagal Tone

Cardiac vagal tone is a measure of nervous system variability that specifically indexes infants' ability to regulate their physiological activity during social situations. It has been associated with individual differences in expression and regulation of emotion. Vagal tone is measured as heart rate variability. Lower levels of vagal tone may reflect infants' efforts to cope with inadequate environmental support (Porges, Doussard-Roosevelt, & Maiti, 1994), including the lower levels of responsiveness found in depressed compared to nondepressed mothers (Field, 2002). Field, Fox, Nawrocki, and Gonzalez (1995) found lower vagal tone in 3- to 6-month-old infants of depressed mothers than in infants with nondepressed mothers. Moreover, whereas infants with nondepressed mothers showed a developmental increase in vagal tone between ages 3 and 6 months, infants with depressed mothers did not. Among 6-month-olds, lower vagal tone was correlated with fewer vocalizations and facial expressions during interactions. The failure to show the developmental increase in vagal tone may reflect cumulative effects of infants' agitated states in trying to elicit responses from their mothers. A tendency toward lower vagal tone could also be inherited or be a function of *in utero* environmental-based physiological differences in neural regulation.

Regardless of the origins, lower vagal tone is associated with poorer emotion regulation abilities and less expression of positive affect. Among infants of nondepressed mothers or unselected samples, lower vagal tone is associated with poorer abilities to self-soothe, less expressed joy and interest, more emotional withdrawal and inhibition, and less exploration of novel stimuli (Pickens & Field, 1993; Porges et al., 1994). Any of these deficits could serve as vulnerabilities in a transactional model of pathways to depression (Porges, 2001).

Frontal Lobe Development

Postnatal brains undergo significant continued development beyond that which occurs during fetal development. Of particular concern with regard to potential influence on depression is the rapid development during the first year of life of the frontal lobes, the interhemispheric connections, and the neurotransmitter systems that mediate emotional behavior (Chugani, Phelps, & Mazziotta, 2002). Each of these structures or systems is related to the experience and regulation of affect. Increasing evidence indicates that quality of caregiving relates to the manner in which these systems develop. Specifically, Field and colleagues' studies of infants in the first few months of life, and Dawson and colleagues' studies of 11- to 18-month-old children, showed links between inadequate parenting and abnormal development of the frontal lobe (Dawson et al., 1999; Field, Fox, Pickens, & Nawrocki, 1995; Jones, Field, Fox, Lundy, & Davalos, 1997). These abnormalities were reflected in hemispheric asymmetries, as measured by EEG. Infants with depressed mothers exhibited atypical patterns of frontal EEG asymmetry: Compared to infants of nondepressed mothers, infants of depressed mothers exhibited reduced left frontal brain activity during playful interactions with their mothers. When the children were 4–5 years old, their frontal brain activation, along with the family's contextual risk level, mediated associations between mothers' depression and children's behavior problems (Dawson et al., 2003).

In studies of unselected infants and adults, right-brain activation is associated with the experience of the negative emotions of sadness and distress, whereas activation of the left frontal region is associated with positive emotions of joy and interest (Davidson & Fox, 1982). In addition, the atypical pattern exhibited by children with depressed mothers has been found to be predictive of an infants' vulnerability to the experience of negative affect (Davidson & Fox, 1989) and may be a marker of current or chronic depressed mood state (Field, Fox, et al., 1995). In depressed adults, reduced left frontal activity was not only present during episodes but also persisted into remission (Henriques & Davidson, 1990). Thus, early experience with a depressed mother may lead to abnormal brain functions that are specifically associated with vulnerability to depressive mood states.

Inherited Vulnerabilities

Genetics undoubtedly play a role in explaining the risk for depression in association with early experience. Several possible roles of genetics have been considered. Until recently, most studies emphasized heritability of depression *per se*. Family studies, behavioral studies, and molecular genetics studies all have strongly supported the heritability of depression in adults, although the genes may differ in men and women (Caspi et al., 2003; Kendler, Gardner, Neale, & Prescott, 2001). In contrast, the evidence for heritability of depression in children and adolescents is mixed (Harrington, 1996).

An alternative to the notion that children may inherit likelihood for depression *per se* is that heritability contributes significantly to vulnerabilities to depression. In tests of this notion, high levels of heritability, based on behavior genetics studies, are found for behavioral inhibition and shyness (Cherny, Fulker, Corley, Plomin, & DeFries, 1994), low self-esteem (Loehlin & Nichols, 1976), neuroticism (Tellegen et al., 1988), sociability (Plomin et al., 1993), subjective well-being (Lykken & Tellegen, 1996), expression of negative emotion (Plomin et al., 1993) and even the tendency to experience negative events (Plomin, 1994). This body of research is consistent with the notion of genetic transmission of affective, cognitive, and interpersonal vulnerabilities for the development of psychopathology. Further work along these lines might benefit from borrowing the notion of endophenotypes, which has primarily been applied to the study of schizophrenia (Gottesman & Gould, 2003). We discuss the ways in which genes and adverse early environments might work together to increase risk for depression later in this chapter.

Attachment System

Theories of attachment and accumulating empirical evidence support a strong case for the idea that disturbances in the attachment relationship as a function of early adverse experiences contribute to vulnerability to the development of depression (Cummings & Cicchetti, 1990; Sroufe, Egeland, Carlson, & Collins, 2005). With insecure attachment, children are likely to experience negative feelings about themselves and others, and to be particularly sensitive to loss. The emotional unavailability or unresponsiveness of a depressed mother, or the experience of maltreatment or loss could increase an infant's risk for both insecure attachment and depression. Insecure attachment could mediate the association among maternal depression, maltreating caregivers, and other early adversities, and the later development of depression. Specifically, insecure attachment leads children to have negative expectancies for other relationships and negative self-perceptions, leaving them vulnerable to depression. Insecure attachment has also been found to be associated with reduce left frontal brain activity, whether or not the mother had been depressed (Dawson et al., 2001). Thus, the developmental course for infants of depressed mothers is likely to be even more complicated than that for other infants. On the positive side, security of mother–child attachment is associated with maternal ability to inhibit cortisol increases among toddlers exposed to stressors, including brief separations, inoculations, and strange events (Gunnar, Brodersen, Nachmias, Buss, & Rigatuso, 1996; Spangler & Grossman, 1993).

Support for the association between maternal depression and insecure attachment in infants is strong but not unequivocal. A meta-analysis showed that clinically significant mater-

nal depression is significantly associated with lower rates of secure attachment and, marginally, with higher rates of avoidant and disorganized attachment (from 17 to 28%, on
average) (Martins & Gaffan, 2000). When clinical samples are compared to community
samples, significantly higher effect sizes are found in the clinical samples, perhaps due to the
chronic nature of clinical depression, along with the accompanying dysfunction between episodes (Atkinson et al., 2000). In individual studies, associations between maternal postnatal
depression and infant insecure attachment are also found to be stronger among mothers
with insecure states of mind (McMahon, Barnett, Kowalenko, & Tennant, 2006), and
among infants born preterm (even after researchers controlled for level of neonatal health
complications) (Poehlmann & Fiese, 2001). Notably, at least among toddlers, contextual
risks did not account for the association between depression in mothers and higher rates of
insecure attachment relative to others (Cicchetti, Rogosch, & Toth, 1998).

Dawson and colleagues (1992) reported the surprising finding that securely attached infants of mothers with high levels of depression, compared to securely attached infants of
nondepressed mothers, showed reduced left frontal activation when exposed to neutral or
positive emotions. This pattern, typical of findings with depressed adults, was not found for
insecurely attached infants (most of whom were classified as avoidant) of depressed mothers. If replicated with a larger sample, the findings fail to support the idea that insecure attachment mediates the association between maternal depression and adverse outcomes in
the children. Instead, as suggested by Dawson and colleagues, children who have avoidant
relationships with their depressed mothers may in fact be protected, in that they are less
likely than children who have secure attachment relationships to model their mothers.

Consistent support has emerged for the association between physical abuse of infants
by their caregivers and insecure attachment. Compared to nonmaltreated infants, a higher
percentage of maltreated infants are classified as insecure, the most common classification
being "disorganized" (Carlson, Cicchetti, Barnett, & Braunwald, 1989; Cicchetti &
Barnett, 1991).

In summary, the findings from at least the most severely depressed mothers and from
infants who experienced maltreatment are consistent with a role of disturbed attachment relationships as a mechanism to explain the association between early adverse experiences and
the later development of depression. Children who experience these adversities early in life
may develop insecure attachment relationships. These insecure attachments, with their associated internalized negative views of the self and the world, serve to organize how children
perceive and behave in interpersonal relationships, and are carried forward in development
beyond the early adversities. Children may become increasingly unable to deal with challenges, and subsequent difficulties may precipitate depression.

Cognitive Vulnerabilities and Self System

Early adverse experiences may also be linked to later depression through the mechanism of
depressotypic cognitions. Early childhood, beginning in the second year of life, is a critical
period for the construction of the sense of self and self in relation to others and the world
(Thompson & Goodvin, 2005). As with secure attachment, a healthy sense of oneself is facilitated by warm, responsive parenting. The early adverse experiences we discuss in this
chapter are associated with cognitive distortions, such as a sense of oneself as unlovable, as
unworthy of others' positive interest, and as unlikely to get one's needs met (Garber & Martin, 2002). Children may develop a sense of hopelessness and helplessness, and may be deficient in administering self-reinforcements. For example, depressed mothers expose their

children to more of their own self-criticism, as well as criticism of the child than do nondepressed mothers (Radke-Yarrow, Belmont, Nottelmann, & Bottomly, 1990). Children who experience inadequate parenting or early life traumas may develop distorted views of themselves and the world. These children may set high, unrealistic standards for themselves, leading to negative self-views.

Researchers are beginning to provide support for the mediational role of depressotypic cognitions in associations between early adverse experiences and the development of depression. For example, even 5-year old children of recently depressed mothers were found to exhibit more depressive cognitions relative to other children, an association that was also partly explained by maternal hostility (Murray, Woolgar, Cooper, & Hipwell, 2001). In another study, the extent of conflictual representations from narratives in preschool-age children who had been maltreated partially mediated the association between child maltreatment and externalizing behavior problems (Toth, Cicchetti, Macfie, Rogosch, & Maughan, 2000). Cicchetti's group has recently built on that work to design preventive interventions that are showing promise in treating toddlers whose mothers are depressed (Toth, Rogosch, Manly, & Cicchetti, 2006).

Kovacs, Akiskal, Gatsionis, and Parrone (1994) described cognitive characteristics, such as self-deprecation and negative self-esteem, as one of two prominent features of dysthymia in children, along with mood features. However, cognitive vulnerability–stress interactions prospectively predicted elevations in depression symptoms, with effect sizes that were small in children but moderately large in adolescents (Lakdawalla, Hankin, & Mermelstein, 2007). Thus, models of the role of cognitive vulnerabilities in associations between early adverse experiences and later development of depression need to be sensitive to these developmental shifts.

Affect: Emotional Expression and Regulation

Another model to explain the association between early adverse experiences and the later emergence of depression is that the early stressors contribute to deficits and delays in emotional expression or regulation. Affective dysregulation is a prominent feature of dysthymia in children, including persistent gloomy mood, as well as irritability and anger (Kovacs et al., 1994). Garber, Braafladt, and Zeman (1991) provided strong support for the role of abnormalities in the regulation of sad affect in the development of depression in children.

Given that caregivers play an essential role in the socialization of their children's emotions, children with depressed mothers are of particular concern. Infants have been observed to imitate their depressed mothers' negative affect (Field, 1994). Moreover, because depressed mothers less often reinforce their infants' positive affect with displays of interest, they likely discourage infants' expressions of positive affect (Pickens & Field, 1993). Similar connections may be drawn between other aspects of early adverse experiences and affective dysregulation.

Essentially, emotion regulation is at the core of many of the vulnerabilities in infancy that have been associated with early adverse experiences, including the stress response system that comprises the autonomic nervous system (ANS; heart rate variability) and the neuroendocrine system (HPA axis), cortical activity (relative right frontal activation and abnormal event-related potential [ERP] patterns), and behavioral indices of emotion regulation. These deficits are among the core vulnerabilities for affective and other disorders.

Integrative Models

Clearly, emergence of depression is not solely (directly or inevitably) determined by any childhood experience in a main effects–type model. Thus, we are challenged to develop and test integrative models that take into account the likely complexities. Two models proposed in the past are now considered too simplistic: the *early experience model* and the *main effects model*. A more recent model, the *vulnerability model,* forms the building block for two other models that yield supportive findings and generate testable hypotheses: *diathesis–stress models* and *transactional models*. In vulnerability models, individuals inherit or acquire deficits or dysfunctions, or abnormalities, that thereby increase their likelihood of developing psychopathology. However, although vulnerabilities acquired as a function of early adverse experience are likely to be a liability, they are unlikely to be singular, linear causes of depression. Diathesis–stress models and transactional models are needed to elaborate on the role of vulnerabilities in explaining associations between early adverse experience and risk for the development of depression.

Diathesis–Stress Models

As reviewed by Monroe and Simons (1991), diathesis–stress models explain that a vulnerability manifests itself only in the context of stress or, more broadly, maladaptive environments. Thus, this model tries to correct for the oversimplification of early experience models, or even vulnerability models, by proposing the conditions under which a vulnerability, or diathesis, would or would not lead to disorder, revealing both exacerbating and resilience or protective factors. In this way of thinking, the stress is a moderator variable. The model has been proposed as a way to explain why some people with the diathesis develop disorder, whereas others do not, and why some people remain disorder-free until a certain point in time, then emerge with the disorder.

Although originally developed to explain the development of schizophrenia in individuals with genetic predisposition, several variations on diathesis–stress models can be developed for the issues discussed in this chapter. As reviewed here, strong support from empirical findings suggests that children who experience early adverse experiences develop one or more diatheses for depression, including a dysregulated HPA system, lower vagal tone, reduced left frontal EEG activation, insecure attachment, dysfunctional cognitions, and deficits and delays in emotional expression or regulation. Children who acquire one or more of these diatheses would be expected to be more sensitive to the effects of additional stressors relative to their less vulnerable counterparts. Longitudinal studies would be required to test these predictions from the model.

Diathesis–stress models in which genetic factors are the primary diatheses also hold tremendous promise for contributing to an understanding of the role of early adverse experiences in the later development of depression. Recent studies of carriers of the short (S) allele of the serotonin transporter gene, 5HTTLPR, reveal this potential of gene–environment interactions influencing vulnerability to stressful life events. Caspi and colleagues (2003) found that carriers of the S allele are more vulnerable to major depression induced by stress. In a large prospective study following individuals from ages 3–26, they found that whereas no main effect of *5HTTLPR* genotype could be detected on depressive symptoms, there was a significant interaction, such that in S carriers, but not long (LL) homozygotes, stressful events predicted onset of new and recurrent episodes of major depression. At least six independent studies have replicated these findings, including studies of children who had experienced maltreatment and/or lack of social support (Grabe et al., 2005; Kaufman et al., 2004). One group reported opposite effects of the S allele in female versus male adolescents (Sjoberg et al., 2005). In the two studies that failed to replicate this statistical interaction (Gillespie, Whitfield, Williams, Heath, & Martin, 2005; Surtees et al., 2006), both involved secondary analyses of studies that were not designed to detect depression. Of most direct relevance to the topic of this chapter, two studies indicated that this polymorphism may influence the susceptibility of the infant to prenatal maternal milieu, reporting associations between the L (long) allele and sudden infant death syndrome (SIDS) (Narita et al., 2001; Weese-Mayer et al., 2003). The role of S allele carrier status in potentially increasing the vulnerability of infants to stressful prenatal environments is also the topic of research currently underway in our lab.

Transactional Models

Goodman and Gotlib (1999) asserted the need for a developmentally sensitive, transactional, integrated model to best understand risk for depression in one population, children with depressed parents. The case for such a model is at least as strong with regard to all aspects of early adverse experience. Considering biological and psychosocial models within an integrative transactional model offers great potential for understanding the role of early adverse experience in the emergence of depression.

In early stages of development, children must develop mechanisms to regulate affect, arousal, and attention; secure attachment relationships; and a differentiated sense of self and self in relation to others, any aberration of which could propel a child onto a pathway to depression (Cicchetti & Toth, 1998). Underlying all of these developmental challenges are not only the socioemotional environment (i.e., good-quality parenting) but also genetic influences, the still-maturing brain, and neuroendocrine mechanisms that influence affective and behavioral regulation, as well as the influence of parenting on the behavioral manifestations of the latter (Dawson et al., 1992).

From these early beginnings, the transactional model not only integrates the multiple potential pathogenic processes but also takes into account the continuous processes of child and environment mutually influencing each other (Sameroff, 1975). Simply put, environmental characteristics influence the child's course of development, and the child's characteristics influence the nature of the environment. Over time, these processes may be adaptive or maladaptive, or may vary from one to the other. For example, children with vulnerability of a pattern of frontal EEG abnormalities, who are likely to experience a predominance of negative emotions, may engage the environment less actively or less positively. Similarly, children who acquire cognitive vulnerabilities may selectively attend to, or be more sensitive to, negative aspects of their environment; conversely, others are likely to interact with the child in ways that are evoked by the child's affective, interpersonal, and cognitive styles. Other studies reveal biological or cognitive vulnerabilities that engender greater sensitivity to environmental stressors relative to children with fewer of the vulnerabilities. As an example, child characteristics such as shyness and poor self-control were related to increases in cortisol over the course of the day in day care, although not at home (Dettling, Parker, Lane, Sebanc, & Gunnar, 2000).

In these ways, children's developmental course will be influenced by their vulnerability traits or tendencies. Transactional models take into account both vulnerabilities, such as the ones in these examples, and diathesis–stress considerations. In addition, developmental processes are given serious consideration and include accounting for stage-specific influences and adaptive or "self-righting" influences inherent in growth and development (Cicchetti & Rogosch, 1997).

The transactional model provides a theoretical context within which one can ask questions that help to explain the alternative courses of development of children who are exposed early to adverse experiences. In the final two sections of this chapter, we present ideas for some of the influences on alternative pathways and suggestions for research that promises to further knowledge of the roles of early adverse experiences in the development of depression.

ALTERNATIVE DEVELOPMENTAL PATHWAYS

Early experiences may link with the later emergence of depression and other outcomes, including healthy outcomes, by following many different pathways. Even if depression is the ultimate outcome, the particular pathways may relate to the relative degree of involvement of cognitive, socioemotional, representational, or biological domains in the depression that emerges (Cicchetti & Toth, 1998).

First, some of the alternative pathways reflect the tremendous differences in the nature of any of the adverse experiences described in this chapter; that is, there is no single characterization of abuse, loss, a depressed mother, and so forth. Each of these situations is associated with a set of experiences that varies for individual children. For example, as Field (2002) has shown, depressed mothers who might be characterized as predominantly withdrawn or as more hostile–intrusive may have infants who follow widely diverging pathways. Field provides converging evidence that suggests infants with predominantly withdrawn mothers may be more vulnerable to depression as a function of developing a withdrawn style themselves, and of having a lower capacity to experience pleasure, whereas infants with predominantly intrusive mother may be more vulnerable to depression in response to stress. Similarly, neither parents who abuse their young children nor the children who have been abused can be characterized in a single way. Crittenden (1998) describes two groups of abused children that, even as toddlers, differ from each other, with one group being exceedingly compliant, vigilantly attentive to parents' cues, quiet and withdrawn, and displaying false positive affect, and the other being angry and aggressive, demanding, negative, and noncompliant, possibly as a strategy to get parents' attention. These two patterns may differentially predict depression and externalizing disorders. Moreover, the timing of any of the early adverse experiences will influence the developmental course, a theme that is woven through the material reviewed in this chapter. Furthermore, the transactional processes that unfold over time add even more variation in alternative pathways. Clearly, more process-oriented research will help to elucidate the patterns of adaptation and maladaptation that may unfold over time (Cicchetti & Sroufe, 2000).

FUTURE DIRECTIONS

Considering the role of early experience in the emergence of depression within an integrative, developmentally sensitive, transactional model raises many important questions requiring further study. A few examples are mentioned here.

First, for the diathesis–stress models to further fulfill their promise of being applicable to the issues regarding early adversity and risk for depression, many aspects of the model need further elaboration and testing. For example, it would be important to note whether the moderating processes operate similarly over the course of development. It is not clear whether children would remain vulnerable to depression equally over the course of their development or whether they might, for example, accomplish some developmental tasks that would reduce the potential triggering mechanism of later-occurring stressors. Support for consideration of different developmental processes comes from Hammen's (1992) analysis of longitudinal data. She found that, for young children, adverse experiences alone predict depression. In contrast, for older children, the model for predicting depression also includes negative attributional style. Thus, although a diathesis–stress model adds to our understanding of associations between early adverse experiences and the development of depression, it also leaves unexplained many of the complexities of causal pathways, processes, and multiple determinants of outcome that are needed for a transactional model. As one example of work that is beginning to elucidate underlying mechanisms, neuroimaging of healthy adult S allele carriers has revealed alterations in the anatomy and function of brain regions associated with processing negative emotions (Pezawas et al., 2005). When interpreted within a developmental perspective on emotion regulation, and in the context of genetic susceptibility for depression for a subset of people, these findings are very promising.

Second, researchers might benefit from borrowing the behavior genetics notion of active/evocative gene × environment interaction and other aspects of gene–environment interplay (Rutter, Moffitt, & Caspi, 2006). Silberg and Rutter (2002) expanded on this idea relative to children with depressed parents. As applied to the study of early adverse experiences, the vulnerabilities acquired as a function of the early adverse experiences might be considered the equivalent of an active/evocative gene; that is, children's abnormal stress reactivity, relative right frontal EEG activation, lower vagal tone, cognitive vulnerabilities, and so forth, might be expressed in ways that evoke particular reactions from others. Infants and young children with these characteristics might be less responsive, expressive, and attentive. Others might find these children to be particularly challenging, and might react with harshness or withdrawal. Although we acknowledge the complexities of the required research designs, research is needed to examine the extent to which children's biological and cognitive vulnerabilities are expressed in behavioral tendencies that in turn influence the patterns of parent–child interaction that emerge over children's early years of development.

Third, promising research in terms of the earliest adverse experiences is pursuing the notion of fetal programming (Egliston, McMahon, & Austin, 2007; Van den Bergh, Mulder, Mennes, & Glover, 2005). Initially developed to explain associations among poor nutrition during pregnancy, newborn birthweight, and adult health outcomes, such as heart disease, this relatively new area of study has generated interesting findings in both animals and humans relevant to a range of outcomes. The basic premise is that adverse conditions at particular periods of fetal development may lead to the later development of problems. New research may reveal, for example, that fetal experiences associated with maternal stress or depression alter brain development, with consequences that only emerge over time. Also intriguing is how fetal exposures may alter gene expression in ways that increase the likelihood of the development of depression or other disorders.

Fourth, with a lens on early adverse experience as an entry point to study the development of depression in young people, the notion of endophenotype is appealing (Gottesman & Gould, 2003). Much of the research described here suggests that early adverse experiences are likely to be associated with endophenotypes rather than with a specific phenotype, such as major depression (Hasler, Drevets, Manji, & Charney, 2004). An example of work that is consistent with this idea is studies of frontal EEG asymmetry (Anokhin, Heath, & Myers, 2006) and temperamental fearfulness (Goldsmith & Lemery, 2000; Gonda et al., 2006). Studies that examined prenatal anxiety show similar promise in this regard (Van den Bergh et al., 2005).

Finally, although not the emphasis of this chapter, the ideas presented here have important implications for interventions. For example, research that furthers our understanding of the neurobiology of the stress response could lead to the development of both biological and behavioral interventions. An important step will be to establish the extent of contribution of any of the aspects of the fetal environment to the later emergence of depression. If a significant role is found, such individuals could be studied for other signs of vulnerability. For example, for those identified early as having abnormal stress responses, the goal would be to decrease their vulnerability to develop depression, including increasing environmental supports. Some work is already being conducted along these lines (Chaffin et al., 2006; Dozier et al., 2006). This is only one of many implications for preventive and therapeutic interventions that might be developed from the research exploring associations between early adverse experiences and depression.

ACKNOWLEDGMENTS

This work was partially funded by an Emory University Research Committee Grant and the Silvio O. Conti Center for the Neurobiology of Mental Disease National Institutes of Health Grant No. MH58922.

REFERENCES

Adamson, L. B., & Frick, J. E. (2003). The still face: A history of a shared experimental paradigm. *Infancy, 4*, 451–473.

Anokhin, A. P., Heath, A. C., & Myers, E. (2006). Genetic and environmental influences on frontal EEG asymmetry: A twin study. *Biological Psychology, 71*, 289–295.

Arborelius, L., Owens, M. J., Plotsky, P. M., & Nemeroff, C. B. (1999). The role of corticotropin-releasing factor in depression and anxiety disorders. *Journal of Endocrinology, 160*(1), 1–12.

Atkinson, L., Paglia, A., Coolbear, J., Niccols, A., Parker, K. C. H., & Guger, S. (2000). Attachment security: A meta-analysis of maternal mental health correlates. *Clinical Psychology Review, 20*, 1019–1040.

Bandura, A. (1986). *Social foundations of thought and action: A social cognitive theory.* Englewood Cliffs, NJ: Prentice-Hall.

Barnett, D., Ganiban, J., & Cicchetti, D. (1999). Maltreatment, negative expressivity, and the development of Type D attachments from 12- to 24-months of age. *Monographs of the Society for Research in Child Development, 64*(3), 97–118.

Belsky, J. (1993). Etiology of child maltreatment: A developmental–ecological analysis. *Psychological Bulletin, 114*, 413–434.

Byrne, G., & Suomi, S. J. (1999). Social separation in infant *Cebus appella*: Patterns of behavioral and cortisol response. *International Journal of Developmental Neuroscience, 17*, 265–274.

Carlson, V., Cicchetti, D., Barnett, D., & Braunwald, K. (1989). Disorganized/disoriented attachment relationships in maltreated infants. *Developmental Psychology, 25*, 382–393.

Caspi, A., Sugden, K., Moffitt, T. E., Taylor, A., Craig, I. W., Harrington, H., et al. (2003). Influence of life stress on depression: Moderation by a polymorphism in the 5-HTT gene. *Science, 301*, 386–389.

Cerel, J. P., Fristad, M. A., Verducci, J., Weller, R. A., & Weller, E. B. (2006). Childhood bereavement: Psychopathology in the 2 years postparental death. *Journal of the American Academy of Child and Adolescent Psychiatry, 45*(6), 681–690.

Chaffin, M., Hanson, R., Saunders, B. E., Nichols, T., Barnett, D., Zeanah, C., et al. (2006). Report of the APSAC Task Force on Attachment Therapy, Reactive Attachment Disorder, and Attachment Problems. *Child Maltreatment, 11*(1), 76–89.

Cherny, S. S., Fulker, D. W., Corley, R. P., Plomin, R., & DeFries, J. C. (1994). Continuity and change in infant shyness from 14 to 20 months. *Behavior Genetics, 24,* 365–379.

Chorpita, B. F. (2001). *Control and the development of negative emotion.* New York: Oxford University Press.

Chugani, H. T., Phelps, M. E., & Mazziotta, J. C. (2002). Positron emission tomography study of human brain functional development. In M. H. Johnson, Y. Munakata, & R. O. Gilmore (Eds.), *Brain development and cognition: A reader* (2nd ed., pp. 101–116). Malden, MA: Blackwell.

Cicchetti, D., & Barnett, D. (1991). Attachment organization in maltreated preschoolers. *Development and Psychopathology, 3,* 397–411.

Cicchetti, D., & Rogosch, F. A. (1996). Equifinality and multifinality in developmental psychopathology. *Development and Psychopathology, 8,* 597–600.

Cicchetti, D., & Rogosch, F. A. (1997). The role of self-organization in the promotion of resilience in maltreated children. *Development and Psychopathology, 9,* 799–817.

Cicchetti, D., Rogosch, F. A., & Toth, S. L. (1998). Maternal depressive disorder and contextual risk: Contributions to the development of attachment insecurity and behavior problems in toddlerhood. *Development and Psychopathology, 10,* 283–300.

Cicchetti, D., & Sroufe, L. A. (2000). The past as prologue to the future: The times, they've been a-changin.' *Development and Psychopathology, 12*(3), 255–264.

Cicchetti, D., & Toth, S. (1998). The development of depression in children and adolescents. *American Psychologist, 53,* 221–241.

Clark, L. A. (1989). The anxiety and depressive disorders: Descriptive psychopathology and differential diagnoses. In P. C. Kendall & D. Watson (Eds.), *Anxiety and depression: Distinctive and overlapping features* (pp. 83–129). San Diego, CA: Academic Press.

Cohn, J. F., Matias, R., Tronick, E., Lyons-Ruth, K., & Connell, D. B. (1986). Face-to-face interactions, spontaneous and structured, of mothers with depressive symptoms. *New Directions for Child Development, 34,* 31–46.

Cole, D. A., & Rehm, L. P. (1986). Family interaction patterns and childhood depression. *Journal of Abnormal Child Psychology, 14,* 297–314.

Crittenden, P. M. (1998). Dangerous behavior and dangerous contexts: A 35-year perspective on research on the developmental effects of child physical abuse. In P. K. Trickett & C. J. Schellenbach (Eds.), *Violence against children in the family and the community* (pp. 11–38). Washington, DC: American Psychological Association Press.

Cummings, E. M., & Cicchetti, D. (1990). Toward a transactional model of relations between attachment and depression. In M. T. Greenberg, D. Cicchetti, & E. M. Cummings (Eds.), *Attachment in the preschool years: Theory, research, and intervention* (pp. 339–372). Chicago: University of Chicago Press.

Dadds, M. R., Sanders, M. R., Morrison, M., & Rebgetz, M. (1992). Childhood depression and conduct disorder: II. An analysis of family interaction patterns in the home. *Journal of Abnormal Psychology, 101,* 505–513.

Davidson, R. J., & Fox, N. (1982). Asymmetrical brain activity discriminates between positive and negative affective stimuli in human infants. *Science, 218,* 1235–1237.

Davidson, R. J., & Fox, N. A. (1989). Frontal brain asymmetry predicts infants' response to maternal separation. *Journal of Abnormal Psychology, 98,* 127–131.

Davidson, R. J., Pizzagalli, D., & Nitschke, J. B. (2002). The representation and regulation of emotion in depression: Perspectives from affective neuroscience. In I. H. Gotlib & C. Hammen (Eds.), *Handbook of depression* (pp. 219–244). New York: Guilford Press.

Davies, P. T., & Cummings, E. M. (1994). Marital conflict and child adjustment: An emotional security hypothesis. *Psychological Bulletin, 116,* 387–411.

Dawson, G., Ashman, S. B., Hessl, D., Spieker, S., Frey, K., Panagiotides, H., et al. (2001). Autonomic and brain electrical activity in securely- and insecurely-attached infants of depressed mothers. *Infant Behavior and Development, 24*, 135–149.

Dawson, G., Ashman, S. B., Panagiotides, H., Hessl, D., Self, J., Yamada, E., et al. (2003). Preschool outcomes of children of depressed others: Role of maternal behavior, contextual risk, and children's brain activity. *Child Development, 74*, 1158–1175.

Dawson, G., Frey, K., Self, J., Panagiotides, H., Hessl, D., Yamada, E., et al. (1999). Frontal brain electrical activity in infants of depressed and nondepressed mothers: Relation to variations in infant behavior. *Development and Psychopathology, 11*, 589–605.

Dawson, G., Grofer Klinger, L., Panagiotides, H., Hill, D., & Spieker, S. (1992). Frontal lobe activity and affective behavior of infants of mothers with depressive symptoms. *Child Development, 63*, 725–737.

Dettling, A. C., Parker, W. W., Lane, S., Sebanc, A., & Gunnar, M. (2000). Quality of care and temperament determine changes in cortisol concentrations over the day for young children in childcare. *Psychoneuroendocrinology, 25*, 819–836.

Devane, C. L., Stowe, Z. N., Donovan, J. L., Newport, D. J., Pennell, P. B., Ritchie, J. C., et al. (2006). Therapeutic drug monitoring of psychoactive drugs during pregnancy in the genomic era: Challenges and opportunities. *Journal of Psychopharmacology, 20*(Suppl. 4), 54–59.

DiPietro, J. A., Bornstein, M. H., Costigan, K. A., Pressman, E. K., Hahn, C.-S., Painter, K., et al. (2002). What does fetal movement predict about behavior during the first two years of life? *Developmental Psychobiology, 40*, 358–371.

DiPietro, J. A., Irizarry, R. A., Costigan, K. A., & Gurewitsch, E. D. (2004). The psychophysiology of the maternal–fetal relationship. *Psychophysiology, 41*, 510–520.

Dozier, M., Peloso, E., Lindheim, O., Gordon, M. K., Manni, M., Sepulveda, S., et al. (2006). Developing evidence-based interventions for foster children: An example of a randomized clinical trial with infants and toddlers. *Journal of Social Issues, 62*(4), 767–785.

Egeland, B., Pianta, R., & O'Brian, M. (1993). Maternal intrusiveness in infancy and child maladaptation in early school years. *Development and Psychopathology, 5*, 359–370.

Egliston, K.-A., McMahon, C. A., & Austin, M. P. (2007). Stress in pregnancy and infant HPA axis functioning: Conceptual and methodological issues relating to the use of salivary cortisol as an outcome measure. *Psychoneuroendocrinology, 32*, 1–13.

Essex, M. J., Klein, M. H., Cho, E., & Kalin, N. H. (2002). Maternal stress beginning in infancy may sensitize children to later stress exposure: Effects on cortisol and behavior. *Biological Psychiatry, 52*, 776–784.

Field, T. (1985). Attachment as psychological attunement: Being on the same wavelength. In M. Reite & T. Field (Ed.), *Psychobiology of attachment* (pp. 415–454). New York: Academic Press.

Field, T. (1994). The effects of mother's physical and emotional unavailability on emotion regulation. *Monographs of the Society for Research in Child Development, 59*(2–3), 208–227, 250–283.

Field, T. (2002). Prenatal effects of maternal depression. In S. H. Goodman & I. H. Gotlib (Eds.), *Children of depressed parents* (pp. 59–88). Washington, DC: American Psychological Association.

Field, T., Diego, M., Dieter, J., Hernandez-Reif, M., Schanberg, S., Kuhn, C., et al. (2004). Prenatal depression effects on the fetus and the newborn. *Infant Behavior and Development, 27*(2), 216–229.

Field, T., Diego, M., & Hernandez-Reif, M. (2006). Prenatal depression effects on the fetus and newborn: A review. *Infant Behavior and Development, 29*(3), 445–455.

Field, T., Estroff, D. B., Yando, R., del Valle, C., Malphurs, J., & Hart, S. (1996). "Depressed" mothers' perceptions of infant vulnerability are related to later development. *Child Psychiatry and Human Development, 27*(1), 43–53.

Field, T., Fox, N., Nawrocki, T., & Gonzalez, J. (1995). Vagal tone in infants of depressed mothers. *Development and Psychopathology, 7*, 227–231.

Field, T., Fox, N., Pickens, J., & Nawrocki, T. (1995). Relative right frontal EEG activation in 3- to 6-month-old infants of "depressed" mothers. *Developmental Psychology, 31*, 358–363.

Field, T., Healy, B., Goldstein, S., & Guthertz, M. (1990). Behavior-state matching and synchrony in mother–infant interactions of nondepressed versus depressed dyads. *Developmental Psychology, 26*, 7–14.

Garber, J., Braafladt, N., & Zeman, J. (1991). The regulation of sad affect: An information-processing perspective. In J. Garber & K. A. Dodge (Eds.), *The development of emotion regulation and dysregulation* (pp. 208–242). Cambridge, UK: Cambridge University Press.

Garber, J., & Martin, N. C. (2002). Negative cognitions in offspring of depressed parents: Mechanisms of risk. In S. H. Goodman & I.H. Gotlib (Eds.), *Children of depressed parents: Mechanisms of risk and implications for treatment* (pp. 121–154). Washington, DC: American Psychological Association.

Gelles, R. J. (1998). The youngest victims: Violence toward children. In R. K. Berger (Ed.), *Issues in intimate violence* (pp. 5–24). Thousand Oaks, CA: Sage.

Gillespie, N. A., Whitfield, J. B., Williams, B., Heath, A. C., & Martin, N. G. (2005). The relationship between stressful life events, the serotonin transporter (5-HTTLPR) genotype and major depression. *Psychological Medicine, 35*, 101–111.

Glover, V. (1999). Mechanisms by which maternal mood in pregnancy may affect the fetus. *Contemporary Reviews in Obstetrics and Gynecology, 11*, 155–160.

Goldsmith, H., & Lemery, K. S. (2000). Linking temperamental fearfulness and anxiety symptoms: A behavior-genetic perspective. *Biological Psychiatry, 48*(12), 1199–1209.

Gonda, X., Rihmer, Z., Zsombok, T., Bagdy, G., Akiskal, K. K., & Akiskal, H. S. (2006). The 5HTTLPR polymorphism of the serotonin transporter gene is associated with affective temperaments as measured by TEMPS-A. *Journal of Affective Disorders, 91*(2–3), 125–131.

Goodman, S. H., & Gotlib, I. H. (1999). Risk for psychopathology in the children of depressed mothers: A developmental model for understanding mechanisms of transmission. *Psychological Review, 106*, 458–490.

Goodman, S. H., & Tully, E. C. (in press). Recurrence of depression during pregnancy: Psychosocial and personal functioning correlates. *Depression and Anxiety.*

Gottesman, I. I., & Gould, T. D. (2003). The endophenotype concept in psychiatry: Etymology and strategic intentions. *American Journal of Psychiatry, 160*, 636–645.

Gottman, J. M., & Katz, L. F. (2002). Children's emotional reactions to stressful parent–child interactions: The link between emotion regulation and vagal tone. *Marriage and Family Review, 34*, 265–283.

Grabe, H. J., Lange, M., Wolff, B., Volzke, H., Lucht, M., Freyberger, H. J., et al. (2005). Mental and physical distress is modulated by a polymorphism in the 5-HT transporter gene interacting with social stressors and chronic disease burden. *Molecular Psychiatry, 10*, 220–224.

Graham, Y. P., Heim, C., Goodman, S. H., Miller, A. H., & Nemeroff, C. B. (1999). The effects of neonatal stress on brain development: Implications for psychopathology. *Development and Psychopathology, 11*, 545–565.

Grych, J., & Fincham, F. D. (1990). Marital conflict and children's adjustment: A cognitive–contextual framework. *Psychological Bulletin, 108*, 267–290.

Gunnar, M., & van Dulmen, M. H. (2007). Behavior problems in postinstitutionalized internationally adopted children. *Developmental Psychopathology, 19*(1), 129–148.

Gunnar, M. R., Brodersen, L., Nachmias, M., Buss, K., & Rigatuso, J. (1996). Stress reactivity and attachment security. *Developmental Psychobiology, 29*(3), 191–204.

Gunnar, M. R., & Vazquez, D. M. (2001). Low cortisol and a flattening of expected daytime rhythm: Potential indices of risk in human development. *Development and Psychopathology, 13*, 515–538.

Haley, D. W., & Stansbury, K. (2003). Infant stress and parent responsiveness: Regulation of physiology and behavior during still-face and reunion. *Child Development, 74*(5), 1534–1546.

Hamilton, E. B., Asarnow, J. R., & Tompson, M. C. (1999). Family interaction styles of children with depressive disorders, schizophrenia-spectrum disorders, and normal controls. *Family Process, 38*, 463–476.

Hammen, C. (1992). Cognitive, life stress, and interpersonal approaches to a developmental psychopathology model of depression. *Development and Psychopathology, 4*, 189–206.

Handley, S. L., Dunn, T. L., Waldron, G., & Baker, J. M. (1980). Tryptophan, cortisol and puerperal mood. *British Journal of Psychiatry, 136*, 498–508.

Hane, A. A., & Fox, N. A. (2006). Ordinary variations in maternal caregiving influence human infants' stress reactivity. *Psychological Science, 17*(6), 550–556.

Harrington, R. (1996). Family–genetic findings in child and adolescent depressive disorders. *International Review of Psychiatry, 8,* 355–368.

Hart, J., Gunnar, M., & Cicchetti, D. (1996). Altered neuroendocrine activity in maltreated children related to symptoms of depression. *Development and Psychopathology, 8,* 201–214.

Hasler, G., Drevets, W. C., Manji, H. K., & Charney, D. S. (2004). Discovering endophenotypes for major depression. *Neuropsychopharmacology, 29*(10), 1765–1781.

Heim, C., Newport, D. J., Heit, S., Graham, Y. P., Wilcox, M., Bonsall, R., et al. (2000). Pituitary–adrenal and autonomic responses to stress in women after sexual and physical abuse in childhood. *Journal of the American Medical Association, 284*(5), 592–597.

Henriques, J. B., & Davidson, R. J. (1990). Regional brain electrical asymmetries discriminate between previously depressed subjects and healthy controls. *Journal of Abnormal Psychology, 99,* 22–31.

Hernandez-Reif, M., Field, T. F., Diego, M. A., & Ruddock, M. (2006). Greater arousal and less attentiveness to face/voice stimuli by neonates of depressed mothers on the Brazelton Neonatal Behavioral Assessment Scale. *Infant Behavior and Development, 29*(4), 594–598.

Hooley, J. M., & Gotlib, I. H. (2000). A diathesis–stress conceptualiztion of expressed emotion and clinical outcome. *Applied and Preventative Psychology, 9,* 135–152.

Jones, N. A., Field, T., Fox, N. A., Lundy, B. L., & Davalos, M. (1997). EEG activation in 1-month-old infants of depressed mothers. *Development and Psychopathology, 9*(3), 491–505.

Jungmeen, K., & Cicchetti, D. (2006). Longitudinal trajectories of self-system processes and depressive symptoms among maltreated and nonmaltreated children. *Child Development, 77*(3), 624–639.

Kaffman, A., & Meaney, M. J. (2007). Neurodevelopmental sequelae of postnatal maternal care in rodents: Clinical and research implications of molecular insights. *Journal of Clinical Psychology and Psychiatry, 48,* 224–244.

Kaufman, J., & Charney, D. (2001). Effects of early stress on brain structure and function: Implications for understanding the relationship between child maltreatment and depression. *Development and Psychopathology, 13,* 451–471.

Kaufman, J., Yang, B. Z., Douglas-Palumberi, H., Houshyar, S., Lipschitz, D., Krystal, J. H., et al. (2004). Social supports and serotonin transporter gene moderate depression in maltreated children. *Proceedings of the National Academy of Sciences USA, 101,* 17316–17321.

Kay, G., Tarcic, N., Poltyrev, T., & Weinstock, M. (1998). Prenatal stress depresses immune function in rats. *Physiology and Behavior, 63*(3), 397–402.

Kelly, R. H., Danielsen, B. H., Golding, J. M., Anders, T. F., Gilbert, W. M., & Zatzick, D. F. (1999). Adequacy of prenatal care among women with psychiatric diagnoses giving birth in California in 1994 and 1995. *Psychiatric Services, 50*(12), 1584–1590.

Kendler, K. S., Gardner, C. O., Neale, M. C., & Prescott, C. A. (2001). Genetic risk factors for major depression in men and women: Similar or different heritabilities and same or partly distinct genes? *Psychological Medicine, 31,* 605–616.

Kinard, E. M. (1995). Mother and teacher assessments of behavior problems in abused children. *Journal of the American Academy of Child and Adolescent Psychiatry, 34,* 1043–1053.

King, S. (2007, April). *Prenatal maternal stress from a disaster affects physical, cognitive, and behavioral development in children: Project Ice Storm.* Presentation at the annual meeting of the Society for Research in Child Development, Boston.

King, S., & Laplante, D. P. (2005). The effects of prenatal maternal stress on children's cognitive development: Project Ice Storm. *Stress: The International Journal on the Biology of Stress, 8*(1), 35–45.

Kovacs, M., Akiskal, H. S., Gatsionis, C., & Parrone, P. L. (1994). Childhood-onset dysthymic disorder: Clinical features and prospective naturalistic outcome. *Archives of General Psychiatry, 51,* 365–374.

Lakdawalla, Z., Hankin, B. L., & Mermelstein, R. (2007). Cognitive theories of depression in children and adolescents: A conceptual and quantitative review. *Clinical Child and Family Psychology Review, 10*(1), 1–24.

Loehlin, J. C., & Nichols, R. C. (1976). *Heredity, environment, and personality.* Austin: University of Texas Press.

Loughhead, A. M., Stowe, Z. N., Newport, D. J., Ritchie, J. C., DeVane, C. L., & Owens, M. J. (2006). Placental passage of tricyclic antidepressants. *Biological Psychiatry, 59*(3), 287–290.

Lykken, D. T., & Tellegen, A. (1996). Happiness is a stochatic phenomenon. *Psychological Science, 7,* 186–189.

Lyons-Ruth, K., Lyubchik, A., Wolfe, R., & Bronfman, E. (2002). Parental depression and child attachment: Hostile and helpless profiles of parent and child behavior among families at risk. In S. H. Goodman & I. H. Gotlib (Eds.), *Children of depressed parents* (pp. 89–120). Washington, DC: American Psychological Association.

Marcus, S. M., Flynn, H. A., Blow, F. C., & Barry, K. L. (2003). Depressive symptoms among pregnant women screened in obstetrics settings. *Journal of Women's Health, 12*(4), 373–380.

Martins, C., & Gaffan, E. (2000). Effects of early maternal depression on patterns of infant–mother attachment: A meta-analytic investigation. *Journal of Child Psychology and Psychiatry, 41*(6), 737–746.

McLeod, B. D., Wood, J. J., & Weisz, J. R. (2007). Examining the association between parenting and childhood anxiety: A meta-analysis. *Clinical Psychology Review, 27*(2), 155–172.

McMahon, C. A., Barnett, B., Kowalenko, N. M., & Tennant, C. C. (2006). Maternal attachment state of mind moderates the impact of postnatal depression on infant attachment. *Journal of Child Psychology and Psychiatry, 47*(7), 660–669.

Milberger, S., Biederman, J., Faraone, S. V., Chen, L., & Jones, J. (1996). Is maternal smoking during pregnancy a risk factor for attention deficit hyperactivity disorder in children? *American Journal of Psychiatry, 153,* 1138–1142.

Monk, C., Sloan, R., Myers, M., & Ellman, L. (2004). Fetal heart rate reactivity differs by women's psychiatric status: An early marker for developmental risk? *Journal of the American Academy of Child and Adolescent Psychiatry, 43*(3), 283–290.

Monroe, S. M., & Simons, A. D. (1991). Diathesis–stress theories in the context of life-stress research: Implications for depressive disorders. *Psychological Bulletin, 110,* 406–425.

Moore, G. A., & Calkins, S. D. (2004). Infants' vagal regulation in the still-face paradigm is related to dyadic coordination of mother–infant interaction. *Developmental Psychology, 40*(6), 1068–1080.

Murray, L., Woolgar, M., Cooper, P., & Hipwell, A. (2001). Cognitive vulnerability to depression in 5-year-old children of depressed mothers. *Journal of Child Psychology and Psychiatry, 42*(7), 891–899.

Narita, N., Narita, M., Takashima, S., Nakayama, M., Nagai, T., & Okado, N. (2001). Serotonin transporter gene variation is a risk factor for sudden infant death syndrome in the Japanese population. *Pediatrics, 107,* 690–692.

Nemeroff, C. B. (2004). Neurobiological consequences of childhood trauma. *Journal of Clinical Psychiatry, 65*(Suppl. 1), 18–28.

O'Connor, T. G., Caprariello, P., Blackmore, E. R., Gregory, A. M., Glover, V., Fleming, P., et al. (2007). Prenatal mood disturbance predicts sleep problems in infancy and toddlerhood. *Early Human Development, 83*(7), 451–458.

O'Connor, T. G., Heron, J., Golding, J., Beveridge, M., & Glover, V. (2002). Maternal antenatal anxiety and children's behavioural/emotional problems at 4 years: Report from the Avon Longitudinal Study of Parents and Children. *British Journal of Psychiatry, 180*(6), 502–508.

O'Connor, T. G., Heron, J., Golding, J., & Glover, V. (2003). Maternal antenatal anxiety and behavioural/emotional problems in children: A test of a programming hypothesis. *Journal of Child Psychology and Psychiatry, 44*(7), 1025–1036.

O'Connor, T. G., Rutter, M., & the English & Romanian Adoptees Study Team. (2000). Attachment disorder behavior following early severe deprivation: Extension and longitudinal follow-up. *Journal of the American Academy of Child and Adolescent Psychiatry, 39,* 703–712.

Oberlander, T. F., Misri, S., Fitzgerald, C. E., Kostaras, X., Rurak, D., & Riggs, W. (2004). Pharmacologic factors associated with transient neonatal symptoms following prenatal psychotropic medication exposure. *Journal of Clinical Psychiatry, 65,* 230–237.

Pezawas, L., Meyer-Lindenberg, A., Drabant, E. M., Verchinski, B. A., Munoz, K. E., Kolachana, B. S., et al. (2005). 5-HTTLPR polymorphism impacts human cingulate–amygdala interactions: A genetic susceptibility mechanism for depression. *Nature Neuroscience, 8*(6), 828–834.

Pfeffer, C. R. (1996). *Severe stress and mental disturbance in children.* Washington, DC: American Psychiatric Press.

Pickens, J., & Field, T. (1993). Facial expressivity in infants of "depressed" mothers. *Developmental Psychology, 29,* 986–988.

Pihoker, C., Owens, M. J., Kuhn, C., Schanberg, S., & Nemeroff, C. B. (1993). Maternal separation in neonatal rats elicits activation of the hypothalamic–pituitary–adrenocortical axis: A putative role for corticotropin-releasing factor. *Psychoneuroendocrinology, 7,* 485–493.

Plomin, R. (1994). *Genetics and experience: The interplay between nature and nurture.* Thousand Oaks, CA: Sage.

Plomin, R., Emde, R. N., Braungart, J. M., Campos, J., Corley, R. P., Fulker, D. W., et al. (1993). Genetic change and continuity from fourteen to twenty months: The MacArthur Longitudinal Twin Study. *Child Development, 64,* 1354–1376.

Plotsky, P. M., Thrivikraman, K. V., Nemeroff, C. B., Caldji, C., Sharma, S., & Meaney, M. J. (2005). Long-term consequences of neonatal rearing on central corticotropin-releasing factor systems in adult male rat offspring. *Neuropsychopharmacology, 30*(12), 2192–2204.

Poehlmann, J., & Fiese, B. H. (2001). The interaction of maternal and infant vulnerabilities on developing attachment relationships. *Development and Psychopathology, 13*(1), 1–11.

Porges, S. W. (2001). The polyvagal theory: Phylogenetic substrates of a social nervous system. *International Journal of Psychophysiology, 42,* 123–146.

Porges, S. W., Doussard-Roosevelt, J. A., & Maiti, A. K. (1994). Vagal tone and the physiological regulation of emotion. *Monographs of the Society for Research in Child Development, 59*(2–3, Serial No. 240), 167–186.

Racusin, G. R., & Kaslow, N. J. (1991). Assessment and treatment of childhood depression. In P. A. Keller & S. R. Hyman (Eds.), *Innovations in clinical practice: A sourcebook* (Vol. 10, pp. 223–243). Sarasota, FL: Professional Resource Exchange.

Radke-Yarrow, M., Belmont, B., Nottelmann, E., & Bottomly, L. (1990). Young children's self-conceptions: Origins in the natural discourse of depressed and normal mothers and their children. In D. Cicchetti & M. Beeghly (Eds.), *The self in transition: Infancy to childhood* (pp. 345–361). Chicago: University of Chicago Press.

Rutter, M., Colvert, E., Kreppner, J., Beckett, C., Castle, J., Groothues, C., et al. (2007). Early adolescent outcomes for institutionally deprived and non-deprived adoptees: I. Disinhibited attachment. *Journal of Child Psychology and Psychiatry and Allied Disciplines, 48*(1), 17–30.

Rutter, M., Moffitt, T. E., & Caspi, A. (2006). Gene-environment interplay and psychopathology: Multiple varieties but real effects. *Journal of Child Psychology and Psychiatry, and Allied Disciplines, 47*(3–4), 226–261.

Sameroff, A. J. (1975). Transactional models in early social relations. *Human Development, 18,* 65–79.

Schmiege, S. J., Khoo, S. T., Sandler, I. N., Ayers, T. S., & Wolchik, S. A. (2006). Symptoms of internalizing and externalizing problems: Modeling recovery curves after the death of a parent. *American Journal of Preventive Medicine, 31*(6, Suppl. 1), 152–160.

Schneider, M. L., Moore, C. F., & Kraemer, G. W. (2003). On the relevance of prenatal stress to developmental psychopathology: A primate model. In D. Cicchetti & E. Walker (Eds.), *Neurodevelopmental mechanisms in psychopathology* (pp. 155–186). New York: Cambridge University Press.

Shamir-Essakow, G., Ungerer, J. A., Rapee, R. M., & Safier, R. (2004). Caregiving representations of mothers of behaviorally inhibited and uninhibited preschool children. *Developmental Psychology, 40*(6), 899–910.

Silberg, J., & Rutter, M. (2002). Nature–nurture interplay in the risks associated with parental depression. In S. H. Goodman & I. H. Gotlib (Eds.), *Children of depressed parents: Mechanisms of risk and implications for treatment* (pp. 13–36). Washington, DC: American Psychological Association.

Sjoberg, R. L., Nilsson, K. W., Nordquist, N., Ohrvik, J., Leppert, J., Lindstrom, L., et al. (2005). Development of depression: Sex and the interaction between environment and a promoter polymorphism of the serotonin transporter gene. *International Journal of Neuropsychopharmacology,* 1–7.

Smith, R., Cubis, J., Brinsmead, M., Lewin, T., Singh, B., Owens, P., et al. (1990). Mood changes, obstetrical experience and alterations in plasma cortisol, beta-endorphin and corticotrophin releasing hormone during pregnancy and the puerperium. *Journal of Psychosomatic Research, 34*, 53–69.

Spangler, G., & Grossman, K. E. (1993). Biobehavioral organization in securely and insecurely attached infants. *Child Development, 64*, 1439–1450.

Sroufe, L. A., Egeland, B., Carlson, E. A., & Collins, W. A. (2005). *The development of the person: The Minnesota study of risk and adaptation from birth to adulthood* New York: Guilford Press.

Surtees, P. G., Wainwright, N. W., Willis-Owen, S. A., Luben, R., Day, N. E., & Flint, J. (2006). Social adversity, the serotonin transporter (5-HTTLPR) polymorphism and major depressive disorder. *Biological Psychiatry, 59*, 224–229.

Teixeira, J. M., Fisk, N. M., & Glover, V. (1999). Association between maternal anxiety in pregnancy and increased uterine artery resistance index: Cohort based study. *British Medical Journal, 318*, 153–157.

Tellegen, A., Lykken, D. T., Bouchard, T. J., Wilcox, K. J., Segal, N. L., & Rich, S. (1988). Personality similarity in twins reared apart and together. *Journal of Personality and Social Psychology, 54*, 1031–1039.

Thompson, R. A., & Goodvin, R. (2005). The individual child: Temperament, emotion, self, and personality. In M. H. Bornstein & M. E. Lamb (Eds.), *Developmental science: An advanced textbook* (5th ed., pp. 391–428). Mahwah, NJ: Erlbaum.

Toth, S. L., Cicchetti, D., Macfie, J., Rogosch, F. A., & Maughan, A. (2000). Narrative representations of moral-affiliative and conflictual themes and behavioral problems in maltreated preschoolers. *Journal of Clinical Child Psychology, 29*, 307–318.

Toth, S. L., Rogosch, F. A., Manly, J. T., & Cicchetti, D. (2006). The efficacy of toddler–parent psychotherapy to reorganize attachment in the young offspring of mothers with major affective disorder: A randomized preventive trial. *Journal of Consulting and Clinical Psychology, 74*(6), 1006–1016.

Tronick, E. Z., & Gianino, A. F., Jr. (1986). The transmission of maternal disturbance to the infant. In E. Z. Tronick & T. Field (Eds.), *Maternal depression and infant disturbance* (pp. 5–11). San Francisco: Jossey-Bass.

Van den Bergh, B. R. H., Mulder, E. J., Mennes, M., & Glover, V. (2005). Antenatal maternal anxiety and stress and the neurobehavioural development of the fetus and child: Links and possible mechanisms: A review. *Neuroscience and Biobehavioral Reviews, 29*(2), 237–258

Wadhwa, P. D., Glynn, L., Hobel, C. J., Garite, T. J., Porto, M., Chicz-DeMet, A., et al. (2002). Behavioral perinatology: Biobehavioral processes in human fetal development. *Regulatory Peptides, 108*, 149–157.

Weese-Mayer, D. E., Berry-Kravis, E. M., Maher, B. S., Silvestri, J. M., Curran, M. E., & Marazita, M. L. (2003). Sudden infant death syndrome: Association with a promoter polymorphism of the serotonin transporter gene. *American Journal of Medical Genetics A, 117*, 268–274.

Weinberg, K. M., & Tronick, E. (1998). The impact of maternal psychiatric illness on infant development. *Journal of Clinical Psychiatry, 59*, 53–61.

Weinberg, K. M., & Tronick, E. Z. (1996). Infant affective reactions to the resumption of maternal interaction after the still-face. *Child Development, 67*, 905–914.

Williams, M. T., Hennessy, M. B., & Davis, H. N. (1998). Stress during pregnancy alters rat offspring morphology and ultrasonic vocalizations. *Physiological Behavior, 63*(3), 337–343.

Zagron, G., & Weinstock, M. (2006). Maternal adrenal hormone secretion mediates behavioural alterations induced by prenatal stress in male and female rats. *Behavioural Brain Research, 175*(2), 323–328.

Zuckerman, B., Amorao, H., Bauchner, H., & Cabral, H. (1989). Depressive symptoms during pregnancy: Relationships to poor health behaviors. *American Journal of Obstetrics and Gynecology, 160*, 1107–1111.

Zuckerman, B., Bauchner, H., Parker, S., & Cabral, H. (1990). Maternal depressive symptoms during pregnancy, and newborn irritability. *Journal of Developmental and Behavioral Pediatrics, 11*(4), 190–194.

Zuckerman, B., & Bresnahan, K. (1991). Developmental and behavioral consequences of prenatal drug and alcohol exposure. *Pediatric Clinics of North America, 38*(6), 1387–1406.

CHAPTER 12

Children of Depressed Parents

Constance L. Hammen

Research on the link between parental depression, and depression and other forms of psychopathology in offspring has grown from a trickle to a large volume of studies in recent years. Initially the research largely served the goals of simply describing the association between parental and offspring disorders or exploring familial patterns consistent with genetic mediation. More commonly in recent years, the studies, like high-risk research in general, have attempted to explore the mechanisms accounting for the development of depression in offspring. The shift from demonstrating an association between parental and child disorders to exploring the mechanisms is an important development, but excellent reviews of such research have revealed the enormous complexity of such an undertaking (Goodman, 2007; Goodman & Gotlib, 1999; Joorman, Eugene, & Gotlib, in press). These reviews identify and discuss a variety of theoretical perspectives and multivariable models, developmental considerations, and diverse ages of samples based on a wide array of sampling, design, and measurement strategies.

In an attempt to avoid duplicating the excellent reviews, I attempt in this chapter to take stock of what we know and what remains to be clarified. The first section is a discussion of significant methodological problems that affect the interpretation and meaning of offspring studies. It is followed by a selective review of the research on outcomes of offspring of depressed parents. For methodological reasons, this section is largely based on longitudinal studies and on studies based on procedures that establish clinical significance of parental depression. Many important studies that were based only on self-reported subclinical symptoms are omitted. An effort is made to include research on parental factors that may modify children's outcomes, such as parent gender, single- and dual-parent depression, and clinical features. The final segment is a selective review of promising mechanisms and mediators of the effects of parental depression, factors that are likely to be candidates for inclusion in emerging comprehensive models.

METHODOLOGICAL ISSUES IN STUDIES
OF CHILDREN'S RISK DUE TO PARENTAL DEPRESSION

A number of methodological issues involving research designs, definitions of depression, and, of course, the vastly complex array of potential risk factors and mechanisms hamper firm conclusions in many aspects of the field. The methodological issues are particularly pertinent, because differences in key design and assessment methods may obscure the meaning of results in terms of etiological and treatment implications. Although there is little doubt that parents' depression is a significant risk factor for the development of affective and other disorders in their children, it is likely that different, multiple etiological factors are operative. An important challenge to the field, therefore, is to refine conclusions about what is currently known or what is unclear, and to develop more differentiated models of mechanisms of risk that may apply to different forms of depression.

Design Issues

Research on high-risk of disorder traditionally focuses on the children of psychiatrically disordered parents before they develop disorder, but in the case of depression, cross-sectional studies that commonly include older children and adolescents have discovered that many youth have diagnosable problems by the time the study begins. Thus, it becomes impossible to characterize accurately the temporal and causal sequence of parent and child disorders (although many investigators have emphasized the transactional, bidirectional nature of parent–child effects). Truly high-risk designs that can follow children of depressed parents from pregnancy or birth to the development of diagnosable disorders are rare. Studies of infants and young children of depressed parents are vitally important but frequently are limited by not following the children long enough to determine whether behavioral and emotional symptoms noted early in development actually portend diagnosable mood disorders. At a minimum, longitudinal studies are needed to determine that parental depressive episodes temporally precede youth negative outcomes, and to evaluate the effects of specific variables on later outcomes consistent with causal mechanisms.

Sample selection and recruitment methods are also significant challenges. Although both cross-sectional and longitudinal studies have important contributions to make to research on offspring of depressed parents, both types of studies commonly obscure the current status of the parent's depression when samples are recruited based on a history of depression or treatment. Many studies compared "depressed" and "control" groups without clarification of current status. There is no question that *current* parental depression is a potent influence on children's adjustment. Indeed, the recent findings from the Sequenced Treatment Alternatives to Relieve Depression (STAR*D) trial demonstrated the impact of effective treatment of maternal depression on children's current diagnoses (Weissman et al., 2006). The Weissman and colleagues (2006) study indicated that remission of maternal depression substantially reduced rates of diagnoses in children; thus, the patterns underscore the critical role of current psychosocial determinants of children's outcomes. However, offspring studies vary widely in both the prevalence or inclusion of current depression in parents, and the nature and clinical features of past depression. Thus, whereas important questions about the role of stable features and mechanisms of parental depression may be overlooked in parents who are not currently depressed, effects of transient adverse conditions may be accentuated in parents with current depression. Complete etiological models require consideration of both state-dependent and state-independent factors.

Another crucial design issue is the sample source and recruitment method. It has often been observed that samples drawn from those who are currently or recently in treatment for depression are likely to be more severely depressed and to have complications such as comorbid Axis I and II psychopathology correlated with help seeking. Depression is well known to afflict far more people than those who actually seek treatment for it. Thus, findings based on clinically ascertained samples of parents may be less generalizable to the typical population of persons with depressive disorders in the community. Randomly selected community samples may be desirable but expensive, leaving many investigators with the option of recruiting self-selected volunteers whose characteristics may vary considerably from sample to sample. It is vital to characterize and, when appropriate, to evaluate the effects of sample characteristics, including histories of depression and comorbid disorders, as well as sociodemographic factors.

Definitions of Depression

A critical question in studies of children of depressed parents is how the parental depression is defined and what it means. As Goodman and Gotlib (1999) noted, it is likely that different aspects of parental depression are related to the relative contributions of genetic factors in the transmission of depression (i.e., some depression subtypes may have a greater genetic component than others). Particular caution is warranted in interpreting the findings of studies based on parental depression defined by self-reported questionnaire measures, such as the Beck Depression Inventory or the Center for Epidemiologic Studies Depression Scale (CES-D). Elevated scores may be transitory and reflect conditions not specific to depression (low self-esteem, medical symptoms, stress and worries about life conditions or specific events, demoralization due to life conditions such as poverty or burdens and responsibilities), or traits and temperaments, such as low-positive affectivity. Although any of these conditions may indeed have a detrimental effect on children, do we benefit by attributing such outcomes to "depression"? Instead, in nonclinical samples it seems fruitful to determine more precisely which features of the parent's symptoms are associated with which kinds of offspring difficulties. *Depression* includes heterogeneous features even when diagnosed by DSM criteria, but reliance on elevated scores of self-report scales, especially if only one testing is included, stretches the term beyond its useful limits and may add uninterpretable noise.

As noted, even when diagnosed by currently accepted criteria for major depressive disorder (MDD), the construct of depression is enormously heterogeneous. At the simplest level, depression varies in chronicity, severity, and impairment—all of which may affect children's outcomes but are rarely explored. At more complex levels, depression may also have important etiological subtypes that may manifest as differences in age of onset, frequency of recurrence, familiality, differing symptom profiles (melancholia, psychosis), and comorbidities (e.g., anxiety disorders, substance use disorders). Although the field has not progressed very far in identification of etiological subtypes, it stands to reason that not all depressions are alike in their impact on children or on the mechanisms by which adverse effects may occur.

OUTCOMES OF CHILDREN OF DEPRESSED PARENTS

In view of the issues raised regarding sampling, designs, and definitions of depression, the following sections focus largely on relatively recent longitudinal studies designed to study offspring at risk due to *parental depression*, defined as meeting diagnostic criteria or some meaningful criteria establishing clinical significance. Such studies may include both clinical and community samples.

Overall Effects Associated with Parental Diagnosed Depression

Outcomes of Children and Adolescents

Many of the studies that meet the methodological criteria noted earlier have included a wide age range of offspring, including both school-age and adolescent children, which makes it difficult to separate results by developmental stage. A small number of longitudinal studies based on *clinically ascertained samples* have included direct diagnostic evaluations of the parents and children. Weissman and her colleagues, for example, reported on 10-year (Weissman, Warner, Wickramaratne, Moreau, & Olfson, 1997) and 20-year (Weissman et al., 2006) follow-ups of offspring of samples of depressed and control parents ($n = 151$ at 20 years; mean age, 35). At 10 years, 78% of the offspring of depressed parents had diagnoses compared with 47% of controls (56 vs. 25% major depression, respectively). At 20 years, the investigators found three times higher rates of major depression, substance dependence, and anxiety disorders in the high-risk offspring than in controls. The children of depressed parents also had significantly higher levels of psychosocial impairment, treatment seeking, and physical illnesses. Hammen, Burge, Burney, and Adrian (1990) followed a sample of 8- to 17-year-old offspring of mothers with unipolar, bipolar, or medical disorders, and controls. At the 3-year follow-up, children of women with unipolar depression had the highest cumulative probability of major depression (45%) of any group, and also of conduct, over-anxious, and substance use disorders. It should be noted that children of women with bipolar disorders and medical illnesses also experienced somewhat elevated rates of disorder and impairment, but at significantly lower levels of frequency or severity compared to offspring of depressed women (e.g., Hammen et al., 1990). Children of mothers with unipolar depression were also significantly more likely than children in the other groups to have social and academic impairment (Anderson & Hammen, 1993).

Billings and Moos (1983) originally identified 133 families with a parent with unipolar depression seeking treatment and demographically matched control families with children age 18 or under. At a 10-year follow-up, Timko, Cronkite, Berg, and Moos (2002) included the offspring of depressed parents who still lived at home, and reported that they had significantly more psychological distress, psychosocial disturbance, and physical problems than did control offspring, with high rates among offspring of parents with both unremitted and remitted depression. Their study did not include diagnostic assessments of the offspring, relying instead on parent questionnaire reports. A relatively small-scale longitudinal study of offspring by Williamson, Birmaher, Axelson, Ryan, and Dahl (2004) is noteworthy, because it included families of treated patients only if 3- to 13-year-old children (or siblings) of the proband had no history of mood disorder at entry. Follow-ups over 4 or 5 years revealed a threefold increased risk for developing first-onset major depression in the high-risk group compared with a low-risk control group. Mother's lifetime history of anxiety disorders and youth's history of behavioral disorders were predictors of major depression beyond effects of family risk status. Unfortunately, a limitation of the study was inclusion of families with bipolar probands, so that the effects due only to unipolar depression are unclear. In one of few tests of the specificity of effects of parental depression (see also Hammen et al., 1990), a 5-year longitudinal study of offspring of patients with depression or panic disorder (PD) was recently reported by Biederman and colleagues (2006), who compared children of parent groups with PD only, depression only, both PD and depression, or no disorder. These investigators found that PD in parents was associated with a wide variety of anxiety disorders in offspring, but parental depression was associated with increased risk of depression and disruptive behavior disorders. Children's impairment was also greater in groups with parental depression, regardless of PD status. Definitive conclusions await additional follow-ups, because the majority of children were 12 years or younger.

Among *community samples*, whereas several large-scale studies were initially designed as high-risk studies targeting depressed parents, several others were designed more generally to focus on adolescents, with later supplemental studies examining whether parents were depressed. Of the former, Beardslee, Keller, Lavori, Staley, and Sacks (1993) conducted a 4-year follow-up on 81 families of parents with depressive disorder, nonaffective disorder, and no disorder. At follow-up the rate of major depression was 26% in children of parents with mood disorders compared with 10% in non-ill parents. Hammen and Brennan (2001) identified a sample of over 800 families with differing histories of maternal depression (or no history), and found that 20% of youth of depressed mothers had a diagnosable depressive disorder by age 15 compared to 10% in those with never-depressed mothers. By the 5-year follow-up at age 20, rate of depressive disorder was 36 vs. 26%, respectively. However, as Hammen, Brennan, and Keenan-Miller (in press) reported, the association between maternal and child depression by age 20 was accounted for by whether the child was depressed by age 15, and whether the youth experienced social dysfunction at 15. Youth with recurrent major depression by age 20 were especially likely to show social impairment, hypothesized to contribute to further risk for depression.

Lieb, Isensee, Hofler, Pfister, and Wittchen (2002) reported on baseline and 4-year follow-up outcomes of 2,427 community adolescents and young adults as a function of parental depression. Offspring of parents with lifetime major depression were nearly three times more likely than offspring of nondepressed parents to experience depression, and they also had elevated rates of substance use and anxiety disorders. Klein, Lewinsohn, Rohde, Seeley, and Olino (2005) followed community adolescents to age 24, and they also found that maternal depression was associated with greater offspring risk for depression, as well as anxiety and substance use disorders—even when they controlled for parental sociodemographic factors and comorbidity. The offspring of depressed parents also experienced significant impairment in various forms, even after researchers controlled for offspring psychopathology (Lewinsohn, Olino, & Klein, 2005).

A study that is unique for its 13-year follow-up was based on a small sample of children of postnatally depressed community women. Researchers found that maternal depression was associated with 23% rates in youth with depressive disorder compared with 7% of youth with nondepressed mothers (Halligan, Murray, Martins, & Cooper, 2007). The children of depressed women also had more anxiety and behavioral disorders than did children of nondepressed women.

Taken together, the studies of both clinical and community samples of offspring of depressed parents indicate up to two or three times the rate of depressive and other disorders compared to offspring of nondepressed samples. These disorders typically arise by early adolescence and are often accompanied by psychosocial and medical problems. In subsequent sections, several moderators of the effects are explored, but note that among the relatively few longitudinal studies, attention to crucial factors such as parents' current or typical mood state and comorbid conditions, and the specificity of parental depression effects, has been limited.

Outcomes of Infants to Preschoolers

Several studies with parental samples based on diagnostic or clinically meaningful depression criteria (e.g., stability of elevated symptoms) and longitudinal designs have assessed outcomes in infants and toddlers. These studies have generally focused on three targets: emotion regulation and behavioral disruption, cognitive/intellectual functioning, and attachment. The largest observational study, the National Institute of Child Health and Human Development (NICHD) Early Child Care Research Network (1999) study of 1,215 women with infants, assessed children's cognitive–linguistic and behavioral functioning in relation to mothers' depression symptoms and behaviors during tasks with them over five testing sessions between 1 and 36 months. Compared with children of nondepressed women, children of women with the most chronically elevated depressive symptoms had lower cognitive–linguistic performance and reported more behavioral problems. Other studies have also reported decrements in intellectual performance. One example is a study of nearly 5,000 five-year-olds whose mothers' depression severity and chronicity was assessed multiple times from pregnancy to age 5 (Brennan et al., 2000). These investigators found that both severity and chronicity of maternal depression symptoms predicted children's lower vocabulary scores and greater reports of behavior problems. Other longitudinal studies have also indicated that very young children of chronically dysphoric women display or are reported to have more social and behavioral difficulties than children of nondepressed women (e.g., Dawson et al., 2003; Field et al., 1996; Murray, Sinclair, Cooper, Ducournau, & Turner, 1999).

A number of investigations have focused on the issue of attachment security, although relatively few have been longitudinal. Attachment insecurity is theoretically central to many formulations of the effects of maternal depression, because it may mediate the maladaptive effects of maternal depression, and also because it likely portends stable patterns of disrupted emotion regulation, negative self-perceptions, and social dysfunction that contribute to later diagnosable psychological disorders in offspring. Interestingly, the attachment patterns of infants of depressed women have been found to be variable across studies. Martins and Gaffan (2000), in a meta-analysis of seven studies that included diagnosed maternal samples, assessed four categories of attachment using the Strange Situation procedure and included families that were generally free of potentially confounding factors, such as marital dissolution or child maltreatment. They found that, after removing one outlying study, the aggregated results showed a significant effect of maternal depression being associated with fewer children classified as securely attached, and marginally greater classification as insecure–avoidant or disorganized attachment, with greater consistency among the latter type. Variability in outcomes and the contributors to the disorganized-insecure attachment type remain important questions for further study.

Moderators of Effects of Parental Depression

Effects of Fathers' Depression

Consequences of paternal depression have been examined in a limited number of studies. The findings of these studies are mixed, likely due to the variations in samples, design, and methods of assessing psychopathology in parents and offspring. Connell and Goodman (2002), for example, conducted a general meta-analysis of effects of maternal and paternal disorders on children's internalizing and externalizing disorders and symptoms. They found that depression in either parent was associated with children's internalizing and externalizing pathology. However, mothers' depression was significantly more strongly related to children's internalizing disorders than was fathers' depression. In general (among subjects not tested specifically for depression), larger effect sizes were obtained for studies based on symptoms in parents and children rather than on diagnoses. Kane and Garber (2004) conducted a specific meta-analysis of effects of fathers' depression on offspring but did not compare mothers and fathers' depression. Like Connell and Goodman, Kane and Garber found significant but modest associations between fathers' depression and children's internalizing and externalizing psychopathology. They, too, noted that effect sizes for internalizing problems were greater for measures based on symptoms rather than diagnoses, as well as for studies based on community rather than clinical samples. They did not report specific analyses for child gender and age.

Among relatively large studies that used diagnostic assessments of parental depression and youth disorders but varied in sample selection, results are somewhat equivocal. In Weissman and colleagues' (1997) clinically ascertained sample of parents, Nomura, Warner, and Wickramaratne (2001) reported that when only the mother was depressed, offspring were significantly more likely to experience depression, anxiety disorder, or substance dependence than when no parent was depressed; in contrast, when only the father was depressed, youth did not have a significantly elevated risk for any disorder except anxiety. The effects for depression in offspring were qualified by gender of the depressed parent: A girl was significantly more likely to be depressed if her father was depressed, whereas a boy was more likely to be depressed if his mother was depressed. Billings and Moos (1983) also studied the offspring of parents with clinically ascertained depression, although children's diagnostic outcomes were not obtained, and symptoms and outcomes were reported by parents. They found that fathers' and mothers' depression affected children equally, and there were no child gender or age effects.

Lieb and colleagues (2002) interviewed a large representative community sample of youth, obtaining diagnostic information about the parents mainly from the youth or the mothers as informants. Maternal and paternal major depressions were equally associated with depressive disorders in youth. Maternal depression was significantly associated with more substance use and anxiety disorders in offspring than was paternal depression, but fathers' depression was as likely as mothers' depression to be associated with youth generalized anxiety disorder. For the most part, there were no interactions with gender of the offspring.

The Oregon Adolescent Depression Project, a longitudinal community study of youth, added a parent component in which researchers conducted direct interviews with 75% of mothers and 46% of fathers, with informants providing diagnostic information on those not interviewed (Klein et al., 2005). Klein and colleagues (2005) found that maternal, but not paternal, major depression was associated with offspring depression and anxiety disorders by age 24. Importantly, these findings were qualified by clinical characteristics of youth and parental depression. Both mothers' and fathers' early-onset major depression (and fathers' recurrent depression) predicted youth major depression. Also, when youth depression was defined as moderate or severe major depression (excluding mild depression), both mothers' and fathers' depressions were significantly predictive.

A high-risk community sample based on maternal histories of depression examined youth outcomes by age 15. Brennan, Hammen, Katz, and LeBrocque (2002) reported on 522 families using direct diagnostic interviews with mothers, fathers, and youth. They found that maternal depression was associated with diagnoses of youth depression, externalizing, and nondepressive internalizing disorders. However, fathers' depression was related only to youth externalizing disorders. The most significant combination of parental disorders in the prediction of youth depression was maternal depression and paternal substance abuse.

Exposure to One versus Two Depressed Parents

The mental health status of the coparent in studies of children of depressed parents has commonly been ignored, but the likelihood of nonrandom mating may greatly affect outcomes and implications. For instance, several studies have shown assortative mating in which depressed individuals are married to others with mood disorders, and depressed women often have husbands with antisocial and substance abuse problems (e.g., Dierker, Merikangas, & Szatmari, 1999; Kim-Cohen, Moffitt, Taylor, Pawlby, & Caspi, 2005; Mathews & Reus, 2001). A few studies have examined the effects of two-parent depression on risk for youth disorders. Nomura and colleagues (2001) found a twofold greater risk of MDD in offspring if both parents (compared to one parent) had depression. In contrast, Brennan and colleagues (2002) found that two depressed parents increased rates of youth externalizing disorders but not of MDD. This finding is similar to that reported by Lieb and colleagues (2002), who also found no differential risk for depression in youth with one versus two parents with depression. Finally, Nomura and colleagues found that the combination of nondepressed mother and depressed father was associated with earlier age of onset of youth conduct disorder.

Effects of Mother and Father Depression on Youth Course of Depression

Limited research on this topic suggests that additional studies would be fruitful. For instance, Rohde, Lewinsohn, Klein, and Seeley (2005) found that among youth with recurrent major depression, maternal, but not paternal, depression was associated with more youth depression recurrence, chronicity, and severity; anxiety disorders; and lower psychosocial functioning. Paternal depression was associated only with lower psychosocial functioning. Several of the effects were moderated by gender, such that, among those with recurrent depression, worse outcomes occurred among sons than among daughters. Compared with maternal depression, paternal depression was notably associated with sons' suicidal ideation and attempts in this sample of youth with recurrent depression (see also Lewinsohn et al., 2005).

Taken together, data on youth depressive symptoms and relatively sparse research based on diagnoses suggest that maternal depression is more robustly associated with youth psychopathology, especially depression, than is paternal depression. Paternal depression does, however, have adverse effects on youth. Further descriptive research on combinations of parental pathology, on possible differential effects due to current versus past parental depression, on gender of offspring, and on parental comorbidity with depression will help to clarify whether fathers' and mothers' depressive experiences have unique effects on offspring (e.g., see Kim-Cohen et al., 2005).

Features of Parental Depression

Parental Depression and Youth Depression Characteristics

The importance of distinguishing among clinical features and subtypes of parental depression is supported by several studies that have reported associations between these constructs and youth outcomes, including both presence and characteristics of disorder. Key features of parental depression include clinical course status, severity, chronicity, age of onset, timing of child's exposure, clinical subtypes or symptom features, and comorbidity. Two clinically ascertained samples and several community-based samples reported on the association between parental depression features and youth outcomes. Billings and Moos (1985) were among the first to report on the enduring effects of parental depression despite remission: At a 4-year follow-up they found that parents whose depression had remitted nonetheless had children with greater problems in functioning than children in control families (although fewer problems than children of parents with continuing depression). In a recent clinical sample, the STAR*D trial, Pilowsky and colleagues (2006) found that mothers with the atypical depression subtype had the highest rates of offspring with depressive or anxiety disorders. Moreover, they found that history of maternal suicide attempts, comorbid PD with agoraphobia, and substance abuse was also associated with increased risk of depression in offspring, and irritable depression was linked to youth with "any disorder." Interestingly, severity of depression was not associated with youth outcomes, although the sample had relatively severely depressed women with limited variability. Chronicity features, such as maternal depression age of onset, years of youth exposure, and number of major depression episodes per year of exposure, were unrelated to children's outcomes.

Similar results were reported in the Oregon Adolescent Depression Project based on analyses of depressed youth. Rohde and colleagues (2005) found that there were no main age-of-onset effects of parental depression and recurrence on clinical outcomes of the depressed offspring. In further analyses, Klein, Lewinsohn, Rohde, Seeley, and Durbin (2002) did not find familial similarity in parental and offspring depression severity, recurrence, chronicity, age of onset, melancholia, and suicidality. Partially in contrast, in their large adolescent community sample in Munich, Schreier, Höfler, Wittchen, and Lieb (2006), after controlling for sociodemographic characteristics, observed that maternal and adolescent offspring depression shared several clinical features, including severity, melancholia, and elevated number of major depression symptoms. Like Klein and colleagues, however, they did not find similarity in recurrence, age of onset, or suicidality.

A goal of the large community sample study by Hammen and Brennan (2003) was to elucidate the contribution of maternal depression severity, chronicity, and timing to outcomes in 15-year-old youth. Considering that the three features are typically confounded, a large and diverse sample is needed to disentangle the effects of each. Based on the experience of parental depression during the first 10 years of the child's life, the investigators found that severity of depression, even if relatively brief, was predictive of diagnosable depression in youth, whereas chronic but nonsevere parental depression increased risk of youth depression only if it persisted for more than 20 months. However, chronicity of maternal depression was predictive of youth nondepressive disorders. Timing of maternal depression in relation to youth age, based on samples unconfounded with persistence and severity, was not differentially predictive. Because several investigators had speculated that exposure to maternal depression during infancy might be especially disruptive of healthy development, these results suggest that experiencing maternal depression only during the first 2 years of life was no more predictive of youth depression than when the exposure occurred at a later point. Halligan and colleagues (2007) also observed the confounding of postpartum depression with later depression, and found that maternal depression in the postpartum period only was not predictive of youth depression. Maternal depression was associated with youth depression over a 13-year follow-up only if the postpartum depression was also associated with later episodes of maternal depression.

Other studies of the effects of chronicity of depression have used various definitions. Campbell, Cohn, and Meyers (1995) found that women with postpartum depression that persisted for only 2 months did not differ from nondepressed women in interactions with their infants, but depression persisting over 6 months was associated with less positive interactions between infants and mothers compared with those with mothers who had remitted. Brennan and colleagues (2000) found an interaction between chronicity and severity of maternal depression symptoms during the first 5 years in predicting children's behavioral problems and lower vocabulary scores. The NICHD Early Child Care Research Network (1999) compared a large community sample of women and infants tested five times over a 36-month period, and found that women who had chronically elevated depression symptoms, compared to those who were only sometimes or never depressed, performed less sensitively in interactions; moreover, infants of women with chronically elevated symptoms had more impaired cognitive and linguistic performances and behavior problems. Dawson and colleagues (2003) assessed infants of depressed mothers at 14 months and 3½ years, and found that children whose mothers were chronically depressed over the children's lives displayed significantly lower frontal and parietal brain activation than did children of never-depressed and remitted-depressed mothers. Children's frontal brain activation was a mediator of the association between maternal depression and behavioral problems.

Hammen and colleagues (1987) noted that discussions of the independent variable maternal depression typically obscure the roles of three interrelated features: current mood status, history of depression (severity and chronicity), and impairment. Each of these features was measured and probed in a sample of women with unipolar depression, bipolar depression, medical disorder, and no disorder in relation to children's outcomes. Impairment of functioning in the depressed parent in key roles (e.g., employment, marital, parental, and social)—even when not in a depressed episode—may be an important moderator or mediator of offspring outcomes. Hammen and colleagues found that both ongoing maternal difficulties in roles and current depressed symptoms were independent predictors of various measures of children's disorders and adjustment, whereas lifetime diagnostic status was less predictive. Several of these individual roles, such as parenting and marital functioning, have been studied extensively, as I discuss later, but information on multiple role functioning is rarely reported or evaluated in relation to the effects of clinical history of depression.

Taken together, most, but not all, of the studies indicate that chronicity of maternal depression is an important determinant of more adverse outcomes in offspring. An implication is that because measuring depression symptomatology at only one time in cross-sectional studies cannot distinguish between parents with only transitory versus repeated elevations of dysphoric mood, it may obscure the meaning of results. Further clarification is needed also to distinguish between different contributory roles, if any, of chronic and current depression, and how the effects may be modified by the child's age and outcomes measured.

Comparisons of Depressed Youth of Depressed and Nondepressed Parents

Another fruitful way of exploring effects of parental depression is to compare depressed youth who have parents with, versus without, depression. The question is whether there are unique characteristics of depression in youth whose parents have depression. Beardslee and colleagues (1993) found that depressed offspring of depressed parents had longer episodes of major depression, earlier onset, and more comorbid conditions than did depressed youth of nondepressed parents. Weissman and colleagues (1997) made similar comparisons in their 10-year follow-up of a clinical sample of depressed parents and their offspring. They compared youth who had been depressed at an earlier point on their outcomes at the 10-year follow-up, and reported that offspring of depressed parents had significantly more persisting depression, greater severity, and more work and interpersonal impairment than did the depressed offspring of nondepressed parents. At the 20-year follow-up of the youth, Weissman and colleagues (2006) found that depression was first evident at a mean of 16 years in the high-risk group, compared with 19 years in the low-risk group.

Lieb and colleagues (2002) also found that both greater recurrence of major depression and greater impairment, especially social, were associated with parental depression in the Munich youth sample. Also, youth with severe depression, compared to mild or moderate depression, were more likely to come from families with parental depression. Similarly, analyses by Rohde and colleagues (2005) indicated that depressed youth in the Oregon sample who came from families with depressed mothers were more likely to have recurrent depression, comorbid anxiety disorders, greater severity and chronicity of depression, and lower psychosocial functioning than were depressed offspring of nondepressed parents. Hammen and Brennan (2001) found that 15-year-old offspring with histories of depressive disorders did not differ in age of onset or number of episodes as a function of maternal depression status, but the depressed children of depressed mothers were more likely to experience dysthymic disorder and comorbid conditions overall than were depressed offspring of nondepressed mothers. Most significantly, depressed offspring of depressed mothers were more impaired on a variety of interpersonal—but not academic—functioning measures at age 15 than were depressed offspring of nondepressed mothers.

Taken together, the limited number of relevant studies of clinical features of parental depression and parental depression status relative to features of youth depression and other outcomes strongly suggests that these topics are important to pursue. It appears that aspects of both parental depression chronicity and severity, and possibly symptom subtypes, predict variability in youth outcomes. Also, youth depression that occurs in the context of parental depression appears to be marked by greater social dysfunction and more severe, chronic, or recurrent depressions than youth depression in the context of no parental depression. Studies also need to investigate whether the variability in offspring outcomes is associated with parental depression and clinical features as such, or with correlated features such as impaired functioning, sociodemographic disadvantage, disruptions in parenting and family functioning, and genetic or biological characteristics.

Mechanisms of Effects of Parental Depression

Research has focused on several variables that are hypothesized to account for the association between parental and offspring depression, including problematic interpersonal relationships (parenting, marital discord), transmission of maladaptive cognitions, exposure to stressors, and biological factors. There is widespread recognition that these variables commonly overlap and are associated with both the state of depression and the risk for developing depression. Several studies for each of the major topics are very briefly reviewed in this section to highlight key findings and research strategies.

Biological Factors

There is ample evidence that unipolar depression is moderately heritable (e.g., Levinson, Chapter 8, this volume), but it is unlikely that there is a genetically transmitted disease of depression. Rather, it is speculated (e.g., Joorman et al., in press) that heritable traits such as temperament, expression of negative emotions, shyness and inhibition, and emotion regulation are among many characteristics that constitute risk factors for depression (see also Gotlib, Joormann, Minor, & Hallmayer, 2008). The possibilities are numerous and complex. For example, Durbin, Klein, Hayden, Buckley, and Moerk (2005) found a specific association between maternal depression and low positive emotionality (PE) in preschool-age children. They speculated that such temperamental traits may operate via various pathways to increase risk for depression—such as eliciting fewer protective and positive relationships, or reducing responsiveness to rewarding stimuli.

Research suggests that dysfunctional neuroregulatory mechanisms (Goodman, 2007; Goodman & Gotlib, 1999), arising from genetic factors, and adverse parenting quality and stress, may underlie problems in emotion regulation that predict maladaptive symptoms. For instance, infants, children, and adolescents of depressed mothers have been shown to display EEG asymmetries (left frontal hypoactivation) similar to those shown by depressed adults (e.g., Dawson, Frey, Panagiotides, Osterling, & Hessl, 1997; Dawson, Klinger, Panagiotides, Hill, & Spieker, 1992; Field, Fox, Pickens, & Nawrocki, 1995; Forbes et al., 2006; Tomarken, Dichter, Garber, & Simien, 2004). Notably, Shankman and colleagues (2005) found that low PE in children is associated with EEG asymmetry. Further follow-up of the offspring with EEG asymmetries would be hypothesized to reveal emergence of depression and related behavioral impairments.

Maladaptive neurobiological processes are well known to occur in infants and young children exposed to adverse conditions, presumably including dysfunctional parenting due to depression (e.g., see Goodman & Brand, Chapter 11, this volume). Current research in adult depression emphasizes the role of such processes as contributors to abnormal reactions to stressors (e.g., see Thase, Chapter 9, and Monroe, Slavich, & Georgiades, Chapter 15, this volume; for studies of children, see Goodman & Brand, Chapter 11, this volume). Neuroendocrine dysfunction in the form of hypothalamic–pituitary–adrenocortical (HPA) axis dysregulation has rarely been studied in children of depressed mothers. Ashman, Dawson, Panadiotides, Yamada, and Wilkinson (2002) found that maternal depression moderated the association between internalizing symptoms and abnormal cortisol responses to a mild stressor in young children. Interestingly, exposure to maternal depression during the first 2 years of life was the best predictor of elevated cortisol levels (although the authors note that the effect may be due to greater exposure during that period rather than timing as such). Essex, Klein, Cho, and Kalin (2002) found that exposure to maternal stress in both infancy and preschool, compared to exposure during either alone, was associated with higher levels of cortisol in children. The authors interpreted the results as being consistent with a model in which children are sensitized to stress in early childhood (show higher cortisol levels when exposed to stress) and also found that exposure to maternal depression beginning in infancy was a potent predictor of cortisol levels. Children with higher cortisol levels also had higher levels of mental health symptoms in first grade.

Stressors

There are several ways in which stressors play a key role in the intergenerational transmission of depression. Virtually all models of depression are diathesis–stress models, in which stressors play a triggering role in depression, affecting the timing, and possibly the severity and duration, of symptoms through various cognitive, neurobiological, and social vulnerability mechanisms. Children of depressed parents are typically exposed to highly stressful environments, in part because the parent's depression syndrome is itself aversive to the child (see Hammen, 2002). Additionally, however, depression is typically accompanied by chronically stressful conditions that contribute to or result from symptomatology. Moreover, women with histories of depression, even when not currently depressed, have been shown to contribute to the occurrence of stressful life events in part through their behaviors and characteristics, as well as through consequences of the environments they create or select. This process, termed *stress generation* (Hammen, 1991), is also seen in the offspring of depressed mothers (Hammen & Brennan, 2001). An unresolved question concerns the possible role of abnormalities in the neurobiological responses to stressors, as noted previously, and whether they are due to genetic factors or to acquired dysfunctions stemming from excessive stress during sensitive developmental periods (see Gotlib et al., 2008). Further studies of children's cognitive and behavioral coping and problem-solving strategies are needed. One issue is whether children's skills are deficient or simply overwhelmed by the magnitude of adverse environmental and interpersonal stressors in families with a depressed parent.

A factor representing exposure to stress that has attracted specific study is marital discord. Research has consistently shown a significant association between depression and marital distress (e.g., Beach, Jones, & Franklin, Chapter 27, this volume). Marital discord may be a stable feature of the lives of many depressed women, occurring even in periods of remission from depression (Hammen & Brennan, 2002). Downey and Coyne (1990) speculated that marital distress plays an important role as a mechanism in disorders of offspring, and suggested that parental depression and marital distress may create different pathways to different forms of psychopathology in offspring. The hypothesis was specifically tested by Davies, Dumenci, and Windle (1999) in nonclinically depressed women in families with adolescent children. They found that maternal depressive symptoms mediated the association between marital distress and youth depression, but that marital distress mediated the link between maternal depression and youth externalizing symptoms. In samples of kindergarten children, Cummings, Keller, and Davies (2005) found that marital conflict partially mediated the association between maternal depression symptoms and children's internalizing and externalizing symptoms. Studying a community high risk sample of adolescents, Hammen, Shih, and Brennan (2004) found that marital discord was more strongly associated with offspring depression diagnoses and nondepressive disorders in families with a depressed compared to a nondepressed mother.

Several theorists have speculated about the unique effects of marital distress as a stressor for children. For example, Davies and colleagues (1999; see also Cummings & Davies, 1994) proposed several possible explanations for the association between parental discord and offspring disorders, including social learning of dysfunctional emotional and interpersonal coping, internalization of blame and other maladaptive cognitions, emotional contagion, modeling of hostile interpersonal styles, and sensitization through repeated exposure, leading to lower thresholds of aggression and emotional dysregulation.

Parent–Child Relationships

Both general episodic and chronic stressors, and the stress of marital discord in particular, may be highly disruptive of optimal parent–child relations. Much of the research on mechanisms of intergenerational transmission of depression has posited that children's adverse outcomes stem in large part from impaired parenting. An extensive body of work based on observational studies of parent–child interaction quality was summarized by Lovejoy, Graczyk, O'Hare, and Neuman (2000), whose examination of studies published from 1974 to 1996 yielded 46 studies of depressed women interacting with their children. They found that the largest effect associated with maternal depression was expression of negative affect and behaviors toward offspring (e.g., hostility, anger, intrusiveness, coercion), with moderate associations with disengaged behavior (e.g., withdrawal), and small effects associated with reduced levels of positive behaviors. Moreover, although effects were strongest for current maternal depression, even those with past lifetime histories of depression showed similar patterns, suggesting that some of the effects may be stable, likely reflecting enduring mood, stress, and personal characteristics. Furthermore, the negative effects were strongest for infants and young children—and effect sizes were similar in studies based on diagnoses or elevated self-reported symptoms.

Goodman's (2007) review identified a number of studies indicating that maternal parenting quality does indeed mediate the association between maternal depression and children's adverse outcomes (see also Joorman et al., in press). The mechanisms of effects of maladaptive parenting are likely highly developmentally specific, for example, affecting attachment and emotion regulation in very young children, and acquisition of accurate self- and social perceptions and role enactments in older children. Research has suggested that infants of depressed mothers display greater frequency of insecure attachment (e.g., Cicchetti, Rogosch, & Toth, 1998; Teti, Gelfand, Messinger, & Isabella, 1995; see also Siefer, Sameroff, Dickstein, Keitner, & Miller [1996] for an exception). As reviewed by Goodman, parenting qualities are also predictive in older children of a variety of maladaptive cognitions and behaviors that either are associated with depression itself or serve as vulnerabilities to later depression. These maladaptive outcomes are speculated to result from both inadequate parenting, resulting in diminished acquisition of social and cognitive skills, and modeling and learning depressive affect, cognitions, and behaviors.

Two additional points about quality of relationships and interactions in families of a depressed parent are significant. First is that the large amount of research documenting struggles of the depressed person with close relationships (spouse and children), plus the fact that these difficulties are persistent despite remission of depressive episodes, suggests *relational pathology* (Lyons-Ruth, Zoll, Connell, & Grunebaum, 1986) as a core construct in depression transmission. The difficulties in relating sensitively, warmly, and reciprocally are aspects of an interpersonal approach to depression (e.g., Gotlib & Hammen, 1992; Hammen, 1992) that emphasizes recurring depression due to the generation of stressors and being ensnared in stressful interpersonal contexts. Thus, it is noteworthy that depressed adolescent offspring of depressed mothers displayed significantly more interpersonal difficulties than did equally depressed offspring of never-depressed mothers (Hammen & Brennan, 2003), and that such interpersonal problems were predictive of recent depressive symptoms and future depressive episodes (Hammen, Brennan, Keenan-Miller, & Herr, 2008; Hammen, Shih, Altman, & Brennan, 2003). Furthermore, maternal depression was a significant predictor of young women's perpetration of severe intimate partner violence by age 20 (Keenan-Miller, Hammen, & Brennan, 2007).

Second, and relatedly, relationship problems in families of depressed parents are likely highly reciprocal. The bidirectional association between depression and marital difficulties is well known, but the effect of children's negative affect and behaviors on parents' moods and parenting must also be acknowledged. Nelson, Hammen, Brennan, and Ullman (2003) found that maternal depression and expressed emotion (criticism expressed in descriptions of the adolescent child) separately predicted youth externalizing symptoms and role impairment, but it was speculated that children's externalizing behaviors likely elicited criticism from the mother. It might also be hypothesized that children's behavioral difficulties are highly stressful and even depression-provoking for mothers (see also Frye & Garber, 2005).

Cognitive Vulnerability

Maladaptive information-processing style and cognitive content, leading to negativity in views of the self and others, have long been conceptualized as important mechanisms of depression, particularly in diathesis–stress models. Researchers studying the effects of parental depression have hypothesized that social learning processes, including both modeling and the effects of negative parenting style, contribute to the acquisition of dysfunctional cognitions (e.g., Goodman, 2007). For example, Garber and Flynn (2001) found significant associations between maternal depression history and adolescents' low self-worth, depressive attributional style, and hopelessness, and these associations, depending on type of cognition, were related to mothers' own negative cognitions, perceived parenting style, and negative life events. Measures of interpersonal cognitions reflecting dysfunctional attitudes about the self in relation to others, such as insecure attachment cognitions and excessive reassurance seeking, have also shown associations with youth depression in at-risk samples (e.g., Abela, Hankin, Haigh, Adams, Vinokuroff, & Trayhern, 2005; Hammen & Brennan, 2003).

Several approaches to the study of cognitive vulnerability emphasize the need for experimental methods that do not rely on self-report questionnaires that might be biased by current mood state. For instance, Taylor and Ingram (1999) administered a self-reference encoding task for recall of positive and negative self-descriptive words, following a mood induction procedure, to a sample of 8- to 12-year-old children of outpatient depressed women. As predicted, in the negative mood condition, high-risk children recalled higher levels of negative self-descriptors compared to the control mood condition, suggesting that dysfunctional cognitions may be latent in children at risk, potentially contributing to depression vulnerability. Joorman, Talbot, and Gotlib (2007) studied 9- to 14-year-old daughters of women with histories of recurrent major depression or no depression, who themselves had no history of depressive episodes. The investigators used a dot probe task to assess selective attention to emotional stimuli, following a mood induction task to prime negative schemas. Results supported the prediction that the daughters of depressed mothers would attend selectively to negative facial expressions, whereas daughters of never-depressed women attended selectively to positive faces.

MODELS OF INTERGENERATIONAL
TRANSMISSION OF DEPRESSION

The previous sections have briefly reviewed the status of several promising factors hypothesized to account for the association between parental depression and offspring disorder. As we have seen, these variables tend to overlap with each other, thus attesting to the complexity of mechanisms of intergenerational transmission. Increasingly, investigators in recent years have formulated models in which multiple determinants act in concert to predict youth outcomes (e.g., Garber & Martin, 2002; Hammen, 1991). An example of such a model was described by Goodman and Gotlib (1999) and more recently by Goodman (2007), in which the child's hereditary and neuroregulatory characteristics, along with exposure to the affect, cognitions, and behaviors of a depressed mother and stressors in the environment, are mechanisms that mediate the effects of maternal depression and predict vulnerabilities (psychological dysfunctions, including deficits in cognitive, affective, behavioral, and interpersonal skills) for the development of depression and other negative outcomes. Various additional features of the child's and mother's clinical attributes further affect the mother's depression, the mechanisms, and child outcomes. This model captures several features that are recognized as critical to comprehensive models, and that are increasingly incorporated into empirical attempts to account more fully for the intergenerational transmission of depression.

One essential feature of comprehensive models of mechanisms of the effects of parental depression is the idea that depression in the parent occurs in a context of adverse environmental and family factors, and that such factors—which may both result from and/or cause parental depression—may affect the development and functioning of the child, including risk for depression (e.g., see Cummings, DeArth-Pendley, Du Rocher, Schudlich, & Smith, 2001; Hammen, 1991; Rutter, 1990). A second feature is inclusion of multivariable and integrative components, making the assumption that single, main effects models are ill-suited to capturing the effects of multiple contributors. A third feature is an emphasis on transactional processes in which components and outcomes may have bidirectional effects, acknowledging not only the complexity of associations among variables but also the interactive and interrelated effects of depression, interpersonal (parental and marital) discord, biological variables, cognitions, and stressors. A fourth important feature of emerging models of intergenerational transmission of risk for depression is their developmental perspective, emphasizing the role of different variables and mechanisms of transmission of forms of maladjustment at different stages of development, as well as the cumulative consequences for subsequent development. Somewhat different models may therefore have different features, depending on the age of the child and the nature of outcomes evaluated.

Not surprisingly, complex models are very difficult to test, ideally requiring expensive longitudinal designs with sufficiently large numbers of participants to reveal effects of interactions, and sensitivity to detection of unique effects of correlated variables. They also require assessment of a wide array of variables, ideally assessed with multiple measures and informants. There are limited empirical tests based on complex models to date, with notable studies in progress but not yet completed. Several published examples are noted.

Hammen (1991) tested and found support for a model of depression outcomes based on children of depressed, bipolar, medically ill, and healthy mothers. Maternal clinical background was hypothesized to predict maternal chronic and contextual stress, and both variables were hypothesized to predict parenting quality, and children's stress and social competence; the latter in turn were the proximal predictors of depression. An expanded similar model, called an *interpersonal stress model of intergenerational transmission of depression*, was tested in a large community sample of adolescent offspring of depressed and nondepressed mothers (Hammen et al., 2004). Consistent with the emphasis on maladaptive interpersonal processes in depression, the model indicated that maternal depression is associated with maternal interpersonal discord with the spouse and others, with the adverse family context predicting both parent–child discord and the youth's own negative social life events. Parent–child problems also contributed to youth social competence, and also to youth stressful life events; the youth stress served as the proximal predictor of depression. The association between the mothers' (and grandmothers') depression and offspring depression was entirely mediated by the interpersonal and stress factors. Although having the advantage of a large sample, the model did not include biological factors and was based on a cross-sectional design. Further analyses with a longitudinal design are underway.

Several projects specifically examined "contextual" factors such as parenting/marital functioning and socioeconomic status, but did not examine processes by which such factors predict youth depression. Seifer and colleagues (1996) reported on a longitudinal study of 14-month-old infants of women with psychopathology (mostly major depression). The study included a variety of measures of family functioning, home environment, stress, and economic status, as well as clinical variables. The authors hypothesized that an aggregate measure of contextual risk based on presence–absence of 10 indicators of adverse conditions (e.g., presence of maternal mental illness, poor family functioning, father absence, low maternal education) would be stronger predictors of children's social competence than would clinical variables. The results supported their prediction that the multiple risk-indicator score was the strongest predictor, with modest contributions by a dimensional measure of parent mental illness, and virtually no predictive effect due to categorical diagnosis. The study suggests that nonspecific factors, such as maternal impairment of functioning and presence of general psychological distress, may be crucial factors in child maladjustment. A 16-month follow-up indicated that variability in severity of maternal depression symptoms was predictive of child and family functioning, even when diagnosis was controlled (Seifer, Dickstein Sameroff, Magee, & Hayden, 2001). Because the study included women with various diagnoses besides major depression (e.g., bipolar disorder, anxiety and substance use disorders), it is difficult to generalize results to other populations. Nevertheless, the research raises the important point that overreliance on diagnostic classification may obscure important patterns, and that it is important to characterize the clinical histories and impairment of parents in relation to outcomes.

Cicchetti and colleagues (1998) also evaluated the role of adverse contextual factors in the association between maternal depressive disorder, and toddlers' attachment status and behavior problems. The contextual factors were mother-reported perceived stress, parenting hassles, social support, marital quality, and level of conflict in the home—variables found to be significantly more negative for depressed compared to nondepressed women. Child attachment insecurity was significantly related to maternal depression status but not to scores on the contextual risk factor composite, whereas contextual risk, but not maternal depression, predicted mothers' reports of child total behavior problems. The latter effect appeared to be specific to externalizing symptomatology, with no significant association between contextual factors and internalizing symptoms. The authors speculated that negative contextual factors may contribute to inadequate limit setting and consistency in managing children's problem behaviors. Although the depressed sample was selected by Diagnostic Interview Schedule–based diagnoses of unipolar major depression, it was unclear whether both current and lifetime diagnoses were assessed—presumably, it was the latter—but current depression status was not defined.

Fergusson, Horwood, and Lynskey (1995) examined associations between adolescent and maternal depression symptoms, and measures of social and contextual disadvantage in a large-community birth-cohort sample. They found that girls', but not boys', depression was associated with maternal symptoms. Maternal depression symptoms no longer predicted girls' symptoms, once the significant effects of marital conflict, adverse family life events, and lower family social position were accounted for. Furthermore, longitudinal analyses suggested that mothers' depression symptoms when their children were ages 8–10 predicted increased family adversity 3 years later. Their model suggested that family adversity factors mediate the association between mothers' and daughters' depressive symptoms. There was no measure of parenting quality, and specific mechanisms accounting for girls' symptoms were not tested. The authors interpreted the results to suggest that the association between maternal depression and youth depression is spurious, but other investigators, as noted earlier, have cast similar results in a different light, arguing that the role of maternal depression is important, not spurious, and that negative effects on offspring are likely due to parenting behaviors and family qualities that are adversely affected by (as well as causes of) depression.

Boyle and Pickles (1997) used structural equation modeling to test the effects of contextual factors in a large community sample of children, examining maternal depression defined by self-reported symptoms. Like Fergusson and colleagues (1995), they found that maternal depression symptoms were related to girls', but not boys', depression symptoms. Unlike Fergusson et al., however, they found that controlling for contextual factors (economic disadvantage and a measure of family functioning) weakened but did not eliminate the association between mothers' and daughters' depression symptoms.

The complex models reviewed represent a variety of goals and methods, including general identification of factors that put children at risk, clarifying specific mechanisms of transmission of depression, testing whether context factors are "confounds" or whether parental depression effects are "spurious." The models also differed considerably in samples and methods of assessment of parental and youth depression, as well as variables included. These studies provide a starting point for both further empirical investigation and conceptual development to address the many unresolved issues of how and under what conditions parental depression leads to youth depression and other maladjustment.

FUTURE DIRECTIONS

After more than two decades of research on the intergenerational transmission of risk for depression, considerable advances have been made in validating children's risk for depression and other forms of maladjustment. Youth of depressed parents are not only more likely to experience depression but their depression also is commonly more severe and recurrent than depression occurring in offspring of never-depressed parents. However, research that has successfully described outcomes and illuminated some of the likely mechanisms of such risk has also succeeded in underscoring the complexity of the task of synthesizing results from diverse samples and designs, and of integrating variables from different domains into comprehensive models. As a result, there is a sense of knowing more and knowing less at the same time.

My goal in this review was to highlight methodological challenges to the field, emphasizing the need to conduct studies that examine the unfolding, in a developmental and causal sense, of processes prior to onset of depression in the offspring, and to consider the heterogeneity of depression. Depression is not only heterogeneous in its presentation, but it is also terribly common and often secondary to other conditions and life circumstances. The heterogeneity issue is enormously important, raising issues that range from the identification of possibly different models of depression risk, depending on features and subtypes of parental depression, to the very question of whether depression is unique and specific in its effects and, if so, which of its elements have negative effects on children. Different models, for example, may be needed for parental chronic depression compared to episodic depression with comorbid disorders of different kinds, or depression with marked anhedonia and low positivity, or irritability, or impaired interpersonal functioning. Even simpler questions require further study, such as the extent to which youth outcomes depend on status of parents' past depression independent of current depression.

A growing body of research has recently raised questions about possible moderators of the effects of parental depression, and further studies are needed to clarify the sometimes inconsistent findings. For example, issues concerning the gender of the depressed parent require additional research and are made more complex by considerations of timing and current status of depression, the coparent's status, and gender and age of the child. Nonrandom mating not only complicates genetic studies but also portends a cascade of social and environmental challenges that may be very difficult to disentangle to study the effects of depression. The age of the child studied and the developmental context are enormously complex matters that are made more challenging by the need to study developmentally salient outcomes that themselves may determine different outcomes as the child matures into young adulthood.

Another major goal of this review was both to highlight the relatively extensive evidence indicating that parental depression is associated with numerous correlated risk factors, and to point out the paucity of empirical studies of integrative models. Stress (including socioeconomic context), parenting, marital/family, cognitive, and biological factors have attracted considerable attention and merit additional focus on their effects and the processes by which they operate to result in maladaptive outcomes in youth. Much is to be gained from increasingly detailed studies of each of the risk factors, and perhaps other, yet to be revealed factors. At the same time, it is evident that the different risk factors interact, overlap, and co-occur, necessitating complex longitudinal studies. Such studies are essential to address not only the scientific aim of understanding the processes of transmission of depression from parents to children but also the practical goals of treatment and preventive intervention. Such complex, longitudinal, high-risk research is expensive and never as extensive or flexible as would be ideal. It is my hope, however, that the challenge will continue to be undertaken, so that many of the unresolved issues of the field identified in this chapter will yield answers in the next generation of research.

REFERENCES

Abela, J. R. Z., Hankin, B. L., Haigh, E. A. P., Adams, P., Vinokuroff, T., & Trayhern, L. (2005). Interpersonal vulnerability to depression in high-risk children: The role of insecure attachment and reassurance seeking. *Journal of Clinical Child and Adolescent Psychology, 34*(1), 182–192.

Anderson, C. A., & Hammen, C. L. (1993). Psychosocial outcomes of children of unipolar depressed, bipolar, medically ill, and normal women: A longitudinal study. *Journal of Consulting and Clinical Psychology, 61*(3), 448–454.

Ashman, S. B., Dawson, G., Panagiotides, H., Yamada, E., & Wilkinson, C. W. (2002). Stress hormone levels of children of depressed mothers. *Development and Psychopathology, 14*, 333–349.

Beardslee, W. R., Keller, M. B., Lavori, P. W., Staley, J. E., & Sacks, N. (1993). The impact of parental affective disorder on depression in offspring: A longitudinal follow-up in a nonreferred sample. *Journal of the American Academy of Child and Adolescent Psychiatry, 32*(4), 723–730.

Biederman, J., Petty, C., Hirshfeld Becker, D. R., Henin, A., Faraone, S. V., Dang, D., et al. (2006). A controlled longitudinal 5-year follow-up study of children at high and low risk for panic disorder and major depression. *Psychological Medicine, 36*, 1141–1152.

Billings, A. G., & Moos, R. (1983). Comparison of children of depressed and nondepressed parents: A social environmental perspective. *Journal of Abnormal Child Psychology, 11*, 483–486.

Billings, A. G., & Moos, R. H. (1985). Psychosocial processes of remission in unipolar depression: Comparing depressed patients with matched community controls. *Journal of Consulting and Clinical Psychology, 53*, 314–325.

Boyle, M. H., & Pickles, A. (1997). Maternal depressive symptoms and ratings of emotional disorder symptoms in children and adolescents. *Journal of Child Psychology and Psychiatry, and Allied Disciplines, 38*(8), 981–992.

Brennan, P. A., Hammen, C., Andersen, M. J., Bor, W., Najman, J. M., & Williams, G. M. (2000). Chronicity, severity, and timing of maternal depressive symptoms: Relationships with child outcomes at age 5. *Developmental Psychology, 36*(6), 759–766.

Brennan, P. A., Hammen, C., Katz, A. R., & Le Brocque, R. M. (2002). Maternal depression, paternal psychopathology, and adolescent diagnostic outcomes. *Journal of Consulting and Clinical Psychology, 70*(5), 1075–1085.

Campbell, S. B., Cohn, J. F., & Meyers, T. (1995). Depression in first-time mothers: Mother–infant interaction and depression chronicity. *Developmental Psychology, 31*(3), 349–357.

Cicchetti, D., Rogosch, F. A., & Toth, S. L. (1998). Maternal depressive disorder and contextual risk: Contributions to the development of attachment insecurity and behavior problems in toddlerhood. *Development and Psychopathology, 10*, 283–300.

Connell, A. M., & Goodman, S. H. (2002). The association between psychopathology in fathers versus mothers and children's internalizing and externalizing behavior problems: A meta-analysis. *Psychological Bulletin, 128*, 746–773.

Cummings, E. M., & Davies, P. T. (1994). Maternal depression and child development. *Journal of Child Psychology and Psychiatry, and Allied Disciplines, 35*, 73–112.

Cummings, E. M., DeArth-Pendley, G., Du Rocher Schudlich, T., & Smith, D. A. (2001). Parental depression and family functioning: Toward a process-oriented model of children's adjustment. In S. R. H. Beach (Ed.), *Marital and family processes in depression: A scientific foundation for clinical practice* (pp. 89–110). Washington, DC: American Psychological Association.

Cummings, E. M., Keller, P. S., & Davies, P. T. (2005). Towards a family process model of maternal and paternal depressive symptoms: Exploring multiple relations with child and family functioning. *Journal of Child Psychology and Psychiatry, 46*(5), 479–489.

Davies, P. T., Dumenci, L., & Windle, M. (1999). The interplay between maternal depressive symptoms and marital distress in the prediction of adolescent adjustment. *Journal of Marriage and the Family, 61*(1), 238–254.

Dawson, G., Ashman, S. B., Panagiotides, H., Hessl, D., Self, J., & Yamada, E., et al. (2003). Preschool outcomes of children of depressed mothers: Role of maternal behavior, contextual risk, and children's brain activity. *Child Development, 74*(4), 1158–1175.

Dawson, G., Frey, K., Panagiotides, H., Osterling, J., & Hessl, D. (1997). Infants of depressed mothers exhibit atypical frontal brain activity: A replication and extension of previous findings. *Journal of Child Psychology and Psychiatry, and Allied Disciplines, 38*(2), 179–186.

Dawson, G., Klinger, L. G., Panagiotides, H., Hill, D., & Spieker, S. (1992). Frontal lobe activity and affective behavior of infants of mothers with depressive symptoms. *Child Development, 63*(3), 725–737.

Dierker, L. C., Merikangas, K. R., & Szatmari, P. (1999). Influence of parental concordance for psychiatric disorders on psychopathology in offspring. *Journal of the American Academy of Child and Adolescent Psychiatry, 38*(3), 280–288.

Downey, G., & Coyne, J. C. (1990). Children of depressed parents: An integrative review. *Psychological Bulletin, 108*(1), 50–76.

Durbin, C. E., Klein, D. N., Hayden, E. P., Buckley, M. E., & Moerk, K. C. (2005). Temperamental emotionality in preschoolers and parental mood disorders. *Journal of Abnormal Psychology, 114*, 28–37.

Essex, M. J., Klein, M. H., Cho, E., & Kalin, N. H. (2002). Maternal stress beginning in infancy may sensitize children to later stress exposure: Effects on cortisol and behavior. *Biological Psychiatry, 52*, 776–784.

Fergusson, D. M., Horwood, L. J., & Lynskey, M. T. (1995). Maternal depressive symptoms and depressive symptoms in adolescents. *Journal of Child Psychology and Psychiatry, and Allied Disciplines, 36*(7), 1161–1178.

Field, T., Fox, N. A., Pickens, J., & Nawrocki, T. (1995). Relative right frontal EEG activation in 3- to 6-month-old infants of "depressed" mothers. *Developmental Psychology, 31*(3), 358–363.

Field, T., Lang, C., Martinez, A., Yando, R., Pickens, J., & Bendell, D. (1996). Preschool follow-up of infants of dysphoric mothers. *Journal of Clinical Child Psychology, 25*(3), 272–279.

Forbes, E. E., Shaw, D. S., Fox, N. A., Cohn, J. F., Silk, J. S., & Kovacs, M. (2006). Maternal depression, child frontal asymmetry, and child affective behavior as factors in child behavior problems. *Journal of Child Psychology and Psychiatry, and Allied Disciplines, 47*(1), 79–87.

Frye, A. A., & Garber, J. (2005). The relations among maternal depression, maternal criticism, and adolescents' externalizing and internalizing symptoms. *Journal of Abnormal Child Psychology, 33*(1), 1–11.

Garber, J., & Flynn, C. (2001). Predictors of depressive cognitions in young adolescents. *Cognitive Therapy and Research, 25,* 353–376.

Garber, J., & Martin, N. C. (2002). Negative cognitions in offspring of depressed parents: Mechanisms of risk. In S. H. Goodman & I. H. Gotlib (Eds.), *Children of depressed parents: Mechanisms of risk and implications for treatment* (pp. 121–153). Washington, DC: American Psychological Association.

Goodman, S. H. (2007). Depression in mothers. *Annual Review of Clinical Psychology, 3,* 107–135.

Goodman, S. H., & Gotlib, I. H. (1999). Risk for psychopathology in the children of depressed mothers: A developmental model for understanding mechanisms of transmission. *Psychological Review, 106,* 458–490.

Gotlib, I. H., & Hammen, C. L. (1992). *Psychological aspects of depression: Toward a cognitive–interpersonal integration.* Oxford, UK: Wiley.

Gotlib, I. H., Joormann, J., Minor, K. L., & Hallmayer, J. (2008). HPA-axis reactivity may underlie the associations among the 5-HTTLPR polymorphism, stress, and risk for depression. *Biological Psychiatry, 63,* 847–851.

Halligan, S. L., Murray, L., Martins, C., & Cooper, P. J. (2007). Maternal depression and psychiatric outcomes in adolescent offspring: A 13-year longitudinal study. *Journal of Affective Disorders, 9,* 145–154.

Hammen, C. (1991). Generation of stress in the course of unipolar depression. *Journal of Abnormal Psychology, 100*(4), 555–561.

Hammen, C. (1992). Cognition, life stress, and interpersonal approaches to a developmental psychopathology model of depression. *Development and Psychopathology, 4,* 189–206.

Hammen, C. (2002). The context of stress in families of children with depressed parents. In S. Goodman & I. Gotlib (Eds.), *Children of depressed parents: Mechanisms of risk and implications for treatment* (pp. 175–199). Washington, DC: American Psychological Association.

Hammen, C., Adrian, C., Gordon, D., Burge, D., Jaenicke, C., & Hiroto, D. (1987). Children of depressed mothers: Maternal strain and symptom predictors of dysfunction. *Journal of Abnormal Psychology, 96*(3), 190–198.

Hammen, C., & Brennan, C. (2002). Interpersonal dysfunction in depressed women: Impairments independent of depressive symptoms. *Journal of Affective Disorders, 72,* 145–156.

Hammen, C., Brennan, P., & Keenan-Miller, D. (in press). Patterns of adolescent depression to age 20: The role of maternal depression and youth interpersonal dysfunction. *Journal of Abnormal Child Psychology.*

Hammen, C., Brennan, P., Keenan-Miller, D., & Herr, N. (2008). Early onset recurrent subtype of adolescent depression: Clinical and psychosocial correlates. *Journal of Child Psychology and Psychiatry, and Allied Disciplines, 49,* 440–443.

Hammen, C., & Brennan, P. A. (2001). Depressed adolescents of depressed and nondepressed mothers: Tests of an interpersonal impairment hypothesis. *Journal of Consulting and Clinical Psychology, 69*(2), 284–294.

Hammen, C., & Brennan, P. A. (2003). Severity, chronicity, and timing of maternal depression and risk for adolescent offspring diagnoses in a community sample. *Archives of General Psychiatry, 60,* 253–258.

Hammen, C., Burge, D., Burney, E., & Adrian, C. (1990). Longitudinal study of diagnoses in children of women with unipolar and bipolar affective disorder. *Archives of General Psychiatry, 47*(12), 1112–1117.

Hammen, C., Shih, J., Altman, T., & Brennan, P. (2003). Interpersonal impairment and the prediction of depressive symptoms in children of depressed and nondepressed mothers. *Journal of the Academy of Child and Adolescent Psychiatry, 42,* 571–577.

Hammen, C., Shih, J. H., & Brennan, P. A. (2004). Intergenerational transmission of depression: Test of an interpersonal stress model in a community sample. *Journal of Consulting and Clinical Psychology, 72,* 511–522.

Joormann, J., Eugene, F., & Gotlib, I. (in press). Parental depression: Impact on children and mechanisms underlying transmission of risk. In S. Nolen-Hoeksema & L. Hilt (Eds.), *Handbook of adolescent depression.* Mahwah, NJ: Erlbaum.

Joormann, J., Talbot, L., & Gotlib, I. H. (2007). Biased processing of emotional information in girls at risk for depression. *Journal of Abnormal Psychology*, 116(1), 135–143.

Kane, P., & Garber, J. (2004). The relations among depression in fathers, children's psychopathology, and father–child conflict: A meta-analysis. *Clinical Psychology Review*, 24, 339–360.

Keenan-Miller, D., Hammen, C., & Brennan, P. (2007). Adolescent psychosocial risk factors for severe intimate partner violence in young adulthood. *Journal of Consulting and Clinical Psychology*, 75, 456–463.

Kim-Cohen, J., Moffitt, T. E., Taylor, A., Pawlby, S. J., & Caspi, A. (2005). Maternal depression and children's antisocial behavior: Nature and nurture effects. *Archives of General Psychiatry*, 62(2), 173–181.

Klein, D. N., Lewinsohn, P. M., Rohde, P., Seeley, J. R., & Durbin, C. E. (2002). Clinical features of major depressive disorder in adolescents and their relatives: Impact on familial aggregation, implications for phenotype definition, and specificity of transmission. *Journal of Abnormal Psychology*, 111(1), 98–106.

Klein, D. N., Lewinsohn, P. M., Rohde, P., Seeley, J. R., & Olino, T. M. (2005). Psychopathology in the adolescent and young adult offspring of a community sample of mothers and fathers with major depression. *Psychological Medicine*, 35, 353–365.

Lewinsohn, P. M., Olino, T. M., & Klein, D. N. (2005). Psychosocial impairment in offspring of depressed parents. *Psychological Medicine*, 35(10), 1493–1503.

Lieb, R., Isensee, B., Hofler, M., Pfister, H., & Wittchen, H. U. (2002). Parental major depression and the risk of depression and other mental disorders in offspring: A prospective–longitudinal community study. *Archives of General Psychiatry*, 59, 365–374.

Lovejoy, M. C., Graczyk, P. A., O'Hare, E., & Neuman, G. (2000). Maternal depression and parenting behavior: A meta-analytic review. *Clinical Psychology Review*, 20, 561–592.

Lyons-Ruth, K., Zoll, D., Connell, D., & Grunebaum, H. U. (1986). The depressed mother and her one-year-old infant: Environment, interaction, attachment, and infant development. *New Directions for Child Development*, 34, 61–82.

Martins, C., & Gaffan, E. A. (2000). Effects of early maternal depression on patterns of infant–mother attachment: A meta-analytic investigation. *Journal of Child Psychology and Psychiatry, and Allied Disciplines*, 41, 737–746.

Mathews, C. A., & Reus, V. I. (2001). Assortative mating in the affective disorders: A systematic review and meta-analysis. *Comprehensive Psychiatry*, 42, 257–262.

Murray, L., Sinclair, D., Cooper, P., Ducournau, P., & Turner, P. (1999). The socioemotional development of 5-year-old children of postnatally depressed mothers. *Journal of Child Psychology and Psychiatry, and Allied Disciplines*, 40, 1259–1271.

Nelson, D. R., Hammen, C., Brennan, P. A., & Ullman, J. B. (2003). The impact of maternal depression on adolescent adjustment: The role of expressed emotion. *Journal of Consulting and Clinical Psychology*, 71, 935–944.

NICHD, Early Child Care Research Network. (1999). Chronicity of maternal depressive symptoms, maternal sensitivity, and child functioning at 36 months. *Developmental Psychology*, 35(5), 1297–1310.

Nomura, Y., Warner, V., & Wickramaratne, P. (2001). Parents concordant for major depressive disorder and the effect of psychopathology in offspring. *Psychological Medicine*, 31(7), 1211–1222.

Pilowsky, D. J., Wickramaratne, P. J., Rush, A. J., Hughes, C. W., Garber, J., Malloy, E., et al. (2006). Children of currently depressed mothers: A STAR*D ancillary study. *Journal of Clinical Psychiatry*, 67, 126–136.

Rohde, P., Lewinsohn, P. M., Klein, D. N., & Seeley, J. R. (2005). Association of parental depression with psychiatric course from adolescence to young adulthood among formerly depressed individuals. *Journal of Abnormal Psychology*, 114, 409–420.

Rutter, M. (1990). Commentary: Some focus and process considerations regarding effects of parental depression on children. *Developmental Psychology*, 26(1), 60–67.

Schreier, A., Höfler, M., Wittchen, H., & Lieb, R. (2006). Clinical characteristics of major depressive disorder run in families: A community study of 933 mothers and their children. *Journal of Psychiatric Research*, 40(4), 283–292.

Seifer, R., Dickstein, S., Sameroff, A. J., Magee, K. D., & Hayden, L. C. (2001). Infant mental health and variability of parental depression symptoms. *Journal of the American Academy of Child and Adolescent Psychiatry, 40*(12), 1375–1382.

Seifer, R., Sameroff, A. J., Dickstein, S., Keitner, G., & Miller, I. (1996). Parental psychopathology, multiple contextual risks, and one-year outcomes in children. *Journal of Clinical Child Psychology, 25*(4), 423–435.

Shankman, S. A., Tenke, C. E., Bruder, G. E., Durbin, C. E., Hayden, E. P., & Klein, D. N. (2005). Low positive emotionality in young children: Association with EEG asymmetry. *Development and Psychopathology, 17*(1), 85–98.

Taylor, L., & Ingram, R. E. (1999). Cognitive reactivity and depressotypic information processing in children of depressed mothers. *Journal of Abnormal Psychology, 108*, 202–208.

Teti, D. M., Gelfand, D. M., Messinger, D. S., & Isabella, R. (1995). Maternal depression and the quality of early attachment: An examination of infants, preschoolers, and their mothers. *Developmental Psychology, 31*(3), 364–376.

Timko, C., Cronkite, R. C., Berg, E. A., & Moos, R. H. (2002). Children of parents with unipolar depression: A comparison of stably remitted, partially remitted, and nonremitted parents and nondepressed controls. *Child Psychiatry and Human Development, 32*, 165–185.

Tomarken, A. J., Dichter, G. S., Garber, J., & Simien, C. (2004). Resting frontal brain activity: Linkages to maternal depression and socio-economic status among adolescents. *Biological Psychology, 67*, 77–102.

Weissman, M. M., Warner, V., Wickramaratne, P., Moreau, D., & Olfson, M. (1997). Offspring of depressed parents: 10 years later. *Archives of General Psychiatry, 54*(10), 932–940.

Weissman, M. M., Wickramaratne, P., Nomura, Y., Warner, V., Pilowsky, D., & Verdeli, H. (2006). Offspring of depressed parents: 20 years later. *American Journal of Psychiatry, 163*, 1001–1008.

Williamson, D., Birmaher, B., Axelson, D., Ryan, N., & Dahl, R. (2004). First episode of depression in children at low and high familial risk for depression. *Journal of the American Academy of Child Psychiatry, 43*, 291–297.

CHAPTER 13

Cognitive Aspects of Depression

Jutta Joormann

Ⓞne of the most important topics in depression research is the question of vulnerability versus resilience. How can we explain why some people respond to what we would consider to be minor stressors with increasingly negative affect that can spiral into a full-blown depressive episode, whereas others seem never to become depressed, even when they face major adversity? Cognitive theories of depression propose that people's thoughts, inferences, attitudes, and interpretations, and the way in which they attend to and recall these events determine their emotional responses. Consequently, cognitions play a crucial role in how much people are affected by negative experiences and determine whether these events will be followed by quick recovery or by recurring depressive episodes. These models, therefore, make the important assumption that investigating the content of cognition and the nature of cognitive processes in depression is crucial for our understanding of the onset and maintenance of this disorder. Indeed, most cognitive theories of depression propose vulnerability–stress hypotheses, which posit that the onset and recurrence of this disorder is due to the interaction of a psychological vulnerability (e.g., certain cognitions or particular ways of processing information) and a precipitating stressor (e.g., a life event or some other environmental factor).

Studies investigating the interaction of cognition and emotion have a long tradition in depression research. Early studies focused primarily on demonstrating that the thought contents of depressed and nondepressed people differ, and that depressed individuals exhibit cognitive deficits and biased processing of emotional material. These studies employed a variety of self-report measures and experimental tasks, and generally provided consistent evidence that depression is characterized by negative, automatic thoughts about the self, the future, and the world (Ingram, Miranda, & Segal, 1998; Mathews & MacLeod, 2005). Indeed, one of the most successful interventions for depression, cognitive-behavioral therapy, focuses on modifying biased interpretations and dysfunctional automatic thoughts (Beck, 1976). Similarly, other theorists highlight cognitive biases as possible vulnerability markers for depression (e.g., Ingram et al., 1998). Fewer studies, however, have explicitly tested the underlying vulnerability–stress model or examined how deficits in recall, attentional biases toward negative material, and mood-congruent memory are related to each other and, more importantly, to the hallmark feature of depression—sustained negative affect.

In this chapter I provide a brief review of the literature on cognition in unipolar depression (see Johnson, Cuellar, & Miller, Chapter 7, this volume, for a discussion of cognitive aspects of bipolar disorder and of differences in cognition between unipolar and bipolar depression). I discuss the major models for explaining the role of cognition in this disorder and review evidence indicating that depression is characterized by general cognitive deficits (e.g., concentration difficulties, working memory impairments) and by preferential processing of negative material. My primary goal in this chapter, however, is to summarize recent research focusing on mechanisms that might underlie depression-related changes in cognitive content and processing and, more importantly, on the consequence of these changes for depressive affect. Recent models of the interaction of cognition and emotion underscore the critical role that cognitive processes play in the regulation of emotion and mood (e.g., Larsen, 2000). Indeed, in recent years, depression has been conceptualized as a disorder of emotion dysregulation. Theorists have suggested that it is not so much an abnormal initial response to a stressor, such as a stressful life event, that characterizes individuals who are vulnerable to depression; rather, it is an inability to regulate the duration and intensity of the ensuing negative affect (e.g., Teasdale, 1988).

Numerous studies demonstrate, for example, that people who respond to negative life events and negative mood states with rumination are prone to experience recurrent depressive episodes (e.g., Nolen-Hoeksema, 2000; Nolen-Hoeksema, Wisco, & Lyubomirsky, in press). But why do people ruminate? Negative mood is generally associated with, or in part comprises, the activation of mood-congruent representations in working memory (e.g., Siemer, 2005). Thus, negative mood has been found to be related to more frequent negative thoughts, to selective attention to negative stimuli, and to greater accessibility of negative memories (Blaney, 1986; Mathews & MacLeod, 2005). These changes in cognition are likely related to the way in which people respond to negative affect; indeed, theorists have posited that maladaptive responses such as rumination maintain negative mood (Nolen-Hoeksema et al., in press). This research has also demonstrated, however, that negative mood alone does not necessarily lead to prolonged rumination. In fact, changes in cognition due to negative mood are usually transient, and mood-congruent cognitions are often replaced quite quickly by thoughts and memories that serve to regulate and repair the mood state (e.g., Rusting & DeHart, 2000). A critical question, therefore, is why, in response to negative mood, do some people initiate a self-defeating cycle of increasingly negative ruminative thinking and intensifying negative affect? Given that sustained negative affect and anhedonia are the defining symptoms of a major depressive episode, it is imperative that we identify the processes that lead to rumination, and that hinder effective mood and emotion regulation in depression.

COGNITIVE MODELS OF DEPRESSION

Depressive Schemas and Attributional Style

Research on cognition in depression has been guided primarily by three models: the *helplessness model*, which subsequently was refined to take into account attributional style and is now referred to as the *hopelessness model* (Abramson, Metalsky, & Alloy, 1989; Alloy,

Abramson, Walshaw, & Neeren, 2006); Beck's (1976) *schema theory of depression*; and Bower's (1981) *network theory of cognition and emotion.* The helplessness/hopelessness model of depression has its roots in Seligman's (1975) concept of *learned helplessness*, which states that expectancies about the lack of control over events lead to depressive episodes. This model has been refined by Abramson and colleagues (1989), who proposed that *hopelessness* (i.e., the expectation that highly desired outcomes will not occur, or that highly aversive outcomes are certain) is a proximal sufficient cause of depressive symptoms. Hopelessness is the consequence of attributing negative life events to stable and global causes. Moreover, attributions of these events to internal causes lead to lowered self-esteem and feelings of worthlessness, which further strengthen the symptoms of hopelessness depression. Abramson and colleagues point out that the hopelessness model may not apply to all forms of depression; rather, it may represent an important subtype of depressive disorders (e.g., Alloy et al., 2006).

Beck (1976) postulates that existing memory representations, or *schemas,* lead individuals to filter stimuli from the environment, such that their attention is directed toward information that is congruent with their schemas. Beck theorizes that the schemas of depressed persons include themes of loss, separation, failure, worthlessness, and rejection; consequently, depressed individuals exhibit a systematic bias in their processing of environmental stimuli or information that is relevant to these themes. Because of this bias, depressed people attend selectively to negative stimuli in their environment, and interpret neutral and ambiguous stimuli in a schema-congruent way. Moreover, dysfunctional schema and processing biases are presumed to endure beyond the depressive episode, representing stable vulnerability factors for depression onset and recurrence. When the dysfunctional schemas are activated by stressors, specific negative cognitions are generated that take the form of automatic thoughts and revolve around pessimistic views about the self, the world, and the future—the cognitive triad. Schemas and biases can remain latent, which means that they are less accessible and do not influence cognition and affect as long as they are not activated by a stressful event. Once activated, however, schema-influenced negative thoughts and processing biases initiate and maintain depressed mood through a vicious cycle of increasingly negative thinking and negative affect. In more recent forms of this model, Beck differentiates between schemas that involve social relationships (*sociotropy*) and schemas that concern achievement (*autonomy*; Beck, Epstein, & Harrison, 1983). Finally, Beck's *cognitive specificity hypothesis* posits that these schemas are likely to be activated by "congruent" life events, thereby starting the vicious cycle of negative automatic thoughts, processing biases, and depressed mood.

Bower (1981) similarly postulates that *associative networks* lead to cognitive biases in depressed individuals. These associative networks comprise numerous nodes, each containing specific semantic representations that can be activated by environmental stimuli. The activation of any one node causes the partial activation, or *priming,* of all the other nodes within its associative network through a process of *spreading activation.* Consequently, the representations of the primed nodes require less activation for access to occur than do the representations of nonprimed nodes, resulting in a processing advantage for stimuli that are related to these primed representations. Like Beck, Bower also postulates that associative networks are stable constructs; the attentional biases of depressed individuals are expected to endure beyond the depressive episode. Even though Bower's model is a general model of the interaction of cognition and emotion, and not specifically a model of depression, habitually lowered thresholds for activation or habitually strengthened connections between nodes nevertheless might be used to explain vulnerability to depression. Indeed, Ingram (1984) and Teasdale (1988) both have drawn on Bower's theory in explaining the onset, maintenance, and recurrence of depressive disorders.

In summary, while the hopelessness model makes assumptions about the content of depressive cognition, or what Ingram and colleagues (1998) termed *cognitive products*, Beck and Bower add assumptions about cognitive processes. Taken together, Beck and Bower postulate that depressed individuals are characterized by cognitive biases in all aspects of information processing, including perception, attention, memory, and reasoning, all of which serve to facilitate the processing of negatively valenced information. Moreover, because these biases are hypothesized to endure beyond discrete episodes of depression, they should also characterize the functioning of individuals who, although not currently depressed, are vulnerable to experiencing episodes of depression.

Resource Allocation and Affective Interference

The cognitive theories of depression discussed thus far focus on only one aspect of depressive cognition: preferential processing of mood-congruent stimuli. Two distinct patterns of cognitive correlates of depression and dysphoria, however, are frequently reported: Although depressed people report concentration difficulties and impairments in recalling neutral stimuli (Burt, Zembar, & Niederehe, 1995), they easily concentrate on negative, self-focused thoughts and exhibit enhanced recall of mood-congruent memories (Mathews & MacLeod, 2005). Thus, whereas some researchers focus on examining "cognitive symptoms" of depression, such as concentration difficulties, distractibility, attention deficits, and impaired recall of information independent of valence, other researchers have focused on examining biased processing of emotional information. Few attempts have been made to integrate the findings obtained in these separate lines of research (Ellis & Ashbrook, 1988; Hertel, 2004; Williams, Watts, MacLeod, & Mathews, 1997).

The *resource allocation hypothesis* postulates that, because their cognitive capacity is reduced, depressed individuals have deficits in remembering and in engaging in other effortful cognitive procedures (e.g., Ellis & Ashbrook, 1988). The general assumption is that there is a limit on the amount of resources available for cognitive operations, and that depression either occupies or functionally reduces these resources (Ellis & Ashbrook, 1988). Thus, deficits should become evident in effortful tasks and should be detectable in effortful, resource-demanding components of memory tasks, but not in automatic aspects of these tasks. Similarly, the *affective interference hypothesis* posits that because depressed persons are preoccupied with the processing of emotional material, their performance on other tasks will not be impaired if they need to process emotional aspects of stimuli, but it will suffer if they have to ignore the emotional aspects and respond to other aspects of the material (Siegle, Ingram, & Matt, 2002). For example, if depressed individuals have to make valence judgments about words, their tendency to prioritize the processing of emotional material will aid them. If, however, they are instructed to ignore the emotional content of words while making a lexical decision judgment, their processing priorities will interfere, and their performance will be impaired (Siegle et al., 2002).

Inhibition and Cognitive Control

One of the most troubling aspects of depression is the frequent occurrence of ruminative, unintentional, and often uncontrollable negative thoughts and memories. Rumination has been found to increase the risk of onset of depression, to maintain depressive episodes, and to increase the risk of recurrence. But why do people ruminate? Inhibition, working memory, and cognitive control are important concepts in understanding the dysfunctional cognitive processes that may underlie sustained processing of negative information and rumination in depression. *Working memory* is commonly described as a system for the active maintenance and manipulation of information, and for the control of attention (Baddeley & Hitch, 1994). An important characteristic of working memory, and one that differentiates it from long-term memory, is its capacity-limited focus of attention (see Cowan, 1995). Given this capacity limitation, executive control processes and, in particular, cognitive inhibition, are critical for updating working memory content efficiently and are therefore essential for engaging in goal-directed planning and maintaining a coherent stream of thought. Thus, Hasher and Zacks (1988) propose that the efficient functioning of working memory depends on inhibitory processes that both limit the access of information into working memory and update its contents by removing information that is no longer relevant.

What happens when these processes malfunction? As Hasher and Zacks (1988) have pointed out, too much irrelevant information gets into working memory. As a consequence, links between relevant and irrelevant information are created and stored in long-term memory, setting the stage for slow and less accurate retrieval of relevant information and enhanced retrieval of irrelevant information. In addition, irrelevant information in working memory is sustained longer. Thus, individuals who exhibit an inhibitory deficit are easily distracted by irrelevant information and thoughts. As the central function of working memory, impaired inhibitory processes might have severe cognitive and emotional consequences, including rumination. If changes in mood are in fact associated with activations of mood-congruent material in working memory, the ability to control the contents of working memory might play an important role in the development of rumination and, therefore, in recovery from negative mood.

Indeed, Hertel (2004) has proposed that depression is characterized by reduced cognitive control that impairs the override of automatic, prepotent response tendencies. Hertel has further proposed that rumination and negative, self-focused thoughts are prepotent responses for depressed individuals. Overriding prepotent responses and focusing attention on the demands of the current task are roles of inhibitory processes and cognitive control. Thus, dysfunction in inhibitory processes in depression might be responsible for the lack of self-controlled attention to the task at hand. In a similar model, Beevers (2005) proposed that cognitive vulnerability occurs when negatively biased automatic processing is not corrected by reflective processing. Considered collectively, these models propose that individuals who exhibit a reduced ability to exert cognitive control are vulnerable to rumination and to experiencing depressive episodes. Therefore, it appears that the constructs of cognitive control and inhibition are important in explaining general cognitive deficits in depression and preferential processing of depression-relevant material. Cognitive control may also play an important role in emotion regulation more broadly, which is discussed below (e.g., Joormann, Yoon, & Zetsche, 2007).

EMPIRICAL TESTS OF COGNITIVE MODELS OF DEPRESSION

Depressive Cognition: Dysfunctional Attitudes and Attributional Style

Researchers investigating the role of dysfunctional attitudes and attributional style have relied almost exclusively on self-report measures, specifically, the Dysfunctional Attitudes

Scale (DAS) and the Cognitive Styles Questionnaire (CSQ). The DAS is a 40-item self-report measure that assesses maladaptive cognitions such as perfectionist standards and concerns about being evaluated by others (Weissman & Beck, 1978). The CSQ is a modified version of the Attributional Styles Questionnaire (ASQ; Peterson et al., 1982) that assesses the tendency to respond to positive and negative events with internal, stable, and global attributions (Alloy et al., 2000). Numerous cross-sectional studies in which these and other questionnaires were administered to depressed and nondepressed participants have reported associations among dysfunctional attitudes, attributional styles, and other negative cognitions in currently depressed adults (Alloy, Abramson, & Francis, 1999; Fresco, Alloy, & Reilly-Harrington, 2006), adolescents, and children (for a recent review, see Ingram, Nelson, Steidtmann, & Bistricky, 2007).

These findings are interesting; given that negative thinking is a defining symptom of depressive episodes, however, it is impossible to determine whether depressed participants endorse these cognitions because they are currently depressed, or whether these cognitions precipitate the onset of depression and play a role in increasing people's vulnerability (Barnett & Gotlib, 1988; Haaga, Dyck, & Ernst, 1991). To investigate this important question, a number of studies have used remission designs (for a review, see Ingram et al., 1998; Ingram & Siegle, Chapter 4, this volume). The reasoning behind these designs is that if cognitions are not only symptoms of depression but also vulnerability factors, they should remain stable beyond the depressive episode; any cognitive pattern that is not found in remitted depressed participants is less likely to be a vulnerability factor for this disorder. Remission designs have produced mixed findings. In a review of these studies, for example, Haaga and colleagues (1991) stated that there is only limited evidence that depressive cognitions remain stable (see also Ingram et al., 1998; Just, Abramson, & Alloy, 2001). As previously discussed, however, vulnerability–stress models hypothesize that prior activation of latent dysfunctional schemas is necessary before negative cognitions can be observed. Therefore, subsequent research on cognitive reactivity has used mood inductions and has attempted to heighten self-focus, self-relevance, and other priming designs to activate negative schemas before assessing dysfunctional cognitions in remitted participants. This research has painted a more positive picture (for a recent review, see Scher, Ingram, & Segal, 2005). Gemar, Segal, Sagrati, and Kennedy (2001), for example, reported that, compared to never-depressed participants, formerly depressed participants demonstrate a greater change in dysfunctional attitudes after a negative mood induction (see also Miranda, Persons, & Byers, 1990). It should be noted, though, that other studies did not find a relation between DAS scores and depression history, even when priming procedures were employed (e.g., Brosse, Craighead, & Craighead, 1999). Haeffel and colleagues (2005) have pointed out that some of the negative findings in previous remission studies might be due to design features (e.g., small samples and assessment of dysfunctional attitudes and attributional style directly after a treatment that focused on modifying these cognitions). These authors, therefore, used a remission design, in which they recruited a large sample of remitted participants but excluded participants who had remitted in response to a treatment that targeted the negative cognitions. Haeffel and colleagues reported that CSQ scores, but not DAS scores, were higher in the remitted-depressed than in the control participants. Remission designs have also been criticized because they cannot differentiate between vulnerability factors and consequences or "scars" of having experienced a past depressive episode (Just et al., 2001; Lewinsohn, Steinmetz, Larson, & Franklin, 1981).

More promising are longitudinal studies. Few researchers have examined the ability of self-report measures of cognitive functioning to predict recovery and improvements in symptom severity. Interestingly, whereas some investigators have found self-reported cognitions to predict symptomatic improvement (e.g., Lewinsohn, Rohde, Seeley, Klein, & Gotlib, 2000), others have not (e.g., Lara, Klein, & Kasch, 2000). Other prospective studies have investigated the prediction of depression onset. Brown, Hammen, Craske, and Wickens (1995), for example, reported that DAS scores interacted with exam performance to predict depressive symptoms. Joiner, Metalsky, Lew, and Klocek (1999) and Hankin, Abramson, Miller, and Haeffel (2004) found that dysfunctional attitudes interacted with the discrepancy between acceptable and actual exam scores to predict depressive symptoms after receipt of the grade. Gibb, Beevers, Andover, and Holleran (2006) reported that negative attributional style in interaction with negative events predicted subsequent depressive symptoms (see also Fresco et al., 2006; Gibb & Alloy, 2006). Similarly, Lewinsohn, Joiner, and Rohde (2001) reported that dysfunctional attitudes interacted with stress to predict onset of a depressive episode during a 1-year interval in high school students.

Recently, longitudinal studies have focused on high-risk samples. These studies are particularly promising when they assess participants before the first onset of psychopathology. There are different ways of identifying someone as "high-risk for depression." High-risk samples can be relatives of depressed individuals or participants who are at high risk because of other factors (e.g., a certain socioeconomic status or cognitive profile). Abela and Skitch (2007), for example, found an interaction between daily hassles and DAS scores in children at high risk for depression due to their parent's psychopathology. Alloy and colleagues (2006) recruited never-depressed college students who demonstrated depressive cognitive styles, defined by elevated scores on the DAS and the CSQ. In a 2.5-year follow-up, these investigators found support for Beck's model and for the hopelessness model. Nondepressed individuals who exhibited negative attributional styles and dysfunctional attitudes were more likely than control participants who scored low on measures of cognitive vulnerability to experience first onsets of depression. Indeed, the risk of depression in the high-risk group was about seven times higher than it was in the low-risk group (Alloy et al., 2006). Therefore, longitudinal studies largely support the formulation that cognitive factors interact with acute stressors to play an important role in the onset, maintenance, and recurrence of depressive episodes.

Cognitive Deficits and Processing Biases in Depression

Cognitive Deficits

Depressed people often complain about concentration difficulties (Watts & Sharrock, 1985); indeed, "difficulty concentrating" is a symptom of a major depressive episode in the fourth edition of the *Diagnostic and Statistical Manual of Mental Disorders* (DSM-IV; American Psychiatric Association, 1994). In addition, a large literature strongly suggests that depressed individuals are impaired in their recall of nonemotional information (for reviews, see Burt et al., 1995; Mathews & MacLeod, 2005). In the frequently cited meta-analysis by Burt and colleagues (1995), however, memory impairments were reported more consistently for inpatients than for outpatients. Moreover, these kinds of memory impairments were also reported in other psychological disorders. Burt et al. proposed, therefore, that memory deficits are associated with psychopathology in general rather than with a specific disorder. Moreover, in a series of studies, Hertel (1998; Hertel & Rude, 1991) presented evidence indicating that depression-related impairments are not observed in all components of memory, but are found primarily in free recall tasks and in controlled aspects of recognition.

Overall, studies thus far provide evidence that depression is associated with greater memory impairment in contexts in which (1) attention is not constrained by the task (e.g., Hertel & Rude, 1991); (2) increased cognitive effort is required (see review by Hartlage, Alloy, Vazquez, & Dykman, 1993); and (3) attention is easily allocated to personal concerns and other thoughts that are irrelevant to the task (Ellis & Ashbrook, 1988). Interestingly, Hertel and Rude (1991) were able to eliminate a depressive deficit by providing instructions that focused participants on the task and did not allow task-irrelevant thoughts. Hertel (1998) also reported that students with dysphoria who had to wait in an unconstrained situation (without being given any instructions regarding what to do during the waiting period) and students with dysphoria who were instructed to rate self-focused material designed to induce rumination showed comparable recall deficits. In contrast, no deficit was found for students with dysphoria who were told what to do during the waiting period (rating self-irrelevant and task-irrelevant material).

These results suggest that, at least with respect to memory deficits, depressed people might have the ability to perform at the level of nondepressed people in structured situations but have problems doing this on their own initiative in unconstrained situations (Hertel, 2004). Moreover, these results suggest that eliminating the opportunity to ruminate also eliminated the impairment in the memory task, a result that might explain why unconstrained tasks lead to impaired performance in the depressed group. Unconstrained situations call for cognitive flexibility and goal-oriented behavior, and require cognitive control, that is, focal attention to relevant stimuli, as well as inhibition of irrelevant material (Hertel, 2004). Thus, these performance deficits in the recall of neutral information do not seem to reflect a generalized deficit or a lack of resources on the part of depressed individuals but might be due instead to depression-related inhibitory dysfunctions in the processing of irrelevant information.

Other studies have investigated depression-related deficits in attention tasks and in tasks that assess executive functioning. Channon, Baker, and Robertson (1993) found few differences between depressed and nondepressed participants on a variety of working memory tasks (i.e., only on the backward digit span; see also Barch, Sheline, Csernansky, & Snyder, 2003). Recently, Rose and Ebmeier (2006) reported that depressed patients were slower and less accurate than controls on an n-back task, but that task difficulty did not influence this effect. These findings replicate results reported by Harvey and colleagues (2004), who reported further that performance deficit on the n-back task was correlated with number of hospitalizations and longitudinal course of the disorder. Importantly, Harvey and colleagues did not find differences between their depressed and nondepressed groups on a number of other tasks assessing working memory functioning, including a digit span. Consistent with these findings, Egeland and colleagues (2003) concluded from the results of their study that reduced performance on working memory tasks in depression is due not to a specific deficit in executive functioning, but to a nonspecific speed reduction and a loss of vigilance that is consistent with a lack of effort. Grant, Thase, and Sweeney (2001) administered a battery of cognitive tasks to 123 depressed outpatients and noted the surprising absence of cognitive deficits in their sample. The only indications of deficits were fewer completed categories, increased perseveration, and impaired maintenance of set on the Wisconsin Card Sorting Task (WCST), a widely used measure of executive control and cognitive flexibility. These results suggest the presence of depression-related deficits in the generation and maintenance of problem-solving strategies and difficulties in set switching (see also Harvey et al., 2004). Importantly, though, there was no evidence of deficits in executive functioning on any of the other tasks administered by the authors. Grant and colleagues

(2001) concluded that pervasive cognitive deficits most likely characterize depressed older adults and severely depressed inpatients who present with psychotic features (for similar conclusions, see Harvey et al., 2004; Rose & Ebmeier, 2006).

To summarize, surprisingly little empirical support has been found so far for pervasive depressive deficits in the processing of neutral information. Indeed, the bulk of evidence points to depressive deficits in the control of attention rather than to limited processing capacities. When depressed participants' attention is well controlled by the demands of the task, and they have no opportunity to ruminate, no depressive deficits are found. Focusing attention requires the inhibition of task-irrelevant thoughts. Thus, these findings support the affective interference hypothesis and the proposition that depressed individuals are characterized by reduced cognitive control. These results also suggest that examining how depressed individuals process emotional information may help us understand their difficulties in processing neutral material.

Cognitive Biases in Memory

Cognitive models of depression posit that depressed individuals exhibit cognitive biases in all aspects of information processing, including attention, memory, and interpretation (Mathews & MacLeod, 2005). Although these theoretical predictions are straightforward, the empirical results are not. A current controversy in cognitive theories of emotional disorders, for example, concerns the existence of attentional biases and interpretation biases in depression. Overall, there is strong evidence for biased memory processes (Mathews & MacLeod, 2005; Williams et al., 1997). In fact, biased memory for negative, relative to positive, information represents perhaps the most robust cognitive finding associated with major depression (Blaney, 1986; Matt, Vasquez, & Campbell, 1992). In a meta-analysis of studies assessing recall performance, Matt and colleagues found that people with major depression remembered 10% more negative words than positive words. Nondepressed controls, in contrast, demonstrated a memory bias for positive information in 20 of 25 studies. It should be noted, however, that memory biases are found most consistently in free-recall tasks and may also be restricted to explicit memory tasks. Results using recognition or implicit memory measures have been much less conclusive. In his review of the implicit memory literature, Watkins (2002; see also Barry, Naus, & Lynn, 2004) reported that, across studies, no bias is found in depressed participants when the encoding and/or the recall of the emotional material depend purely on perceptual processing. For example, if depressed participants are asked to count the letters in emotional words at encoding and to complete word stems or word fragments at recall, no evidence of an implicit memory bias is obtained (Watkins, Martin, & Stern, 2000). If, however, participants are asked to rate the recency of their experience with the word, or to imagine themselves in a scene involving the word at encoding, and are asked to freely associate to a cue word or to provide a word that fits a given definition, implicit memory biases are obtained more consistently. Encoding and recall in these latter studies are conceptual instead of perceptual. This suggests that depressive deficits are due mostly to differences in the elaboration of emotional material between depressed individuals and their nondepressed counterparts.

Three prospective studies have focused on biases in recall. These studies examined responses to the self-referential encoding task, in which participants are presented with a list of words, are asked to indicate whether each word is self-descriptive, then, in an incidental memory test, are asked to recall the words. The proportion of the negative self-referential words recalled is used an index of negative bias in recall. Two studies in which this measure was used with samples of undergraduates yielded contradictory results: whereas Reilly-Harrington, Alloy, Fresco, and Whitehouse (1999) found that this index predicted increases in depressive symptoms following stressful life events, Hammen, Marks, DeMayo, and Mayol (1985) did not. Bellew and Hill (1991) found that incidental recall of negative words assessed in a sample of pregnant women predicted depressive symptoms 3 months after the birth of the child. In addition, two studies demonstrated that biased recall of positive material predicts recovery from a depressive episode in a 1-year follow-up (e.g., Rottenberg, Joormann, Brozovich, & Gotlib, 2005).

In a recent review, Williams and colleagues (2007) presented evidence that overgeneral memory is characteristic of patients diagnosed with major depressive disorder (MDD). In the Autobiographical Memory Test (AMT), depressed participants respond to positive and negative cues with memories that summarize a category of similar events. Importantly, this research has demonstrated that overgeneral memories are associated with difficulties in problem solving and in imaging specific future events, and delayed recovery from episodes of depression (Peeters, Wessel, Merckelbach, & Boon-Vermeeren, 2002; Raes et al., 2005). Moreover, overgeneral memories remain stable outside of episodes of the disorder (Mackinger, Pachinger, Leibetseder, & Fartacek, 2000) and have been shown to predict later onset of depressive episodes in postpartum depression following students' negative life events, and after unsuccessful *in vitro* fertilization (van Minnen, Wessel, Verhaak, & Smeenk, 2005). Brittlebank, Scott, Williams, and Ferrier (1993) found that overgeneral recall of autobiographical memories, particularly for positive memories, predicted less complete recovery from depression at a 7-month follow-up among 22 patients diagnosed with major depression. In contrast, Brewin, Reynolds, and Tata (1999) found that overgeneral recall of autobiographical memories did not predict recovery from depression, although intrusive memories of life events did predict recovery. Finally, in a series of experimental studies, Dalgleish and colleagues (2007) further demonstrated that deficits in executive control and cognitive inhibition may underlie overgeneral memory deficits in depression. These authors propose that reduced specificity is the result of deficits in executive control and inhibition, leading to impoverished retrieval strategies during memory search and/or problems with inhibiting inappropriate candidate memory responses in the AMT. Indeed, the authors found a significant relation between reduced specificity of autobiographical memories in depression and poor performance on tasks assessing executive control. An important explanation of this relation is that a reduced ability to inhibit prepotent responses (i.e., negative self-referent, ruminative responses) makes it difficult for individuals to focus on the goal of retrieving a specific event.

Cognitive Biases in Interpretation and Attention

Results with regard to whether depression is characterized by an interpretation bias have been mixed (Lawson, MacLeod, & Hammond, 2002). Butler and Mathews (1983), for example, presented clinically depressed participants with ambiguous scenarios and found that, compared to nondepressed participants, depressed individuals ranked negative interpretations higher than they did other possible interpretations. In a study assessing biases using response latencies to target words presented after ambiguous sentences, no interpretation bias was found (Lawson & MacLeod, 1999). Lawson and colleagues (2002) also examined startle magnitude during imagery elicited by emotionally ambiguous tests. Using this measure, these authors reported evidence for more negative interpretations in their depressed sample and concluded that the failure to find a bias in their previous study was due to the use of response latencies. Rude, Wenzlaff, Gibbs, Vane, and Whitney (2002) found that a measure of interpretation bias, the Scrambled Sentences Test, predicted increases in depressive symptoms after 4–6 weeks in a large sample of undergraduate students, especially when administered under cognitive load. Clearly, further studies are needed that investigate interpretive biases in depression.

Some studies have failed to find attentional biases in depression (e.g., Mogg, Bradley, Williams, & Mathews, 1993). Most studies have used either the Modified Stroop Task or an attentional allocation paradigm, such as the dot-probe task. In the dot-probe task, paired stimuli (words or faces) are presented simultaneously: One stimulus is neutral, and the other is emotional. Participants are asked to respond to a probe that replaces either the neutral or the emotional stimulus. Allocation of attention to the spatial position of the stimuli is determined from response latencies to the probes. Most studies using the Stroop task do not find differences between depressed participants and controls (e.g., Mogg et al., 1993). Bradley, Mogg, Millar, and White (1995), for example, found that depression was not associated with increased Stroop interference, and the well-replicated interference effect in anxiety was not present in patients with depression and comorbid generalized anxiety disorder (GAD). Several investigators have used the dot-probe task with supraliminal stimuli, and also with briefly presented and masked emotional words, to investigate processing biases in depression. Here, too, results have not been encouraging (e.g., Mogg, Bradley, & Williams, 1995). Strikingly, no study using these experimental tasks has found a bias in clinically depressed participants when the stimuli have been masked to investigate unconscious processing (for a recent review, see Mathews & MacLeod, 2005). Furthermore, no attentional biases were found in participants who had previously been depressed (e.g., Gilboa & Gotlib, 1997; Hedlund & Rude, 1995). Based on such findings, Williams and colleagues (1997) proposed that depressed persons are not characterized by biases in attentional functioning, but by biases in postattentional elaboration. These authors suggested that anxiety-congruent biases are observed in tasks that assess the early, orienting stage of processing, prior to awareness (e.g., selective attention and priming tasks). In contrast, depressive biases are observed in strategic elaboration; therefore, they would be found in recall tasks but not in selective attention tasks.

Although this formulation seems plausible, it may be premature to conclude that depressed persons are not characterized by an attentional bias. Recent studies using the dot-probe task, for example, have reported selective attention in depression. Interestingly, these biases were found under conditions of long stimuli exposures (Bradley, Mogg, & Lee, 1997; Gotlib, Krasnoperova, Yue, & Joormann, 2004; Joormann & Gotlib, 2007; Mogg et al., 1995). Mogg and colleagues (1995) reported a mood-congruent bias in depressed participants, but only under supraliminal conditions. Similarly, Bradley and colleagues (1997) reported a mood-congruent bias on the dot-probe task for both induced and naturally occurring dysphoria when stimuli were presented for 500 or 1000 msec, but not when they were presented for brief durations (14 msec). Using a dot-probe task with emotional faces as stimuli, Gotlib and colleagues (2004) found an attentional bias for negative faces that were presented for 1000 msec in clinically diagnosed depressed participants. In two recent studies, Joormann, Talbot, and Gotlib (2007) replicated these findings in samples of remitted depressed adults and nondisordered girls at high risk for depression due to their mothers' psychopathology (see also Joormann & Gotlib, 2007). These findings suggest that rather than being simply a symptom of depression or a scar of a previous depressive episode, attentional biases may play an important role in the vulnerability to depression. Indeed, Beevers and Carver (2003) demonstrated that changes in attentional bias for negative, but not for positive, words following a negative mood induction interacted with life stress to predict onset of depressive symptoms in college students.

Overall, these results suggest that depressed individuals do not direct their attention to negative information more frequently than do control participants, but once it captures their attention, they exhibit difficulties disengaging from it. Similar difficulties in disengaging attention from negative material have been demonstrated in an exogenous cueing task (Koster, Leyman, DeRaedt, & Crombey, 2006). Rinck and Becker (2005) reported that depressed participants did not show enhanced detection of depression-related words in a visual search task, but they were more easily distracted by negative words. In a recent study, Eizenman and colleagues (2003) used eye-tracking technology to monitor point of gaze continuously. Depressed individuals spent significantly more time looking at pictures featuring sadness and loss (longer total fixation time) and had significantly longer average glance durations for these pictures than did nondepressed controls; the two groups did not differ, however, in fixation frequency.

In summary, these results suggest that depression is characterized by a selective bias for negative information, but that this bias does not operate throughout all aspects of selective attention. Depressed individuals may not automatically orient their attention toward negative information in the environment, but once such information has become the focus of their attention, they may have greater difficulty disengaging from it. These results are consistent with recent research suggesting that selective attention is not a unitary concept, and that it is important to distinguish among different components (e.g., orienting vs. maintenance–disengagement) and underlying mechanisms of selective attention (LaBerge, 1995; Posner, 1995). Selective attention involves at least two mechanisms: (1) activation of selected, relevant information; and (2) active inhibition of unselected, irrelevant information (Hasher & Zacks, 1988; Tipper, 1985). Depression is not associated with differential initial activation levels of negative, compared to neutral, stimulus representations. Instead, dysfunctional inhibitory mechanisms in the processing of negative stimuli might explain the observed difficulties in disengaging attention from negative material and, consequently, the increased elaboration of negative material associated with this disorder.

Cognitive Inhibition

As outlined in previous sections, there is emerging evidence that depression is characterized by deficits in the inhibition of mood-congruent material. These deficits may result in prolonged processing of negative, goal-irrelevant aspects of presented information, thereby hindering recovery from negative mood and leading to the sustained negative affect that characterizes depressive episodes. Indeed, it has been suggested that deficits in cognitive inhibition lie at the heart of memory and attention biases in depression, and set the stage for ruminative responses to negative events and negative mood states. Over the last 15–20 years, a number of emergent experimental methodologies have the potential to test inhibition models (Anderson & Bjork, 1994). Some of these designs, such as negative priming (Tipper, 1985) and directed forgetting (Bjork, 1972), are discussed below.

The negative affective priming (NAP) task was designed to assess inhibition in the processing of emotional information (Joormann, 2004). This task assesses response times to positive and negative material that participants are instructed to ignore. Joormann (2004) found that dysphoric participants and participants with a history of depressive episodes exhibited reduced inhibition of negative material. Thus, these participants responded faster when a negative target was presented after a to-be-ignored negative distractor on the previous trial. As predicted, no group difference was found for the positive adjectives. In a related study, participants who scored high on a self-report measure of rumination exhibited a reduced ability to inhibit the processing of emotional distractors, a finding that remained significant even after the researcher controlled for level of depressive symptoms (Joormann, 2006). Importantly, researchers replicated these findings using a negative priming task with emotional faces (Goeleven, De Raedt, Baert, & Koster, 2006).

Negative priming tasks assess only one aspect of inhibition, that is, the ability to control the access of relevant and irrelevant material to working memory. Although these studies suggest that depression, and probably also rumination, involve difficulties in keeping irrelevant emotional information from *entering* working memory, no studies have examined whether depression and rumination are also associated with difficulties in *removing* previously relevant negative material from working memory. Difficulties in inhibiting the processing of negative material that was, but is no longer, relevant might explain why people respond to negative mood states and negative life events with recurring, uncontrollable, and unintentional negative thoughts. To test this hypothesis, Joormann and Gotlib (2008) used a Modified Sternberg Task that combines a short-term recognition task with instructions to ignore a previously memorized list of words to assess inhibition of irrelevant positive and negative stimuli. They found that participants diagnosed with major depression exhibited difficulties in removing irrelevant negative material from working memory. Specifically, compared to never-depressed controls, depressed individuals exhibited longer decision latencies to an intrusion probe (i.e., a probe from the irrelevant list) than to a new probe (i.e., a completely new word), reflecting the strength of the residual activation of the contents of working memory that were declared to be no longer relevant. Importantly, this pattern was not found for positive material. Joormann and Gotlib also found that difficulty in removing negative, irrelevant words from working memory was highly correlated with self-reported rumination, even after they controlled for level of depressive symptoms. In summary, therefore, these findings indicate that depression and rumination are associated with inhibitory impairments in the processing of emotional material, specifically, with difficulties in removing irrelevant negative material from working memory.

Similar findings have been reported in directed-forgetting tasks (Bjork, 1972). Using positive and negative words, Power, Dalgleish, Claudio, Tata, and Kentish (2000), reported differential directed-forgetting effects for depressed and nondepressed participants. Specifically, the depressed participants exhibited a facilitation effect for negative words after the "forget" instruction. In a recent study, Hertel and Gerstle (2003) found that, compared with controls, participants with dysphoria recalled more words that they were supposed to suppress, with a tendency toward increased recall of to-be-suppressed negative words. Moreover, the degree of forgetting was significantly correlated with self-report measures of rumination and unwanted thoughts. Using a slightly modified version of this task, in which participants were instructed to remember or to forget positive and negative nouns, Joormann, Hertel, Brozovich, and Gotlib (2005) investigated intentional forgetting of positive and negative adjectives that depressed and control participants had learned to associate with neutral nouns. Importantly, the authors provided multiple opportunities for participants to practice the active suppression of the items to examine whether forgetting would increase in relation to the suppression training. The results indicated that depressed participants could be trained to forget negative words, and the authors offered several implications of this research for interventions.

In summary, these findings suggest that depression is associated with difficulties in inhibiting negative irrelevant material. As the central function of working memory, impaired inhibitory processes might have severe cognitive and emotional consequences, including rumination. In the final section of this chapter, I discuss possible links between cognitive aspects of depression and dysfunctional emotion regulation.

COGNITIVE ASPECTS OF EMOTION AND MOOD REGULATION

Depression has been conceptualized as a disorder of emotion dysregulation. The construct of *emotion regulation*, which evolved from the broader concept of coping with stress, involves the utilization of behavioral and cognitive strategies in an effort to modulate affect intensity and duration (Thompson, 1994). Investigators have identified a number of strategies that people commonly use to regulate negative moods and emotions. Although some of these strategies involve overt behavior, people frequently attempt to alter their affect through cognitive processes (e.g., reappraisal, generating distracting thoughts, making downward social comparisons, engaging in positive counterfactual thinking). Only recently, however, have researchers begun to examine how and why these strategies work, whether regulation strategies are uniformly successful at improving negative mood (Larsen, 2000), and whether there are reliable individual differences in the use and effectiveness of these strategies (e.g., Joormann & Siemer, 2004).

The research reviewed in this chapter on cognitive aspects of depression has important implications for our understanding of emotion and mood regulation in this disorder. Certainly, there are a number of ways in which deficits in cognitive control, inhibitory dysfunction, cognitive biases, and depressive cognitions affect the ability to recover from negative affect. For example, mood-congruent cognitive biases that are activated when one experiences a negative event can lead to a vicious cycle of increasingly negative thoughts and negative affect. Difficulties in cognitive control, and in inhibiting activated but goal-irrelevant negative thoughts, memories, and interpretations, can make it impossible to employ self-regulatory strategies that aid mood and emotion regulation, such as reappraisal of the emotion-eliciting situation or recall of mood-incongruent memories and thoughts. The investigation of cognitive aspects of emotion and mood regulation in depression promises to be an exciting field of future research for a number of reasons. We now know that cognitive processes play an important role in the onset and maintenance of emotional disorders, and previous studies have successfully described cognitive aspects of depression. We know far less, however, about the functional role of these processes. For example, we do not fully understand the nature of the relation among different cognitive biases or how cognitive aspects of depression affect emotion dysregulation. Furthermore, recent advances in research on biological aspects of depression have sparked interest in the question of the relation between cognition and emotion regulation. Contemporary accounts of neural aspects of emotion regulation posit a top-down modulation of ventral limbic structures, such as the amygdala, by more dorsal structures, such as the dorsolateral prefrontal cortex (DLPFC) (e..g., Ochsner & Gross, 2005). Interestingly, these regions have also been found to be activated in tasks that involve the cognitive inhibition of prepotent responses, an observation that led Ochsner and Gross (2005) and other researchers to propose that an overlapping set of prefrontal regions may play an important role in the cognitive control of emotion, for example, through effortful cognitive strategies such as reappraisal or the cognitive suppression of emotional responses. Importantly, using positron emission tomography (PET) and functional magnetic resonance imaging (fMRI), investigators have identified abnormalities in limbic and prefrontal cortical areas in depression that largely overlap with regions implicated in emotion regulation (e.g.,

Mayberg, 1997; see Davidson, Pizzagalli, & Nitschke, Chapter 10, this volume). Although relevant research is still in its infancy, investigators have suggested that limbic–cortical dysregulation might result in sustained negative affect, rumination, and impaired reward processing—formulations that parallel behavioral findings in depression of biased processing of negative information, rumination, and a lack of responsivity to positive stimuli. In the remainder of this chapter, I discuss two possible mediators of the relation between basic cognitive dysfunctions and individual differences in emotion regulation: the tendency to ruminate and the inability to use memories to repair a negative mood state.

Ruminative Response Style

According to Nolen-Hoeksema and her collaborators (in press), rumination is a particularly detrimental response to negative affect that hinders recovery from negative mood and prolongs depressive episodes. What characterizes rumination and differentiates it from negative automatic thoughts is that it is a *style* of thought rather than just negative *content* (Nolen-Hoeksema, 1991; Nolen-Hoeksema et al., in press). Thus, *rumination* is defined by the process of recurring thoughts and ideas, often described as a "recycling" of thoughts, and not necessarily by the content of these recurring thoughts. The majority of studies on rumination to date have been concerned with consequences of ruminative responses. In an extensive program of experimental and correlational studies, Nolen-Hoeksema and colleagues investigated ruminative response styles in depression and dysphoria, and analyzed how these response styles exacerbate sad moods and predict future depressive episodes (Morrow & Nolen-Hoeskema, 1990). Self-reported levels of ruminative response style have been found to predict higher levels of dysphoria over time in prospective studies with nonclinical samples, even after researchers control for initial differential depression levels (e.g., Nolen-Hoeksema & Morrow, 1991). Moreover, studies have shown that rumination predicts higher levels of depressive symptoms and onset of major depressive episodes, and mediates the gender difference in depressive symptoms (Nolen-Hoeksema, 2000; Nolen-Hoeksema, Stice, Wade, & Bohon, 2007). Research also indicates that rumination enhances cognitive biases in information-processing tasks and impairs mood regulation, resulting in sustained negative mood states (e.g., Lyubomirksy & Nolen-Hoeksema, 1995). Thus, when participants with dysphoria who were induced to ruminate, they endorsed more negative interpretations of hypothetical situations, generated less effective problem-solving strategies (Lyubomirsky & Nolen-Hoeksema, 1995), and showed increased recall of negative autobiographical memories (Lyubomirsky, Caldwell, & Nolen-Hoeksema, 1998).

Although this line of research informs us about the devastating effects of rumination, it does not particularly help us in determining why it is so difficult for some people to redirect their thoughts and control their attention, before it becomes dysfunctional. Finding an answer to this question might increase our understanding of cognitive processes in depression and inform our interventions. As outlined in previous sections, deficits in inhibitory processes may play a central role in the occurrence of ruminative responses. Davis and Nolen-Hoeksema (2000) recently reported that ruminators made more errors on the WCST than did nonruminators. Because the WCST measures executive control and cognitive flexibility, these results provide empirical support for the hypothesis that rumination is related to the executive control component of working memory. In addition, Joormann (2006) reported a correlation between rumination and deficits in cognitive inhibition, as assessed by negative priming, and Joormann and Gotlib (2008) found a correlation between rumination and the ability to remove irrelevant negative material from working memory. These findings suggest that deficits in executive control and inhibition are related to sustained processing of negative material and rumination, which in turn maintains the negative mood state and hinders recovery from negative affect. Further evidence for this proposition comes from recent brain imaging studies. Using fMRI, investigators have found that the combination of DLPFC hypoactivity and sustained amygdala activity was related to self-reported rumination in a study that examined prolonged elaborative processing of emotional information in depression (Siegle, Steinhauer, Thase, Stenger, & Carter, 2002). In this study, whereas nondepressed individuals' amygdalar responses to all stimuli decayed quickly after offset, depressed individuals were characterized by sustained amygdalar responses to negative words. This sustained response lasted throughout the following nonemotional processing trials for depressed, but not for control, participants. Moreover, the difference in sustained amygdalar activity to negative and positive words was related to self-reported rumination. Clearly, more studies are needed to investigate processes that underlie this dysfunctional emotion regulation strategy and that investigate neural correlates of inhibition and rumination in depression.

In this context, it is important to note that there are at least two broad but distinct classes of cognitive affect regulation strategies. One class of strategies reduces negative affect by generating thoughts and appraisals that directly alter the perceptions of the situation that elicited the emotion or the experience of the negative affect (e.g., reappraisal). In contrast, a different class of strategies alleviates negative affect less directly by strengthening mood-incongruent (i.e., positive) thoughts, memories, and associations, and by evoking competing affective states. Importantly, these latter strategies may be useful in modulating affective states that have no identifiable triggers or cause; consequently, they may be particularly effective in regulating the normal fluctuations in mood states that people experience throughout the day. Memory might play an important role in these indirect attempts to regulate mood and emotion.

Memory and Mood Repair

Memories affect emotion regulation in important ways. Investigators have demonstrated that memories of unpleasant events fade faster than do memories of pleasant events, and that this differential fading is associated with happiness (Walker, Skowronski, & Thompson, 2003). Researchers have also found that recalling positive autobiographical memories can repair an induced negative mood state (Joormann & Siemer, 2004), and that the process of remembering positive events and forgetting negative events is associated with increased well-being over the lifespan (Charles, Mather, & Carstensen, 2003). Indeed, the literature on mood regulation suggests that mood-incongruent recall is often used as a mood-repair strategy in response to a negative mood induction (e.g., Rusting & DeHart, 2000). Studies investigating the use and effectiveness of mood regulation strategies in depression suggest that in contrast to nondepressed persons, depressed individuals are unable to use positive autobiographical memories to regulate induced negative mood states (Joormann & Siemer, 2004; Joormann, Siemer, & Gotlib, 2007). In two studies, we examined the formulation that dysphoria and rumination are critical factors in determining whether mood-congruent memory retrieval, as opposed to mood-repair processes, occurs (Joormann & Siemer, 2004). Whereas nondysphoric participants' mood ratings improved under distraction, as well as under mood-incongruent recall instructions, participants with dysphoria did not benefit from the recall of positive memories, and distraction seemed to alleviate their sad mood. In a recent study, we replicated these findings in a sample of currently depressed participants. Interestingly, previously depressed participants exhibited similar difficulties in repairing their negative mood with positive memories (Joormann et al., 2007).

Cooney, Joormann, Atlas, Eugene, and Gotlib (2007) investigated the neural correlates of mood-incongruent recall. These investigators induced sad mood in participants and had them use positive autobiographical memories to regulate that negative affect. Cooney and colleagues found less involvement of dorsal brain regions, such as the DLPFC and dorsal anterior cingulate cortex (ACC), in recovery from the sad mood; instead, activation was found in orbitofrontal and ventromedial prefrontal cortex. These findings are consistent with the formulation that different emotion regulation strategies are associated with activation in different brain areas. Whereas voluntary suppression of affect and strategic reappraisal of the emotion-eliciting situation might be more strongly associated with dorsal areas of the PFC that have traditionally been linked to cognitive control and working memory, more automatic regulation strategies, such as changes in the accessibility of mood-congruent thoughts, may be associated with activation in more ventral areas of the PFC that have traditionally been linked to emotional processing and associative learning. Given the importance of these brain regions in neural models of depression, future research is needed to investigate this proposition more explicitly.

Taken together, these results indicate that people who experience a negative mood state can enter into a self-defeating cycle, in which their negative mood primes unpleasant memories that in turn exacerbate their distress. People sometimes attempt to break this maladaptive cycle by actively recruiting pleasant memories, thereby repairing their sad mood. The inhibition of negative irrelevant information might play a crucial role in these processes. The accessibility of specific, mood-incongruent memories may depend on the individual's ability to inhibit mood-congruent memories activated by the sad mood. These processes might operate on an automatic level and might explain how, usually in nondepressed individuals, sad mood dissipates, even though these individuals do not actively take steps to repair their mood. Inasmuch as depressed individuals are not able to inhibit mood-congruent activation, mood-incongruent memories remain less accessible, a process that stabilizes rather than repairs negative mood. In addition, reported impairments in the processing of positive stimuli in depression might add to the difficulties in mood and emotion regulation.

SUMMARY AND FUTURE DIRECTIONS

Studies examining cognitive aspects of depression are beginning to elucidate the nature of the relations among cognition, emotion regulation, and depression. Depressed individuals have difficulties disengaging from negative material; consequently, they exhibit sustained processing and increased elaboration of negative content. Because the experience of negative mood states and negative life events is associated with the activation of mood-congruent cognitions in working memory, the ability to control the contents of working memory may be critical in differentiating people who recover easily from negative affect from those who initiate a vicious cycle of increasingly negative ruminative thinking and deepening sad mood. Investigating individual differences in executive functions and, specifically, in the inhibitory control of the contents of working memory, has the potential to provide important insights into the maintenance of negative affect and vulnerability to experience depressive episodes.

Clearly, future studies are needed that investigate more explicitly and systematically the underlying mechanisms of depressive cognition and the role of cognition in emotion and mood regulation. Other important areas of future research include studies on developmental aspects of depressive cognition and emotion dysregulation in high-risk populations, and on the transmission of these vulnerabilities from depressed parents to their offspring. As outlined in the previous section, the integration of biological and psychological research on stress reactivity and emotion regulation will be important to improve our understanding of depressive disorders and to identify factors that increase vulnerability to these disorders. Recent fMRI studies, for example, have examined neural correlates of memory biases (Ramel et al., 2007), attentional biases (Monk et al., 2008), and rumination (Siegle et al., 2002) in depression and in high-risk samples. Using a dot-probe task in the scanner, for example, Monk and colleagues (2008) demonstrated that offspring of depressed parents exhibit increased amygdalar activation in response to negative facial expressions. Similarly, Ellenbogen, Schwartzman, Stewart, and Walker (2006), who recently investigated the relation between cognitive biases and cortisol response to stressful challenges in depressed and control participants, reported that attentional disengagement from emotional faces is associated with poststress mood and cortisol levels.

Finally, recent studies have investigated genetic factors that may affect cognitive aspects of depression and emotion dysregulation. Importantly, these studies suggest a relation between brain regions involved in affect regulation and variations in the serotonin transporter gene, which has been associated with increased risk for depression (Pezawas et al., 2005). As described in the previous section, medial and dorsolateral prefrontal brain areas are implicated in the cognitive modulation of emotion processing areas, such as the amygdala and the orbitofrontal cortex. Interestingly, recent genetic studies have shown that carriers of the short allele of a functional 5′ promoter polymorphism of the serotonin transporter gene (5-HTT), a genetic variation that has been associated with increased risk for depression, show reduced gray-matter volume in limbic regions that are critical for the processing of negative emotion, such as the amygdala, and less connectivity between the amygdala and regions of the PFC (Pezawas et al., 2005). Moreover, short allele carriers have been found to exhibit an exaggerated amygdalar response to negative stimuli (Hariri et al., 2005; Pezawas et al., 2005). This is an exciting new area of research, and two studies so far have investigated whether this polymorphism is associated with cognitive biases in depression. Beevers, Gibb, McGeary, and Miller (2007) reported an association of the short allele of the 5-HTT with dot-probe attentional allocation in psychiatric inpatients, while Hayden and colleagues (2008) reported that the short allele is associated with biased recall in the self-referential encoding task following a negative mood induction in girls at risk for depression. These findings are exciting and represent first steps toward a more comprehensive model of how psychological and biological factors interact to facilitate or hinder emotion regulation, thereby affecting individuals' vulnerability to experiencing depressive episodes.

REFERENCES

Abela, J. R. Z., & Skitch, S. A. (2007). Dysfunctional attitudes, self-esteem, and hassles: Cognitive vulnerability to depression in children of affectively ill parents. *Behaviour Research and Therapy, 45,* 1127–1140.

Abramson, L. Y., Metalsky, G. I., & Alloy, L. B. (1989). Hopelessness depression: A theory-based subtype of depression. *Psychological Review, 96,* 358–372.

Alloy, L. B., & Abramson, L. Y. (1999). The Temple–Wisconsin Cognitive Vulnerability to Depression Project: Conceptual background, design, and methods. *Journal of Cognitive Psychotherapy, 13,* 227–262.

Alloy, L. B., Abramson, L. Y., & Francis, E. L. (1999). Do negative cognitive styles confer vulnerability to depression? *Current Directions in Psychological Science, 8,* 128–132.

Alloy, L. B., Abramson, L. Y., Hogan, M. E., Whitehouse, W. G., Rose, D. T., Robinson, M. S., et al. (2000). The Temple–Wisconsin Cognitive Vulnerability to Depression Project: Lifetime history of Axis I psychopathology in individuals at high and low cognitive risk for depression. *Journal of Abnormal Psychology, 109,* 403–418.

Alloy, L. B., Abramson, L. Y., Walshaw, P. D., & Neeren, A. M. (2006). Cognitive vulnerability to unipolar and bipolar mood disorders. *Journal of Social and Clinical Psychology, 25,* 726–754.

American Psychiatric Association. (1994). *Diagnostic and statistical manual of mental disorders* (4th ed.). Washington, DC: Author.

Anderson, M. C., & Bjork, R. A. (1994). Mechanisms of inhibition in long-term memory: A new taxonomy. In D. Dagenbach & T. Carr (Eds.), *Inhibitory processes in attention, memory, and language* (pp. 265–325). San Diego, CA: Academic Press.

Baddeley, A. D., & Hitch, G. J. (1994). Developments in the concept of working memory. *Neuropsychology, 8,* 485–493.

Barch, D. M., Sheline, Y. I., Csernansky, J. G., & Snyder, A. Z. (2003). Working memory and prefrontal cortex dysfunction: Specificity to schizophrenia compared with major depression. *Biological Psychiatry, 53,* 376–384.

Barnett, P. A., & Gotlib, I. H. (1988). Psychosocial functioning and depression: Distinguishing among antecedents, concomitants, and consequences. *Psychological Bulletin, 104,* 97–126.

Barry, E. S., Naus, M. J., & Lynn, P. R. (2004). Depression and implicit memory: Understanding mood congruent memory bias. *Cognitive Therapy and Research, 28,* 387–414.

Beck, A. T. (1976). *Cognitive therapy and the emotional disorders.* New York: International Universities Press.

Beck, A. T., Epstein, N., & Harrison, R. (1983). Cognitions, attitudes and personality dimensions in depression. *British Journal of Cognitive Psychotherapy, 1,* 1–16.

Beevers, C. G. (2005). Cognitive vulnerability to depression: A dual process model. *Clinical Psychology Review, 25,* 975–1002.

Beevers, C. G., & Carver, C. S. (2003). Attentional bias and mood persistence as prospective predictors of dysphoria. *Cognitive Therapy and Research, 27,* 619–637.

Beevers, C. G., Gibb, B. E., McGeary, J. E., & Miller, I. W. (2007). Serotonin transporter genetic variation and biased attention for emotional word stimuli among psychiatric inpatients. *Journal of Abnormal Psychology, 116,* 208–212.

Bellew, M., & Hill, A. B. (1991). Schematic processing and the prediction of depression following childbirth. *Personality and Individual Differences, 12,* 943–949.

Bjork, R. A. (1972). Theoretical implications of directed forgetting. In A. W. Melton & E. Martin (Eds.), *Coding processes in human memory.* Washington, DC: Winston.

Blaney, P. H. (1986). Affect and memory: A review. *Psychological Bulletin, 99,* 229–246.

Bower, G. H. (1981). Mood and memory. *American Psychologist, 36,* 129–148.

Bradley, B. P., Mogg, K., & Lee, S. C. (1997). Attentional biases for negative information in induced and naturally occurring dysphoria. *Behaviour Research and Therapy, 35,* 911–927.

Bradley, B. P., Mogg, K., Millar, N., & White, J. (1995). Selective processing of negative information: Effects of clinical anxiety, concurrent depression, and awareness. *Journal of Abnormal Psychology, 104,* 532–536.

Brewin, C. R., Reynolds, M., & Tata, P. (1999). Autobiographical memory processes and the course of depression. *Journal of Abnormal Psychology, 108,* 511–517.

Brittlebank, A. D., Scott, J., Williams, J. M., & Ferrier, I. N. (1993). Autobiographical memory in depression: State or trait marker? *British Journal of Psychiatry, 162,* 118–121.

Brosse, A. L., Craighead, L. W., & Craighead, W. E. (1999). Testing the mood-state hypothesis among previously depressed and never-depressed individuals. *Behavior Therapy, 30,* 97–115.

Brown, G. P., Hammen, C. L., Craske, M. G., & Wickens, T. D. (1995). Dimensions of dysfunctional attitudes as vulnerabilities to depressive symptoms. *Journal of Abnormal Psychology, 104,* 431–435.

Burt, D. B., Zembar, M. J., & Niederehe, G. (1995). Depression and memory impairment: A meta-analysis of the association, its pattern, and specificity. *Psychological Bulletin, 117,* 285–305.

Butler, G., & Mathews, A. (1983). Cognitive processes in anxiety. *Advances in Behaviour Research and Therapy, 5,* 51–62.

Channon, S., Baker, J. E., & Robertson, M. M. (1993). Working memory in clinical depression: An experimental study. *Psychological Medicine, 23,* 87–91.

Charles, S. T., Mather, M., & Carstensen, L. L. (2003). Aging and emotional memory: The forgettable nature of negative images for older adults. *Journal of Experimental Psychology: General, 132,* 310–324.

Cooney, R. E., Joormann, J., Atlas, L. Y., Eugene, F., & Gotlib, I. H. (2007). Neural correlates of affect regulation through mood-incongruent recall. *NeuroReport, 18,* 1771–1774.

Cowan, N. (1995). *Attention and memory: An integrated framework.* New York: Oxford University Press.

Dalgleish, T., Williams, J. M. G., Golden, A. M. J., Perkins, N., Barrett, L. F., Barnard, P. J., et al. (2007). Reduced specificity of autobiographical memory and depression: The role of executive control. *Journal of Experimental Psychology: General, 136,* 23–42.

Davis, R. N., & Nolen-Hoeksema, S. (2002). Cognitive inflexibility among ruminators and nonruminators. *Cognitive Therapy and Research, 24,* 699–711.

Egeland, J., Rund, B. R., Sundet, K., Landro, N. I., Asbjornsen, A., Lund, A., et al. (2003). Attention profile in schizophrenia compared with depression: Differential effects of processing speed, selective attention and vigilance. *Acta Psychiatrica Scandinavica, 108,* 276–284.

Eizenman, M., Yu, L. H., Grupp, L., Eizenman, E., Ellenbogen, M., Gemar, M., et al. (2003). A naturalistic visual scanning approach to assess selective attention in major depressive disorder. *Psychiatry Research, 118,* 117–128.

Ellenbogen, M. A., Schwartzman, A. E., Stewart, J., & Walker, C. D. (2006). Automatic and effortful emotional information processing regulates different aspects of the stress response. *Psychoneuroendocrinology, 31,* 373–387.

Ellis, H. C., & Ashbrook, P. W. (1988). Resource allocation model of the effects of depressed mood states on memory. In K. Fiedler & J. P. Forgas (Eds.), *Affect, cognition, and social behavior* (pp. 25–43). Göttingen: Hogrefe.

Fresco, D. M., Alloy, L. B., & Reilly-Harrington, N. (2006). Association of attributional style for negative and positive events and the occurrence of life events with depression and anxiety. *Journal of Social and Clinical Psychology, 25,* 1140–1159.

Gemar, M. C., Segal, Z. V., Sagrati, S., & Kennedy, S. J. (2001). Mood-induced changes on the Implicit Association Test in recovered depressed patients. *Journal of Abnormal Psychology, 110,* 282–289.

Gibb, B. E., & Alloy, L. B. (2006). A prospective test of the hopelessness theory of depression in children. *Journal of Clinical Child and Adolescent Psychology, 35,* 264–274.

Gibb, B. E., Beevers, C. G., Andover, M. S., & Holleran, K. (2006). The hopelessness theory of depression: A prospective multi-wave test of the vulnerability–stress hypothesis. *Cognitive Therapy and Research, 30,* 763–772.

Gilboa, E., & Gotlib, I. H. (1997). Cognitive biases and affect persistence in previously dysphoric and never-dysphoric individuals. *Cognition and Emotion, 11,* 517–538.

Goeleven, E., De Raedt, R., Baert, S., & Koster, E. H. W. (2006). Deficient inhibition of emotional information in depression. *Journal of Affective Disorders, 93,* 149–152.

Gotlib, I. H., Krasnoperova, E., Yue, D. L., & Joormann, J. (2004). Attentional biases for negative interpersonal stimuli in clinical depression. *Journal of Abnormal Psychology, 113,* 127–135.

Grant, M. M., Thase, M. E., & Sweeney, J. A. (2001). Cognitive disturbances in outpatient depressed younger adults: Evidence of modest impairment. *Biological Psychiatry, 50,* 35–43.

Haaga, D. A., Dyck, M. J., & Ernst, D. (1991). Empirical status of cognitive theory of depression. *Psychological Bulletin, 110,* 215–236.

Haeffel, G. J., Abramson, L. Y., Voelz, Z. R., Metalsky, G. I., Halberstadt, L., Dykman, B. M., et al. (2005). Negative cognitive styles, dysfunctional attitudes, and the remitted depression paradigm: A search for the elusive cognitive vulnerability to depression factor among remitted depressives. *Emotion, 5,* 343–348.

Hammen, C., Marks, T., DeMayo, R., & Mayol, A. (1985). Self-schemas and risk for depression: A prospective study. *Journal of Personality and Social Psychology, 49,* 1147–1159.

Hankin, B. L., Abramson, L. Y., Miller, N., & Haeffel, G. J. (2004). Cognitive vulnerability–stress theories of depression: Examining affective specificity in the prediction of depression versus anxiety in three prospective studies. *Cognitive Therapy and Research, 28*, 309–345.

Hariri, A. R., Drabant, E. M., Munoz, K. E., Kolachana, B. S., Mattay, V. S., Egan, M. F., et al. (2005). A susceptibility gene for affective disorders and the response of the human amygdala. *Archives of General Psychiatry, 62*, 146–152.

Hartlage, S., Alloy, L. B., Vazquez, C., & Dykman, B. (1993). Automatic and effortful processing in depression. *Psychological Bulletin, 113*, 247–278.

Harvey, P. O., Le Bastard, G., Pochon, J. B., Levy, R., Allilaire, J. F., Dubois, B., et al. (2004). Executive functions and updating of the contents of working memory in unipolar depressions. *Journal of Psychiatric Research, 38*, 567–576.

Hasher, L., & Zacks, R. T. (1988). Working memory, comprehension, and aging: A review and a new view. In G. H. Bower (Ed.), *The psychology of learning and motivation* (Vol. 22, pp. 193–225). San Diego, CA: Academic Press.

Hayden, E. P., Dougherty, L. R., Maloney, B., Olino, T. M., Sheikh, H., Durbin, C. E., et al. (2008). Early-emerging cognitive vulnerability to depression and the serotonin transporter promoter region polymorphism. *Journal of Affective Disorders, 107*, 227–230.

Hedlund, S., & Rude, S. S. (1995). Evidence of latent depressive schemas in formerly depressed individuals. *Journal of Abnormal Psychology, 104*, 517–525.

Hertel, P. T. (1998). The relationship between rumination and impaired memory in dysphoric moods. *Journal of Abnormal Psychology, 107*, 166–172.

Hertel, P. T. (2004). Memory for emotional and nonemotional events in depression: A question of habit? In D. Reisberg & P. Hertel (Eds.), *Memory and emotion* (pp. 186–216). New York: Oxford University Press.

Hertel, P. T., & Gerstle, M. (2003). Depressive deficits in forgetting. *Psychological Science, 14*, 573–578.

Hertel, P. T., & Rude, S. S. (1991). Depressive deficits in memory: Focusing attention improves subsequent recall. *Journal of Experimental Psychology: General, 120*, 301–309.

Ingram, R. E. (1984). Toward an information-processing analysis of depression. *Cognitive Therapy and Research, 8*, 443–477.

Ingram, R. E., Miranda, J., & Segal, Z. V. (1998). *Cognitive vulnerability to depression*. New York: Guilford Press.

Ingram, R. E., Nelson, T., Steidtmann, D. K., & Bistricky, S. L. (2007). Comparative data on child and adolescent cognitive measures associated with depression. *Journal of Consulting and Clinical Psychology, 75*, 390–403.

Joiner, T. E. J., Metalsky, G. I., Lew, A., & Klocek, J. (1999). Testing the causal mediation component of Beck's theory of depression: Evidence for specific mediation. *Cognitive Therapy and Research, 23*, 401–412.

Joormann, J. (2004). Attentional bias in dysphoria: The role of inhibitory processes. *Cognition and Emotion, 18*, 125–147.

Joormann, J. (2006). The relation of rumination and inhibition: Evidence from a negative priming task. *Cognitive Therapy and Research, 30*, 149–160.

Joormann, J., & Gotlib, I. H. (2007). Selective attention to emotional faces following recovery from depression. *Journal of Abnormal Psychology, 116*, 80–85.

Joormann, J., & Gotlib, I. H. (2008). Updating the contents of working memory in depression: Interference from irrelevant negative material. *Journal of Abnormal Psychology, 117*, 206–213.

Joormann, J., Hertel, P. T., Brozovich, F., & Gotlib, I. H. (2005). Remembering the good, forgetting the bad: Intentional forgetting of emotional material in depression. *Journal of Abnormal Psychology, 114*, 640–648.

Joormann, J., & Siemer, M. (2004). Memory accessibility, mood regulation, and dysphoria: Difficulties in repairing sad mood with happy memories? *Journal of Abnormal Psychology, 113*, 179–188.

Joormann, J., Siemer, M., & Gotlib, I. H. (2007). Mood regulation in depression: Differential effects of distraction and recall of happy memories on sad mood. *Journal of Abnormal Psychology, 116*, 484–490.

Joormann, J., Talbot, L., & Gotlib, I. H. (2007). Biased processing of emotional information in girls at risk for depression. *Journal of Abnormal Psychology, 116*, 135–143.

Joormann, J., Yoon, K. L., & Zetsche, U. (2007). Cognitive inhibition in depression. *Applied and Preventive Psychology, 12*, 128–139.

Just, N., Abramson, L. Y., & Alloy, L. B. (2001). Remitted depression studies as tests of the cognitive vulnerability hypotheses of depression onset: A critique and conceptual analysis. *Clinical Psychology Review, 21*, 63–83.

Koster, E. H. W., Leyman, L., DeRaedt, R., & Crombey, G. (2006). Cueing of visual attention by emotional facial expressions: The influence of individual differences in anxiety and depression. *Personality and Individual Differences, 41*, 329–339.

LaBerge, D. (1995). *Attentional processing: The brain's art of mindfulness.* Cambridge, MA: Harvard University Press.

Lara, M. E., Klein, D. N., & Kasch, K. L. (2000). Psychosocial predictors of the short-term course and outcome of major depression: A longitudinal study of a nonclinical sample with recent-onset episodes. *Journal of Abnormal Psychology, 109*, 644–650.

Larsen, R. J. (2000). Toward a science of mood regulation. *Psychological Inquiry, 11*, 129–141.

Lawson, C., & MacLeod, C. (1999). Depression and the interpretation of ambiguity. *Behaviour Research and Therapy, 37*, 463–474.

Lawson, C., MacLeod, C., & Hammond, G. (2002). Interpretation revealed in the blink of an eye: Depressive bias in the resolution of ambiguity. *Journal of Abnormal Psychology, 111*, 321–328.

Lewinsohn, P. M., Rohde, P., Seeley, J. R., Klein, D. N., & Gotlib, I. H. (2000). Natural course of adolescent major depressive disorder in a community sample: Predictors of recurrence in young adults. *American Journal of Psychiatry, 157*, 1584–1591.

Lewinsohn, P. M., Steinmetz, J. L., Larson, D. W., & Franklin, J. (1981). Depression-related cognitions: Antecedent or consequence? *Journal of Abnormal Psychology, 90*, 213–219.

Lyubomirsky, S., Caldwell, N. D., & Nolen-Hoeksema, S. (1998). Effects of ruminative and distracting responses to depressed mood on retrieval of autobiographical memories. *Journal of Personality and Social Psychology, 75*, 166–177.

Lyubomirsky, S., & Nolen-Hoeksema, S. (1995). Effects of self-focused rumination on negative thinking and interpersonal problem solving. *Journal of Personality and Social Psychology, 69*, 176–190.

Mackinger, H. F., Pachinger, M. M., Leibetseder, M. M., & Fartacek, R. R. (2000). Autobiographical memories in women remitted from major depression. *Journal of Abnormal Psychology, 109*, 331–334.

Mathews, A., & MacLeod, C. (2005). Cognitive vulnerability to emotional disorders. *Annual Review of Clinical Psychology, 1*, 167–195.

Matt, G. E., Vazquez, C., & Campbell, W. K., (1992). Mood-congruent recall of affectively toned stimuli: A meta-analytic review. *Clinical Psychology Review, 12*, 227–255.

Mayberg, H. S. (1997). Limbic–cortical dysregulation: A proposed model of depression. *Journal Professional Neuropsychiatry and Clinical Neurosciences, 9*(3), 471–481.

Miranda, J., Persons, J. B., & Byers, C. N. (1990). Endorsement of dysfunctional beliefs depends on current mood state. *Journal of Abnormal Psychology, 99*, 237–241.

Mogg, K., Bradley, B. P., & Williams, R. (1995). Attentional bias in anxiety and depression: The role of awareness. *British Journal of Clinical Psychology, 34*, 17–36.

Mogg, K., Bradley, B. P., Williams, R., & Mathews, A. (1993). Subliminal processing of emotional information in anxiety and depression. *Journal of Abnormal Psychology, 102*, 304–311.

Monk, C. S., Klein, R. G., Telzer, E. H., Schroth, B. A., Mannuzza, S., Moulton, J. L., et al. (2008). Amygdala and nucleus accumbens activation to emotional facial expressions in children and adolescents at risk for major depression. *American Journal of Psychiatry, 165*, 90–98.

Morrow, J., & Nolen-Hoeksema, S. (1990). Effects of responses to depression on the remediation of depressive affect. *Journal of Personality and Social Psychology, 58*, 519–527.

Nolen-Hoeksema, S. (1991). Responses to depression and their effects on the duration of depressive episodes. *Journal of Abnormal Psychology, 100*, 569–582.

Nolen-Hoeksema, S. (2000). The role of rumination in depressive disorders and mixed anxiety/depressive symptoms. *Journal of Abnormal Psychology, 109,* 504–511.

Nolen-Hoeksema, S., & Morrow, J. (1991). A prospective study of depression and posttraumatic stress symptoms after a natural disaster: The 1989 Loma Prieta earthquake. *Journal of Personality and Social Psychology, 61,* 115–121.

Nolen-Hoeksema, S., Stice, E., Wade, E., & Bohon, C. (2007). Reciprocal relations between rumination and bulimic, substance abuse, and depressive symptoms in female adolescents. *Journal of Abnormal Psychology, 116,* 198–207.

Nolen-Hoeksema, S., Wisco, B. E., & Lyubomirsky, S. (in press). Rethinking rumination. *Perspectives on Psychological Science.*

Ochsner, K. N., & Gross, J. J. (2005). The cognitive control of emotion. *Trends in Cognitive Sciences, 9,* 242–249.

Peeters, F., Wessel, I., Merckelbach, H., & Boon-Vermeeren, M. (2002). Autobiographical memory specificity and the course of major depressive disorder. *Comprehensive Psychiatry, 43,* 344–350.

Peterson, C., Semmel, A., von Baeyer, C., Abramson, L. Y., Metalsky, G. I., & Seligman, M. E. P. (1982). The Attributional Style Questionnaire. *Cognitive Therapy and Research, 6,* 287–299.

Pezawas, L., Meyer-Lindenberg, A., Drabant, E. M., Verchinski, B. A., Munoz, K. E., Kolachana, B. S., et al. (2005). 5-HTTLPR polymorphism impacts human cingulate–amygdala interactions: A genetic susceptibility mechanism for depression. *Nature Neuroscience, 8,* 828–834.

Posner, M. I. (1995). Attention in cognitive neuroscience: An overview. In M. S. Gazzaniga (Ed.), *The cognitive neurosciences* (pp. 615–624). Cambridge, MA: MIT Press.

Power, M. J., Dalgleish, T., Claudio, V., Tata, P., & Kentish, J. (2000). The directed forgetting task: Application to emotionally valent material. *Journal of Affective Disorders, 57,* 147–157.

Raes, F., Hermans, D., Williams, J. M. G., Demyttenaere, K., Sabbe, B., Pieters, G., et al. (2005). Reduced specificity of autobiographical memory: A mediator between rumination and ineffective social problem-solving in major depression? *Journal of Affective Disorders, 87,* 331–335.

Ramel, W., Goldin, P. R., Eyler, L. T., Brown, G. G., Gotlib, I. H., & McQuaid, J. R. (2007). Amygdala reactivity and mood-congruent memory in individuals at risk for depressive relapse. *Biological Psychiatry, 61,* 231–239.

Reilly-Harrington, N. A., Alloy, L. B., Fresco, D. M., & Whitehouse, W. G. (1999). Cognitive styles and life events interact to predict bipolar and unipolar symptomatology. *Journal of Abnormal Psychology, 108,* 567–578.

Rinck, M., & Becker, E. S. (2005). A comparison of attentional biases and memory biases in women with social phobia and major depression. *Journal of Abnormal Psychology, 114,* 62–74.

Rose, E. J., & Ebmeier, K. P. (2006). Pattern of impaired working memory during major depression. *Journal of Affective Disorders, 90,* 149–161.

Rottenberg, J., Joormann, J., Brozovich, F., & Gotlib, I. H. (2005). Emotional intensity of idiographic sad memories in depression predicts symptom levels 1 year later. *Emotion, 5,* 238–242.

Rude, S. S., Wenzlaff, R. M., Gibbs, B., Vane, J., & Whitney, T. (2002). Negative processing biases predict subsequent depressive symptoms. *Cognition and Emotion, 16,* 423–440.

Rusting, C. L., & DeHart, T. (2000). Retrieving positive memories to regulate negative mood: Consequences for mood-congruent memory. *Journal of Personality and Social Psychology, 78(4),* 737–752.

Scher, C. D., Ingram, R. E., & Segal, Z. V. (2005). Cognitive reactivity and vulnerability: Empirical evaluation of construct activation and cognitive diatheses in unipolar depression. *Clinical Psychology Review, 25,* 487–510.

Seligman, M. E. P. (1975). *Helplessness: On depression, development, and death.* New York: Freeman.

Siegle, G. J., Ingram, R. E., & Matt, G. E. (2002). Affective interference: An explanation for negative attention biases in dysphoria? *Cognitive Therapy and Research, 26,* 73–87.

Siegle, G. J., Steinhauer, S. R., Thase, M. E., Stenger, A., & Carter, C. S. (2002). Can't shake that feeling: Event-related fMRI assessment of sustained amygdala activity in response to emotional information in depressed individuals. *Biological Psychiatry, 51,* 693–707.

Siemer, M. (2005). Mood-congruent cognitions constitute mood experience. *Emotion, 5,* 296–308.

Teasdale, J. D. (1988). Cognitive vulnerability to persistent depression. *Cognition and Emotion, 2*, 247–274.

Thompson, R. A. (1994). Emotion regulation: A theme in search of definition. *Monographs of the Society for Research in Child Development, 59*(2–3), 25–52, 250–283.

Tipper, S. P. (1985). The negative priming effect: Inhibitory processes by ignored objects. *Journal of Experimental Psychology, 37*, 571–590.

van Minnen, A., Wessel, I., Verhaak, C., & Smeenk, J. (2005). The relationship between autobiographical memory specificity and depressed mood following a stressful life event: A prospective study. *British Journal of Clinical Psychology, 44*, 405–415.

Walker, W. R., Skowronski, J. J., & Thompson, C. P. (2003). Life is pleasant—and memory helps to keep it that way! *Review of General Psychology, 7*, 203–210.

Watkins, P. C. (2002). Implicit memory bias in depression. *Cognition and Emotion, 16*, 381–402.

Watkins, P. C., Martin, C. K., & Stern, L. D. (2000). Unconscious memory bias in depression: Perceptual and conceptual processes. *Journal of Abnormal Psychology, 109*, 282–289.

Watts, F., & Sharrock, R. (1985). Description and measurement of concentration problems in depressed patients. *Psychological Medicine, 15*, 317–326.

Weissman, A. N., & Beck, A. T. (1978, November). *Development and validation of the Dysfunctional Attitude Scale: A preliminary investigation.* Paper presented at the annual meeting of the American Educational Research Association, Toronto.

Williams, J. M., Watts, F. N., MacLeod, C., & Mathews, A. (1997). *Cognitive psychology and emotional disorder.* Chichester, UK: Wiley.

Williams, J. M. G., Barnhofer, T., Crane, C., Herman, D., Raes, F., Watkins, E., et al. (2007). Autobiographical memory specificity and emotional disorder. *Psychological Bulletin, 133*, 122–148.

CHAPTER 14

Depression in Its Interpersonal Context

Thomas E. Joiner, Jr. *and* Katherine A. Timmons

We are a gregarious species; thus, it is unsurprising that interpersonal analyses have long been a feature of intellectual discourse. For example, from Plato to Rousseau and beyond, political philosophers have emphasized the importance of accounting for—and perhaps even taking advantage of—the powerful influence of the interpersonal context on human affairs. For Plato's philosopher–ruler, for example, interpersonal relations and processes are to be managed confidently and engineered so that the state, and the individual, will be well.

Historically, however, clinical approaches to the study of depression have minimized or overlooked the complex interpersonal context of the disorder. Depression is expressed in the way individuals behave and interact, and, in turn, their interpersonal characteristics shape their risk for, and experiences of, the disorder. Not surprisingly, depression also impacts others' thoughts, feelings, and behaviors in response to the depressed person. Perhaps this last fact explains why clinical views of depression have not shared the confidence of philosophers in the ability to manage the interpersonal context. Instead, their descriptions view the interpersonal processes related to depression as mysterious, annoying, and recalcitrant. Consider a sampling regarding depressed people:

> Their complaints are really "plaints" in the legal sense of the word. . . . [E]verything derogatory that they say of themselves at bottom relates to someone else. . . . [T]hey give a great deal of trouble, perpetually taking offence and behaving as if they had been treated with great injustice. (Freud, 1917/1951, p. 247)

> The physician tends to shun such persons since they threaten not only his need for professional gratification but, even worse, may affect his own spirits by contagion. (Berblinger, 1970, in a statement that foreshadows later work on *depression contagion*, cited in Akiskal, 1983, p. 12)

Quite a litany. One wonders whether the clinicians might have benefited from the efficacious and analytical approach of the philosophers. Perhaps it is possible, in light of recent work on the interpersonal aspects of depression, to achieve this partly, such that depressotypic interpersonal behavior is demystified and loses the distress and frustration evident in the words of the clinicians.

To this end, our goal in this chapter is to survey work examining the interpersonal context of depression. Depression in its interpersonal domain is discussed in three distinct but highly overlapping areas. First, interpersonal characteristics and features of depressed people are summarized. Second, these and other interpersonal characteristics are examined in their role as vulnerability factors for the disorder, and recent research attempting to integrate these risk factors is discussed. Third, the interpersonal consequences of depressotypic interpersonal behaviors are summarized. Finally, we discuss an interpersonal model of depression chronicity, one that incorporates much of the material on the interpersonal characteristics, causes, and consequences of depression.

INTERPERSONAL–BEHAVIORAL CHARACTERISTICS OF DEPRESSED PEOPLE

Social Skills and Depression

There is considerable consensus that depression is associated with social skills problems (see Segrin, 2001, which informs several sections below, for a thorough review). People with depression consistently evaluate their own social skills more negatively than do nondepressed people (e.g., Youngren & Lewinsohn, 1980). It is not particularly surprising that depressed people evaluate their social skills negatively. But are their negative views of their social skills simply a function of a negative self-evaluation bias, or do others also rate their social skills negatively? Segrin's (1990) meta-analysis concluded that depressed–nondepressed differences on partner or observer ratings of social skills are real, but not as strong as depressed–nondepressed differences on self-reported social skills.

Basic Behavioral Features of Depression

Related to the noted problems with social skills, some of depressed people's interpersonal difficulties may stem from basic differences between depressed and nondepressed people on factors such as facial expressions, eye contact, posture, gesturing, and so forth. There is evidence to suggest that the facial expressions of depressed people are more animated than those of other people when expressing sadness; otherwise, depressed people's facial expressions are generally less animated than those of others (Schwartz, Fair, Salt, Mandel, & Klerman, 1976). Several studies have also demonstrated that depressed people engage in less eye contact than do nondepressed people (e.g., Kazdin, Sherick, Esveldt-Dawson, & Rancurello, 1985; Youngren & Lewinsohn, 1980). Interestingly, these features have been shown to improve with successful treatment (Ellgring, 1986). Similar findings have emerged with regard to posture and nonverbal gestures. For example, depressed individuals may hold their heads in a downward position more than do nondepressed persons, and may engage in more self-touching (e.g., rubbing, scratching—possible indicators of distress and discomfort) than do nondepressed people (e.g., Ranelli & Miller, 1981). Kazdin and colleagues (1985) found that depressed children may not use illustrators (speech-accompanying gestures) as much as do nondepressed children. Interestingly, as with facial expressions, it appears that as the symptoms of depression remit, the tendency to use illustrators increases (e.g., Ekman & Friesen, 1972).

Communication Behaviors and Depression

Another, related line of research has examined the communication behaviors of depressed versus nondepressed people. For example, compared to nondepressed people, depressed people speak more slowly, and with less volume and voice modulation (e.g., Youngren & Lewinsohn, 1980). Because factors such as voice modulation, rate of speech, and verbal responses account for the animated and appealing qualities of speech, it is not surprising that the voices of depressed people are perceived negatively by others (e.g., Tolkmitt, Helfrich, Standke, & Scherer, 1982).

In addition to the *quality* of speech, investigators have also examined the *content* of speech in depression. In studies of married couples with a depressed member, themes involving dysphoric feelings and negative self-evaluation were likely to emerge in conversations (e.g., Hautzinger, Linden, & Hoffman, 1982). There is some evidence that negativity in social interactions is particularly likely to emerge between depressed people and intimate relationship partners as opposed to strangers or nonintimate acquaintances. For example, Segrin and Flora (1998) studied depressed and nondepressed students discussing "events of the day" with either a friend or a stranger. They reported that depressed students tended to withhold negative verbal content when talking with strangers but were more likely to disclose negative topics when talking with a friend.

Interpersonal Feedback Seeking and Depression

One specific type of communication behavior in depressed people that appears to be highly aversive to others involves the inappropriate solicitation of interpersonal feedback. Two such feedback-seeking behaviors have been consistently associated with depression: excessive reassurance seeking and negative feedback seeking.

Excessive reassurance seeking is associated with the interpersonal theory of depression, in which Coyne (1976) proposed a process through which dysphoric or depressed individuals behave in a way that contributes to an interpersonal environment that can lead to, and maintain, depression. Initially, mildly depressed or dysphoric individuals seek reassurance from others to alleviate doubts about their self-worth. Although reassurance is often provided, these individuals doubt its truth and may attribute it to others' sense of obligation. Faced with this uncertainty, the individual continues to seek from others reassurance as to his or her worth. As this cycle progresses, others become frustrated with this constant need for reassurance and reject the individual, leading to an environment that promotes the development or maintenance of depression. A number of studies have demonstrated that adults with symptoms of depression (Davila, 2001; Joiner & Metalsky, 2001) or diagnoses of depression (Joiner & Metalsky, 2001; Joiner, Metalsky, Gencoz, & Gencoz, 2001) have higher scores on a measure of excessive reassurance seeking. Similar results have also been found in children (Abela et al., 2005; Joiner et al., 2001). Notably, in a study of youth and adult psychiatric inpatients, Joiner and colleagues (2001) found that reassurance seeking appears specifically to characterize the interpersonal behavior of depressed individuals as opposed to those with other psychiatric diagnoses.

The opposite type of feedback-seeking behavior, negative feedback seeking, also characterizes depressed individuals. *Negative feedback seeking*, defined as the tendency to solicit actively criticism and other negative interpersonal feedback from others, derives from self-verification theory (Swann, 1990), which argues that the need to attain self-consistent and self-verifying information is powerful enough that it may override the pain of seeking and receiving negative feedback. Thus, for people with negative self-views, including depressed people, negative feedback is sought even at the expense of the pain it may cause. Giesler, Josephs, and Swann (1996) examined self-verification theory among clinically depressed participants and reported that when presented with a choice between negative and positive feedback, 82% of clinically depressed adults chose unfavorable over favorable feedback, compared to 64% of nondepressed participants with low self-esteem and 25% of non-depressed participants with high self-esteem. Joiner, Katz, and Lew (1997) extended this work to children and adolescents, and found that depressed youth psychiatric inpatients expressed more interest in negative feedback than did nondepressed youth psychiatric inpatients.

Summary

To summarize, depressed people, compared to their nondepressed counterparts, have been characterized as lower in self-rated and actual social skills, as more negative in speech quality and content, as more likely to engage in aversive feedback-seeking behavior, as less likely to have animated facial expressions (except when sad), as exhibiting less eye contact, and as demonstrating fewer nonverbal gestures that indicate interest in others. The effects of these characteristics on the interpersonal environment are likely to be negative.

One important consideration is whether these characteristics represent stable, trait-like characteristics of depressed individuals or whether they are simply concomitants of depressed mood. As noted, the behavioral characteristics of depressed people seem to improve with remission (Ekman & Friesen, 1972; Ellgring, 1986), but a number of the characteristics described earlier have also been found to predate the development of the disorder. Therefore, these characteristics may represent stable individual traits that serve as risk factors for depression rather than simple correlates of depressed mood.

INTERPERSONAL RISK FACTORS FOR DEPRESSION

Generally speaking, work on interpersonal vulnerability to depression falls into two broad, nonexclusive categories. First, many of the interpersonal–behavioral characteristics of depressed people discussed previously have also been examined as specific risk factors. Second, broader conceptualizations of interpersonal styles taken from personality or cognitive approaches have been examined as risk factors. Specific examples from both areas are reviewed in turn, and integrative studies examining both types of risk factors are then summarized.

Interpersonal Behaviors as Risk Factors for Depression

Social Skills Impairment

Although there is some support in the literature for the view that social skills problems are antecedents of depression, it appears that a majority of the evidence does not support this view, suggesting that social skills deficits may be more state- than trait-like. Studies with strong methodological features, such as inclusion of structured clinical interviews for mood disorders among large samples, have failed to find an effect (e.g., Lewinsohn et al., 1994). More recently, a study of the interpersonal origins of depression in young adults found that neither self-reported nor interview-assessed interpersonal problem-solving skills were associated with increased depressive symptoms over a 6-month interval, nor was the onset of a major depressive episode over a 2-year interval, although interpersonal relationships with family and peers were significant predictors of depression (Eberhart & Hammen, 2006). The extent to which these relationship difficulties might have been influenced by impaired social skills or whether other, unmeasured social skills may be associated with depression is unclear. Overall, however, evidence for the main effect of social skills problems on later depression is relatively weak.

Nonetheless, this leaves open the possibility that social skills deficits operate as a risk factor for depression *only under certain circumstances*, such as in the presence of negative life events. Although this possibility has not yet received abundant research attention, Segrin and Flora (2000) have provided evidence in support of this view. For example, in a study of college freshmen who had moved a long distance from home to attend college (conceived as a stressful experience), Segrin and Flora found that social skills problems assessed during the senior year of high school predicted depressive symptoms at the end of the first college semester. From this perspective, social skills problems may comprise a diathesis that leads to depression only when it is activated by stress. Further studies are needed to replicate this effect and to determine what type of social skills may be related to risk for depression, and whether these are different from the social skills deficits observed in depressed individuals.

Excessive Reassurance Seeking

Recently, Joiner, Metalsky, and colleagues have extended the construct of excessive reassurance seeking to argue that it represents a vulnerability factor for depression. In empirical tests of this perspective, Joiner and Metalsky reported that adults who develop future depressive symptoms (compared to those who remain symptom-free) obtained elevated reassurance-seeking scores at baseline, whereas all participants who were symptom-free did not obtain elevated scores on other interpersonal variables. Similarly, Davila (2001) found that excessive reassurance-seeking scores prospectively predicted increases in depressive symptoms in a sample of young adults who were transitioning to college.

A number of studies have also supported a diathesis–stress model, and have found that excessive reassurance seeking confers vulnerability for depression following diverse experiences of life stress, including academic and interpersonal stress (Joiner & Metalsky, 2001) and basic training for Air Force cadets (Joiner & Schmidt, 1998), and that excessive reassurance seeking is specific to depression, but not anxiety, symptom increases. A number of recent studies that have examined the role of excessive reassurance seeking as a risk factor for depression in children and adolescents have found similar results. In a multiwave study of children of affectively ill parents, Abela, Zuroff, Ho, Adams, and Hankin (2006) found that older children who scored high in reassurance seeking and experienced high levels of hassles or parental depression showed increases in depressive symptoms. In summary, converging evidence supports the theory that excessive reassurance seeking increases risk for depression.

Negative Feedback Seeking

In addition to examining feedback-seeking preferences and behavior of depressed individuals, researchers have begun to explore the role of negative feedback seeking as a potential risk factor for the disorder. In their initial application of self-verification theory specifically to depression, Swann, Wenzlaff, Krull, and Pelham (1992) proposed that depressed people elicit interpersonal rejection because they gravitate to persons who evaluate them negatively (a form of negative feedback seeking). Consistent with this view, these researchers found that, compared to nondepressed students, depressed students sought more negative feedback from others and were more rejected by others. This process may lead directly to increases in depressive symptoms. For example, Joiner (1995) found that requests for negative feedback, if honored (i.e., negative feedback is provided), predisposed college students to future depressive reactions. Pettit and Joiner (2001) examined the effects of negative feedback seeking under conditions of noninterpersonal stress, specifically, exam failure. They found that when individuals who initially scored high in negative feedback seeking received what they considered to be a failing exam grade, they were more likely to exhibit increased depressive symptoms. Borelli and Prinstein (2006) also found that negative feedback seeking was related to increased depression in adolescents over an 11-month interval, although these results were reduced to statistical nonsignificance in the context of a path model that included a number of related variables, such as global self-worth, social anxiety, and peer rejection. The mechanisms behind this process are unclear; the authors suggest that negative feedback seeking, when honored, is likely to lead to increasingly negative self-concepts and negative affect, which might make an individual more vulnerable to depression following negative events. Future research is needed to determine whether the actual behavior of feedback seeking per se or some more global characteristic leads to risk for depression.

Interpersonal Styles as Risk Factors for Depression

In addition to behavioral characteristics, certain kinds of broader interpersonal styles have been associated with depression. These interpersonal styles representing personality traits or broad, cognitive patterns related to interpersonal functioning may be associated with depression.

Interpersonal Inhibition

Although the possibility has not received enough empirical attention, there are at least some reasons to suspect that interpersonal inhibition (e.g., avoidance, withdrawal, shyness) represents a risk factor for depression. Ball, Otto, Pollack, and Rosenbaum (1994) found that lack of assertiveness is a predictor of major depression, even beyond the variance accounted for by a very strong clinical predictor: past history of depression. Various reports have also demonstrated that shyness is associated with depression (e.g., Alfano, Joiner, Perry, & Metalsky, 1994). In addition, there is some evidence that shyness and withdrawal serve as vulnerability factors for future depression. For example, in a study of temperament and depression, Elovainio and colleagues (2004) found that several temperament subscales, including shyness with strangers, predicted depression increases over a 4-year period. Joiner (1997) found that shy undergraduates were prone to increases in depression symptoms in the absence, but not in the presence, of social support, as a function of increases in loneliness. Boivin, Hymel, and Burkowski (1995) reported that among children, social withdrawal is a risk factor for the subsequent occurrence of depressive symptoms.

In this context, it is interesting to note that Price, Sloman, Gardner, Gilbert, and Rohde (1994) have argued from an evolutionary–psychological perspective that depression may represent an evolved form of a primordial *involuntary subordinate strategy* that arose as a means to cope with social competition and conflict, particularly with the losses therein. These authors contend that the primary function of depression is to facilitate *withdrawal* in threatening situations of interpersonal conflict, so that people can "cut their losses," "live to fight another day," and, relatedly, communicate a "no threat" signal to others. Consistent with this model, Shively, Laber-Laird, and Anton (1997) reported that manipulations of social status among female cynomolgus monkeys, such that previously dominant animals became subordinate, produced behavioral and hormonal depressive reactions (e.g., fearful scanning of the environment, hypersecretion of cortisol). Notably, a key behavioral feature of newly subordinate animals was decreased social affiliation (cf. interpersonal avoidance). From a conceptual standpoint, it stands to reason that interpersonal inhibition and avoidance may lead to future depression, because they involve diminution of social reinforcement and social support. As Lewinsohn (1974) and others have persuasively argued, a lack of positive reinforcement is involved in maintaining depression.

An alternative possibility, however, is that interpersonal inhibition and avoidance are characteristics of anxiety disorders, which have been shown to overlap closely with depression. In a review of research on the overlap between anxiety and depression, Watson (2005) proposed that mood and anxiety disorders should be combined into an overarching class of emotional disorders. One such overarching model, the tripartite model of depression and anxiety (Clark & Watson, 1991), proposes that depression and anxiety can be described by three factors. The first, *negative affectivity*, is the shared, general distress component of both disorders. The second, *positive affectivity*, is associated with depression, such that only depressed individuals have low positive affect. Finally, the third factor, *physiological arousal*, has been related specifically to anxiety. It may be that any relation between interpersonal inhibition and depression may be explained by this relationship and accounted for by the general negative affectivity component of both disorders. Social anxiety disorder, which is most closely related to interpersonal inhibition, has been found to be a risk factor for depression in a longitudinal study of adolescents and young adults in Germany (Stein et al., 2001). However, social anxiety disorder also has been associated with the second factor of depression, low positive affect, which is unique among anxiety disorders (Brown, Chorpita, & Barlow, 1998). Future studies are needed to elaborate fully the relationship among anxiety disorders, interpersonal inhibition, and depression.

Interpersonal Dependency

A reasonably well-established empirical tradition, especially in psychiatry and personality psychology, identifies interpersonal dependency as a risk factor for depression (e.g., Blatt, Quinlan, Chevron, McDonald, & Zuroff, 1982). In this regard, a similar line of thought regarding interpersonal vulnerability has emerged from the cognitive approach. Beck's notion of sociotropy indicates that excessive need for and doubt about interpersonal attachment (e.g., acceptance, support, guidance, admiration; see Beck, 1983, p. 272) lead to behaviors (e.g., obsequiousness) that cause and maintain depression. Both sociotropy and dependency have been examined as risk factors for depression (see Zuroff, Mongrain, & Santor, 2004, for a review and discussion of the relation between the two constructs).

Evidence suggests that interpersonal dependency may directly predict the onset of depressive diagnoses. In a cross-sectional, case–control study, Mazure, Bruce, Maciejewski, and Jacobs (2000) found that sociotropy was related to depression onset. Similarly, Sanathara, Gardner, Prescott, and Kendler (2003) found that interpersonal dependency was prospectively related to the onset of major depressive disorder in a large, population-based study of twins. Studies have also examined the prospective prediction of depressive symptoms rather than diagnoses, and have shown that dependency (Mongrain, Lubbers, &

Struthers, 2004) and sociotropy (Shih, 2006) predict increased depressive symptoms over time.

More frequently, dependency and sociotropy have been examined as risk factors within a diathesis–stress framework, such that individuals who have higher interpersonal dependency are most likely to become depressed following interpersonal stressors. This hypothesis has received some support, particularly when studies have examined increases in depressive symptoms. For example, recent studies have found that dependency interacts with stress to predict increased depression in college students (Priel & Shahar, 2000; Shahar, Joiner, Zuroff, & Blatt, 2004). There is also some evidence that sociotropy may represent a more general vulnerability factor, because it has been found to predict increased depression in interaction with noninterpersonal events as well (e.g., Fresco, Sampson, Craighead, & Koons, 2001). The interaction between sociotropy or dependency and interpersonal stress has not been as well supported in the prediction of depressive diagnoses. For example, although they found sociotropy to be related to depression onset, Mazure and colleagues (2000) did not find a significant interaction between sociotropy and life events. Similarly, Frewen and Dozois (2006) found that sociotropy was not a significant predictor alone or in interaction with negative life events when they controlled for other, related personality variables.

Attachment Style

Recently, researchers have begun to examine attachment style as a risk factor for depression. This work derives from Bowlby's (1973) theory of attachment, which proposes that infant attachment to a primary caregiver leads to internal working models that form a basis for the individual's future relationships with others and emotion regulation abilities. Different prototypes for attachment styles, initially described by Ainsworth, Blehar, Waters, and Wall (1978), were later extended to adult relationships (Hazan & Shaver, 1987). Although different theorists have proposed different categories for attachment, all categorical systems can be divided into secure and insecure types of attachment. As one example of the categorization of attachment styles, Hazan and Shaver (1987) described secure, anxious, and avoidant attachment styles in adults. They stated that securely attached adults are generally confident, socially skilled, and able to form stable close relationships. Anxiously attached adults tend to seek close relationships but are prone to worry about rejection and abandonment, may have problems with jealousy, and generally experience unstable relationships. Adults with an avoidant attachment style are inhibited, uncomfortable with closeness, and less socially skilled—a number of the interpersonal characteristics associated with depression.

A number of researchers have examined attachment styles in relationship to depression. Although these studies have used a variety of different categorizations of attachment style, an association between general, insecure attachment and depression has been well-established in adults for both depressive symptoms (e.g., Roberts, Gotlib, & Kassel, 1996) and diagnoses (e.g., Reinecke & Rogers, 2001). An anxious attachment style, as opposed to other attachment styles, may be particularly related to depression (Roberts et al., 1996). In addition to their concurrent relationship with depression, insecure attachment styles also appear to increase risk for depression. Again, insecure attachment was found to be significantly related to both increases in depressive symptoms (Hankin, Kassel, & Abela, 2005) and onset of the disorder (Eberhart & Hammen, 2006). One study to date extended the research on attachment style as a risk factor by examining a diathesis–stress framework and found that interpersonal attachment cognitions combine with interpersonal stress to predict depression and other symptoms (Hammen et al., 1995).

Integrations of Interpersonal Risk Factors for Depression

Considering the range of interpersonal behaviors and interpersonal styles that have been explored as risk factors for depression and the conceptual overlap among the constructs, it is not surprising that researchers have begun to examine the interrelations between these variables. To date, the behavioral characteristics of excessive reassurance seeking and social skills have been examined in relation to the interpersonal styles of interpersonal dependency and insecure attachment. Each of these areas is explored in turn.

Most of the integrative studies to date have focused on excessive reassurance seeking. Cross-sectionally, it appears that reassurance seeking is related to sociotropy (Beck, Robbins, Taylor, & Baker, 2001) and dependency (Shahar et al., 2004). Shahar and colleagues (2004) examined potential mediating and moderating effects in the prospective prediction of depression, and found that when dependency was included in the equation, reassurance seeking did not show a significant predictive effect alone or in combination with life stress. Instead, the interaction between dependency and life stress was the only significant predictor of increased depression. Thus, it is unclear whether excessive reassurance seeking leads to depression independent of dependency.

Three studies have examined the relationship between excessive reassurance seeking and insecure attachment styles. Davila (2001) examined the relationship between the two variables and depressive symptoms, both concurrently and prospectively, in a sample of young adults transitioning to college. Both insecure attachment and reassurance seeking were related to concurrent depressive symptoms when the other variable was controlled, and reassurance seeking was a significant predictor of future depressive symptoms when researchers controlled for attachment variables. In a similar study with children, Abela and colleagues (2005) found that both insecure attachment and reassurance seeking were related to depression, but this effect was qualified by a significant interaction, such that insecurely attached children who also scored high in reassurance seeking were the most depressed. In contrast to these results, Shaver, Schachner, and Mikulincer (2005) argued that reassurance seeking is better conceptualized as a facet of insecure attachment, and they found that attachment anxiety mediated the relationship between reassurance seeking and concurrent depressive symptoms in a sample of college students in romantic relationships. Again, therefore, more research is needed to clarify the nature of the relationship between reassurance seeking and insecure attachment.

Research on the relation between social skills and depressive interpersonal styles has been more sparse. Two studies have found a significant association between self-reported social skills and insecure attachment (Deniz, Hamarta, & Ari, 2005; DiTommaso, Brannen-McNulty, Ross, & Burgess, 2003). Although not specifically examining the relationship to depression, DiTommaso and colleagues (2003) did find that the relationship between attachment and loneliness was partially mediated by low social expressiveness. A similar cross-sectional study found a significant relation between social skills and dependency, such that dependent individuals with higher levels of social skills were less depressed, but it also found that the skills of social expressiveness, social sensitivity, and social control had main effects as predictors of depressive symptoms, independent of dependency (Huprich, Clancy, Bornstein, & Nelson-Gray, 2004). Finally, although not precisely measuring social skills, Connor-Smith and Compas (2002) found that individuals high in sociotropy had poorer coping skills. They also reported that coping skills moderated the relationship between sociotropy and depression, such that those with poor coping skills and high levels of sociotropy had more severe symptoms of depression.

INTERPERSONAL CONSEQUENCES OF DEPRESSION

Given that depression may be associated with negative feedback seeking, impaired social skills, interpersonal avoidance, and excessive reassurance seeking *premorbidly*, and given that current symptoms are clearly associated with social skills problems, negative verbal and nonverbal parameters, and so forth, it is not surprising that the personal relationships of depressed people are affected. In fact, the relationships of depressed people are characterized by dimensions such as rejection, dissatisfaction, low intimacy, and decreased activity and involvement (e.g., Gotlib & Lee, 1989). Evidence suggests that intimate relationships, including marital and parental relationships, may be particularly disrupted by depression (see Davila, Stroud, & Starr, Chapter 20, this volume).

In addition to relationship problems, there is some evidence that one interpersonal consequence of depression is *contagious depression*, the spread of depressive symptoms form one person to another. Recall Berblinger's (cited in Akiskal, 1983, p. 12) earlier statement about depressed people: "The physician tends to shun such persons since they threaten not only his need for professional gratification but, even worse, may affect his own spirits by contagion." In a meta-analysis on contagion of depressive symptoms and mood from 36 studies ($n = 4,952$), Joiner and Katz (1999) reached the following conclusions:

1. There was substantial support for the view that depressive symptoms and mood are contagious, but the phenomenon was most pronounced in studies of depressive symptoms (vs. depressive mood).
2. Contagion of depressive mood depended on the methodological approach, with strongest to weakest results in the following order: transcript studies, audiotape/videotape studies, studies using actual friends/acquaintances, and confederate studies.
3. Contagion of depressed mood/symptoms held across combinations of target × respondent gender.
4. There was some tentative evidence that contagion was specific to depressive versus other symptoms and moods.

In a study designed specifically to address contagion of depressive symptoms, Joiner (1994) demonstrated that the roommates of depressed college students tended to experience increased depressive symptoms themselves over the course of a few weeks. Shared negative life stress was ruled out as an explanation of the finding. This effect was particularly pronounced among roommate dyads in which there were high levels of reassurance seeking, a finding consistent with the view that excessive reassurance seeking may serve as an "interpersonal vehicle" that carries the distress and desperation of depressive symptoms from one person to another. In fact, this same line of reasoning appears to apply to interpersonal rejection (just as it may apply to contagion of depressive symptoms). Specifically, Joiner and Metalsky found that those with depressive symptoms do *not* elicit interpersonal rejection *unless* they *also* excessively seek reassurance (Joiner, 1999; Joiner & Metalsky, 1995). This line of research also indicates that persons with depressive symptoms who engage in multiple depressotypic interpersonal behaviors (e.g., excessive reassurance seeking and negative feedback seeking) are especially likely to disaffect others (e.g., Joiner & Metalsky, 1995). Notably, in these studies, although neither depression nor depressotypic interpersonal behavior was related *individually* to indices of interpersonal rejection, they were in combination. Thus, an interesting question emerges: Why are depression and, for example, reassurance seeking, not sufficient in themselves to induce rejection from others? It may be that without the urgency and desperation associated with depressive symptoms, reassurance seeking alone may be relatively tolerable to others (Joiner & Metalsky, 1995). Conversely, others may tolerate depression, unless it is persistently "taken to them" through excessive reassurance seeking.

AN INTEGRATIVE INTERPERSONAL FRAMEWORK FOR THE STUDY OF DEPRESSION AND ITS CHRONICITY

Two important features of depression are that it persists and recurs. In the DSM-IV Mood Disorders Field Trial (Keller et al., 1995), the most frequent diagnostic course among several hundred patients with current major depression was "recurrent, with antecedent dysthymia, without full interepisode recovery." Indeed, it is quite common for subclinical depressive symptoms to persist in the wake of a remitted depressive episode (Judd et al., 2000). Thus, depression is persistent within acute episodes and recurrent across substantial portions of people's lives. Chronicity is a feature of depression about which a useful explanatory model should have something to say.

Joiner's (2000) argument that interpersonal self-propagatory processes are involved in generating and maintaining depression may partly explain the chronicity of depression. Joiner defines a *self-propagatory process* as a complex of psychological and behavioral factors that (1) represents depression-related, initiated, and active behaviors that (2) serve to prolong or exacerbate existing symptoms or to induce the recurrence of past symptoms. The general logic of this perspective is that several depression-related mechanisms actively produce an array of interpersonal and other problems; these problems, in turn, are strong predictors of lengthened and/or future depression. The framework borrows heavily from Hammen and colleagues' (e.g., Hammen, 1991) work on *stress generation* (contributing to the occurrence of one's own negative interpersonal events). Stress generation is viewed as a higher-order concept that may subsume several specific mechanisms for the generation of stress and the propagation of depression. Several of these specific behavioral mechanisms have been mentioned already (e.g., negative feedback seeking, excessive reassurance seeking, interpersonal avoidance). Each of these mechanisms was claimed to propagate depression through diminution of social reinforcement and social support.

For example, excessive reassurance seeking is an active and motivated behavior on the part of the depressed person, in keeping with the definition for a self-propagatory process. Moreover, excessive reassurance seeking is involved in the generation of interpersonal stress (e.g., rejection—Pothoff, Holahan, & Joiner, 1995; "contagious" depression—Joiner, 1994). As described earlier, there is evidence that excessive reassurance seeking is implicated in the development of depression itself (e.g., Joiner & Metalsky, 2001). Overall, then, excessive reassurance seeking, interpersonal stress, and depression are all reciprocally involved, with one behavior often leading to the others in serial fashion. In this light, the chronicity of depression is a consequence of this serial, unfolding process in people's lives. Similar arguments can be made for variables such as negative feedback seeking and interpersonal avoidance.

Although they are more distal and trait-like in nature, and may not function directly as self-propagatory processes, several other interpersonal risk factors for depression also contribute to depression's chronicity through the generation of stress. Poor social skills, for example, have been found to predict the recurrence of depression through the generation of stressful life events (Bos, Bouhuys, Geerts, van Os, & Ormel, 2007). Insecure attachment has also been found to contribute to the generation of interpersonal stress, which mediates the relationship between insecure attachment and depression (Hankin et al., 2005). Similarly, sociotropy has been found to be related to stress generation in women (Shih, 2006). In this way, individuals with interpersonal deficits or vulnerable interpersonal styles may have a chronic risk for generating negative social environments, placing them at increased risk for depression. It is likely that active, self-propagatory processes compound this preexisting risk and lead to increased depression severity.

Borrowing from the work of Sacco (1999), Joiner (2000) noted an additional process that deserves mention and future research, namely, *blame maintenance,* defined as the development of negatively tinged and autonomous perceptions of the depressed person in the minds of others. Once developed, these perceptions take on an independent and autonomous quality, in that they selectively guide attention to confirm themselves. Importantly, negative person perceptions can be viewed as an antecedent of blaming and otherwise negative communications from others to the depressed person. It has been documented that these negative communications in turn predict various forms of depression and its chronicity (Hooley & Teasdale, 1989). Ironically, due to the pressure of self-verification needs, depressed patients may actively solicit these negative communications; even if they do not, these communications may nonetheless be forthcoming because of the influence of blame maintenance processes.

FUTURE DIRECTIONS

Depression, depressotypic interpersonal behaviors (social skills problems, negative verbal and nonverbal behaviors, excessive reassurance seeking, negative feedback seeking, etc.), interpersonal styles (e.g., interpersonal avoidance, dependency, and insecure attachment), interpersonal rejection (along with other types of stress), and contagious depression comprise intertwining threads that together make up the fabric of the depressive social environment. Each category of variables may act as a vulnerability factor for the others. Each class may serve as an entrée into a circular and self-amplifying pathway featuring the others.

A more textured understanding of the threads of this pathway, and how they relate to noninterpersonal risk factors for depression, represents a major avenue for future research from an interpersonal perspective. Researchers have begun to examine the interconnections between these variables, particularly in the overlap of the interpersonal behaviors and interpersonal styles that serve as risk factors for depression. At this time, it is clear that there are significant relationships between most of these risk factors, but the connections between them and their interaction in the development or maintenance of depression remain elusive. One important consideration in future studies of the interpersonal context of depression is to determine to what extent depressotypic interpersonal behaviors represent normal interpersonal processes as opposed to purely pathological behavior. It may be that behaviors such as reassurance seeking or negative feedback seeking serve adaptive functions under certain circumstances, and only become problematic for certain individuals (e.g., those with insecure attachment or dependency needs). Alternatively, these behavioral processes may escalate in most people given the right combination of mood and stressful life events. A full theoretical understanding of these processes will need to take into account the variations in these behaviors among both clinical and nonclinical populations.

For this reason, an important direction for future research involves the simultaneous empirical scrutiny of the interpersonal characteristics and processes summarized here. Although there is reason to believe that each of these variables is associated with depression in substantive ways, a large-scale project clearly documenting involvement in the onset or maintenance of clinical, diagnosed depression would prove illuminating. Examining the contribution of interpersonal factors to the development of depression could clarify whether each risk factor has an effect that is independent of the other risk factors and other, related features of depression, such as comorbid anxiety. Especially if conducted longitudinally, this project could delineate some particulars of the self-propagatory processes described by Joiner (2000), including their interplay with one another. For example, in the case of interpersonal inhibition and excessive reassurance seeking, it is possible that interpersonal avoidance may focus the effects of reassurance seeking and negative feedback seeking on just one or two relationships, thus damaging those relationships and leaving the person bereft of depression-buffering social support.

Importantly, we do not claim here that interpersonal factors account for most aspects of depression. Additional factors are clearly at play, including noninterpersonal, stable vulnerability factors that maintain risk over time. Examples of persistent vulnerabilities may include genetic and neurobiological risk factors, as well as cognitive style risk factors (Abramson, Metalsky, & Alloy, 1989; Beck, 1983; Nolen-Hoeksema, 1991). The interplay of interpersonal and noninterpersonal risks for depression is an understudied question, although research on the association between factors such as attachment style and cognitive distortions holds promise (Hankin et al., 2005; Reinecke & Rogers, 2001; Roberts et al., 1996). Overall, however, large questions remain: Do these factors interact with one another to amplify risk? Does an interpersonal factor lead to depression *because* it exacerbates underlying cognitive or neurobiological variables, or vice versa?

As one example, Nolen-Hoeksema, Morrow, and Fredrickson (1993) have proposed that a ruminative response style represents a stable vulnerability to depression (see Nolen-Hoeksema & Hilt, Chapter 17, this volume). Specifically, they have argued that the duration of depressive symptoms is influenced by the manner in which individuals respond to their own symptoms. Ruminative response styles include persistent attention to one's negative emotions; this attention is focused on one's symptoms, as well as on the causes, meanings, and consequences of those symptoms. Although speculative, one possibility for an integration of interpersonal and cognitive views is that rumination drives behaviors such as excessive reassurance seeking and negative feedback seeking. With respect to reassurance seeking, it is the case that dysphoric ideation and mood fuel excessive reassurance seeking. Because rumination may sustain negative ideation and dysphoric mood, it could also drive reassurance seeking. Reassurance seeking, in turn, has been shown to lead to outcomes such as increased depression, interpersonal rejection, and "depression contagion." Similarly, because rumination may maintain focus on feelings of inadequacy or social incompetence, it may induce negative feedback seeking and interpersonal avoidance.

Another research direction involves the tailoring of psychotherapeutic approaches based on findings from an interpersonal perspective. Interestingly, on the surface, interpersonal psychotherapy (IPT) for depression (Klerman, Weissman, Rousaville, & Chevron, 1984) seems to flow naturally from viewing depression in its interpersonal context (and, crucially, the treatment seems effective; e.g., see Weissman & Klerman, 1993; Beach, Jones, & Franklin, Chapter 27, this volume). There is clear compatibility, but nonetheless real discontinuity between basic research on the interpersonal aspects of depression on the one hand, and the development and application of IPT on the other. Specifically, the emphasis of IPT on the interpersonal domains of grief, role transitions, role disputes, and social skills does not rely heavily and specifically on the detailed research on, for example, verbal and nonverbal behaviors, or on excessive reassurance seeking and negative feedback seeking. This is less a criticism of IPT (which has proved its merit) than an underscoring of an area for future work that could significantly refine and improve IPT. This point applies as well to other empirically supported psychotherapies.

Although research has revealed the interpersonal characteristics of, and risk factors for, depression, a number of methodological limitations need to be addressed in future studies. First, many of the proposed interpersonal behaviors associated with depression, such as excessive reassurance seeking and negative feedback seeking, are measured with brief self-report questionnaires. For this reason, it is not clear whether these behaviors, the participant's perception of these behaviors, or some other psychological characteristic is driving the observed effects. Future work is needed to continue the process of construct validation of these interpersonal variables to truly understand their role in depression. Second, many of the studies on interpersonal behaviors as risk factors for depression have been conducted on college students and have measured depressive symptom increases rather than more severe symptoms or depressive diagnoses. Again, future research is needed to clarify these processes in clinical samples, and longitudinal studies would be the best way to elaborate the role of interpersonal processes in the onset and maintenance of depression. Third, the broader interpersonal styles, such as interpersonal inhibition, dependency, and insecure attachment, may be associated with both anxiety and depression. Studies are needed to determine whether these styles maintain an association with depression after researchers control for anxious symptoms.

Despite these limitations, a growing body of evidence supports the importance of interpersonal processes in depression. Without knowledge of the characteristics, motivations, and consequences of depressotypic interpersonal behavior, depression and its social vicissitudes would seem bewildering. Considered in this light, the frustrated reactions of many theoreticians and clinicians to depressed patients, highlighted at the beginning of the chapter, become understandable. With knowledge from an interpersonal perspective, they become remediable.

REFERENCES

Abela, J. R. Z., Hankin, B. L., Haigh, E. A. P., Adams, P., Vinokuroff, T., & Trayhern, L. (2005). Interpersonal vulnerability to depression in high-risk children: The role of insecure attachment and reassurance seeking. *Journal of Clinical Child and Adolescent Psychology, 34*, 182–192.

Abela, J. R. Z., Zuroff, D. C., Ho, M. R., Adams, P., & Hankin, B. L. (2006). Excessive reassurance-seeking, hassles, and depressive symptoms in children of affectively ill patients: A multiwave longitudinal study. *Journal of Abnormal Child Psychology, 34*, 171–187.

Abramson, L. Y., Metalsky, G. I., & Alloy, L. B. (1989). Hopelessness depression: A theory-based subtype of depression. *Psychological Review, 96*, 358–372.

Ainsworth, M. D. S., Blehar, M. C., Waters, E., & Wall, S. (1978). *Patterns of attachment: A psychological study of the strange situation.* Hillsdale, NJ: Erlbaum.

Akiskal, H. S. (1983). Dysthymic disorder: Psychopathology of proposed chronic depressive subtypes. *American Journal of Psychiatry, 140*, 11–20.

Alfano, M. S., Joiner, T. E., Jr., Perry, M., & Metalsky, G. I. (1994). Attributional style: A mediator of the shyness–depression relationship? *Journal of Research in Personality, 28*, 287–300.

Ball, S. G., Otto, M. W., Pollack, M. H., & Rosenbaum, J. F. (1994). Predicting prospective episodes of depression in patients with panic disorder: A longitudinal study. *Journal of Consulting and Clinical Psychology, 62*, 359–365.

Beck, A. T. (1983). Cognitive therapy of depression: New perspectives. In P. Clayton & J. E. Barret (Eds.), *Treatment of depression: Old controversies and new approaches* (pp. 265–290). New York: Raven Press.

Beck, R., Robbins, M., Taylor, C., & Baker, L. (2001). An examination of sociotropy and excessive reassurance seeking in the prediction of depression. *Journal of Psychopathology and Behavioral Assessment*, *23*, 101–105.

Blatt, S. J., Quinlan, D., Chevron, E., McDonald, C., & Zuroff, D. (1982). Dependency and self-criticism: Psychological dimensions of depression. *Journal of Consulting and Clinical Psychology*, *50*, 113–124.

Boivin, M., Hymel, S., & Burkowski, W. M. (1995). The roles of social withdrawal, peer rejection, and victimization by peers in predicting loneliness and depressed mood in childhood. *Development and Psychopathology*, *7*, 765–785.

Borelli, J. L., & Prinstein, M. J. (2006). Reciprocal, longitudinal associations among adolescents' negative feedback seeking, depressive symptoms, and peer relations. *Journal of Abnormal Child Psychology*, *34*, 159–169.

Bos, E. H., Bouhuys, A. L., Geerts, E., van Os, T. W., & Ormel, J. (2007). Stressful life events as a link between problems in nonverbal communication and recurrence of depression. *Journal of Affective Disorders*, *97*, 161–169.

Bowlby, J. (1973). *Attachment and loss: Vol. 2. Separation: Anxiety and anger.* New York: Basic Books.

Brown, T. A., Chorpita, B. F., & Barlow, D. H. (1998). Structural relationships among dimensions of the DSM-IV anxiety and mood disorders and dimensions of negative affect, positive affect, and autonomic arousal. *Journal of Abnormal Psychology*, *107*, 179–192.

Clark, L. A., & Watson, D. (1991). Tripartite model of anxiety and depression: Psychometric evidence and taxonomic implications. *Journal of Abnormal Psychology*, *100*, 316–336.

Connor-Smith, J. K., & Compas, B. E. (2002). Vulnerability to social stress: Coping as a mediator or moderator of symptoms of anxiety and depression. *Cognitive Therapy and Research*, *26*, 39–55.

Coyne, J. C. (1976). Toward an interactional description of depression. *Psychiatry*, *39*, 28–40.

Davila, J. (2001). Refining the association between excessive reassurance seeking and depressive symptoms: The role of related interpersonal constructs. *Journal of Social and Clinical Psychology*, *20*, 538–559.

Deniz, M. E., Hamarta, E., & Ari, R. (2005). An investigation of social skills and loneliness levels of university students with respect to their attachment styles in a sample of Turkish students. *Social Behavior and Personality*, *33*, 19–32.

DiTommaso, E., Brannen-McNulty, C., Ross, L., & Burgess, M. (2003). Attachment styles, social skills, and loneliness in young adults. *Personality and Individual Differences*, *35*, 303–312.

Eberhart, N. K., & Hammen, C. L. (2006). Interpersonal predictors of onset of depression during the transition to adulthood. *Personal Relationships*, *13*, 195–206.

Ekman, P., & Friesen, W. V. (1972). Hand movements. *Journal of Communication*, *22*, 353–374.

Ellgring, H. (1986). Nonverbal expression of psychological studies in psychiatric patients. *European Archives of Psychiatry and Neurological Sciences*, *236*, 31–34.

Elovainio, M., Kivimäki, M., Puttonen, S., Heponiemi, T., Pulkki, L., & Keltikangas-Järvinen, L. (2004). Temperament and depressive symptoms: A population-based longitudinal study on Cloninger's psychobiological temperament model. *Journal of Affective Disorders*, *83*, 227–232.

Fresco, D. M., Sampson, W. S., Craighead, L. W., & Koons, A. N. (2001). The relationship of sociotropy and autonomy to symptoms of depression and anxiety. *Journal of Cognitive Psychotherapy*, *15*, 17–31.

Freud, S. (1951). Mourning and melancholia. In J. Strachey (Ed. & Trans.), *The standard edition of the complete psychological works of Sigmund Freud* (Vol. 14, pp. 237–260). London: Hogarth Press. (Original work published 1917)

Frewen, P. A., & Dozois, D. J. A. (2006). Self-worth appraisal of life events and Beck's congruency model of depression vulnerability. *Journal of Cognitive Psychotherapy*, *20*, 231–240.

Giesler, R. B., Josephs, R. A., & Swann, W. B. (1996). Self-verification in clinical depression: The desire for negative evaluation. *Journal of Abnormal Psychology*, *105*, 358–368.

Gotlib, I. H., & Lee, C. M. (1989). The social functioning of depressed patients: A longitudinal assessment. *Journal of Social and Clinical Psychology*, *8*, 223–237.

Hammen, C. (1991). Generation of stress in the course of unipolar depression. *Journal of Abnormal Psychology*, *100*, 551–561.

Hammen, C. L., Burge, D., Daley, S. E., Davila, J., Paley, B., & Rudolph, K. D. (1995). Interpersonal attachment cognitions and prediction of symptomatic responses to interpersonal stress. *Journal of Abnormal Psychology, 104,* 436–443.

Hankin, B. L., Kassel, J. D., & Abela, J. R. Z. (2005). Adult attachment dimensions and specificity of emotional distress symptoms: Prospective investigations of cognitive risk and interpersonal stress generation as mediating mechanisms. *Personality and Social Psychology Bulletin, 31,* 136–151.

Hautzinger, M., Linden, M., & Hoffman, N. (1982). Distressed couples with and without a depressed partner: An analysis of their verbal interaction. *Journal of Behavior Therapy and Experimental Psychiatry, 13,* 307–314.

Hazan, C., & Shaver, P. (1987). Romantic love conceptualized as an attachment process. *Journal of Personality and Social Psychology, 52,* 511–524.

Hooley, J. M., & Teasdale, J. D. (1989). Predictors of relapse in unipolar depressives: Expressed emotion, marital distress, and perceived criticism. *Journal of Abnormal Psychology, 98,* 229–235.

Huprich, S. K., Clancy, C., Bornstein, R. F., & Nelson-Gray, R. O. (2004). Do dependency and social skills combine to predict depression?: Linking two diatheses in mood disorders research. *Individual Differences Research, 2,* 2–16.

Joiner, T., Metalsky, G., Gencoz, F., & Gencoz, T. (2001). The relative specificity of excessive reassurance-seeking to depression in clinical samples of adults and youth. *Journal of Psychopathology and Behavioral Assessment, 23,* 35–42.

Joiner, T. E., Jr. (1994). Contagious depression: Existence, specificity to depressed symptoms, and the role of reassurance-seeking. *Journal of Personality and Social Psychology, 67,* 287–296.

Joiner, T. E., Jr. (1995). The price of soliciting and receiving negative feedback: Self-verification theory as a vulnerability to depression theory. *Journal of Abnormal Psychology, 104,* 364–372.

Joiner, T. E., Jr. (1997). Shyness and low social support as interactive diatheses, and loneliness as mediator: Testing an interpersonal-personality view of depression. *Journal of Abnormal Psychology, 106,* 145–151.

Joiner, T. E., Jr. (1999). A test of interpersonal theory of depression among youth psychiatric inpatients. *Journal of Abnormal Child Psychology, 27,* 75–84.

Joiner, T. E., Jr. (2000). Depression's vicious scree: Self-propagatory and erosive factors in depression chronicity. *Clinical Psychology: Science and Practice, 7,* 203–218.

Joiner, T. E., Jr., & Katz, J. (1999). Contagion of depressive symptoms and mood: Meta-analytic review and explanations from cognitive, behavioral, and interpersonal viewpoints. *Clinical Psychology: Science and Practice, 6,* 149–164.

Joiner, T. E., Jr., Katz, J., & Lew, A. (1997). Self-verification and depression in youth psychiatric inpatients. *Journal of Abnormal Psychology, 106,* 608–618.

Joiner, T. E., Jr., & Metalsky, G. I. (1995). A prospective test of an integrative interpersonal theory of depression: A naturalistic study of college roommates. *Journal of Personality and Social Psychology, 69,* 778–788.

Joiner, T. E., Jr., & Metalsky, G. I. (2001). Excessive reassurance-seeking: Delineating a risk factor involved in the development of depressive symptoms. *Psychological Science, 12,* 371–378.

Joiner, T. E., Jr., & Schmidt, N. B. (1998). Excessive reassurance-seeking predicts depressive but not anxious reactions to acute stress. *Journal of Abnormal Psychology, 107,* 533–537.

Judd, L. L., Paulus, M. J., Schettler, P. J., Akiskal, H. S., Endicott, J., Leon, A. C., et al. (2000). Does incomplete recovery from first lifetime major depressive episode herald a chronic course of illness? *American Journal of Psychiatry, 157,* 1501–1504.

Kazdin, A. E., Sherick, R. B., Esveldt-Dawson, K., & Rancurello, M. D. (1985). Nonverbal behavior and childhood depression. *Journal of the American Academy of Child Psychiatry, 24,* 303–309.

Keller, M. B., Klein, D. N., Hirschfeld, R. M. A., Kocsis, J. H., McCullough, J. P., Miller, I., et al. (1995). Results of the DSM-IV mood disorders field trial. *American Journal of Psychiatry, 152,* 843–849.

Klerman, G. L., Weissman, M. M., Rousaville, B. J., & Chevron, E. S. (1984). *Interpersonal therapy for depression.* New York: Basic Books.

Lewinsohn, P. M. (1974). A behavioral approach to depression. In R. J. Friedman & M. M. Katz (Eds.), *The psychology of depression: Contemporary theory and research* (pp. 54–77). Washington, DC: Winston-Wiley.

Lewinsohn, P. M., Roberts, R. E., Seeley, J. R., Rohde, P., Gotlib, I. H., & Hops, H. (1994). Adolescent psychopathology: II. Psychosocial risk factors for depression *Journal of Abnormal Psychology, 103*, 302–315.

Mazure, C. M., Bruce, M. L., Maciejewski, P. K., & Jacobs, S. C. (2000). Adverse life events and cognitive–personality characteristics in the prediction of major depression and antidepressant response. *American Journal of Psychiatry, 157*, 896–903.

Mongrain, M., Lubbers, R., & Struthers, W. (2004). The power of love: Mediation of rejection in roommates of dependents and self-critics. *Personality and Social Psychology Bulletin, 30*, 94–105.

Nolen-Hoeksema, S. (1991). Responses to depression and their effects on the duration of depressive episodes. *Journal of Abnormal Psychology, 100*, 569–582.

Nolen-Hoeksema, S., Morrow, J., & Fredrickson, B. L. (1993). Response styles and the duration of episodes of depressed mood. *Journal of Abnormal Psychology, 102*, 20–28.

Pettit, J., & Joiner, T. E., Jr. (2001). Negative-feedback seeking leads to depressive symptom increases under conditions of stress. *Journal of Psychopathology and Behavioral Assessment, 23*, 69–74.

Potthoff, J. G., Holahan, C. J., & Joiner, T. E., Jr. (1995). Reassurance-seeking, stress generation, and depressive symptoms: An integrative model. *Journal of Personality and Social Psychology, 68*, 664–670.

Price, J., Sloman, L., Gardner, R., Jr., Gilbert, P., & Rohde, P. (1994). The social competition hypothesis of depression. *British Journal of Psychiatry, 164*, 309–315.

Priel, B., & Shahar, G. (2000). Dependency, self-criticism, social context and distress: Comparing moderating and mediating models. *Personality and Individual Differences, 28*, 515–525.

Ranelli, C. J., & Miller, R. E. (1981). Behavioral predictors of amitriptyline response in depression. *American Journal of Psychiatry, 138*, 30–34.

Reinecke, M. A., & Rogers, G. M. (2001). Dysfunctional attitudes and attachment style among clinically depressed adults. *Behavioural and Cognitive Psychotherapy, 29*, 129–141.

Roberts, J. E., Gotlib, I. H., & Kassel, J. D. (1996). Adult attachment security and symptoms of depression: The mediating roles of dysfunctional attitudes and low self-esteem. *Journal of Personality and Social Psychology, 70*, 310–320.

Sacco, W. P. (1999). A social-cognitive model of interpersonal processes in depression. In T. Joiner & J. C. Coyne (Eds.), *The interactional nature of depression* (pp. 329–362). Washington, DC: American Psychological Association Press.

Sanathara, V. A., Gardner, C. O., Prescott, C. A., & Kendler, K. S. (2003). Interpersonal dependence and major depression: Aetiological inter-relationship and gender differences. *Psychological Medicine, 33*, 927–931.

Schwartz, G. E., Fair, P. L., Salt, P., Mandel, M. R., & Klerman, G. (1976). Facial expression and imagery in depression: An electromyographic study. *Psychosomatic Medicine, 38*, 337–347.

Segrin, C. (1990). A meta-analytic review of social skill deficits in depression. *Communication Monographs, 57*, 292–308.

Segrin, C. (2001). *Interpersonal processes in psychological problems.* New York: Guilford Press.

Segrin, C., & Flora, J. (1998). Depression and verbal behavior in conversation with friends and strangers. *Journal of Language and Social Psychology, 11*, 43–70.

Segrin, C., & Flora, J. (2000). Poor social skills are a vulnerability factor in the development of psychosocial problems. *Human Communication Research, 26*, 489–514.

Shahar, G., Joiner, T. E., Jr., Zuroff, D. C., & Blatt, S. J. (2004). Personality, interpersonal behavior, and depression: Co-existence of stress-specific moderating and mediating effects. *Personality and Individual Differences, 36*, 1583–1596.

Shaver, P. R., Schachner, D. A., & Mikulincer, M. (2005). Attachment style, excessive reassurance seeking, relationship processes, and depression. *Personality and Social Psychology Bulletin, 31*, 343–359.

Shih, J. H. (2006). Sex differences in stress generation: An examination of sociotropy/autonomy, stress, and depressive symptoms. *Personality and Social Psychology Bulletin, 32*, 434–446.

Shively, C. A., Laber-Laird, K., & Anton, R. F. (1997). Behavior and physiology of social stress and depression in female cynomolgus monkeys. *Biological Psychiatry, 41*, 871–882.

Stein, M. B., Fuetsch, M., Müller, N., Höfler, M., Lieb, R., & Wittchen, H. (2001). Social anxiety disorder and the risk of depression: A prospective community study of adolescents and young adults. *Archives of General Psychiatry, 58,* 251–256.

Swann, W. B., Jr. (1990). To be or to be adored known?: The interplay of self-enhancement and self-verification. In E. T. Higgins & R. M. Sorrentino (Eds.), *Handbook of motivation and cognition: Vol. 2. Foundations of social behavior* (pp. 408–448). New York: Guilford Press.

Swann, W. B., Wenzlaff, R. M., Krull, D. S., & Pelham, B. W. (1992). Allure of negative feedback: Self-verification strivings among depressed persons. *Journal of Abnormal Psychology, 101,* 293–305.

Tolkmitt, F., Helfrich, H., Standke, R., & Scherer, K. R. (1982). Vocal indicators of psychiatric treatment effects in depressives and schizophrenics. *Journal of Communication Disorders, 15,* 209–222.

Watson, D. (2005). Rethinking the mood and anxiety disorders: A quantitative hierarchical model for DSM-IV. *Journal of Abnormal Psychology, 114,* 522–536.

Weissman, M., & Klerman, G. (Eds.). (1993). *New applications of interpersonal psychotherapy.* Washington, DC: American Psychiatric Press.

Youngren, M. A., & Lewinsohn, P. M. (1980). The functional relation between depression and problematic interpersonal behavior. *Journal of Abnormal Psychology, 89,* 333–341.

Zuroff, D. C., Mongrain, M., & Santor, D. A. (2004). Conceptualizing and measuring personality vulnerability to depression: Comment on Coyne and Whiffen (1995). *Psychological Bulletin, 130,* 489–511.

CHAPTER 15

The Social Environment and Life Stress in Depression

Scott M. Monroe, George M. Slavich, *and* Katholiki Georgiades

It has long been suspected that the social environment plays an important role in depression. Depressed individuals, clinicians, and theorists commonly assume that depression is intimately intertwined with the stressors and strains of people's social worlds. There can be little doubt about the general truth of these assumptions. However, such views are far too sweeping and nonspecific. There are many forms of life stress, numerous "roles" for life stress in depression, and a number of pathways via which depression and stress may be intertwined. It is within these more refined relations between particular dimensions of life stress and aspects of depression that theoretically trivial and fertile effects can be distinguished.

This chapter examines these important issues and related topics. We begin by breaking down the nonspecific notions of *social environment* and *life stress* into more explicit and useful concepts. In a similar manner, we disaggregate depression into its specific features and clinical course to then distinguish the various "roles" that life stress may play with different aspects of the disorder (e.g., the onset vs. clinical course of an episode). We next provide an overview of empirical findings, and key theoretical and methodological issues involving life stress and depression. Throughout this discussion, we emphasize requirements for satisfactorily handling an expanding framework of dynamic interrelations between life stress and depression over time. Then, having reviewed the general research literature on life stress and depression, we venture on to topics that are more debatable and controversial in nature, and discuss unresolved issues, empirical gaps, and emerging themes. By approaching these topics from a life stress perspective, we are able to advance lines of inquiry that may be useful in resolving the issues and closing the gaps. We conclude with a discussion of directions for future theory and research.

PRELIMINARY CONSIDERATIONS AND CLARIFICATIONS

People tend to think very globally about the *social environment*, *adversity*, and *life stress*, and about how such factors relate to *depression*. It is helpful to begin by restricting what is to be considered within the broad scope of these terms. First, what aspects of the social environment are relevant for depression? At a *distal level*, the social environment reflects aspects of cultural variation and differences in socioeconomic status (SES); at a more *proximal level*, the social environment reflects individual differences in exposure to major life events (e.g., deaths, relationship breakups) and chronic difficulties (e.g., ongoing health, financial, or relationship problems); and at the most *immediate level*, the social environment reflects the quotidian details and vicissitudes of everyday life. Which of these levels might be most relevant for understanding depression? Second, what aspects of depression are under the influence of the social environment and life stress? Does life stress contribute to the onset of depression in general, to the development of different types of depression, or to the clinical course of depression? By attending first to these distinctions, we can focus attention on the most promising areas for understanding which elements of the social environment and life stress play particular roles with regard to specific features of depression.

What Features of the Social Environment Are Relevant for Depression?

The social environment encompasses a variety of concepts of potential relevance for depression, such as SES, geography, and cultural factors. Research on SES and screening scale scores of depressive symptoms, for example, has consistently demonstrated an inverse linear association, with lower SES correlating with higher depressive symptomatology (Kohn, Dohrenwend, & Mirotznik, 1998). Findings for SES and major depression have been more complex, possibly varying by gender, geography, ethnicity, and diagnostic interview procedures (cf. DSM-IV-TR; American Psychiatric Association, 2000). However, in a recent meta-analysis including both symptom and diagnostic measures of depression, low SES individuals were at greater risk initially for incurring depression (odds ratio [OR] = 1.24) and at even greater risk for persisting depression (OR = 2.06; Lorant et al., 2003). Furthermore, quasi-experimental research has tried to disentangle competing explanations for the association between SES and psychopathology by attempting to determine whether adversity related to lower SES leads to depression (i.e., social causation), or whether depression leads to lower SES over time (i.e., social selection). Here, the findings point convincingly toward social causation of depression, at least for women (Dohrenwend, 2000). Finally, recent research on changes over time in socioeconomic circumstances also implicates low SES as a causal factor for increases in depressive symptoms and caseness of major depression (Lorant et al., 2007).

These general lines of research linking SES and depression provide clues about proximal and more specific mechanisms that account for the SES–depression relationship. A favored interpretation is that low SES inherently involves greater life stress, which represents a process through which SES translates into individual risk (Dohrenwend, 2000). But *life stress* is a term that is overly general and nonspecific. Based on research and theory over the past several years, we make the case for a critical role of major life events in the onset of major depression (Hammen, 2005; Mazure, 1998; Paykel, 2003; Tennant, 2002).

In What Ways Is Depression Influenced by the Social Environment?

Social factors and life stress may influence the onset, clinical course, and clinical characteristics of a depressive episode. These separate relations may be of interest on their own; yet if they are not taken into active consideration, they may obscure or confuse the causal picture between social factors and depression. A comprehensive account of the role that life stress plays in depression requires attention to these broader issues involving depression and its dynamic nature over time.

LIFE STRESS AND DEPRESSION: RESEARCH ISSUES AND EMPIRICAL FINDINGS

Reviews of research on life stress and depression unanimously conclude that major life events precede the onset of many, if not the majority of, depressive episodes (Hammen, 2005; Kessler, 1997; Mazure, 1998; Paykel, 2003; Tennant, 2002). Despite strong consensus about the consistency of these findings, however, questions remain about what the findings indicate specifically about the nature of depression (Hammen, 2005; Kessler, 1997). For example, do major stressors lead to particular types of depression, or can less major forms of adversity trigger a depressive episode? Some intriguing methodological challenges are posed when we try to resolve such questions. How these challenges have been handled in the past has implications for evaluating the reported findings, particularly with respect to the sensitivity and potential biases of the procedures employed.

Conceptualization and Measurement of Life Stress

Attributing illnesses of unknown origins to stress, adversity, and negative emotions is a recurrent theme in the history of medicine and psychiatry, and should give one pause when invoking psychosocial factors as causes of disorders of unknown origin (Sontag, 1978). It is against this backdrop of psychological preconceptions that modern research on life stress must be examined and evaluated. Psychological stressors are very popular explanations for unwanted emotional and physical states. As a result of their intuitive appeal and social legitimacy, they possess unwarranted explanatory power that exceeds their scientific utility. These tendencies to rely on life stress explanations often infiltrate the procedures adopted by researchers to measure and test hypotheses, permitting biased results to elude critical commentary. The challenge is to translate the productive ideas about psychological stress into more precise concepts, definitions, and operational procedures, thereby providing an appropriate empirical platform for scientific inquiry (Monroe & Slavich, 2007).

Self-Report Checklist Procedures

Research on life stress proliferated in the late 1960s and 1970s as a result of methodological innovations in measurement of life events (Paykel, 2001). Holmes and colleagues' development of the Schedule of Recent Experiences (SRE) (Hawkins, Davies, & Holmes, 1957; Rahe, Meyer, Smith, Kjaer, & Holmes, 1964) introduced the idea of measuring individual differences in exposure to life stress, with the potential to do so in a standard and objective manner. The SRE was a brief 43-item self-report checklist of common life events "empirically observed to occur just prior to the time of onset of disease" (Holmes, 1979, p. 46).

These investigators later developed standard weights for the degree of readjustment required by these events and subsequently published the well-known Social Readjustment Rating Scale (SRRS; Holmes & Rahe, 1967).

Innovation and expediency, however, outweighed rigor in the early development of these methods, and eventually serious deficiencies in the self-report checklist approach were recognized, including confounds between life events and actual symptoms of depression (e.g., inclusion of items such as sexual difficulties, changes in sleeping and eating habits) and between life events as consequences (not causes) of depression (trouble with a boss, divorce, marital separation, being fired at work, change in recreation, etc.). Despite early recognition of these major limitations (Brown, 1974; Paykel, 2001), as well as mounting empirical evidence that documented many other problems with self-report checklists (Dohrenwend, 2006; McQuaid et al., 1992; McQuaid, Monroe, Roberts, Kupfer, & Frank, 2000), measures of this type continue to predominate in research on life stress and depression (Grant, Compas, Thurm, McMahon, & Gipson, 2004; Monroe, 2008).

Investigator-Based Methods

Fortunately other researchers developed more scientifically sound procedures for assessing life stress (Brown & Harris, 1978; Dohrenwend, 2006; Hammen, 1991; Paykel, 2001). Probably the most elaborate system for assessing, defining, and rating life stress is the Life Events and Difficulties Schedule (LEDS), developed by Brown and Harris. Using a comprehensive manual, the LEDS incorporates explicit rules and operational criteria for defining acute and chronic stressors, for distinguishing between complex constellations of such stressors, and for rating these experiences (Brown & Harris, 1978). The unique biographical circumstances of the person are taken into account when rating each life event, so that the stressor experience is judged in light of what it might mean for that person given the context. The interview-based information can be presented in a separate meeting to raters who are blind to the subjective reactions of the particular individual to prevent confounding of reaction with possible depression status.

Other investigators have developed or adapted stress assessment procedures that are consistent with the LEDS philosophy and incorporate many of the same methodological advantages (Dohrenwend, 2006; Hammen, 1991; Paykel, 2001). Importantly, these investigator-based approaches have been found to be superior to self-report measures with respect to their psychometric properties, ability to control for potential sources of bias, and capacity to predict depression (Brown & Harris, 1989; Hammen, 2005; Mazure, 1998; McQuaid et al., 1992, 2000; Paykel, 2003; Tennant, 2002).

Life Stress and the Onset of Depression

As recent reviews of the topic uniformly indicate, there is a strong relation between major life stress and the onset of depression, with little doubt about the consistency or theoretical importance of the basic finding (Hammen, 2005; Mazure, 1998; Paykel, 2003; Tennant, 2002). In one review of over 20 studies, Mazure (1998) noted that the consistency and strength of the association between life stress and depression is not simply a generic stress effect; rather, it is specifically related to the "occurrences that are defined as *undesirable, major* life events" (p. 294; original emphasis). Kessler (1997) came to a comparable conclusion that "there is a consistently documented association between exposure to major stressful life events and subsequent onset of episodes of major depression" (p. 193), and that life stress associations are "generally stronger when 'contextual' measures are used rather than simple life event checklists" (p. 193).

In particular, one class of contextually rated life events, termed *severe events*, has been found to predict the onset of depression most consistently (Brown & Harris, 1989). These events represent highly aversive experiences, generally involving serious threats to core relationships or occupation, and sometimes involving acute economic or health changes (Brown & Harris, 1989). Indeed, the presence of a single, severe life event has been found to predict depression in the majority of cases; when these major events are taken into account, the less severe stressors, alone or in combination, are typically not predictive of depression (Brown & Harris, 1978, 1989; Monroe & Simons, 1991). Although more minor forms of life stress may on occasion play a role in depression (Hammen, Henry, & Daley, 2000; Kendler, Hettema, Butera, Gardner, & Prescott, 2003; Monroe et al., 2006), a strong case can be made that the dominant effect is attributable to a major, severe life event.

If major negative life events are of particular relevance for depression, then these forms of stress can provide a focal point and clues about the processes that eventuate in an episode of the disorder. The general and nonspecific idea of stress obviously is narrowed considerably. However, further specification of the nature and qualities of particular types of severe life events could enhance the prediction of the onset of depression. Indeed, recent findings suggest that particular types of major stress are especially potent in precipitating depression. Such events include humiliation and entrapment (Brown, Harris, & Hepworth, 1995; Kendler et al., 2003), social defeat (Gilbert, Allan, Brough, Melley, & Miles, 2002), loss and danger (Kendler et al., 2003), and targeted rejection and social exclusion (Allen & Badcock, 2003; Slavich, Thornton, Torres, Monroe, & Gotlib, in press). Progress along these lines could ultimately provide a conceptual basis for a taxonomy of life stress in depression (Allen & Badcock, 2006; Nesse, 2000).

Life Stress and the Clinical Characteristics of Depression

A major issue facing depression researchers is how to explain the substantial heterogeneity in the clinical presentation of depression. Why do individuals with depression exhibit such different combinations of signs and symptoms? Clearly a full account of depression must be capable of explaining such variability in phenotypes across, as well as within, depressed persons over time. Several lines of research have attempted to explain individual differences in clinical characteristics of depression in relation to life stress, and this research can be categorized into (1) studies of symptom severity and symptom profiles, and (2) studies of depressive subtypes.

Life Stress, Symptom Severity, and Symptom Profiles

Depressed people with major life stress have been found to have more severe depressive symptomatology compared to depressed people without such stress (e.g., Monroe, Harkness, Simons, & Thase, 2001; Tennant, 2002). Interestingly, these effects have been primarily attributable to preonset, as opposed to postonset, major life events (e.g., Monroe et al., 2001). That the preonset events are more removed in time relative to the postonset events suggests that the effect reflects matters of etiological relevance.

Few explanations have been offered as to why life stress is related to greater overall symptom severity in depressed people. Are individuals with prior stress elevated "across the board" for all depressive symptoms? Or are the associations with stress primarily accounted for by particular types of symptoms (e.g., cognitive–affective vs. somatic)? Research suggests that stress–severity associations often hold for symptoms assessed with the Beck Depression Inventory (BDI; Beck, Steer, & Garbin, 1988), but not for those assessed with the Hamilton Rating Scale for Depression (HRSD; Hamilton, 1960). Due to the different loadings of cognitive (BDI) versus somatic (HRSD) symptoms on the two instruments, these findings suggest some degree of symptom specificity. Alternatively, method variance may account for the differences between the self-reported BDI and the interview-based HRSD. Monroe and colleagues (2001) found life stress to be associated principally with cognitive–affective symptoms. Across different assessment methods there also was a consistent positive association between severe life events and suicidal ideation. Overall, research on life stress and the symptoms of depression is relatively sparse, and this is especially true for chronic stressors and depression symptoms. However, the existing clues suggest that a better understanding of such associations may be of use for clarifying the role of life stress in depression.

Life Stress and Subtypes of Depression

Many of the earliest accounts of depression refer to a syndrome of "sadness without reason" (Klibansky, Panofsky, & Saxl, 1964; Monroe & Depue, 1991). Kraepelin (1921), and others suggested that some forms of depression "may be to an astonishing degree largely *independent of external influences*" (p. 181, original emphasis). Others, addressing similar concepts, invoke terms such as *excessive depression*, *unjustified depression*, and *depression disproportionate to causative factors* (Jackson, 1986, p. 316). All of these observations reflect the central idea that social circumstances cannot fully explain the onset of *some* forms of depression. As a result of these observations and writings, it is often assumed that there exists an *endogenous* subtype of depression that is biologically based and arises independent of environmental circumstances. This viewpoint simultaneously implies that other forms of depression are due to adverse social circumstances, indicating a nonendogenous, or reactive, form of depression (Jackson, 1986).

The general distinction between stress-related and biologically based subtypes of depression has stimulated a number of related classification schemes and distinctions. Dichotomies such as *endogenous–reactive*, *neurotic–psychotic*, and *endogenous–neurotic* have been proposed and investigated. Many other terms loosely reflect one or the other of the two hypothesized etiological distinctions (e.g., situational, secondary, and nonendogenous for the stress-based concept; melancholic, retarded, and vital for the biologically based concept). Unfortunately, adding to the confusion, such terms have been used to describe differences between depressed persons in their presenting symptomatic and syndromal features, irrespective of social versus biological assumptions about cause. For instance, people exhibiting psychomotor retardation, unreactive mood, and pervasive anhedonia have been considered to represent an endogenous or melancholic subtype of the disorder (Rush & Weissenburger, 1994). Overall, despite the appeal of such typologies, inconsistency and confusion in their usage have hampered progress toward identifying potential subtypes of depression (Hammen, 2005; Katschnig, Pakesch, & Egger-Zeidner, 1986; Monroe & Depue, 1991).

Notwithstanding definitional difficulties, attempts to validate subtype distinctions based on the presence of life stress have been numerous over many decades, producing an extensive and often contentious debate (Mapother, 1926). Several reviews of literature from the past 25 years have suggested that life stress appears to be more common prior to the onset of almost *any* depressive subtype based on symptomatic differences (relative to the rate for nondepressed populations; Mazure, 1998). Yet some of these studies also suggest that there is a weak relationship between life events and a particular symptom pattern or depressive subtype (Katschnig et al., 1986; Mazure, 1998; Monroe & Depue, 1991; Tennant, 2002). Again, some of these inconsistencies can be ascribed to the lack of standardization for defining both stress and the endogenous and nonendogenous forms of depression (Hammen, 2005; Katschnig et al., 1986). Also, the relation of major life stress to different subtypes of depression may depend on whether the depressive episode is a first onset or recurrence. For example, patients with a recurrence who presented with an endogenous symptom pattern reported fewer severe events relative to first-onset patients, recurrence patients with nonendogenous symptoms, and community controls (Brown et al., 1995; Frank, Anderson, Reynolds, Ritenour, & Kupfer, 1994). Further work incorporating other symptoms or factors that distinguish subtypes may be of use to clarify the utility of such distinctions (Parker et al., 1999).

Life Stress and the Clinical Course of Depression

A number of studies have examined the association between life stress and the course of a depressive episode. Owing to the dynamic and changing nature of both stress and depression over time, this area of study is methodologically challenging. Whereas research on life stress and the onset of depression has one focal point for prediction, research on life stress and the clinical course of depression has many possible points of interest over time (e.g., remission, relapse, recurrence). And whereas the timing of life stress vis-à-vis onset is fixed by the nature of the question (i.e., stress precedes onset), important questions about the clinical course of a depressive episode involve stress at any point in time, pre- and postonset.

Compared to research on life stress and the onset of depression, research on life stress and the clinical course of depression has not been as common, mostly due to a general lack of attention to clinical course issues, as well as to diffusion of the existing attention across the different components that comprise the topic (i.e., remission, relapse, recurrence). Variations in design (e.g., definitions of the relevant outcomes for remission, relapse, recurrence), populations (community depressives, patients in different forms of treatment), and methods (self-report checklists and investigator-based stress assessments) further reduce the number of studies within any topic area, despite considerable potential for this area of research to uncover and resolve important clinical and conceptual matters.

Remission

With regard to remission, two related considerations are apparent: the timing of recovery and the absolute likelihood of recovery. Do stress-related depressions remit more or less quickly than depressions that are unrelated to major stress? And, do stress-related depressions have a better or worse overall likelihood of recovery? Although a few studies have addressed these issues, once again, the variability in methods and the heterogeneity of depressed populations complicate the interpretive picture. The major concerns are the timing of life stress (preonset vs. postonset), the nature of life stress (severe life events vs. other indices of stress), the nature of the population of participants studied (first onset, recurrences, severity, age), and the presence or type of treatment (natural course, psychotherapy, pharmacotherapy).

In terms of events prior to onset and *time to recovery*, inconsistent findings have been reported. Whereas some studies suggest a more rapid resolution of depression following preonset stress (e.g., Kendler, Walters, & Kessler, 1997; Parker & Blignault, 1985), other data suggest a slower response time to remission (Karp et al., 1993). In terms of life events following onset, recovery appears to be delayed considerably when stressors occur during treatment (e.g., Monroe, Roberts, Kupfer, & Frank, 1996). Again, however, caution is warranted owing to the relatively few studies on the topic, the diversity of methods; and the definitions, designs, and populations employed.

Research on life stress and the overall *likelihood of recovery* from depression has been somewhat more plentiful. Reviews underscore the inconsistent findings across studies, with some reporting that life events prior to onset forecast a better outcome, and others reporting a worse outcome (Mazure, 1998; Paykel, 2003; Tennant, 2002). Occurrence of major events during the course of the episode appears to prevent recovery (Mazure, 1998). Some of the discrepancies in this literature, again, may be due to differences in methods and populations studied. For example, some studies suggest that life stress prior to onset forecasts a lower likelihood of recovery for people with severe forms of depression (e.g., recurrent depression) compared to those with less severe forms (e.g., first onset; Monroe et al., 1996). Also, although the presence of chronic stressors has rarely been taken into account (Hammen, 2005), such forms of stress have been found to make recovery less likely (Tennant, 2002). Overall, whereas questions about preonset events, chronic stressors, and clinical course remain unanswered, there is more consistency about the adverse effects of concurrent stressors on overall recovery.

Relapse

Once recovery is achieved, previously depressed persons are at risk for slipping back into the previous episode. Can life stress help to explain why some individuals relapse and others do not during this vulnerable period? With regard to preonset stressors (i.e., Does stress prior to onset predict vulnerability to relapse?), the evidence is mixed (Mazure, 1998; Paykel, 2003; Tennant, 2002). Theoretically, however, the question is central to understanding depression over the life course: Does a stress-related episode imply that, once recovered, the psychobiological system will be more or less vulnerable to depression reemerging? This question hinges on two additional questions, which we address in turn. First, does the initial stress abate or continue? And second, does the psychobiological system change as a consequence of prior stress or depression?

Life stress occurring prior to the onset of a depressive episode may signify the likelihood of continuing stress given that depressed persons often generate life events, even when they are not actively depressed (Hammen, 2005). In light of this evidence for stressors occurring concurrently with an episode of depression, it seems reasonable to consider that continuation of stress after remission represents a proximal and potent trigger of relapse. Thus, the continuation of preonset stressors, the occurrence of new stressors, and the presence of chronic stressors after remission is achieved all might contribute to a social vulnerability to relapse. Research to date has not taken into consideration these dynamic, interactive stress processes over time, even though such information might be of considerable theoretical and clinical value.

In addition to changes in life stress over time, there may be psychobiological changes consequent to major stress or depression that render the person more susceptible to recurrence (Monroe & Harkness, 2005; Post, 1992). These social and biological processes may be especially important for understanding individual differences in the lifetime course of major depression and the problem of recurrence. We address this topic in detail next.

Recurrence

Over the past several years, concern about the long-term course of depression over the lifespan has moved from the periphery to the center of research and clinical interests. In one of the early reviews of the topic, Belsher and Costello (1988) concluded that about 50% of patients have a recurrence within 2 years following successful treatment. Since then, estimates of long-term morbidity owing to recurrence have steadily risen. Most recently, DSM-IV-TR (American Psychiatric Association, 2000) reported, "At least 60% of individuals with Major Depressive Disorder, Single Episode, can be expected to have a second episode. Individuals who have had two episodes have a 70% chance of having a third, and individuals who have had three episodes have a 90% chance of having a fourth" (p. 372).

In terms of clinical observations, Kraepelin remarked many years ago that one of his patients became depressed "after the death first of her husband, next of her dog, and then of her dove" (1921, p. 179). This suggests that repeated exposure to losses and experiences of depression result in a progressive lowering of the threshold for stress needed to trigger subsequent recurrences. More recently, Post (1992) provided a more formal conceptual premise for such observations, developing the *kindling* hypothesis for life stress and the recurrence of depression. The relation of stress to subsequent episodes of depression is hypothesized to change over time, such that progressively less severe doses of stress are required to bring about onset; eventually, after many episodes, recurrences may appear apparently spontaneously, independent of psychosocial origins. These intriguing ideas are derived from animal laboratory work on electrophysiological kindling and behavioral sensitization, paradigms that demonstrate the plausibility of transitions from precipitated episodes to episodes independent, or autonomous, of psychosocial origins (Post, 1992).

There is ambiguity, however, about the implications for understanding the role of life stress within this conceptual premise. For example, does stress become *more* or *less* relevant for successive recurrences? On the one hand, one might reason that stress becomes progressively less important over time, with nonstress factors beginning to predominate in causing a recurrence episode (the *stress autonomy hypothesis*). On the other hand, one might reason that life stress becomes progressively *more* important in triggering recurrence episodes as vulnerability to stress increases over successive episodes (the *stress sensitization hypothesis*); that is, with an accruing history of prior episodes, less severe life events acquire the capability to trigger a recurrence of depression. Because severe life events occur relatively infrequently compared to events of lesser magnitude, these latter, more frequent and common stressors increase the probability, and hasten the onset, of recurrence (see Monroe & Harkness, 2005).

Fortunately, the stress sensitization and stress autonomy hypotheses can readily be tested. For example, if severe stress is essential for the onset of early episodes, it seems probable from the stress sensitization point of view that severe stress would still bring about recurrence in a sensitized system (see Monroe, Slavich, Torres, & Gotlib, 2007a). Thus, although proportionately fewer people with many episodes of depression will have experienced a severe event before the onset of their most recent recurrence, those people who do incur severe stress should have a very high likelihood of breakdown. Alternatively, if longitudinal studies of life stress and recurrence of depression find that people with more lifetime episodes are less likely to succumb following a major life event, then the evidence would support the stress autonomy premise (Monroe & Harkness, 2005).

There are noteworthy gaps between these ideas about life stress and depression recurrence, and epidemiological data on the recurrence of depression. If depression researchers are indeed largely studying samples of people with recurrent depression, then why do severe events remain the strongest stress-related predictor of episode onset? Specifically, if 91% of depressed persons in the community report a prior episode of depression (Kessler, 1997), then how do we account for up to 80% of depressed persons in the community reporting a recent, major life event (Mazure, 1998)? Why is there relatively little firm evidence available for lesser severities of stressors triggering onset of a recurrence (cf. Monroe et al., 2006)? Researchers have begun to study different facets of these ideas (Hammen et al., 2000; Kendler, Kuhn, Vittum, Prescott, & Riley, 2005; Monroe et al., 2006), and the relations also may be moderated by genetic or other factors (Kendler, Thornton, & Gardner, 2001).

EMPIRICAL INCONSISTENCIES AND RESEARCH GAPS

Compared to other risk indices, major life events represent one of the strongest predictors of the onset of depression (Kendler, Gardner, & Prescott, 2002, 2006). Major life events also have significant implications for understanding the clinical course of an episode and the lifetime course of the disorder. These wide-ranging findings provide the foundation for moving toward a better understanding of the nature and course of depression. However, there is relatively little discussion about what these findings specifically suggest about depression. We suspect that part of the problem harkens back to the intuitive appeal of stress as a culturally accepted and nonspecific explanation. Stress "makes sense" and possesses high face validity, which can deflect attention from asking deeper questions about the processes involved (Monroe, 2008). Without further analysis, however, such an unquestioning attitude undermines the search for underlying mechanisms, and leads investigators to overlook important inconsistencies and research gaps. Yet by considering more fully the research on life stress and depression, there is considerable potential for researchers to develop insights into central questions about the nature of this disorder.

Despite consensus about the broad diagnostic status of depression, its variations, and public health significance, less agreement exists concerning its core features, possible subtypes, and underlying causes. That debate continues about the dimensional versus categorical nature of the disorder alone, despite decades of extensive research and deliberations, underscores the complexity of the problem and the challenges facing investigators (Kendell, 1976). Attempts to explain the causes of depression are particularly hindered in light of problems in understanding the basic nature of the disorder. It is in this context that the magnitude and consistency of findings for major life events in relation to the onset of an episode of depression are useful for expanding thinking about the disorder's origins and its many features, and for addressing inconsistencies and gaps in current knowledge.

Not all people with depression report prior severe events, and not all people who experience severe events develop depression. Approximately 50% or more of depressed patients have experienced recent stress, as have about 80% of community depressives (compared to approximately 24% in nondepressed samples; see Table 1 in Mazure, 1998); between 20 and 50% of persons experiencing a recent major life stress succumb to depression (Brown & Harris, 1989; Monroe & Simons, 1991). From a life stress perspective, then, one needs to explain why some people become depressed following major life events, whereas others do not, and why some depressed persons apparently have not experienced a recent major life event. The most readily apparent explanations include the following: (1) Depression is a heterogeneous class of disorders with regard to clinical and presentation etiology; (2) stress is one factor in a multifactorial model of depression; and finally, and less obviously, (3) depression is a dimensional disorder in which stress plays a graded role.

Life Stress, Clinical Heterogeneity, and Depression Subtypes

Although the available evidence for a distinct subtype of stress-related depression is modest, creative approaches may yet uncover a form of depression that is largely, if not uniquely, linked to major life stress. This optimism is warranted by findings that indicate the following: (1) A substantial proportion of (but not all) depressed people relative to nondepressed controls experience severe stress prior to depression; (2) preonset severe stress predicts the clinical course of depressed persons; and (3) preonset severe stress predicts greater levels of depressive symptoms, specificity of symptoms, and, possibly, symptom profiles. Whereas one can debate the findings within any of these three literatures, the broad and emerging picture is that major stress is an intrinsically important causal factor for a large proportion of depressed persons.

One obstacle to isolating a hypothetical, stress-induced subtype of depression is the significant heterogeneity of the signs, symptoms, and presentations of major depression. Different people diagnosed with major depression often present with different symptoms and permutations of the requisite criteria and features. Life stress may influence the presenting features of depression, and these influences may occur in addition to any etiological role for stress. For instance, stress might have a causal role for one subtype of depression and a *pathoplastic* (i.e., symptom modification) role for another. Awareness of such *dual roles* associated with life stress may be required to explain individual differences in depressive features and the detection of distinctive syndromes.

There are additional sources of clinical heterogeneity that, if taken into account, could enhance our ability to detect unique patterns of stress influences on specific syndromes or particular symptom expressions. With respect to psychosocial factors, the early loss experiences of separation from or death of a loved one have been reported to distinguish between neurotic and psychotic depressive features (Brown & Harris, 1978). Personality characteristics also have been implicated as creating variability in symptomatic expression of depression (Clark, Vittengl, Kraft, & Jarrett, 2003; Hirschfeld & Shea, 1992). Another intriguing possibility is that severe life events are equally important for people incurring a first episode of depression, regardless of whether they meet symptom criteria for endogenous or nonendogenous depression. However, for subsequent recurrences of depression, severe events may be associated predominantly with nonendogenous presentations of depression (Brown et al., 1995; Frank et al., 1994).

Finally, an underappreciated advantage of a life stress perspective on the heterogeneity of depression is the potential for isolating a non-stress-related form of the disorder. The classic endogenous depression subtype has been distinguished throughout time by a stark and severe clinical presentation in people who otherwise appear to be relatively stress-free and to have advantaged situations and attractive social worlds (Jackson, 1986; Monroe & Depue, 1991). Cases of classic endogenous depression may be easily overlooked in contemporary society, with ubiquitous and specious explanation of "stress" helping to obscure the true origins of the disorder. These superficial and biased explanations based on life stress are minimized when rigorous stress assessment procedures are adopted, with precise definitions of major stressors and accurate dating of preonset stressors. Use of such methods would increase capability to isolate a hypothetical subtype of depression that develops independent of life circumstances.

Life Stress, Multifactorial Models, and Depression Subtypes

The etiology of depression has long been thought to be due to a variety of factors operating together to precipitate a depressive episode (Jackson, 1986). The central importance of life stress has typically been formalized within these conceptual schemes (e.g., diathesis–stress models of depression; Abramson, Metalsky, & Alloy, 1989; Monroe & Simons, 1991; Zuckerman, 1999). Within these approaches, life stress is an important component in the cause of depression (or subtype of depression), yet necessarily operates in concert with other vulnerability factors (or *diatheses*). Major life stress activates, or interacts with, the underlying diathesis, transforming predisposition into manifest depression. Returning to the theme of severe events as a pivotal focus for depression onset, we pose the following questions: What other forms of vulnerability do severe events require to precipitate depression? What additional susceptibilities are sufficient to allow severe stress to eventuate in depression?

Investigators might proceed in a number of ways to determine how severe life stress operates with other vulnerability factors in depression. Initially, a better understanding of how severe stress is related to other vulnerability factors would be useful. For example, how are severe events related to cognitive vulnerability, or to genetic and familial liability? Patient samples provide a useful starting point for testing severe stress associations with other vulnerability factors, and for testing predictions in relation to other validating considerations (e.g., clinical characteristics, clinical course, and outcome). Because patient samples typically report approximately 50% incidence of recent severe stress, there is an optimal level of variability in severe stress occurrence to probe associations with other vulnerability factors. Next, interactions between severe stress and other risk factors can be evaluated within depressed samples to determine whether there are further associations of particular theoretical interest. Does the pairing of severe events with other vulnerability factors predict a distinctive symptom profile or clinical course (see Monroe, Slavich, Torres, & Gotlib, 2007b)? Once the nature of severe stress, other risk factors, and their interactions are better modeled and validated, the groundwork will be laid for research on the stress processes that influence depression onset and course.

Along these lines, it is helpful to distinguish between two different models for life stress and diatheses coactions. On the one hand, traditional diathesis–stress theory posits an ipsative or inverse relationship between severe stress and the diathesis: The greater the allotment of one factor, the less of the other is required (Abramson et al., 1989; Ingram & Price, 2001; Monroe & Simons, 1991). The sum of the two factors is critical, not the relative loading of either. This additive model parsimoniously accounts for many diverse findings in the research literature, including the concerns that (1) not all people with severe stress develop depression, and (2) not all depressed people report recent life stress.

On the other hand, if there is something of particular etiological importance about severe life events, then a second model is important to consider. Recognizing, again, that not all people with severe stress succumb to depression, other factors are required to explain why some people break down under stress and others do not. Within this conceptualization, severe life events are associated with one (or more) additional vulnerability indices in a *permissive* manner. In direct contrast to the ipsative model, severe stress is associated with *heightened* cognitive vulnerability, or with *greater* genetic predisposition. Consistent with this *interactive* or *multiplicative model*, Kendler and colleagues (1995) found that the likeli-hood of depression onset was greatest for women with heightened genetic liability *and* a re-cent major life event. There are two noteworthy implications of this model. First, it implic-itly specifies that the class of major depression is heterogeneous. Because not all people with major depression have prior severe life events, alternative causal explanations are required for the nonstress depressive conditions. Second, this perspective readily incorporates many popular concepts as moderators of the impact of stress in the genesis of depression (Hammen, 2005). Thus, social support (or lack thereof), coping efficacy, personality attrib-utes, biological factors, and so on, all are easily integrated into the framework, further ex-plaining why some people may succumb to stress and others do not.

Of course, variants of these two basic models also might be considered. For example, one could extrapolate to three or more subtypes of depression, each with different arrange-ments of vulnerability factors and interrelations. The two models proposed, though, provide a reasonable starting point for testing competing hypotheses and for learning about how se-vere stress interacts with other indicators of risk.

Life Stress and Dimensional Models of Depression

Categorical models of psychopathology possess many advantages. They simplify thinking about the disorder in question (i.e., it is either present or absent), have clinical benefits (e.g., facilitate treatment decisions), and provide distinct practical benefits (e.g., public health planning, treatment reimbursement). Indeed, this perspective has been extraordinarily suc-cessful in leading to the discovery of the causes of many diseases, thereby alleviating sundry scourges of humankind (Gordon, 1993). With such victories and virtues in its favor, it is easy to understand why a categorical approach continues to dominate conceptual systems in psychopathology.

Alternatively, dimensional approaches to depression have their advocates, and there has been a recent resurgence of interest in such models of disorder (Ruscio & Ruscio, 2000; Widiger & Clark, 2000). These models assume that disorder is distributed along a continuum, without natural *break points*, or thresholds for differentiating people with and without the problem (Kendell, 1976; Lewis, 1934). In this context, the debate be-tween categorical and dimensional viewpoints has stimulated thought and controversy, but little research has been aimed at resolving the matter. Might the particular importance of severe life events in depression be useful for moving research on this topic along pro-ductive lines?

Perhaps, most generally, a basic misunderstanding about life stress in relation to psy-chological disorders biases thinking in subtle ways against dimensional approaches. From DSM-III through DSM-IV-TR, the criteria for mental disorders require that the "syndrome or pattern must not be merely an expectable and culturally sanctioned response to a particu-lar event" (American Psychiatric Association, 2000, p. xxi). There are at least three major concerns with this criterion. First, it presumes knowledge about what constitutes the range of expectable responses under particular environmental and cultural conditions (as well as a reliable means for evaluating the matter). Second, it is not theoretically clear why an expectable response to an event—if the response meets the indicated diagnostic criteria and impairment requirements—would *necessarily* be dismissed on such a basis alone (Wakefield, Schmitz, First, & Horwitz, 2007). Finally, the addition of the dismissive adverb *merely* to the official diagnostic nomenclature undermines the clinical gravity and perceived impor-tance of an event-related psychological problem.

These matters may be complicated by the overvalued explanatory potential of life stress and major events. Comments and attitudes, such as those in DSM, imply that clinical science possesses firm knowledge about the range of human reactions to the vicissitudes of life, that for a given situation X the range of normal responses is Y, and the range of abnormal responses is Z (and that Y and Z do not overlap). While the argument possesses plausibility at the extremes (e.g., depression emerging under completely tranquil circumstance or under extreme trauma), many people—and quite possibly the majority of people with major depression—inhabit social worlds filled with dilemmas and hardships that exist in a gray area of suspected environmental determination for which the "expectable" responses are simply not known (or are so varied as to render meaningless the notion of *expectable*). By directly addressing the issue conceptually and empirically, researchers might develop (1) better ways of thinking about adversity, emotion, and depression and (2) an empirical basis for specifying the expectable response range to diverse forms of life stress (Wakefield et al., 2007).

Traditional thinking based on a categorical model may obscure alternative ways to consider the matter. Viewing the stress process in terms of a more finely tuned fit between environmental challenge and individual response, however, suggests the possibility of graded reactions in proportion to varying degrees of challenge (Weiner, 1992). In other words, depression may not represent a dichotomous breakdown under major stress, but a complex and graded mixture of adaptation and maladaptation to specific, psychologically meaningful environmental challenges (Allen & Badcock, 2006; de Kloet, Joëls, & Holsboer, 2005; Nesse, 2000). This way of viewing the stress process in depression is more consistent with the dimensional approach to depression.

At first glance, though, such speculation appears to contradict a central premise of our discussion that something particularly useful about major life events can lead to fresh insights about depression. But, again, by focusing on major events as a pivotal piece of information, novel directions for research may be brought to light. For example, the findings for major life events and depression onset could inform us about a possible artifact of the categorical systems used to define major depression; that is, by arbitrarily constraining the information on depression into two categories (depressed or nondepressed), the role of life stress in depression may be underestimated. Could the "average" reaction to a severe event simply be what is needed to push most people over the definitional threshold for a diagnosis of major depression? Could less severe life events perhaps precipitate psychobiological responses that typically fall just below what is required for a clinical diagnosis? It may be, as well, that other factors moderate the average reaction range between life stress and depression in a dimensional manner (e.g., early life stress increases the likelihood of exceeding the threshold in the face of major stress, or availability of social support lessens the likelihood of exceeding the threshold). Pursuing this line of thinking further, we note that there has been little systematic study of people with severe stress who do *not* meet full criteria for major depression; available information suggests that these people suffer, too, yet from somewhat milder forms of the disorder (Brown, 1991). More generally, it is noteworthy that these ways of thinking about relations between stress and depression help to explain why not all people who have experienced severe events necessarily develop depression; a substantial proportion suffer from debilitating, but subthreshold, depressive conditions (Gotlib, Lewinsohn, & Seeley, 1995).

Last, it is worth considering why an expectable response to adversity would be summarily dismissed with the adverb *merely*, suggesting that it does not merit full consideration as a syndrome or mental disorder. In addressing this point, we hesitantly shift from matters of science to matters of values in the recognition and remediation of human suffering. What forms of misery and malady are sanctioned by a society? Which dysphoric and debilitated groups are accorded social legitimacy and allowed to be considered "ill," to adopt the sick role, and to not be held accountable or blamed for their incapacity? From this vantage point, a categorical approach to defining psychopathology lends a shorthand legitimacy to depression: It is consistent with a medical viewpoint and, importantly, provides the appearance of clearly demarcating the normal from the abnormal. A dimensional approach is less desirable in this regard: It is difficult to discern who is deserving of the sick role from who is undeserving, and there is no "natural" reference point or cultural anchor to guide important decisions. When and where depression shades into demoralization—when and where clinical entities and subsyndromal conditions merge into, or overlap with, expressions of the miseries of everyday life—are poorly understood at present, perhaps are ultimately indeterminate. It is the frank reluctance of clinical science to address directly the question of "an expectable response" to adversity in its many forms that belies a great gap in our understanding of so-called "normal responses," the limits of normal functioning, and the beginnings of psychopathology. Without such a knowledge base, discussions and definitions of the abnormal, demarcating the boundaries of the pathological, possess an inevitably arbitrary element that is grounded both in society's values and in current science (Wakefield, 1992).

Our intent is not to advocate for a categorical or dimensional model of depression, but to provide examples of life stress research that might be useful for research on these models of depression. It is quite conceivable that the dimensional issues play into the previously discussed problem of subtypes of depression, yielding even more complex frameworks that incorporate distinct categorical subtypes and dimensional typologies (Kendell, 1976). In all likelihood, the category of depression, as currently defined, will turn out to be a complex and cumbersome mélange of categorical and dimensional subgroup distinctions, with different, yet possibly overlapping, etiological factors and arrangements. Finding solutions to the riddle of depression's causes may depend as much on intelligent and creative probing of the boundaries of the disorder as on seeking answers within the currently accepted definition of the phenotype.

FUTURE DIRECTIONS

Although psychosocial and biological approaches to depression often emphasize the central importance of stress, there is remarkably little common ground in what actually constitutes "stress" and relatively few efforts to draw linkages across the two levels of analysis. The paucity of translational ideas and research between the literatures, however, is by no means a necessary state of affairs. Each perspective can inform the other, and bridging the psychosocial and biological approaches represents one of the most promising areas for understanding how social adversity impacts biological processes in ways that may lead to major depression. Three topics for future research possess particularly strong potential for integrating ideas across these two levels of analysis, and for furthering understanding of the causal pathways leading to depression.

Translating the Psychology of Stress into the Biology of Depression

One of the most consistently replicated biological findings in psychiatry is the overactivity of the hypothalamic–pituitary–adrenal (HPA) axis in depressed patients (Goodwin & Jamison, 2007). At a very general level, the human life stress and human neuroendocrine research appear to converge: One might expect cortisol, a key stress hormone, to be elevated in depressed persons suffering from recent major stress. Indeed, the approximate proportion of the depressed samples with prior stress (50%) nicely parallels the approximate proportion of patients with HPA axis dysregulation and excessive cortisol secretion (50%; Young, Lopez, Murphy-Weinberg, Watson, & Akil, 2000). However, there are fundamental gaps and inconsistencies in the literature for determining how research on naturally occurring major life events translates to the research on HPA axis dysfunction in depression (van Praag, de Kloet, & van Os, 2004).

In fact, few studies have examined directly the association between major life events and cortisol dysregulation in depressed patients. Of the little work conducted, at least one study reported elevated cortisol in depressed persons with recent major stress (e.g., Dolan, Calloway, Fonagy, De Souza, & Wakeling, 1985) whereas another study reported HPA axis dysfunction for depressed persons *without* recent stress (Roy, Pickar, Linnoila, Doran, & Paul, 1986). Other, more recent studies also have yielded discrepant findings regarding cortisol's relation to life events and depression onset (Hammen, 2005). Inconsistencies in this literature may be attributable to differences across studies in the measurement of life stress or in the method of assessment for HPA functioning. Clarifying how major life stress and HPA axis disturbances operate in relation to one another is an obvious next step, the results of which will guide further inquiry into the nature of the associations involved with regard to depression. For example, if the high-stress group exhibits HPA irregularities, is it due to continuation of the environmental stress or to more centrally mediated "breakdown" in regulation of the HPA axis? Given the theoretical importance of stress and cortisol, as well as the adverse effects of excessive cortisol on brain structure and function, all possible contributing factors to HPA axis overdrive are worthy of exploration (Sapolsky, 2000).

Finally, HPA disturbance has been associated with poor treatment response and risk of relapse (de Kloet et al., 2005). Greater risk of relapse has also been reported in patients with residual symptoms (Judd, Schettler, & Akiskal, 2002), as well as patients with life stress (Mazure, 1998). A tempting interpretation is that these separate findings work in a unified manner: Continued social adversity and life stress drive HPA activity and symptomatology, which collectively eventuate in relapse. More generally, these observations point to the need to evaluate each domain of risk, and their independent and combined contributions to treatment response, relapse, and recurrence.

In general, there are several empirical gaps with respect to HPA axis functioning, current environmental stress, and depression. This raises further questions as to what factors influence the integrity of the HPA regulatory system, particularly with regard to the sensitivity of HPA function and susceptibility to dysregulation. We address this topic next.

Early Adversity and the Developmental Neurobiology of Stress Regulation

Recent animal laboratory research has highlighted the formative influences of prenatal and early life experiences for the development of individual differences in HPA axis function and stress sensitivity. Differences in early stress exposure also forecast the development of behavioral problems in the animals as they mature (Huizink, Mulder, & Buitelaar, 2004; Meaney, 2001). These animal laboratory studies complement a literature implicating early adversity as a general vulnerability factor for a wide range of problems later in life for humans, including depression (Heim, Plotsky, & Nemeroff, 2004).

An integration of these findings may suggest that early stress exposure renders the organism more vulnerable to the deleterious effects of subsequent stressors by setting in motion alterations in stress-sensitive neurobiological systems. For example, individuals exposed to early adversity may be more likely to develop hyperresponsive threat/stress systems, which may in turn sensitize them (or increase susceptibility) to subsequent stressors. Alternatively, the vital biological regulatory systems of individuals exposed to early adversity may be more prone to dysregulation as a result of repeated activations of these systems (Repetti, Taylor, & Seeman, 2002). Overall, exposure to early adversity points toward changes in key neurobiological regulatory systems that may modulate adaptation to stressful circumstances, which may in turn help to explain further why some people faced with major stressors develop depression and others do not.

Recent work has begun to explore the intervening mechanisms linking early adversity to later morbidity, with advances in understanding how early adversity contributes to stress sensitization and the pathophysiology of depression (Gunnar & Quevedo, 2007; Heim et al., 2004). Noteworthy, too, is that early adversity broadens and adds another layer to the types of stress that can explain depression. Future studies on early development, neurobiological indicators of stress regulatory systems, and current life events may help to specify better the pathophysiology of depression and the possibility of distinctive subtypes (Heim et al., 2004). The reliable measurement of early adversity in adults adds another challenging area given that these experiences occurred far back in time (Brewin, Andrews, & Gotlib, 1993).

Life Stress and the Molecular Genetics of Depression

Another explanation for why only some people develop depression in the face of life stress involves the role of specific vulnerability genes. This area of research recently has become quite attractive given topical advances in the mapping of the human genome and the development of powerful molecular genetics techniques for detecting specific allelic variations in genes. In a landmark study, Caspi and colleagues (2003) reported that individuals with one or two copies of the short allele of the serotonin transporter (5-HTT) gene promoter polymorphism are especially susceptible to developing depression following stressful life events. As a result of these and other findings, a new generation of studies is emerging on life stress, genes, and depression. One can anticipate considerable effort and output over the next several years testing interactions between life stress and specific genes in depression.

In this context, a major challenge for future research will be to ensure that the life stress component of the gene–environment interaction is assessed in as sophisticated and competent a manner as is the genetics component. It is quite possible that techniques for addressing the genetics will overshadow those for life stress, and that careful conceptualization and measurement of stress will be neglected. For instance, to date, the majority of studies attempting to replicate the original findings of Caspi and colleagues (2003) have used varied procedures for indexing life stress, with no two studies using the same or, arguably, even similar measures; only one of 11 studies to date (i.e., Kendler et al., 2005) has adopted measurement procedures in keeping with preferred practices for life stress assessment (Monroe & Reid, in press).

The promise of research on gene–environment interactions depends on proper specification of both the genetic and environmental components of the interaction. Optimal measurement of the particular environmental factor, though costly at times, enhances the statistical power of the research design and increases the ability to discover genes of causal relevance (Moffitt, Caspi, & Rutter, 2005). The successful replication by Kendler and colleagues (2005) of an interaction between major life events and the serotonin transporter gene in depression onset bears testimony to the importance of taking the assessment of life stress as seriously as the assessment of genetic vulnerability. More generally, these studies provide exciting leads for future research on life stress and its role in the development of major depression.

REFERENCES

Abramson, L. Y., Metalsky, G. I., & Alloy, L. B. (1989). Hopelessness depression: A theory-based subtype of depression. *Psychological Review, 96,* 358–372.

Allen, N. B., & Badcock, P. B. T. (2003). The social risk hypothesis of depressed mood: Evolutionary, psychosocial, and neurobiological perspectives. *Psychological Bulletin, 129,* 887–913.

Allen, N. B., & Badcock, P. B. T. (2006). Darwinian models of depression: A review of evolutionary accounts of mood and mood disorders. *Progress in Neuropsychopharmacology and Biological Psychiatry, 30,* 815–826.

American Psychiatric Association. (2000). *Diagnostic and statistical manual of mental disorders* (4th ed., text revision). Washington, DC: American Psychiatric Association.

Beck, A. T., Steer, R. A., & Garbin, M. G. (1988). Psychometric properties of the Beck Depression Inventory: Twenty-five years of evaluation. *Clinical Psychology Review, 8,* 77–100.

Belsher, G., & Costello, C. G. (1988). Relapse after recovery from unipolar depression: A critical review. *Psychological Bulletin, 104,* 84–96.

Brewin, C. R., Andrews, B., & Gotlib, I. H. (1993). Psychopathology and early experience: A reappraisal of retrospective reports. *Psychological Bulletin, 113,* 82–98.

Brown, G. W. (1974). Meaning, measurement, and stress of life events. In B. S. Dohrenwend & B. P. Dohrenwend (Eds.), *Stressful life events: Their nature and effects* (pp. 217–243). New York: Wiley.

Brown, G. W. (1991). Aetiology of depression: Something of the future? In P. E. Bebbington (Ed.), *Social psychiatry: Theory, methodology, and practice* (pp. 35–63). New Brunswick, NJ: Transaction.

Brown, G. W., & Harris, T. O. (1978). *Social origins of depression: A study of psychiatric disorder in women.* New York: Free Press.

Brown, G. W., & Harris, T. O. (Eds.). (1989). *Life events and illness.* New York: Guilford Press.

Brown, G. W., Harris, T. O., & Hepworth, C. (1995). Loss, humiliation and entrapment among women developing depression: A patient and non-patient comparison. *Psychological Medicine, 25,* 7–21.

Caspi, A., Sugden, K., Moffitt, T. E., Taylor, A., Craig, I. W., Harrington, H., et al. (2003). Influence of life stress on depression: Moderation by a polymorphism in the 5-HTT gene. *Science, 301,* 386–389.

Clark, L. A., Vittengl, J., Kraft, D., & Jarrett, R. B. (2003). Separate personality traits from states to predict depression. *Journal of Personality Disorders, 17,* 152–172.

de Kloet, E. R., Joëls, M., & Holsboer, F. (2005). Stress and the brain: From adaptation to disease. *Nature Reviews: Neuroscience, 6,* 463–475.

Dohrenwend, B. P. (2000). The role of adversity and stress in psychopathology: Some evidence and its implications for theory and research. *Journal of Health and Social Behavior, 41,* 1–19.

Dohrenwend, B. P. (2006). Inventorying stressful life events as risk factors for psychopathology: Toward resolution of the problem of intracategory variability. *Psychological Bulletin, 132,* 477–495.

Dolan, R. J., Calloway, S. P., Fonagy, P., De Souza, F. V., & Wakeling, A. (1985). Life events, depression and hypothalamic–pituitary–adrenal axis function. *British Journal of Psychiatry, 147,* 429–433.

Frank, E., Anderson, B., Reynolds, C. F., Ritenour, A., & Kupfer, D. J. (1994). Life events and the research diagnostic criteria endogenous subtype: A confirmation of the distinction using the Bedford College methods. *Archives of General Psychiatry, 51,* 519–524.

Gilbert, P., Allan, S., Brough, S., Melley, S., & Miles, J. N. (2002). Relationship of anhedonia and anxiety to social rank, defeat and entrapment. *Journal of Affective Disorders, 71,* 141–151.

Goodwin, F. K., & Jamison, K. R. (2007). *Manic–depressive illness: Bipolar disorders and recurrent depression* (2nd ed.). New York: Oxford University Press.

Gordon, R. (1993). *The alarming history of medicine: Amusing anecdotes from Hippocrates to heart transplants*. New York: St. Martin's Press.

Gotlib, I. H., Lewinsohn, P. M., & Seeley, J. R. (1995). Symptoms versus a diagnosis of depression: Differences in psychosocial functioning. *Journal of Consulting and Clinical Psychology, 63*, 90–100.

Grant, K. E., Compas, B. E., Thurm, A. E., McMahon, S. D., & Gipson, P. Y. (2004). Stressors and child and adolescent psychopathology: Measurement issues and prospective effects. *Journal of Clinical Child and Adolescent Psychology, 33*, 412–425.

Gunnar, M., & Quevedo, K. (2007). The neurobiology of stress and development. *Annual Review of Psychology, 58*, 145–173.

Hamilton, M. (1960). A rating scale for depression. *Journal of Neurology, Neurosurgery, and Psychiatry, 23*, 56–62.

Hammen, C. (1991). Generation of stress in the course of unipolar depression. *Journal of Abnormal Psychology, 100*, 555–561.

Hammen, C. (2005). Stress and depression. *Annual Review of Clinical Psychology, 1*, 293–319.

Hammen, C., Henry, R., & Daley, S. E. (2000). Depression and sensitization to stressors among young women as a function of childhood adversity. *Journal of Consulting and Clinical Psychology, 68*, 782–787.

Hawkins, N. G., Davies, R., & Holmes, T. H. (1957). Evidence of psychosocial factors in the development of pulmonary tuberculosis. *American Review of Tuberculosis, 75*, 768–780.

Heim, C., Plotsky, P. M., & Nemeroff, C. B. (2004). Importance of studying the contributions of early adverse experience to neurobiological findings in depression. *Neuropsychopharmacology, 29*, 641–648.

Hirschfeld, R. M. A., & Shea, M. T. (1992). Personality. In E. S. Paykel (Ed.), *Handbook of affective disorders* (2nd ed., pp. 149–170). New York: Guilford Press.

Holmes, T. H. (1979). Development and application of a quantitative measure of life change magnitude. In J. E. Barrett, R. M. Rose, & G. L. Klerman (Eds.), *Stress and mental disorder* (pp. 37–53). New York: Raven Press.

Holmes, T. H., & Rahe, R. H. (1967). The Social Readjustment Rating Scale. *Journal of Psychosomatic Research, 11*, 213–218.

Huizink, A. C., Mulder, E. J., & Buitelaar, J. K. (2004). Prenatal stress and risk for psychopathology: Specific effects or induction of general susceptibility? *Psychological Bulletin, 130*, 115–142.

Ingram, R. E., & Price, J. M. (2001). The role of vulnerability in understanding psychopathology. In R. E. Ingram & J. M. Price (Eds.), *Vulnerability to psychopathology: Risk across the lifespan* (pp. 3–19). New York: Guilford Press.

Jackson, S. W. (1986). *Melancholia and depression*. New Haven, CT: Yale University Press.

Judd, L. L., Schettler, P. J., & Akiskal, H. S. (2002). The prevalence, clinical relevance, and public health significance of subthreshold depressions. *Psychiatric Clinics of North America, 25*, 685–698.

Karp, J. F., Frank, E., Anderson, B., George, C. J., Reynolds, C. F. I., Mazumdar, S., et al. (1993). Time to remission in late-life depression: Analysis of effects of demographic, treatment, and life-events measures. *Depression, 1*, 250–256.

Katschnig, H., Pakesch, G., & Egger-Zeidner, E. (1986). Life stress and depressive subtypes: A review of present diagnostic criteria and recent research results. In H. Katschnig (Eds.), *Life events and psychiatric disorders: Controversial issues* (pp. 201–245). Cambridge, UK: Cambridge University Press.

Kendell, R. E. (1976). The classification of depressions: A review of contemporary confusion. *British Journal of Psychiatry, 129*, 15–28.

Kendler, K. S., Gardner, C. O., & Prescott, C. A. (2002). Toward a comprehensive developmental model for major depression in women. *American Journal of Psychiatry, 159*, 1133–1145.

Kendler, K. S., Gardner, C. O., & Prescott, C. A. (2006). Toward a comprehensive developmental model for major depression in men. *American Journal of Psychiatry, 163*, 115–124.

Kendler, K. S., Hettema, J. M., Butera, F., Gardner, C. O., & Prescott, C. A. (2003). Life event dimensions of loss, humiliation, entrapment, and danger in the prediction of onsets of major depression and generalized anxiety. *Archives of General Psychiatry, 60*, 789–796.

Kendler, K. S., Kessler, R. C., Walters, E. E., MacLean, C. J., Sham, P. C., Neale, M. C., et al. (1995). Stressful life events, genetic liability and onset of an episode of major depression in women. *American Journal of Psychiatry, 152*, 833–842.

Kendler, K. S., Kuhn, J. W., Vittum, J., Prescott, C. A., & Riley, B. (2005). The interaction of stressful life events and a serotonin transporter polymorphism in the prediction of episodes of major depression: A replication. *Archives of General Psychiatry, 62*, 529–535.

Kendler, K. S., Thornton, L. M., & Gardner, C. O. (2001). Genetic risk, number of previous depressive episodes, and stressful life events in predicting onset of major depression. *American Journal of Psychiatry, 158*, 582–586.

Kendler, K. S., Walters, E. E., & Kessler, R. C. (1997). The prediction of length of major depressive episodes: Results from an epidemiological of female twins. *Psychological Medicine, 27*, 107–117.

Kessler, R. C. (1997). The effects of stressful life events on depression. *Annual Review of Psychology, 48*, 191–214.

Klibansky, R., Panofsky, E., & Saxl, F. (1964). *Saturn and melancholy: Studies in the history of natural philosophy religion and art.* New York: Basic Books.

Kohn, R., Dohrenwend, B. P., & Mirotznik, J. (1998). Epidemiological findings on selected psychiatric disorders in the general population. In B. Dohrenwend (Ed.), *Adversity, stress, and psychopathology* (pp. 235–284). New York: Oxford University Press.

Kraepelin, É. (1921). *Manic–depressive insanity and paranoia.* Edinburgh, UK: Livingstone.

Lewis, A. J. (1934). Melancholia: A historical review. *Journal of Mental Science, 80*, 1–42.

Lorant, V., Croux, C., Weich, S., Deliege, D., Mackenbach, J., & Ansseau, M. (2007). Depression and socio-economic risk factors: 7-year longitudinal population study. *British Journal of Psychiatry, 190*, 293–298.

Lorant, V., Deliege, D., Eaton, W., Robert, A., Philippo, P., & Ansseau, M. (2003). Socioeconomic inequalities in depression: A meta-analysis. *American Journal of Epidemiology, 157*, 98–112.

Mapother, E. (1926). Discussion on manic–depressive psychosis. *British Medical Journal, 2*, 872–879.

Mazure, C. M. (1998). Life stressors as risk factors in depression. *Clinical Psychology: Science and Practice, 5*, 291–313.

McQuaid, J. R., Monroe, S. M., Roberts, J. E., Kupfer, D. J., & Frank, E. (2000). A comparison of two life stress assessment approaches: Prospective prediction of treatment outcome in recurrent depression. *Journal of Abnormal Psychology, 109*, 787–791.

McQuaid, J. R., Monroe, S. M., Roberts, J. R., Johnson, S. L., Garamoni, G., Kupfer, D. J., et al. (1992). Toward the standardization of life stress assessment: Definitional discrepancies and inconsistencies in methods. *Stress Medicine, 8*, 47–56.

Meaney, M. J. (2001). Maternal care, gene expression, and the transmission of individual differences in stress reactivity across generations. *Annual Review of Neuroscience, 24*, 1161–1192.

Moffitt, T. E., Caspi, A., & Rutter, M. (2005). Strategy for investigating interactions between measured genes and measured environments. *Archives of General Psychiatry, 62*, 473–481.

Monroe, S. M. (2008). Modern approaches to conceptualizing and measuring human life stress. *Annual Review of Clinical Psychology, 4*, 33–52.

Monroe, S. M., & Depue, R. A. (1991). Life stress and depression. In J. Becker & A. Kleinman (Eds.), *Psychosocial aspects of depression* (pp. 101–130). New York: Erlbaum.

Monroe, S. M., & Harkness, K. L. (2005). Life stress, the "kindling" hypothesis, and the recurrence of depression: Considerations from a life stress perspective. *Psychological Review, 112*, 417–445.

Monroe, S. M., Harkness, K., Simons, A. D., & Thase, M. E. (2001). Life stress and the symptoms of major depression. *Journal of Nervous and Mental Disease, 189*, 168–175.

Monroe, S. M., & Reid, M. W. (in press). Gene–environment interactions in depression: Genetic polymorphisms and life stress polyprocedures. *Psychological Science.*

Monroe, S. M., Roberts, J. E., Kupfer, D. J., & Frank, E. (1996). Life stress and treatment course of recurrent depression: II. Postrecovery associations with attrition, symptom course, and recurrence over 3 years. *Journal of Abnormal Psychology, 105*, 313–328.

Monroe, S. M., & Simons, A. D. (1991). Diathesis–stress in the context of life stress research: Implications for the depressive disorders. *Psychological Bulletin, 110*, 406–425.

Monroe, S. M., & Slavich, G. M. (2007). Psychological stressors, overview. In G. Fink (Ed.), *Encyclopedia of stress, second edition* (Vol. 3, pp. 278–284). Oxford, UK: Academic Press.

Monroe, S. M., Slavich, G. M., Torres, L. D., & Gotlib, I. H. (2007a). Major life events and major chronic difficulties are differentially associated with history of major depressive episodes. *Journal of Abnormal Psychology, 116*, 116–124.

Monroe, S. M., Slavich, G. M., Torres, L. D., & Gotlib, I. H. (2007b). Severe life events predict specific patterns of change in cognitive biases in major depression. *Psychological Medicine, 37,* 863–871.

Monroe, S. M., Torres, L. D., Guillaumot, J., Harkness, K. L., Roberts, J. E., Frank, E., et al. (2006). Life stress and the long-term treatment course of recurrent depression: III. Nonsevere life events predict recurrence for medicated patients over 3 years. *Journal of Consulting and Clinical Psychology, 74,* 112–120.

Nesse, R. M. (2000). Is depression an adaptation? *Archives of General Psychiatry, 57,* 14–20.

Parker, G., & Blignault, I. (1985). Psychosocial predictors of outcome in subjects with untreated depressive disorder. *Journal of Affective Disorders, 8,* 73–81.

Parker, G., Roy, K., Wilhelm, K., Mitchell, P., Austin, M. P., Hadzi-Pavlovic, D., et al. (1999). Sub-grouping non-melancholic depression from manifest clinical features. *Journal of Affective Disorders, 53,* 1–13.

Paykel, E. S. (2001). The evolution of life events research in psychiatry. *Journal of Affective Disorders, 62,* 141–149.

Paykel, E. S. (2003). Life events and affective disorders. *Acta Psychiatrica Scandinavica, 108*(Suppl. 418), 61–66.

Post, R. (1992). Transduction of psychosocial stress into the neurobiology of recurrent affective disorder. *American Journal of Psychiatry, 149,* 999–1010.

Rahe, R. H., Meyer, M., Smith, M., Kjaer, G., & Holmes, T. H. (1964). Social stress and illness onset. *Journal of Psychosomatic Research, 54,* 35–44.

Repetti, R. L., Taylor, S. E., & Seeman, T. E. (2002). Risky families: Family social environments and the mental and physical health of offspring. *Psychological Bulletin, 28,* 330–366.

Roy, A., Pickar, D., Linnoila, M., Doran, A. R., & Paul, S. M. (1986). Cerebrospinal fluid monoamine and monoamine metabolite levels and the dexamethasone suppression test in depression: Relationship to life events. *Archives of General Psychiatry, 43,* 356–360.

Ruscio, J., & Ruscio, A. M. (2000). Informing the continuity controversy: A taxometric analysis of depression. *Journal of Abnormal Psychology, 109,* 473–487.

Rush, A. J., & Weissenburger, J. E. (1994). Melancholic symptom features and DSM-IV. *American Journal of Psychiatry, 151,* 489–98.

Sapolsky, R. M. (2000). Glucocorticoids and hippocampal atrophy in neuropsychiatric disorders. *Archives of General Psychiatry, 57,* 925–935.

Slavich, G. M., Thornton, T., Torres, L. D., Monroe, S. M., & Gotlib, I. H. (in press). Targeted rejection predicts hastened onset of major depressive disorder. *Journal of Social and Clinical Psychology.*

Sontag, S. (1978). *Illness as metaphor.* New York: Farrar, Straus & Giroux.

Tennant, C. (2002). Life events, stress and depression: A review of recent findings. *Australian and New Zealand Journal of Psychiatry, 36,* 173–182.

van Praag, H. M., de Kloet, E. R., & van Os, J. (2004). *Stress, the brain and depression.* New York: Cambridge University Press.

Wakefield, J. C. (1992). The concept of mental disorder: On the boundary between biological facts and social values. *American Psychologist, 47,* 373–388.

Wakefield, J. C., Schmitz, M. F., First, M. B., & Horwitz, A. V. (2007). Extending the bereavement exclusion for major depression to other losses: Evidence from the National Comorbidity Survey. *Archives of General Psychiatry, 64,* 433–440.

Weiner, H. W. (1992). *Perturbing the organism: The biology of stressful experience.* Chicago: University of Chicago Press.

Widiger, T. A., & Clark, L. A. (2000). Toward DSM-V and the classification of psychopathology. *Psychological Bulletin, 126,* 946–963.

Young, E. A., Lopez, J. F., Murphy-Weinberg, V., Watson, S. J., & Akil, H. (2000). Hormonal evidence for altered responsiveness to social stress in major depression. *Neuropsychopharmacology, 23,* 411–418.

Zuckerman, M. (1999). *Vulnerability to psychopathology: A biosocial model.* Washington, DC: American Psychological Association.

PART III

DEPRESSION IN SPECIFIC POPULATIONS

Although depressive disorders occur in all demographic groups, cultures, and ages, their manifestations, meanings, treatments, and possible causes may differ importantly from one population to another. The seven chapters in this section detail considerations about the experience of depression in particular groups. Chentsova-Dutton and Tsai (Chapter 16) discuss a growing body of research on cultural differences in the expression and experience of depression. The well-documented gender differences in the experience of depression, reviewed by Nolen-Hoeksema and Hilt (Chapter 17), continue to challenge simple unitary explanations of this disorder. Depression in children, discussed by Garber, Gallerani, and Frankel (Chapter 18), and depression in adolescents, discussed by Rudolph (Chapter 19), are presented as separate chapters in recognition of both the unique features of these groups and the enormous body of recent research on these topics. Davila, Stroud, and Starr (Chapter 20) provide an overview of the literature on depression in the context of couple and family relationships, and highlight conceptual themes in this area of research. Blazer and Hybels (Chapter 21) review the experience of depression in later life, a topic of increasing social concern. Finally, although suicide is not uniquely associated with depressive disorders, Berman (Chapter 22) addresses the relatively common experience of suicidality in depressed individuals and discuss its management.

CHAPTER 16

Understanding Depression across Cultures

Yulia E. Chentsova-Dutton *and* Jeanne L. Tsai

Major depression is associated with significant global economic burden, disability, and diminished quality of life (Murray & Lopez, 1997). Clearly, studying this affliction across cultures continues to be an important goal for researchers. Despite significant advances in this field, however, we are still grappling with fundamental questions. Imagine a young woman living in the United States who experiences profound feelings of distress and worthlessness, and who no longer enjoys spending time with friends, has significant trouble falling asleep, feels tired much of the time, and has difficulty concentrating. These symptoms are easily identified by psychologists and psychiatrists as the syndrome of major depression. But how does this syndrome translate across cultures? Do individuals reporting similar symptoms in other cultural contexts also suffer from major depression? Conversely, do individuals reporting different symptoms, such as Chinese suffering from fatigue, weakness, and bodily aches and pains (Kleinman, 1982); Puerto Ricans reporting crying jags, difficulty sleeping, and visions and hallucinations (Koss-Chioino, 1999); or rural Nepalese complaining of numbness and tingling (Kohrt et al., 2005) suffer from other disorders or from "indigenous" forms of major depression? What role does culture play in shaping depression? Are some aspects of depression more or less culturally shaped? In this chapter, we review the extant evidence accumulated over several generations by anthropologists, psychiatrists, and psychologists using different research approaches to address these questions. Before we begin this review, we briefly define what we mean by *culture* and by *depression*.

DEFINING CULTURE

In Kroeber and Kluckhohn's (1952) classic definition, *culture* is described as

> patterns, explicit and implicit, of and for behaviour acquired and transmitted by symbols . . . including their embodiment in artifacts; the essential core of culture consists of traditional . . . ideas and especially their attached values; culture systems may, on the one hand, be considered as products of action, on the other, as conditional elements of future action. (p. 181)

This definition stresses that culture exists in the heads of its members (e.g., values and norms), as well as in the world, as embodied in daily patterns of behavior and in cultural artifacts (e.g., daily interaction patterns, songs). Furthermore, this definition highlights the mutual constitution of culture and psychological processes; that is, culture shapes behavior, thought, and emotions of individuals and is in turn shaped by them. Individuals are not merely passive recipients of culture, but are active contributors to change or stability in their cultural worlds. For example, lyrics of popular songs, such as "Just put on a happy face," from the popular musical *Bye Bye Birdie*, communicate to the listener that certain ways of experiencing and expressing emotional distress, such as trying to act as if one is happy, are desirable in the mainstream American culture. At the same time, listeners create demand for certain songs, and not for others, thus contributing to cultural selection and maintenance.

DEFINITION OF DEPRESSION

According to the fourth, text revision edition of the *Diagnostic Manual of Mental Disorders* (DSM-IV-TR; American Psychiatric Association, 2000), major depression is characterized by the prolonged presence of either depressed mood or *anhedonia*, a markedly diminished interest or pleasure in response to previously enjoyable activities. This definition focuses on symptoms that are experienced subjectively and are emotional rather than physical in nature. Of course, this definition did not develop in a cultural vacuum. Western cultural contexts emphasize the uniqueness and autonomy of each individual and the importance of personal goals, values, and preferences. In these contexts, key markers of healthy functioning include promotion of the self, positive views of the self, a focus on personal accomplishments, and open expression of one's emotions to signal personal preferences (Heine, Lehman, Markus, & Kitayama, 1999). The symptoms of major depression (e.g., feelings of worthlessness and failure to experience pleasure) reflect deviations from these cultural norms. Also, in Western cultures, diseases of the mind and the body are considered to be distinct. Although criteria for major depression, a mental illness, include both emotional and physical symptoms, a diagnosis of major depression cannot be made in the absence of its key emotional symptoms (i.e., depression and/or anhedonia). Thus, Western criteria for major depression (and other mental disorders) reflect cultural biases of viewing emotional distress as characterizing individuals rather than groups, and as fundamentally distinct from physical distress. These biases are reflected in the multiaxial assessment system used by DSM, in which emotional, social, and physical aspects of functioning are recorded on separate axes.

These norms of socioemotional functioning, however, are not universally shared by other cultures. For instance, in East Asian cultures (e.g., Japan), individuals are viewed as inherently interdependent with others and defined by their social context. Healthy emotional functioning in East Asian cultural contexts is marked by self-criticism, ability to avoid interpersonal tension, and moderation of open expression of emotions in an effort to preserve interpersonal harmony. In these cultural contexts, interpersonal symptoms of depression, such as social withdrawal or failure to maintain interpersonal obligations, may be more salient and exact a greater toll on a person's daily functioning than intrapersonal symptoms. Thus, reporting that one feels negatively about one's abilities or that one experiences excessive levels of negative emotions may not serve as useful markers of depression in these cultural settings. In addition, in many non-Western cultures, mind and body are not viewed as separate and distinct entities, but are seen as intimately connected and mutually constitutive. As a result, patients in some cultures may talk about their distress as an integrated psychobiological phenomenon, without making distinctions between bodily pain and feelings of despair.

How do we study cultural variation in a disorder whose very definition is culturally constructed? Researchers have approached this challenge in several different ways. We briefly describe a number of these research approaches, then review empirical findings for each. We review studies that rely on indigenous conceptions of depression, on the standardized DSM or *International Classification of Diseases* (ICD) criteria for the syndrome of major depression, and on self-report measures of depressive symptoms. Throughout the chapter we use the terms *indigenous forms of distress*, *prevalence rates of major depression*, and *levels of depressive symptoms*, respectively, to refer to these distinct ways of conceptualizing and assessing depression. We focus on studies examining unipolar depression and also describe the few studies that have examined cultural shaping of bipolar spectrum disorders.

RESEARCH APPROACHES TO STUDYING DEPRESSION ACROSS CULTURES

Three key approaches have been influential in the field of cultural psychopathology. The *ethnographic* approach assumes that even if members of a particular culture experience the symptoms defined by Western culture as depression, the meanings and implications of these symptoms may vary considerably across cultures. Following Kleinman's (1977) article urging researchers who study mental illness across cultures to consider carefully not only the symptoms of the disorder but also the personal and culturally shaped interpretation of these symptoms, several generations of psychiatrists and psychologists have used ethnographic methods in their quest to understand the cultural underpinnings of depression. Proponents of the ethnographic approach utilize local construction of depression by focusing on the structures, norms, and values that shape the meaning of the depressive symptoms within a particular cultural context. Most of the work that falls under this approach is based on ethnographic interviews and behavioral observations.

In contrast, the *biomedical* approach assumes that, regardless of the cultural context, the disorder exists if individuals report having the familiar symptoms of depression, and if associated factors show similar relations to the disorder across cultural contexts. To date, the bulk of the research employing a biomedical approach focuses on the prevalence rates of major depression, and risk and protective factors in various nations and cultural groups. Most of this work is based on epidemiological data using structured diagnostic interviews or self-report surveys.

Finally, an emerging *cultural* approach seeks to understand meaningful connections between culture and the psychology of individuals living in it. The cultural approach uses both descriptive and experimental methods to identify specific factors, such as the ways selves are constructed across cultures, that contribute to cultural variation in major depression. Thus, researchers are beginning to operationalize aspects of culture that may shape the expression of depression.

Each of these research traditions contributes unique strengths to the study of culture and depression. It is by comparing and pooling the findings from each of these approaches

.t we minimize their shortcomings and maximize their strengths. In this chapter, we present research findings from each of these approaches, highlight consistent themes that emerge from these bodies of literature, and propose other ways of studying depression across cultures that we believe will advance our current knowledge base.

Ethnographic Approach: Examining the Meaning of Depression across Cultures

Ethnographic studies typically focus on one culture at a time. Working closely with local informants, researchers examine local ways of experiencing and expressing emotional distress, and relate them to the ideas and practices of that culture.

Indigenous Forms of Distress

Over several decad , ethnographers have accumulated from diverse cultures rich accounts of indigenous forms of distress that resemble depression in some of their features. In some cases, the resemblance is very close, and it is easy to become convinced that the indigenous disorder is indeed depression. For example, Tousignant and Maldonaldo (1989) described the illness of *pena*, the word that translates as "suffering" in highland Ecuador. In its severe form, *pena* is characterized by crying spells, problems with concentration, anhedonia, social withdrawal, sleep and appetite disturbances, gastrointestinal symptoms, and heart pain. Thus, symptoms of *pena* closely resemble those of major depression. Another similarity is that *pena* is often experienced in response to personal loss. However, Tousignant and Maldonaldo argue that unlike depression, *pena* is primarily an interpersonal strategy to appeal to others "for payment of an incurred loss" (p. 900). Thus, *pena* serves as a signal to others to act to restore equity and ensure reciprocity among individuals in a small community. An injured party in a conflict may signal distress by withdrawing from others and displaying symptoms characteristic of *pena*. In turn, the party's social circle may attempt to remedy the situation by sharing feelings with the sufferer, and by bringing him or her back into the social network. Thus, although *pena* looks very similar to depression, its personal and social implications, and its management, differ from those of depression in Western cultures. *Pena* provides an example of an indigenous depressive disorder for which the symptoms, but not their meanings, closely match Western criteria for depression.

Other indigenous disorders do not resemble depression as closely in their key symptoms. Examples of these disorders include *ataque de nervios* in Puerto Rico (Guarnaccia, Rivera, Franco, & Neighbors, 1996), *hwa-byung* in Korea (Lin et al., 1992), *jhum-jhum* in Nepal (Kohrt et al., 2005), and *neurasthenia* in China (Kleinman, 1982). Key complaints that characterize many of these disorders are somatic rather than emotional. For example, *hwa-byung* (Lin et al., 1992) is distinguished by constricted sensations in the chest, and *jhum-jhum* (Kohrt et al., 2005), by numbness or a tingling sensation. Despite these unique features, some scholars have suggested that these culture-bound syndromes may be subtle variants of depression. Consistent with this notion, studies show that individuals with indigenous disorders, such as Korean patients with *hwa-byung* (Lin et al., 1992) and Nepalese patients with *jhum-jhum* (Kohrt et al., 2005), have higher levels of depressive symptoms than do those without the disorder. It is important to note, however, that the association between indigenous disorders and depression, as measured by Western criteria, is far from perfect. For instance, only half of self-defined *hwa-byung* sufferers actually meet criteria for major depression. Thus, indigenous disorders may better map onto a broader cluster of disorders that includes major depression, as well as other mental disorders that frequently co-occur with depression, such as anxiety or somatization disorders.

Conceptions of Depression across Cultural Contexts

In addition to examining indigenous forms of distress, recent ethnographic studies have turned to documenting the conception of depressive symptoms across cultures. In these studies, researchers interview individuals with symptoms of major depression and their friends, family, or physicians about the manifestation, perceived causes, and preferred coping and treatment strategies for depressive symptoms.

EMPHASIS ON SOMATIC FEATURES OF DEPRESSION

Consistent with research on indigenous forms of distress, somatic features of depression are commonly emphasized in non-Western settings. For instance, Puerto Ricans and African immigrants to the United States (Koss-Chioino, 1999; Sellers, Ward, & Pate, 2006) identify symptoms such as heart pounding, body aches, tiredness, and headaches as key features of their depression. The physical complaints can overshadow psychological ones: Puerto Rican patients produce less frequent and less varied reports of psychological than of physical symptoms of depression, and embed them in physical symptoms (Koss-Chioino, 1999). In some cases, such as among South Asian women in the United States, there is even an expectation that depression is merely a prelude to more serious physical ailments (Karasz, 2005b). Given this emphasis on somatic symptoms of depression, it is hardly surprising that South Asian immigrants in the United States are less likely than European Americans to recognize and label a vignette based on emotional features (e.g., crying, sadness and lack of interest in previously enjoyable activities) as depression (Karasz, 2005a). Thus, despite exposure to North American culture, somatic rather than emotional presentation continues to match more closely the South Asian cultural conception of depression.

On the other hand, the choice to report distress in somatic terms may be quite deliberate and shaped by the notion that it is more appropriate to reveal physical symptoms to others than to reveal psychological symptoms. In many cultural contexts, psychological symptoms of depression are construed as stigmatizing and socially disadvantageous. For example, although focus groups of South Asian immigrant women in England recognize that depression is characterized by both psychological and somatic symptoms, they feel that physical symptoms have greater legitimacy in their community and are more appropriate to disclose to medical professionals than are psychological symptoms (Burr & Chapman, 2004). In some cases, patients may also tailor their reports of symptoms to satisfy their clinicians. Caribbean older adults in England perceive that their general practitioners prioritize physical complains in an effort to "cure your pains and then think about the depression later on" (Lawrence et al., 2006, p. 1380).

Finally, somatic reports of depression may be encoded in the local language, creating a culture-specific *idiom of distress*. Emotional distress may be verbalized as physical pain depending on the terms and metaphors available in a particular language, and on the local codes for communication of emotions. For instance, in Chinese, somatic terms such as *heart discomfort* serve as shared metaphors for affective states or emotions (Tung, 1994).

EMPHASIS ON INTERPERSONAL FEATURES OF DEPRESSION

In addition to emphasizing bodily complaints, conceptions of depression in non-Western cultural groups often focus on social causes. For example, based on semistructured interviews,

Pang (1995) reported that many older Korean immigrants did not report feeling depressed; instead, they explained and communicated their distress in terms of loneliness and family dynamics, as well as somatic complaints. Studies indicate that although the British (Jadhav, Weiss, & Littlewood, 2001), European Americans (Karasz, 2005a), and South Asians (Karasz, 2005a, 2005b; Raguram, Weiss, Keval, & Channabasavanna, 2001) recognize that interpersonal stressors have an important role in etiology of depression, interpersonal causes are emphasized more heavily by Asian individuals. For instance, South Asian women in the United States are more likely than their European American counterparts to believe that depression is caused by interpersonal stressors, such as marital conflict (Karasz, 2005a, 2005b); in contrast, European American individuals are more likely to endorse the Western biopsychiatric model of depression and attribute depression to biological causes. These differences occur against a backdrop of cultural similarities in other aspects of etiological theories of depression. For example, British and Indian individuals similarly endorse cognitive causes of depression, such as worrying or thinking too much (Jadhav et al., 2001; Raguram et al., 2001).

Documenting etiological theories of distress is important, because patients' choices of coping and treatment strategies are closely tied to the perceived causes of their depression. Consistent with their view of depression as interpersonal in origin, South Asian immigrants are more likely than European Americans to endorse interpersonal strategies for managing their depressive symptoms, such as turning to family and close friends for help (Karasz, 2005a). In contrast, consistent with their view of depression as biological in origin, European Americans are more likely than South Asian immigrants to recommend professional interventions by a psychiatrist or psychologist (Karasz, 2005a). When European Americans suggest self-management strategies for alleviating distress, the strategies they suggest also tend to be physical (e.g., exercise), rather than social (e.g., conversation with a close friend) in nature. Future studies need to examine whether choice of therapies that match cultural conceptions of depression would increase compliance. It is also important to investigate whether the common perception that depression is caused by thinking patterns and worrying would make cognitively based therapies more acceptable than biological therapies in non-Western cultural settings.

In summary, ethnographic studies provide compelling evidence that cultural norms and beliefs shape views of the causes, manifestations, and ways of coping with depressive symptoms. Although these studies contribute to our understanding of depression across cultures, they have a number of serious limitations. Because of their in-depth nature, most ethnographic studies are based on very few participants, which limits the generalizability of their findings. Moreover, although researchers have firsthand knowledge about the cultures they are studying, it is unclear to what extent their observations are influenced by their own cultural biases. Finally, because most of these studies are not comparative (i.e., do not include direct comparisons of data collected in more than one culture), it is unclear whether the meaning and consequences of depressive symptoms differ as drastically across cultures as these accounts suggest. The few studies that provide such comparisons (Karasz, 2005a) are still the exception rather than the rule. Thus, it is important to complement the ethnographic approach with cross-cultural examinations of the construct of depression across cultures.

Biomedical and Cross-Cultural Approaches:

Examining the Construct of Depression across Cultures

Biomedical and cross-cultural studies of depression have used standardized instruments to assess prevalence of symptoms of major depression and to identify factors associated with depression across cultures. This research approach requires an enormous investment of time and resources to orchestrate coordinated data collection across many cultural contexts. Cross-cultural studies typically boast large sample sizes, allowing researchers to examine the contribution of a number of risk factors to the etiology and progression of major depression. We briefly review the cross-cultural data on the prevalence of major depression, examine whether somatic versus psychological presentation of depression depends on a cultural setting, and identify factors known to be associated with depression across cultures.

Cross-Cultural Differences in the Prevalence Rates of Major Depression

Epidemiological studies show that prevalence rates of major depressive disorder vary dramatically across cultures. Figure 16.1 shows 12-month prevalence rates reported in recent epidemiological studies using standardized structured clinical interviews assessing DSM-IV criteria for major depressive disorder. As is evident from Figure 16.1, in Ukraine or Canada, 1 in roughly 10 adults reports experiencing major depression in the past year, compared with only 1 in roughly 50 adults in China or Korea. Epidemiological studies show consistent patterns of differences in rates of depression across nations. Depression rates among teens and adults are consistently higher in countries with rapidly changing economic and political conditions, such as Chile (Simon, Goldberg, Von Korff, & Ustün, 2002), and the post-Soviet states (Bromet et al., 2005; Pikhart et al., 2004) than in countries with stable economic and political conditions. Prevalence rates of major depression in the United States and Canada are consistently higher (Kessler et al., 2005; Vasiliadis, Lesage, Adair, Wang, & Kessler, 2007) than rates of depression in East Asian countries (Inaba et al., 2005; Kawakami et al.,

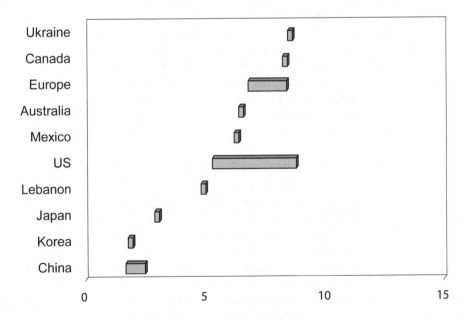

FIGURE 16.1. Twelve-month prevalence estimates for DSM-IV major depressive disorder by nation. Prevalence rates were obtained from Ayuso-Mateos et al. (2001); Bromet et al. (2005); Cho et al. (2007); Henderson, Andrews, and Hall (2000); Hasin, Goodwin, Stinson, and Grant (2005); Karam et al. (2006); Kawakami et al. (2005); Lee (2001); Ohayon and Hong (2006); Slone et al. (2006); Vasiliadis, Lesage, Adair, Wang, and Kessler (2007); World Health Organization World Mental Health Survey Consortium (2004).

2005; Simon et al., 2002). In addition to differences in prevalence rates, depression has higher recurrence rates in Western and Latin American cultural contexts than in Asian cultural contexts (Simon et al., 2002). For example, 33–44% of patients in Western and Latin American cultural contexts experience recurrence of their depressive symptoms after 1 year, compared to only 9% of patients in Asian cultural contexts. In contrast, prevalence rates for bipolar spectrum disorders are remarkably similar across cultures (Weissman et al., 1996).

Although cultural biases in the use of standardized diagnostic instruments have been documented, it is unlikely that these differences are due entirely to methodological differences across epidemiological studies. Notably, even studies using standardized sampling and assessment procedures across countries obtain widely different prevalence rates of major depression across nations (Simon et al., 2002). Thus, it is unlikely that national differences in prevalence rates can be entirely explained by factors such as methodological and sampling differences across studies.

SOMATIZATION OF DEPRESSIVE SYMPTOMS

Based on ethnographic evidence of non-Western cultures that place greater emphasis on somatic symptoms of depression, researchers have long questioned whether the disparities in prevalence of major depression are due to the tendency of individuals in non-Western cultures to *somatize*, or to report depression in physical rather than in psychological terms. Consistent with ethnographic data, cross-cultural studies show that in many non-Western, as well as in South and Eastern European countries, depression is associated with somatic complaints (Bhui, Bhugna, Goldberg, Sauer, & Tylee, 2004; Burr & Chapman, 2004; Gutkovich et al., 1999; Mak & Zane, 2004; Pang, 1995; Takeuchi, Chun, Gong, & Shen, 2002; Waza, Graham, Zyzanski, & Inoue, 1999). Patients from non-Western cultural settings and minority patients are less likely to report psychological symptoms of depression, such as worthlessness, delusions of guilt, and suicidal ideation, and more likely to report somatic symptoms of depression, such as poor appetite, lack of sleep, and headaches, relative to Western samples (Brown, Schulberg, & Madonia, 1996; Slone et al., 2006; Stompe et al., 2001). For example, Waza and colleagues (1999) reviewed medical charts of Japanese and American primary care patients who had received new diagnoses of depression. They found that whereas Japanese patients were more likely to present with exclusively physical symptoms, American patients were more likely to present with exclusively psychological symptoms.

In sharp contrast to these findings are recent reports that challenge the notion that Western cultures foster an overemphasis on psychological symptoms at the expense of somatic symptoms. These studies show that depression is often reported in somatic terms and associated with unexplained medical complaints in the United States and England (Bhui et al., 2004; Keyes & Ryff, 2003). Levels of acculturation and time spent in a Western cultural context are not associated with diminished levels of somatization among immigrants (Mak & Zane, 2004). It is also not the case that psychological symptoms of depression are reported at the expense of physical symptoms in Western settings. In a study conducted across 14 countries, Simon, Von Korff, and colleagues (1999) reported that, contrary to the notion that patients in non-Western cultures somatize their psychological symptoms, the proportion of somatic symptoms to psychological symptoms does not differ across countries. Moreover, somatization is more likely to be maladaptive and to be associated with depression in Western cultures, such as the United States, than in non-Western cultures, such as Korea (Keyes & Ryff, 2003).

What factors account for inconsistencies in the findings of these sets of studies? Somatic presentation may in part reflect the quality of relationships between medical doctors and their patients. Simon, Von Korff, and colleagues (1999) found that, across cultures, patients were more likely to initially report somatic symptoms when they used walk-in clinics and did not have an ongoing relationship with their physicians. Studies reporting that individuals in non-Western cultural settings present with somatic symptoms tend to rely on initial clinical presentation of patients who have not developed strong rapport with their clinicians. Thus, somatization may reflect initial reluctance to report symptoms that are less salient or more stigmatizing in a particular culture rather than an absence of these symptoms. This tendency to report some types of symptoms preferentially may be conditioned by verbal and nonverbal reinforcement of psychological versus somatic responses by clinicians. Lam, Marra, and Salzinger (2005) demonstrated that verbal and nonverbal reinforcement of psychological versus somatic responses to vignettes of stressful life events resulted in conditioned preference for particular types of reports. It is possible that social interactions in different cultural contexts condition responses that are culturally normative.

The initial tendency of individuals to selectively report some symptoms of depression but not others may be overcome with careful probing during the assessment. For example, in England, patients report psychological symptoms spontaneously but acknowledge somatic symptoms when probed by clinicians. In contrast, in India, patients report somatic symptoms spontaneously but report psychological symptoms upon being probed (Jadhav et al., 2001; Raguram et al., 2001). Thus, patients across cultures are aware of both their physical and psychological symptoms but may fail to attend to or may feel reluctant to report some of them.

In summary, cross-cultural studies of somatization indicate that both somatic and emotional symptoms are a part of depression across cultural contexts, and that patients tend to make initial somatic complaints to their physicians when they do not feel comfortable disclosing information about their emotional distress, or vice versa. The literature on somatization underscores the need to establish that standardized Western assessment instruments are capturing similar constructs of depression across cultural settings. We turn now to an examination of whether cultural similarities in risk and protective factors, and patterns of comorbid disorders across cultures, are sufficient to allow us to conclude that the same concept is assessed by epidemiological studies despite large differences in prevalence of major depression.

Risk Factors for Major Depression across Cultures

A number of risk factors show remarkable similarity in their association with depression across cultures. We briefly review evidence suggesting that women, individuals who are under high levels of stress, and those who are poor, disadvantaged, and unmarried experience disproportionately high levels of depression across diverse cultural settings.

GENDER

Ample evidence shows that across countries of North America (Inaba et al., 2005; Ohayon, 2007), Western and Eastern Europe (Bromet et al., 2005; Pikhart et al., 2004), the Caribbean, Central and South America (Almeida-Filho et al., 2004; Slone et al., 2006), and East Asia (Inaba et al., 2005), women are more vulnerable than men to depression. In the United

States, this pattern holds for minority groups, such as Chinese Americans (Mak & Zane, 2004; Takeuchi et al., 2002), Hispanic Americans (Oquendo, Lizardi, Greenwald, Weissman, & Mann, 2004), and Native Americans (Sawchuk et al., 2005). Only a few studies fail to replicate this pattern. For example, gender differences are not evident in some East Asian contexts, such as among South Koreans (Ohayon & Hong, 2006). Future studies need to reveal the sociocultural factors that may explain why gender differences do not emerge for these cultural contexts.

STRESS

Country-level stressors, such as rapid economic and political changes, are known to be risk factors for increased prevalence of depression. For example, recession in Greece in the early 1980s was associated with increased prevalence of mood disorders (Madianos & Stefanis, 1992). Across countries, government stability is associated with lower levels of depressive symptoms (Van Hemert, Van de Vijver, & Poortinga, 2002). On the individual level, stressful and traumatic life events are associated with depressive symptoms across cultures (Kanazawa, White, & Hampson, 2007; Ohayon & Hong, 2006; Slone et al., 2006; Takeuchi et al., 2002; Unger et al., 2001). For example, negative life events similarly predict levels of depressive symptoms for teens from the United States, China, Korea, and the Czech Republic (Dmitrieva, Chen, Greenberger, & Gil-Rivas, 2004).

SOCIOECONOMIC DISADVANTAGE

Van Hemert and colleagues (2002) examined country-level associations between self-reported depressive symptoms and economic factors. They found that individuals in richer countries tend to report lower levels of depressive symptoms. Individual-level factors, such as poverty, unemployment, and lack of education, are consistently associated with depression across countries (Almeida-Filho et al., 2004; Bahar, Henderson, & Mackinnon, 1992; Bromet et al., 2005; Dressler et al., 2004; Ohayon, 2007; Oquendo et al., 2004; Pikhart et al., 2004). Because these variables are likely to be associated with a perceived failure to follow the cultural norm for a desirable lifestyle (Dressler et al., 2004), as well as with chronic life stress and lack of financial resources to manage negative life events and obtain health care, it is not surprising that, across cultures, low socioeconomic status is associated with depression. Interestingly, specific indices of socioeconomic disadvantage show cross-cultural differences in their association with emotional distress. For example, one study showed that lack of education did not emerge as a risk factor in Japan (Inaba et al., 2005). It appears that reliance on a conservative seniority stratification system in the workplace diminishes the association between education levels and professional promotion. In this cultural setting, other markers of financial stability may predict depression better than education.

MARITAL STATUS AND INTERPERSONAL FUNCTIONING

In addition to gender, stress, and socioeconomic status, ability to maintain healthy relationships is associated with depression across diverse cultural contexts. The odds of developing major depression or reporting depressive symptoms are heightened among unmarried relative to married adults across cultures (Inaba et al., 2005; Kawakami et al., 2005; Pikhart et al., 2004). The heightened risk is driven by individuals who are divorced, separated, or widowed (Almeida-Filho et al., 2004; Bromet et al., 2005; Ohayon, 2007; Slone et al., 2006).

More generally, the lack of stable and supportive social relationships is associated with heightened levels of depressive symptoms and increased prevalence of major depression across cultural groups in the United States (Whitbeck, McMorris, Hoyt, Stubben, & LaFromboise, 2002), as well as in other countries (Calvete & Connor-Smith, 2006). This is not a surprise considering that healthy interpersonal functioning plays an important role in buffering the effects of stress on levels of depressive symptoms across diverse cultural contexts (Calvete & Connor-Smith, 2006).

In summary, numerous studies lend support to the notion that despite large differences in prevalence rates, the construct of depression is associated with similar risk factors across countries. Another step in determining whether depression is similar across cultures involves examining the comorbidity of depression with other common forms of mental illness.

Patterns of Comorbidity across Cultures

Although depression traditionally has been conceptualized as a category that is independent of other forms of psychopathology, this assumption is not true. Clinicians and researchers have long observed that psychiatric comorbidity is the rule rather than the exception in Western cultures, including North America (Hasin, Goodwin, Stinson, & Grant, 2005), Finland (Melartin et al., 2002), and Australia (Henderson, Andrews, & Hall, 2000). These studies tell us that a patient with major depressive disorder and panic disorder in these cultures is not affected by two independent maladies. Rather, this patient demonstrates vulnerability to the broader cluster of disorders that includes both depression and panic disorder.

Research demonstrates that common forms of psychological distress systematically co-occur in both children and adults (Achenbach & Edelbrock, 1984; Krueger, Caspi, Moffitt, & Silva, 1998). For example, mood disorders, anxiety disorders, and somatization (what have been described as *internalizing disorders* in the child clinical literature) often co-occur at rates significantly higher than chance. Similarly, substance use and antisocial behavior (what has been described as *externalizing disorders*) also co-occur at rates significantly higher than chance. In addition, there is a weaker, albeit still significant, association between clusters of internalizing and externalizing disorders (Hasin et al., 2005). Thus, depression shows high rates of comorbidity with other internalizing disorders, such as anxiety disorders, and moderate rates of comorbidity with externalizing disorders, such as alcohol dependence.

Do these patterns of comorbidity generalize to other cultural contexts? An emerging body of literature suggests that the answer is "yes." High comorbidity rates have been documented for major depression and other internalizing disorders in countries as diverse as India (Raguram et al., 2001), Mexico (Slone et al., 2006), Poland (Malyszczak & Szechinski, 2004), and Saudi Arabia (Becker, 2004). In the United States, this association holds for minority groups, such as African Americans, Hispanic Americans, and Native Americans (Brown et al., 1996; Lagomasino et al., 2005; Sawchuk et al., 2005). A handful of studies report that major depression also shows significant association with externalizing disorders, such as alcohol use and/or abuse and antisocial behavior across cultural groups, such as Native American tribes in the United States (Sawchuk et al., 2005; Whitbeck et al., 2002) and adolescents in China (Unger et al., 2001).

Unfortunately, these studies do not formally compare patterns of comorbidity across cultures. Small-scale comparisons based on samples of primary care patients in the United States have yielded differences in rates of comorbidity of major depression and other common psychiatric disorders across ethnic groups (Brown et al., 1996; Lagomasino et al.,

2005). For example, depressed African Americans have higher rates of panic disorder, somatization disorder, and alcohol dependence than do European Americans (Brown et al., 1996). Similarly, Merikangas and colleagues (1996) found that although patterns of association between depression and other disorders are similar, the degree of association differs substantially across cultures. For example, the odds ratio (OR) for the association of depression and anxiety disorder ranged widely, from about 3 in Switzerland to about 15 in Puerto Rico. On the other hand, Krueger and colleagues (2003) examined comorbidity patterns of common mental disorders among patients in primary care centers across 14 countries and found that the patterns of association between depression and other common psychiatric syndromes held across cultures. As expected, depression was highly associated with internalizing syndromes, such as symptoms of anxiety and somatic distress, and moderately associated with externalizing syndromes, such as hazardous use of alcohol. Thus, emerging evidence suggests that depression reflects a broader internalizing tendency across cultures, although cultural factors may influence the strength of its association with other internalizing disorders.

Despite cross-cultural differences in prevalence of major depression, extant research suggests that epidemiological studies are capturing a comparable construct across diverse cultural settings. An important strength of cross-cultural studies is their attention to experimental, sampling, and linguistic similarity in methods employed across cultures. One tradeoff is that relatively less attention is given to cross-cultural similarity in conceptual meanings and the behavioral context of symptoms of depression. Another weakness of this research approach is that epidemiological studies rarely attempt to measure cultural factors such as ideas and practices. Instead, they rely on country as a proxy for culture. As a result, when cross-national differences are detected, it is often difficult to know which of the many specific cultural, demographic, or biological factors may account for higher levels of depression in some countries, such as the United States, and lower levels of depression in other countries, such as Japan. Complementing a cross-cultural approach with more culturally nuanced approaches may allow researchers to identify and examine closely the association of specific cultural factors, such as self-enhancement tendency or cultural norms regarding emotions, and the occurrence and expression of depression.

Cultural Approach: Examining Cultural Factors Associated with Depression

In this section, we describe emerging studies that use a cultural approach to studying depression. Because this research approach is a relative newcomer to the field of cultural psychopathology, these studies examine fewer cultural contexts than is the case with other approaches. Most of the studies that we describe in this section are based on comparison of North American (i.e., United States and Canada) and East Asian (i.e., Japan, Korea, China) cultural settings. Despite this limitation in scope, however, the cultural approach promises to provide us with a more sophisticated and empirically based understanding of the ways in which depression is culturally shaped.

The Role of Positivity Biases

Symptoms of depression, such as depressed mood, loss of interest in pleasurable activities, and decreases in self-esteem, are more likely to be viewed as abnormal in cultural settings such as North America (Heine, 2001; Mesquita & Karasawa, 2002; Tsai, Knutson, & Fung,

2006) and Puerto Rico (Koss-Chioino, 1999, p. 335) that promote the assumption that the "preferred ethos of euphoria" and feeling good about oneself is a healthy way of being. In these cultural settings, positivity biases, such as a tendency to view oneself and one's life and one's future in unrealistically positive light, and sense of control over one's life, serve as useful tools to motivate the independent self to pursue important goals. Indeed, displays of positivity biases are associated with increasing engagement with these cultural settings. For example, levels of reported self-esteem steadily increase with East Asian individuals' increasing acculturation to Western culture (Heine et al., 1999).

East Asian cultures provide an interesting cultural contrast. In these cultures, self-criticism and moderation are valued as a path to self-improvement and a way to maintain interpersonal harmony. Consistent with this cultural imperative, healthy individuals from East Asian cultures are less likely to self-enhance (Arnault, Sakamoto, & Moriwaki, 2005) and display lower levels of unrealistic optimism (Chang, Asakawa, & Sanna, 2001) than do individuals of European descent from the United States and Canada.

Implications of positivity biases for mental health may differ across cultures. Because North American cultures place a premium on feeling good about the self, the future, and life, individuals in these cultural contexts who fail to develop this worldview tend to be at risk for developing depressive symptoms. In contrast, positivity biases do not reflect a culturally normative worldview in East Asian cultures. In these cultural settings, low levels of positivity biases may not be associated with heightened levels of depressive symptoms, but may simply reflect reluctance to endorse positive items on depression questionnaires. For instance, Japanese individuals are less likely than European Americans to report that they feel happy or enjoy life, even though these groups do not differ in their reports of negative affect and somatic symptoms of depression (Iwata & Buka, 2002; Kanazawa et al., 2007). Studies examining cultural models of the self and the future, and perceptions of control have garnered support for the notion that positivity biases show different patterns of associations with levels of depressive symptoms across cultures.

MODELS OF THE SELF

A number of investigators have examined individuals' perceptions of the actual self (how one is), and their relation to levels of depressive symptoms across cultural contexts. They reported that negative descriptions of the actual self show stronger associations with levels of depressive symptoms for U.S., Korean, and Spanish samples, compared to samples from Japan, China, and the Czech Republic (Arnault et al., 2005; Calvete & Connor-Smith, 2005; Farruggia, Chen, Greenberger, Dmitrieva, & Macek, 2004).

It may not be enough to examine descriptions of the actual self alone. Instead, the greater the discrepancy between the actual self and the ideal self (how one would ideally like to be), the more susceptible one may be to depression. A large distance between ideal and actual selves represents a failure to fulfill a cultural imperative to self-enhance. Heine and Lehman (1999) found that the relation between levels of depressive symptoms and discrepancies between ideal and actual selves is stronger for European Canadians than for Japanese, with a bicultural Asian Canadian sample falling in between the two groups. In contrast, actual-undesired self-discrepancy predicts levels of depressive symptoms equally well for Asian American and European American students (Hardin & Leong, 2005). These data suggest that for European American samples, depression is associated with both failure to achieve the ideal self and inability to distance oneself from undesirable outcomes. In contrast, heightened levels of depressive symptoms among individuals in East Asian cultures are uniquely associated with failure to escape the undesirable self (Cheung, 1997), consistent with a notion that self-criticism rather than self-enhancement is an important cultural imperative in East Asian cultures.

MODELS OF THE FUTURE AND THE WORLD

Studies examining individuals' positive view of the future and their lives show a similar pattern. Although pessimism and hopelessness are associated with depressive symptoms across national groups, this association is stronger for European Americans than for individuals in Hong Kong (Stewart et al., 2005), as well as for Asian Americans (Hardin & Leong, 2005) and African Americans (Kennard, Stewart, Hughes, Patel, & Emslie, 2006). In addition, Calvete and Connor-Smith (2005) reported that although symptoms of depression are predicted by dissatisfaction with life circumstances for Spanish and U.S. students alike, the link between dissatisfaction with circumstances and heightened levels of depressive symptoms is stronger for the U.S. students than for the Spaniards.

ATTRIBUTIONAL STYLES

Another line of research has examined negative perceptions of the self, the world, and the future in the wake of negative life events. According to the hopelessness theory of depression (Abramson, Metalsky, & Alloy, 1989), individuals who tend to attribute negative events to internal, stable, and global causes are at increased risk for depression. Studies with primarily European American samples support this theory (Abela, 2002). Given an emphasis on positive self-presentation in European American cultural contexts, negative attributional style may represent a failure to interpret life stressors in a culturally normative way. Although negative attributions following negative life events have been found to be associated with depressed mood for U.S., Russian, French, and Chinese adults and children (Ameli, Swendsen, Campagnone, & Grillon, 2002; Anderson, 1999; Gutkovich et al., 1999), this association is weaker for Japanese students (Sakamoto & Kambara, 1998), and minority groups in the United States (Cardemil, Kim, Pinedo, & Miller, 2005; Rieckmann, Wadsworth, & Deyhle, 2004). Additional studies examining the association between negative explanatory style and the etiology and maintenance of depression across cultures are needed to examine the validity of attributional theory of depression across cultural groups.

LOCUS OF CONTROL

Finally, having an *external locus of control*, or believing that life events are out of one's personal control, is thought to be a risk factor for depression (Neff & Hoppe, 1993). For example, Mirowsky and Ross (1984) found that among Mexican Americans and Mexicans, being fatalistic (i.e., having an external locus of control) was predictive of higher levels of depression. However, the association between external locus of control (or fatalism) and depression is not universal. Although having an external locus of control was positively correlated with levels of depression for American and Turkish college students, such was not the case for Nigerian or Filipino college students (Akande & Lester, 1994; Lester, Castromayor, & Icli, 1991). Similarly, Sastry and Ross (1998) found that although believing in personal control is related to lower levels of depression across cultural groups, the magnitude of the correlation is weaker for East and South Asians than for non-Asians.

To summarize, viewing oneself, one's future, and one's life negatively; attributing negative life events to internal, stable, and global causes; and believing that they are not under one's control are known to be harmful or "depressogenic" beliefs. The cultural approach challenges this notion, and suggests that these beliefs and attributional styles are greater risk factors for depression for individuals from Western cultural settings, such as European Americans, than for individuals from cultures that place less emphasis on promoting the self, such as East Asians. This pattern of findings helps us understand how East Asians can appear depressed due to their failure to endorse positive assessments of themselves and their lives, yet remain surprisingly resilient to major depression, in part due to their tendency to persevere under stress.

Cultural Norms Regarding Negative Emotions

Another cultural factor that may shape the impact of depression on emotional responding is adherence to cultural norms regarding emotions. Different cultures endorse different norms regarding the experience and expression of negative emotions. For example, healthy emotional functioning is associated with open expression of emotions in European American cultural contexts, and with emotional balance and moderation in East Asian cultural contexts. Abnormal emotional functioning can also be expected to vary relative to these culture-specific norms of emotional functioning; that is, emotional symptoms of psychopathology may represent deviations from culturally specific norms of emotional expression rather than from culturally universal patterns of healthy emotional functioning. For example, Okazaki and Kallivayalil (2002) found that levels of depressive symptoms among Asian American students were associated with deviations from a culturally normative belief that it is inappropriate to express and experience depression.

Studies of European Americans indicate that individuals with major depressive disorder exhibit diminished reactivity to a variety of standard emotional cues (Gehricke & Shapiro, 2000; Sloan, Strauss, Quirk, & Sajatovic, 1997). Diminished emotional reactivity represents deviation from the European American cultural norm of open, or even exaggerated, emotional responding. Depression may reduce attention to, or concern with, cultural norms of emotional responding, resulting in emotional responses that contradict these norms; that is, in European American cultural contexts, a depressed individual may fail to express his or her feelings openly. In contrast, in Asian cultural contexts, a depressed individual may fail to moderate his or her emotions.

To test this hypothesis, we presented depressed and nondepressed European Americans and Asian Americans with sad and amusing films (Chentsova-Dutton et al., 2007). Consistent with previous studies, whereas major depression was associated with *diminished* emotional responding to the sad film for European Americans, it was associated with *enhanced* emotional responding for Asian Americans. In other words, within each cultural group, depressed participants demonstrated the culturally inappropriate negative emotional response. Being depressed may result in a failure to endorse and enact cultural norms of emotional expression. Alternatively, deviating from cultural norms may result in depression. Regardless, these findings suggest that the impact of depression on emotional responding varies depending on the dominant cultural model of healthy emotional functioning.

CONCLUSIONS AND FUTURE DIRECTIONS

Recent decades have seen a growing interest in understanding the role of culture in shaping depression. Nearly 1,000 studies on culture and depression have been published in the last

15 years alone. These studies use different research approaches to examine whether the Western body of knowledge about major depression generalizes to other cultural contexts, and, increasingly, to identify specific cultural factors associated with resilience and vulnerability to major depression.

In this chapter, we have reviewed recent evidence gathered in ethnographic, biomedical, and cultural approaches to the study of cultural shaping of depression. Despite differences in these theoretical and methodological approaches, all have demonstrated the various ways in which culture may influence depression—from concepts of depression and illness to prevalence rates across countries, to the association of positivity biases with levels of depressive symptoms. These approaches have also identified important similarities—from similar conceptualization of depression as caused by worrying too much to risk factors and comorbidity, to the patterns of emotional responding that represent deviations from cultural norms regarding experience and expression of emotions. Despite these advances, it is sobering to realize how little we know about depression across cultures. It is important that future researchers move beyond the approaches described here by studying depression in more cultural contexts and combining multiple research approaches to examine more explicitly how culture influences other aspects of depression, such as its biological and genetic markers, and its treatment.

Combining Diverse Approaches

In particular, more studies are needed that combine research tools developed by ethnographic, biomedical, and cultural approaches. Only by combining these research approaches can we uncover the extent of cultural similarities and differences in depression. One recent example of this is the study by Kohrt and colleagues (2005). They studied *jhum-jhum*, a common illness in rural Nepal that is characterized by numbness and tingling sensations. The study combined ethnographic and biomedical approaches to investigate the relationship between *jhum-jhum* and depression, measuring levels of depression in patients with *jhum-jhum* and conducting medical exams to identify cases of *jhum-jhum* caused by medical conditions, such as arthritis or diabetes. This study demonstrated that the presence of somatic symptoms in this non-Western cultural setting was associated with higher levels of depressive symptoms, regardless of medical explanation for the somatic symptoms. The study benefited from combining different approaches. Limiting this study to a single approach, such as the ethnographic interview, would not have allowed researchers to examine whether the biological and cultural factors interacted in shaping the expression of distress among rural Nepalese.

Behavioral, Physiological, and Genetic Markers of Depression

A recent set of studies has begun to examine interactions between ethnicity and physiological markers of depression, such as hormonal responses to stress, and genetic markers for depression (Gallagher-Thompson et al., 2006; Zintzaras, 2006). For example, Gallagher-Thompson and colleagues (2006) showed that physiological responses to stress differ for Hispanic and non-Hispanic caregivers. Regardless of their stress levels, Hispanic women had flatter daytime cortisol slopes than did their European American counterparts. This study suggests that we cannot take for granted that physiological markers of depression identified in European American samples hold universally for other cultural and ethnic groups. Future examinations of cultural differences in behavioral, physiological, and genetic markers of depression and their interactions with stress would open a new frontier in the research on cultural shaping of depression.

Barriers to Treatment

As the numbers of ethnic/minority and immigrant populations in Western countries skyrocket, the crisis in providing effective mental health services to these individuals is more apparent than ever. Mounting evidence suggests that evidence-based care for depression improves outcomes for these individuals (for a review, see Miranda et al., 2005). Despite these promising data, individuals from non-Western cultural settings face countless barriers in obtaining effective treatment for depression. These barriers range from low rates of treatment seeking (Lagomasino et al., 2005; Ohayon & Hong, 2006; Williams et al., 2007; Wittchen & Jacobi, 2005) to low likelihood of detection of depressive symptoms by clinicians (Simon, Goldberg, et al., 1999). Once in treatment, barriers include unwillingness of patients to engage in a biological treatment strategy for an ailment they believe to be of an interpersonal or spiritual nature, and some patients' inability to tolerate standard doses of antidepressants, resulting in lower likelihood of taking antidepressants (Cooper et al., 2003). In addition, some patients may feel hesitant to engage in therapies requiring disclosure of feelings, due to their belief that it is inappropriate to discuss personal and family problems with strangers (Lawrence et al., 2006). It is no surprise that these factors result in high treatment dropoff rates for individuals from non-Western cultural settings and minority patients (Organista, Muñoz, & Gonzalez, 1994). It is likely that cultural factors, such as fatalism, acceptance of suffering, stigma, and cultural conceptions of depression as being interpersonally based contribute to these barriers. Given these challenges in recruiting, accurately diagnosing, and delivering effective treatment modalities to culturally diverse populations, future research needs to utilize our knowledge of cultural conceptions of depression to design more effective recruitment, assessment, and treatment programs.

Indigenous Forms of Treatment

A final, promising future direction is to explore the effects of non-Western treatment approaches, such as acupuncture, yoga, and meditative practices, on depression in Western populations. These practices may be particularly useful for treating individuals who cannot take some antidepressant medications, such as pregnant women or individuals who do not respond to antidepressants. For example, studies suggest that acupuncture provides relief to depressed individuals and appears to be comparable to other treatments in terms of response and relapse rates (Gallagher, Allen, Hitt, Schnyer, & Manber, 2001).

Similarly, a number of studies support the use of meditation, mindfulness practices, and yoga for treating depression (Segal, Williams, & Teasdale, 2002; Woolery, Myers, Sternlieb, & Zeltzer, 2004). For example, patients with mood and anxiety disorders undergoing mindfulness-based therapy show reduced *rumination*, or maladaptive tendency to focus on symptoms of depression, compared to waiting-list controls (Ramel, Goldin, Carmona, & McQuaid, 2004). Reduced rumination can help patients predisposed to depression manage negative affect in their lives. Consistent with this notion, treatment with mindfulness-based cognitive therapy, a meditation-based psychotherapeutic intervention, reduced risk of relapse among patients with a history of multiple previous episodes of major depression (Teasdale et al., 2000). Future studies need to examine whether these practices are particularly beneficial within the context of East Asian and Southeast Asian cultural values and norms.

REFERENCES

Abela, J. R. Z. (2002). A test of the diathesis–stress and causal mediation components of Beck's cognitive theory of depression. *British Journal of Clinical Psychology, 41,* 111–128.

Abramson, L. Y., Metalsky, G. I., & Alloy, L. B. (1989). Hopelessness depression: A theory-based subtype of depression. *Psychological Review, 96,* 358–372.

Achenbach, T. M., & Edelbrock, C. (1984). Psychopathology of childhood. *Annual Review of Psychology, 35,* 227–256.

Akande, A., & Lester, D. (1994). Suicidal preoccupation, depression and locus of control in Nigerians and Americans. *Personality and Individual Differences, 16*(6), 979.

Almeida-Filho, N., Lessa, I., Magalhaes, L., Araujo, M. J., Aquino, E., James, S. A., et al. (2004). Social inequality and depressive disorders in Bahia, Brazil: Interactions of gender, ethnicity, and social class. *Social Science and Medicine, 59*(7), 1339–1353.

Ameli, R., Swendsen, J., Compagnone, P., & Grillon, C. (2002). Cross-cultural validity of the cognitive theory of depression: A French–American comparison. *Annales Médico-Psychologiques, 160*(5–6), 362–368.

American Psychiatric Association. (2000). *Diagnostic and statistical manual of mental disorders* (4th ed., text rev.). Washington, DC: Author.

Anderson, C. A. (1999). Attributional style, depression, and loneliness: A cross-cultural comparison of American and Chinese students. *Personality and Social Psychology Bulletin, 25*(4), 482–499.

Arnault, D. S., Sakamoto, S., & Moriwaki, A. (2005). The association between negative self-descriptions and depressive symptomology: Does culture make a difference? *Archives of Psychiatric Nursing, 19*(2), 93–100.

Ayuso-Mateos, J. J., Vázquez, J. L., Dowrich, C., Lehtinen, V., Dalgard, O. S., Casey, P., et al. (2001). Depressive disorders in Europe: Prevalence figures from the ODIN study. *British Journal of Psychiatry, 179,* 308–316.

Bahar, E., Henderson, A. S., & Mackinnon, A. J. (1992). An epidemiological study of mental health and socioeconomic conditions in Sumatra, Indonesia. *Acta Psychiatrica Scandinavica, 85*(4), 257–263.

Becker, S. M. (2004). Detection of somatization and depression in primary care in Saudi Arabia. *Social Psychiatry and Psychiatric Epidemiology, 39*(12), 962–966.

Bhui, K., Bhugra, D., Goldberg, D., Sauer, J., & Tylee, A. (2004). Assessing the prevalence of depression in Punjabi and English primary care attendees: The role of culture, physical illness and somatic symptoms. *Transcultural Psychiatry, 41*(3), 307–322.

Bromet, E. J., Gluzman, S. F., Paniotto, V. I., Webb, C. P. M., Tintle, N. L., Zakhozha, V., et al. (2005). Epidemiology of psychiatric and alcohol disorders in Ukraine: Findings from the Ukraine World Mental Health Survey. *Social Psychiatry and Psychiatric Epidemiology, 40*(9), 681–690.

Brown, C., Schulberg, H. C., & Madonia, M. J. (1996). Clinical presentations of major depression by African Americans and whites in primary medical care practice. *Journal of Affective Disorders, 41*(3), 181–191.

Burr, J., & Chapman, T. (2004). Contextualizing experiences of depression in women from South Asian communities: A discursive approach. *Sociology of Health and Illness, 26*(4), 433–452.

Calvete, E., & Connor-Smith, J. K. (2005). Automatic thoughts and psychological symptoms: A cross-cultural comparison of American and Spanish students. *Cognitive Therapy and Research, 29*(2), 201–217.

Calvete, E., & Connor-Smith, J. K. (2006). Perceived social support, coping, and symptoms of distress in American and Spanish students. *Anxiety, Stress and Coping: An International Journal, 19*(1), 47–65.

Cardemil, E. V., Kim, S., Pinedo, T. M., & Miller, I. W. (2005). Developing a culturally appropriate depression prevention program: The Family Coping Skills program. *Cultural Diversity and Ethnic Minority Psychology, 11,* 99–112.

Chang, E. C., Asakawa, K., & Sanna, L. J. (2001). Cultural variations in optimistic and pessimistic bias: Do Easterners really expect the worst and Westerners really expect the best when predicting future life events? *Journal of Personality and Social Psychology, 81,* 476–491.

Chentsova-Dutton, Y., Chu, J. P., Tsai, J. L., Rottenberg, J., Gross, J. J., & Gotlib, I. H. (2007). Depression and emotional reactivity: Variations among Asian American and European Americans. *Journal of Abnormal Psychology, 116,* 776–785.

Cheung, S. K. (1997). Self-discrepancy and depressive experiences among Chinese early adolescents: Significance of identity and the undesirable self. *International Journal of Psychology, 32*(5), 347–359.

Cho, M. J., Kim, J. K., Jeon, H. J., Suh, T., Chung, I. W., Hong, J. P., et al. (2007). Lifetime and 12-month prevalence of DSM-IV psychiatric disorders among Korean adults. *Journal of Nervous and Mental Disease, 195,* 203–210.

Cooper, L. A., Gonzales, J. J., Gallo, J. J., Rost, K. M., Meredith, L. S., Rubenstein, L. V., et al. (2003). The acceptability of treatment for depression among African-American, Hispanic, and white primary care patients. *Medical Care, 41*(4), 479–489.

Dmitrieva, J., Chen, C., Greenberger, E., & Gil-Rivas, V. (2004). Family relationships and adolescent psychosocial outcomes: Converging findings from Eastern and Western cultures. *Journal of Research on Adolescence, 14*(4), 425–447.

Dressler, W. W., Ribeiro, R. P., Balieiro, M. C., Oths, K. S., & Dos Santos, J. E. (2004). Eating, drinking and being depressed: The social, cultural and psychological context of alcohol consumption and nutrition in a Brazilian community. *Social Science and Medicine, 59*(4), 709–720.

Farruggia, S. P., Chen, C., Greenberger, E., Dmitrieva, J., & Macek, P. (2004). Adolescent self-esteem in cross-cultural perspective: Testing measurement equivalence and a mediation model. *Journal of Cross-Cultural Psychology, 35*(6), 719–733.

Gallagher, S. M., Allen, J. J. B., Hitt, S. K., Schnyer, R. N., & Manber, R. (2001). Six-month depression relapse rates among women treated with acupuncture. *Complementary Therapies in Medicine, 9,* 216–218.

Gallagher-Thompson, D., Shurgot, G. R., Rider, K., Gray, H. L., McKibbin, C. L., Kraemer, H. C., et al. (2006). Ethnicity, stress, and cortisol function in Hispanic and non-Hispanic white women: A preliminary study of family dementia caregivers and noncaregivers. *American Journal of Geriatric Psychiatry, 14*(4), 334–342.

Gehricke, J., & Shapiro, D. (2000). Reduced facial expression and social context in major depression: Discrepancies between facial muscle activity and self-reported emotion. *Psychiatry Research, 95,* 157–167.

Guarnaccia, P. J., Rivera, M., Franco, F., & Neighbors, C. (1996). The experiences of *ataques de nervios*: Towards an anthropology of emotions in Puerto Rico. *Culture, Medicine and Psychiatry, 20,* 343—367.

Gutkovich, Z., Rosenthal, R. N., Galynker, I., Muran, C., Batchelder, S., & Itskhoki, E. (1999). Depression and demoralization among Russian-Jewish immigrants in primary care. *Psychosomatics: Journal of Consultation Liaison Psychiatry, 40*(2), 117–125.

Hardin, E. E., & Leong, F. T. L. (2005). Optimism and pessimism as mediators of the relations between self-discrepancies and distress among Asian and European Americans. *Journal of Counseling Psychology, 52*(1), 25–35.

Hasin, D. S., Goodwin, R. D., Stinson, F. S., & Grant, B. F. (2005). Epidemiology of major depressive disorder: Results from the national epidemiologic survey on alcoholism and related conditions. *Archives of General Psychiatry, 62*(10), 1097–1106.

Heine, S. J. (2001). Self as cultural product: An examination of East Asian and North American selves. *Journal of Personality, 69,* 881–905.

Heine, S. J., & Lehman, D. R. (1999). Culture, self-discrepancies, and self-satisfaction. *Personality and Social Psychology Bulletin, 25*(8), 915–925.

Heine, S. J., Lehman, D. R., Markus, H. R., & Kitayama, S. (1999). Is there a universal need for positive self-regard? *Psychological Review, 106,* 766–794.

Henderson, S., Andrews, G., & Hall, W. (2000). Australia's mental health: An overview of the general population survey. *Australian and New Zealand Journal of Psychiatry, 34*(2), 197–205.

Inaba, A., Thoits, P. A., Ueno, K., Gove, W. R., Evenson, R. J., & Sloan, M. (2005). Depression in the United States and Japan: Gender, marital status, and SES patterns. *Social Science and Medicine, 61*(11), 2280–2292.

Iwata, N., & Buka, S. (2002). Race/ethnicity and depressive symptoms: A cross-cultural/ethnic comparison among university students in East Asia, North and South America. *Social Science and Medicine*, 55(12), 2243–2252.

Jadhav, S., Weiss, M. G., & Littlewood, R. (2001). Cultural experience of depression among White Britons in London. *Anthropology and Medicine*, 8(1), 47–70.

Karam, E. G., Mneimneh, Z. N., & Karam, A. N. (2006). 12-month prevalence and treatment of mental disorders in Lebanon: A national epidemiologic survey. *Lancet*, 367, 1000–1006.

Kanazawa, A., White, P. M., & Hampson, S. E. (2007). Ethnic variation in depressive symptoms in a community sample in Hawaii. *Cultural Diversity and Ethnic Minority Psychology*, 13(1), 35–44.

Karasz, A. (2005a). Cultural differences in conceptual models of depression. *Social Science and Medicine*, 60(7), 1625–1635.

Karasz, A. (2005b). Marriage, depression and illness: Sociosomatic models in a South Asian immigrant community. *Psychology and Developing Societies*, 17(2), 161–180.

Kawakami, N., Takeshima, T., Ono, Y., Uda, H., Hata, Y., Nakane, Y., et al. (2005). Twelve-month prevalence, severity, and treatment of common mental disorders in communities in Japan: Preliminary finding from the World Mental Health Japan Survey 2002–2003. *Psychiatry and Clinical Neurosciences*, 59(4), 441–452.

Kennard, B. D., Stewart, S. M., Hughes, J. L., Patel, P. G., & Emslie, G. J. (2006). Cognitions and depressive symptoms among ethnic minority adolescents. *Cultural Diversity and Ethnic Minority Psychology*, 12(3), 578–591.

Kessler, R. C., Berglund, P., Demler, O., Jin, R., Merikangas, K. R., & Walters, E. E. (2005). Lifetime prevalence and age-of-onset distributions of DSM-IV disorders in the National Comorbidity Survey Replication. *Archives of General Psychiatry*, 62, 593–602.

Keyes, C. L. M., & Ryff, C. D. (2003). Somatization and mental health: A comparative study of the idiom of distress hypothesis. *Social Science and Medicine*, 57(10), 1833–1845.

Kleinman, A. (1977). Depression, somatization, and the new cross-cultural psychiatry. *Social Science and Medicine*, 11, 3–10.

Kleinman, A. (1982). Neurasthenia and depression: A study of somatization and culture in China. *Culture, Medicine and Psychiatry*, 6(2), 117–190.

Kohrt, B. A., Kunz, R. D., Baldwin, J. L., Koirala, N. R., Sharma, V. D., & Nepal, M. K. (2005). "Somatization" and "comorbidity": A study of *jhum-jhum* and depression in rural Nepal. *Ethos*, 33(1), 125–147.

Koss-Chioino, J. D. (1999). Depression among Puerto Rican women: Culture, etiology and diagnosis [Special issue]. *Hispanic Journal of Behavioral Sciences*, 21(3), 330–350.

Kroeber, A. L., & Kluckhohn, C. (1952). *Culture: A critical review of concepts and definitions*. Cambridge, MA: Harvard University, Peabody Museum of Archaeology and Ethnology.

Krueger, R. F., Caspi, A., Moffitt, T. E., & Silva, P. E. (1998). The structure and stability of common mental disorders (DSM-III-R): A longitudinal–epidemiological study. *Journal of Abnormal Psychology*, 107, 216–227.

Krueger, R. F., Chentsova-Dutton, Y. E., Markon, K. E., Goldberg, D., & Ormel, J. (2003). A cross cultural study of the structure of comorbidity among common psychopathological syndromes in the general health care setting. *Journal of Abnormal Psychology*, 112, 437–447.

Lagomasino, I. T., Dwight-Johnson, M., Miranda, J., Zhang, L., Liao, D., Duan, N., et al. (2005). Disparities in depression treatment for Latinos and site of care. *Psychiatric Services*, 56(12), 1517–1523.

Lam, K., Marra, C., & Salzinger, K. (2005). Social reinforcement of somatic versus psychological description of depressive events. *Behaviour Research and Therapy*, 43(9), 1203–1218.

Lawrence, V., Banerjee, S., Bhugra, D., Sangha, K., Turner, S., & Murray, J. (2006). Coping with depression in later life: A qualitative study of help-seeking in three ethnic groups. *Psychology Medicine*, 36, 1375–1383.

Lee, C. K. (2001). *The epidemiological survey of psychiatric illnesses in Korea*. Seoul, Korea: Ministry of Health and Welfare.

Lester, D., Castromayor, I. J., & Icli, T. (1991). Locus of control, depression, and suicidal ideation among American, Philippine, and Turkish students. *Journal of Social Psychology, 131*(3), 447–449.

Lin, K.-M., Lau, J. K., Yamamoto, J., Zheng, Y.-P., Kim, H.-S., Cho, K.-H., et al. (1992). Hwa-Byung: A community study of Korean Americans. *Journal of Nervous and Mental Disease, 180*(6), 386–391.

Madianos, M. G., & Stefanis, C. N. (1992). Changes in the prevalence of symptoms of depression and depression across Greece. *Social Psychiatry and Psychiatric Epidemiology, 27*, 211–219.

Mak, W. W. S., & Zane, N. W. (2004). The phenomenon of somatization among community Chinese Americans. *Social Psychiatry and Psychiatric Epidemiology, 39*(12), 967–974.

Malyszczak, K., & Szechinski, M. (2004). Comorbidity of different forms of anxiety disorders and depression. *Psychiatria Polska, 38*(4), 603–609.

Melartin, T. K., Rytsälä, H. J., Leskelä, U. S., Lestelä-Mielonen, P. S., Sokero, T. P., & Isometsä, E. T. (2002). Current comorbidity of psychiatric disorders among DSM-IV major depressive disorder patients in psychiatric care in the Vantaa Depression Study. *Journal of Clinical Psychiatry, 63*(2), 126–134.

Merikangas, K. R., Angst, J., Eaton, W., Canino, G., Rubio-Stipec, M., Wacker, H., et al. (1996). Comorbidity and boundaries of affective disorders with anxiety disorders and substance misuse: Results of an international task force. *British Journal of Psychiatry, 30*, 58–67.

Mesquita, B., & Karasawa, M. (2002). Different emotional lives. *Cognition and Emotion, 16*, 127–141.

Miranda, J., Bernal, G., Lau, A., Kohn, L., Hwang, W.-C., & LaFromboise, T. (2005). State of the science on psychosocial interventions for ethnic minorities. *Annual Review of Clinical Psychology, 1*(1), 113–142.

Mirowsky, J., & Ross, C. E. (1984). Mexican culture and its emotional contradictions. *Journal of Health and Social Behavior, 25*(1), 2–13.

Murray, C. J. L., & Lopez, A. D. (1997). Alternative projections of mortality and disability by cause 1990–2020: Global Burden of Disease Study. *Lancet, 349*, 1498–1504.

Neff, J. A., & Hoppe, S. K. (1993). Race/ethnicity, acculturation, and psychological distress: Fatalism and religiosity as cultural resources. *Journal of Community Psychology, 21*, 3–20.

Ohayon, M. M. (2007). Epidemiology of depression and its treatment in the general population. *Journal of Psychiatric Research, 41*(3–4), 207–213.

Ohayon, M. M., & Hong, S.-C. (2006). Prevalence of major depressive disorder in the general population of South Korea. *Journal of Psychiatric Research, 40*(1), 30–36.

Okazaki, S., & Kallivayalil, D. (2002). Cultural norms and subjective disability as predictors of symptom reports among Asian Americans and white Americans. *Journal of Cross-Cultural Psychology, 33*(5), 482–491.

Oquendo, M. A., Lizardi, D., Greenwald, S., Weissman, M. M., & Mann, J. J. (2004). Rates of lifetime suicide attempt and rates of lifetime major depression in different ethnic groups in the United States. *Acta Psychiatrica Scandinavica, 110*(6), 446–451.

Organista, K. C., Muñoz, R. F., & Gonzalez, G. (1994). Cognitive-behavioral therapy for depression in low-income and minority medical outpatients: Description of a program and exploratory analyses. *Cognitive Therapy and Research, 18*, 241–259.

Pang, K. Y. (1995). A cross-cultural understanding of depression among elderly Korean immigrants: Prevalence, symptoms and diagnosis. *Clinical Gerontologist, 15*(4), 3–20.

Pikhart, H., Bobak, M., Pajak, A., Malyutina, S., Kubinova, R., Topor, R., et al. (2004). Psychosocial factors at work and depression in three countries of central and Eastern Europe. *Social Science and Medicine, 58*(8), 1475–1482.

Raguram, R., Weiss, M. G., Keval, H., & Channabasavanna, S. M. (2001). Cultural dimensions of clinical depression in Bangalore, India. *Anthropology and Medicine, 8*(1), 31–46.

Ramel, W., Goldin, P. R., Carmona, P. E., & McQuaid, J. R. (2004). The effects of mindfulness meditation on cognitive processes and affect in patients with past depression. *Cognitive Therapy and Research, 28*(4), 433–455.

Rieckmann, T. R., Wadsworth, M. E., & Deyhle, D. (2004). Cultural identity, explanatory style, and depression in Navajo adolescents. *Cultural Diversity and Ethnic Minority Psychology, 10*(4), 365–382.

Sakamoto, S., & Kambara, M. (1998). A longitudinal study of the relationship between attributional style, life events, and depression in Japanese undergraduates. *Journal of Social Psychology, 138*(2), 229–240.

Sastry, J., & Ross, C. E. (1998). Asian ethnicity and the sense of personal control. *Social Psychology Quarterly, 61*(2), 101–120.

Sawchuk, C. N., Roy-Byrne, P., Goldberg, J., Manson, S., Noonan, C., Beals, J., et al. (2005). The relationship between post-traumatic stress disorder, depression and cardiovascular disease in an American Indian tribe. *Psychological Medicine, 35*(12), 1785–1794.

Segal, Z. V., Williams, J. M. G., & Teasdale, J. D. (2002). *Mindfulness-based cognitive therapy for depression: A new approach to preventing relapse.* New York: Guilford Press.

Sellers, S. L., Ward, E. C., & Pate, D. (2006). Dimensions of depression: A qualitative study of wellbeing among black African immigrant women. *Qualitative Social Work: Research and Practice, 5*(1), 45–66.

Simon, G. E., Goldberg, D., Tiemens, B. G., & Ustün, T. B. (1999). Outcomes of recognized and unrecognized depression in an international primary care study. *General Hospital Psychiatry, 21,* 97–105.

Simon, G. E., Goldberg, D. P., Von Korff, M., & Ustün, T. B. (2002). Understanding cross-national differences in depression prevalence. *Psychological Medicine, 32,* 585–594.

Simon, G. E., Von Korff, M., Picvinelli, M., Fullerton, C., & Ormel, J. (1999). An international study of the relation between somatic symptoms and depression. *New England Journal of Medicine, 18,* 1329–1335.

Sloan, D. M., Strauss, M. E., Quirk, S. W., & Sajatovic, M. (1997). Subjective and expressive emotional responses in depression. *Journal of Affective Disorders, 46,* 135–141.

Slone, L. B., Norris, F. H., Murphy, A. D., Baker, C. K., Perilla, J. L., Diaz, D., et al. (2006). Epidemiology of major depression in four cities in Mexico. *Depression and Anxiety, 23*(3), 158–167.

Stewart, S. M., Kennard, B. D., Lee, P. W. H., Mayes, T., Hughes, C., & Emslie, G. (2005). Hopelessness and suicidal ideation among adolescents in two cultures. *Journal of Child Psychology and Psychiatry, and Allied Disciplines, 46*(4), 364–372.

Stompe, T., Ortwein-Swoboda, G., Chaudhry, H. R., Friedmann, A., Wenzel, T., & Schanda, H. (2001). Guilt and depression: A cross-cultural comparative study. *Psychopathology, 34*(6), 289–298.

Takeuchi, D. T., Chun, C.-A., Gong, F., & Shen, H. (2002). Cultural expressions of distress. *Health: An Interdisciplinary Journal for the Social Study of Health, Illness and Medicine, 6*(2), 221–235.

Teasdale, J. D., Segal, Z. V., Williams, J. M. G., Ridgeway, V. A., Soulsby, J. M., & Lau, M. A. (2000). Prevention of relapse, recurrence in major depression by mindfulness-based cognitive therapy. *Journal of Consulting and Clinical Psychology, 68*(4), 615–623.

Tousignant, M., & Maldonaldo, M. (1989). Sadness, depression and social reciprocity in highland Ecuador. *Social Science and Medicine, 28*(9), 899–904.

Tsai, J. L., Knutson, B., & Fung, H. H. (2006). Cultural variation in affect valuation. *Journal of Personality and Social Psychology, 90,* 288–307.

Tung, M. P. M. (1994). Symbolic meanings of the body in Chinese culture and "somatization." *Culture, Medicine and Psychiatry, 18,* 483–492.

Unger, J. B., Li, Y., Johnson, C. A., Gong, J., Chen, X., Li, C. Y., et al. (2001). Stressful life events among adolescents in Wuhan, China: Associations with smoking, alcohol use, and depressive symptoms. *International Journal of Behavioral Medicine, 8*(1), 1–18.

Van Hemert, D. A., Van de Vijver, F. J. R., & Poortinga, Y. H. (2002). The Beck Depression Inventory as a measure of subjective well-being: A cross-national study. *Journal of Happiness Studies, 3*(3), 257–286.

Vasiliadis, H.-M., Lesage, A., Adair, C., Wang, P. S., & Kessler, R. C. (2007). Do Canada and the United States differ in prevalence of depression and utilization of services? *Psychiatric Services, 58,* 63–71.

Waza, K., Graham, A. V., Zyzanski, S. J., & Inoue, K. (1999). Comparison of symptoms in Japanese and American depressed primary care patients. *Family Practice, 16*(5), 528–533.

Weissman, M. M., Bland, R., Canino, G. J., Faravelli, C., Greenwald, S., Hwu, H.-G., et al. (1996). Cross-national epidemiology of major depression and bipolar disorder. *Journal of the American Medical Association, 24,* 293–299.

Whitbeck, L. B., McMorris, B. J., Hoyt, D. R., Stubben, J. D., & LaFromboise, T. (2002). Perceived discrimination, traditional practices, and depressive symptoms among American Indians in the upper Midwest. *Journal of Health and Social Behavior, 43*(4), 400–418.

Williams, D. R., Gonzalez, H., Neighbors, H., Nesse, R., Abelson, J. M., Sweetman, J., et al. (2007). Prevalence and distribution of major depressive disorder in African Americans, Caribbean blacks, and non-Hispanic whites: Results from the National Survey of American Life. *Archives of General Psychiatry, 64*(3), 305–315.

Wittchen, H.-U., & Jacobi, F. (2005). Size and burden of mental disorders in Europe—a critical review and appraisal of 27 studies [Special issue]. *European Neuropsychopharmacology, 15*(4), 357–376.

Woolery, A., Myers, H., Sternlieb, B., & Zeltzer, L. K. (2004). A yoga intervention for young adults with elevated symptoms of depression. *Alternative Therapies in Health and Medicine, 10*, 60–63.

World Health Organization World Mental Health Survey Consortium. (2004). Prevalence, severity, and unmet need for treatment of mental disorders in the World Health Organization World Mental Health Surveys. *Journal of the American Medical Association, 291*, 2581–2590.

Zintzaras, E. (2006). *C677t* and *a1298c* methylenetetrahydrofolate reductase gene polymorphisms in schizophrenia, bipolar disorder and depression: A meta-analysis of genetic association studies. *Psychiatric Genetics, 16*(3), 105–115.

CHAPTER 17

Gender Differences in Depression

Susan Nolen-Hoeksema *and* Lori M. Hilt

Unipolar depression is a relatively common psychiatric problem, but it is even more common among women than among men. About twice as many women as men meet the criteria for major depressive disorder (MDD) or dysthymic disorder at some time in their lives (Kessler et al., 2003). For example, the National Comorbidity Survey found a lifetime prevalence for major depressive disorder of 21.3% in women and 12.7% in men (Kessler, McGonagle, Swartz, Blazer, & Nelson, 1993; Kessler et al., 2003). The absolute prevalence of depression varies substantially across cultures and nations, but the gender difference in depression remains significant across most demographic and cultural groups (Andrade et al., 2003). The World Health Organization estimated that depression is the leading cause of disease-related disability for women in the world today (Murray & Lopez, 1996).

We review the epidemiology of gender differences in depression, then describe the most prominent explanations for this difference, including biological, psychological and social explanations. Finally, we present a model integrating the best-supported explanations and suggest future directions for research.

EPIDEMIOLOGICAL DATA

Epidemiological studies of children often find no gender difference in depression, or that boys are somewhat more prone to depression than girls (Twenge & Nolen-Hoeksema, 2002). At about age 12 or 13 years, however, girls' rates of depression begin to increase sharply, whereas boys' rates remain stable or increase much less. By late adolescence, girls are twice as likely as boys to be diagnosed with unipolar depression, and score significantly higher on continuous measures of depressive symptoms (Galambos, Leadbeater, & Barker, 2004; Hankin et al., 1998). The absolute prevalence of diagnosable depression varies across the adult age span, but the gender difference remains significant (Kessler et al., 2003).

The gender difference in depression is found across racial/ethnic groups in the United States and, indeed, may be even more pronounced among black and Hispanic adults than among white adults (Blazer, Kessler, McGonagle, & Swartz, 1994; Williams et al., 2007). Among adolescents, Hispanic girls appear to be at particularly high risk for depressive symptoms. In a study of 1,065 young adolescents from a low-income community, we found that Hispanic girls had significantly higher depressive symptom scores than white or black girls, or any group of boys (McLaughlin, Hilt, & Nolen-Hoeksema, 2007).

The observed greater prevalence of depression among women compared to men may be due to women having a greater number of first onsets, longer depressive episodes, a greater recurrence of depression than men, or all of these. Data from several studies of adults (Eaton et al., 1997; Keller & Shapiro, 1981; Kessler et al., 1993) and children or adolescents (Hankin et al., 1998; Kovacs, 2001) suggest that the gender difference is primarily due to a greater number of first onsets of depression, and not to gender differences in the duration or recurrence of depression.

This suggests that factors associated with gender contribute to more women than men "crossing the line" from dysphoria into a major depressive episode, but once individuals are in an episode, factors unrelated to gender determine the duration of episodes. In his *kindling model* of depression, Post (1992) argued that major stressors trigger first onsets of depression, but then biological changes create autonomous processes that maintain depression and trigger recurrences. Several neurobiological processes appear to be state-dependent in major depression, including elevated peripheral levels of norepinephrine metabolites, increased phasic rapid eye movement (REM) sleep, poor sleep maintenance, hypercortisolism, decreased cerebral blood flow and glucose metabolism within anterior cortical structures, and increased blood flow and glucose metabolism in paralimbic regions (Thase, Jindal, & Howland, 2002). These processes may help to maintain the symptoms of depression once they begin, even if they did not trigger the symptoms initially.

In addition, Hammen (1991) argued that depression leads people to generate their own stress, which then maintains their depression. In studies of adolescents and adults, Hammen and colleagues found that depressed individuals do experience more "dependent" stressors of their own making, such as choosing less satisfying mates, failing to meet educational or career goals, and creating more interpersonal conflict (for a review, see Hammen, 2003). Unfortunately, very few studies have examined predictors of first onset of depression and predictors of the duration or recurrence of depression separately. We highlight the few that have done so as we review the literature.

Depression is highly comorbid with many other disorders, but patterns of comorbidity vary with gender. Depressed women are more likely than depressed men to have a history of anxiety disorders (Breslau, Schultz, & Peterson, 1995; Kessler, 2000). Furthermore, Kendler, Gardner, Gatz, and Pedersen (2007) found that depression and generalized anxiety disorder are more strongly genetically related to each other in women than in men. Substance abuse is also frequently comorbid with depression (Marcus et al., 2005), but women are more likely to report having developed depression before they developed an alcohol use disorder, whereas men are more likely to have developed an alcohol use disorder before they developed depression (Kessler et al., 1997; Sannibale & Hall, 2001). This suggests that substance use is more often secondary to depression in women than in men, but depression is more often secondary to substance use in men than in women.

Suicide attempts and suicide completion, which frequently occur in the context of depression, also show complex gender patterns. Women are much more likely than men to report suicide attempts (Brockington, 2001; Lewinsohn, Rohde, & Seeley, 1996). Men, however, are much more likely than women to complete suicide (Centers for Disease Control and Prevention [CDC], 2004). Men's greater rate of completed suicide may be due to the fact that they tend to choose more lethal means of suicide than do women (Canetto & Sakinofsky, 1998; Crosby, Cheltenham, & Sacks, 1999).

BIOLOGICAL EXPLANATIONS

The fact that, among adults, women are more prone to depression than men across many nations and cultures suggests that biological factors play a role in the gender difference in depression. Most biological explanations have focused on the effects of gonadal hormones, especially estradiol and progesterone, on women's moods. Recently, several studies have investigated whether women may carry a greater genetic vulnerability to depression than men.

Hormonal Explanations

Hormones have long been thought to play a role in women's depressions, because some women experience new onsets of depression, or significant exacerbation of existing depressions, during periods when levels of their gonadal hormones are undergoing substantial change, specifically, puberty, the premenstrual phase of the menstrual cycle, the postpartum period, and menopause. The literature on hormones and moods among women is vast (for detailed reviews see DeRose, Wright, & Brooks-Gunn, 2006; Korszun, Altemus, & Young, 2006; Somerset, Newport, Ragan, & Stowe, 2007). We summarize the major trends in the literatures on each of the periods of the lifecycle during which women are thought to be especially prone to depression.

Puberty

As noted earlier, the gender difference in depression does not emerge until early adolescence. Some investigators have suggested that the activation of gonadal hormone systems in puberty plays a role in the increase in rates of depression in girls. The evidence that hormonal changes play a direct role in the emergence of gender differences in depression in early adolescence is inconsistent. In a report on 1,073 U.S. children ages 9 to 13 years, depression levels in girls rose significantly in midpuberty, whereas boys' depression levels did not (Angold, Costello, & Worthman, 1998). In analyses of hormonal data from only the girls in this study, testosterone and estradiol levels better accounted for increases in depressive symptoms in the girls than did pubertal stage or age (Angold, Costello, Erklani, & Worthman, 1999). Several other studies have found no relationship between pubertal stage, or hormonal levels, and mood in girls or boys going through puberty (for reviews, see Buchanan, Eccles, & Becker, 1992; DeRose et al., 2006).

The normal hormonal changes of puberty may only trigger depression in girls with a genetic vulnerability to the disorder. In genetically vulnerable girls, normal hormonal cycling, which begins in puberty, may trigger dysregulation of neurotransmitter systems, leading to increases in depressive symptoms. If this is correct, we would not expect to see consistent relationships between hormone levels and mood in nonselected community samples of girls. Instead, only among genetically vulnerable girls should a relationship between hormones and mood be apparent.

Several researchers have found that the *timing* of puberty (compared to that of a girl's or boy's peers) rather than a specific stage of puberty is associated with risk for several types of psychopathology. Girls who go through the peak pubertal changes (e.g., menarche, weight gain, development of secondary sex characteristics) several months or more before their female peer group are more likely than girls who mature around the same time as their peer group to show depression, anxiety disorders, eating disorders, substance abuse, and delinquent symptoms (e.g., Graber, Lewinsohn, Seeley, & Brooks-Gunn, 1997; Kaltiala-Heino, Kosunen, & Rimpela, 2003; Petersen, Sarigiani, & Kennedy, 1991; Rierdan & Koff, 1991; Siegel, Yancey, Aneshensel, & Schuler, 1999; Stattin & Magnusson, 1990; Stice, Presnell, & Bearman, 2001), although other studies have found no effects of early maturation for girls (e.g., Angold et al., 1998; Paikoff, Brooks-Gunn, & Warren, 1991). For boys, it may be that late maturation is a risk factor for increases in depressive symptoms (e.g., Siegel et al., 1999), although two other studies found that both early and late perceived timing predicted higher depressive symptoms for boys (Graber et al., 1997; Kaltiala-Heino et al., 2003). The mixed findings on the effects of pubertal timing may be due to differences in measurement method (e.g., informant, retrospective recall, perceived vs. actual timing; see Dorn, Dahl, Woodward, & Biro, 2006).

The reasons for these differences in the impact of pubertal timing on girls' and boys' vulnerabilities are not entirely clear, but several investigators have suggested that the meanings associated with pubertal changes are very different for boys and girls (see Brooks-Gunn, 1988). Girls are much more likely than boys to dislike the physical changes that accompany puberty, particularly the weight gain in fat and the loss of the long–lithe, prepubescent look idealized in modern fashions (Dornbusch et al., 1984; Siegel et al., 1999). Girls who reach menarche considerably earlier than their peers (e.g., in sixth grade) are particularly dissatisfied and unhappy with their bodies (Rierdan & Koff, 1991). In turn, several studies have shown that more negative body image is associated with increased levels of depressive symptoms in girls compared to boys (Allgood-Merten, Lewinsohn, & Hops, 1990).

In addition to timing, there may be individual differences in the effects of pubertal change among adolescents regardless of timing. As Angold and Worthman (1993) note, the onset of puberty is likely to have very different personal and social meanings to a 12-year-old girl who gains considerable body fat and is teased for it compared to that of an athletic 12-year-old girl who gains useful muscle mass as a result of puberty. Similarly, cultures view pubertal changes differently, so the meaning of these changes to European American, Latina, and African American adolescents may be different (Smolak & Striegel-Moore, 2001). In fact, in one study, pubertal status was a better predictor of depressive symptoms than age among European American adolescents, but not among Hispanic or African American adolescents (Hayward, Gotlib, Schraedley, & Little, 1999).

The Premenstrual Phase of the Menstrual Cycle

The fourth edition of the *Diagnostic and Statistical Manual of Mental Disorders* (DSM-IV), defines *premenstrual dysphoric disorder* (PMDD) as the presence, during most menstrual cycles in the last year, of five or more symptoms representing a significant mood disturbance, which emerge during the last week of the luteal phase of the menstrual cycle and begin to remit a few days after the onset of menses. Although many women self-report that they have mild-to-moderate physical symptoms (e.g., bloating and breast tenderness) during the premenstrual phase of the menstrual cycle, many fewer women (approximately 3–8%) have symptoms meeting the criteria for PMDD (see Somerset et al., 2007).

Evidence that PMDD is heritable (Chang, Holroyd, & Chau, 1995) and that premenstrual complaints can be eliminated with suppression of ovarian activity or surgical menopause (Casper & Hearn 1990) suggests that the disorder has biological roots. For years investigators searched for hormonal imbalances in women with PMDD, with few consistently positive findings (Somerset et al., 2007; Steiner & Born, 2000). The current consensus in the field is that normal hormonal fluctuations trigger biochemical events within the central nervous system and other target tissues that unleash premenstrual symptoms in vulnerable women (Steiner, Dunn, & Born, 2003). In particular, serotonin systems may be dysregulated by normal hormonal changes in vulnerable women, leading to changes in their moods. The selective serotonin reuptake inhibitors (SSRIs) are effective in treating premenstrual symptoms, even when the drugs are taken only around the premenstrual phase (Steiner & Born, 2000).

The Postpartum Phase

Over half of all women experience the postpartum blues (dysphoria, mood lability, crying, anxiety, insomnia, poor appetite, and irritability) in the first few weeks after giving birth. Although annoying and sometimes confusing, these symptoms are usually not debilitating and typically subside within 2–3 weeks postpartum. *Postpartum depression* is the term used for an episode of major depression that occurs within the first several weeks after giving birth. Major depression with postpartum onset can be very debilitating and, if not treated, can linger for months or more (Flynn, 2005).

A meta-analysis of studies of postpartum depression found that 13% of women experience a depressive episode severe enough to qualify for a diagnosis of major depression in the first few weeks after giving birth, a rate not significantly higher than the approximately 12% of nonpostpartum women who are depressed in the same time period (O'Hara & Swain, 1996). A very large Danish study, however, found that postpartum women were at increased risk for depression compared to women who were not in the postpartum period (Munk-Olsen, Laursen, Pedersen, Mors, & Mortensen, 2006). The researchers compared 1,117,804 adults who had become new parents during a designated period to over 1 million adults who had not become parents during the same period on rates of hospital admissions or outpatient visits for mental disorders. New mothers had a much higher risk of unipolar depressive disorders in the first 5 months after birth, and of any mental disorder in the first 3 months, compared to women who were not new mothers. Interestingly, men had a lower risk of mental disorders if they were new fathers (although see Goodman, 2004, for evidence that men experience postpartum depression). Thus, it appears that motherhood can trigger episodes of not only depression but also other mental disorders.

Since the onset of major depression during the postpartum phase coincides with large changes in levels of estrogen, progesterone, and several other hormones, these changes have been thought to play a causal role (Steiner & Dunn, 1996). Studies comparing women with and without postpartum depression have failed to find consistent hormonal differences, however (Somerset et al., 2007). Family-history studies show that women with postpartum depression often have a family history of depression (Steiner & Tam, 1999). These women also tend to have a personal history of depression prior to becoming pregnant or are depressed during pregnancy (O'Hara & Swain, 1996). Thus, it may be primarily women who carry some underlying vulnerability to depression who tend to develop postpartum depressions.

Menopause

Perimenopause is the period immediately before menopause, from the time when the hormonal and clinical features of approaching menopause begin until the end of the first year after menopause. During menopause, estrogen levels decline gradually. Symptoms associated with this decline include hot flashes, night sweats, and vaginal dryness. The 1996 Cross-National Study demonstrated an increase in the onset of depression in women ages 45 to 49 (Weissman, 1996). Because this is around the age of perimenopause for many women, this increase may be attributable to the biological changes of perimenopause. Some studies comparing women known to be in perimenopause or menopause to women who are not undergoing these biological changes have found that perimenopausal or menopausal women have higher levels of depressive symptoms or general negative mood (Avis, Brambilla, McKinlay, & Vass, 1994; Bromberger et al., 2001). Most studies, including longitudinal ones that follow the same women as they transition into perimenopause and menopause, do not find an association between menopausal status and depression (e.g., Avis et al., 1994; Matthews, 1992; Matthews et al., 1990; see review by Avis, 2003).

Summary

The hormonal changes of puberty, the menstrual cycle, the postpartum period, and menopause may only trigger depression in women with a genetic or other biological vulnerability to the disorder (Steiner et al., 2003; Young & Korszun, 1999). There are multiple, complex relationships between gonadal hormones and the neurotransmitters that regulate mood, including serotonin. Estrogens, in specific, have profound effects on serotonergic function, from modulating pre- and postsynaptic serotonin receptors and serotonin reuptake to enhancing and diminishing serotonin synthesis and catabolism, respectively (Amin, Canli, & Epperson, 2005; Steiner et al., 2003). In vulnerable women, normal hormonal cycling may trigger dysregulation of neurotransmitter systems, leading to increases in depressive symptoms.

Genetic Factors

Family-history studies clearly show that depression runs in families, particularly among female members (MacKinnon, Jamison, & DePaulo, 1997). Several studies show greater genetic effects of major depression among females than among males (Bierut et al., 1999; Boomsma et al., 2000; Happonen et al., 2002; Jacobson & Rowe, 1999; Jansson et al., 2004; Kendler, Gatz, Gardner, & Pedersen, 2006; Scourfield et al., 2003; Silberg et al., 1999; van der Valk, van den Oord, Verhulst, & Boomsma, 2003). Other studies find greater genetic effects in males than in females (Rice, Harold, & Thapar, 2002), or no sex differences in genetic effects (Bartels et al., 2003; Eaves et al., 1997; Gjone & Stevenson, 1997; Hewitt, Silberg, Neale, Eaves, & Erickson, 1992; Kendler & Prescott, 1999; Lau, Eley, & Rijsdijk, 2006; Rutter, Silberg, O'Connor, & Simonoff, 1999; Thapar & McGuffin, 1994; van der Valk et al., 2003). Unfortunately, the discrepancies in findings are not easily attributable to the age of the participants or the methods of studies (Lau & Eley, in press). Thus, there is at best mixed evidence that women's greater vulnerability to depression is genetically based. It may be that women have a greater genetic vulnerability to certain risk factors for depression (e.g., experiencing stressful life events) rather than a greater genetic vulnerability to depression per se (e.g., Silberg et al., 1999).

PSYCHOLOGICAL EXPLANATIONS

As with the biological explanations, psychological explanations for the gender difference in depression have evolved over the last few decades. Early psychoanalytic explanations attributed women's excessive vulnerability to depression to masochism and psychological dependency (Deutsch, 1944). In the 1960s and 1970s, women were said to be more vulnerable to depression because they had low self-esteem and tended to make self-defeating attributions (Dweck & Gilliard, 1975; Radloff, 1975). New perspectives on gender role development, introduced by authors such as Gilligan (1982) and Chodorow (1978), led to theories that girls were silenced during their adolescent years as they were socialized to play subservient roles to male partners and to focus their attention solely on becoming a good wife and mother (Chevron, Quinlan, & Blatt, 1978; Helgeson, 1994; Hill & Lynch, 1983; Jack, 1991). Across several decades, a theme in the psychological literature has been that women are less assertive than men and more prone to helplessness, which contributes to their higher rates of depression (see Nolen-Hoeksema, 1990; Radloff, 1975).

A review of the literatures on all these psychological variables is beyond the scope of this chapter (see Nolen-Hoeksema [1990] and Nolen-Hoeksema & Girgus [1994] for more detailed reviews). Instead, we focus on two psychological variables that in the last several years have been studied extensively in relation to the gender difference in depression: interpersonal orientation and rumination.

Interpersonal Orientation

One of the most consistent psychological differences between women and men is in interpersonal orientation (Feingold, 1994). Women are more likely than men to feel strong emotional ties with a wide range of people in their lives, to see their roles vis-à-vis others (i.e., mother, daughter, wife/partner) as central to their self-concepts, to care what others think of them, and to be emotionally affected by events in the lives of other people.

An interpersonal orientation leads women to develop strong social support networks that can buffer them against adversity. Some women, however, cross a line from an interpersonal orientation to an excessive concern about their relationships with others, which leads them to silence their own wants and needs in favor of maintaining a positive emotional tone in the relationships, and to feel too responsible for the quality of the relationship (Helgeson, 1994; Jack, 1991). This leads these women to have less power and to obtain less benefit from relationships. Women do score higher than men on measures of excessive concern with relationships, and high scores on these measures have been correlated with depression (Helgeson & Fritz, 1996; Nolen-Hoeksema & Jackson, 2001). Similarly, studies of children and adolescents find that girls score higher than boys on need for social approval, reassurance seeking, and social-evaluative concerns, and high scorers on these measures are more prone to develop symptoms of depression (Little & Garber, 2005; Prinstein, Borelli, Cheah, Simon, & Aikins, 2005; Rudolph, Caldwell, & Conley, 2004; Rudolph & Conley, 2005). For example, Rudolph and Conley (2005) found that social-evaluative concerns fully mediated the gender difference in depression in a group of adolescents. Thus, women may be more likely than men to overvalue relationships as sources of self-worth, which interpersonal theories of depression have identified as a risk factor for depression (e.g., Barnett & Gotlib, 1988; Joiner & Coyne, 1999).

Rumination

Rumination is the tendency to focus on one's symptoms of distress, and the possible causes and consequences of these symptoms, in a repetitive and passive manner rather than in an active, problem-solving manner (Nolen-Hoeksema, 1991; Nolen-Hoeksema, Wisco, &

Lyubomirsky, in press). When people ruminate, they have thoughts such as "Why am I so unmotivated? I just can't get going. I'm never going to get my work done feeling this way." Although some rumination may be a natural response to distress and depression, there are stable individual differences in the tendency to ruminate (Nolen-Hoeksema & Davis, 1999). People who ruminate a great deal in response to their sad or depressed moods have longer periods of depressive symptoms and are more likely to be diagnosed with MDD (Nolen-Hoeksema, 2000). The effects of rumination on depression over time remain significant even after researchers control for baseline levels of depression.

Women are more likely than men to ruminate in response to sad, depressed, or anxious moods (Nolen-Hoeksema & Jackson, 2001; Nolen-Hoeksema, Larson, & Grayson, 1999). The gender difference in rumination is found both in self-report survey and interview studies, and in laboratory studies in which women's and men's responses to sad moods are observed (Butler & Nolen-Hoeksema, 1994). In turn, when researchers control statistically for gender differences in rumination, the gender difference in depression becomes nonsignificant, suggesting that rumination helps to account for the gender difference in depression (Nolen-Hoeksema et al., 1999).

We noted earlier that the gender difference in depression is found for onsets but not in the duration of episodes. Interestingly, several researchers have found that rumination predicts new onsets of major depression but does not predict the duration of episodes of major depression (see the review in Nolen-Hoeksema et al., in press). Although this contradicts the original formulation of the rumination model (Nolen-Hoeksema, 1991), it parallels the findings that women have more onsets but not longer episodes of depression than men. Thus, a greater tendency to ruminate may lead more women than men to cross the line from dysphoria to major depression, but once a woman (or a man) has crossed that line, other processes may influence the duration of episodes.

SOCIAL EXPLANATIONS

The social explanations for women's greater rates of depression compared to men's have focused on negative events and conditions that women face more often than men. Some of these events and conditions are tied to women's social roles, others are independent of these roles, and still others may emerge from women's greater interpersonal orientation.

Traumatic Events

The traumatic events most consistently linked to women's high rates of depression are physical and sexual abuse (for a review, see Weiss, Longhurst, & Mazure, 1999). As many as 1 woman in 3 globally has been beaten, coerced into sex, or otherwise abused in her lifetime (Heise, Ellsburg, & Gottemuller, 1999). Large, nationally representative studies of rape suggest that about 13–15% of women are the victims of completed rape at some time in their lives (Kilpatrick, Edmunds, & Seymour, 1992; Kilpatrick & Saunders, 1996; Koss, Gidycz, & Wisniewski, 1987; Tjaden & Thoennes, 1998). Men are the victims of sexual and physical abuse as well, but women represent 85% of the victims of the nonfatal intimate assaults that occur in the United States each year (Greenfield et al., 1998).

Sexual and physical assault have been linked both retrospectively and prospectively to depression. For example, the National Women's Study (NWS; Saunders, Kilpatrick, Hanson, Resnick, & Walker, 1999) found that women who had been the victims of completed rape in childhood had a lifetime prevalence of depression of 52% compared to 27% in nonvictimized women. Similarly, the Epidemiologic Catchment Area (ECA) study found that rape during childhood or adulthood increased a woman's risk of depression by 2.4 (Burnam et al., 1988).

Childhood sexual assault appears to be an especially potent predictor of depression, both during childhood and continuing into adulthood (e.g., Kendler, Kuhn, & Prescott, 2004). Girls are much more likely to be the victims of childhood sexual assault than boys (Laumann, Gagnon, Michael, & Michaels, 1994). In fact, one review estimated that 35% of the gender difference in adult depression could be attributed to the higher rate of childhood sexual assault experienced by girls (Cutler & Nolen-Hoeksema, 1991). Although most of the studies in this area are retrospective, one recent prospective study of several hundred children and matched controls followed through early adulthood found that child abuse predicted current and lifetime MDD (Widom, DuMont, & Czaja, 2007); furthermore, this study found that abused children had earlier onset of MDD compared to controls. Thus, the higher rate of child sexual abuse may place women at increased risk for depression.

Childhood Adversity

There are, unfortunately, many other adversities children can suffer in addition to abuse, including parental separation or loss, neglect, and poverty. Early childhood adversity is a risk factor for depression, perhaps particularly in girls and women (Daley, Hammen, & Rao, 2000). For example, Rudolph and Flynn (2007) found that early childhood adversity sensitized pubertal girls, but not pubertal boys, to subsequent stress, increasing their risk for depressive symptoms.

Children whose mothers are frequently depressed are exposed to a variety of adversities, including separation from the mother, increased family conflict, and disruptions in daily routines (Goodman, 2007). Children of depressed mothers are at increased risk for many forms of psychopathology, including depression. Girls appear to be more affected than boys by maternal depression, and more generally, family discord and disruption (Downey & Coyne, 1990; Goodman, Brogan, Lynch, & Fielding, 1993; Hops, Sherman, & Biglan, 1990).

Recall that women show more first onsets of depression but not necessarily more persistence or duration of depression. Daley and colleagues (2000) found that childhood adversity, including family violence, predicts first onsets of depression in women in their early adult years but not recurrence of depression. Thus, childhood adversity may set the stage for a girl or woman eventually to develop depression; then, other factors come into play to determine the duration and recurrence of her depression.

Interpersonal Stress

Women's greater interpersonal orientation may create more interpersonal stress in their lives, leading to more depression (Hammen, 2003). Having many people to whom one feels emotionally close may increase the chance that tragedy will befall one of these people and have a negative emotional impact on one's own well-being, a hypothesis that Kessler, McLeod, and Wetherington (1985) term *the cost of caring*. Kessler and McLeod (1984) found that women reported a greater number of negative events occurring among people in their social network than did men, presumably because this network was larger for women than men. Adolescent girls also report more interpersonal stressors than do boys (e.g., Ge,

Lorenz, Conger, Elder, & Simons, 1994; Rudolph & Hammen, 1999; Shih, Eberhart, Hammen, & Brennan, 2006). In one study, girls' higher rate of interpersonal stressors partially accounted for the gender difference in subjective distress (Liu & Kaplan, 1999), and in another study, the higher levels of stress experienced by girls was largely due to their higher levels of interpersonal stressors (Shih et al., 2006).

Chronic interpersonal stress often comes in the form of discord with one's partner. In intimate heterosexual relationships, some women face inequities in the distribution of power over making important decisions, such as the decision to move to a new city, or how to spend the family's income (Nolen-Hoeksema et al., 1999). Even when they voice their opinions, women may feel these opinions are not taken seriously, or that their viewpoints on important issues are not respected and affirmed by their partners. Nolen-Hoeksema and colleagues (1999) grouped inequities in workload and in heterosexual relationships under a variable labeled *chronic strain*, and showed that chronic strain predicted increases in depression over time and partially mediated the gender difference in depression.

Hammen and colleagues (e.g., Daley et al., 2000) have differentiated between this type of chronic interpersonal strain and episodic interpersonal stress (e.g., the breakup of a relationship, a close friend moves away). In studies of young adult women, they find that whereas chronic interpersonal stress predicts first onsets, but not recurrence, of depression, episodic interpersonal stress predicts both first onsets and recurrence of depression.

Women's interpersonal orientation also appears to make them more sensitive to interpersonal stressors when they occur. Adult women, more than adult men, report that interpersonal stressors impact their well-being (Leadbeater, Blatt, & Quinlan, 1995). Similarly, in a study of pubertal girls and boys, Rudolph and Flynn (2007) found that interpersonal stressors were more likely to lead to depression in the girls than in the boys (see also Ge et al., 1994).

Some of the excess interpersonal stressors women experience may be created by themselves. Hammen's (1991) model of stress generation conceptualizes certain stressors as dependent (i.e., contributed to, in part or in whole, by the individual), and Hammen finds that women are more likely than men to experience dependent stressors. Women who overvalue relationships may seek reassurance to an extent that is excessive and annoys others (Joiner, Metalsky, Katz, & Beach, 1999). This can lead to rejection by others, or at least conflict in relationships, which then only feeds a woman's worries about the status of the relationships. Adolescent girls are more likely to report dependent stressors (especially within the interpersonal domain; e.g., peer conflict) compared to adolescent boys (Rudolph & Hammen, 1999; Shih et al., 2006). Furthermore, Shih and colleagues (2006) found that dependent interpersonal stress mediated the gender difference in adolescent depression. There was also evidence in this study of higher stress reactivity among the adolescent girls, who were more likely than adolescent boys to become depressed when experiencing stressful life events.

AN INTEGRATIVE MODEL

Although each of the factors we discuss in this chapter could independently might contribute to women's higher rates of depression compared to men, these factors likely interact in complex ways to produce depression in women. The major stressors that are more common in women's than in men's lives, particularly early abuse experiences, could contribute to a greater reactivity to stress in women compared to men. Studies of survivors of child sexual abuse show that, even as adults, they have a more poorly regulated biological response to stress, as measured by cortisol levels, adrenocorticotropic hormone levels, and cardiac measures, compared to people who did not suffer child sexual abuse (Heim et al., 2000; Zahn-Waxler, 2000). In turn, this greater biological reactivity is associated with a greater adult prevalence of major depression. On the other hand, women who have more poorly regulated biological responses to stress find it more difficult to engage in efficacious behavioral responses to new stressors, raising the likelihood that they will experience chronic and frequent stressors.

The stresses in women's lives also may contribute to a greater psychological reactivity to stress. For example, people who have a history of sexual abuse are more likely to engage in rumination, perhaps because they remain hypervigilant for new threats (Nolen-Hoeksema, 1998). In addition, women who face chronic stressors because of inequities in their heterosexual relationships become more ruminative over time (Nolen-Hoeksema et al., 1999). In turn, rumination impairs problem solving, increasing the likelihood of new stressors.

Depression has its own effects on biological and psychological stress reactivity. Depression may increase biological reactivity to stress by sensitizing the neurotransmitter and neuroendocrine systems linked to depression (Post, 1992; Post & Weiss, 1995). In turn, this lowers the threshold for new depressive episodes, so that milder and milder stressors can trigger a new episode. Depression may also increase the tendency to ruminate by activating and strengthening associative networks of negative cognitions (Teasdale, 1988). With each new depressive episode, these networks are more interconnected and more easily primed, increasing the probability of rumination.

Depression also appears to increase the social stress in individuals' lives. Depressed women are even more likely than nondepressed women to generate interpersonal stress in their lives (Hammen, 1991). For example, depressed women have lower quality interactions and communications with their children, even though they may fervently desire to be good mothers. The problems these women show in parenting may be a direct result of their symptoms of depression, such as irritability, apathy, and poor concentration. The children of depressed mothers are often themselves distressed, oppositional, and critical, and trigger or exacerbate irritability and criticality in their mothers (Hammen, Burge, & Adrian, 1991).

Depression is also often associated with dysfunctional marital or romantic relationships (see Downey & Coyne, 1990; Gotlib & Beach, 1995), some of which are a consequence of depression. Depression elicits discomfort and rejection from others (Joiner & Coyne, 1999). In addition, depressed women often marry men with psychopathology (Hammen, Rudoph, Weisz, Rao, & Burge, 1999). Even in teenage years, depressed adolescent women have more stressful romantic relationships, including more experiences of physical and psychological coercion in romantic relationships, and are more likely to pair with adolescent boys with symptoms of personality disorders (Rao, Hammen, & Daley, 1999). Thus, depression may contribute to poor interpersonal skills and choices, increasing a woman's vulnerability to interpersonal stressors.

As noted, girls appear to be even more sensitive than boys to family discord and other consequences of their mothers' depressions. Thus, the rate of intergenerational transmission of depression from mother to daughter may be very high for psychosocial, if not genetic, reasons; that is, depression in mothers creates chronic and episodic interpersonal stress in the lives of their children, but daughters are more affected by this stress than are sons. Maternal depression creates early adversity that sensitizes daughters to the experience of stressors as they grow older.

The complex interrelationships among stress, stress reactivity, and depression call for comprehensive interventions that address the variety of problems a depressed woman might face in overcoming her depression and preventing new depressions. Simply relieving her depressive symptoms, for example, through medication, is unlikely to break the negative interpersonal and cognitive cycles that maintain depression and keep a woman at risk for new episodes of depression.

FUTURE DIRECTIONS FOR RESEARCH

A number of the risk factors for depression identified in this chapter require further research before conclusions can be drawn about their contributions to the gender difference in depression. First, it is unlikely that direct effects of genetic or hormonal factors on women's depression will be found, but there may be complex interactions between genetic predispositions and normative hormonal change that help to account for women's excessive rates of depression. More research investigating these interactive effects is needed. Second, the long history of theory on women's interpersonal orientation as a contributor to their vulnerability to depression, and recent evidence favoring these theories, makes this an important target for future research. This research should use both longitudinal and experimental designs to try to establish the predictive and causal relationships between excessive interpersonal orientation and depression.

Third, a critical focus for new research is the emergence of gender differences in depression in adolescence. Many questions remain to be answered. What is the time course for the emergence of this gender difference in different ethnic and cultural groups, and why does the time course differ across these groups? Is it only girls with preadolescent risk factors for depression who become depressed in adolescence, or do many girls develop depression in adolescence with no preexisting risk factors? What are the critical biological, psychological, and social contributors to the increase in depression in girls in adolescence? How do these variables interact with one another over time? All of the risk factors for depression discussed in this chapter may show increases in prevalence in early adolescence, or may interact with the many changes of adolescence, leading girls to be more vulnerable to depression. For example, a genetic vulnerability to depression, or more broadly to neurotransmitter or hypothalamic–pituitary–adrenal (HPA) axis dysregulation, may be triggered by the hormonal changes of puberty in girls. An excessive interpersonal orientation or a tendency to ruminate may interact with changes at puberty, such as the beginning of romantic dating, to contribute to depression in some girls. Some social risk factors for depression in girls, especially sexual abuse, increase in prevalence at puberty. Understanding the emergence of gender differences in depression in adolescence will be crucial to the design of effective prevention and intervention programs for adolescent girls.

Finally, the evidence that women have more first onsets of depression, but not longer or more recurrent depressions, has largely been ignored by researchers of gender differences in depression. Yet most of the theories of why women are more vulnerable to depression than men imply that they should have longer and more recurrent depressions, as well as more first onsets. If this set of epidemiological trends continues to be supported by future research, it will be important to understand why this pattern of results is found. We noted in our integrative model that many biological, psychological, and interpersonal processes are changed or exacerbated by depression. These processes may then perpetuate depression, even if they were not the cause of the onset of depression. It will be critical for future research to determine what processes make depression self-perpetuating once it begins, and to focus new interventions on these processes.

What is clear from the existing literature on the gender differences in depression is that no single factor is likely to explain these differences. Instead, the differences may be overdetermined by a confluence of social, psychological, and biological differences between women and men.

REFERENCES

Allgood-Merten, B., Lewinsohn, P. M., & Hops, H. (1990). Sex differences and adolescent depression. *Journal of Abnormal Psychology, 99,* 55–63.

Amin, Z., Canli, T., & Epperson, C. N. (2005). Effect of estrogen–serotonin interactions on mood and cognition. *Behavioral and Cognitive Neuroscience Reviews, 4,* 43–58.

Andrade, L., Caraveo-Anduaga, J. J., Berglund, P., Bijl, R. V., DeGraaf, R., Volbergh, W., et al. (2003). The epidemiology of major depressive episodes: Results from the International Consortium of Psychiatric Epidemiology (ICPE) surveys. *International Journal of Methods in Psychiatric Research, 12,* 3–21.

Angold, A., Costello, E. J., Erkanli, A., & Worthman, C. M. (1999). Pubertal changes in hormones of adolescent girls. *Psychological Medicine, 29,* 1043–1053.

Angold, A., Costello, E. J., & Worthman, C. M. (1998). Puberty and depression: The roles of age, pubertal status and pubertal timing. *Psychological Medicine, 28,* 51–61.

Angold, A., & Worthman, C. W. (1993). Puberty onset of gender differences in rates of depression: A developmental, epidemiological, and neuroendorcrine perspective. *Journal of Affective Disorders, 29,* 145–158.

Avis, N. E. (2003). Depression during the menopausal transition. *Psychology of Women Quarterly, 27,* 91–100.

Avis, N. E., Brambilla, D., McKinlay, S., & Vass, K. (1994). A longitudinal analysis of the association between menopause and depression: Results from the Massachusetts Women's Health Study. *Annals of Epidemiology, 4,* 214–220.

Barnett, P. A., & Gotlib, I. H. (1988). Psychosocial functioning and depression: Distinguishing among antecedents, concomitants, and consequences. *Psychological Bulletin, 104*(1), 97–126.

Bartels, M., Hudziak, J. J., Boomsma, D. I., Rietveld, M. J., Van Beijsterveldt, T. C., & van den Oord, E. J. (2003). A study of parent ratings of internalizing and externalizing problem behavior in 12-year-old twins. *Journal of the American Academy of Child and Adolescent Psychiatry, 42,* 1351–1359.

Bierut, L. J., Heath, A. C., Bucholz, K. K., Dinwiddie, S. H., Madden, P. A. F., Statham, D. J., et al. (1999). Major depressive disorder in a community-based twin sample: Are there different genetic and environmental contributions for men and women? *Archives of General Psychiatry, 57,* 557–563.

Blazer, D. G., Kessler, R. C., McGonagle, K. A., & Swartz, M. S. (1994). The prevalence and distribution of major depression in a national community sample: The National Comorbidity Survey. *American Journal of Psychiatry, 151,* 979–986.

Boomsma, D. I., Beem, A. L., van den Berg, M., Dolan, C. V., Koopmans, J. R., Vink, J. M., et al. (2000). Netherlands twin family study of anxious depression (NETSAD). *Twin Research, 3,* 323–334.

Breslau, N., Schultz, L., & Peterson, E. (1995). Sex differences in depression: A role for preexisting anxiety. *Psychiatry Research, 58,* 1–12.

Brockington, I. (2001). Suicide in women. *International Clinical Psychopharmacology, 16*(Suppl. 12), 7–19.

Bromberger, J. T., Meyer, P. M., Kravitz, H. M., Sommer, B., Cordal, A., Powell, L., et al. (2001). Dysphoric mood and natural menopause: A multi-ethnic community study. *American Journal of Public Health, 91,* 1435–1442.

Brooks-Gunn, J. (1988). Antecedents and consequences of variations in girls maturational timing. *Journal of Adolescent Health Care, 9,* 365–373.

Buchanan, C. M., Eccles, J. S., & Becker, J. B. (1992). Are adolescents the victims of raging hormones: Evidence for activational effects of hormones on moods and behavior at adolescence. *Psychological Bulletin, 111,* 62–107.

Burnam, M. A., Stein, J. A., Golding, J. M., Siegel, J. M., Sorensen, S. B., Forsythe, A. B., et al. (1988). Sexual assault and mental disorders in a community population. *Journal of Consulting and Clinical Psychology*, *56*, 843–850.

Butler, L. D., & Nolen-Hoeksema, S. (1994). Gender differences in responses to a depressed mood in a college sample. *Sex Roles*, *30*, 331–346.

Canetto, S. S., & Sakinofsky, I. (1998). The gender paradox in suicide. *Suicide and Life-Threatening Behavior*, *28*, 1–23.

Casper, R. F., & Hearn, M. T. (1990). The effect of hysterectomy and bilateral oophorectomy in women with severe premenstrual syndrome. *American Journal of Obstetrics and Gynecology*, *162*, 105–109.

Centers for Disease Control and Prevention (CDC), National Center for Injury Prevention and Control. (2004). Web-based injury statistics query and reporting system. Retrieved on September 1, 2007, from *www.cdc.gov/ncipc/wisquars/default.htm*

Chang, A. M., Holroyd, E., & Chau, J. P. C. (1995). Premenstrual syndrome in employed Chinese women in Hong Kong. *Health Care for Women International*, *16*, 551–561.

Chevron, E. S., Quinlan, D. M., & Blatt, S. J. (1978). Sex roles and gender differences in the expression of depression. *Journal of Abnormal Psychology*, *87*, 680–683.

Chodorow, N. (1978). *The reproduction of mothering*. Berkeley: University of California Press.

Crosby, A. E., Cheltenham, M. P., & Sacks, J. J. (1999). Incidence of suicidal ideation and behavior I the United States, 1994. *Suicide and Life-Threatening Behavior*, *29*, 131–140.

Cutler, S. E., & Nolen-Hoeksema, S. (1991). Accounting for sex differences in depression through female victimization: Childhood sexual abuse. *Sex Roles*, *24*, 425–438.

Daley, S. E., Hammen, C., & Rao, U. (2000). Predictors of first onset and recurrence of major depression in young women during the 5 years following high school graduation. *Journal of Abnormal Psychology*, *109*, 525–533.

DeRose, L. M., Wright, A. J., & Brooks-Gunn, J. (2006). Does puberty account for the gender differential in depression? In C. L. M. Keyes & S. H. Goodman (Eds.), *Women and depression* (pp. 89–128). New York: Cambridge University Press.

Deutsch, H. (1944). *The psychology of women*. New York: Grune & Stratton.

Dorn, L. D., Dahl, R. E., Woodward, H. R., & Biro, F. (2006). Defining the boundaries of early adolescence: A user's guide to assessing pubertal status and pubertal timing in research with adolescents. *Applied Developmental Science*, *10*, 30–56.

Dornbusch, S. M., Carlsmith, J. M., Duncan, P. D., Gross, R. T., Martin, J. A., Ritter, P. L., et al. (1984). Sexual maturation, social class, and the desire to be thin among adolescent females. *Developmental and Behavioral Pediatrics*, *5*, 308–314.

Downey, G., & Coyne, J. C. (1990). Children of depressed parents: An integrative review. *Psychological Bulletin*, *108*, 50–76.

Dweck, C. S., & Gilliard, D. (1975). Expectancy statements as determinants of reactions to failure: Sex differences in persistence and expectancy change. *Journal of Personality and Social Psychology*, *32*, 1077–1084.

Eaton, W., Anthony, J., Gallo, J., Cai, G., Tien, A., Romanoski, A., et al. (1997). Natural history of Diagnostic Interview Schedule/DSM-IV major depression. *Archives of General Psychiatry*, *54*, 993–999.

Eaves, L. J., Silberg, J. L., Meyer, J. M., Maes, H. H., Simonoff, E., Pickles, A., et al. (1997). Genetics and developmental psychopathology: 2. The main effects of genes and environment on behavioral problems in the Virginia Twin Study of Adolescent Behavioral Development. *Journal of Child Psychology and Psychiatry*, *38*, 965–980.

Eckenrode, J., & Gore, S. (1981). Stressful live events and social supports: The significance of context. In B. H. Gottlieb (Ed.), *Social networks and social support*. Beverly Hills, CA: Sage.

Feingold, A. (1994). Gender differences in personality: A meta-analysis. *Psychological Bulletin*, *116*, 429–456.

Flynn, H. A. (2005). Epidemiology and phenomenology of postpartum mood disorders. *Psychiatric Annals*, *35*, 522–551.

Galambos, N. L., Leadbeater, B. J., & Barker, E. T. (2004). Gender differences in and risk factors for depression in adolescent: A 4-year longitudinal study. *International Journal of Behavior Development*, *28*, 16–25.

Ge, X., Lorenz, F. O., Conger, R. D., Elder, G. H., & Simons, R. L. (1994). Trajectories of stressful life events and depressive symptoms during adolescence. *Developmental Psychology, 30*, 467–483.

Gilligan, C. (1982). *In a different voice: Psychological theory and women's development.* Cambridge, MA: Harvard University Press.

Gjone, H., & Stevenson, J. (1997). The association between internalizing and externalizing behaviour in childhood and early adolescence: Genetic or environmental common influences. *Journal of Abnormal Child Psychology, 54*, 277–286.

Goodman, J. H. (2004). Parental postpartum depression, its relationship to maternal postpartum depression, and implications for family health. *Journal of Advanced Nursing, 45*, 26–35.

Goodman, S. H. (2007). Depression in mothers. *Annual Review of Clinical Psychology, 3*, 107–135.

Goodman, S. H., Brogan, D., Lynch, M. E., & Fielding, B. (1993). Social and emotional competence in children of depressed mothers. *Child Development, 64*, 516–531.

Gotlib, I., & Beach, S. (1995). A marital/family discord model of depression: Implications for therapeutic intervention. In N. S. Jacobson & A. S. Gurman (Eds.), *Clinical handbook of couple therapy* (pp. 411–436). New York: Guilford Press.

Graber, J. A., Lewinsohn, P. M., Seeley, J. R., & Brooks-Gunn, J. (1997). Is psychopathology associated with the timing of pubertal development? *Journal of the American Academy of Child Adolescent Psychiatry, 36*, 1768–1776.

Greenfield, L. A., Rand, M. R., Craven, D., Klaus, P. A., Perkins, C. A., et al. (1998). *Violence by intimates: Analysis of data on crimes by current or former spouses, boyfriends, and girlfriends* (NCJ-167237). Washington, DC: U.S. Department of Justice.

Hammen, C. (2003). Social stress and women's risk for recurrent depression. *Archives of Women's Mental Health, 6*, 9–13.

Hammen, C., Burge, D., & Adrian, C. (1991). Timing of mother and child depression in a longitudinal study of children at risk. *Journal of Consulting and Clinical Psychology, 59*, 341–345.

Hammen, C., Rudolph, K., Weisz, J., Rao, U., & Burge, D. (1999). The context of depression in clinic-referred youth: Neglected areas in treatment. *Journal of the American Academy of Child and Adolescent Psychiatry, 38*, 64–71.

Hammen, C. L. (1991). *Depression runs in families: The social context of risk and resilience in children of depressed mothers.* New York: Springer-Verlag.

Hankin, B. L., Abramson, L. Y., Moffitt, T. E., McGee, R., Silva, P., & Angell, K. E. (1998). Development of depression from preadolescence to young adulthood: Emerging gender differences in a 10-year longitudinal study. *Journal of Abnormal Psychology, 107*, 128–140.

Happonen, M., Pulkkinen, L., Kaprio, J., Van der Meere, M. J., Viken, R. J., & Rose, R. J. (2002). The heritability of depressive symptoms: Multiple informants and multiple measures. *Journal of Child Psychology and Psychiatry, 43*, 471–479.

Hayward, C., Gotlib, I. H., Schraedley, P. K., & Little, I. F. (1999). Ethnic differences in the association between pubertal status and symptoms of depression in adolescent girls. *Journal of Adolescent Health, 25*, 143–149.

Heim, C., Newport, J., Heit, S., Graham, Y., Wilcox, M., Bonsall, R., et al. (2000). Pituitary–adrenal and autonomic responses to stress in women after sexual and physical abuse in childhood. *Journal of the American Medical Association, 284*, 592–596.

Heise, L., Ellsberg, M., & Gottenmuller, M. (1999). Ending violence against women. *Population Reports, 11*(Series L), 1–43.

Helgeson, V. (1994). Relation of agency and communion to well-being: Evidence and potential explanations. *Psychological Bulletin, 116*, 412–428.

Helgeson, V., & Fritz, H. (1996). Implications of communion and unmitigated communion for adolescent adjustment to Type I diabetes. *Women's Health: Research on Gender, Behavior, and Policy, 2*, 169–194.

Hewitt, J. K., Silberg, J. L., Neale, M. C., Eaves, L. J., & Erickson, M. (1992). The analysis of parental ratings of children's behavior using LISREL. *Behavior Genetics, 22*, 293–317.

Hill, J. P., & Lynch, M. E. (1983). The intensification of gender-related role expectations during early adolescence. In J. Brooks-Gunn & A. C. Petersen (Eds.), *Girls at puberty* (pp. 201–228). New York: Plenum Press.

Hops, H., Sherman, L., & Biglan, A. (1990). Maternal depression, marital discord, and children's behavior: A developmental perspective. In Gerald R. Patterson (Ed.), *Depression and aggression in family interaction* (pp. 185–208). Hillsdale, NJ: Erlbaum.

Jack, D. C. (1991). *Silencing the self: Women and depression.* New York: HarperPerennial.

Jacobson, K. C., & Rowe, D. C. (1999). Genetic and environmental influences on the relationships between family connectedness, school connectedness, and adolescent depressed mood: Sex differences. *Developmental Psychology, 35,* 926–939.

Jansson, M., Gatz, M., Berg, S., Johansson, B., Malberg, B., McClearn, G. E., et al. (2004). Gender differences in the heritability of depressive symptoms in the elderly. *Psychological Medicine, 34,* 471–479.

Joiner, T., & Coyne, J. C. (1999). *The interactional nature of depression: Advances in interpersonal approaches.* Washington, DC: American Psychological Association.

Joiner, T., Metalsky, G., Katz, J., & Beach, S. R. (1999). Depression and excessive reassurance-seeking. *Psychological Inquiry, 10,* 269–278.

Kaltiala-Heino, R., Kosunen, E., & Rimpela, M. (2003). Pubertal timing, sexual behaviour and self reported depression in middle adolescence. *Journal of Adolescence, 26,* 531–545.

Keller, M., & Shapiro, R. (1981). Major depressive disorder: Initial results from a one-year prospective naturalistic follow-up study. *Journal of Nervous Mental Disorders, 169,* 761–768.

Kendler, K. S., Gardner, C. O., Gatz, M., & Pedersen, N. L. (2007). The sources of comorbidity between major depression and generalized anxiety disorder in a Swedish National Twin sample. *Psychological Medicine, 37,* 453–462.

Kendler, K. S., Gatz, M., Gardner, C. O., & Pedersen, N. L. (2006). A Swedish National Twin Study of lifetime major depression. *American Journal of Psychiatry, 163,* 109–114.

Kendler, K. S., Kuhn, J., & Prescott, C. A. (2004). The interrelationship of neuroticism, sex, and stressful life events in the prediction of episodes of major depression. *American Journal of Psychiatry, 161,* 631–636.

Kendler, K. S., & Prescott, C. A. (1999). A population based twin study of lifetime major depression in men and women. *Archives of General Psychiatry, 56,* 39–44.

Kessler, R. C. (2000). Gender differences in major depression: Epidemiological findings. In E. Frank (Ed.), *Gender and its effects on psychopathology* (pp. 61–84). Washington, DC: American Psychiatric Publishing.

Kessler, R. C., Berglund, P., Demler, O., Jin, R., Koretz, D., Merikangas, K. R., et al. (2003). The epidemiology of major depressive disorder: Results from the National Comorbidity Survey Replication (NCS-R). *Journal of the American Medical Association, 289,* 3095–4105.

Kessler, R. C., Crum, R. M., Warner, L. A., Nelson, C. B., Schulenberg, J., & Anthony, J. C. (1997). Lifetime co-occurrence of DSM-III-R alcohol abuse and dependence with other psychiatric disorders in the National Comorbidity Survey. *Archives of General Psychiatry, 54,* 313–321.

Kessler, R. C., McGonagle, K. A., Swartz, M., Blazer, D. G., & Nelson, C. B. (1993). Sex and depression in the National Comorbidity Survey I: Lifetime prevalence, chronicity, and recurrence. *Journal of Affective Disorders, 29,* 85–96.

Kessler, R. C., McLeod, J., & Wethington, E. (1985). The costs of caring: A perspective on the relationship between sex and psychological distress. In I. G. Sarason & B. R. Sarason (Eds.), *Social support: Theory, research and applications* (pp. 491–506). Dordrecht: Martinus Nijhoff.

Kessler, R. C., & McLeod, J. D. (1984). Sex differences in vulnerability to undesirable life events. *American Sociological Review, 49,* 620–631.

Kilpatrick, D. G., Edmunds, C., & Seymour, A. (1992). *Rape in America: A report to the nation.* Charleston, SC: National Victims Center and the Crime Victims Research and Treatment Center, Medical University of South Carolina.

Kilpatrick, D. G., & Saunders, B. E. (1996). *Prevalence and consequences of child victimization: Results from the National Survey of Adolescents* (Grant No. 93-IJ-CX-0023). Washington, DC: U.S. Department of Justice, Office of Justice Programs, National Institute of Justice.

Korszun, A., Altemus, M., & Young, E. A. (2006). The biological underpinnings of depression. In C. L. M. Keyes & S. H. Goodman (Eds.), *Women and depression* (pp. 41–61). New York: Cambridge University Press.

Koss, M. P., Gidycz, C. A., & Wisniewski, N. (1987). The scope of rape: Incidence and prevalence of sexual aggression and victimization in a national sample of higher education students. *Journal of Consulting and Clinical Psychology, 55,* 162–170.

Kovacs, M. (2001). Gender and the course of major depressive disorder through adolescence in clinically referred youngsters. *Journal of the American Academy of Child and Adolescent Psychiatry, 40,* 1079–1085.

Lau, J. Y. F., & Eley, T. C. (in press). The genetics of adolescent depression. In S. Nolen-Hoeksema & L. M. Hilt (Eds.), *Handbook of depression in adolescents.* New York: Routledge.

Lau, J. Y. F., Eley, T. C., & Rijsdijk, F. (2006). I think, therefore I am: A twin study of attributional style in adolescents. *Journal of Child Psychology and Psychiatry, 47,* 696–703.

Laumann, E. O., Gagnon, J. H., Michael, R. T., & Michaels, S. (1994). *The social organization of sexuality: Sexual practices in the United States.* Chicago: University of Chicago Press.

Leadbeater, B. J., Blatt, S. J., & Quinlan, D. M. (1995). Gender-linked vulnerabilities to depressive symptoms, stress, and problem behaviors in adolescents. *Journal of Research on Adolescence, 5,* 1–29.

Lewinsohn, P. M., Rohde, P., & Seeley, J. R. (1996). Adolescent suicidal ideation and attempts: Prevalence, risk factors, and clinical implications. *Clinical Psychology: Science and Practice, 3,* 25–46.

Little, S. A., & Garber, J. (2005). The role of social stressors and interpersonal orientation in explaining the longitudinal relation between externalizing and depressive symptoms. *Journal of Abnormal Psychology, 114,* 432–443.

Liu, X., & Kaplan, H. B. (1999). Explaining gender differences in symptoms of subjective distress in young adolescents. *Stress Medicine, 15,* 41–51.

MacKinnon, D., Jamison, K. R., & DePaulo, J. R. (1997). Genetics of manic depressive illness. *Annual Review of Neuroscience, 20,* 355–373.

Marcus, S. M., Young, E. A., Kerber, K. B., Kornstein, S., Farabaugh, A. H., Mitchell, J., et al. (2005). Gender differences in depression: Findings from the STAR*D study. *Journal of Affective Disorders, 87,* 141–150.

Matthews, K. A. (1992). Myths and realities of the menopause. *Psychosomatic Medicine, 54,* 1–9.

Matthews, K. A., Wing, R., Lewis, H., Meilahn, E., Kelsey, S., Costello, E., et al. (1990). Influences of natural menopause on psychological characteristics and symptoms of middle-aged healthy women. *Journal of Consulting and Clinical Psychology, 58,* 345–351.

McLaughlin, K., Hilt, L., & Nolen-Hoeksema, S. (2007). Racial/ethic differences in internalizing and externalizing symptoms in adolescents. *Journal of Abnormal Child Psychology, 35,* 801–806.

Munk-Olsen, T., Laursen, T. M., Pedersen, C. B., Mors, O., & Mortensen, P. B. (2006). New parents and mental disorders: A population-based register study. *Journal of the American Medical Association, 296,* 2582–2589.

Murray, C., & Lopez, E. (Eds.). (1996). *The global burden of disease, injuries and risk factors in 1990 and projected to 2020.* Cambridge, MA: Harvard University Press.

Nolen-Hoeksema, S. (1990). *Sex differences in depression.* Stanford, CA: Stanford University Press.

Nolen-Hoeksema, S. (1991). Responses to depression and their effects on the duration of depressive episodes. *Journal of Abnormal Psychology, 100,* 569–582.

Nolen-Hoeksema, S. (1998, August). *Contributors to the gender difference in rumination.* Paper presented at the annual meeting of the American Psychological Association, San Francisco.

Nolen-Hoeksema, S. (2000). The role of rumination in depressive disorders and mixed anxiety/depressive symptoms. *Journal of Abnormal Psychology, 109,* 504–511.

Nolen-Hoeksema, S., & Davis, C. G. (1999). "Thanks for sharing that": Ruminators and their social support networks. *Journal of Personality and Social Psychology, 77,* 801–814.

Nolen-Hoeksema, S., & Girgus, J. S. (1994). The emergence of gender differences in depression in adolescence. *Psychological Bulletin, 115,* 424–443.

Nolen-Hoeksema, S., & Jackson, B. (2001). Mediators of the gender difference in rumination. *Psychology of Women Quarterly, 25,* 37–47.

Nolen-Hoeksema, S., Larson, J., & Grayson, C. (1999). Explaining the gender difference in depression. *Journal of Personality and Social Psychology, 77,* 1061–1072.

Nolen-Hoeksema, S., Wisco, B., & Lyubomirsky, S. (in press). Rethinking rumination. *Perspectives on Psychological Science.*

O'Hara, M. W., & Swain, A. M. (1996). Rates and risk of postpartum depression: A meta-analysis. *International Review of Psychiatry, 8,* 37–54.

Paikoff, R. L., Brooks-Gunn, J., & Warren, M. P. (1991). Effects of girls' hormonal status on depressive and aggressive symptoms over the course of one year. *Journal of Youth and Adolescence, 20,* 191–215.

Petersen, A. C., Sarigiani, P. A., & Kennedy, R. E. (1991). Adolescent depression: Why more girls? *Journal of Youth and Adolescence, 20,* 247–271.

Post, R. M. (1992). Transduction of psychosocial stress into the neurobiology of recurrent affective disorder. *American Journal of Psychiatry, 149,* 999–1010.

Post, R. M., & Weiss, S. R. B. (1995). The neurobiology of treatment-resistant mood disorders. In F. E. Bloom & D. J. Kupfer (Eds.), *Psychopharmacology: The fourth generation of progress* (pp. 1155–1170). New York: Raven Press.

Prinstein, M. J., Borelli, J. L., Cheah, C. S. L., Simon, V. A., & Aikins, J. W. (2005). Adolescent girls' interpersonal vulnerability to depressive symptoms: A longitudinal examination of reassurance-seeking and peer relationships. *Journal of Abnormal Psychology, 114,* 676–688.

Radloff, L. S. (1975). Sex differences in depression: The effects of occupational and marital status. *Sex Roles, 1,* 249–265.

Rao, U., Hammen, C., & Daley, S. (1999). Continuity of depression during the transition to adulthood: A 5-year longitudinal study of young women. *Journal of the American Academy of Child and Adolescent Psychiatry, 38,* 908–915.

Rice, F., Harold, G. T., & Thapar, A. (2003). Negative life events as an account of age-related differences in the genetic aetiology of depression in childhood and adolescence. *Journal of Child Psychology and Psychiatry, 44,* 977–987.

Rierdan, J., & Koff, E. (1991). Depressive symptomatology among very early maturing girls. *Journal of Youth and Adolescence, 20,* 415–425.

Rudolph, K. D., Caldwell, M. S., & Conley, C. S. (2005). Need for approval and children's well-being. *Child Development, 76,* 309–323.

Rudolph, K. D., & Conley, C. S. (2005). The socioemotional costs and benefits of social-evaluative concerns: Do girls care too much? *Journal of Personality, 73,* 115–137.

Rudolph, K. D., & Flynn, M. (2007). Childhood adversity and youth depression: Influence of gender and pubertal status. *Development and Psychopathology, 19,* 497–521.

Rudolph, K. D., & Hammen, C. (1999). Age and gender as determinants of stress exposure, generation, and reactions in youngsters: A transactional perspective. *Child Development, 70,* 660–677.

Rutter, M., Silberg, J., O'Connor, T., & Simonoff, E. (1999). Genetics and child psychiatry: II. Empirical research findings. *Journals of Child Psychology and Psychiatry, 40,* 19–55.

Sannibale, C., & Hall, W. (2001). Gender-related symptoms and correlates of alcohol dependence among men and women with a lifetime diagnosis of alcohol use disorders. *Drug and Alcohol Review, 20,* 369–383.

Saunders, B. E., Kilpatrick, D. G., Hanson, R. F., Resnick, H. S., & Walker, M. E. (1999). Prevalence, case characteristics, and long-term psychological correlates of child rape among women: A national survey. *Child Maltreatment, 4,* 607–613.

Scourfield, J., Rice, F., Thapar, A., Harold, G. T., Martin, N., & McGuffin, P. (2003). Depressive symptoms in children and adolescents: Changing aetiological influences with development. *Journal of Child Psychology and Psychiatry, 44,* 968–976.

Shih, J. H., Eberhart, N. K., Hammen, C. L., & Brennan, P. A. (2006). Differential exposure and reactivity to interpersonal stress predict sex differences in adolescent depression. *Journal of Clinical Child and Adolescent Psychology, 35,* 103–115.

Siegel, J. M., Yancey, A. K., Aneshensel, C. S., & Schuler, R. (1999). Body image, perceived pubertal timing, and adolescent mental health. *Journal of Adolescent Health, 25,* 155–165.

Silberg, J., Pickles, A., Rutter, M., Hewitt, J., Simonoff, E., Maes, H., et al. (1999). The influence of genetic factors and life stress on depression among adolescent girls. *Archives of General Psychiatry, 56,* 225–232.

Smolak, L., & Striegel-Moore, R. H. (2001). Challenging the myth of the golden girl: Ethnicity and eating disorders. In R. H. Striegel-Moore & L. Smolak (Eds.), *Eating disorders: Innovative directions in research and practice* (pp. 111–132). Washington, DC: American Psychological Association.

Somerset, W., Newport, D. J., Ragan, K., & Stowe, Z. N. (2007). Depressive disorders in women: From menarche to beyond the menopause. In C. L. M. Keyes & S. H. Goodman (Eds.), *Women and depression* (pp. 62–88). New York: Cambridge University Press.

Stattin, H., & Magnusson, D. (1990). *Pubertal maturation in female development.* Hillsdale, NJ: Erlbaum.

Steiner, M., & Born, L. (2000). Advances in the treatment of premenstrual dysphoria. *CNS Drugs, 13,* 286–304.

Steiner, M., Dunn, E., & Born, L. (2003). Hormones and mood: From menarche to menopause and beyond. *Journal of Affective Disorders, 74,* 67–83.

Steiner, M., & Tam, W. Y. K. (1999). Postpartum depression in relation to other psychiatric disorders. In L. Miller (Ed.), *Postpartum mood disorders* (pp. 47–63). Washington, DC: American Psychiatric Press.

Stice, E., Presnell, K., & Bearman, S. K. (2001). Relation of early menarche to depression, eating disorders, substance abuse, and comorbid psychopathology among adolescent girls. *Developmental Psychology, 37,* 608–619.

Teasdale, J. (1988). Cognitive vulnerability to persistent depression. *Cognition and Emotion, 2,* 247–274.

Thapar, A., & McGuffin, P. (1994). A twin study of depressive symptoms in childhood. *British Journal of Psychiatry, 165,* 259–265.

Thase, M. E., Jindal, R., & Howland, R. H. (2002). Biological aspects of depression. In I. H. Gotlib & C. L. Hammen (Eds.), *Handbook of depression* (pp. 192–218). New York: Guilford Press.

Tjaden, P., & Thoennes, N. (1998). *Prevalence, incidence and consequence of violence against women: Findings from the National Violence Against Women Survey: Research in brief.* Washington, DC: National Institute of Justice, U.S. Department of Justice.

Twenge, J. M., & Nolen-Hoeksema, S. (2002). Age, gender, race, SES, and birth cohort differences on the Children's Depression Inventory: A meta-analysis. *Journal of Abnormal Psychology, 111,* 578–588.

van der Valk, J. C., van den Oord, E. J., Verhulst, F. C., & Boomsma, D. I. (2003). Genetic and environmental contributions to stability and change in children's internalizing and externalizing problems. *Journal of the American Academy of Child and Adolescent Psychiatry, 42,* 1212–1220.

Weiss, E. L., Longhurst, J. G., & Mazure, C. M. (1999). Childhood sexual abuse as a risk factor for depression in women: Psychosocial and neurobiological correlates. *American Journal of Psychiatry, 156,* 816–828.

Weissman, M. (1996, May). *Epidemiology of major depression in women.* Paper presented at the annual meeting of the American Psychiatric Association, New York.

Widom, C. S., DuMont, K., & Czaja, S. J. (2007). A prospective investigation of major depressive disorder and comorbidity in abused and neglected children grown up. *Archives of General Psychiatry, 64,* 49–56.

Williams, D. R., Gonzalez, H. M., Neighbors, H., Nesse, R., Abelson, J. M., Sweetman, J., et al. (2007). Prevalence and distribution of major depressive disorder in African Americans, Caribbean blacks, and Non-Hispanic whites. *Archives of General Psychiatry, 64,* 305–315.

Young, E., & Korszun, A. (1999). Women, stress, and depression: Sex differences in hypothalamic–pituitary–adrenal axis regulation. In E. Leibenluft (Ed.), *Gender differences in mood and anxiety disorders: From bench to bedside* (pp. 31–52). Washington, DC: American Psychiatric Press.

Zahn-Waxler, C. (2000). The development of empathy, guilt, and internalization of distress: Implications for gender differences in internalizing and externalizing problems. In R. Davidson (Ed.), *Anxiety, depression, and emotion: Wisconsin Symposium on Emotion* (Vol. 1, pp. 222–265). Oxford, UK: Oxford University Press.

CHAPTER 18

Depression in Children

Judy Garber, Catherine M. Gallerani, *and* Sarah A. Frankel

$\mathbf{D}$o children experience depression? The answer to this question is complex, and depends on the definition of depression and the age of the child. Depression can be a symptom, syndrome, and nosologic disorder. The single symptom of sadness is a common subjective state experienced by most individuals at various points in their lives, and by itself is not necessarily pathological. The syndrome of depression comprises more than an isolated dysphoric mood and occurs in combination with other symptoms to form a symptom complex, or *syndrome*. When this clinical syndrome is characterized by a particular symptom picture with a specifiable course, outcome, treatment response, and etiological correlates, then it is considered a distinct nosological disorder.

There is now general consensus among clinicians and researchers that children can and do experience depressive symptoms, and can be diagnosed with depressive disorders. This chapter reviews the prevalence, phenomenology, course and outcome, comorbidity, assessment, and etiology of depression in children. Bipolar depression and treatment are not addressed here, because they are covered more extensively in other chapters in this volume. We focus primarily on children (i.e., infants, preschoolers, and preadolescents), although we discuss some findings with adolescents that are relevant for comparisons with younger children or when studies included children ranging from childhood through adolescence.

PREVALENCE

Major depressive disorder (MDD) rarely has been assessed in infants, is very uncommon in young children, and is still relatively infrequent during middle childhood, with rates increasing significantly during adolescence (Costello, Foley, & Angold, 2006). In their meta-analysis, Costello and colleagues (2006) concluded that the overall prevalence estimate of depression in children is 2.8%, ranging from .03 to 3.0%. This rate varies, however, by age, informant, and type of depression (i.e., MDD, dysthymia). Among very young children (i.e., ages 2–5), prevalence rates have been found to be 1.4% for MDD, .6% for dysthymic disorder (DD), and .7% for depression not otherwise specified (NOS)/minor depression, with rates significantly higher in older preschoolers (3.0%) than in toddlers (.3%) (Egger & Angold, 2006). In children ages 9, 11, and 13, Costello and colleagues (1996) reported 3-month prevalence to be .03% for MDD, .13% for DD, and 1.45% for depression NOS. Thus, the rates of diagnosed depressive disorders in preadolescents are relatively low, although they are higher when based on children's compared to parents' report about children's depressive symptoms (Rubio-Stipec, Fitzmaurice, Murphy, & Walker, 2003). Also, inclusion of impairment criteria, emphasized in the fourth edition of the *Diagnostic and Statistical Manual of Mental Disorders* (DSM IV; American Psychiatric Association, 1994), results in lower rates of depression (3.4%) compared to when impairment is not included (4.1%, Canino et al., 2004).

In adults, the prevalence of depression in females is about two times that of males (Weissman & Olfson, 1995). This gender difference, however, has not been found in prepubertal children. Some researchers have shown that the rate of MDD is about equal in preadolescent girls and boys (e.g., Angold & Rutter, 1992), whereas others have found higher rates among preadolescent boys than among girls (e.g., Angold, Costello, & Worthman, 1998; Steinhausen & Winkler, 2003). Angold and colleagues (1998) showed that girls had higher rates of depressive disorders after Tanner Stage III, whereas boys had higher rates before this stage. A meta-analysis of 310 studies using the Children's Depression Inventory (CDI) found no significant sex differences in self-reported depressive symptoms for children ages 8–12, although boys in this age range reported slightly higher scores than girls (Twenge & Nolen-Hoeksema, 2002).

PHENOMENOLOGY

Infants have been observed to experience sadness, irritability, sleep and eating problems, fatigue, withdrawal, apathy, abnormal reactions to strangers, fussiness, and tantrums (Guedeney, 2007). The precise age at which other symptoms of depressive disorder emerge (e.g., anhedonia, psychomotor changes, low self-worth, guilt, concentration problems, hopelessness, suicidality) is less clear. Moreover, the extent to which manifestations of depressive symptoms in very young children have continuity with adolescent- and adult-onset mood disorders is still a matter of debate.

Spitz and Wolf (1946) first proposed that infants could become depressed, and others (e.g., Guedeney, 2007; Trad, 1994) continue to argue that depression in infants exists. The five-axis classification system (Diagnostic Classification [DC]: 0–3) for mental health and developmental disorders in infancy includes infant depression as an Axis I mood disorder (Zero to Three, 2005); evidence of the reliability and validity of this classification system has been reported (Cordeiro, Caldeira Da Silva, & Goldschmidt, 2003; Guedeney et al., 2003).

Failure to thrive (FTT), which has several similarities to depression, is defined as having a weight below the 3rd percentile on Gairdner–Pearson growth charts or body weight that decreases over 2 major centiles. Infants with FTT show psychomotor delay, iron deficiency, behavioral difficulties, and feeding problems (Raynor & Rudolf, 1996); no identified organic disease accounts for these symptoms, however. Risk factors for FTT and depression are similar, and include poverty, parental psychopathology, maternal isolation, poor parent–child interactions, family dysfunction, and inadequate parental knowledge (Raynor & Rudolf, 1996). Low appetite, inadequate feeding skills, shyness, and undemandingness can be maladaptive in feeding situations (Wright & Birks, 2000) and lead to less responsiveness from parents, which then can contribute to FTT (Frank & Drotar, 1994). This in turn can lead to more withdrawal by the infant, thereby creating a vicious cycle of maladaptive parent–child interactions. Thus, FTT in babies may be one manifestation of depression in infants.

For children from preschool through adolescence, DSM IV criteria are used to define depressive disorders similarly, regardless of age. Two minor developmental variations in these criteria are that for children and adolescents, irritability is a symptom of dysphoric mood, and the duration of dysthymia is 1 rather than 2 years. Thus, according to DSM-IV, few real developmental differences exist in the symptoms of depressive disorders.

In research with preschool-age children, however, Luby, Heffelfinger, Mrakotsky, and colleagues (2002) identified a specific symptom constellation characterized by developmentally modified symptoms of MDD (e.g., substituting changes in "work" with changes in activities and play), and removing the 2-week duration criterion due to the normative fluctuations in mood associated with this young age group. Luby, Mrakotsky, Heffelfinger, and colleagues (2003) found that the most severely impaired preschoolers were identified using unmodified DSM criteria, but the modified criteria identified a large number of seriously impaired children missed by the existing DSM-IV criteria. Finally, Luby, Mrakotsky, Heffelfinger, Brown, and Spitznagel (2004) reported in preschool-age children evidence of a melancholic-like subtype of depression consistent with that identified for adults.

Manifestations of depression might depend on an individual's level of cognitive, social, and physiological development; therefore, the symptoms of depression might not be isomorphic across the lifespan (Weiss & Garber, 2003). Indeed, evidence consistent with this assertion has been reported (Avenevoli & Steinberg, 2001; Kovacs, Obrosky, & Sherrill, 2003). Although there may exist a core set of common depressive symptoms across all ages, other symptoms might be uniquely associated with the syndrome at different developmental levels.

Developmental differences in depressive symptoms may be seen in at least two ways. First, children and adults might have the same symptom but differ in how it is expressed. Second, symptoms that comprise the syndrome could differ developmentally (i.e., different combinations of symptoms would define the syndrome at different ages). This would appear as developmental differences in the rates of particular symptoms and in the composition of the syndrome. In a meta-analysis of 16 empirical studies comparing the rates of depressive symptoms in different age groups, Weiss and Garber (2003) found that more developmentally advanced individuals had higher levels of anhedonia, hopelessness, hypersomnia, weight gain, and social withdrawal, and lower levels of energy (see also Sorensen, Nissen, Mors, & Thomsen, 2005). Weiss and Garber also reviewed studies comparing the structure of depression at different age levels and found that two studies reported a similar factor structure across ages, two found developmental differences, and one found mixed results. Although some have argued against the existence of developmental differences in depressive symptoms (e.g., Ryan et al., 1987), "The suggestion that the clinical presentation of major depression varies with age is far from resolved and more developmentally sensitive studies are required" (Goodyer, 1996, p. 407).

COURSE AND OUTCOME

Childhood-onset MDD is a chronic and recurrent illness associated with poor psychosocial outcomes (Birmaher et al., 2004). The duration of a major depressive episode (MDE) in children is on average 7–9 months (Kovacs et al., 1984b). Approximately 90% of depressed child outpatients and inpatients recover from an MDE by 1.5–2 years after onset (Birmaher, Arbelaez, & Brent, 2002). Kovacs and colleagues (1984a, 1984b) reported that among 8- to 13-year-old children with dysthymia, 91% eventually recovered, although this took almost 9 years. The median episode length for dysthymia was 4 years.

Recurrence, or the onset of a new depressive episode, is high for children (Kennard, Emslie, Mayes, & Hughes, 2006). Early-onset depressions tend to recur, and younger age of onset significantly predicts relapse (e.g., Birmaher et al., 1996). Longitudinal studies of youth consistently have found that major depression has a cumulative probability of recurrence of 40% by 2 years, and 70% by 5 years (Emslie, Rush, Weinberg, Gullion, et al., 1997). In a 9-year follow-up, Kovacs (1996a) reported that 80% of the children with prior dysthymia and 50% of children with prior MDD had subsequent episodes of depression.

Regarding the long-term course of childhood-onset depression, longitudinal studies indicate a mixed picture. Some studies (e.g., Harrington, Fudge, Rutter, Pickles, & Hill, 1990; Weissman et al., 1999) found that prepubertal-onset depression did not show continuity into adulthood, but was sometimes followed by behavioral problems and impaired functioning. Other studies (e.g., Dunn & Goodyer, 2006; Geller, Zimerman, Williams, Bolhofner, & Craney, 2001b; Kovacs, 1996b; Weissman et al., 1999) showed that depression during childhood recurs into adulthood. Still others (e.g., Weissman et al., 1999) reported that early-onset depression appears to have a bipolar course emerging over time. One predictor of the recurrence and continuity of childhood depression into adulthood is a positive family history of MDD. Weissman and colleagues (1999) reported that patients with prepubertal-onset MDD who experienced a recurrence had higher rates of depressive disorders in their first-degree relatives.

Depressive symptoms in children also have been found to be stable (e.g., Cole, Martin, Powers, & Truglio, 1996; Hofstra, van der Ende, & Verhulst, 2000). Cole and colleagues (1996) reported high stability of depression over a 6-month period for both third- and sixth-grade children based on self-, teacher, parent, and peer report. In contrast, a prospective study of 3- to 12-year-old children showed a lack of stability in depressive symptoms from very early childhood to preadolescence based on self- and parent report (Pihlakoski et al., 2006). The issues of continuity, stability, and change in depressive symptoms and disorders in individuals with varying ages of onset from infancy through adulthood need further study (Avenevoli & Steinberg, 2001).

Factors associated with the onset, duration, and recurrence of childhood depression include demographic (e.g., age, gender), individual (e.g., preexisting diagnosis, negative cognitive style), family (e.g., parental psychopathology), biological (e.g., neurobiological dysregulation), and psychosocial factors (e.g., poor support, stressful life events) (Birmaher et al., 2004; Timbremont & Braet, 2004). Birmaher and colleagues (2004) showed that for girls, higher levels of guilt, more prior depressive episodes, and greater parental psychopathology predicted a more severe clinical course of depression.

Recurrence of depression may result from *kindling*, sensitization, or *scarring* (Lewinsohn, Steinmetz, Larson, & Franklin, 1981; Monroe & Harkness, 2005; Post, 1992); that is, prior MDEs may increase vulnerability to subsequent episodes, and as the number of past depressive episodes increases, so does the probability of future episodes. Moreover, significant impairment in interpersonal relationships, school and work settings, and overall quality of life has been found among individuals with prepubertal-onset MDD (Geller, Zimerman, Williams, Bolhofner, & Craney, 2001b).

COMORBIDITY

Comorbidity between depression and other disorders in childhood is the rule rather than the exception, with rates of comorbidity ranging from 30 to between 80 and 95% (e.g., Kovacs, 1996b; Sorensen et al., 2005). Dysthymia is the most common comorbid disorder with MDD; 30% of children with MDD had underlying dysthymia, and 70% of those with early-onset dysthymia had a subsequent MDD (Kovacs, 1994). Children with such *double-depression* have more severe and longer depressive episodes, a higher rate of other comorbid disorders (e.g., generalized anxiety disorder), more suicidality, less social competence, and less parental monitoring (Goodman, Schwab-Stone, Lahey, Shaffer, Jensen, 2000).

Other common comorbid diagnoses with MDD include anxiety disorders, oppositional defiant disorder, conduct disorder (CD), attention-deficit/hyperactivity disorder (ADHD), substance abuse, and enuresis or encopresis (Wagner, 2003). The median odds ratio (OR) of an association between CD and depression has been found to be 6.6 and between anxiety and depression, 8.2 (Angold, Costello, & Erkanli, 1999). Indeed, in terms of heterotypic comorbidity, anxiety and depression are the most commonly co-occurring conditions, with estimates ranging from 16 to 75% (Angold et al., 1999; Seligman & Ollendick, 1998); overanxious disorder and generalized anxiety disorder account for most of the comorbidity with MDD (Costello et al., 2006). In depressed clinical samples, children's rates of comorbid anxiety disorders are about two- to threefold higher than rates of comorbid CD (Kovacs & Devlin, 1998).

Comorbidity of depression and anxiety disorders is so high that some researchers (e.g., Patterson, Greising, Hyland, & Burger, 1994) have challenged the discriminant validity of the two diagnoses. Others (e.g., Watson & Clark, 1984) have suggested that anxiety and depression share a single underlying process, referred to as *negative affectivity*. Cole, Truglio, and Peeke (1997) showed that anxiety and depression in young children (third graders) formed a unified, indistinguishable construct, whereas in older children (sixth graders), they yielded a dual-factor or tripartite model. Moreover, anxiety has been found to precede depression in children temporally (Cole, Peeke, Martin, Truglio, & Seroczynski, 1998; Kovacs, Gatsonis, Paulaukas, & Richards, 1989). Concurrent comorbidity, as well as homotypic and heterotypic continuity, have been found to be more common in girls than in boys (Costello, Mustillo, Erkanli, Keeler, & Angold, 2003).

Comorbidity affects risk for recurrent depression, duration of depressive episodes, suicide attempts, utilization of mental health services, and functional impairment (Ezpeleta, Domenech, & Angold, 2006). Angold and colleagues (1999) argued that comorbidity is not simply the result of methodological problems, arbitrary groupings of symptoms into diagnoses, or an artifact. Rather, comorbidity is a real phenomenon, adding to the complexity of depressive disorders in children. Possible mechanisms for such comorbidity include negative affectivity, a common genetic diathesis, and/or shared risk factors. Other important questions in need of further study include the following: What explains concurrent versus sequential comorbidity? What is the trajectory of different comorbid conditions across development, and what accounts for these changes? What is the temporal relation between depression and comorbid disorders? How can intervention strategies effectively reduce comorbidity?

ASSESSMENT AND DIAGNOSIS

Methods of assessing depression in children include self-report, others' reports, clinical interviews, naturalistic behavioral observations, and laboratory tasks (e.g., Garber & Kaminski, 2000; Kendall, Cantwell, & Kazdin, 1989; Klein, Dougherty, & Olino, 2005). Several challenges arise in the attempt to assess depression accurately in young children, because their language, reading, and cognitive abilities typically are not yet fully developed. Multiple informants (e.g., child, parents, teachers, peers) can provide a more comprehensive picture of the psychological state of the child, although these individuals often have different perspectives, resulting in low interinformant agreement (Achenbach, McConaughy, & Howell, 1987; De Los Reyes & Kazdin, 2005). This discrepancy has been related to parental psychopathology; actual differences in behaviors across settings; and the difficulty of observing subjective symptoms of depression, such as sadness, hopelessness, guilt, and worthlessness. Using more than one source to assess depression in children requires determining who is the "best" informant about particular symptoms, and resolving discrepancies between informants. Children are likely to know more about their own internal states (i.e., mood, guilt, hopelessness), whereas others (e.g., parents, teachers) might be better reporters about observable symptoms (i.e., changes in eating patterns, concentration difficulties) (e.g., Kazdin & Marciano, 1998). Given that in the individual case we do not know who is the more accurate informant, the best strategy may be to interview both children and parents about all depressive symptoms.

Although use of multiple sources when assessing depression in children is generally recommended, reasons for analyzing parents' and children's reports separately include the following: (1) correlations between children's and parents' ratings of depression tend to be small (Herjanic & Reich, 1997); (2) child- and parent-report measures of children's depression have different factor structures (Cole, Hoffman, Tram, & Maxwell, 2000); (3) the relation of children's depression to stressful life events (Compas, Howell, Phares, Williams, & Ledoux, 1989; Stanger, McConaughy, & Achenbach, 1992) and perceived control (Weisz, Southam-Gerow, & McCarty, 2001) tends to be stronger for children's compared to parents' reports; and (4) heritability estimates are greater in parents' than in children's self-reports of children's depression (e.g., Eaves, et al., 1997).

A highly structured interview for assessing depression in children age 6 or older is the Diagnostic Interview for Children and Adolescents (DICA; Reich, 2000). Although it has good interrater reliability and moderate validity, the DICA tends to overdiagnose depression and has low parent–child agreement. Other psychometrically adequate structured interviews are the Children's Interview for Psychiatric Syndromes (ChIPS; Weller, Weller, Fristad, Rooney, & Schecter, 2000), for children as young as age 6, and the Diagnostic Interview Schedule for Children (DISC; Shaffer, Fisher, Lucas, Dulcan, & Schwab-Stone, 2000) for children age 9 and older.

The Schedule for Affective Disorders and Schizophrenia for School-Age Children (K-SADS) is a widely used, semistructured interview for diagnosing mood disorders (Kaufman, Birmaher, Brent, et al., 1997). The K-SADS can be used with children as young as age 8, and it has adequate reliability and validity (Ambrosini, 2000). Other good semi-structured interviews for assessing depression in children are the Child and Adolescent Psychiatric Assessment (CAPA; Angold & Costello, 2000) for age 9 and above, the Child Assessment Schedule (CAS; Hodges, Cools, & McKnew, 1989) for children as young as age 5, and the Interview Schedule for Children and Adolescents (ISCA; Kovacs, 1986) for children age 8 and above. A commonly used clinician-rated measure of depressive symptoms for children is the Children's Depression Rating Scale—Revised (CDRS-R; Poznanski, Mokros, Grossman, & Freeman, 1985).

A frequently used self-report measure of depressive symptoms is the CDI (Kovacs, 1981), which has adequate reliability and validity (e.g., Saylor, Finch, Spirito, & Bennett, 1984), differentiates between normal and clinic-referred children (Carey, Faulstich, Gresham, Ruggiero, & Enyart, 1987), and correlates moderately with parent report of children's depression (Garber, 1984). Other self-report measures are the Center for Epidemiologic Studies Depressive Scale for Children (CES-DC; Radloff, 1977), the Mood and Feelings Questionnaire (Angold et al., 1995), the Depression Self-Rating Scale (Birleson, 1981), the Dimensions of Depression Profile for Children and Adolescents (Harter & Nowakowski, 1987), and the Multiscore Depression Inventory for Children (Berndt, Petzel, & Berndt, 1980).

Parent-report measures of children's depressive symptoms include the Parent version of the CDI (P-CDI; Cole et al., 2000; Garber, 1984) and the Anxious/Depressed subscale of the Child Behavior Checklist (CBCL; Achenbach & Edelbrock, 1991). The Child Behavior Checklist—Teacher Report Form (CBCL TRF; Achenbach & Edelbrock, 1986), the teacher version of the CBCL, yields a similar Anxious/Depressed subscale. A peer measure of depression is the Peer Nomination Inventory for Depression (Lefkowitz & Tesiny, 1980). Laboratory behavioral measures also may be used to assess depressive symptoms in children (Garber & Kaminski, 2000).

Finally, measures created to evaluate depressive symptoms in young children include pictorial instruments such as the Preschool Symptom Self-Report (PRESS; Martini, Strayhorn, & Puig-Antich, 1990), the Pictorial Instrument for Children and Adolescents–III—Revised (PICA-III-R; Ernst, Cookus, & Moravec, 2000), and the Dominic-R and the Terry Questionnaires (Valla, Bergeron, & Smolla, 2000). The Berkeley Puppet Interview (BPI; Measelle, Ablow, Cowan, & Cowan, 1998) uses puppets to assess young children's perceptions of their academic and social competence, achievement motivation, peer acceptance, depression/anxiety, and aggression/hostility. Parent and teacher questionnaires paralleling the BPI, such as the MacArthur Health and Behavior Questionnaire (HBQ), assess physical and mental health of young children, validly screen children under age 9, and identify internalizing disorders (Lemery-Chalfant et al., 2007; Luby, Heffelfinger, & Measelle, 2002).

ETIOLOGY

Much of the research on the etiology of depression in children has been based on the downward extension of theories developed to explain depression in adults. If depression is essentially the same construct across development, then similar causal processes should underlie the disorder at any age. Rather than having different theories of child and adult depression, theories need to explain developmental variation in the characteristics of depression (e.g., prevalence, course). Conversely, if child and adult depression are not the same, then different theories may be appropriate (e.g., Cole, 1991). Similar to juvenile- and adult-onset types of diabetes, which share some commonalities but also have important differences in course, correlates, and treatment, if distinct child- and adult-onset types of depression exist, then different theories would be needed. Although many theories of depression exist, we highlight here the factors with the most empirical support: genes, neurobiology, stressful life events, negative cognitions, self-regulation, and interpersonal relationships, as well as interactions among these factors.

Genes

Family, twin, and adoption studies have yielded varying results regarding genetic contributions to individual differences in depression (Lau & Eley, 2008). In a meta-analysis of family studies of childhood depression, Rice, Harold, and Thapar (2002a) reported that for children with MDD, the likelihood of a first-degree relative having MDD was 2.3 times higher than that for children without MDD, and 1.85 times higher than that for psychiatric controls. Additionally, offspring of depressed parents were four times more likely than normal controls, and 1.7 times more likely than psychiatric controls, to have MDD; were at increased risk of experiencing early-onset depression; had longer episodes; and had particularly negative outcomes when their depression began in childhood (Weissman et al., 1987). A family history of MDD also is associated with greater recurrence rates and continuity into adulthood for childhood-onset, but not for adolescent- or adult-onset, MDD (Wickramaratne, Greenwald, & Weissman, 2000). Family studies, however, confound genetic and environmental effects, such as maladaptive parenting styles, marital dysfunction, and stress (Goodman & Gotlib, 1999).

Twin studies with children report heritability estimates comparable to those found in adults (Rice et al., 2002a). Some studies (e.g., Gjone, Stevenson, Sundet, & Eilertsen, 1996) have indicated that childhood-onset depression is associated with a greater genetic contribution, whereas others (Rice, Harold, & Thapar, 2002a) have found environmental factors to be more important. Heritability estimates in twin studies of childhood depression vary by informant, sex, and age. Parent reports of children's depressive symptoms showed modest to high estimates of genetic effects (30–80%), whereas self-reported depressive symptoms generated lower estimates (15–80%). Girls show larger genetic effects than boys (Happonen et al., 2002; Scourfield et al., 2003), although some studies have not replicated this (Hewitt et al., 1997; van der Valk, van den Oord, Verhulst, & Boomsma, 2003), and other studies have found no sex differences in the heritability of depression in children (Bartels et al., 2004; Gjone & Stevenson, 1997). In a study of pre- and postpubertal twins, Silberg and colleagues (1999) found evidence of genetic heritability only for postpubertal girls. In contrast, Eley and Stevenson (1999) reported that genetic effects decreased with age in females but increased with age in males. Genes also have been found to play a larger role in the relation between negative life events and depression in older adolescents (ages 12–17 years) than in children (ages 8–11 years) (Rice, Harold, & Thapar, 2003). Moreover, age-related changes in heritability estimates can result from different gene effects at different ages, from the same genes impacting the phenotypical expression of a trait at different ages, or from environmental influences that vary with development (Lau & Eley, 2008).

Studies identifying genetic risk factors that interact with negative life events to predict depressive symptoms highlight the importance of gene–environment interactions in risk for depression. Caspi and colleagues (2003) showed that the relation between childhood maltreatment and adult depression is moderated by the serotonin transporter (5-HTTLPR) gene for individuals possessing one or two copies of the short allele (s) compared to individuals homozygous for the long allele. Kaufman, Yang, Douglas-Palumberi, Grasso, and colleagues (2004) reported that maltreated children with the s/s genotype had significantly higher depression scores than children with the same genotype who had not been maltreated. In another study, Kaufman, Yang, Douglas-Palumberi, Houshyar, and colleagues (2004) reported that an interaction between the s/s allele of the 5-HTTLPR gene, the MET allele of the brain-derived neurotropic factor (BDNF) val66met polymorphism, and child history of maltreatment predicted the highest depression scores.

Thus, estimates of heritability tend to be moderate, shared environment effects tend to be small, and nonshared environmental effects emerge as the largest environmental influence on individual differences in childhood depression. Vulnerability to depression clearly has a genetic component, but the exact genetic mechanisms underlying depression are still unclear.

Genes likely influence risk for depression through such endophenotypes as temperament, cognitive style, stress reactivity, and/or hormone and neurotransmitter levels (Thapar & Rice, 2006). Moreover, multiple genetic loci likely contribute to the risk for depression (e.g., Holmans et al., 2007). Recent genetic research has focused on identifying specific candidate genes associated with systems involved in depression, and using genetic linkage studies to identify common genes in families at high risk for depression (see Levinson, this volume).

Neurobiology

Psychobiological studies of depression, which have been extended to children (e.g., Kaufman & Charney, 2003; Zalsman et al., 2006), have focused on dysregulation in neuroendocrine and neurochemical systems, and in disturbances in sleep architecture. In addition, structural and functional brain differences in depressed and high-risk children increasingly are being investigated (e.g., Field, Fox, Pickens, & Nawrocki, 1995; Thomas et al., 2001).

Psychoneuroendocrinology

As discussed by Thase (Chapter 9, this volume), depressed individuals show dysregulation of the human stress response in the limbic–hypothalamic–pituitary–adrenocortical (LHPA) system. The LHPA axis is active from birth (Gunnar, 1989). Large increases in cortisol levels during infancy are correlated with stress, and tremendous variability in the magnitude of cortisol response to stress has been found among infants. Some neuroendocrine changes have been associated with depression-like symptoms in infants, such as prolonged crying, withdrawal, and eventual apathy in response to stress, particularly separation (Trad, 1994).

Most studies have not found differences in basal cortisol secretion between depressed and nondepressed children, as has been found in adults (Feder et al., 2004; Kaufman, Martin, King, & Charney, 2001), although some studies have shown elevated cortisol secretion near sleep onset in suicidal or depressed adolescent inpatients (Dahl, Ryan, Puig-Antich, et al., 1991). Recently, Forbes, Williamson, and colleagues (2006) reported that depressed adolescents have significantly higher cortisol around sleep onset than do depressed children, which suggests a possible influence of puberty on LHPA dysregulation. Additionally, a series of studies of 8- to 16-year-olds found evening cortisol hypersecretion and morning dehydroepiandrosterone (DHEA) hyposecretion (Goodyer et al., 1996), a pattern that increased risk for persistent MDEs at 1-year follow-up (Goodyer, Herbert, & Altham, 1998).

Studies of the dexamethasone suppression test (DST) as an indicator of abnormalities in LHPA response in children have found greater sensitivity in inpatients compared to outpatients (61 vs. 29%) and in children compared to adolescents (58 vs. 44%), although comparisons with psychiatric controls were stronger in adolescent samples (85%) than in child samples (60%; Dahl et al., 1992; Dahl & Ryan, 1996). Depressed and nondepressed children also have not been found to differ in baseline or post corticotropin-releasing hormone (CRH) levels of cortisol or adrenocorticotropic hormone (ACTH) (Birmaher, Dahl, et al., 2000).

Growth hormone (GH) regulation also may be a biological marker of central noradrenergic and serotoninergic processes (Birmaher et al., 2000). GH, normally secreted by the pituitary gland, functions as a growth-promoting agent throughout the body and is mostly secreted during sleep in children (Ryan & Dahl, 1993). Some studies report an increase in unstimulated GH secretion at night in depressed children (e.g., Kutcher et al.,

1991), whereas others report blunted GH secretion throughout the day (e.g., Meyer et al., 1991). Compared to nondepressed controls, children with MDD have a blunted GH response to stimulation with insulin-induced hypoglycemia and growth hormone–releasing hormone (GHRH) (e.g., Ryan et al., 1994), which continues even after remission (Dahl et al., 2000). Blunted GH response to GHRH also has been found in children with no personal history of depression but with high rates of affective illness in their families (Birmaher et al., 2000). Bonari and colleagues (2004) demonstrated that children of depressed mothers had increased stress hormone levels at baseline and in response to laboratory stressors. Thus, GH system dysregulation may be a trait vulnerability marker for depression (Dinan, 1998). Such at-risk children need to be followed to determine whether their blunted GH response predicts onset of depressive episodes.

Neurotransmitters

Biological dysregulation has been found in the neurochemistry of depressed individuals, with serotonin, norepinephrine, and acetylcholine particularly implicated in the pathophysiology of mood disorders (see Thase, Chapter 9, this volume). Depressed girls show a blunted cortisol response and an increased prolactin response after administration of L-5-hydroxytryptophan (L-5HTP) (Ryan et al., 1992). Similar results have been found in never-depressed children with high familial loading for depression (Birmaher et al., 1997), suggesting a possible serotoninergic system marker for depression. Also paralleling results in adults, children with recurrent depression secreted significantly less prolactin than did children with a single episode of depression, which suggests that the course of the disorder over time may be related to neurobiological functioning. Kaufman and colleagues (1998) reported that depressed abused children had a greater prolactin response after administration of L-5HTP compared to depressed nonabused children and nondepressed nonabused controls, thus highlighting the possible role of early childhood adversity on neurobiological functioning.

Investigation into the effectiveness of selective seratonin reuptake inhibitors (SSRIs) in reducing depressive symptoms in children also has implicated serotoninergic system dysregulation in childhood depression (Emslie, Rush, Weinberg, Kowatch, et al., 1997). The effect of SSRIs on the developing brain needs further study. Overall, children, adolescents, and adults exhibit serotoninergic system dysregulation, although the nature of the abnormalities varies depending on age, gender, and history of trauma. Moreover, serotoninergic system dysregulation may be a risk factor for depression, in that it has been found in both high-risk and currently depressed children (Birmaher et al., 1997).

Functional and Anatomical Brain Differences

Structural magnetic resonance imaging (sMRI) studies of depressed adults have shown various case-control differences (see Thase, Chapter 9, this volume). sMRI studies in depressed children have found a smaller left subgenual prefrontal cortex (PFC), lower frontal lobe volumes, and greater ventricular volumes compared to nondepressed psychiatric controls (Botteron, Raichle, Drevets, Heath, & Todd, 2002; Nolan et al., 2002; Steingard et al., 2002). Smaller left subgenual PFC in depressed female adolescent twins suggests the possibility of genetic transmission of structural abnormalities (Todd & Botteron, 2001). Reduced amygdalar, but not hippocampal, volume has been reported in depressed youth compared to nondepressed controls, although no significant association was found between amygdalar volume reduction and severity, duration, or age of onset of depression (Rosso et al., 2005).

Studies that use fMRI with children are still rare. Depressed children (ages 8–16) have been found to have a blunted amygdalar response to fearful faces compared to nondepressed controls and anxious youth (Thomas et al., 2001). Another study, however, found increased amygdalar activity during successful memory encoding of evocative faces in depressed youth compared to nondepressed controls and anxious youth (Roberson-Nay et al., 2006). Using single-photon emission computed tomography (SPECT), Bonte and colleagues (2001) showed that depressed children had decreased activity in the occipital region.

Studies of brain asymmetry have revealed greater left frontal hypoactivation in infant (Dawson, Frey, Pangiotides, Osterling, & Hessl, 1997; Field et al., 1995) and young adolescent (Tomarken, Dichter, Garber, & Simien, 2004) offspring of depressed mothers compared to offspring of nondepressed mothers. Davidson, Pizzagalli, Nitschke, and Putman (2002) proposed that decreased left frontal activation reflects an underactivation of the approach system and reduced positive emotionality. Neuroimaging studies of depressed adults indicate disruption in structure and function of several reward-related areas, which may influence the reduced positive affect that is characteristic of many depressed patients (Drevets, 2001). Similarly, depressed youth (ages 9–17) show more disrupted neural responses to rewarding events than do nondepressed youth (Forbes, May, et al., 2006); abnormalities occurred in both reward decision/anticipation and reward outcome phases of processing. Ladouceur and colleagues (2005) reported that depressed children process emotional information differently than do nondepressed controls, and recommended examining the neural mechanisms behind these processing differences. Brain imaging research in children, particularly of the nucleus accumbens, amygdala, and medial and ventral PFC regions, may help provide a better understanding of the neural correlates of early-onset depression (Ernst, Pine, & Hardin, 2006).

Sleep Architecture Abnormalities

Although depressed children subjectively report sleep disturbances, sleep electroencephalographic (EEG) results are less consistent in children than in adults (Ryan & Dahl, 1993). Depressed children show sleep anomalies such as prolonged sleep latencies; reduced REM latencies, especially in more severely depressed patients (Dahl, Ryan, Puig-Antich, et al., 1991); increased REM density; and decreased sleep efficiency, although results are inconsistent across studies. Some studies have failed to find differences between depressed and nondepressed children in EEG sleep patterns (Bertocci et al., 2005). Sleep polysomnography measures have been shown to predict recurrence of depression in children, particularly in boys (Armitage et al., 2002; Emslie et al., 2001).

The absence of consistent patterns of sleep abnormalities in depressed youth compared to the robust findings in adults has been attributed to the role of maturational changes, suggesting differences in the nature and function of sleep across development (Kaufman et al., 2001). Dahl and Ryan (1996) noted that because young children are deep sleepers, their sleep is difficult to disrupt. As children get older, this protective aspect of sleep begins to decrease. Thus, the sleep disturbances associated with depression may not become evident until adolescence or young adulthood.

In summary, research with children has sometimes, although not always, yielded results consistent with those found in depressed adults (Kaufman & Charney, 2003; Zalsman et al., 2006). The inconsistencies could be a function of developmental factors, state of the illness (i.e., single episode vs. recurrent), or severity. Moreover, the underlying neurobiology may be different in those with a history of trauma and abuse (e.g., Kaufman et al., 1998). The neurobiological literature on depression in children often diverges from that of adolescents and adults, thus highlighting the importance of placing affective neuroscience within a developmental framework, taking into account evolving neurological systems across the lifespan (Cicchetti & Posner, 2005).

Temperament

Temperament refers to a behavioral, emotional, and/or cognitive style that is relatively stable across time and consistent across situations (Rothbart & Bates, 1998; Shiner, 1998). Temperament is thought to have a genetic or biological basis (e.g., Gray, 1987), although experience, particularly within the social context, can affect its development (Caspi, Henry, McGee, Moffitt, & Silva, 1995; Hartup & van Lieshout, 1995). Personality traits linked particularly with depression in children are negative and positive emotionality, and constraint and attentional control (Compas, Connor-Smith, & Jaser, 2004).

Negative emotionality (NE), the propensity to experience negative emotions (e.g., anxiety, fear, sadness, anger), is characterized by sensitivity to negative stimuli, increased wariness, vigilance, physiological arousal, and emotional distress. *Positive emotionality* (PE), or *surgency*, is characterized by sensitivity to reward cues, approach, energy, involvement, sociability, and adventurousness. NE and PE, respectively, are conceptually related to negative (NA) and positive affectivity (PA; Clark & Watson, 1991), neuroticism and extraversion (Eysenck & Eysenck, 1985), the behavioral inhibition and activation systems (Gray, 1991), difficult temperament and activity/approach (Thomas & Chess, 1977), and harm avoidance and novelty seeking (Cloninger, 1987). Although different terms are used, these constructs share much conceptual and empirical overlap (see Klein, Durbin, & Shankman, Chapter 5, this volume).

The *tripartite model of anxiety and depression* (Clark & Watson, 1991) asserts that high levels of NA are associated with both depression and anxiety, whereas low levels of PA are uniquely related to depression, particularly anhedonia. Evidence consistent with this model has been found in children (e.g., Lonigan, Phillips, & Hooe, 2003; Phillips, Lonigan, Driscoll, & Hooe, 2002) and across different ethnic groups (Austin & Chorpita, 2004). In both clinical and nonclinical samples of children, low PA has been found to be a significant risk factor for depression, and low extraversion and low emotional stability predict internalizing problems (Van Leeuwen, Mervielde, De Clercq, & De Fruyt, 2007).

The *vulnerability model*, which posits that temperament places individuals at risk for depression, has found some empirical support in children (e.g., Caspi, Moffitt, Newman, & Silva, 1996; Goodwin, Fergusson, & Horwood, 2004; Nigg, 2006). For example, Caspi and colleagues (1996) reported that children rated as inhibited, socially reticent, and easily upset at age 3 had elevated rates of depressive disorders at age 21. Thus, temperamental characteristics, such as low positive mood and inhibition, have a direct relation with depressive symptoms in children.

The association between temperament and mood disorders differs by gender. Gjerde (1995) reported that shy and withdrawn behavior in girls and higher levels of undercontrolled behaviors in boys at ages 3 and 4 predicted chronic depression during adulthood. Parenting behaviors, such as rejection or inconsistent discipline, also moderate the relation between temperament and depression. In girls, the link between fearful temperament and depressive symptoms was stronger for those whose parents were rejecting, whereas parental warmth buffered against the relation between child frustration and internalizing problems (Oldehinkel, Veenstra, Ormel, de Winter, & Verhuls, 2006). Similarly, in a study of families undergoing divorce, among children experiencing high levels of parental rejection, low PE predicted higher levels of depressive symptoms, and impulsivity and depression were significantly associated in children receiving inconsistent parental discipline (Lengua, Wolchik, Sandler, & West, 2000). Interestingly, high levels of PE served as a buffer against the adverse effects of parental rejection on depression.

A bidirectional relation between child temperament and parenting also has been found, such that parental rejection and inconsistent discipline each predicted increases in children's NE (fear and irritability), child irritability predicted increases in inconsistent discipline by parents, higher effortful control predicted decreases in parental rejection (Lengua, 2006; Lengua & Kovacs, 2005), and high withdrawal predicted more negative interactions with parents and peers (Finch & Graziano, 2001). Lengua (2006) concluded that child temperament and parenting predicted changes in each other and in subsequent adjustment. Thus, the relation between child temperament and parenting may be best characterized as a transactional model of mutual influence that can contribute to the development of depression.

Temperament itself can be a *diathesis* that moderates the effect of other risk factors (e.g., stress) on depression. Under conditions of stress, negative affectivity has been shown to lead to greater emotional arousal, more difficulty modulating emotional reactivity to stress, and a greater likelihood of using avoidance coping (Compas et al., 2004). For example, among girls with more reactive temperament, peer rejection significantly predicted an increasing trajectory of depressed mood (Brendgen, Wanner, Morin, & Vitaro, 2005).

Temperament also may contribute to the development of the cognitive vulnerability to depression (e.g., Garber, 2007; Hankin & Abramson, 2001). Mezulis, Hyde, and Abramson (2006) reported that higher levels of withdrawal measured at ages 1 and 4 interact with recent life events to predict more negative cognitions in children at age 11. Similarly, low PE in early childhood predicted depressive cognitions in middle childhood (Hayden, Klein, & Durbin, 2005).

In summary, evidence is consistent with both the *vulnerability* (direct) and *pathoplasty* (indirect, interactional) models of the relation between temperament and depression. Any single model is not likely to capture fully the complex interplay between temperament and depression, and different dimensions of temperament (e.g., frustration, fear, shyness) may each fit different models of this relation (Ormel et al., 2005). Research focused on the biological and genetic components of temperament and psychopathology is needed.

Stressful Life Events and Trauma

Stress has a prominent role in most theories of depression, and a clear empirical association exists between stressful life events and depression in children (Grant et al., 2006). Indeed, the link between stress and depression emerges even before birth, as indicated by animal models showing that both antenatal and prepartum stress impact the developing physiology of the fetus, and later physiological and behavioral outcomes in offspring of stressed animals (see Goodman & Brand, Chapter 11, this volume).

In human infants, stress in the fetal environment can affect birthweight and the development of the LHPA axis, both of which may increase risk for depression (Austin, Leader, & Reilly, 2005; Gale & Martyn, 2004). Infants born to prenatally depressed mothers have been found to display high irritability and excessive crying (Lundy et al., 1999). Although the mechanisms by which stress impacts the developing fetus are not entirely understood, stress-induced hormonal changes in mothers, including elevated levels of CRH and cortisol, may lead to increased LHPA fetal activity, difficulty habituating to stimuli, temperamental difficulties, reduced birthweight, and slowed growth (Kapoor, Dunn, Kostaki, Andrews, & Matthews, 2006; Weinstock, 2005), making these infants more sensitive to stress and predisposing them to depression as they mature.

Depressive symptoms in babies, although rare, are associated with a stressful and changing environment, particularly separation from the mother between the ages of 6 and 8 months (Moreau, 1996). Infants' responses to separation are characterized by negative changes in sleep patterns, heart rate, activity, temperature, monoamine systems, and immune and endocrine function (Kalin & Carnes, 1984). *Hospitalism*, defined as infants subjected to long and frequent hospital stays, and earlier age of entering the hospital have been associated with more depressive symptoms in infants (Moreau, 1996).

In school-age children, depressive symptoms and disorders are significantly associated with both major and minor undesirable life events, particularly cumulative or chronic stressors, and negative life events are more prevalent among depressed compared to nondepressed children (e.g., Goodyer, Herbert, Tamplin, & Altham, 2000; Grant et al., 2006). Two models of this potentially bidirectional relation are *stress exposure* and *stress generation*. Whereas the stress exposure model posits that individuals who experience stressors are more likely to be depressed than those who have not (Brown, 1993), the stress generation model asserts that depressed individuals generate many of the stressors they encounter as a function of their own behavior, and these stressors serve to exacerbate and maintain depressive symptoms (Hammen, 1991). Indeed, some studies (Carter, Garber, Ciesla, & Cole, 2006; Cole, Nolen-Hoeksema, Girgus, & Paul, 2006; Gibb & Alloy, 2006) have found a reciprocal relation between stress and depression, incorporating both the stress generation and stress exposure models, and highlighting the "vicious cycle" between them.

Stress also has been found to predict the onset of both depressive symptoms in previously asymptomatic adolescents (Aseltine, Gore, & Colton, 1994) and clinically significant depressive episodes, controlling for prior symptom levels in children and adolescents (Garber, Martin, & Keiley, 2002; Goodyer et al., 2000; McFarlane, Bellissimo, Norman, & Lange, 1994; Monroe, Rohde, Seeley, & Lewinsohn, 1999). Only three of these studies (Aseltine et al., 1994; Garber et al., 2002; Monroe et al., 1999), however, controlled for lifetime history of MDD to rule out the possibility that earlier depressive disorder contributed to onset subsequently.

Stressful life events increase from childhood through adolescence, with girls reporting greater increases than boys (Garber, 2007; Ge, Lorenz, Conger, Elder, & Simons, 1994), paralleling increases in rates of depression during adolescence (Hankin, Abramson, Moffitt, Silva, & McGee, 1998). Few studies, however, have found that gender moderates the relation between stress and depression (although see Eberhart, Shih, Hammen, & Brennan, 2006). Ge and colleagues (1994) showed that an increasing trajectory of stressful life events predicted growth in depressive symptoms for girls but not for boys.

Although no specific stressful event invariably leads to depression, events occurring during childhood, such as loss, disappointment, separation, interpersonal conflict, and rejection (Goodyer et al., 2000; Monroe et al., 1999; Rueter, Scaramella, Wallace, & Conger, 1999), as well as parents' marital conflict and divorce, family violence, maltreatment, and economic disadvantage are particularly depressogenic (Eley & Stevenson, 2000; Gilman, Kawachi, Fitzmaurice, & Buka, 2003; Hankin, 2005; Reinherz, Paradis, Giaconia, Stashwick, & Fitzmaurice, 2003; Uhrlass & Gibb, 2007). Juvenile-onset depression also has been linked to childhood stressors such as more perinatal insults, parental criminal convictions, parental psychopathology, parent figure changes, and peer problems (before age 9), whereas adult-onset depression has been found to be associated with more residence changes and un-wanted sexual contact during childhood (Jaffee et al., 2002). Moreover, the relation between a family history of mood disorders and depression in preschoolers has been found to be mediated by stress (Luby, Belden, & Spitznagel, 2006).

Children facing multiple stressors are particularly at risk. A study of inner-city, low income, African American families revealed high rates of both neglect and conflict, and both were associated with depression in the children (Sagrestano, Paikoff, Holmbeck, & Fendrich, 2003). Possible mediators between sociocultural and economic disadvantage and depression include lack of access to adequate health care and educational opportunities, fewer social resources, and greater exposure to violence. Indeed, children living in lower SES conditions are most likely to witness violence and to be the victims of abuse themselves (Buka, Stichick, Birdthistle, & Earls, 2001).

Interpersonal stressors (e.g., rejection) are especially depressogenic for individuals who tend to be more socially dependent, or *sociotropic*. According to the *specific vulnerability hypothesis* (e.g., Beck, 1983), individuals who derive their self-esteem predominantly from interpersonal relationships (*sociotropy*) are at increased risk for depression when they experience stressors within the social domain. Evidence consistent with this hypothesis has been found in children (e.g., Hammen & Goodman-Brown, 1990; Little & Garber, 2000, 2005). For example, Little and Garber (2005) showed that youth who placed a high level of importance on interpersonal relationships were more susceptible to depressive symptoms following dependent social stressors than were those for whom interpersonal issues were less salient.

Another moderator of the stress–depression relation is social support. The interaction between genes and childhood maltreatment significantly predicts higher levels of depressive symptoms in children with low versus high social support, indicating that support may buffer against the vulnerability to depression resulting from this gene–environment interaction (Kaufman, Yang, Douglas-Palumberi, Grasso, et al., 2004; Kaufman, Yang, Douglas-Palumberi, Houshyar, et al., 2004). Moreover, in a sample of African American youth, Natsuaki and colleagues (2007) found that for children living in highly disordered neighborhoods (i.e., child exposure to gangs, harassment, drug dealing), supportive parenting (i.e., use of inductive reasoning) served as a protective factor for depressive symptoms.

Thus, stress often precedes mood disorders, although not all individuals exposed to the same stressors become depressed; that is, there is not a perfect correspondence between exposure to negative life events and the onset of depression. Rather, genetic vulnerability, as well as how individuals interpret and respond to events, differentiates who does and who does not become depressed. Some of this individual variability is due to differences in appraisals of the meaning of the events with regard to the self and future. Such appraisal processes are central to cognitive theories of depression.

Negative Cognitions

Consistent with cognitive-stress models of depression in adults (Abramson, Metalsky, & Alloy, 1989; Beck, 1967; see also Joorman, Chapter 13, this volume), depressed children report more hopelessness, cognitive distortions, cognitive errors, and more negative attributional styles compared to nondepressed children (Abela & Hankin, 2008). However, such concurrent covariation between negative cognitions and depression does not indicate whether cognitions are a concomitant, cause, and/or consequence of depression. Reviews of over 30 prospective studies (Abela & Hankin, 2008; Lakdawalla, Hankin, & Mermelstein,

2007) have found a small effect size for the relation between the cognitive vulnerability–stress interaction and elevations in depression among children (ages 8–12; partial correlation = .15) and a somewhat larger effect (partial correlation = .22) among adolescents (ages 13–19). Thus, the cognition × stress interaction may be a stronger predictor of depression in adolescents than children. This is consistent with the developmental hypothesis that depressive cognitions do not emerge until later childhood/early adolescence, when formal operational thinking is developing, and that the relation of the cognitive vulnerability to depression becomes stronger with increasing age (e.g., Abela, 2001; Cole et al., 2008; Turner & Cole, 1994; Weisz et al., 2001). In addition, mixed evidence regarding the applicability of cognitive/diathesis–stress models of depression to children likely is partially due to use of assessment methods that do not consider sufficiently the cognitive developmental level of the children being studied. For example, questionnaires that require metacognitive skills, self-reflection, or perspective taking may not be appropriate for young children.

Evidence also is inconsistent regarding the stability of negative cognitions, particularly after recovery from a depressive episode (e.g., Just, Abramson, & Alloy, 2001). Whereas some studies have not found differences in the cognitive styles of remitted versus nondepressed children (Asarnow & Bates, 1988; McCauley, Mitchell, Burke, & Moss, 1988), studies using priming techniques have shown evidence of a stable cognitive vulnerability in children (e.g., Scher, Ingram, & Segal, 2005; Timbremont & Braet, 2004). Priming negative affect in children may be important for accessing latent maladaptive cognitive structures that contribute to depression.

The relation of cognitive vulnerability to depression also may depend on the specific type of cognitions. Abela (2001) suggested that inferential styles about consequences and the self may develop earlier than causal attributions, which require more abstract, higher-order thinking. In addition, Abela (Abela & Payne, 2003; Abela & Sarin, 2002) proposed the *weakest link hypothesis*, which asserts that individuals are as vulnerable to depression as their most negative inferential style makes them. Indeed, Abela and Payne (2003) showed that children's most depressive inferential style—about causes, consequences, or the self—interacted with negative events to predict increases in depressive symptoms. The weakest link approach may explain some of the inconsistencies in past research on cognitive–stress models of depression in children.

Cognitive vulnerability also has been found in high-risk offspring of depressed parents. Children of depressed mothers report significantly lower self-worth and a more negative attributional style than do children of nondepressed mothers (e.g., Garber & Robinson, 1997; Murray, Woolgar, Cooper, & Hipwell, 2001). Garber and Robinson (1997) showed that offspring of mothers with more chronic depression reported significantly more negative cognitions than did children of mothers with no history of psychiatric disorders, even when children's current level of depressive symptoms was controlled. Thus, children who have not yet experienced depression themselves, but who are at risk, report more negative cognitions that likely serve as a vulnerability to the onset of depression.

Possible mechanisms through which negative cognitions develop include modeling of parents' negative beliefs, dysfunctional parent–child relationships, exposure to stressful life events, and feedback from others (Garber & Martin, 2002). Several studies (Bruce et al., 2006; Garber & Flynn, 2001; Gibb & Alloy, 2006; Mezulis et al., 2006) have found that negative life events, as well as interpersonal difficulties, predict depressive cognitions. For example, in a study of children followed from infancy through fifth grade, peer harassment predicted negative cognitions, and a significant interaction between mothers' negative attributions and negative life events predicted children's negative cognitions (Mezulis et al., 2006).

The experience of depression itself also can lead to depressive cognitions (Haines, Metalsky, Cardamone, & Joiner, 1999; Nolen-Hoeksema, Girgus, & Seligman, 1992). Nolen-Hoeksema and colleagues (1992) suggested that depression during childhood can lead to the development of a pessimistic explanatory style, which remains even after the depression has remitted. Consistent with this perspective, Cole, Martin, Peeke, Seroczynski, and Hoffman (1998; Hoffman, Cole, Martin, Tram, & Seroczynski, 2000) showed that the relation between depressive symptoms and perceived competence in children is bidirectional.

Identification of the specific types of cognitive vulnerabilities that contribute to the onset, maintenance, and recurrence of depressive episodes in children require further study. In addition, more research is needed that maps out the origins of cognitive vulnerability and the developmental trajectories of various negative cognitions and their relation to depression over the life course.

Self-Regulation

Self-regulation is the way in which one stimulates, modifies, or manages thoughts, affects and behaviors through biological, cognitive, social, and/or behavioral means (Calkins, 1994; Thomson, 1994). In infancy, caregivers provide initial regulation until children begin to learn self-soothing behaviors (e.g., sucking, head turning). As children develop, they acquire gross motor skills and cognitive abilities that improve self-regulation by facilitating their ability to monitor and exert control over their behaviors (Cole, Martin, & Dennis, 2004).

Coping is a form of self-regulation activated in times of stress (Compas, Connor-Smith, Saltzman, Thomsen, & Wadsworth, 2001; Eisenberg, Fabes, & Guthrie, 1997). Eisenberg and colleagues (1997) distinguished among three categories of coping: emotion regulation, problem-focused coping, and behavioral regulation. *Emotion regulation* refers to direct attempts to manage affect; *problem-focused coping* includes attempts to regulate the situation; and *behavioral regulation* involves managing behaviors resulting from emotional arousal. Compas and colleagues (2001) expanded this definition of coping to incorporate attempts to regulate emotion, cognition, behavior, physiology, and the environment, and emphasized that coping involves volitional and intentional responses to stress, whereas involuntary or automatic reactions reflect individual differences in temperament. Compas and colleagues also distinguished between *engagement coping* (i.e., problem solving, cognitive restructuring, positive reappraisal, distraction) and *disengagement coping* (i.e., avoidance, self-blame, emotional discharge, rumination).

Eisenberg, Fabes, Guthrie, and Reiser (2000; Eisenberg et al., 2004) showed that (1) behavior regulation predicted socially appropriate behavior, (2) this relation was moderated by negative emotionality, and (3) two dimensions of self-regulation—effortful control and impulsivity—predicted resiliency 2 years later in children ages 4–8. Moreover, low attention regulation and low impulsivity were associated with internalizing symptoms, whereas high impulsivity, low attention focusing, and low inhibitory control were associated with externalizing symptoms (Eisenberg et al., 2001). Lengua and Sandler (1996) similarly showed that attention regulation and inhibitory control are related to higher social competence. Children with stronger self-regulation skills may be better able to delay maladaptive responses and to use active coping strategies in response to stressful situations.

In their review, Compas and colleagues (2001) reported that engagement coping is associated with lower internalizing and externalizing symptoms, whereas disengagement coping is associated with higher symptom levels. For example, in a sample of children ages 9–12, active coping predicted fewer depressive symptoms, whereas avoidant coping predicted higher levels of depressive symptoms (Lengua, Sandler, West, Wolchick, & Curran, 1999). Many studies have been cross-sectional, however, limiting our ability to draw conclusions about the direction of the coping–depression relation. Just as coping can reduce emotional distress, emotional distress can affect coping. For example, children who are less depressed may be better at generating solutions to problems and maintaining a positive outlook when faced with stress.

Studies examining the relation between self-regulation and depression in children have highlighted the importance of examining gender and context. Garber, Braafladt, and Weiss (1995) found that depressed girls reported using problem solving in interpersonal situations less than did nondepressed girls. In achievement situations, depressed children of both genders reported using fewer support-seeking, cognitive, and affect change strategies than did nondepressed children. In a sample of 4- to 7-year-old children at risk for depression, Silk, Shaw, Forbes, Lane, and Kovacs (2006) showed that positive reward anticipation in the context of a negative emotion–inducing task was associated with lower internalizing problems, and this link was stronger for children of depressed compared to nondepressed mothers. This latter result highlights the potential protective effect of self-regulatory behavior for children at risk for depression.

In summary, deficiencies in self-regulatory skills have been associated with a range of adverse outcomes in children. Prospective research is needed to characterize the direction of the relation between self-regulation and depression, and to identify deficits in self-regulation that are specific to different outcomes.

Interpersonal Relationships

Parents

Interpersonal perspectives on depression emphasize the importance of the social environment (Gotlib & Hammen, 1992). According to attachment theory (Bowlby, 1980), children with caretakers who are consistently accessible and supportive develop cognitive representations, or *working models*, of the self and others as positive and trustworthy. In contrast, unresponsive or inconsistent caretakers produce insecure attachments, leading to working models that include abandonment, self-criticism, and excessive dependency. Such insecure attachment increases the child's vulnerability to depression, particularly when exposed to new interpersonal stressors. Securely attached toddlers have been found to be more cooperative, persistent, enthusiastic, and higher functioning (Matas, Arend, & Sroufe, 1978), and when exposed to stress show lower levels of depressive symptoms as children (Abela et al., 2005).

Beyond attachment, other kinds of dysfunctional interpersonal patterns, especially serious abuse and neglect, are associated with depression in infants and children (Kaslow, Deering, & Racusin, 1994; Trad, 1994). Maltreatment leads to avoidant or resistant attachments and withdrawal behaviors in infants, self-esteem deficits in childhood, and increased risk of subsequent abuse (e.g., Lamb, Gaensbauer, Malkin, & Schultz, 1985). Moreover, a consistent relation has been found between childhood emotional abuse and depressive cognitive styles (Gibb, 2002).

Parenting dimensions particularly associated with depression in children are control–autonomy and acceptance–rejection (e.g., Barber, 1996). Currently depressed children describe their parents as controlling, rejecting, and unavailable (e.g., Stein et al., 2000), and perceive their families to have less cohesion and greater conflict than do nondepressed youth (e.g., Garrison, Jackson, Marsteller, McKeown, & Addy, 1990). Children's ratings of parents' psychologically controlling behavior predict children's depressive symptoms over and above prior depression levels (Barber, 1996). Children's prior depressive symptoms, however, also predict their ratings of parents' behavior. Mothers of depressed children similarly describe themselves as more rejecting, less communicative, and less affectionate than do mothers of both nondepressed and psychiatric controls (e.g., Puig-Antich et al., 1985a), and maternal hostile childrearing attitudes predict increases in children's depression (Katainen, Raikkonen, Keskivaara, & Keltikangas-Jarvinen, 1999).

Observational studies have shown that lower levels of parental warmth and higher levels of maternal hostility predict higher levels of internalizing symptoms in youth (Ge, Best, Conger, & Simons, 1996), and escalating parent–child conflict predicts increases in adolescents' internalizing symptoms (Rueter et al., 1999). Mothers of depressed children also have been observed to be less rewarding (Cole & Rehm, 1986), and more dominant and controlling (Amanat & Butler, 1984) than mothers of nondepressed children. Levels of maternal criticism of children have been coded to be highest for mothers of depressed children compared to mothers of children with ADHD or healthy controls (Asarnow, Tompson, Woo, & Cantwell, 2001). Thus, convergence among children's, parents', and observers' ratings indicates that families of depressed children are characterized by considerable dysfunction.

Interpersonal difficulties persist even after depression has resolved. Some improvement in the mother–child relationship has been found with remission, although even without symptoms, children continue to have interpersonal difficulties, particularly with siblings (Puig-Antich et al., 1985b). Social adversities, such as persistent poor friendships, low involvement of fathers, stressful family environments, and lack of responsiveness to maternal discipline, contribute to the maintenance or relapse of depressive disorders in youth (e.g., McCauley et al., 1993) and negative attitudes by family members toward depressed children predict relapse (Asarnow, Goldstein, Tompson, & Guthrie, 1993).

Some evidence is consistent with a transactional perspective on the relation between parenting and children's depression; that is, children's and parents' behaviors influence each other reciprocally (Elgar, Curtis, McGrath, Waschbusch, & Stewart, 2003; Sagrestano et al., 2003). For example, a 4-year, cross-lagged panel study of children ages 0–14 found that maternal depressive symptoms often precede child aggression and hyperactivity, whereas child emotional problems precede maternal depressive symptoms (Elgar et al., 2003).

Relationships between depressed parents and their children consistently have been found to be disrupted (Hammen, Chapter 12, this volume). Such difficulties are one important mechanism of the intergenerational transmission of depression (Goodman & Gotlib, 1999). Bifulco and colleagues (2002) showed that the relation between maternal and child depression was mediated by children's report of neglect and abuse (see also Hammen, Shih, & Brennan, 2004; Leinonen, Solantaus, & Punamaki, 2003). In contrast, Kim, Capaldi, and Stoolmiller (2003; see also Frye & Garber, 2005; Jones, Forehand, & Neary, 2001) found that observed parenting practices did not mediate the effects of parental depression on the development of depressive symptoms in young men 10 years later, when earlier behavior problems were controlled.

Finally, children's depressive cognitions may mediate the relation between parenting behaviors and child depression (Abela, Skitch, Adams, & Hankin, 2006; Gibb & Alloy, 2006; Gibb et al., 2001; McGinn, Cukor, & Sanderson, 2005). McGinn and colleagues (2005) found that self-reported childhood experiences of parental abuse and neglect were associated with higher depressive symptoms, and dysfunctional cognitive style partially mediated this relation. Similarly, Gibb and colleagues (2001) reported that negative cognitive style partially mediated the relation between emotional maltreatment in childhood and episodes of depression during young adulthood.

Peers

Depressed children have significant peer difficulties and social skills deficits (e.g., Altmann & Gotlib, 1988), have poorer friendships (Goodyer, Wright, & Altham, 1990), view themselves as less socially competent (Rudolph, Hammen, & Burge, 1997), are rated by teachers as being rejected by their peers more than are nondepressed children (Rudolph, Hammen & Burge, 1994), and are rated more negatively by their peers (Peterson, Mullins, & Ridley-Johnson, 1985). Rejection by peers has been found to predict higher levels of self-reported depressive symptoms among antisocial, but not among nonantisocial, youth (French, Conrad, & Turner, 1995).

Cole, Martin, and colleagues (1998) showed that depressed children perceived their social acceptance more unfavorably than did their peers. Moreover, *perceived* rejection, even more than actual peer rejection, predicts increases in depressive symptoms in elementary school children (e.g., Kistner, Balthazor, Risi, & Burton, 1999; Panak & Garber, 1992). In addition, regardless of how well a child is actually liked by peers, those with high levels of rejection sensitivity are more likely to experience internalizing problems (Sandstrom, Cillessen, & Eisenhower, 2003).

These studies are consistent with a *cognitive distortion model of depression*, in which depressed children perceive themselves and their peer relationships more negatively than the actual situation warrants. Depressed children not only think that they are less accepted by their peers and have a lower friendship quality with their best friends, but they also have a more negative and biased view of their social acceptance and friendship quality compared to their friends (Brendgen, Vitaro, Turgeon, & Poulin, 2002). In a sample of children in grades 5 and 6, Rudolph and Clark (2001) found actual social skills deficits (e.g., withdrawal) in depressed children, as well as overly negative views of their social status. The perception of rejection and negative cognitive bias may result in withdrawn or hostile behavior (Renouf & Harter, 1990), which may in turn elicit actual negative interactions with peers. This then reinforces the depressed child's negative perceptions, thereby creating a self-perpetuating cycle of cognitive distortions, negative social interactions, and depression.

The types of friends with whom children associate also may contribute to the development and course of depression. In a sample of children followed from third to fifth grade, children's self-reported friendships with highly aggressive children were associated with higher levels of depression across the 2 years, controlling for initial depression levels (Mrug, Hoza, & Bukowski, 2004). Connell and Dishion (2006) also showed that spending time with peers who engaged in delinquent behaviors predicted elevations in self-reported depressive symptoms assessed monthly. Depressed children might associate with delinquent peers for a sense of belonging not found in their broader social network, but this deviant peer group typically gives low positive feedback, which then may further increase their depression (Brendgen, Vitaro, & Bukowski, 2000).

Overall, families with a depressed member tend to be characterized by less support and more conflict, and such family dysfunction increases children's risk of developing depression. Moreover, depressed children often are themselves more interpersonally difficult, which can exacerbate problems in their social network. Thus, the relation between child depression and interpersonal dysfunction is bidirectional. Family and peer environments clearly are important and sometimes stressful contexts in which children develop schemas about themselves and others that can then serve as a vulnerability to depression. Stice, Ragan, and Randall (2004), in a prospective study of children ages 11–15, found that deficits in perceived parental support, but not peer support, predicted increases in depressive symptoms, and depressive symptoms in turn predicted decreases in peer, but not parental, support. Depressed children's reactions to their environments can exacerbate and perpetuate negative social exchanges, which furthers the interpersonal vicious cycle, thereby resulting in more rejection and depression (Coyne, 1976). Thus, a transactional model of mutual influence probably best characterizes the association between depressed individuals and their social environment.

CONCLUSIONS AND FUTURE DIRECTIONS

Depressive symptoms and disorders are an important concern even during childhood. Although diagnosed mood disorders are relatively rare in young children, symptoms of depression can be found from infancy through preadolescence. During middle childhood, depressive disorders can be diagnosed, but are still less prevalent than during adolescence. Although many symptoms that comprise the syndrome of depression are similar at all ages, noteworthy differences in the phenomenology and structure of depressive syndrome can be found in children and adults. Nevertheless, depressive episodes during childhood tend to show a course similar to that found in adults. Also, during childhood, comorbidity of depression with other forms of psychopathology is the rule rather than the exception.

Several important questions remain with regard to depression in children. First, do infants and toddlers actually experience full depressive episodes? Epidemiological studies are needed that not only assess diagnoses but also measure a range of symptoms that may be age-appropriate manifestations of mood disorders in children. Whether such symptom patterns represent depressive disorders would then need to be determined by examining both their continuity across time and their construct validity; that is, their relation to theoretically derived etiological correlates (e.g., neurobiological dysregulation, stress). Additionally, what accounts for increases in depression from pre- to postadolescence? What changes from childhood to adolescence, or what protects children? What accounts for the shift in the sex ratio around puberty? Are there ethnic/racial and cultural differences in the rates of mood disorders in children, and if so, why?

With regard to phenomenology, what is the structure of depression in children, and how does this differ from that of adolescents and adults? What accounts for changes in this structure over time? What is the normative developmental trajectory of depressive symptoms (e.g., irritability, anhedonia, fatigue), and how do such changes affect the syndrome of depression in children versus adolescents? What influences the course and outcome of depressive disorders across development? What sustains depressive symptoms, and why do they remit? Are early-onset depressions more or less severe, recurrent, and familial than later-onset depressions? Do the same processes that underlie first-onset mood disorders explain relapses and recurrences? What accounts for the high rate of comorbidity of depression with other psychopathology during childhood? What are the best methods for assessing depressive symptoms at different ages, and how should discrepancies across informants be resolved?

With regard to etiology, some evidence is consistent with the various biological and psychosocial models of depression. One way to deal with such etiological heterogeneity has been to suggest specific subtypes that map onto different causal processes (Abramson et al., 1989; Winokur, 1997). Winokur (1997) proposed that unipolar depression can be divided into endogenous, reactive, and emotionally unstable forms on the basis of differences on clinical, follow-up, personality, familial, and treatment variables. Another approach has been to formulate integrated models of depression that include the additive or interactive effects of multiple risk factors (e.g., Akiskal & McKinney, 1975; Kendler, Gardner, & Prescott, 2002). Akiskal and McKinney suggested that most distal causal processes (e.g., stress, low rates of positive reinforcement) went through a common final neuroanatomical pathway. Diathesis–stress models highlight that person characteristics, such as genetic or cognitive vulnerability, interact with environmental stressors to produce depression (Abramson et al., 1989; Beck, 1967; Caspi et al., 2003; Kendler et al., 1995; Monroe & Simons, 1991). Interpersonal cognitive approaches (e.g., Gotlib & Hammen, 1992) suggest that cognitions about important social relationships may be a risk for depression when negative interpersonal events occur. Negative cognitive schemas about the self and others may be the result of earlier attachment and interpersonal difficulties. Conversely, Ingram, Miranda, and Segal (1998) posited that cognitive processes are the common final pathway through which all social and nonsocial information is processed and linked to depression.

A broad, reciprocal, and dynamic biopsychosocial model of depression that incorporates the various etiological processes discussed here needs to be tested further (Garber, 2007). According to this perspective, children are born with certain biological propensities, such as stress reactivity or an irritable temperament, that make them more vulnerable to the effects of negative life events or less able to obtain help from others to deal with them. As children grow, they learn in part through interactions with others the extent to which they are capable of coping effectively with stressors, and whether others can be counted on for support. Children also learn through such interactions whether they are worthy of others' love and support. Exposure to stressful life events can activate negative affective structures that connect with developing negative schemas about the self and others (Ingram et al., 1998). A cycle begins in which children develop some symptoms of depression (e.g., low self-esteem, anhedonia), which then lead to their being exposed to further stressors, such as interpersonal rejection and academic failure. Also, exposure to chronic or severe stressors can produce biological changes that further maintain or exacerbate the depressive symptoms. Thus, this is a *mediated moderation model* (Baron & Kenny, 1986). Individual diatheses moderate the relation between stress and depression, and contribute to the manner in which the child responds to negative life events; such specific responses to stress then mediate the effect of the individual diatheses on subsequent depression. Individuals with particular biological and/or psychological "depressogenic" vulnerabilities who encounter stressful events and respond ineffectively, so that the stressor is not adequately managed, then develop depression. Once present, depressive symptoms can feed back to the person's biology and cognitions, as well as alter the context in such a way as to generate even more stressors, and so the cycle continues. This *scarring* (Lewinsohn, Allen, Seeley, & Gotlib, 1999) or *kindling* hypothesis (Post, 1992), results in dynamic changes in these biopsychosocial systems over time.

What needs to be done next? First, future studies should test multivariate etiological models. Such investigations should not simply examine the independent contribution of individual risk factors, but should test more complex moderator and mediator models that explore how these various vulnerability factors synergistically combine to explain the onset of depression. Second, testing such multivariate *models* will allow us to examine specificity. Just because a particular risk factor (e.g., stress) predicts more than one disorder (e.g., anxiety and depression) does not mean that the risk factor cannot be part of a more complex causal model (Garber & Hollon, 1991). The issue of specificity only can be addressed by comparing multivariate models rather than individual risk factors.

Third, multiple research strategies should be used. For example, studies can compare currently depressed, remitted, high-risk, and never-depressed children with regard to these multilevel models, then follow these groups over time to examine temporal precedence in the relations among the hypothesized etiological variables to the onset, maintenance, and recurrence of depression. Finally, experimental designs that randomly assign children from each of these groups (i.e., currently depressed, remitted, high-risk, never-depressed) to both singular and multimodal interventions can be used to examine processes of change. In addition, laboratory analogue studies that experimentally manipulate specific processes are needed to understand causal mechanisms.

One final fundamental question is whether depressive vulnerabilities are permanent characteristics of individuals, and by what internal and external mechanisms are they turned on and off? That is, what biological, psychosocial, and/or environmental processes set off vulnerabilities to produce depressive symptoms and episodes, and conversely, how do we explain the remission of symptoms? Do vulnerable individuals no longer have the risk factor(s), or do they develop mechanisms that compensate for them?

ACKNOWLEDGEMENTS

This work was supported in part by grants from the National Institute of Mental Health (Nos. K02 MH66249, R01MH64735, and R01MH57822) and from the William T. Grant Foundation (No. 961730).

REFERENCES

Abela, J. R. Z. (2001). The hopelessness theory of depression: A test of the diathesis-stress model and causal mediation of components in third and seventh grade children. *Journal of Abnormal Child Psychology, 29,* 241–254.

Abela, J. R. Z., & Hankin, B. L. (2008). Cognitive vulnerability to depression in children and adolescents: A developmental perspective. In J. R. Z. Abela & B. L. Hankin (Eds.), *Handbook of depression in children and adolescents* (pp. 35–78). New York: Guilford Press.

Abela, J. R. Z., Hankin, B. L., Haigh, E. A. P., Adams, P., Vinokuroff, T., & Trayhern, L. (2005). Interpersonal vulnerability to depression in high-risk children: The role of insecure attachment and reassurance seeking. *Journal of Clinical Child and Adolescent Psychology, 34,* 182–192.

Abela, J. R. Z., & Payne, A. V. L. (2003). A test of the integration of the hopelessness and self-esteem theories of depression in school children. *Cognitive Therapy and Research, 27,* 519–535.

Abela, J. R. Z., & Sarin, S. (2002). Cognitive vulnerability to hopelessness depression: A chain is only as strong as its weakest link. *Cognitive Therapy and Research, 26,* 811–829.

Abela, J. R. Z., Skitch, S. A., Adams, P., & Hankin, B. L. (2006). The timing of parent and child depression: A hopelessness theory perspective. *Journal of Clinical Child and Adolescent Psychology, 35,* 253–263.

Abramson, L. Y., Metalsky, G. I., & Alloy, L. B. (1989). Hopelessness depression: A theory-based subtype of depression. *Psychological Review, 96,* 358–372.

Achenbach, T. M., & Edelbrock, C. S. (1986). *Manual for the Teacher's Report Form and Teacher Version of the Child Behavior Profile.* Burlington: University of Vermont.

Achenbach, T. M., & Edelbrock, C. S. (1991). *Manual for the Child Behavior Checklist and 1991 Profile.* Burlington: University of Vermont.

Achenbach, T. M., McConaughy, S. H., & Howell, C. T. (1987). Child/adolescent behavioral and emotional problems: Implications of cross-informant correlations for situational specificity. *Psychological Bulletin, 101*, 213–232.

Akiskal, H. S., & McKinney, W. T. (1975). Overview of recent research in depression: Integration of ten conceptual models into a comprehensive clinical framework. *Archives of General Psychiatry, 32*, 285–305.

Altmann, E. O., & Gotlib, I. H. (1988). The social behavior of depressed children: An observational study. *Journal of Abnormal Child Psychology, 16*, 29–44.

Amanat, E., & Butler, C. (1984). Oppressive behaviors in the families of depressed children. *Family Therapy, 11*, 65–75.

Ambrosini, P. J. (2000). Historical development and present status of the Schedule for Affective Disorders and Schizophrenia for School-Age Children (K-SADS). *Journal of the American Academy of Child and Adolescent Psychiatry, 39*, 49–58.

American Psychiatric Association. (1994). *Diagnostic and statistical manual of mental disorders* (4th ed.). Washington, DC: American Psychiatric Association.

Angold, A., & Costello, E. J. (2000). The Child and Adolescent Psychiatric Assessment (CAPA). *Journal of the American Academy of Child and Adolescent Psychiatry, 39*, 39–48.

Angold, A., Costello, E. J., & Erkanli, A. (1999). Comorbidity. *Journal of Child Psychology and Psychiatry and Allied Disciplines, 40*, 57–87.

Angold, A., Costello, E. J., Pickles, A., Messer, S. C., Winder, F., & Silver, D. (1995). The development of a short questionnaire for use in epidemiological studies of depression in children and adolescents. *International Journal of Methods in Psychiatric Research, 5*, 237–249.

Angold, A., Costello, E. J., & Worthman, C. M. (1998). Puberty and depression: The roles of age, pubertal status and pubertal timing. *Psychological Medicine, 28*, 51–61.

Angold, A., & Rutter, M. (1992). Effects of age and pubertal status on depression in a large clinical sample. *Development and Psychopathology, 4*, 5–28.

Armitage, R., Hoffmann, R. F., Emslie, G. J., Weinberg, W. A., Mayes, T. L., & Rush, A. J. (2002). Sleep microarchitecture as a predictor of recurrence in children and adolescents with depression. *International Journal of Neuropsychopharmacology, 5*, 217–228.

Asarnow, J. R., & Bates, S. (1988). Depression in child psychiatric inpatients: Cognitive and attributional patterns. *Journal of Abnormal Child Psychology, 16*, 601–615.

Asarnow, J. R., Goldstein, M. J., Tompson, M., & Guthrie, D. (1993). One-year outcomes of depressive disorders in child psychiatric in-patients: Evaluation of the prognostic power of a brief measure of expressed emotion. *Journal of Child Psychology and Psychiatry and Allied Disciplines, 34*, 129–137.

Asarnow, J. R., Tompson, M., Woo, S., & Cantwell, D. P. (2001). Is expressed emotion a specific risk factor for depression or a nonspecific correlate of psychopathology? *Journal of Abnormal Child Psychology, 29*(6), 573–583.

Aseltine, R., Gore, S., & Colton, M. E. (1994). Depression and the social developmental context of adolescence. *Journal of Personality and Social Psychology, 67*, 252–263.

Austin, A. A., & Chorpita, B. F. (2004). Temperament, anxiety, and depression: Comparisons across five ethnic groups of children. *Journal of Clinical Child and Adolescent Psychology, 33*, 216–226.

Austin, M. P., Leader, L. R., & Reilly, N. (2005). Prenatal stress, the hypothalamic–pituitary–adrenal axis, and fetal and infant neurobehaviour. *Early Human Development, 81*, 917–926.

Avenevoli, S., & Steinberg, L. (2001). The continuity of depression across the adolescent tradition. In H. Reese & R. Kail (Eds.), *Advances in child development and behavior* (pp. 139–173). San Diego, CA: Academic Press.

Barber, B. K. (1996). Parental psychological control: Revisiting a neglected construct. *Child Development, 67*, 3296–3319.

Baron, R. M., & Kenny, D. A. (1986). The moderator-mediator variable distinction in social psychological research: Conceptual, strategic, and statistical considerations. *Journal of Personality and Social Psychology, 51*, 1173–1182.

Bartels, M., van den Oord, E. J., Hudziak, J. J., Rietveld, M. J., van Beijsterveldt, C. E., & Boomsma, D. I. (2004). Genetic and environmental mechanisms underlying stability and change in problem behaviors at ages 3, 7, 10 and 12. *Developmental Psychology, 40*, 852–867.

Beck, A. T. (1967). *Depression: Clinical, experiential, and theoretical aspects.* New York: Harper & Row.

Beck, A. T. (1983). Cognitive therapy of depression: New perspectives. In P. J. Clayton & J. E. Barrett (Eds.), *Treatment of depression: Old controversies and new approaches* (pp. 265–290). New York: Raven Press.

Berndt, D. J., Petzel, T. P., & Berndt, S. M. (1980). Development and initial evaluation of a multiscore depression inventory. *Journal of Personality Assessment, 44,* 396–403.

Bertocci, M. A., Dahl, R. E., Williamson, D. E., Iosif, A., Birmaher, B., Axelson, D., et al. (2005). Subjective sleep complaints in pediatric depression: A controlled study and comparison with EEG measures of sleep and waking. *Journal of the American Academy of Child and Adolescent Psychiatry, 44,* 1158–1166.

Bifulco, A. T., Moran, P. M., Ball, C., Jacobs, C., Bains, R., Bunn, A., et al. (2002). Child adversity, parental vulnerability and disorder: Examination of inter-generational transmission of risk. *Journal of Child Psychology and Psychiatry and Allied Disciplines, 43,* 1075–1086.

Birleson, P. (1981). The validity of depressive disorder in childhood and the development of a self-rating scale: A research report. *Journal of Child Psychology and Psychiatry, 22,* 73–88.

Birmaher, B., Arbelaez, C., & Brent, D. (2002). Course and outcome of child and adolescent major depressive disorder. *Child and Adolescent Psychiatric Clinics of North America, 11,* 619–637.

Birmaher, B., Dahl, R. E., Williamson, D. E., Perel, J. M., Brent, D. A., Axelson, D. A., et al. (2000). Growth hormone secretion in children and adolescents at high risk for major depressive disorder. *Archives of General Psychiatry, 57,* 867–872.

Birmaher, B., Kaufman, J., Brent, D. A., Dahl, R. E., Perel, J. M., Al-Shabbout, M., et al. (1997). Neuroendocrine response to 5-hydroxy-L-tryptophan in prepubertal children at high risk of major depressive disorder. *Archives of General Psychiatry, 54,* 1113–1119.

Birmaher, B., Ryan, N. D., Williamson, D. E., Brent, D. A., Kaufman, J., Dahl, R. E., et al. (1996). Childhood and adolescent depression: A review of the past 10 years. Part I. *Journal of the American Academy of Child and Adolescent Psychiatry, 35,* 1427–1439.

Birmaher, B., Williamson, D., Dahl, R. E., Axelson, D. A., Kaufman, J., Dorn, L. D., et al. (2004). Clinical presentation and course of depression in youth: Does onset in childhood differ from onset in adolescence? *Journal of the American Academy of Child and Adolescent Psychiatry, 43,* 63–70.

Bonari, L., Pinto, N., Ahn, E., Einarson, A., Steiner, M., & Koren, G. (2004). Perinatal risks of untreated depression during pregnancy. *Canadian Journal of Psychiatry, 49,* 726–735.

Bonte, F. J., Trivedi, M. H., Devous, M. D., Sr., Harris, T. S., Payne, J. K., Weinberg, W. A., et al. (2001). Occipital brain perfusion deficits in children with major depressive disorder. *Journal of Nuclear Medicine, 42,* 1059–1061.

Botteron, K. N., Raichle, M. E., Drevets, W. C., Heath, A. C., & Todd, R. D. (2002). Volumetric reduction in left subgenual prefrontal cortex in early onset depression. *Biological Psychiatry, 51,* 342–344.

Bowlby, J. (1980). *Attachment and loss: Vol. 3. Loss, sadness, and depression.* New York: Basic Books.

Brendgen, M., Vitaro, F., & Bukowski, W. (2000). Deviant friends and early adolescents' emotional and behavioral adjustment. *Journal of Research on Adolescence, 10,* 173–189.

Brendgen, M., Vitaro, F., Turgeon, L., & Poulin, F. (2002). Assessing aggressive and depressed children's social relations with classmates and friends: A matter of perspective. *Journal of Abnormal Child Psychology, 30,* 609–624.

Brendgen, M., Wanner, B., Morin, A. J. S., & Vitaro, F. (2005). Relations with parents and with peers, temperament, and trajectories of depressed mood during early adolescence. *Journal of Abnormal Child Psychology, 33,* 579–594.

Brown, G. W. (1993). Life events and affective disorder: Replications and limitations. *Psychosomatic Medicine, 55,* 248–259.

Bruce, A. E., Cole, D. A., Dallaire, D. H., Jacquez, F. M., Pineda, A. Q., & LaGrange, B. (2006). Relations of parenting and negative life events to cognitive diatheses for depression in children. *Journal of Abnormal Child Psychology, 34,* 321–333.

Buka, S. L., Stichick, T. L., Birdthistle, I., & Earls, F. J. (2001). Youth exposure to violence: Prevalence, risks, and consequences. *American Journal of Orthopsychiatry, 71,* 298–310.

Calkins, S. (1994). Origins and outcomes of individual differences in emotion regulation. *Monographs of the Society for Research in Child Development, 59,* 53–72.

Canino, G., Shrout, P. E., Rubio-Stipec, M., Bird, H. R., Bravo, M. Ramirez, R., et al. (2004). DSM-IV rates of child and adolescent disorders in Puerto Rico. *Archives of General Psychiatry, 61*, 85–93.

Carey, M. P., Faulstich, M. E., Gresham, F. M., Ruggiero, L., & Enyart, P. (1987). Children's Depression Inventory: Construct and discriminant validity across clinical and nonreferred (control) populations. *Journal of Consulting and Clinical Psychology, 55*, 755–761.

Carter, J. S., Garber, J., Ciesla, J. A., & Cole, D. A. (2006). Modeling relations between hassles and internalizing and externalizing symptoms in adolescents: A four-year prospective study. *Journal of Abnormal Psychology, 115*, 428–442.

Caspi, A., Henry, B., McGee, R. O., Moffitt, T. E., & Silva, P. A. (1995). Temperamental origins of child and adolescent behavior problems: From age three to age fifteen. *Child Development, 66*, 55–68.

Caspi, A., Moffitt, T. E., Newman, D. L., & Silva, P. A. (1996). Behavioral observations at age 3 years predict adult psychiatric disorders: Longitudinal evidence from a birth cohort. *Archives of General Psychiatry, 53*, 1033–1039.

Caspi, A., Sugden, K., Moffitt, T. E., Taylor, A., Craig, I. W., Harrington, H., et al. (2003). Influence of life stress on depression: Moderation by a polymorphism in the 5-HTT gene. *Science, 301*, 386–389.

Cicchetti, D., & Posner, M. I. (2005). Cognitive and affective neuroscience and developmental psychopathology *evelopment and Psychopathology, 17*, 569–575.

Clark, L. A., & Watson, D. (1991). Tripartite model of anxiety and depression: Psychometric evidence and taxonomic implications. *Journal of Abnormal Psychology, 100*, 316–336.

Cloninger, C. R. (1987). A systematic method for clinical description and classification of personality variants: A proposal. *Archives of General Psychiatry, 44*, 573–588.

Cole, D. A. (1991). Preliminary support for a competency based model of depression in children. *Journal of Abnormal Psychology, 100*, 181–190.

Cole, D. A., Ciesla, J., Dallaire, D. H., Jacquez, F. M., Pineda, A., LaGrange, B., et al. (2008). Emergence of attributional style and its relation to depressive symptoms. *Journal of Abnormal Psychology, 117*, 16–31.

Cole, D. A., Hoffman, K., Tram, J. M., & Maxwell, S. E. (2000). Structural differences in parent and child reports of children's symptoms of depression and anxiety. *Psychological Assessment, 12*, 174–185.

Cole, D. A., Martin, J. M., Peeke, L. G., Seroczynski, A. D., & Hoffman, K. (1998). Are cognitive errors of underestimation predictive or reflective of depressive symptoms in children?: A longitudinal study. *Journal of Abnormal Psychology, 107*, 481–496.

Cole, D. A., Martin, J. M., Powers, B., & Truglio, R. (1996). Modeling causal relations between academic and social competence and depression: A multitrait–multimethod longitudinal study of children. *Journal of Abnormal Psychology, 105*, 258–270.

Cole, D. A., Nolen-Hoeksema, S., Girgus, J., & Paul, G. (2006). Stress exposure and stress generation in child and adolescent depression: A latent trait–state–error approach to longitudinal analyses. *Journal of Abnormal Psychology, 115*, 40–51.

Cole, D. A., Peeke, L. G., Martin, J. M., Truglio, R., & Seroczynski, A. D. (1998). A longitudinal look at the relation between depression and anxiety in children and adolescents. *Journal of Consulting and Clinical Psychology, 66*, 451–460.

Cole, D. A., & Rehm, L. P. (1986). Family interaction patterns and childhood depression. *Journal of Abnormal Child Psychology, 14*, 297–314.

Cole, D. A., Truglio, R., & Peeke, L. (1997). Relation between symptoms of anxiety and depression in children: A multitrait–multimethod–multigroup assessment. *Journal of Consulting and clinical Psychology, 65*, 110–119.

Cole, P. M., Martin, S. E., & Dennis, T. A. (2004). Emotion regulation as a scientific construct: Methodological challenges and directions for child development research. *Child Development, 75*, 317–333.

Compas, B. E., Connon-Smith, J., & Jaser, S. S. (2004). Temperament, stress reactivity, and coping: Implications for depression in childhood and adolescence. *Journal of Clinical Child and Adolescent Psychology, 33*, 21–31.

Compas, B. E., Connor-Smith, J. K., Saltzman, H., Thomsen, A. H., & Wadsworth, M. E. (2001). Coping with stress during childhood and adolescence: Problems, progress, and potential in theory and research. *Psychological Bulletin, 127*, 87–127.

Compas, B. E., Howell, D. C., Phares, V., Williams, R. A., & Ledoux, N. (1989). Parent and child stress and symptoms: An integrative analysis. *Developmental Psychology, 25*, 550–559.

Connell, A. M., & Dishion, T. J. (2006). The contribution of peers to monthly variation in adolescent depressed mood: A short-term longitudinal study with time-varying predictors. *Development and Psychopathology, 18*, 139–154.

Cordeiro, M. J., Caldeira Da Silva, P., & Goldschmidt, T. (2003). Diagnostic classification: Results from a clinical experience of three years with DC: 0–3. *Infant Mental Health Journal, 24*, 349–364.

Costello, E. J., Angold, A., Burns, B. J., Stangl, D. K., Tweed, D. L., Erkanli, A., et al. (1996). The Great Smoky Mountains study of youth: Goals, design, methods, and the prevalence of DSM-III-R disorders. *Archives of General Psychiatry, 53*, 1129–1136.

Costello, E. J., Foley, D. L., & Angold, A. (2006). 10-year research update review: The epidemiology of child and adolescent psychiatric disorders: II. Developmental epidemiology. *American Academy of Child and Adolescent Psychiatry, 45*, 8–25.

Costello, E. J., Mustillo, S., Erkanli, A., Keeler, G., & Angold, A. (2003). Prevalence and development of psychiatric disorders in childhood and adolescence. *Archives of General Psychiatry, 60*, 837–844.

Coyne, J. C. (1976). Toward an interactional description of depression. *Psychiatry, 39*, 28–40.

Dahl, R. E., Birmaher, B., Williamson, D. E., Dorn, L., Perel, J., Kaufman, J., et al. (2000). Low growth hormone response to growth-hormone-releasing hormone in child depression. *Biological Psychiatry, 48*, 981–988.

Dahl, R. E., Kaufman, J., Ryan, N. D., Perel, J., Al-Shabbout, M., Birmaher, B., et al. (1992). The dexamethasone suppression test in children and adolescents: A review and a controlled study. *Biological Psychiatry, 32*, 109–126.

Dahl, R. E., & Ryan, N. D. (1996). The psychobiology of adolescent depression. In D. Cicchetti & S. L. Toth (Eds.), *Rochester symposium on developmental psychopathology: Vol. 7. Adolescence: Opportunities and challenges* (pp. 197–232). Rochester, NY: Rochester University Press.

Dahl, R. E., Ryan, N. D., Puig-Antich, J., Nguyen, N. A., Al-Shabbout, M., Myer, V. A., et al. (1991). 24-hour cortisol measures in adolescents with major depression: A controlled study. *Biological Psychiatry, 30*, 25–36.

Davidson, R. J., Pizzagalli, D., Nitschke, J. B., & Putnam, K. (2002). Depression: Perspectives from affective neuroscience. *Annual Review of Psychology, 53*, 545–574.

Dawson, G., Frey, K., Panagiotides, H., Osterling, J., & Hessl, D. (1997). Infants of depressed mothers exhibit atypical frontal brain activity: A replication and extension of previous findings. *Journal of Child Psychology and Psychiatry and Allied Disciplines, 38*, 179–186.

De Los Reyes, A., & Kazdin, A. E. (2005). Informant discrepancies in the assessment of childhood psychopathology: A critical review, theoretical framework, and recommendations for further study. *Psychological Bulletin, 131*, 483–509.

Dinan, T. G. (1998). Neuroendocrine markers: Role in the development of antidepressants. *CNS Drugs, 10*, 145–157.

Drevets, W. C. (2001). Neuroimaging and neuropathological studies of depression: Implications for the cognitive-emotional features of mood disorders. *Current Opinion in Neurobiology, 11*, 240–249.

Dunn, V., & Goodyer, I. M. (2006). Longitudinal investigation into childhood- and adolescence-onset depression: Psychiatric outcome in early adulthood. *British Journal of Psychiatry, 188*, 216–222.

Eaves, L. J., Silberg, J. L., Meyer, J. M., Maes, H. H., Simonoff, E., Pickles, A., et al. (1997). Genetics and developmental psychopathology: 2. The main effects of genes and environment on behavioral problems in the Virginia Twin Study of Adolescent Behavioral Development. *Journal of Child Psychology and Psychiatry and Allied Disciplines, 38*, 965–980.

Eberhart, N. K., Shih, J. H., Hammen, C. L., & Brennan, P. A. (2006). Understanding the sex difference in vulnerability to adolescent depression: An examination of child and parent characteristics. *Journal of Abnormal Child Psychology, 34*, 495–508.

Egger, H. L., & Angold, A. (2006). Common emotional and behavioral disorders in preschool children: Presentation, nosology, and epidemiology. *Journal of Child Psychology and Psychiatry and Allied Disciplines, 47*, 313–337.

Eisenberg, N., Cumberland, A., Spinrad, T. L., Fabes, R. A., Shepard, S. A., Reiser, M., et al. (2001). The relations of regulation and emotionality to children's externalizing and internalizing problem behavior. *Child Development, 72,* 1112–1134.

Eisenberg, N., Fabes, R. A., & Guthrie, I. K. (1997). Coping with stress: The roles of regulation and development. In I. N. Sandler & S. A. Wolchick (Eds.), *Handbook of children's coping with common stressors: Linking theory, research and intervention* (pp. 41–70). New York: Plenum Press.

Eisenberg, N., Fabes, R. A., Guthrie, I. K., & Reiser, M. (2000). Dispositional emotionality and regulation: Their role in predicting quality of social functioning. *Journal of Personality and Social Psychology, 78,* 136–157.

Eisenberg, N., Spinrad, T. L., Fabes, R. A., Reiser, M., Cumberland, A., Shepard, S. A., et al. (2004). The relations of effortful control and impulsivity to children's resiliency and adjustment. *Child Development, 75,* 25–46.

Eley, T. C., & Stevenson, J. (1999). Exploring the covariation between anxiety and depression. *Journal of Child Psychology and Psychiatry and Allied Disciplines, 40,* 1273–1282.

Eley, T. C., & Stevenson, J. (2000). Specific life events and chronic experiences differentially associated with depression and anxiety in young twins. *Journal of Abnormal Child Psychology, 28,* 383–394.

Elgar, F. J., Curtis, L. J., McGrath, P. J., Waschbusch, D. A., & Stewart, S. H. (2003). Antecedent-consequence conditions in maternal mood and child adjustment: A four-year cross-lagged study. *Journal of Clinical Child and Adolescent Psychology, 32,* 362–374.

Emslie, G. J., Armitage, R., Weinberg, W. A., Rush, A. J., Mayes, T. L., & Hoffman, R. F. (2001). Sleep polysomnography as a predictor of recurrence in children and adolescents with major depression. *International Journal of Neuropsychopharmocology, 4,* 159–168.

Emslie, G. J., Rush, A. J., Weinberg, W. A., Gullion, C. M., Rintelmann, J., & Hughes, C. W. (1997). Recurrence of major depressive disorder in hospitalized children and adolescents. *Journal of the American Academy of Child and Adolescent Psychiatry, 36,* 785–792.

Emslie, G. J., Rush, A. J., Weinberg, W. A., Kowatch, R. A., Hughes, C. W., Carmody, T., et al. (1997). A double-blind, randomized, placebo-controlled trial of fluoxetine in children and adolescents with depression. *Archives of General Psychiatry, 54,* 1031–1037.

Ernst, M., Cookus, B. A., & Moravec, B. C. (2000). Pictorial Instrument for Children and Adolescents (PICA-III-R). *Journal of the American Academy of Child and Adolescent Psychiatry, 39,* 94–99.

Ernst, M., Pine, D. S., & Hardin, M. (2006). Triadic model of the neurobiology of motivated behavior in adolescence. *Psychological Medicine, 36,* 299–312.

Eysenck, H. J., & Eysenck, M. W. (1985). *Personality and individual differences: A natural science approach.* New York: Plenum Press.

Ezpeleta, L., Domenech, J. M., & Angold, A. (2006). A comparison of pure and comorbid CD/ODD and depression. *Journal of Child Psychology and Psychiatry, 47,* 704–712.

Feder, A., Coplan, J. D., Goetz, R. R., Mathew, S. J., Pine, D. A., Dahl, R. E., et al. (2004). Twenty-four-hour cortisol secretion patterns in prepubertal children with anxiety or depressive disorders. *Biological Psychiatry, 56,* 198–204.

Field, T., Fox, N. A., Pickens, J., & Nawrocki, T. (1995). Relative frontal EEG activation in 3- to 6-month-old infants of "depressed" mothers. *Developmental Psychology, 31,* 358–363.

Finch, J. F., & Graziano, W. G. (2001). Predicting depression from temperament, personality, and patterns of social relations. *Journal of Personality, 69,* 27–55.

Forbes, E. E., May, J. C., Siegle, G. J., Ladouceur, C. D., Ryan, N. D., Carter, C. S., et al. (2006). Reward-related decision-making in pediatric major depressive disorder: An fMRI study. *Journal of Child Psychology and Psychiatry and Allied Disciplines, 47,* 1031–1040.

Forbes, E. E., Williamson, D. E., Ryan, N. D., Birmaher, B., Axelson, D. A., & Dahl, R. E. (2006). Peri-sleep-onset cortisol levels in children and adolescents with affective disorders. *Biological Psychiatry, 59,* 24–30.

Frank, D. A., & Drotar, D. (1994). Failure to thrive. In R. M. Reece (Ed.), *Child abuse: Medical diagnosis and management* (pp. 298–324). Philadelphia: Lea & Febiger.

French, D. C., Conrad, J., & Turner, T. M. (1995). Adjustment of antisocial and nonantisocial rejected adolescents. *Development and Psychopathology, 7,* 857–874.

Frye, A. A., & Garber, J. (2005). The relations among maternal depression, maternal criticism, and adolescents' externalizing and internalizing symptoms. *Journal of Abnormal Child Psychology, 33,* 1–11.

Gale, C. R., & Martyn, C. N. (2004). Birthweight and later risk of depression in a national birth cohort. *British Journal of Psychiatry, 184,* 28–33.

Garber, J. (1984). The developmental progression of depression in female children. In D. Cicchetti & K. Schneider-Rosen (Eds.), *New directions for child development* (pp. 29–58). San Francisco: Jossey-Bass.

Garber, J. (2006). Depression in children and adolescents: Linking risk research and prevention. *American Journal of Preventive Medicine, 31,* S104–S125.

Garber, J. (2007). Depression in youth: A developmental psychopathology perspective. In A. Masten & A. Sroufe (Eds.), *Multilevel dynamics in developmental psychopathology: Pathways to the future* (Vol. 34, pp. 181–242). New York: Erlbaum.

Garber, J., Braafladt, N., & Weiss, B. (1995). Affect regulation in depressed and nondepressed children and young adolescents. *Development and Psychopathology, 7,* 93–115.

Garber, J., & Flynn, C. (2001). Predictors of depressive cognitions in young adolescents. *Cognitive Therapy and Research, 25,* 353–376.

Garber, J., & Hollon, S. D. (1991). What can specificity designs say about causality in psychopathology research? *Psychological Bulletin, 110,* 129–136.

Garber, J., & Kaminski, K. M. (2000). Laboratory and performance-based measures of depression in children and adolescents. *Journal of Clinical Child Psychology, 29,* 509–525.

Garber, J., Keiley, M. K., & Martin, N. C. (2002). Developmental trajectories of adolescents' depressive symptoms: Predictors of change. *Journal of Consulting and Clinical Psychology, 70,* 79–95.

Garber, J., & Martin, N. C. (2002). Negative cognitions in offspring of depressed parents: Mechanisms of risk. In S. H. Goodman & I. H. Gotlib (Eds.), *Children of depressed parents: Mechanisms of risk and implications for treatment* (pp. 121–153). Washington, DC: American Psychological Association.

Garber, J., Martin, N. C., & Keiley, M. K. (2002, September). *Predictors of the first onset of major depressive disorder.* Paper presented at the annual meeting of the Society for Research on Psychopathology, San Francisco.

Garber, J., & Robinson, N. S. (1997). Cognitive vulnerability in children at risk for depression. *Cognition and Emotion, 11,* 619–635.

Garrison, C., Jackson, K., Marsteller, F., McKeown, R., & Addy, C. (1990). A longitudinal study of depressive symptomatology in young adolescents. *Journal of Child and Adolescent Psychiatry and Allied Disciplines, 29,* 581–585.

Ge, X., Best, K. M., Conger, R. D., & Simons, R. L. (1996). Parenting behaviors and the occurrence and co-occurrence of adolescent depressive symptoms and conduct problems. *Developmental Psychology, 32,* 717–731.

Ge, X., Lorenz, F., Conger, R., Edler, C., & Simons, R. L. (1994). Trajectories of stressful life events and depressive symptoms during adolescence. *Developmental Psychopathology, 30,* 467–483.

Geller, B., Zimerman, B., Williams, M., Bolhofner, K., & Craney, J. L. (2001a). Adult psychosocial outcome of prepubertal major depressive disorder. *Journal of the American Academy of Child and Adolescent Psychiatry, 40,* 673–677.

Geller, B., Zimerman, B., Williams, M., Bolhofner, K., & Craney, J. L. (2001b). Bipolar disorder at prospective follow-up of adults who had prepubertal major depressive disorder. *American Journal of Psychiatry, 158,* 125–127.

Gibb, B. E. (2002). Childhood maltreatment and negative cognitive styles: A quantitative and qualitative review. *Clinical Psychology Review, 22,* 223–246.

Gibb, B. E., & Alloy, L. B. (2006). A prospective test of the hopelessness theory of depression in children. *Journal of Clinical Child and Adolescent Psychology, 35,* 264–274.

Gibb, B. E., Alloy, L. B., Abramson, L. Y., Rose, D. T., Whitehouse, W. G., Donovan, P., et al. (2001). History of childhood maltreatment, negative cognitive styles, and episodes of depression in adulthood. *Cognitive Therapy and Research, 25,* 425–446.

Gilman, S. E., Kawachi, I., Fitzmaurice, G. M., & Buka, S. L. (2003). Family disruption in childhood and risk of adult depression. *American Journal of Psychiatry, 160,* 939–946.

Gjerde, P. F. (1995). Alternative pathways to chronic depressive symptoms in young adults: Gender differences in developmental trajectories. *Child Development*, 66, 1277–1300.

Gjone, H., & Stevenson, J. (1997). A longitudinal twin study of temperament and behavior problems: Common genetic or environmental influences? *Journal of the American Academy of Child and Adolescent Psychiatry*, 36, 1448–1456.

Gjone, H., Stevenson, J., Sundet, J. M., & Eilertsen, D. E. (1996). Changes in heritability across increasing levels of behavior in young twins. *Behavior Genetics*, 4, 419–426.

Goodman, S. H., & Gotlib, I. H. (1999). Risk for psychopathology in the children of depressed mothers: A developmental model for understanding mechanisms of transmission. *Psychological Review*, 106, 458–490.

Goodman, S. H., Schwab-Stone, M., Lahey, B. B., Shaffer, D., & Jensen, P. S. (2000). Major depression and dysthymia in children and adolescents: Discriminant validity and differential consequences in a community sample. *Journal of the American Academy of Child and Adolescent Psychiatry*, 39, 761–770.

Goodwin, R. D., Fergusson, D. M., & Horwood, L. J. (2004). Early anxious/withdrawn behaviours predict later internalizing disorders. *Journal of Child Psychology and Psychiatry and Allied Disciplines*, 45, 874–883.

Goodyer, I. M. (1996). Physical symptoms and depressive disorders in childhood and adolescence. *Journal of Psychosomatic Research*, 41, 405–408.

Goodyer, I. M., Herbert, J., & Altham, P. M. E. (1998). Adrenal steroid secretion and major depression in 8- to 16-year-olds: III. Influence of cortisol/DHEA ratio at presentation on subsequent rates of disappointing life events and persistent major depression. *Psychological Medicine*, 28, 265–273.

Goodyer, I. M., Herbert, J., Altham, P. M. E., Pearson, J., Secher, S. M., & Shiers, H. M. (1996). Adrenal secretion during major depression in 8- to 16-year-olds: I. Altered diurnal rhythms in salivary cortisol and dehyrepiandrosterone (DHEA) at presentation. *Psychological Medicine*, 26, 245–256.

Goodyer, I. M., Herbert, J., Tamplin, A., & Altham, P. M. E. (2000). Recent life events, cortisol, dehydroepiandrosterone and the onset of major depression in high-risk adolescents. *British Journal of Psychiatry*, 177, 499–504.

Goodyer, I., Wright, C., & Altham, P. M. E. (1990). The friendships and recent life events of anxious and depressed school-age children. *British Journal of Psychiatry*, 156, 689–698.

Gotlib, I. H., & Hammen, C. L. (1992). *Psychological aspects of depression: Toward a cognitive interpersonal integration*. Chichester, UK: Wiley.

Grant, K. E., Compas, B. E., Thurm, A. E., McMahon, S. D., Gipson, P. Y., Campbell, A. J., et al. (2006). Stressors and child and adolescent psychopathology: Evidence of moderating and mediating effects. *Clinical Psychology Review*, 26, 257–283.

Gray, J. A. (1987). The neuropsychology of emotion and personality. In S. D. Iversen & S. M. Stahl (Eds.), *Cognitive neurochemistry* (pp. 171–190). London: Oxford University Press.

Gray, J. A. (1991). The neuropsychology of temperament. In J. Strelau & A. Angleitner (Eds.), *Explorations in temperament: International perspectives on theory and measurement* (pp. 105–128). New York: Plenum Press.

Guedeney, N. (2007). Withdrawal behavior and depression in infancy. *Infant Mental Health Journal*, 28, 393–408.

Guedeney, N., Guedeney, A., Rabouam, C., Mintz, A. S., Danon, G., Huet, M. M., et al. (2003). The Zero-to-Three diagnostic classification: A contribution to the validation of this classification from a sample of 85 under-threes. *Infant Mental Health Journal*, 24, 313–336.

Gunnar, M. R. (1989). Studies of the human infant's adrenocortical response to potentially stressful events. *New Directions for Child Development*, 45, 3–18.

Haines, B. A., Metalsky, G. I., Cardamone, A. L., & Joiner, T. (1999). Interpersonal and cognitive pathways into the origins of attributional style: A developmental perspective. In T. Joiner & J. C. Coyne (Eds.), *The interactional nature of depression* (pp. 65–92). Washington, DC: American Psychological Association.

Hammen, C. L. (1991). The generation of stress in the course of unipolar depression. *Journal of Abnormal Psychology*, 100, 555–561.

Hammen, C. L., & Goodman-Brown, T. (1990). Self schemas and vulnerability to specific life stress in children at risk for depression. *Cognitive Therapy and Research, 14,* 215–227.

Hammen, C. L., Shih, J. H., & Brennan, P. A. (2004). Intergenerational transmission of depression: Test of an interpersonal stress model in a community sample. *Journal of Consulting and Clinical Psychology, 72,* 511–522.

Hankin, B. L. (2005). Childhood maltreatment and psychopathology: Prospective tests of attachment, cognitive vulnerability, and stress as mediating processes. *Cognitive Therapy and Research, 29,* 645–671.

Hankin, B. L., & Abramson, L. (2001). Development of gender differences in depression: An elaborated cognitive vulnerability-transactional stress theory. *Psychological Bulletin, 127,* 773–796.

Hankin, B. L., Abramson, L. Y., Moffitt, T. E., Silva, P. A., & McGee, R. (1998). Development of depression from preadolescence to young adulthood: Emerging gender differences in a 10-year longitudinal study. *Journal of Abnormal Psychology, 107,* 128–140.

Happonen, M., Pulkkinen, L., Kaprio, J., Van der Meere, J., Viken, R. J., & Rose, R. J. (2002). The heritability of depressive symptoms: Multiple informants and multiple measures. *Journal of Child Psychology and Psychiatry, 43,* 471–480.

Harrington, R., Fudge, H., Rutter, M., Pickles, A., & Hill, J. (1990). Adult outcomes of childhood and adolescent depression. *Archives of General Psychiatry, 47,* 465–473.

Harter, S., & Nowakowski, M. (1987). *Manual for the Dimensions of Depression Profile for Children and Adolescents.* Denver, CO: University of Denver.

Hartup, W. W., & van Leishout, C. F. M. (1995). Personality development in social context. *Annual Review of Psychology, 46,* 655–687.

Hayden, E. P., Klein, D. N., & Durbin, C. E. (2005). Parent reports and laboratory assessments of child temperament: A comparison of their associations with risk for depression and externalizing disorders. *Journal of Psychopathology and Behavioral Assessment, 27,* 89–100.

Herjanic, B., & Reich, W. (1997). Development of a structured psychiatric interview for children: Agreement between child and parent on individual symptoms. *Journal of Abnormal Child Psychology, 25,* 21–31.

Hewitt, J. K., Silberg, J. L., Rutter, M., Simonoff, E., Meyer, J. M., Maes, H., et al. (1997). Genetics and developmental psychopathology: 1. Phenotypic assessment in the Virginia twin study of adolescent behavioral development. *Journal of Child Psychology and Psychiatry, 38,* 943–963.

Hodges, K., Cools, J., & McKnew, D. (1989). Test-retest reliability of a clinical research interview for children: The Child Assessment Scale. *Psychological Assessment, 1,* 317–322.

Hoffman, K. B., Cole, D. A., Martin, J. M., Tram, J., & Serocynski, A. D. (2000). Are the discrepancies between self- and others' appraisals of competence predictive or reflective of depressive symptoms in children and adolescents?: A longitudinal study, Part II. *Journal of Abnormal Psychology, 109,* 651–662.

Hofstra, M. B., van der Ende, J., & Verhulst, F. C. (2000). Continuity and change in psychopathology from childhood into adulthood: A 14-year follow-up study. *Journal of the American Academy of Child and Adolescent Psychiatry, 39,* 850–858.

Holmans, P., Weissman, M. M., Zubenko, G. S., Scheftner, W. A., Crowe, R. R., DePaulo, J. R., et al. (2007). Genetics of recurrent early-onset major depression (GenRED): Final genome scan report. *American Journal of Psychiatry, 164,* 248–258.

Ingram, R. E., Miranda, J., & Segal, Z. V. (1998). *Cognitive vulnerability to depression.* New York: Guilford Press.

Jaffee, S. R., Moffitt, T. E., Caspi, A., Fombonne, E., Poulton, R., & Martin, J. (2002). Differences in early childhood risk factors for juvenile-onset and adult-onset depression. *Archives of General Psychiatry, 58,* 215–222.

Jones, D. J., Forehand, R., & Neary, E. M. (2001). Family transmission of depressive symptoms: Replication across Caucasian and African American mother–child dyads. *Behavior Therapy, 32,* 123–138.

Just, N., Abramson, L. Y., & Alloy, L. B. (2001). Remitted depression studies as tests of the cognitive vulnerability hypothesis of depression onset: A critique and conceptual analysis. *Clinical Psychology Review, 21,* 63–83.

Kalin, N. H., & Carnes, M. (1984). Biological correlates of attachment bond disruption in humans and nonhuman primates. *Neuropsychopharmacology and Biological Psychiatry, 8*, 459–469.

Kapoor, A., Dunn, E., Kostaki, A., Andrews, M. H., & Matthews, S. G. (2006). Fetal programming of hypothalamo–pituitary–adrenal function: Prenatal stress and glucocorticoids. *Journal of Physiology, 572*, 31–44.

Kaslow, N. J., Deering, C. G., & Racusin, G. R. (1994). Depressed children and their families. *Clinical Psychology Review, 14*, 39–59.

Katainen, S., Raikkonen, K., Keskivaara, P., & Keltikangas-Jarvinen, L. (1999). Maternal child-rearing attitudes and role satisfaction and children's temperament as antecedents of adolescent depressive tendencies: Follow-up study of 6- to 15-year-olds. *Journal of Youth and Adolescence, 28*, 139–163.

Kaufman, J., Birmaher, B., Brent, D., Rao, U., Flynn, C., Moreci, P. et al. (1997). The Schedule for Affective Disorders and Schizophrenia for School-Aged Children: Present and Lifetime Version (K-SADS-PL): Initial reliability and validity data. *Journal of the American Academy of Child and Adolescent Psychiatry, 36*, 980–988.

Kaufman, J., Birmaher, B., Perel, J., Dahl, R. E., Stull, S., Brent, D., et al. (1998). Serotonergic functioning in depressed abused children: clinical and familial correlates. *Biological Psychiatry, 44*, 973–981.

Kaufman, J., & Charney, D. (2003). The neurobiology of child and adolescent depression: Current knowledge and future directions. In D. Cicchetti & E. Walker (Eds.), *Neurodevelopmental mechanisms in psychopathology* (pp. 461–490). New York: Cambridge University Press.

Kaufman, J., Martin, A., King, R. A., & Charney, D. (2001). Are child-, adolescent-, and adult-onset depression one and the same disorder? *Biological Psychiatry, 49*, 980–1001.

Kaufman, J., Yang, B. Z., Douglas-Palumberi, H., Grasso, D., Lipschitz, D., Housyar, S., et al. (2004). Brain-derived neurotrophic factor-5-HTTLPR gene interaction and environmental modifiers of depression in children. *Biological Psychiatry, 59*, 673–680.

Kaufman, J., Yang, B. Z., Douglas-Palumberi, H., Houshyar, S., Lipschitz, D., Krystal, J. H., et al. (2004). Social supports and serotonin transporter gene moderate depression in maltreated children. *Proceedings of the National Academy of Sciences of the United States of America, 101*, 17316–17321.

Kazdin, A. E., & Marciano, P. L. (1998). Childhood and adolescent depression. In R. A. Barkley & E. J. Mash (Eds.), *Treatment of childhood disorders* (2nd ed., pp. 211–248). New York: Guilford Press.

Kendall, P. C., Cantwell, D. P., & Kazdin, A. E. (1989). Depression in children and adolescents: Assessment issues and recommendations. *Cognitive Therapy and Research, 13*, 109–146.

Kendler, K. S., Gardner, C. O., & Prescott, C. A. (2002). Toward a comprehensive developmental model for major depression in women. *American Journal of Psychiatry, 159*, 1133–1145.

Kendler, K. S., Kessler, R. C., Walters, E. E., MacLean, C., Neale, M. C., Heath, A. C., et al. (1995). Stressful life events, genetic liability, and onset of an episode of major depression in women. *American Journal of Psychiatry, 152*, 833–842.

Kennard, B. D., Emslie, G. J., Mayes, T. L., & Hughes, J. L. (2006). Relapse and recurrence in pediatric depression. *Child and Adolescent Psychiatric Clinics of North America, 15*, 1057–1079.

Kim, H. K., Capaldi, D. M., & Stoolmiller, M. (2003). Depressive symptoms across adolescence and young adulthood in men: Predictions from parental and contextual risk factors. *Development and Psychopathology, 15*, 469–495.

Kistner, J., Balthazor, M., Risi, S., & Burton, C. (1999). Predicting dysphoria in adolescence from actual and perceived peer acceptance in childhood. *Journal of Clinical Child Psychology, 28*, 94–104.

Klein, D. N., Dougherty, L. R., & Olino, T. M. (2005). Toward guidelines for evidence-based assessment of depression in children and adolescents. *Journal of Clinical Child and Adolescent Psychology, 34*, 412–432.

Kovacs, M. (1981). Rating scales to assess depression in school-aged children. *Acta Paedopsychiatrica, 46*, 305–315.

Kovacs, M. (1986). A developmental perspective on methods and measures in the assessment of depressive disorders: The clinical interview. In M. Rutter, C. Izard, & P. Read (Eds.), *Depression in young people: Developmental and clinical perspectives* (pp. 435–468). New York: Guilford Press.

Kovacs, M. (1994). Childhood-onset dysthymic disorder: Clinical features and prospective naturalistic outcome. *Archives of General Psychology, 51*, 365–374.

Kovacs, M. (1996a). The course of childhood-onset depressive disorders. *Psychiatric Annals, 26,* 326–330.

Kovacs, M. (1996b). Presentation and course of major depressive disorder during childhood and later years of the life span. *Journal of the American Academy of Child and Adolescent Psychiatry, 35,* 705–715.

Kovacs, M., & Devlin, B. (1998). Internalizing disorders in childhood. *Journal of Child Psychology and Psychiatry and Allied Disciplines, 39,* 47–63.

Kovacs, M., Feinberg, T. L., Crouse-Novak, M. A., Paulauskas, S. L., & Finkelstein, R. (1984a). Depressive disorders in childhood: I. A longitudinal prospective study of characteristics and recovery. *Archives of General Psychiatry, 41,* 229–237.

Kovacs, M., Feinberg, T. L., Crouse-Novak, M., Paulauskas, S. L., Pollock, M., & Finkelstein, R. (1984b). Depressive disorders in childhood: II. A longitudinal study of the risk for a subsequent major depression. *Archives of General Psychiatry, 41,* 653–649.

Kovacs, M., Gatsonis, C., Paulauskas, S. L., & Richards, C. (1989). Depressive disorders in childhood: IV. A longitudinal study of comorbidity with and risk for anxiety disorders. *Archives of General Psychiatry, 46,* 776–782.

Kovacs, M., Obrosky, D. S., & Sherrill, J. (2003). Developmental changes in the phenomenology of depression in girls compared to boys from childhood onward. *Journal of Affective Disorders, 74,* 33–48.

Kutcher, S., Malkin, D., Silverberg, J., Marton, P., Williamson, P., Malkin, A., et al. (1991). Nocturnal cortisol, thyroid stimulating hormone, and growth hormone secretory profiles in depressed adolescents. *Journal of the American Academy of Child and Adolescent Psychiatry, 30,* 407–414.

Ladouceur, C. D., Dahl, R. E., Williamson, D. E., Birmaher, B., Ryan, N. D., & Casey, B. J. (2005). Altered emotional processing in pediatric anxiety, depression, and comorbid anxiety-depression. *Journal of Abnormal Child Psychology, 33,* 165–177.

Lakdawalla, Z., Hankin, B. L., & Mermelstein, R. (2007). Cognitive theories of depression in children and adolescents: A conceptual and quantitative review. *Clinical Child and Family Psychology Review, 10,* 1–24.

Lamb, M. E., Gaensbauer, T. J., Malkin, C. M., & Schultz, L. A. (1985). The effects of child maltreatment on security of infant–adult attachment. *Infant Behavior and Development, 8,* 35–45.

Lau, J. Y. F., & Eley, T. C. (2008). Disentangling gene–environment correlations and interactions in adolescent depression. *Journal of Child Psychology and Psychiatry, 49,* 142–150.

Lefkowitz, M. M., & Tesiny, E. P. (1980). Assessment of childhood depression. *Journal of Consulting and Clinical Psychology, 48,* 43–50.

Leinonen, J. A., Solantaus, T. S., & Punamaki, R. L. (2003). Parental mental health and children's adjustment: The quality of marital interaction and parenting as mediating factors. *Journal of Child Psychology and Psychiatry and Allied Disciplines, 44,* 227–241.

Lemery-Chalfant, K., Schreiber, J. E., Schmidt, N. L., Van Hulle, C. A., Essex, M. J., & Goldsmith, H. H. (2007). Assessing internalizing, externalizing, and attention problems in young children: Validation of the Macarthur HBQ. *Journal of the American Academy of Child and Adolescent Psychiatry, 46,* 1315–1323.

Lengua, L. J. (2006). Growth in temperament and parenting as predictors of adjustment during children's transition to adolescence. *Developmental Psychology, 42,* 819–832.

Lengua, L. J., & Kovacs, E. A. (2005). Bidirectional associations between temperament and parenting and the prediction of adjustment problems in middle childhood. *Applied Developmental Psychology, 26,* 21–38.

Lengua, L. J., & Sandler, I. N. (1996). Self-regulation as a moderator of the relation between coping and symptomatology in children of divorce. *Journal of Abnormal Child Psychology, 24,* 681–701.

Lengua, L. J., Sandler, I. N., West, S. G., Wolchik, S. A., & Curran, P. J. (1999). Emotionality and self-regulation, threat appraisal, and coping in children of divorce. *Development and Psychopathology, 11,* 15–37.

Lengua, L. J., Wolchik, S. A., Sandler, I. N., & West, S. G. (2000). The additive and interactive effects of parenting and temperament in predicting adjustment problems of children of divorce. *Journal of Clinical Child Psychology, 29,* 232–244.

Lewinsohn, P. M., Allen, N. B., Seeley, J. R., & Gotlib, I. H. (1999). First onset versus recurrence of depression: Differential processes of psychosocial risk. *Journal of Abnormal Psychology, 108*, 483–489.

Lewinsohn, P. M., Steinmetz, J. L., Larson, D. W., & Franklin, J. (1981). Depression related cognitions: Antecedent or consequence? *Journal of Abnormal Psychology, 91*, 213–219.

Little, S. A., & Garber, J. (2000). Interpersonal and achievement orientations and specific hassles predicting depressive and aggressive symptoms in children. *Cognitive Therapy and Research, 24*, 651–671.

Little, S. A., & Garber, J. (2005). The role of social stressors and interpersonal orientation in explaining the longitudinal relation between externalizing and depressive symptoms. *Journal of Abnormal Psychology, 114*, 432–443.

Lonigan, C. J., Phillips, B. M., & Hooe, E. S. (2003). Relations of positive and negative affectivity to anxiety and depression in children: Evidence from a latent variable longitudinal study. *Journal of Consulting and Clinical Psychology, 71*, 465–481.

Luby, J. L., Belden, A. C., & Spitznagel, E. (2006). Risk factors for preschool depression: The mediating role of early stressful life events. *Journal of Child Psychology and Psychiatry and Allied Disciplines, 47*, 1292–1298.

Luby, J. L., Heffelfinger, A. K., & Measelle, J. R. (2002). Differential performance of the MacArthur HBQ and DISC-IV in identifying DSM-IV internalizing psychopathology in young children. *Journal of the American Academy of Child and Adolescent Psychiatry, 41*, 458–466.

Luby, J. L., Heffelfinger, A. K., Mrakotsky, C., Hessler, M. J., Brown, K. M., & Hildebrand, T. (2002). Preschool major depressive disorder: Preliminary validation for developmentally modified DSM-IV criteria. *Journal of the American Academy of Child and Adolescent Psychiatry, 41*, 928–937.

Luby, J. L., Mrakotsky, C., Heffelfinger, A., Brown, K., Hessler, M., & Spitznagel, E. (2003). Modification of DSM-IV criteria for depressed preschool children. *American Journal of Psychiatry, 160*, 1169–1172.

Luby, J. L., Mrakotsky, C., Heffelfinger, A., Brown, K., & Spitznagel, E. (2004). Characteristics of depressed preschoolers with and without anhedonia: Evidence of a melancholic depressive subtype in young children. *American Journal of Psychiatry, 161*, 1998–2004.

Lundy, B. L., Jones, N. A., Field, T., Nearing, G., Davalos, M., Pietro, P. A., et al. (1999). Prenatal depression effects on neonates. *Infant Behavior and Development, 22*, 119–129.

Martini, D. R., Strayhorn, J. M., & Puig-Antich, J. (1990). A symptom self-report measure for preschool children. *Journal of the American Academy of Child and Adolescent Psychiatry, 29*, 594–600.

Matas, L., Arend, R. A., & Sroufe, L. A. (1978). Continuity of adaptation in the second year: The relationship between quality of attachment and later competence. *Child Development, 49*, 547–556.

McCauley, E., Mitchell, J. R., Burke, P., & Moss, S. (1988). Cognitive attributes of depression in children and adolescents. *Journal of Consulting and Clinical Psychology, 56*, 903–908.

McCauley, E., Myers, K., Mitchell, J., Calderon, R., Schloredt, K., & Treder, R. (1993). Depression in young people: Initial presentation and clinical course. *Journal of the American Academy of Child and Adolescent Psychiatry, 32*, 714–722.

McFarlane, A. H., Bellissimo, A., Norman, G. R., & Lange, P. (1994). Adolescent depression in a school-based community sample: Preliminary findings on contributing social factors. *Journal of Youth and Adolescence, 23*, 601–620.

McGinn, L. K., Cukor, D., & Sanderson, W. C. (2005). The relationship between parenting style, cognitive style, and anxiety and depression: Does increased early adversity influence symptom severity through the mediating role of cognitive style? *Cognitive Therapy and Research, 29*(2), 219–242.

Measelle, J. R., Ablow, J. C., Cowan, P. A., & Cowan, C. P. (1998). Assessing young children's views of their academic, social, and emotional lives: An evaluation of the self-perception scales of the Berkeley Puppet Interview. *Child Development, 69*, 1556–1576.

Meyer, W. J., Richards, G. E., Cavallo, A., Holt, K. G., Hejazi, M. S., Wigg, C., et al. (1991). Depression and growth hormone. *Journal of the American Academy of Child and Adolescent Psychiatry, 30*, 335.

Mezulis, A. H., Hyde, J. S., & Abramson, L. Y. (2006). The developmental origins of cognitive vulnerability to depression: Temperament, parenting, and negative life events in childhood as contributors to negative cognitive style. *Developmental Psychology, 42*, 1012–1025.

Monroe, S. M., & Harkness, K. L. (2005). Life stress, the "kindling" hypothesis, and the recurrence of depression: Considerations from a life stress perspective. *Psychological Review, 112*(2), 417–445.

Monroe, S. M., Rohde, P., Seeley, J. R., & Lewinsohn, P. M. (1999). Life events and depression in adolescence: Relationship loss as a prospective risk factor for first onset of major depressed. *Journal of Abnormal Psychology, 108*, 606–614.

Monroe, S. M., & Simons, A. D. (1991). Diathesis-stress theories in the context of life stress research: Implications for the depressive disorders. *Psychological Bulletin, 110*, 406–425.

Moreau, D. (1996). Depression in the young. *Annals of the New York Academy of Sciences, 789*, 31–44.

Mrug, S., Hoza, B., & Bukowski, W. M. (2004). Choosing or being chosen by aggressive-disruptive peers: Do they contribute to children's externalizing and internalizing problems? *Journal of Abnormal Child Psychology, 32*, 53–65.

Murray, L., Woolgar, M., Cooper, P., & Hipwell, A. (2001). Cognitive vulnerability to depression in 5-year-old children of depressed mothers. *Journal of Child Psychology and Psychiatry and Allied Disciplines, 42*, 891–899.

Natsuaki, M. N., Ge, X., Brody, G. H., Simons, R. L., Gibbons, F. X., & Cutrona, C. E. (2007). African American children's depressive symptoms: The prospective effects of neighborhood disorder, stressful life events and parenting. *American Journal of Community Psychology, 39*, 163–176.

Nigg, J. T. (2006) Temperament and developmental psychopathology. *Journal of Child Psychology and Psychiatry and Allied Disciplines, 47*, 395–422.

Nolan, C. L., Moore, G. J., Madden, R., Farchione, T., Bartoi, M., Lorch, E., et al. (2002). Prefrontal cortical volume in childhood-onset major depression: Preliminary findings. *Archives of General Psychiatry, 59*, 173–179.

Nolen-Hoeksema, S., Girgus, J. S., & Seligman, M. E. P. (1992). Predictors and consequences of childhood depressive symptoms: A 5-year longitudinal study. *Journal of Abnormal Psychology, 101*, 405–422.

Oldehinkel, A. J., Veenstra, R., Ormel, J., de Winter, A. F., & Verhulst, F. C. (2006). Temperament, parenting, and depressive symptoms in a population sample of preadolescents. *Journal of Child Psychology and Psychiatry and Allied Disciplines, 47*, 684–695.

Ormel, J., Oldehinkel, A. J., Ferdinand, R. F., Hartman, C. A., de Winter, A. F., Veenstra, R., et al. (2005). Internalizing and externalizing problems in adolescence: General and dimension-specific effects of familial loadings and preadolescent temperament traits. *Psychological Medicine, 35*, 1825–1835.

Panak, W., & Garber, J. (1992). Role of aggression, rejection, and attributions in the prediction of depression in children. *Development and Psychopathology, 4*, 145–165.

Patterson, M. L., Greising, L., Hyland, L. T., & Burger, G. K. (1994). Childhood depression, anxiety, and aggression: A reanalysis of Epkins and Meyers. *Journal of Personality Assessment, 69*, 607–613.

Peterson, L., Mullins, L. L., & Ridley-Johnson, R. (1985). Childhood depression: Peer reactions to depression and life stress. *Journal of Abnormal Child Psychology, 13*, 597–609.

Phillips, B. M., Lonigan, C. J., Driscoll, K., & Hooe, E. S. (2002). Positive and negative affectivity in children: A multitrait-multimethod investigation. *Journal of Clinical Child and Adolescent Psychology, 31*, 465–479.

Pihlakoski, L., Sourander, A., Aromaa, M., Rautava, P., Helenius, H., & Sillanpaa, M. (2006). The continuity of psychopathology from early childhood to preadolescence. *European Child and Adolescent Psychiatry, 15*, 409–417.

Post, R. M. (1992). Transduction of psychosocial stress into the neurobiology of recurrent affective disorder. *American Journal of Psychiatry, 149*, 999–1010.

Poznanski, E., Mokros, B., Grossman, J., & Freeman, L. N. (1985). Diagnostic criteria in childhood depression. *American Journal of Psychiatry, 142*, 1168–1173.

Puig-Antich, J., Lukens, E., Davies, M., Goetz, D., Brennan-Quattrock, J., & Todak, G. (1985a). Psychosocial functioning in prepubertal major depressive disorders: I. Interpersonal relationships during the depressive episode. *Archives of General Psychiatry, 42*, 500–507.

Puig-Antich, J., Lukens, E., Davies, M., Goetz, D., Brennan-Quattrock, J., & Todak, G. (1985b). Psychosocial functioning in prepubertal depressive disorders: II. Interpersonal relationships after sustained recovery from affective episode. *Archives of General Psychiatry, 42*, 511–517.

Radloff, L. S. (1977). The CES-D Scale: A self report depression scale for research in the general population. *Applied Psychological Measurement, 1*, 385–401.

Raynor, P., & Rudolf, M. C. J. (1996). What do we know about children who fail to thrive? *Child: Care, Health and Development, 22*, 241–250.

Reich, W. (2000). Diagnostic Interview for Children and Adolescents (DICA). *Journal of the American Academy of Child and Adolescent Psychiatry, 39*, 59–66.

Reinherz, H. Z., Paradis, A. D., Giaconia, R. M., Stashwick, C. K., & Fitzmaurice, G. (2003). Childhood and adolescent predictors of major depression in the transition to adulthood. *American Journal of Psychiatry, 160*, 2141–2147.

Renouf, A. G., & Harter, S. (1990). Low self-worth and anger as components of the depressive experience in young adolescents. *Development and Psychopathology, 2*, 293–310.

Rice, F., Harold, G. T., & Thapar, A. (2002a). Assessing the effects of age, sex and shared environment on the genetic aetiology of depression in childhood and adolescence. *Journal of Child Psychology and Psychiatry and Allied Disciplines, 43*, 1039–1051.

Rice, F., Harold, G. T., & Thapar, A. (2002b). The genetic aetiology of childhood depression: A review. *Journal of Child Psychology and Psychiatry and Allied Disciplines, 43*, 65–79.

Rice, F., Harold, G. T., & Thapar, A. (2003). Negative life events as an account of age-related differences in the genetic aetiology of depression in childhood and adolescence. *Journal of Child Psychology and Psychiatry, 44*, 977–987.

Roberson-Nay, R., McClure, E. B., Monk, C. S., Nelson, E. E., Guyer, A. E., Fromm, S. J., et al. (2006). Increased amygdala activity during successful memory encoding in adolescent major depressive disorder: An fMRI study. *Biological Psychiatry, 60*, 966–973.

Rosso, I. M., Cintron, C. M., Steingard, R. J., Renshaw, P. F., Young, A. D., & Yurgelun-Todd, D. A. (2005). Amygdala and hippocampus volumes in pediatric major depression. *Biological Psychiatry, 57*, 21–26.

Rothbart, M. K., & Bates, J. E. (1998). Temperament. In W. Damon (Series Ed.) & N. Eisenberg (Vol. Ed.), *Handbook of child psychology: Vol. 3. Social, emotional, and personality development* (5th ed., pp. 105–176). New York: Wiley.

Rubio-Stipec, M., Fitzmaurice, G., Murphy, J., & Walker, A. (2003). The use of multiple informants in identifying the risk factors of depressive and disruptive disorders: Are they interchangeable? *Social Psychiatry and Psychiatric Epidemiology, 38*, 51–58.

Rudolph, K. D., & Clark, A. G. (2001). Conceptions of relationships in children with depressive and aggressive symptoms: Social-cognitive distortion or reality? *Journal of Abnormal Child Psychology, 29*, 41–56.

Rudolph, K. D., Hammen, C., & Burge, D. (1994). Interpersonal functioning and depressive symptoms in childhood: Addressing the issues of specificity and comorbidity. *Journal of Abnormal Child Psychology, 22*, 355–371.

Rudolph, K. D., Hammen, C., & Burge, D. (1997). A cognitive-interpersonal approach to depressive symptoms in preadolescent children. *Journal of Abnormal Child Psychology, 25*, 33–45.

Rueter, M. A., Scaramella, L., Wallace, L. E., & Conger, R. D. (1999). First-onset of depressive or anxiety disorders predicted by the longitudinal course of internalizing symptoms and parent–adolescent disagreements. *Archives of General Psychiatry, 56*, 726–732.

Ryan, N. D., Birmaher, B., Perel, J. M., Dahl, R. E., Meyer, V., Al-Shabbout, M., et al. (1992). Neuroendocrine response to L-5-hydroxytryptophan challenge in prepubertal major depression: Depressed versus normal control. *Archives of General Psychiatry, 49*, 843–851.

Ryan, N. D., & Dahl, R. (1993). The biology of depression in children and adolescents. In J. J. Mann & D. J. Kupfer (Eds.), *Biology of depressive disorders, Part B: Subtypes of depression and comorbid disorders* (pp. 37–58). New York: Plenum Press.

Ryan, N. D., Dahl, R. E., Birmaher, B., Williamson, D. E., Iyengar, S., Nelson, B., et al. (1994). Stimulatory tests of growth hormone secretion in prepubertal major depression: Depressed versus normal children. *Archives of General Psychiatry, 33*, 824–833.

Ryan, N. D., Puig-Antich, J., Ambrosini, P., Rabinovich, H., Robinson, D., Nelson, B., et al. (1987). The clinical picture of major depression in children and adolescents. *Archives of General Psychiatry, 44*, 854–861.

Sagrestano, L. M., Paikoff, R. L., Holmbeck, G. N., & Fendrich, M. (2003). A longitudinal examination of familial risk factors for depression among inner-city African American adolescents. *Journal of Family Psychology, 17,* 108–120.

Sandstrom, M. J., Cillessen, A. H. N., & Eisenhower, A. (2003). Children's appraisal of peer rejection experiences: Impact on social and emotional adjustment. *Social Development, 12,* 530–550.

Saylor, C. F., Finch, A. J., Spirito, A., & Bennett, B. (1984). The Children's Depression Inventory: A systematic evaluation of psychometric properties. *Journal of Consulting and Clinical Psychology, 52,* 955–967.

Scher, C. D., Ingram, R. E., & Segal, Z. V. (2005). Cognitive reactivity and vulnerability: Empirical evaluation of construct activation and cognitive diatheses in unipolar depression. *Clinical Psychology Review, 25,* 487–510.

Scourfield, J., Rice, F., Thapar, A., Harold, G., Martin, N., & McGuffin, P. (2003). Depressive symptoms in children and adolescents: Changing aetiological influences with development. *Journal of Child Psychology and Psychiatry, 44,* 968–976.

Seligman, L. D., & Ollendick, T. H. (1998). Comorbidity of anxiety and depression in children and adolescents: An integrative review. *Clinical Child and Family Psychology Review, 1,* 125–144.

Shaffer, D., Fisher, P., Lucas, C. P., Dulcan, M. K., & Schwab-Stone, M. E. (2000). NIMH Diagnostic Interview Schedule for Children Version IV (NIMH DISC-IV): Description, differences from previous versions and reliability of some common diagnoses. *Journal of the American Academy of Child and Adolescent Psychiatry, 39,* 28–38.

Shiner, R. L. (1998). How shall we speak of children's personalities in middle childhood?: A preliminary taxonomy. *Psychological Bulletin, 124,* 308–332.

Silberg, J., Pickles, A., Rutter, M., Hewitt, J., Simonoff, E., Maes, H., et al. (1999). The influence of genetic factors and life stress on depression among adolescent girls. *Archives of General Psychiatry, 56,* 225–232.

Silk, J. S., Shaw, D. S., Forbes, E. E., Lane, T. L., & Kovacs, M. (2006). Maternal depression and child internalizing: The moderating role of child emotion regulation. *Journal of Clinical Child and Adolescent Psychology, 35,* 116–126.

Sorensen, M. J., Nissen, J. B., Mors, O., & Thomsen, P. H. (2005). Age and gender differences in depressive symptomatology and comorbidity: An incident sample of psychiatrically admitted children. *Journal of Affective Disorders, 84,* 85–91.

Spitz, R. A., & Wolf, K. M. (1946). Anaclitic depression: An inquiry into the genesis of psychiatric conditions in childhood, II. *Psychoanalytic Study of the Child, 2,* 313–342.

Stanger, C., McConaughy, S., & Achenbach, T. M. (1992). Three-year course of behavioral/emotional problems in a national sample of 4- to 16-year-olds: II. Predictors of syndromes. *Journal of the American Academy of Child and Adolescent Psychiatry, 31,* 941–950.

Stein, D., Williamson, D. E., Birmaher, B., Brent, D. A., Kaufman, J., Dahl, R. E., et al. (2000). Parent–child bonding and family functioning in depressed children and children at high risk and low risk for future depression. *Journal of the American Academy of Child and Adolescent Psychiatry, 39,* 1387–1395.

Steingard, R., Renshaw, P. F., Hennen, J., Lenox, M., Cintron, C. B., Young, A. D., et al. (2002). Smaller frontal lobe white matter volumes in depressed adolescents. *Society of Biological Psychiatry, 52,* 413–417.

Steinhausen, H. C., & Winkler, M. C. (2003). Prevalence of affective disorders in children and adolescents: Findings from the Zurich epidemiological studies. *Acta Psychiatrica Scandinavica, 108,* 20–23.

Stice, E., Ragan, J., & Randall, P. (2004). Prospective relations between social support and depression: Differential direction of effects for parent and peer support? *Journal of Abnormal Psychology, 113*(1), 155–159.

Thapar, A., & Rice, F. (2006). Twin studies in pediatric depression. *Child and Adolescent Psychiatric Clinics of North America, 15,* 869–881.

Thomas, A., & Chess, S. (1977). *Temperament and development.* Oxford, UK: Brunner/Mazel.

Thomas, K. M., Drevets, W. C., Dahl, R. E., Ryan, N. D., Birmaher, B., Eccard, C. H., et al. (2001). Amygdala response to fearful faces in anxious and depressed children. *Archives of General Psychiatry, 58,* 1057–1063.

Thomson, R. A. (1994). Emotion regulation: A theme in search of definition. *Monographs of the Society for Research in Child Development, 59,* 25–52.

Timbremont, B., & Braet, C. (2004). Cognitive vulnerability in remitted depressed children and adolescents. *Behaviour Research and Therapy, 42,* 423–437.

Todd, R. D., & Botteron, K. N. (2001). Family, genetic, and imaging studies of early-onset depression. *Child and Adolescent Psychiatric Clinics of North America, 10,* 375–390.

Tomarken, A. J., Dichter, G. S., Garber, J., & Simien, C. (2004). Relative left frontal hypo-activation in adolescents at risk for depression. *Biological Psychology, 67,* 77–102.

Trad, P. V. (1994). Depression in infants. In W. M. Reynolds & H. F. Johnston (Eds.), *Handbook of depression in children and adolescents* (pp. 401–426). New York: Plenum Press.

Turner, J. E., & Cole, D. A. (1994). Developmental differences in cognitive diatheses for child depression. *Journal of Abnormal Child Psychology, 22,* 15–32.

Twenge, J. M., & Nolen-Hoeksema, S. (2002). Age, gender, race, socioeconomic status, and birth cohort differences on the Children's Depression Inventory: A meta-analysis. *Journal of Abnormal Psychology, 111*(4), 578–588.

Uhrlass, D. J., & Gibb, B. E. (2007). Childhood emotional maltreatment and the stress generation model of depression. *Journal of Social and Clinical Psychology, 26,* 119–130.

Valla, J. P., Bergeron, L., & Smolla, N. (2000). The Dominic®: A pictorial interview for 6- to 11-year-old children. *Journal of the American Academy of Child and Adolescent Psychiatry, 39,* 85–93.

van der Valk, J. C., van den Oord, E. J., Verhulst, F. C., & Boomsma, D. I. (2003). Using shared and unique parental views to study the etiology of 7-year-old twins' internalizing and externalizing problems. *Behavior Genetics, 33,* 409–420.

Van Leeuwen, K. G., Mervielde, I., De Clercq, B. J., & De Fruyt, F. (2007). Extending the spectrum idea: Child personality, parenting and psychopathology. *European Journal of Personality, 21,* 63–89.

Wagner, K. D. (2003). Major depression in children and adolescents. *Psychiatric Annals, 33,* 266–270.

Watson, D., & Clark, L. A. (1984). Negative affectivity: The disposition to experience aversive emotional states. *Psychological Bulletin, 96,* 465–490.

Weinstock, M. (2005). The potential influence of maternal stress hormones on development and mental health of the offspring. *Brain, Behavior and Immunity, 19,* 296–308.

Weiss, B., & Garber, J. (2003). Developmental differences in the phenomenology of depression. *Development and Psychopathology, 15,* 403–430.

Weissman, M. M., Gammon, G. D., John, K., Merikangas, K. R., Prusoff, B. A., & Sholomskas, D. (1987). Children of depressed parents: Increased psychopathology and early onset of major depression. *Archives of General Psychiatry, 44,* 847–853.

Weissman, M. M., & Olfson, M. (1995). Depression in women: Implications for health care research. *Science, 269,* 799–801.

Weissman, M. M., Wolk, S., Wickramaratne, P., Goldstein, R. B., Adams, P., Greenwald, S., et al. (1999). Children with prepubertal-onset major depressive disorder and anxiety grown up. *Archives of General Psychiatry, 56,* 794–801.

Weisz, J. R., Southam-Gerow, M. A., & McCarty, C. A. (2001). Control-related beliefs and depressive symptoms in clinic-referred children and adolescents: Developmental differences and model specificity. *Journal of Abnormal Psychology, 110,* 97–109.

Weller, E. B., Weller, R. A., Fristad, M. A., Rooney, M. T., & Schecter, J. (2000). Children's Interview for Psychiatric Syndromes (ChIPS). *Journal of the American Academy of Child and Adolescent Psychiatry,* 76–84.

Wickramaratne, P. J., Greenwald, S., & Weissman, M. M. (2000). Psychiatric disorders in the relatives of probands with prepubertal-onset or adolescent-onset major depression. *Journal of the American Academy of Child and Adolescent Psychiatry, 39,* 1396–1405.

Winokur, G. (1997). All roads lead to depression: Clinically homogeneous, etiologically heterogeneous. *Journal of Affective Disorders, 45,* 97–108.

Wright, C., & Birks, E. (2000). Risk factors for failure to thrive: A population-based survey. *Child: Care, Health and Development, 26,* 5–16.

Zalsman, G., Oquendo, M. A., Greenhill, L., Goldberg, P. H., Kamali, M. K., Martin, A., et al. (2006). Neurobiology of depression in children and adolescents. *Child and Adolescent Psychiatric Clinics of North America, 15,* 843–868.

Zero to Three. (2005). *Diagnostic classification: 0–3R: Diagnostic classification of mental health and developmental disorders of infancy and early childhood: Revised edition.* Washington, DC: Author.

CHAPTER 19

Adolescent Depression

Karen D. Rudolph

Depression is a serious mental health problem that carries significant personal and societal costs. Although early theories viewed depression as a disorder of adulthood, contemporary perspectives highlight adolescence as a particularly high-risk period for the emergence of depression. No longer viewed as reflecting normative storm and stress, adolescent depression is now recognized as a pernicious and recurrent disorder that creates significant impairment in the lives of youth and threatens health and well-being through adulthood. Understanding depression during adolescence can therefore inform theories regarding the etiology, course, and consequences of depression, as well as early identification and intervention efforts designed to alleviate current suffering and prevent a downward spiral of impairment throughout the lifespan.

DESCRIPTION OF ADOLESCENT DEPRESSION

Depression can be conceptualized and measured at several levels—as a symptom (sad mood), a syndrome (a theoretically or empirically derived constellation of associated symptoms), or a clinical disorder (a set of symptoms that meet specific diagnostic criteria). Features of depression, such as its prevalence, course, and correlates, differ depending on the definition of depression, as well as the sample of interest (e.g., clinic-referred vs. community). This section provides an overview of basic features of adolescent depression (for a more comprehensive review, see Rudolph, Hammen, & Daley, 2006).

Epidemiology

Prevalence

Epidemiological research consistently reveals a marked increase in rates of depression during adolescence. By middle to late adolescence, rates of diagnosable depression are comparable to those found in adults. In a summary of six epidemiological studies between 1987 and 2000, Lewinsohn and Essau (2002) reported lifetime prevalence rates of major depressive disorder (MDD) in adolescents ranging from 1.9 to 18.4% (compared to less than 3% in preadolescents). The National Comorbidity Study, an epidemiological survey in the United States, reported a lifetime prevalence rate of 14% for MDD in adolescents (Kessler & Walters, 1998; for comparable rates in community studies, see Lewinsohn, Rohde, Seeley, Klein, & Gotlib, 2000; Rao, Hammen, & Daley, 1999). Prospective community studies similarly reveal a sharp rise in rates of clinical depression from childhood through late adolescence (Costello, Mustillo, Erkanli, Keeler, & Angold, 2003; Hankin et al., 1998).

Subclinical depression affects a large minority of adolescents. Based on diagnostic criteria, 10–20% of youth experience subsyndromal or minor depression (Kessler & Walters, 1998). Based on conventional cutoffs on self-report measures, an even greater percentage of youth (20–50%) experience significant symptoms (Kessler, Avenevoli, & Merikangas, 2001). Moreover, research that tracks self-reports of depressive symptoms over time indicates rising rates during adolescence (Ge, Lorenz, Conger, Elder, & Simons, 1994). These elevated and persistent levels of depressive symptoms are associated with significant functional impairment (Gotlib, Lewinsohn, & Seeley, 1995) and herald the onset of subsequent clinical disorders (Angst, Sellaro, & Merikangas, 2000).

Onset, Clinical Features, and Developmental Course

Prospective research indicates that the peak age of onset for depression occurs during midadolescence, at approximately 13–15 years. For example, in the Oregon Adolescent Depression Project (OADP), the mean age of MDD onset was about 15 years (Lewinsohn & Essau, 2002). In a follow-back analysis of individuals assessed from birth, 75% of adults who had experienced a depressive disorder by age 26 had a history of depression onset during childhood or adolescence (Kim-Cohen et al., 2003).

The length of major depressive episodes (MDEs) during adolescence varies across studies, with longer durations in clinical (e.g., mean duration of 7–9 months; Birmaher, Arbeleaz, & Brent, 2002; Rao et al., 1995) than in community samples (e.g., mean duration of 26 weeks for the OADP; Lewinsohn, Rohde, & Seeley, 1994). The vast majority of MDEs remit within 2 years, whereas dysthymia has a mean duration of 4 years; occurrence of dysthymia predicts the future development of MDD (for a review, see Birmaher et al., 1996).

Despite high rates of remission, depression carries a strong risk for recurrence, with as many as 40% of adolescents experiencing another MDE within 2–5 years after recovery (Birmaher et al., 1996; Rao et al., 1999). Predictors of risk for chronicity and recurrence include symptom severity, personal or family history of MDD, comorbidity, suicidality, negative beliefs, and family adversity (Birmaher et al., 2002; Rohde, Lewinsohn, Klein, & Seeley, 2005). In clinical samples, a significant minority (20–40%) of adolescents with MDD develop bipolar disorder within 5 years (for a review, see Birmaher et al., 1996).

Although there is little doubt that depression is chronic and recurrent, less clarity exists about the continuity of depression across developmental periods. Evidence from both community (e.g., Lewinsohn, Rohde, Klein, & Seeley, 1999) and clinical (e.g., Rao et al., 1995) studies attests that adolescent depression portends depression in adulthood. However, growing evidence suggests a possible discontinuity between depression with an onset prior to, versus following, adolescence, as reflected in differing course, correlates, and etiology. Although some youth with childhood-onset depression experience depression in adolescence and adulthood (Weissman et al., 1999), others experience forms of disorder and impairment other than depression (Harrington, Fudge, Rutter, Pickles, & Hill, 1990). Moreover, several of the predictors and correlates of depression, such as genetic contribution (Thapar & McGuffin, 1996), neurobiological dysfunction (Kaufman, Martin, King, & Charney, 2001), family adversity (Harrington, Rutter, & Fombonne, 1996), and medication response (Kaufman et al., 2001), vary across childhood, adolescence, and adulthood. These findings indicate the need to identify factors that reliably distinguish between depressive disorders with an onset at different developmental stages, as well as to elucidate processes that underlie continuity versus discontinuity over time.

Phenomenology and Developmental Features

The same criteria are used to diagnosis depression across development, with only small differences (in adolescents, but not adults, irritability can be one of the mood changes, and there is a 1-year duration criterion for dysthymia). However, there may be developmental changes in the experience and expression of particular symptoms, driven by the maturation of cognitive, emotional, physiological, and social capabilities (Avenevoli & Steinberg, 2001; Weiss & Garber, 2003). In a meta-analysis comparing the *rates* of particular symptoms across age groups, ranging from early childhood through adulthood, Weiss and Garber (2003) found differences in many of the core symptoms (e.g., agitation, retardation, fatigue, guilt, and sadness) and associated symptoms (e.g., anxiety, somatic complaints). Specific cross-sectional comparisons reveal that depressed adolescents are more likely than preadolescents to experience hopelessness/helplessness, lack of energy, hypersomnia, weight loss, and suicidality (Yorbik, Birmaher, Axelson, Williamson, & Ryan, 2004; for a review, see Avenevoli & Steinberg, 2001). Overall, adolescents appear to experience more vegetative symptoms than do preadolescents. However, these developmental differences vary across studies based on the composition of the sample and the informant (Weiss & Garber, 2003), and are not all supported in longitudinal analyses (Avenevoli & Steinberg, 2001). Evidence is mixed regarding whether a similar *structure* underlies the depressive syndrome across development, with some studies supporting quite substantial developmental differences and others showing few differences (Yorbik et al., 2004; for a review, see Weiss & Garber, 2003).

In summary, although depression shows some homotypic continuity across development, there are also phenomenological differences. These differences may reflect developmentally specific manifestations of the same underlying syndrome (i.e., heterotypic continuity), or they may reflect the possibility that childhood- versus adolescence- or adult-onset depression are different disorders. Regardless of their source, these differences must be taken into account in the conceptualization, assessment, and treatment of adolescent depression.

Comorbidity

Comorbidity between depression and other disorders is common, both within an episode and across the lifetime. A meta-analysis in child and adolescent community samples (Angold, Costello, & Erkanli, 1999) revealed high co-occurrence with anxiety disorders (odds ratio [OR] = 8.2), conduct/oppositional defiant disorders (OR = 6.6), and attention-deficit/hyperactivity disorder (ADHD; OR = 5.5). In adolescents, rates of comorbidity are as high as 42% in community samples (e.g., Rohde, Lewinsohn, & Seeley, 1991), with even higher rates in clinical samples. The specific pattern varies across ages. Compared to depression in preadolescence, adolescent depression is less likely to co-occur with separation anxiety and ADHD (Yorbik et al., 2004), and more likely to co-occur with disruptive behavior and substance use disorders (particularly in males; Lewinsohn, Hops, Roberts, Seeley, & Andrews, 1993; Yorbik et al., 2004), and eating disorders (particularly in females; Lewinsohn et al., 1993).

There are several possible explanations for these high rates of comorbidity (for a review, see Angold, Costello, & Erkanli, 1999). Co-occurrence of symptoms and disorders may reflect an artifact of either inadequate diagnostic systems or overlapping assessment instruments. Alternatively, comorbidity may stem from common etiological influences (e.g., a shared genetic liability for depression and anxiety) or co-occurring risk factors (e.g., co-occurring parental depression and family discord creating a risk for both depression and conduct disorder). Given the frequent sequential association between depression and other disorders (i.e., the onset of anxiety and disruptive behavior disorders typically precedes the onset of depression; Kim-Cohen et al., 2003), comorbidity also may be explained by the developmental progression of one disorder into another.

The developmental progression of disorders can take one of two forms. First, it may reflect the maturation of developmental capabilities or the temporal exposure to socialization experiences and life contexts that influence the expression of disorders. For example, Kovacs and Devlin (1998) proposed that the progression from anxiety to depression reflects a "readiness" (p. 54) to show certain physiological aspects of anxiety (e.g., agitation and hyperarousal) earlier in development, and certain physiological (e.g., vegetative symptoms) and cognitive (e.g., rumination) aspects of depression later in development. The *helplessness/hopelessness model* (Alloy, Kelly, Mineka, & Clements, 1990) proposes a series of stages through which helplessness-driven anxiety symptoms progress to hopelessness-driven depression symptoms through a shift from uncertainty to certainty about one's ability to control future outcomes and the likelihood that future negative outcomes will occur. This shift presumably occurs in the context of exposure to increasing levels of life stress. Behavior genetic analyses (Eaves, Silberg, & Erkanli, 2003) reveal that a genetic vulnerability to anxiety prior to puberty accounts in part for the genetic difference in depression following puberty, suggesting that a shared genetic liability is differentially expressed as anxiety earlier in development and as depression later in development. Alternatively, the sequential unfolding of disorders may reflect a functional association whereby one disorder serves as a risk factor for another. For instance, according to the *dual-failure model* (Patterson & Stoolmiller, 1991), disruptive behavior disorders create academic and social problems that heighten risk for depression. This type of functional association may occur independently or in tandem with the evolution of one disorder into another, as driven by internal or external developmental forces.

Understanding the causes and consequences of comorbidity has profound implications for conceptualizing depression, identifying its correlates, predicting course and future impairment, and determining its etiology. Identifying which explanations account for comorbidity between depression and other disorders would inform diagnosis and classification by providing essential information about the overlap versus distinctiveness among disorders. Moreover, testing alternative theoretical models of comorbidity would elucidate the shared versus specific risk factors for depression and co-occurring disorders, as well as improve prediction regarding how or under what conditions another disorder may progress into depression across development. This knowledge could in turn inform prevention efforts designed to interrupt this developmental progression.

Illustrating the significance of comorbidity, research indicates differences in the course and correlates of depression in youth with and without comorbid disorders. Depression comorbidity is associated with more severe and recurrent depression, and a less favorable response to treatment (for a review, see Birmaher et al., 1996). Youth with comorbid depression and externalizing disorders show more interpersonal impairment (Rudolph & Clark, 2001) and life stress (Daley et al., 1997; Rudolph et al., 2000) than those without comorbid disorders. Moreover, compared to depressed youth without conduct disorder, depressed youth with conduct disorder show lower rates of depression and higher rates of criminality/ antisocial personality disorder and alcohol abuse in adulthood (Harrington, Fudge, Rutter, Pickles, & Hill, 1991), suggesting that comorbidity may provide clues about distinct subtypes of depression that differ in continuity across development. Comorbidity also might obscure certain correlates of depression. For example, depressed adolescents with comorbid anxiety do not show the same pattern of brain functioning as those without comorbid anxiety (Kentgen et al., 2000). Thus, future research must consider how comorbidity influences the nature, course, etiology, consequences, and treatment of depression.

Sex Differences

One of the most robust features of depression is the emerging sex difference during adolescence. Both cross-sectional (Angold, Erkanli, Silberg, Eaves, & Costello, 2002) and longitudinal (Costello et al., 2003; Hankin et al., 1998) studies show that girls begin to show higher levels of depressive symptoms and disorders by early to midadolescence (about 12– 14 years of age); this sex difference increases throughout adolescence (Hankin et al., 1998), until it reaches a 2:1 female to male ratio, which persists throughout the lifespan. There are also some sex differences in the manifestation of depression. Depressed adolescent girls are more likely than boys to experience weight or appetite disturbances, worthlessness or guilt (Lewinsohn, Rohde, & Seeley, 1998), and suicidality (Yorbik et al., 2004). Moreover, Lewinsohn and Essau (2002) reported that adolescent females in the OADP were more likely than males to have recurring major depression, suggesting a more pernicious course.

   Based on pioneering work by Nolen-Hoeksema and Girgus (1994), theoretical models of youth depression increasingly attempt to account for the rising rates of depression and the emerging sex difference in depression during adolescence (Cyranowski, Frank, Young, & Shear, 2000; Hankin & Abramson, 2001; Rudolph, in press). These models typically focus on the interactive contributions of biological, psychological, and contextual changes associated with the transition to adolescence, often with a focus on sex-linked roles, beliefs, and experiences within the context of interpersonal relationships. Later sections on the origins of depression describe these perspectives in more detail.

Short- and Long-Term Impairment and Outcomes Associated with Adolescent Depression

Depressed adolescents experience considerable impairment, including academic and interpersonal difficulties; social-cognitive biases; problems in salient social roles, such as school dropout and early pregnancies; and suicidality (for a review, see Harrington & Dubicka, 2001). Despite some debate about the persistence of impairment beyond acute depressive episodes, research indicates enduring difficulties in relationships and role functioning even following remission; this impairment extends through adulthood (e.g., Gotlib, Lewinsohn, & Seeley, 1998) and is most salient in depressed adolescents who show a recurrent course of depression into adulthood (Rao et al., 1995). Although many comorbid disorders precede the onset of depression, some depressed adolescents also go on to develop new disorders (Lewinsohn et al., 1999). These ongoing and newly emerging disturbances might result from several factors, including the chronicity or recurrence of earlier depression, the persistence of an underlying vulnerability (e.g., genetic liability, cognitive bias), or the consequences of earlier depression.

ORIGINS AND DEVELOPMENT OF ADOLESCENT DEPRESSION

Understanding the origins of adolescent depression requires a developmentally based conceptualization that considers how critical transitions of adolescence serve as a backdrop for rising levels of depression, particularly in girls, at this time. This section reviews key theories of depression and supportive empirical evidence in adolescents. As discussed throughout the section, far from representing unique contributors to depression, many of these vulnerabilities and risks can be integrated into a comprehensive framework that emphasizes interactions and transactions between characteristics of youth and their environments in the onset and progression of depression.

Genetic Influences

The strong family aggregation of depression has generated widespread interest in understanding genetic contributions to depression and identifying genetic models of risk. Most research focuses on a *main effect model*, in which genes are presumed to exert a direct influence on liability to depression. Behavior genetic research in this tradition reveals moderate heritability of depression, with estimates ranging from 30 to 80% for parent reports of youth symptoms, and 15 to 80% for youth self-reports of symptoms (Rice, Harold, & Thapar, 2002). Notably, genetic factors seem to play a larger role in adolescent depression than in childhood depression. A behavior genetic analysis of twin pairs revealed significant shared and nonshared environment effects, but no genetic effects, in children (younger than 11), and significant genetic and nonshared environment effects in adolescents (11 and older), with heritability estimates of 71–83% in the older twins (Thapar & McGuffin, 1996). These findings suggest different origins of childhood and adolescent depression, consistent with the idea that age of onset might be a marker for distinct subtypes of disorder. Moreover, another twin study revealed significant heritability that was specific to pubertal girls, but not pubertal boys or prepubertal children (Silberg et al., 1999).

Taking a diathesis–stress perspective, genes also can influence individual susceptibility to pathogenic environments; that is, a genetic predisposition might increase the likelihood that adolescents experience depression when they are exposed to stress. Both behavior genetic research and, more recently, molecular genetic research, provide evidence for gene × environment interactions in the prediction of adolescent depression. One study of adolescent twin pairs provided evidence that genetic liability increased adolescents' sensitivity to life stress (Eaves et al., 2003). Moreover, a cross-sectional study of adolescents revealed that a functional polymorphism in the promoter region of the serotonin transporter (5-HTT) gene predicted heightened depression in the face of life stress for adolescent girls but not for boys (Eley et al., 2004).

Finally, genes can affect the likelihood that individuals are exposed to depressogenic environments through passive or evocative gene–environment correlations (Eaves et al., 2003). Emerging evidence supports such pathways, as reflected in a shared liability to experiencing both negative life events and depression (Thapar, Harold, & McGuffin, 1998). Moreover, genetic liability to life events accounts in part for the higher rates of depression in girls after puberty (Silberg et al., 1999).

Research suggests, therefore, that genes and the environment jointly enhance risk for depression. Moreover, genetic liability to depression seems to be activated during the adolescent years, particularly in girls. This developmental expression of liability may be triggered by biological changes during the pubertal transition. Alternatively, it may stem from increasing psychological and social challenges during adolescence that create an opportunity for genetically mediated exposure or reactivity to life stress. Future research needs to identify specific genetic markers of risk, to elucidate the intersection between genetic and environmental influences, and to determine the specific biological, psychological, and social mechanisms (e.g., temperamental characteristics, neurobiological dysfunction, cognitive vulnerability, stress exposure or reactivity) through which genetic liability is translated into depression.

Biological Influences

Four primary areas of biological vulnerability have been explored: atypical brain structure and function, neuroendocrine dysregulation (including pubertal hormones), disruptions in neurotransmitter systems, and biological rhythm abnormalities, as reflected in sleep patterns. Despite some similarities in the biological markers of depression in adults and adolescents, important developmental differences also emerge (for a review, see Kaufman et al., 2001). These differences illustrate the importance of considering how maturation of biological systems across development might influence the etiology and/or sequelae of depression across the lifespan.

Neuroimaging studies in depressed adults reveal several consistent anatomical and functional abnormalities in the brain, including reduced amygdalar volume, hippocampal abnormalities, and reduced blood flow and metabolism in the prefrontal cortex (for a review, see Davidson, Pizzagalli, & Nitschke, 2002). Some similar abnormalities have been detected in depressed youth. Youth with MDD show reductions of amygdalar, but not hippocampal, volumes (Rosso et al., 2005; in a mixed sample of preadolescents and adolescents), reductions in white frontal matter volume (Steingard et al., 2002), and reduced blood flow in the prefrontal cortex (Chabrol, Barrere, Guell, Bes, & Moron, 1986). Consistent with possible amygdalar dysfunction, youth with a history of MDD show deficits in memory for fearful faces (Pine et al., 2004). Electrophysiological studies of adult depression reveal relative hypoactivation of the left frontal region of the brain. One prominent model of depression (Davidson et al., 2002) proposes that this pattern reflects an underactivation of the approach system that drives the experience of pleasure, leading to withdrawal from the environment. A similar pattern of hypoactivation has been found in high-risk (i.e., offspring of depressed mothers) infants (Dawson, Frey, Panagiotides, Osterling, & Hessl, 1997) and adolescents (Tomarken, Dichter, Garber, & Simien, 2004), suggesting that this asymmetry may represent a useful biological marker of depression vulnerability. Depressive symptoms in adolescents also have been linked to increased activity in the ventromedial prefrontal cortex and anterior cingulate gyrus during the processing of fearful faces (Killgore & Yurgelun-Todd, 2006).

Psychophysiological and neuropsychological research also suggests an atypical pattern of reduced right posterior brain activity in depressed youth (some of these studies include mixed samples of preadolescents and adolescents). Using electroencephalographic (EEG) recordings, one study found evidence for right parietotemporal hypoactivation (but not left frontal hypoactivation) in depressed female adolescents (Kentgen et al., 2000). Using neuropsychological methods (i.e., assessment of perceptual asymmetry in the processing of emotional expressions), another study found that a reduced posterior right hemisphere bias (PRHB) was associated with depressive symptoms in youth exposed to high but not low levels of interpersonal stress (Flynn & Rudolph, 2007). Moreover, maladaptive responses to stress (i.e., fewer effortful, planful responses and more involuntary, dysregulated responses) accounted for the contribution of a reduced PRHB to depressive symptoms, suggesting that this neuropsychological pattern heightens stress reactivity by interfering with effective coping and emotion regulation (Flynn & Rudolph, 2007). Deviant processing of facial emotions (i.e., selective attention to sad facial expressions) also has been found in the never-depressed daughters of depressed mothers, implicating this pattern as a possible marker of vulnerability (Joormann, Talbot, & Gotlib, 2007).

Research consistently demonstrates dysregulation of the biological stress-response system in adults with depression, as reflected in abnormalities in hypothalamic–pituitary–adrenal (HPA) axis function (for a review, see Thase, Jindal, & Howland, 2002). These abnormalities include higher levels of basal cortisol, abnormal responses to the dexamethasone suppression test (DST), and abnormalities in corticotropin-releasing factor (CRF). Most of these abnormalities are not found in depressed adolescents, except for a small degree of nonsuppression on the DST (for a review, see Kaufman et al., 2001). However, a few studies have found that HPA axis dysfunction (elevations in daytime or evening cortisol) predicts future depression and associated problems, such as suicidality, in adolescents (e.g., Goodyer, Herbert, Tamplin, & Altham, 2000; Mathew et al., 2003). One study also found that youth with heightened cortisol reactivity to a social challenge had higher levels of depressive symptoms 1 year later (Susman, Dorn, Inoff-Germain, Nottelman, & Chrousos, 1997), suggesting that examining reactivity rather than merely baseline HPA axis functioning or response to a pharamacological challenge might be critical to understanding risk for depression. Consistent with this idea, the daughters of depressed mothers show heightened cortisol reactivity in response to stress (Gotlib, Joormann, Minor, & Cooney, 2006). Another neuroendocrine marker of depression in adults is a blunted growth hormone response to pharmacological challenge; although this atypical response has been replicated in depressed preadolescents, adolescents do not show the same response (for a review, see Kaufman et al., 2001).

Hormonal changes during puberty also may contribute to the emerging sex difference in depression during adolescence. In the National Institute of Mental Health study of puberty and psychopathology, levels of follicle-stimulating hormone were linked to negative emotions in girls but not boys (Susman et al., 1985). This pattern did not hold for predicting depression diagnoses in the Great Smoky Mountains Study, but higher levels of androgen and estradiol were associated with depression in girls at puberty (Angold, Costello, Erkanli, & Worthman, 1999). The latter study revealed a threshold effect, such that when sex steroid levels (combined testosterone and estradiol) reached the upper 30th percentile, girls were five times more likely to be depressed than those with lower levels, and when they reached the upper 10%, there was an additional quadrupling in the rates of depression (Angold, Worthman, & Costello, 2003). In addition to hormonal effects on depression, some research suggests that the timing, or even perceived timing, of puberty (i.e., early maturation in girls and late maturation in boys) predicts depression and the sex difference in depression, suggesting that psychological and social aspects of puberty may contribute to the emerging sex difference beyond the effects of hormones (Conley & Rudolph, in press; cf. Angold et al., 2003).

There is limited evidence of abnormalities of the serotonergic neurotransmitter system in depressed youth, but the nature of this dysregulation is inconsistent across developmental stages and studies. Both high-risk and currently depressed prepubertal youth show blunted cortisol and increased prolactin in response to presynaptic probes (e.g., L-5-hydroxytryptophan), whereas two studies of adolescents show opposite patterns of prolactin release (one augmented, the other blunted) in response to postsynaptic probes (for a review, see Kaufman et al., 2001). Abnormalities in the serotonergic system are consistent with molecular genetic research that implicates a polymorphism in the serotonin transporter gene as a marker of depression vulnerability (Eley et al., 2004).

Depressed youth also show characteristic sleep disruption, including reduced rapid eye movement (REM) latency and increased REM density. Although adolescents share these particular sleep abnormalities with depressed adults, other sleep difficulties do not appear in adolescence (e.g., decreased delta sleep; for a review, see Kaufman et al., 2001).

Overall, research suggests that whereas some biological markers of depression are present as early as childhood, others appear in adolescence, and still others do not emerge until adulthood. Understanding the reasons for these developmental differences will provide insight into the etiology and sequelae of depression and, potentially, the rise in depression during adolescence (for a review, see Kaufman et al., 2001). These differences are likely due in part to the maturation of physiological systems, resulting in differing levels or types of biological vulnerability; that is, some biological markers may require maturation of the brain and neuroregulatory processes that is not achieved until adulthood. Biological vulnerability also may be triggered in part by puberty, such that changes in pubertal hormones activate, or interact with, other physiological systems implicated in depression. Moreover, developmental differences in biological vulnerability may reflect differing etiology of depression subtypes that are linked to age of onset. Finally, these differences may reflect variability in the course of depression earlier versus later in life; that is, some biological abnormalities may reflect sequelae rather than predisposing risk factors for depression. Because adolescents are less likely than adults to have experienced recurrent depression, they may not yet show the physiological consequences of prior episodes.

Future research needs to identify the origins of biological vulnerability. It is likely that these characteristics are in part genetically transmitted. However, biological vulnerability also may emerge from stressful physiological and social experiences (e.g., prior episodes of depression, social adversity) that create permanent changes in brain structure and function, thereby sensitizing the stress response system (Post, 1992). Identifying biological vulnerabilities to depression also may require considering interactions with stressful life contexts. Considering the intersection between biological and social processes during the transition through puberty may provide insight into the rising rates of depression and the emerging sex difference at this time.

Cognitive Influences

Cognitive models of depression assert that negative belief systems and maladaptive information processing create a vulnerability to depression. These models typically take a diathesis–stress form, wherein negative cognitions are presumed to interact with heightened stress to predict depression. A critical question regarding these models concerns how cognitive-developmental transformations from childhood through adulthood influence the emergence and consolidation of cognitive vulnerability to depression.

According to Beck's (1967) *cognitive model* of depression, negative cognitive schemas (belief systems focused on loss, failure, and worthlessness) and dysfunctional attitudes are triggered by stressful life events. Once activated, these schemas cause biased interpretations of events, resulting in overly pessimistic views of the self, world, and future, and consequent symptoms of depression. According to the *hopelessness theory* (Abramson, Metalsky, & Alloy, 1989), a maladaptive cognitive style interacts with stressful life events to foster negative inferences about the causes, consequences, and self-implications of events; these inferences contribute to the development of hopelessness (i.e., the expectation that desired outcomes will not occur or that aversive outcomes will occur, and that one cannot change the situation) and consequent symptoms of depression. This maladaptive cognitive style is reflected in three types of inferences, including a tendency (1) to attribute stressful events to stable and global causes, (2) to assume that stressful events will have other aversive consequences, and (3) to construe stressful events as a reflection of one's own unworthiness or deficiency. Other variants of cognitive models involve a similar focus on low perceptions of one's ability to control events (Weisz, Southam-Gerow, & McCarty, 2001) and of one's competence (Cole, Martin, & Powers, 1997).

A large corpus of research supports the idea that depressed adolescents show the hypothesized negative beliefs, maladaptive inferential styles, and biased information processing (for a review, see Rudolph et al., 2006). However, most of these studies do not provide an adequate test of cognitive vulnerability–stress theories, because they fail to examine two key elements: (1) the assumption of a prospective association between cognitive vulnerability and subsequent depression, and (2) the role of context (i.e., negative mood state or stressful life events) in activating cognitive vulnerability. Prospective research reveals that negative cognitions are both antecedents (Robinson, Garber, & Hilsman, 1995; Rudolph, Kurlakowsky, & Conley, 2001) and consequences (Pomerantz & Rudolph, 2003) of depression. Indeed, research suggests a reciprocal process in which an increase in negative cognitive styles predicts growth in depressive symptoms, and growth in depressive symptoms predicts an increase in negative cognitive styles (Garber, Keiley, & Martin, 2002). Research also has garnered support for cognition × stress interactions in the prediction of adolescent depression (Abela, 2001; Hankin & Abramson, 2002; Robinson et al., 1995). Finally, research demonstrates information-processing biases following a negative mood induction procedure in the never-depressed early adolescent daughters of depressed mothers, suggesting that these biases may play a role in depression vulnerability (Gotlib et al., 2006).

Despite this support for cognitive vulnerability–stress models of depression in youth, questions remain about the origins and development of cognitive vulnerability. Of particular relevance to understanding the rise in depressive symptoms during adolescence, it has been suggested that cognitive predispositions do not stabilize into trait-like vulnerability factors until youth acquire the capacity for abstract reasoning, generalization, and formal operational thought. Consistent with this idea, cognition × stress interactions predict depression over time more strongly in adolescence than in preadolescence (for a review, see Lakdawalla, Hankin, & Mermelstein, 2007). This consolidation of cognitive vulnerability during adolescence may in part explain the rise in depression during this stage. More research is needed to determine whether girls are particularly likely to show this pattern of increasing cognitive vulnerability, perhaps accounting in part for the emerging sex difference in depression. Some preliminary evidence does suggest that adolescent girls show a more negative cognitive style than do boys (Hankin & Abramson, 2002); this difference partly mediates the sex difference in depression.

Research also needs to elaborate on the origins of cognitive vulnerability and the factors that shape its development and consolidation. Multiple sources of cognitive vulnerability have been proposed, including genetic liability, temperamental traits, life stressors, and socialization experiences. Some research supports these links, but when and how cognitive styles become fully formed and resistant to change are still open questions. Moreover, identifying stage-specific domains of cognitive risk may clarify salient cognitive contributors to depression in adolescence. Finally, theory and research need to clarify the specific cognitive-developmental and biological transformations of adolescence that provide a context for the emergence of cognitive vulnerability.

Interpersonal Influences: Peer and Romantic Relationships

Interpersonal theories of depression focus on the transactions between individuals and their social contexts. According to these theories, depressed individuals engage in maladaptive behaviors that elicit negative responses from others, generating stress and conflict in their relationships. These relationship difficulties perpetuate or exacerbate symptoms and promote the recurrence of depression (Gotlib & Hammen, 1992; Hammen, 2006; Joiner, Coyne, & Blalock, 1999).

Although interpersonal theories were originally developed to explain adult depression, more recent models consider the developmental context of interpersonal dysfunction and depression (Cyranowski et al., 2000; Rudolph, in press; Rudolph, Flynn, & Abaied, 2008). These developmentally informed perspectives emphasize how normative intrapersonal and social challenges and disruptions associated with the adolescent transition create and interact with interpersonal vulnerability to heighten risk for depression. A specific goal is to account for the sharp rise in depression and the emergence of a sex difference in depression during adolescence. For example, one model (Rudolph, in press) proposes that maladaptive appraisals of relationships (e.g., negative conceptions of relationships and overinvestment in relationships) and social-behavioral deficits (e.g., poor self-regulation, social disengagement) potentiate depressive responses to interpersonal challenges, as well as cause youth to create problems in their relationships. Interpersonal vulnerability is amplified during the adolescent transition as a result of normative social-contextual, physical-maturational, and cognitive-developmental changes; this intensification process is particularly salient in girls, because they show more maladaptive appraisals of relationships and certain social-behavioral deficits, and they are exposed to more social challenges during adolescence. Finally, depression exacerbates interpersonal dysfunction, contributing to the continuity of depression over time.

Research supports many aspects of these developmentally based interpersonal models (for reviews, see Rudolph, in press; Rudolph et al., 2008). Both concurrent and longitudinal studies link negative conceptions of the self and others (e.g., views of the self as ineffective and unworthy; views of peers as hostile and untrustworthy) with depressive symptoms (e.g., Hammen et al., 1995; Rudolph & Clark, 2001). Moreover, a heightened investment in relationships, in the form of social-evaluative concerns (Rudolph & Conley, 2005) and interpersonal sensitivity (Rizzo, Daley, & Gunderson, 2006), predicts depressive symptoms over time.

Depressed adolescents also show social-behavioral deficits that likely interfere with the development and maintenance of high-quality relationships. Research based on self-report, parent report, and behavior observations reveals a pattern of maladaptive self-regulation in relationships. In challenging interpersonal situations, adolescents with depressive symptoms engage in lower levels of effortful engagement responses and higher levels of involuntary responses (Connor-Smith, Compas, Wadsworth, Thomsen, & Saltzman, 2000; Flynn & Rudolph, 2007). Adolescent depression also is associated with social disengagement

(Rudolph & Clark, 2001) and helpless behavior (Nolen-Hoeksema, Girgins, & Seligman, 1992) in peer relationships. Finally, *excessive reassurance seeking* (i.e., repeated attempts to seek assurance about one's self-worth; Prinstein, Borelli, Cheah, Simon, & Aikins, 2005) and *negative-feedback seeking* (i.e., active efforts to solicit feedback that verifies one's negative self-concept; Borelli & Prinstein, 2006) predict adolescent depression. Given these social-behavioral deficits, it is not surprising that depressed adolescents experience considerable disturbances in their peer relationships, such as lower levels of peer acceptance and higher levels of peer rejection (Nolan, Flynn, & Garber, 2003; Rudolph & Clark, 2001), as well as compromised close relationships, including poorer quality friendships (according to youth, but not their friends; Brendgen, Vitaro, Turgeon, & Poulin, 2002) and romantic relationships (according to both youth and their partners; Daley & Hammen, 2002).

Thus, considerable research shows that maladaptive appraisals of relationships, social-behavioral deficits, and relationship disturbances are associated with adolescent depression. Yet relatively few studies use longitudinal designs to examine whether interpersonal dysfunction contributes to prospective increases in depression. The available studies do suggest that some types of interpersonal dysfunction predict subsequent depression. For example, maladaptive responses to stress (Wadsworth & Berger, 2006), excessive reassurance seeking (Prinstein et al., 2005), negative-feedback seeking (in girls only; Borelli & Prinstein, 2006), and disturbances in peer (Nolan et al., 2003) and romantic (Monroe, Rohde, Seeley, & Lewinsohn, 1999) relationships predict subsequent depression. Research also suggests that appraisals of relationships and social-behavioral deficits interact with relationship disturbances to predict adolescent depression. In one study, high levels of interpersonal sensitivity amplified depressive responses to romantic relationship stress in adolescent girls (Rizzo et al., 2006). In another study, early adolescents characterized by anxious–solitary behavior showed stable high or increasing trajectories of depression over time when they faced exclusion by peers, but stable low or decreasing trajectories of depression over time when not excluded (Gazelle & Rudolph, 2004).

Even less research has examined the transactional hypothesis that is integral to most interpersonal theories of depression, namely, that depressive symptoms and associated behaviors elicit interpersonal rejection and disruption. In the short term, research shows that depressed adolescents elicit negative responses from unfamiliar peers (Connolly, Geller, Marton, & Kutcher, 1992) and create stress in their relationships (Daley et al., 1997; Krackow & Rudolph, 2008). Adolescent depressive symptoms also predict relationship difficulties over periods of 3 months to 2 years, including social helplessness (Nolen-Hoeksema et al., 1992), negative feedback seeking (Borelli & Prinstein, 2006), instability and poorer quality of friendships (Prinstein et al., 2005), and romantic relationship stress (Hankin, Mermelstein, & Roesch, 2007). As discussed earlier, adolescent depression also predicts considerable psychosocial maladjustment associated with the transition to adulthood (Gotlib et al., 1998; Rao et al., 1999).

In summary, research supports interpersonal theories of adolescent depression, suggesting that relationship dysfunction operates as both an antecedent and a consequence of depression, although more research is needed to confirm this transactional linkage. These processes may be particularly salient during the adolescent transition, especially in girls, when preexisting individual differences in interpersonal vulnerability interact with normative developmental challenges to contribute to rising rates of depression and the emerging sex difference in depression (for a review, see Rudolph, in press). During this stage, interpersonal relationships undergo significant change (e.g., disruptions in former peer groups and formation of new social networks; entrance into platonic and romantic heterosexual relationships); these changes seem to create particular difficulties for girls. Specifically, girls show increasing exposure to stress in their relationships from preadolescence to adolescence, particularly problems to which they contribute, whereas boys show stable and lower rates of disturbances. Girls also show more depressive reactions to relationship challenges than do boys (Hankin et al., 2007; Rudolph, 2002; Rudolph & Hammen, 1999; Shih, Eberhart, Hammen, & Brennan, 2006). Thus, increasing challenges within interpersonal relationships likely contribute to the emerging sex difference in depression across the adolescent transition.

Interpersonal Influences: Family Relationships

Depression has long been viewed as a disorder that arises within the family context. According to early (Bowlby, 1969; Freud, 1917) and contemporary (Goodman & Gotlib, 1999; Gotlib & Hammen, 1992; Hammen, 1991) theories, family adversity (e.g., parental depression, insecure parent–child attachment bonds, maltreatment, and maladaptive parenting) compromises the emerging biological, psychological, and emotional capabilities of young children (e.g., the maturation of neural circuits involved in the regulation and expression of emotion; the development of a healthy sense of self and internal working models of relationships; the acquisition of adaptive emotion regulation abilities), creating a vulnerability to depression.

In a related vein, *stress sensitization theory* (Monroe & Harkness, 2005) suggests that exposure to early adversity sensitizes individuals to later stressors in their lives, thereby lowering their threshold of reactivity. Two recent studies of adolescents (Hammen, Henry, & Daley, 2000; Harkness, Bruce, & Lumley, 2006) confirmed this pattern, demonstrating that youth with a history of family adversity are more likely than those without a history of family adversity to become depressed when faced with low levels of stress. A third study clarified particular patterns of risk associated with the stress sensitization effect across gender and development. Specifically, stress sensitization occurred in prepubertal boys and pubertal girls; in contrast, prepubertal girls with a history of adversity were more reactive to high levels of stress than those without a history of adversity (Rudolph & Flynn, 2007).

Although intriguing, research on stress sensitization does not explain *why* youth with a history of family adversity show heightened stress reactivity. Other lines of research identify possible modes of transmission, including neurobiological, cognitive, and interpersonal pathways. Essex, Klein, and Kalin (2002) found that preschoolers with a history of maternal stress exposure (particularly maternal depression) in infancy, as well as high levels of concurrent maternal stress, had elevated cortisol, suggesting that exposure to maternal stress sensitized the biological stress response system. Heightened cortisol reactivity also occurs in the adolescent female offspring of depressed mothers (Gotlib et al., 2006). Other research links maternal depression to atypical patterns of brain activity involved in the regulation and expression of emotion in infants (Dawson et al., 1997) and early adolescents (Gotlib et al., 2006); this dysregulation may alter reactivity to subsequent stress. Family adversity also contributes to maladaptive cognitive styles and to negative representations of self and relationships that may heighten future stress reactivity (Hankin, 2005; Rudolph et al., 2001). Providing evidence for an interpersonal pathway linking parent and offspring depression, Hammen, Shih, and Brennan (2004) showed that maternal depression is linked to interpersonal stress in mothers; this stress predicted poor parenting quality, as well as social competence deficits and interpersonal stress in offspring, which were linked to youth depression. Social deficits in the depressed adolescent offspring of depressed mothers are more severe than those in the depressed adolescent offspring of nondepressed mothers (Hammen & Brennan, 2001), suggesting that maternal depression plays a key role in the transmission of interpersonal vulnerability.

When coupled with research confirming the strong heritability of adolescent depression, this research suggests that the family transmission of depression and associated psychosocial adversity is likely due to a complicated interweaving of genetic risk (e.g., expressed in the form of stress reactive temperaments or disrupted patterns of brain functioning), neurobiological and psychological sequelae of *in utero* and early stress exposure, maladaptive cognitive styles, and social deficits (for reviews, see Goodman, 2002; Goodman & Gotlib, 1999; Hammen, 1991).

How is this early adversity translated into risk for depression during adolescence? At a simple level, early adversity is likely to be expressed directly as ongoing family disruption and conflict during adolescence. Indeed, family disturbances (e.g., high levels of criticism, hostility, and control, along with low levels of acceptance, warmth, and intimacy) during adolescence are associated concurrently and over time with depressive symptoms (Garber, Robinson, & Valentiner, 1997; Sheeber, Hops, Alpert, Davis, & Andrews, 1997; Sheeber & Sorensen, 1998). Moreover, preexisting vulnerabilities associated with early family adversity may be activated by normative challenges of the adolescent transition (Rudolph et al., 2006). This transition period produces many changes as youth strive to gain autonomy and develop independent social networks, while maintaining connectedness with their families; these changes, along with increasing parental expectations and concerns, foster family tension (for a review, see Paikoff & Brooks-Gunn, 1991). Youth and families entering this transition with compromised resources and strained relationships are particularly likely to experience difficulties negotiating the changing family context, thereby increasing risk for depression in youth. Some research also suggests that adolescent girls are more susceptible than boys to adverse family influences. Maternal depression is more strongly linked to youth depression in adolescent girls than in boys; moreover, family discord accounts for this link in adolescent girls but not boys (for a review, see Sheeber, Davis, & Hops, 2002). More generally, as discussed earlier, early adversity predicts stress sensitization in pubertal girls but not boys. Thus, family influences likely play a critical role in accounting for rising rates of depression during the transition to adolescence, particularly in girls.

Contextual Influences

Life stress theories view depression as a response to adverse environmental events or circumstances that present an objective threat to individuals' well-being (Brown & Harris, 1978). Research has focused on a wide range of stressors, including acute negative life events, chronic stressful conditions, daily hassles, and broader contextual influences, such as socioeconomic disadvantage. Consistent with life stress theories, a variety of stressors contribute to subsequent depression in adolescents (e.g., Ge et al., 1994; Hankin et al., 2007). As reflected in the earlier section on interpersonal influences, exposure to stress within relationships (e.g., conflict, loss, relationship breakups) seems to be particularly strongly associated with depression (Eley & Stevenson, 2000; Rudolph et al., 2000).

Although stress clearly plays a large role in depression, there are significant individual differences in how youth respond to stress. Therefore, diathesis–stress models consider a range of personal attributes and environmental conditions that either attenuate or amplify stress reactivity. Several possible vulnerabilities were discussed in earlier sections, including genetic liability, physiological dysregulation, negative cognitive styles, and social-behavioral deficits. Overall, research supports the idea that some adolescents are more susceptible to the adverse influence of stress than others (for reviews, see Hankin & Abramson, 2001; Rudolph et al., 2006). Thus, how youth appraise and respond to stressors determines their likelihood of experiencing depression.

Building on stress exposure and diathesis–stress theories that emphasize the influence of "fateful" or independent life events on depression (Brown & Harris, 1978), contemporary perspectives acknowledge the transactions between individuals and their social contexts. Hammen's (2006) *stress generation model* proposes that personality characteristics and behaviors of depressed individuals cause them to create stress, particularly in their relationships, which then contributes to future depression. Indeed, a growing body of research confirms that depressed youth generate stress in their own lives (Daley et al., 1997; Hankin et al., 2007; Krackow & Rudolph, 2008; Rudolph et al., 2000; Shih et al., 2006). Moreover, a recent study that directly examined the reciprocal association between stress and depression across multiple waves in two samples provided support for both stress exposure and stress generation processes in youth depression (Cole, Nolen-Hoeksema, Girgus, & Paul, 2006). Beyond depressive symptoms, other characteristics of depression-prone individuals, such as negative conceptions of relationships (Caldwell, Rudolph, Troop-Gordon, & Kim, 2004) and problematic interpersonal problem-solving styles (Davila, Hammen, Burge, Paley, & Daley, 1995), predict subsequent generation of stress.

Life stress theories have particular relevance for understanding the emergence of depression during adolescence. This transition is marked by normative changes that form a backdrop for greater stress exposure and consequent rising rates of depression. Indeed, cross-sectional research reveals more stress in adolescence than in preadolescence (Rudolph & Hammen, 1999). Moreover, longitudinal research shows growth in the experience of stress beginning at age 13, mirrored by growth in depressive symptoms (Ge et al., 1994). Increasing stress levels also have been implicated in the emerging sex difference in depression. Both cross-sectional and longitudinal research suggest that girls are particularly susceptible to increasing levels of stress during adolescence (Ge et al., 1994), especially in their relationships (Hankin et al., 2007; Rudolph & Hammen, 1999; Shih et al., 2006). Furthermore, girls are more likely than boys to experience depression in the face of stress (Ge et al., 1994; Hankin et al., 2007), particularly interpersonal stress (Rudolph & Hammen, 1999; Shih et al., 2006). In fact, greater exposure and reactivity to stress appear to account in part for heightened depression in adolescent girls compared to boys (Hankin et al., 2007; Rudolph, 2002; Shih et al., 2006). Different patterns of stress reactivity in girls and boys appear to be linked not only to the progression through adolescence but also more specifically to the timing of maturation. Specifically, a recent study revealed that heightened exposure to peer stress predicts depression in girls with *early* actual and perceived pubertal timing, and in boys with *late* actual and perceived pubertal timing (Conley & Rudolph, in press). These findings suggest that biological and/or psychological changes associated with the pubertal transition interact with stressors to influence the emerging sex difference in depression.

Adolescents also may generate more stress in their lives than do preadolescents. During adolescence, youth begin to exert greater control over their lives, and often engage in risky behavior and experimentation (Arnett, 1999) that might increase their likelihood of creating stress. Adolescence also is marked by a shift in social networks and close relationships, which presents unique challenges and allows youth to select risky social contexts, such as deviant peer groups or abusive romantic relationships. Although developmental differences in stress generation have not been well explored, one recent study suggests that the stress generation effect of depression increases from early childhood through adolescence (Cole et al., 2006). Moreover, another recent study indicates that depression predicts the subsequent generation of interpersonal stress in early-maturing, but not late-maturing, youth (Rudolph, in press), suggesting once again that understanding the context of depression during adolescence requires a consideration of not only age but also pubertal development.

In summary, significant evidence attests to the role of stress as a key factor in adolescent depression, and more limited evidence suggests that stress exposure, generation, and reactivity contribute in part to the rise in depression and the emerging sex difference in depression during adolescence. Research also supports diathesis–stress models that propose interactions between individual vulnerabilities (e.g., genetic, biological, cognitive, and interpersonal) and contextual risks, indicating the importance of an integrative model of adolescent depression.

FUTURE DIRECTIONS

Depression is a disorder that often emerges during adolescence and follows a chronic or recurring course through adulthood, often generating significant psychosocial impairment. For the most part, the depressive syndrome shows a large degree of continuity across developmental stages. However, some unique, age-linked characteristics indicate the need to explore more explicitly possible differences in the nature, etiology, correlates, course, and consequences of depressive disorders that arise during different stages. It is possible that the syndrome is essentially comparable across the lifespan, but some vulnerability factors (e.g., negative cognitive styles, HPA axis dysregulation) do not become active contributors to depression until later in development, when physiological, cognitive, and emotional capabilities and social experiences coalesce into more stable and organized systems. Alternatively, depressive disorders with an onset in childhood (i.e., prior to puberty) may differ from those with an onset in adolescence (i.e., following puberty). Some preliminary research suggests that childhood-onset depression, particularly when it co-occurs with externalizing disorders, reflects a less specialized syndrome that often predicts nondepressive psychopathology later in life and does not have a strong genetic component. In contrast, adolescent-onset depression seems to be strongly linked to genetic liability and shares many similarities with adult depression, although there are some differences in the neurobiological correlates of depression in adolescents and adults.

Regardless of questions concerning the continuity of depression across the lifespan, clear evidence for heterogeneity in the etiology of depression indicates the need for an integrative model of adolescent depression that considers the unique, synergistic, and transactional contributions of innate predispositions (e.g., temperamental traits, neurobiological functioning), competencies (e.g., cognitive styles and appraisals of relationships, emotion regulation and coping abilities, social-behavioral skills), and social experiences (e.g., relationship disturbances, life stressors) to the emergence and perpetuation of depression. Many questions remain, however, concerning how these vulnerability and risk factors work together to predict adolescent depression.

First, research needs to investigate whether the multiple contributors to depression reflect distinct versus overlapping risks, as well as to identify the complex mechanisms that link these various risks. For example, are negative cognitive styles and poor emotion regulation strategies the expression of genetic liability to depression, or do they represent independent pathways to depression? Does early exposure to adversity become translated into depression vulnerability through the sensitization of biological, cognitive, and/or emotional pathways? What are the unique genetic versus environmental contributions to youth depression arising from parental depression? How and when are atypical patterns of neuro-biological functioning in high-risk youth translated into psychological or emotional processes that create a vulnerability to depression? What are the processes through which depressed youth create and select stressful environments, and are there individual differences in the extent to which depressed youth generate stress in their lives? Answering these questions has implications for not only theory but also efforts aimed at identifying high-risk youth and preventing the expression of liability for depression later in life.

Another critical direction for future research is continued investigation of the specificity of particular vulnerability and risk factors to adolescent depression versus other forms of psychopathology. Relatedly, significant efforts are needed to investigate alternative explanations for depression comorbidity. Clues may stem from the temporal sequencing of disorders, but more research is needed to determine whether this sequence reflects the developmental unfolding of a generalized vulnerability to negative affect and stress reactivity, a functional association between earlier and later disorders, or some combination of the two.

A third avenue for exploration is to elucidate why depression increases during adolescence, and why girls are particularly susceptible at this time. A growing number of developmentally informed theories incorporate an explicit focus on these two questions (Cyranowski et al., 2000; Hankin & Abramson, 2001; Nolen-Hoeksema & Girgus, 1994; Rudolph, in press; Rudolph et al., 2006). Moreover, empirical advances have identified why individual vulnerability and/or risk is amplified during the adolescent transition. However, much remains to be learned about this transition. For example, relatively little is known about how biological, psychological, and social challenges of the adolescent transition interact to predict depression. Moreover, although the focus on depression in adolescent girls is critical given their elevated risk, some adolescent boys do become depressed. Research is needed to determine whether similar or different processes lead to depression in adolescent girls and boys. It also is unclear whether the adolescent transition creates new vulnerabilities to depression in previously healthy youth, or whether it merely exacerbates risk in youth with a genetic liability or other preexisting vulnerabilities.

Finally, it is important to note that transitions can represent turning points at which some youth progress down a deviant trajectory toward increasing risk and impairment, whereas others move toward a more adaptive trajectory. Understanding the factors that determine developmental trajectories over the course of the adolescent transition would shed considerable light on possible characteristics or experiences that amplify or minimize risk for depression through adolescence and adulthood.

REFERENCES

Abela, J. R. Z. (2001). The hopelessness theory of depression: A test of the diathesis–stress and causal mediation components in third and seventh grade children. *Journal of Abnormal Child Psychology*, 29, 241–254.

Abramson, L. Y., Metalsky, G. I., & Alloy, L. B. (1989). Hopelessness depression: A theory-based subtype of depression. *Psychological Review*, 96, 358–372.

Alloy, L. B., Kelly, K. A., Mineka, S., & Clements, C. M. (1990). Comorbidity of anxiety and depressive disorders: A helplessness–hopelessness perspective. In J. D. Maser & C. R. Cloninger (Eds.), *Comorbidity of mood and anxiety disorders* (pp. 499–543). Washington, DC: American Psychiatric Press.

Angold, A., Costello, E. J., & Erkanli, A. (1999). Comorbidity. *Journal of Child Psychology and Psychiatry*, 40, 57–87.

Angold, A., Costello, E. J., Erkanli, A., & Worthman, C. M. (1999). Pubertal changes in hormones of adolescent girls. *Psychological Medicine, 29*, 1043–1053.

Angold, A., Erkanli, A., Silberg, J., Eaves, L., & Costello, E. J. (2002). Depression scale scores in 8- to 17-year-olds: Effects of age and gender. *Journal of Child Psychology and Psychiatry, 43*, 1052–1063.

Angold, A., Worthman, C., & Costello, E. J. (2003). Puberty and depression. In C. Hayward (Ed.), *Gender differences at puberty* (pp. 137–164). New York: Cambridge University Press.

Angst, J., Sellaro, R., & Merikangas, K. R. (2000). Depressive spectrum diagnoses. *Comprehensive Psychiatry, 41*, 39–47.

Arnett, J. J. (1999). Adolescent storm and stress, reconsidered. *American Psychologist, 54*, 317–326.

Avenevoli, S., & Steinberg, L. (2001). The continuity of depression across the adolescent transition. *Advances in Child Development and Behavior, 28*, 139–173.

Beck, A. T. (1967). *Depression: Clinical, experimental, and theoretical aspects.* New York: Harper & Row.

Birmaher, B., Arbelaez, C., & Brent, D. (2002). Course and outcome of child and adolescent major depressive disorder. *Child and Adolescent Psychiatric Clinics of North America, 11*, 619–638.

Birmaher, B., Ryan, N. D., Williamson, D. E., Brent, D. A., Kaufman, J., Dahl, R. E., et al. (1996). Childhood and adolescent depression: A review of the past 10 years: Part I. *Journal of the American Academy of Child and Adolescent Psychiatry, 35*, 1427–1439.

Borelli, J. L., & Prinstein, M. J. (2006). Reciprocal, longitudinal associations between adolescents' negative feedback-seeking, depressive symptoms, and friendship perceptions. *Journal of Abnormal Child Psychology, 34*, 159–169.

Bowlby, J. (1969). *Attachment and loss: Vol. I. Attachment.* New York: Basic Books.

Brendgen, M., Vitaro, F., Turgeon, L., & Poulin, F. (2002). Assessing aggressive and depressed children's social relations with classmates and friends: A matter of perspective. *Journal of Abnormal Child Psychology, 30*, 609–624.

Brown, G. W., & Harris, T. (1978). *Social origins of depression: A study of psychiatric disorders in women.* New York: Free Press.

Caldwell, M. S., Rudolph, K. D., Troop-Gordon, W., & Kim, D. (2004). Reciprocal influences among relational self-views, social disengagement, and peer stress during early adolescence. *Child Development, 75*, 1140–1154.

Chabrol, H., Barrere, M., Guell, A., Bes, A., & Moron, P. (1986). Hyperfrontality of cerebral blood flow in depressed adolescents. *American Journal of Psychiatry, 143*, 263–264.

Cole, D. A., Martin, J. M., & Powers, B. (1997). A competency-based model of child depression: A longitudinal study of peer, parent, teacher, and self-evaluations. *Journal of Child Psychology and Psychiatry, and Allied Disciplines, 38*, 505–514.

Cole, D. A., Nolen-Hoeksema, S., Girgus, J., & Paul, G. (2006). Stress exposure and stress generation in child and adolescent depression: A latent trait–state-error approach to longitudinal analyses. *Journal of Abnormal Psychology, 115*, 40–51.

Conley, C. S., & Rudolph, K. D. (in press). Sex differences in depression: The interactive role of pubertal development and peer stress. *Development and Psychopathology.*

Connolly, J., Geller, S., Marton, P., & Kutcher, S. (1992). Peer responses to social interaction with depressed adolescents. *Journal of Clinical Child Psychology, 21*, 365–370.

Connor-Smith, J. K., Compas, B. E., Wadsworth, M. E., Thomsen, A. H., & Saltzman, H. (2000). Responses to stress in adolescence: Measurement of coping and involuntary stress responses. *Journal of Consulting and Clinical Psychology, 68*, 976–992.

Costello, E. J., Mustillo, S., Erkanli, A., Keeler, G., & Angold, A. (2003). Prevalence and development of psychiatric disorders in childhood and adolescence. *Archives of General Psychiatry, 60*, 837–844.

Cyranowski, J. M., Frank, E., Young, E., & Shear, K. (2000). Adolescent onset of the gender difference in lifetime rates of depression. *Archives of General Psychiatry, 57*, 21–27.

Daley, S. E., & Hammen, C. (2002). Depressive symptoms and close relationships during the transition to adulthood: Perspectives from dysphoric women, their best friends, and their romantic partners. *Journal of Consulting and Clinical Psychology, 70*, 129–141.

Daley, S. E., Hammen, C., Burge, D., Davila, J., Paley, B., Lindberg, N., et al. (1997). Predictors of the generation of episodic stress: A longitudinal study of late adolescent women. *Journal of Abnormal Psychology, 106,* 251–259.

Davidson, R. J., Pizzagalli, D., & Nitschke, J. (2002). The representation and regulation of emotion in depression: Perspectives from affective neuroscience. In I. H. Gotlib & C. L. Hammen (Eds.), *Handbook of depression* (pp. 219–244). New York: Guilford Press.

Davila, J., Hammen, C., Burge, D., Paley, B., & Daley, S. E. (1995). Poor interpersonal problem solving as a mechanism of stress generation in depression among adolescent women. *Journal of Abnormal Psychology, 104,* 592–600.

Dawson, G., Frey, K., Panagiotides, H., Osterling, J., & Hessl, D. (1997). Infants of depressed mothers exhibit atypical frontal brain activity: A replication and extension of previous findings. *Journal of Child Psychology and Psychiatry, 38,* 179–186.

Eaves, L., Silberg, J., & Erkanli, A. (2003). Resolving multiple epigenetic pathways to adolescent depression. *Journal of Child Psychology and Psychiatry, 44,* 1006–1014.

Eley, T. C., & Stevenson, J. (2000). Specific life events and chronic experiences differentially associated with depression and anxiety in young twins. *Journal of Abnormal Child Psychology, 28,* 383–394.

Eley, T. C., Sugden, K., Corsico, A., Gregory, A. M., Sham, P., McGuffin, P., et al. (2004). Gene–environment interaction analysis of serotonin system markers with adolescent depression. *Molecular Psychiatry, 9,* 908–918.

Essex, M. J., Klein, M. H., & Kalin, N. H. (2002). Maternal stress beginning in infancy may sensitize children to later stress exposure: Effects on cortisol and behavior. *Biological Psychiatry, 52,* 776–784.

Flynn, M., & Rudolph, K. D. (2007). Perceptual asymmetry and youths' responses to stress: Understanding vulnerability to depression. *Cognition and Emotion, 21,* 773–788.

Freud, S. (1917). Mourning and melancholia. In J. Strachey (Ed. & Trans.), *The standard edition of the complete psychological works of Sigmund Freud* (Vol. 14). London: Hogarth Press.

Garber, J., Keiley, M. K., & Martin, N. C. (2002). Developmental trajectories of adolescents' depressive symptoms: Predictors of change. *Journal of Consulting and Clinical Psychology, 70,* 79–95.

Garber, J., Robinson, N. S., & Valentiner, D. (1997). The relation between parenting and adolescent depression: Self-worth as a mediator. *Journal of Adolescent Research, 12,* 12–33.

Gazelle, H., & Rudolph, K. D. (2004). Moving toward and away from the world: Social approach and avoidance trajectories in anxious solitary youth. *Child Development, 75,* 829–849.

Ge, X., Lorenz, F. O., Conger, R. D., Elder, G. G., & Simons, R. L. (1994). Trajectories of stressful life events and depressive symptoms during adolescence. *Developmental Psychology, 30,* 467–483.

Goodman, S. H. (2002). Depression and early adverse experiences. In I. H. Gotlib & C. Hammen (Eds.), *Handbook of depression* (pp. 245–267). New York: Guilford Press.

Goodman, S. H., & Gotlib, I. H. (1999). Risk for psychopathology in the children of depressed mothers: A developmental model for understanding mechanisms of transmission. *Psychological Review, 106,* 458–490.

Goodyer, I. M., Herbert, J., Tamplin, A., & Altham, P. M. E. (2000). Recent life events, cortisol, dehydroepiandrosterone and the onset of major depression in high-risk adolescents. *British Journal of Psychiatry, 177,* 499–504.

Gotlib, I., Lewinsohn, P., & Seeley, J. (1998). Consequences of depression during adolescence: Marital status and marital functioning in early adulthood. *Journal of Abnormal Psychology, 107,* 686–690.

Gotlib, I. H., & Hammen, C. (1992). *Psychological aspects of depression: Toward a cognitive–interpersonal integration.* London: Wiley.

Gotlib, I. H., Joormann, J., Minor, K. L., & Cooney, R. E. (2006). Cognitive and biological functioning in children at risk for depression. In T. Canli (Ed.), *Biology of personality and individual differences* (pp. 353–382). New York: Guilford Press.

Gotlib, I. H., Lewinsohn, P. M., & Seeley, J. R. (1995). Symptoms versus a diagnosis of depression: Differences in psychosocial functioning. *Journal of Consulting and Clinical Psychology, 63,* 90–100.

Hammen, C. (1991). *Depression runs in families: The social context of risk and resilience in children of depressed mothers.* New York: Springer-Verlag.

Hammen, C. (2006). Stress generation in depression: Reflections on origins, research, and future directions. *Journal of Clinical Psychology, 62,* 69–82.

Hammen, C., & Brennan, P. A. (2001). Depressed adolescents of depressed and nondepressed mothers: Tests of an interpersonal impairment hypothesis. *Journal of Consulting and Clinical Psychology, 69*, 284–294.

Hammen, C., Burge, D., Daley, S. E., Davila, J., Paley, B., & Rudolph, K. D. (1995). Interpersonal attachment cognitions and prediction of symptomatic responses to interpersonal stress. *Journal of Abnormal Psychology, 104*, 436–443.

Hammen, C., Henry, R., & Daley, S. E. (2000). Depression and sensitization to stressors among young women as a function of childhood adversity. *Journal of Consulting and Clinical Psychology, 68*, 782–787.

Hammen, C., Shih, J. H., & Brennan, P. A. (2004). Intergenerational transmission of depression: Test of an interpersonal stress model in a community sample. *Journal of Consulting and Clinical Psychology, 72*, 511–522.

Hankin, B. L. (2005). Childhood maltreatment and psychopathology: Prospective tests of attachment, cognitive vulnerability, and stress as mediating processes. *Cognitive Therapy Research, 29*, 645–671.

Hankin, B. L., & Abramson, L. Y. (2001). Development of gender differences in depression: An elaborated cognitive vulnerability–transactional stress theory. *Psychological Bulletin, 127*, 773–796.

Hankin, B. L., & Abramson, L. Y. (2002). Measuring cognitive vulnerability to depression in adolescence: Reliability, validity, and gender differences. *Journal of Child and Adolescent Clinical Psychology, 31*, 491–504.

Hankin, B. L., Abramson, L. Y., Moffitt, T. E., Silva, P. A., McGee, R., & Angell, K. E. (1998). Development of depression from preadolescence to young adulthood: Emerging gender differences in a 10-year longitudinal study. *Journal of Abnormal Psychology, 107*, 128–140.

Hankin, B. L., Mermelstein, R., & Roesch, L. (2007). Sex differences in adolescent depression: Stress exposure and reactivity models in interpersonal and achievement contextual domains. *Child Development, 78*, 279–295.

Harkness, K. L., Bruce, A. E., & Lumley, M. N. (2006). The role of childhood abuse and neglect in the sensitization to stressful life events in adolescent depression. *Journal of Abnormal Psychology, 115*, 730–741.

Harrington, R., & Dubicka, B. (2001). Natural history of mood disorders in children and adolescents. In I. M. Goodyer (Ed.), *The depressed child and adolescent* (2nd ed., pp. 353–381). New York: Cambridge University Press.

Harrington, R., Fudge, H., Rutter, M., Pickles, A., & Hill, J. (1990). Adult outcomes of childhood and adolescent depression: I. Psychiatric status. *Archives of General Psychiatry, 47*, 465–473.

Harrington, R., Fudge, H., Rutter, M., Pickles, A., & Hill, J. (1991). Adult outcomes of childhood and adolescent depression: II. Risk for antisocial disorders. *Journal of the American Academy of Child and Adolescent Psychiatry, 30*, 434–439.

Harrington, R., Rutter, M., & Fombonne, E. (1996). Developmental pathways in depression: Multiple meanings, antecedents, and endpoints. *Development and Psychopathology, 8*, 601–616.

Joiner, T. E., Coyne, J. C., & Blalock, J. (1999). On the interpersonal nature of depression: Overview and synthesis. In T. E. Joiner & J. C. Coyne (Eds.), *The interactional nature of depression* (pp. 3–19). Washington, DC: American Psychological Association.

Joormann, J., Talbot, L., & Gotlib, I. H. (2007). Biased processing of emotional information in girls at risk for depression. *Journal of Abnormal Psychology, 116*, 135–143.

Kaufman, J., Martin, A., King, R. A., & Charney, D. (2001). Are child-, adolescent-, and adult-onset depression one and the same disorder? *Biological Psychiatry, 49*, 980–1001.

Kentgen, L. M., Tenke, C. E., Pine, D. S., Fong, R., Klein, R. G., & Bruder, G. E. (2000). Electroencephalographic asymmetries in adolescents with major depression: Influence of comorbidity with anxiety disorders. *Journal of Abnormal Psychology, 109*, 797–802.

Kessler, R. C., Avenevoli, S., & Merikangas, K. R. (2001). Mood disorders in children and adolescents: An epidemiologic perspective. *Biological Psychiatry, 49*, 1002–1014.

Kessler, R. C., & Walters, E. E. (1998). Epidemiology of DSM-III-R major depression and minor depression among adolescents and young adults in the National Comorbidity Survey. *Depression and Anxiety, 7*, 3–14.

Killgore, W. D. S., & Yurgelun-Todd, D. A. (2006). Ventromedial prefrontal activity correlates with depressed mood in adolescent children. *NeuroReport, 17*, 167–171.

Kim-Cohen, J., Caspi, A., Moffit, T. E., Harrington, H., Milne, B. J., & Poulton, R. (2003). Prior juvenile diagnoses in adults with mental disorder: Developmental follow-back of a prospective–longitudinal cohort. *Archives of General Psychiatry, 60,* 709–717.

Kovacs, M., & Devlin, B. (1998). Internalizing disorders in childhood. *Journal of Child Psychology and Psychiatry, and Allied Disciplines, 39,* 47–63.

Krackow, E., & Rudolph, K. D. (2008). Life stress and the accuracy of cognitive appraisals in depressed youth. *Journal of Clinical Child and Adolescent Psychology, 37,* 376–385.

Lakdawalla, Z., Hankin, B. L., & Mermelstein, R. (2007). Cognitive theories of depression in children and adolescents: A conceptual and quantitative review. *Clinical Child and Family Psychology Review, 10,* 1–24.

Lewinsohn, P. M., & Essau, C. A. (2002). Depression in adolescents. In I. H. Gotlib & C. L. Hammen (Eds.), *Handbook of depression* (pp. 541–559). New York: Guilford Press.

Lewinsohn, P. M., Hops, H., Roberts, R. E., Seeley, J. R., & Andrews, J. A. (1993). Adolescent psychopathology: I. Prevalence and incidence of depression and other DSM-III-R disorders in high school students. *Journal of Abnormal Psychology, 102,* 133–144.

Lewinsohn, P. M., Rohde, P., Klein, D. N., & Seeley, J. R. (1999). Natural course of adolescent major depressive disorder: I. Continuity into young adulthood. *Journal of the American Academy of Child and Adolescent Psychiatry, 38,* 56–63.

Lewinsohn, P. M., Rohde, P., & Seeley, J. R. (1994). Psychosocial risk factors for future adolescent suicide attempts. *Journal of Consulting and Clinical Psychology, 62,* 297–305.

Lewinsohn, P. M., Rohde, P., & Seeley, J. R. (1998). Major depressive disorder in older adolescents: Prevalence, risk factors, and clinical implications. *Clinical Psychology Review, 18,* 765–794.

Lewinsohn, P. M., Rohde, P., Seeley, J. R., Klein, D. N., & Gotlib, I. H. (2000). Natural course of adolescent major depressive disorder in a community sample: Predictors of recurrence in young adults. *American Journal of Psychiatry, 157,* 1584–1591.

Mathew, S. J., Coplan, J. D., Goetz, R. R., Feder, A., Greenwald, S., Dahl, R. E., et al. (2003). Differentiating depressed adolescent 24h cortisol secretion in light of their adult clinical outcome. *Neuropsychopharmacology, 28,* 1336–1343.

Monroe, S. M., & Harkness, K. L. (2005). Life stress, the "kindling" hypothesis, and the recurrence of depression: Considerations from a life stress perspective. *Psychological Review, 112,* 417–445.

Monroe, S. M., Rohde, P., Seeley, J. R., & Lewinsohn, P. M. (1999). Life events and depression in adolescence: Relationship loss as a prospective risk factor for first onset of major depressive disorder. *Journal of Abnormal Psychology, 108,* 606–614.

Nolan, S. A., Flynn, C., & Garber, J. (2003). Prospective relations between rejection and depression in young adolescents. *Journal of Personality and Social Psychology, 85,* 745–755.

Nolen-Hoeksema, S., & Girgus, J. S. (1994). The emergence of gender differences in depression in adolescence. *Psychological Bulletin, 115,* 424–443.

Nolen-Hoeksema, S., Girgus, J. S., & Seligman, M. E. P. (1992). Predictors and consequences of childhood depressive symptoms: A 5-year longitudinal study. *Journal of Abnormal Psychology, 101,* 405–422.

Paikoff, R. L., & Brooks–Gunn, J. (1991). Do parent–child relationships change during puberty? *Psychological Bulletin, 110,* 47–66.

Patterson, G. R., & Stoolmiller, M. (1991). Replications of a dual failure model for boys' depressed mood. *Journal of Consulting and Clinical Psychology, 59,* 491–498.

Pine, D. S., Lissek, S., Klein, R. G., Mannuzza, S., Moulton, J. L., Guardino, M., et al. (2004). Face-memory and emotion: Associations with major depression in children and adolescents. *Journal of Child Psychology and Psychiatry, and Allied Disciplines, 45,* 1199–1208.

Pomerantz, E. M., & Rudolph, K. D. (2003). What ensues from emotional distress?: Implications for competence estimation. *Child Development, 74,* 329–345.

Post, R. M. (1992). Transduction of psychosocial stress into the neurobiology of recurrent affective disorder. *American Journal of Psychiatry, 149,* 999–1010.

Prinstein, M. J., Borelli, J. L., Cheah, C. S. L., Simon, V. A., & Aikins, J. W. (2005). Adolescent girls' interpersonal vulnerability to depressive symptoms: A longitudinal examination of reassurance-seeking and peer relationships. *Journal of Abnormal Psychology, 114,* 676–688.

Rao, U., Hammen, C., & Daley, S. (1999). Continuity of depression during the transition to adulthood: A 5-year longitudinal study of young women. *Journal of the American Academy of Child and Adolescent Psychiatry, 38*, 908–915.

Rao, U., Ryan, N. D., Birmaher, B., Dahl, R. E., Williamson, D. E., Kaufman, J., et al. (1995). Unipolar depression in adolescents: Clinical outcomes in adulthood. *Journal of the American Academy of Child and Adolescent Psychiatry, 34*, 566–578.

Rice, F., Harold, G., & Thapar, A. (2002). The genetic aetiology of childhood depression: A review. *Journal of Child Psychology and Psychiatry, 43*, 65–79.

Rizzo, C. J., Daley, S. E., & Gunderson, B. H. (2006). Interpersonal sensitivity, romantic stress, and the prediction of depression: A study of inner-city, minority adolescent girls. *Journal of Youth and Adolescence, 35*, 444–453.

Robinson, N. S., Garber, J., & Hilsman, R. (1995). Cognitions and stress: Direct and moderating effects on depressive versus externalizing symptoms during the junior high school transition. *Journal of Abnormal Psychology, 104*, 453–463.

Rohde, P., Lewinsohn, P. M., Klein, D. N., & Seeley, J. R. (2005). Association of parental depression with psychiatric course from adolescence to young adulthood among formerly depressed individuals. *Journal of Abnormal Psychology, 114*, 409–420.

Rohde, P., Lewinsohn, P. M., & Seeley, J. R. (1991). Comorbidity of unipolar depression: II. Comorbidity with other mental disorders in adolescents and adults. *Journal of Abnormal Psychology, 100*, 214–222.

Rosso, I. M., Cintron, C. M., Steingard, R. J., Renshaw, P. F., Young, A. D., & Yurgelun-Todd, D. A. (2005). Amygdala and hippocampus volumes in pediatric major depression. *Biological Psychiatry, 57*, 21–26.

Rudolph, K. D. (2002). Gender differences in emotional responses to interpersonal stress during adolescence. *Journal of Adolescent Health, 30*, 3–13.

Rudolph, K. D. (in press). Developmental influences on interpersonal stress generation in depressed youth. *Journal of Abnormal Psychology.*

Rudolph, K. D. (in press). The interpersonal context of adolescent depression. In S. Nolen-Hoeksema & L. M. Hilt (Eds.), *Handbook of depression in adolescents.* New York: Routledge.

Rudolph, K. D., & Clark, A. G. (2001). Conceptions of relationships in children with depressive and aggressive symptoms: Social–cognitive distortion or reality? *Journal of Abnormal Child Psychology, 29*, 41–56.

Rudolph, K. D., & Conley, C. S. (2005). Socioemotional costs and benefits of social-evaluative concerns: Do girls care too much? *Journal of Personality, 73*, 115–137.

Rudolph, K. D., & Flynn, M. (2007). Childhood adversity and youth depression: The role of gender and pubertal status. *Development and Psychopathology, 19*, 497–521.

Rudolph, K. D., Flynn, M., & Abaied, J. L. (2008). A developmental perspective on interpersonal theories of youth depression. In J. R. Z. Abela & B. L. Hankin (Eds.), *Handbook of depression in children and adolescents* (pp. 79–102). New York: Guilford Press.

Rudolph, K. D., & Hammen, C. (1999). Age and gender determinants of stress exposure, generation, and reactions in youngsters: A transactional perspective. *Child Development, 70*, 660–677.

Rudolph, K. D., Hammen, C., Burge, D., Lindberg, N., Herzberg, D., & Daley, S. (2000). Toward an interpersonal life-stress model of depression: The developmental context of stress generation. *Development and Psychopathology, 12*, 215–234.

Rudolph, K. D., Hammen, C., & Daley, S. E. (2006). Mood disorders. In D. A. Wolfe & E. J. Mash (Eds.), *Behavioral and emotional disorders in adolescents: Nature, assessment, and treatment* (pp. 300–342). New York: Guilford Press.

Rudolph, K. D., Kurlakowsky, K. D., & Conley, C. S. (2001). Developmental and social-contextual origins of depressive control-related beliefs and behavior. *Cognitive Therapy and Research, 25*, 447–475.

Sheeber, L., Davis, B., & Hops, H. (2002). Gender-specific vulnerability to depression in children of depressed mothers. In S. H. Goodman & I. H. Gotlib (Eds.), *Children of depressed parents: Mechanisms of risk and implications for treatment* (pp. 253–274). Washington, DC: American Psychological Association.

Sheeber, L., Hops, H., Alpert, A., Davis, B., & Andrews, J. A. (1997). Family support and conflict: Prospective relations to adolescent depression. *Journal of Abnormal Child Psychology, 25*, 333–344.

Sheeber, L., & Sorensen, E. (1998). Family relationships of depressed adolescents: A multimethod assessment. *Journal of Clinical Child Psychology, 27*, 268–277.

Shih, J. H., Eberhart, N. K., Hammen, C. L., & Brennan, P. A. (2006). Differential exposure and reactivity to interpersonal stress predict sex differences in adolescent depression. *Journal of Clinical Child and Adolescent Psychology, 35*, 103–115.

Silberg, J. L., Pickles, A., Rutter, M., Hewitt, J., Simonoff, E., Maes, H., et al. (1999). The influence of genetic factors and life stress on depression among adolescent girls. *Archives of General Psychiatry, 56*, 225–232.

Steingard, R. J., Renshaw, P. F., Hennen, J., Lenox, M., Cintron, C. B., Young, A. D., et al. (2002). Smaller frontal lobe white matter volumes in depressed adolescents. *Biological Psychiatry, 52*, 413–417.

Susman, E., Dorn, L. D., Inoff-Germain, G., Nottelmann, E. D., & Chrousos, G. P. (1997). Cortisol reactivity, distress behavior, and behavioral and psychological problems in young adolescents: A longitudinal perspective. *Journal of Research on Adolescence, 7*, 81–105.

Susman, E. J., Nottelmann, E. D., Inoff, G. E., Dorn, L. D., Cutler, G. B., & Loriaux, D. L., et al. (1985). The relation of relative hormone levels and physical development and social–emotional behavior in young adolescents. *Journal of Youth and Adolescence, 14*, 245–264.

Thapar, A., Harold, G., & McGuffin, P. (1998). Life events and depressive symptoms in childhood—shared genes or shared adversity?: A research note. *Journal of Child Psychology and Psychiatry, and Allied Disciplines, 39*, 1153–1158.

Thapar, A., & McGuffin, P. (1996). The genetic etiology of childhood depressive symptoms: A developmental perspective. *Development and Psychopathology, 8*, 751–760.

Thase, M. E., Jindal, R., & Howland, R. H. (2002). Biological aspects of depression. In I. H. Gotlib & C. L. Hammen (Eds.), *Handbook of depression* (pp. 192–218). New York: Guilford Press.

Tomarken, A. J., Dichter, G. S., Garber, J., & Simien, C. (2004). Resting frontal brain activity: Linkages to maternal depression and socio-economic status among adolescents. *Biological Psychology, 67*, 77–102.

Wadsworth, M. E., & Berger, L. E. (2006). Adolescents coping with poverty-related family stress: Prospective predictors of coping and psychological symptoms. *Journal of Youth and Adolescence, 35*, 57–70.

Weiss, B., & Garber, J. (2003). Developmental differences in the phenomenology of depression. *Development and Psychopathology, 15*, 403–430.

Weissman, M. M., Wolk, S., Wickramaratne, P. J., Goldstein, R., Adams, P., Greenwald, S., et al. (1999). Children with prepubertal-onset major depressive disorder and anxiety grown up. *Archives of General Psychiatry, 56*, 794–801.

Weisz, J. R., Southam-Gerow, M. A., & McCarty, C. A. (2001). Control-related beliefs and depressive symptoms in clinic-referred children and adolescents: Developmental differences and model specificity. *Journal of Abnormal Psychology, 110*, 97–109.

Yorbik, O., Birmaher, B., Axelson, D., Williamson, D. E., & Ryan, N. D. (2004). Clinical characteristics of depressive symptoms in children and adolescents with major depressive disorder. *Journal of Clinical Psychiatry, 65*, 1654–1659.

CHAPTER 20

Depression in Couples and Families

Joanne Davila, Catherine B. Stroud, *and* Lisa R. Starr

As authors of other chapters in this book also attest, depression is associated with significant interpersonal impairment, both as a cause and as a consequence of the disorder (see Beach, Jones, & Franklin, Chapter 27; Joiner & Timmons, Chapter 14; Hammen, Chapter 12). Nowhere has this been more evident than in the context of couple and family relationships. In this chapter, we present an overview of the literature on depression in these contexts, highlight conceptual themes, and provide directions for future research. In addition to the literatures on unipolar depression and depressive symptoms, we review the literature on bipolar disorder, although it is much more limited than the others. The bipolar material is presented separately, but we link it to the other findings, so that readers may see the ways in which the literatures do and do not converge.

DEPRESSION IN THE CONTEXT OF COUPLE RELATIONSHIPS

In this section, we focus on the main processes and components of couple relationships, including how they start, function, and end, and discuss their association with depression. We discuss these associations first among adults, then among adolescents.

Depression and Relationship Formation

Although little empirical attention has been paid to whether depression is associated with relationship formation, a number of findings suggest that the experience of depression has implications for involvement in a relationship and vice versa. First, some data indicate that, for adults, being married or in a relationship is associated with less depression (e.g., Gutierrez-Lobos, Wolfl, & Scherer, 2000; Inaba, Thoits, & Ueno, 2005; for a review, see Umberson & Williams, 1999). There are a variety of ways to interpret these data. For example, romantic relationships may be protective for adults, or depressed individuals may be less likely to enter into or remain in romantic relationships. On the other hand, a number of studies suggest that early-onset depression is associated with early marriage (e.g., Gotlib, Lewinsohn, & Seeley, 1998; Kessler, Walters, & Forthofer, 1998). Also, the lower rates of depression among married/coupled persons may reflect the distress associated with divorce or loss rather than with being single (e.g., DePaulo, 2006; Whisman, Weinstock, & Tolejko, 2006). Supporting this, some studies comparing married and never-married people show no differences in depression (e.g., Kessler et al., 2003), or they find that the never-married people are less depressed (Romanoski et al., 1992). These findings are interesting in light of recent research showing that romantic involvement is associated with depression in adolescence, which we review below. For now, we can conclude only that the nature of the association between depression and formation of, or entry into, relationships in adulthood is unclear.

Depression and Relationship Satisfaction

Perhaps one of the most consistent findings is that depression among dating and married couples is associated with less relationship satisfaction (see Whisman, 2001). The evidence also is clear that this association is bidirectional (e.g., Davila, Karney, Hall, & Bradbury, 2003; Whisman & Bruce, 1999). Because these associations are well documented, research has moved to examining questions that provide a more nuanced understanding of these associations.

For instance, some research has focused on moderators to identify for whom the association will be strongest. For example, partners who are characterized by high levels of neuroticism show a stronger association (Davila et al., 2003), as do people who make blame-oriented attributions about their partners' negative behavior (Gordon, Friedman, & Miller, 2005). Some research has focused on mediators to identify mechanisms of the association. For instance, to the extent that their marital dissatisfaction was manifested in greater self-silencing, women showed higher levels of depressive symptoms (Uebelacker, Courtnage, & Whisman, 2003). Researchers also have begun to examine whether the association between depression and relationship discord is best described as linear, or whether it is more complex. For example, drawing on data suggesting that depression and marital discord may each be *taxonic* (i.e., that people fall into qualitatively different categories rather than along a continuum—Beach & Amir, 2003; Beach, Fincham, Amir, & Leonard, 2005), Beach, Fincham, and Leonard (2006) suggested that change in marital discord may show its strongest connection to depression only at high levels, and may show less powerful connections at other points. Other research has begun to examine the role of comorbidity in the association, which is critical given the high rates. For example, Whisman (1999; Whisman, Uebelacker, Tolejko, Chatav, & McKelvie, 2006) demonstrated that the association between marital discord and depression remains even after controlling for other Axis I disorders and personality pathology. All of these findings represent important steps in the research agenda on relationship discord and depression. For the field to remain vital, questions that refine our understanding of the circumstances under which depression and discord covary will be critical.

Depression and Relationship Functioning

In dating and married couples, depression is associated with poor adaptive functioning in a variety of domains. Research on problem solving in couples with a depressed partner demonstrates negative patterns. For example, during problem-solving discussions, such couples demonstrate more negative behavior, particularly the depressive behaviors exhibited by the depressed person (e.g., complaints, self-derogatory statements; Jackman-Cram, Dobson, & Martin, 2006). Partners of depressed spouses also report using more coercive problem-solving tactics (Hammen & Brennan, 2002). Couples also perceive their interactions as negative; depressed partners report greater self-blame and hopeless following interactions, and show greater increases in depressed mood following such interactions (e.g., McCabe & Gotlib, 1993; Sayers, Kohn, & Fresco, 2001; Whisman, Weinstock, & Uebelacker, 2002). These latter findings may speak to how couple interactions function to exacerbate or maintain depression.

Deficits in social support also are associated with depression. For example, lack of support from a partner predicts increased risk for and onset of major depression (Monroe, Bromet, Connell, & Steiner, 1986; Wade & Kendler, 2000). Similarly, criticism of depressed persons by spouses (and family members) predicts relapse in depression, as the literature on expressed emotion has shown (Hooley & Teasdale, 1989; Uehara, Yokoyama, Goto, & Ihda, 1996). This is important, because partners of depressed persons tend to hold negative views of them (e.g., Birtchnell, 1991; Sacco, Dumont, & Dow, 1993) even when they are not depressed (e.g., Levkovitz, Lamy, Ternachiano, Treves, & Fennig, 2003).

Deficits in support also affect the association between depression and marital satisfaction. A recent 12-year longitudinal study of women with a history of major depression, indicated that having a partner with poor support skills is associated with significant marital distress (Bradbury, 2007). In addition, women's own support skills are impaired by their depressive symptoms, which lead to increases in marital stress and further depressive symptoms (Davila, Bradbury, Cohan, & Tochluk, 1997).

Significant negative relationship events, particularly those associated with humiliation or betrayal, also are related to depression (Christian-Herman, O'Leary, & Avery-Leaf, 2001). Cano and O'Leary (2000) found that women who experienced husbands' infidelity and/or husband-initiated separation were significantly more likely than women without such experiences to experience a major depression. As these findings and those on support suggest, events that threaten people's sense of security or safety in their relationships are associated with depressive symptoms, and depressed individuals may be more likely to view and/or experience relationships as being less secure or more vulnerable. Indeed, research indicates that insecurity in romantic relationships is associated with both depressive symptoms and major depression (e.g., Carnelly, Pietromonaco, & Jaffe, 1994; Whiffen, Kallos-Lilly, & MacDonald, 2001).

Depression and Relationship Dissolution

Not only is depression associated with subsequent divorce (e.g., Kessler et al., 1998), suggesting that depression (or its consequences) might impair relationships to the point of dissolution, but loss of a romantic relationship also confers significant risk for depression. Divorced, separated, and widowed individuals show higher rates of depressive symptoms, are more likely to meet criteria for major depression, and are at higher risk than married individuals of becoming depressed (e.g., Barrett, 2000; Kessler et al., 2003; Maciejewski, Prigerson, & Mazure, 2001). Interestingly, in some cases, depression may be associated with staying in an unhappy marriage. Davila and Bradbury (2001) found that, compared to newlyweds who stayed married over 4 years and those who divorced, newlyweds who stayed in unhappy marriages had higher rates of depressive symptoms at the beginning of, and throughout, their marriage. Whether depressive symptoms were a cause or consequence of the marital distress is not clear, nor do we know whether the unhappy couples went on to divorce, but the data suggest that depressive symptoms sometimes may be associated with holding on to rather than dissolving an unhappy marriage.

Adolescent Romantic Relationships and Depression

Although research on depression among couples has focused on adults, there is growing recognition of the importance of examining the association between depression and romantic functioning at earlier ages. Because depression rates rise in adolescence, depression has the potential early on to impair interpersonal functioning. Adolescent interpersonal experiences, especially romantic ones, may serve important socialization functions and result in learning that guides later relational ability. Therefore, the association between depression and poor romantic functioning may begin early and set the stage for continued impairment across the lifespan.

As alluded to earlier, there is growing evidence that involvement in dating and romantic relationships during adolescence, particularly if frequent or steady, is associated with depressive symptoms, and that this is true among early and late adolescents, particularly girls (Compian, Gowen, & Hayward, 2004; Davila, Steinberg, Kachadourian, Cobb, & Fincham, 2004; Joyner & Udry, 2000; Quatman, Sampson, Robinson, & Watson, 2001). Even engaging in statistically normative romantic behaviors (e.g., flirting, kissing) and feeling sexually attracted to someone is associated with depressive symptoms for early-adolescent girls (Steinberg & Davila, 2007; Yoneda & Davila, 2008). Thus, it appears that formation of, or entry into romantic relationships, in adolescence is related to greater depressive symptoms. However, the reasons for this are unclear.

One possibility is that depressed or dysphoric youth may seek out romantic experiences to meet dependence needs, to compensate for poor family or peer relations, or as a search for mood-regulating experiences. These ideas are speculative (see also Gotlib et al., 1998), because no research exists. It also is possible that adolescent romantic experiences are inherently challenging and put youth at risk for depression, particularly youth with poor coping, support, or personal resources that impair their ability to manage such challenges. Our research group has conducted several studies supporting this. Steinberg and Davila (2007) found that the association between romantic experiences and depressive symptoms is stronger for early-adolescent girls with emotionally unavailable parents. Starr and Davila (in press) found that the association between romantic experiences and increases in depressive symptoms (over 1 year) is stronger for early-adolescent girls who engage in greater corumination with friends (i.e., excessive discussion of problems and heightened focus on negative emotions; Rose, 2002). Davila and colleagues (2004) found that romantic involvement is associated more strongly with increases in depressive symptoms among adolescents with a preoccupied style of relating (i.e., who are needy and fearful of rejection).

A number of other adolescent romantic experiences are associated with depression and are consistent with findings in the adult literature. Notably, the breakup of a relationship is associated with first onset of depression in adolescence (Monroe, Rohde, Seeley, & Lewinsohn, 1999). In terms of relationship qualities, less intimacy is associated with greater depressive mood reactivity among adolescent girls (Williams, Connolly, & Segal, 2001). Lower emotional support and higher relationship stress are associated with depressive symptoms among adolescent girls (Daley & Hammen, 2002), and more negative interactions, as well as inequality in the contribution of emotional resources and in decision making, are associated with depressive symptoms, especially for adolescent girls (Galliher, Rostosky,

Welsh, & Kawaguchi, 1999; La Greca & Harrison, 2005). Depressive symptoms also are associated with romantic partners' ratings of adolescent girls as less interpersonally competent (Daley & Hammen, 2002).

In summary, there is growing evidence that depression and romantic experiences in adolescence are linked. Of course, there is much to be explored about the mechanisms by which they affect one another, including severity of depression (e.g., the most depressed adolescents may not have romantic experiences, which may result in a different type of impairment compared to that resulting from involvement and dysfunctional relationships).

Conceptual Themes and Issues

One theme that emerges across research is that romantic relationships (or even experiences in adolescence) can serve as stressors that increase risk for depression. Although relationships may have protective features when they are supportive and satisfying, when they are not, or when people do not have the resources to manage or cope with their challenges, relationships can increase risk for depression. The emerging literature on adolescents highlights the challenging nature of romantic experiences. Whether this is a developmentally unique experience remains an empirical question. The adult literature has tended to look almost exclusively at within-relationship factors in predicting depression, but closer examination of the personal and external resources that partners bring to their relationships in adulthood may shed further light on when, how, and why romantic relationships can increase risk.

Another theme is that of loss. At all ages, both the loss of a romantic relationship, be it through breakup, separation, divorce, or widowhood, and the loss of trust in a relationship (e.g., via betrayal events) predict onset of and increases in depression. Yet loss of some sort is virtually inevitable in romantic relationships, especially for young people early in their relationship "careers," and for older adults nearing the end of life. Understanding who may be most vulnerable to loss and how they can prepare for and respond adaptively may reduce risk.

Consistent with this position, the protective role of support, both within and outside of the romantic relationship, is another theme that cuts across research. Risk for depression is lower when people feel supported by their partners, have external support to help them manage the challenges of relationships, or can engage in adaptive strategies to cope with relationship experiences.

Although these themes have focused on how relationships put people at risk for depression, depression also impairs key aspects of relational functioning, including those that have the potential to result in the very things that are then depressogenic. For example, to the extent that a depressed person and his or her partner cannot effectively communicate, and to the extent that this results in negative views of the depressed person, the partner may withdraw support. Thus, as the literature indicates, depression can be both a cause and consequence of relationship dysfunction, although the precise and varied ways in which people develop and maintain such maladaptive cycles have not been fully elaborated.

Finally, in this section we have not dealt with three issues that may moderate conclusions about the association between depression and romantic dysfunction. The first, which has received the most attention, is that of gender differences. Although some research suggests that associations are stronger for women, this is not a consistent finding, nor has it been adequately examined, because research has tended to focus on female samples (for a review, see Whisman, Weinstock, et al., 2006). In addition, conceptual models of the association between depression and romantic dysfunction largely have not focused on gender, leaving the field to proceed without the benefit of a theoretical framework from which to explore gender differences. A second issue is that of different types of relationships. The literature has focused almost completely on marital or heterosexual dating relationships. With the growing number and recognition of same-sex relationships, as well as recognition of the unique stressors associated with sexual minority status, it is important to examine associations with depression in the context of such relationships. Finally, the literature also has neglected examination of ethnic/cultural differences that may moderate associations between depression and relationship dysfunction. As we note below, such associations can vary in the context of childhood depression and family relationships. Whether they do so in romantic relationships is largely unknown.

Bipolar Disorder and Couple Relationships

In the case of bipolar disorder, although the research is limited, data exist linking the disorder to aspects of relationship formation. Individuals with bipolar disorder are less likely to be married (Suppes et al., 2001). When they do choose mates, they show elevated rates of marrying someone with a psychiatric illness compared to unipolar patients (Colombo, Cox, & Dunner, 1990; Merikangas & Spiker, 1982) and healthy controls, and this may be particularly true for men (for a review, see Mathews & Reus, 2001). As such, bipolar disorder does appear to affect aspects of relationship formation, perhaps more so than does unipolar depression. There also is some direct evidence that marriage may serve a protective function in bipolar disorder that is not seen directly in unipolar depression. For example, being married is associated with a good response to lithium (e.g., Yazici, Kora, Ucok, Tunali, & Turan, 1999) and those with a partner at disorder onset are more likely to achieve full interepisodic remission (Johnson, Lundstrom, Aberg-Wistedt, & Mathe, 2003). Similarly, being unmarried poses a risk for episode onset (Kessing, Agerbo, & Mortensen, 2004; for a review, see Tsuchiya, Byrne, & Mortensen, 2003). On the other hand, getting married is also associated with increased risk for first admission, perhaps because it may function as a stressor (Kessing et al., 2004).

With regard to marital distress, the literature on bipolar disorder, like that on unipolar depression and depressive symptoms, shows that individuals with bipolar disorder report higher levels of martial distress than do controls (Radke-Yarrow, 1998). Furthermore, this is true even in remission (Bauwens, Tracy, Pardoen, Vander Elst, & Mandlewicz, 1991; cf. Frank et al., 1981); among the psychiatric disorders examined in the National Comorbidity Survey Replication (anxiety disorders, mood disorders, and substance use disorders), bipolar disorder had the strongest association with marital distress (Whisman, 2007). In addition, a consistent finding is that spouses report less satisfaction than do their partners with bipolar disorder, with over half reporting that they would not have entered the relationship/married their spouse with bipolar disorder if they had known more about the disorder (Dore & Romans, 2001; Targum, Dibble, Davenport, & Gershon, 1981). Spouses continue to report high levels of dissatisfaction (compared to controls), even when their partners are in remission (Horesh & Fennig, 2000; Levkovitz, Fennig, Horesh, Barak, & Treves, 2000). However, spousal satisfaction also depends on the nature of the symptoms and spouses' perceptions of partners' ability to control the symptoms. Specifically, depressive (compared to manic) symptoms are associated with less satisfaction (e.g., Hooley, Richters, Weintraub, & Neale, 1987; Lam, Donaldson, Brown, & Malliaris, 2005), as are perceptions of more control (e.g., Lam et al., 2005). The same is true for the experience of caregiver burden. Spouses of patients with bipolar disorder feel burdened in their role as a caregiver, particularly during depressive episodes, and when they believe their partners could control their symptoms (Perlick et al., 1999). This greater perceived burden is in turn associated with increased risk of relapse (Perlick, Rosenheck, Clarkin, Raue, & Sirey, 2001).

Regarding relationship functioning, the literature on bipolar disorder has yielded some findings similar to those in the literature on depression. For instance, social support may be lacking among people with bipolar disorder. For example, in couples, the two partners' perceived support was correlated in a remitted group, in which one partner was diagnosed with bipolar disorder (or unipolar depression), but not in the acute group, suggesting that reciprocity in support provision (or how support is perceived) may collapse during the acute phase (Levkovitz et al., 2003). There is also evidence that relationships of individuals with bipolar disorder are characterized by high levels of conflict. For instance, bipolar (and unipolar) inpatients and their spouses reported higher levels of conflict than did control couples, with inpatients reporting higher levels of conflict than their partners (Hoover & Fitzgerald, 1981). Similarly, partners' (and other caregivers') level of expressed emotion (EE) predicts relapse in treated patients over time (for reviews, see Miklowitz, 2004; Mundt, Kronmuller, & Backenstrass, 2000), although there is some indication that this may be specific to depressive episodes (Yan, Hammen, Cohen, Daley, & Henry, 2004).

Regarding relationship dissolution, people with bipolar disorder have higher rates of divorce than others (Coryell et al., 1993; Suppes et al., 2001), and relationship dissolution may give rise to episode onset. For instance, experiencing a divorce is associated with greater risk of hospitalization for a first manic episode (Kessing et al., 2004).

In summary, although the literature on bipolar disorder in the context of family relationships is less well developed than that on unipolar depression or depressive symptoms, the existing research makes clear that bipolar disorder, like depression, affects and is affected by what happens in people's romantic relationships (for a review, see Goodwin & Jamison, 2007). The literature also provides insight into ways in which the associations with romantic relationship functioning might differ for people with bipolar disorder (e.g., greater assortative mating, more direct protective function), as well as potential issues unique to bipolar disorder (e.g., greater spousal dissatisfaction and burden). Naturally, there is much room for conceptual and empirical development of the literature on bipolar disorder in the context of couple relationships in the areas reviewed, and the issues raised earlier with regard to gender differences, couple types, and ethnic/cultural diversity apply here as well. Future research also should continue to clarify the extent to which unipolar and bipolar disorder function similarly (i.e., whether the effects for bipolar disorder are driven by depression), as well as their unique associations with relationship functioning.

DEPRESSION IN THE CONTEXT OF FAMILY RELATIONSHIPS

In this section, we focus on three issues: the association between childhood depression and family functioning, the association between parental depression and family functioning, and the association between family caregiving and depression.

Childhood Depression and Family Functioning

The association between family factors and depression in children and adolescents is well documented. We review these findings in the domain of parent–child/family environmental factors and parental marital factors, and highlight research investigating mechanisms of the association, factors that influence the strength of the association, and the direction of the effects.

Parent–Child and Family Environment Factors

A number of factors distinguish the childrearing behaviors of parents of depressed and nondepressed youth, with research suggesting that parents of depressed youth are more controlling and less supportive and warm, use more coercion, and communicate less effectively (for reviews, see Kaslow, Deering, & Racusin, 1994; Kaslow, Jones, & Palin, 2005). High levels of parental control may be manifested in perfectionistic behavior in children or low self-esteem, which in turn contributes to increases in depression (Garber, Robinson, & Valentiner, 1997; Kenney-Benson & Pomerantz, 2005). Furthermore, low self-esteem also may account for the negative association between parental acceptance and children's depression (Garber et al., 1997). Interestingly, the strength of these associations may vary by ethnicity and nationality. For instance, the associations among caregiver conflict, openness, warmth, and internalizing symptoms were reduced in African American compared to European American children (Vendlinski, Silk, Shaw, & Lane, 2006), but were stronger for adolescents from China compared to adolescents from the United States (Greenberger, Chen, Tally, & Dong, 2000).

Sequential analyses of observed mother–adolescent interactions speak to the bidirectional, transactional nature of the association between parent behavior and adolescent depression, but they have produced contrary findings. In one study, adolescent depressive behavior elicited supportive/facilitative behavior by mothers, which reinforced the depressive behavior (Sheeber, Hops, Andrews, Alpert, & Davis, 1998). In another study, however, adolescent depressive behavior was followed by withdrawal of support (Pineda, Cole, & Bruce, 2007). Thus, parental behavior and adolescent depression influence each other, but it is not entirely clear how they do so.

In terms of general family environment, research shows that high conflict and low cohesiveness prospectively predict the development of depression in children and adolescents (Kaslow et al., 2005; Reuter, Scaramella, Wallace, & Conger, 1999; Sheeber, Hops, & Davis, 2001). Parent–child conflict exerts part of its influence on depression through parent–child attachment quality, with high conflict predicting attachment insecurity, which in turn predicts depressive symptoms (Constantine, 2006). The influence of family conflict on depression also may vary. For example, the association between family conflict and depression was found to be greater in children and adolescents at high genetic risk for depression (Rice, Harold, Shelton, & Thapar, 2006). Furthermore, some research suggests differences in the strength of the association according to gender of the offspring (Cumsille & Epstein, 1994) and gender of the parent (Cole & McPherson, 1993; cf. Sheeber, Davis, Leve, Hops, & Tildesley, 2007).

In addition to elevated rates of parent–child conflict, elevated rates of sexual, physical, and psychological abuse have been found in depressed children and adolescents (e.g., Kaslow et al., 2005). When forms of maltreatment are compared, emotional maltreatment is the strongest predictor of depressive symptoms (Hankin, 2005). The predictive impact of childhood maltreatment on depressive symptoms in young adulthood is partially explained by insecure attachment, negative life events, and negative cognitive style (Hankin, 2005).

Another aspect of the family environment that contributes to depression is EE (levels of criticism, hostility, and emotional overinvolvement; Leff & Vaughn, 1985). EE is higher in families of depressed youth than in those of psychiatric and normal controls (for reviews, see Kaslow et al., 1994, 2005). In addition, some research indicates that critical EE in mothers shows specificity as a risk factor for depression in youth (e.g., Asarnow, Tompson, Woo, & Cantwell, 2001). Similarly, there is evidence that the impact of high EE in predicting depression may depend on the absence of certain comorbid diagnoses. For example, high EE was predictive of depression persistence only in adolescents without comorbid attention-deficit/hyperactivity disorder (ADHD) (McCleary & Sanford, 2002). Although research documents that EE is higher in parents with a history of depression, investigators have also found that mothers' critical EE influences children's depression independently of parental depression (McCleary & Sanford, 2002; Schwartz, Dorer, Beardslee, Lavori, & Keller, 1990).

Finally, much attention has been given to parent–child attachment insecurity, which is consistently related to depression in youth (for a review, see Davila, Ramsay, Stroud, & Steinberg, 2005). Several longitudinal studies show that insecurity predicts increases in depressive symptoms (e.g., Sund & Wichstrom, 2002), and this may be mediated by factors such as negative models of the self (Kenny, Moilanen, Lomax, & Brabeck, 1993) and the tendency to make negative attributions in response to stress in the mother–daughter relationship (Margolese, Markiewicz, & Doyle, 2005). Secure attachment may reduce risk for development of depression by buffering the negative impact of other risk factors, such as economic hardship (e.g., Graham & Easterbrooks, 2000) and childhood maltreatment (Toth & Cicchetti, 1996).

Parental Marital Factors

In addition to parenting and family environment variables, support for the association between interparental conflict and depression in youth is robust (see Kaslow et al., 1994, 2005). Although children may experience a range of symptoms in response to interparental conflict, several studies suggest it is children's appraisals of self-blame that lead to depression (e.g., Grych, Jouriles, Swank, McDonald, & Norwood, 2000). The mechanisms underlying the impact of interparental conflict have received some attention. Most consistently, interparental conflict seems to exert its influence on depression through strained parent–child relationships and disrupted parenting (e.g., Cole & McPherson, 1993; Fauber, Forehand, Thomas, & Wierson, 1990). However, self-esteem and strain in current romantic relationships have also received support as links between interparental conflict in childhood and future episodes of major depressive disorder (MDD) (Turner & Kopiec, 2006).

Given the links between depression and interparental and family conflict, it is not surprising that children from divorced families are more likely to experience depression and MDD concurrently and in the future (Asteline, 1996; Ge, Natsuaki, & Conger, 2006; Strohschien, 2005). Indeed, elevated family conflict seems to account for preexisting elevations in depression seen in youth whose families eventually divorce compared to those whose families remain intact (Asteline, 1996; Strohschien, 2005). Furthermore, environmental (rather than genetic) influences associated with divorce may account for most of the association between divorce and depression (D'Onofrio et al., 2005). Consistent with this, stressful events around the time of divorce may be one avenue by which divorce has an influence on future depression (Ge et al., 2006). However, mediators of the association also may depend on postdivorce family composition; research indicates that whereas financial problems may mediate the association in single-parent families, family conflict and the parent–child relationship may mediate in intact families (Asteline, 1996). Similarly, the impact of divorce on children appears to be strengthened by high levels of parental conflict (Gilman,

Kawachi, Fitzmaurice, & Buka, 2003) and may be greater in females (Storksen, Roysamb, Holmen, & Tambs, 2006).

Parental Depression and Family Functioning

We described earlier the ways in which childhood depression is associated with family functioning. We now examine how parental depression is associated with family and child functioning.

Effects of Depressed Parents on Children

Research has firmly linked parental depression with emotional and behavioral problems in children (see also Hammen, Chapter 12, this volume). Impaired functioning in children of depressed parents has been identified starting in infancy and continuing into adulthood. Infants are likely to have difficult temperaments and impairments in mental and motor development; toddlers have trouble with emotion regulation and self-soothing; older children and adolescents have higher emotional distress, more school problems, difficulties with peers, and lower self-esteem; and young adults have lower life satisfaction and greater mental health utilization (Gotlib & Goodman, 1999; Lewinsohn, Olino, & Klein, 2005). Furthermore, children of depressed parents, not surprisingly, are at heightened risk for depression and other forms of psychopathology, propagating the scourge of depression across generations (Hammen & Brennan, 2003; Hammen, Burge, Burney, & Adrian, 1990). Given the well-documented, consistent association between parental depression and child difficulties, the focus of research has now shifted to identifying mechanisms. Here we briefly summarize this work, but several thorough reviews are available (see Downey & Coyne, 1990; Goodman & Gotlib, 1999; Whiffen, 2005).

Because mothers are typically primary caregivers and women are more vulnerable to depression (particularly during childbearing years; Weissman & Olfson, 1995), research in this area has focused largely on maternal depression. Indeed, a recent meta-analysis (Connell & Goodman, 2002) indicated that maternal depression is more strongly linked to child problems than is paternal depression. It is important to note, however, that emerging evidence suggests that paternal depression also may have deleterious effects, with one meta-analysis (Kane & Garber, 2004) showing a mean correlation of .24 between paternal depression and child internalizing symptoms. Research also indicates that maternal and paternal depression may be associated with different negative outcomes (Lewinsohn et al., 2005; Rohde, Lewinsohn, Klein, & Seeley, 2005), and that maternal depression interacts with paternal psychopathology to predict youth depression (Brennan, Hammen, Katz, & Le Brocque, 2002).

Several biological mechanisms have been proposed to explain the association between parental depression and childhood problems. For example, because depression has a strong genetic component (Faraone, Kremen, & Tsuang, 1990), parents may pass their genetic vulnerability onto children. Furthermore, maternal depression during pregnancy may affect the fetal environment (e.g., restriction of blood flow to the fetus or increased cortisol levels), possibly leading to abnormal neuroregulatory mechanisms at birth (Field et al., 2004; reviewed in Goodman & Gotlib, 1999), although clearly this cannot explain the association between paternal depression and negative outcomes. Although biological mechanisms may help to explain the relation between parental depression and child difficulties, more research is needed to specify the extent of their role and to disentangle their influence from that of environmental factors.

Indeed, parental depression may adversely affect the family environment. Compared to nondepressed individuals, depressed individuals raise more negative topics in conversations (Gotlib & Robinson, 1982), are more self-focused (Ingram, 1990), and are more likely to provoke negative emotions in others (Coyne, 1976). Parenting is also impaired. Compared to their nondepressed counterparts, depressed parents have been found to be more lax, inconsistent, and ineffective, and are more likely to avoid confrontation (Kochanska, Kuczynski, Radke-Yarrow, & Welsh, 1987), to be less responsive to an infant's crying (Donovan, Leavitt, & Walsh, 1998), and to view themselves as less efficacious as parents (Teti & Gelfand, 1991). Depressed parents also report feeling more negatively about parenthood, and are more rejecting toward their children (Colletta, 1983; Lovejoy, Graczyk, O'Hare, & Neuman, 2000; Webster-Stratton & Hammond, 1988; Whitbeck, Hoyt, Simons, & Conger, 1992). And these findings may not be limited to currently depressed parents; according to one meta-analysis, mothers with lifetime histories of depression are also more negative with their children (Lovejoy et al., 2000). Thus, not surprisingly, parenting deficits accompanied by depression predict negative outcomes in children (Hammen, Shih, & Brennan, 2004). This is consistent with the results of three recent meta-analyses indicating that depression impairs parent–child attachment, with children of depressed mothers less likely to be securely attached than children of nondepressed mothers (Atkinson et al., 2000; Martins & Gaffan, 2000; van IJzendoorn, Schuengel, & Bakermans-Kranenburg, 1999).

Marital and family conflicts also may mediate the relation between parental depression and child maladjustment. As we discussed earlier, depression is strongly and bidirectionally linked to marital distress. In turn, marital conflict is associated with child emotional and behavioral problems (Kelly, 2000). Although some studies support the notion that marital conflict accounts for the relation between parental depression and child maladjustment (Cummings, Keller, & Davies, 2005; Emery, Weintraub, & Neale, 1982), others do not (Essex, Klein, Cho, & Kraemer, 2003). Still other evidence suggests that marital discord moderates the relation between parental depression and child problems, with worse outcomes for children of discordant couples (Fendrich, Warner, & Weissman, 1990). Furthermore, research suggests that parent–child conflict, also linked to internalizing symptoms in children (El-Sheikh & Elmore-Staton, 2004; Sheeber, Hops, Alpert, Davis, & Andrews, 1997; Starr & Davila, in press), may also partially mediate the association between parental depression and child symptoms (Kane & Garber, 2004).

Research also has examined moderating factors that exacerbate or buffer the effects of parental depression on children. Some of it has focused on characteristics of the nondepressed parent. For example, Tannenbaum and Forehand (1994) showed that strong communication and low conflict in the father–child relationship protected against the negative consequences of maternal depression. Other research has examined aspects of the relationship between the child and the depressed parent. Brennan, Le Brocque, and Hammen (2003), for example, found that depressed mothers who were more warm and accepting, and less emotionally involved had more resilient children. Further work has identified aspects of child functioning, such as emotional regulation, that moderate the impact of parental depression (Silk, Shaw, Forbes, Lane, & Kovacs, 2006). Future investigations should continue to delineate the conditions under which parental depression predicts poorly functioning offspring.

The Effects of Child Functioning on Depression in Parents

The majority of research on parental depression has focused on its effects on parenting and children's emotional and behavioral problems. Fewer studies have examined the reverse pattern—how the stressors of parenting may spur or exacerbate parental depression. Some research, however, has examined the possibility that raising children with behavioral or emotional problems may lead to parental depression, although the causal relation remains unclear. Gartstein and Sheeber (2004) found that children's externalizing symptoms longitudinally predicted increases in maternal depression. In contrast, in a diary study, Elgar, Waschbusch, McGrath, Stewart, and Curtis (2004) showed that daily maternal depressed mood preceded child inattention, impulsivity, and hyperactivity, suggesting that maternal depression provokes child externalizing symptoms and not vice versa. In a multiwave cross-lagged study, however, Elgar, Curtis, McGrath, Waschbusch, and Stewart (2003) found that maternal depression preceded child externalizing symptoms but followed child internalizing problems, suggesting that the direction of the relation between maternal depression and child psychopathology may differ for different forms of child symptoms. The relation between parental depression and childhood problems is clearly complex, and more research needs to elucidate causal directions.

Another way to consider how children might affect parental depression is with regard to giving birth and entering parenthood. Postpartum depression has received much attention, both in research literature and in popular media. It is important to note, however, that some evidence suggests that rates of depression are no higher for women following childbirth than for nonchildbearing women of similar demographics (Campbell & Cohn, 1991). As with any other stressor, however, having a child can spur depressive symptoms, particularly among women with poor coping skills, marital distress, previous depression, and other motherhood-related stressors (Gotlib, Whiffen, Wallace, & Mount, 1991; Terry, Mayocchi, & Hynes, 1996). Thus, while it is not clear that the postpartum period is as strong a risk factor for depression as once believed, new mothers with these risk factors should be monitored for depression, especially given the potential for negative outcomes for infants.

Depression in Family Caregivers

Caregivers of family members with health problems are at heightened risk for depression. This is hardly surprising given the multitude of stressors faced by caregivers, coupled with the pain of watching a loved one suffer. The majority of research has focused on caregivers of family members with dementia (see Pinquart & Sörensen, 2005). Similar findings exist, however, for caregivers of family members with other health problems, such as cancer (Pinquart & Duberstein, 2005). Prevalence rates of depressive disorders among caretakers of family members with dementia range from 15 to 32%, considerably higher than among the older adult community population (Cuijpers, 2005). Women are especially at risk, because they are more likely both to act as caregivers and to become depressed while doing so (Pinquart & Sörensen, 2005). Stress and coping models suggest that how caregivers react to stress dictates the likelihood that the caregiver will develop depression. Specifically, research has shown that appraisals of problems, availability of social support, and coping resources mediate the relation between caregiver stress and depression (Haley, Levine, Brown, & Bartolucci, 1987).

Conceptual Themes and Issues

One theme that has emerged is the transactional and bidirectional nature of the association between depression and family factors. Parents (through genetic and environmental contributions) serve as causal agents for depression in their offspring, and depressed offspring affect their parents and the family environment in a cyclical fashion over time. We have highlighted research that illuminates the directions of the effects, but research is to a great extent limited in the conclusions that can be drawn.

Second, there are common family factors that serve as risk factors for or consequences of both parental depression and depression in youth, including disruptions in parenting, parent–child conflict, attachment insecurity, and marital discord. Though we cover the parental and offspring literatures separately in our review, there is clear overlap. Indeed, when these family factors are present, both parents and children are at greater risk for depression, and when parents or children are depressed, these types of dysfunction are amplified, again highlighting the cyclical nature of the association between depression and family dysfunction.

Finally, as shown in research examining mediators and moderators, multiple factors interact within the family system to predict depression. Some factors have a synergistic effect. For example, the adverse impact of parental depression on child outcomes is exacerbated in families with parental conflict (Fendrich et al., 1990). Other factors have a protective effect, such as secure attachment buffering the impact of childhood maltreatment (Toth & Cicchetti, 1996). Longitudinal studies that examine multiple factors in combination have the most potential to illuminate the interplay among factors and the ways in which these interactions vary over time.

A large body of research on depression in the context of families has accumulated, but many important issues remain. For instance, although there are exceptions, research largely fails to disentangle genetic and environmental effects of the family processes discussed, despite consensus that these effects are confounded in most designs. Greater understanding of the nature of effects will allow intervention and prevention efforts to target those factors most amenable to change. For example, recent work suggests that interventions should target postdivorce environmental consequences to reduce risk of psychopathology in children. Specifically, a study of the offspring of twins suggests that it is largely environmental factors following divorce that pose a risk for the development of psychopathology (D'Onofrio et al., 2005).

Investigators also need to attend more explicitly to the course of depression. For example, research needs to distinguish among factors related to the development, maintenance, recovery, and recurrence of depression in youth; to elucidate factors that may be differentially related to first onsets and recurrences in caregivers; and to investigate the differential impact of parental depression based on whether it is a first, recurrent, past, or current episode.

Another issue not adequately addressed is the impact of comorbidity. Because depression is highly comorbid with other disorders (e.g., Kessler et al., 2003), it is critical to examine how comorbidity affects the family environment. For example, it has been suggested in the literature on parental depression that the extent to which current associations are attributable to pure depression or to depression comorbid with anxiety is not clear (Whiffen, 2005).

Finally, stressors likely vary according to family composition for both depressed parents and depressed offspring. With so many different types of families (e.g., heterosexual and same-sex couples and parents, single parents, grandparents parenting grandchildren), it is critical to understand how associations may vary according to the family context. The revealing findings in studies examining the interactional nature of both parents' psychopathology on their offspring (Brennan et al., 2002), as well as the differential impact of divorce in one- versus two-parent families (Asteline, 1996), are examples of the revealing findings that are produced by these types of investigations.

Bipolar Disorder and Family Relationships

Like the literature on couple relationships, the literature on bipolar disorder in the context of family relationships is also more limited than that on unipolar depression or depressive symptoms.

Childhood Bipolar Disorder and Family Functioning

Most research in this area has relied on the retrospective reporting of adults, which limits conclusions about whether recalled information pertains to course or development of bipolar disorder, and whether conclusions pertain to childhood and adolescent onset or to adult onset (see Alloy et al., 2005; Alloy, Abramson, Walshaw, Keyser, & Gerstein, 2006). Therefore, we focus primarily on research involving children and adolescents with bipolar disorder (for additional reviews, see Alloy et al., 2005, 2006).

Regarding parent–child and family environment factors, there is emerging evidence that bipolar disorder in childhood and adolescence may be associated with certain negative parenting practices. For instance, in 2- and 4-year follow-ups of children and adolescent outpatients diagnosed with mania, low maternal warmth predicted faster relapse after recovery from mania (Geller et al., 2002; Geller, Tillman, Craney, & Bolhofner, 2004). Similarly, in a comparison of youth with bipolar disorder, youth with ADHD, and community controls, bipolar youth showed higher levels of parent–child impairment on items relating to mother–child warmth and to maternal and paternal tension compared to both groups (Geller et al., 2000). In addition, in a recent study of young adults, individuals with bipolar spectrum disorders reported more physical abuse from mothers and more emotional abuse from both parents prior to their age of onset compared to controls (as cited in Alloy et al., 2005; Neeren, Alloy, & Abramson, in press). However, another investigation of bipolar youth did not find increased history of sexual abuse (Geller et al., 2000).

Research also documents an association between other family factors and the course of bipolar disorder in adolescents. For instance, in a recent study of adolescents diagnosed with bipolar disorder, higher levels of chronic and episodic stress in family (and romantic) relationships predicted less improvement in depression, mania, and the combined symptoms (depression plus mania) during the year assessed, and this was most true among older adolescents (Kim, Miklowitz, Biuckians, & Mullen, 2007). In addition, bipolar adolescents in high EE families exhibited more mood disorder symptoms over a 2-year period than did bipolar adolescents in low EE families. As noted by the authors of this study, it is important to consider the potential bidirectional relationship of these effects, because adolescents often provoke their parents into high EE behavior that in turn leads to short-term worsening of symptoms (Miklowitz, Biuckians, & Richards, 2006). This is consistent with the work on stress we noted earlier, because many of the life events reported by the adolescents were *dependent* (i.e., caused in part by the symptomatic person; Kim et al., 2007).

Researchers also have begun to explore the mechanisms by which EE may put youth at risk. In a cross-sectional investigation of the offspring of mothers diagnosed with bipolar disorder, the contribution of extreme maternal negativity (a component of EE) to risk for offspring bipolar disorder in young adulthood was mediated by offspring frontal lobe dysfunction, as measured by the Wisconsin Card Sorting Test (Meyer et al., 2006). Although the direction of effects is unclear, these intriguing findings call for further investigation of mechanisms explaining the links between bipolar disorder and family environment factors.

Regarding the impact of parental marital factors on youth bipolar disorder, research is scarce. There is some indication that living with biological parents in an intact marriage is associated with stabilization. In a 2-year follow-up of child and adolescent outpatients with bipolar disorder, those living in intact biological families were over twice as likely to recover from manic episodes relative to those in other living situations (Geller et al., 2002). However, bipolar youth were significantly less likely to be living with both biological parents compared to controls (Geller et al., 2000). The mechanisms underlying these associations are unclear, and it remains to be seen whether divorce precedes the onset of bipolar disorder in youth, or whether caring for a child with the disorder increases risk for parental divorce (Geller et al., 2002).

Parental Bipolar Disorder and Family Functioning

The vast majority of research examining the effects of parental mood disorders on children has focused on unipolar depression, with far less research centering on bipolar disorder. This is an unfortunate oversight, because research has clearly linked parental bipolar disorder with impairments in offspring. For instance, bipolar disorder in parents is strongly linked to higher rates of psychopathology in offspring (e.g., Henin et al., 2005). One meta-analysis showed that children of bipolar parents are nearly twice as likely to develop any mental disorder and are over three times as likely to develop an affective disorder (Lapalme, Hodgins, & LaRoche, 1997). Longitudinal research shows that risk for psychopathology among children of bipolar parents increases over time (Hillegers et al., 2005). In addition, children of bipolar parents show impairments in information processing and neuropsychological functioning that are not present in offspring of parents with major depression. Compared to control children, offspring of bipolar parents display attentional biases toward manic–irritable and social threat words, recall more negative words, and show deficits in sustained attention, perceptual memory, and executive functioning (Gotlib, Traill, Montoya, Joormann, & Chang, 2005; Klimes-Dougan, Ronsaville, Wiggs, & Martinez, 2006).

Twin studies have revealed a strong genetic component in bipolar disorder, more so than in unipolar disorder (McGuffin et al., 2003). Thus, many of the negative outcomes in the offspring of bipolar parents may reflect genetic vulnerability. However, a few studies suggest that bipolar disorder negatively impacts parenting skills and family functioning, perhaps indicating that environmental factors also play a role. For example, Chang, Blasey, Ketter, and Steiner (2001) found that families with a bipolar parent reported less cohesion, independence, and achievement orientation, and more conflict compared to normative data. Furthermore, some evidence suggests that bipolar disorder is associated with dysfunctional mother–infant interactions, although this may improve as episodes remit (Hipwell & Kumar, 1996).

Notably, in some areas, studies have found little impairment in children of bipolar individuals. For example, social functioning of children of bipolar parents seems to be comparable to that of the general population, at least when the children themselves do not have a bipolar spectrum disorder (Klein, Depue, & Krauss, 1986; Reichart et al., 2007). In fact, Anderson and Hammen (1993) found that whereas children of mothers with unipolar depression showed poorer functioning, children of mothers with bipolar disorder did not differ from children of women with no psychiatric disorder. Hipwell, Goossens, Melhuish, and Kumar (2000) found that infants of mothers with bipolar disorder were more likely to be securely attached compared to infants of mothers with unipolar depression. Thus, some evidence suggests that parental bipolar disorder does not have the same deleterious effect on child functioning as unipolar depression (although far more research is needed before firm conclusions can be drawn). Given the impairment associated with bipolar disorder, these findings are somewhat counterintuitive. Hammen (in Goodwin & Jamison, 2007) speculates that because family members may perceive manic episodes as being more outside of the person's control compared to depressive episodes, they may be less likely to react negatively to manic symptoms. Future research should examine this idea and carefully delineate the role of specific mood states in family functioning.

CONCLUSIONS

Our goal in this chapter was to provide an overview of the literature on depression in the context of couples and families, including the findings relevant to unipolar depression, depressive symptoms, and bipolar disorder. Although each relational context has its own unique features, challenges, and rewards that affect and are affected by depression, there are a number of cross-cutting themes and issues in existing knowledge and relevant to the direction of future research.

Regarding existing knowledge, as we hope is apparent, there is clear and consistent evidence that what happens in people's closest relationships can put them at risk for, or protect them from, depression, and that depression can have substantial negative effects on these relationships. This is true for unipolar depression, depressive symptoms, and bipolar disorder. In the language of the stress generation model of depression (Hammen, 1991), couple and family relationships have the potential to act as stressors that increase risk for depression, and depression may result in impairment that renders close relationships more stressful. On the one hand, this may sound obvious. On the other hand, because relationships are ubiquitous and desirable, their challenges may not always be appreciated, and their importance to understanding depression may be underestimated. Moreover, the very things that are natural aspects of close relationships (e.g., the potential for loss and the need to manage conflict, to be available and supportive, and to negotiate the needs of multiple parties) are the things that can be most depressogenic when not dealt with adaptively, and the aspects of relationships that are often most impaired when people are depressed. We see this both in couples and in families.

Regarding future directions, in line with the preceding comments, future research needs to examine the temporal sequence of the transactional nature of depression (unipolar, symptoms, and bipolar) and interpersonal functioning in couples and families. Research should progress with an eye toward refining basic associations, identifying mediating and moderating variables, and developing more sophisticated, multifactorial models. Research is needed that focuses on specificity and comorbidity, and on gender differences, and that captures the diversity of couples and families. And, because what happens in families may translate (via children) into what happens in couples, and then again in families over time and across generations, research must consider models that address the development and course of both depression and interpersonal functioning through the lifespan. One benefit of a chapter that reviews depression in the context of both couples and families is that the connections across close relationships and over the lifespan, we hope, become more evident.

REFERENCES

Alloy, L. B., Abramson, L. Y., Urosevic, S., Walshaw, P. D., Nusslock, R., & Neeren, A. M. (2005). The psychosocial context of bipolar disorder: Environmental, cognitive, and developmental risk factors. *Clinical Psychology Review, 25,* 1043–1075.

Alloy, L. B., Abramson, L. Y., Walshaw, P. D., Keyser, J., & Gerstein, R. K. (2006). A cognitive vulnerability–stress perspective on bipolar spectrum disorders in a normative adolescent brain, cognitive, and emotional development context. *Development and Psychopathology, 18,* 1055–1103.

Anderson, C. A., & Hammen, C. L. (1993). Psychosocial outcomes of children of unipolar depressed, bipolar, medically ill, and normal women: A longitudinal study. *Journal of Consulting and Clinical Psychology, 61,* 448–454.

Asarnow, J., Tompson, M., Woo, S., & Cantwell, D. P. (2001). Is expressed emotion a specific risk factor of depression or a non specific correlate of psychopathology? *Journal of Abnormal Clinical Psychology, 29,* 573–583.

Asteline, R. H., Jr. (1996). Pathways linking parental divorce with adolescent depression. *Journal of Health and Social Behavior, 37,* 133–148.

Atkinson, L., Paglia, A., Coolbear, J., Niccols, A., Parker, K. C. H., & Guger, S. (2000). Attachment security: A meta-analysis of maternal mental health correlates. *Clinical Psychology Review, 20,* 1019–1040.

Barrett, A. E. (2000). Marital trajectories and mental health. *Journal of Health and Social Behavior, 41,* 451–464.

Bauwens, F., Tracy, A., Pardoen, D., Vander Elst, M., & Mandlewicz, J. (1991). Social adjustment of remitted bipolar and unipolar out-patients. *British Journal of Psychiatry, 159,* 239–244.

Beach, S. R. H., & Amir, N. (2003). Is depression taxonic, dimensional, or both? *Journal of Abnormal Psychology, 112,* 228–236.

Beach, S. R. H., Fincham, F. D., Amir, N., & Leonard, K. E. (2005). The taxometrics of marriage: Is marital discord categorical? *Journal of Family Psychology, 19,* 276–285.

Beach, S. R. H., Fincham, F. D., & Leonard, K. E. (2006, November). *Nuances in the connection between marriage and depression.* Paper presented at the 40th annual convention of the Association for Behavioral and Cognitive Therapies, Chicago.

Birtchnell, J. (1991). Negative modes of relating, marital quality, and depression. *British Journal of Psychiatry, 158,* 648–657.

Bradbury, T. N. (2007, March). *Depression and the development of marital distress.* Paper presented at the conference Depression and Close Relationships: New Indications from Basic and Intervention Research, Fribourg University, Fribourg, Switzerland.

Brennan, P. A., Hammen, C., Katz, A. R., & Le Brocque, R. M. (2002). Maternal depression, paternal psychopathology, and adolescent diagnostic outcomes. *Journal of Consulting and Clinical Psychology, 70,* 1075–1085.

Brennan, P. A., Le Brocque, R., & Hammen, C. (2003). Maternal depression, parent–child relationships, and resilient outcomes in adolescence. *Journal of the American Academy of Child and Adolescent Psychiatry, 42,* 1469–1477.

Campbell, S. B., & Cohn, J. F. (1991). Prevalence and correlates of postpartum depression in first-time mothers. *Journal of Abnormal Psychology, 100,* 594–599.

Cano, A., & O'Leary, K. D. (2000). Infidelity and separations precipitate major depressive episodes and symptoms of nonspecific depression and anxiety. *Journal of Consulting and Clinical Psychology, 68,* 774–781.

Carnelley, K. B., Pietromonaco, P. R., & Jaffe, K. (1994). Depression, working models of others, and relationship functioning. *Journal of Personality and Social Psychology, 66,* 127–140.

Chang, K. D., Blasey, C., Ketter, T. A., & Steiner, H. (2001). Family environment of children and adolescents with bipolar parents. *Bipolar Disorders, 3,* 73–78.

Christian-Herman, J. L., O'Leary, K. D., & Avery-Leaf, S. (2001). The impact of severe negative events in marriage on depression. *Journal of Social and Clinical Psychology, 20,* 25–44.

Cole, D. A., & McPherson, A. E. (1993). Relation of family subsystems to adolescent depression: Implementing a new family assessment strategy. *Journal of Family Psychology, 7,* 119–133.

Colletta, N. D. (1983). At risk for depression: A study of young mothers. *Journal of Genetic Psychology, 142,* 301–310.

Colombo, M., Cox, G., & Dunner, D. L. (1990). Assortative mating in affective and anxiety disorders: Preliminary findings. *Psychiatric Genetics, 1,* 35–44.

Compian, L., Gowen, L. K., & Hayward, C. (2004). Peripubertal girls' romantic and platonic involvement with boys: Associations with body image and depression symptoms. *Journal of Research on Adolescence, 14,* 23–47.

Connell, A. M., & Goodman, S. H. (2002). The association between psychopathology in fathers versus mothers and children's internalizing and externalizing behavior problems: A meta-analysis. *Psychological Bulletin, 128,* 746–773.

Constantine, M. G. (2006). Perceived family conflict, parental attachment, and depression in African American female adolescents. *Cultural Diversity and Ethnic Minority Psychology, 12,* 697–709.

Coryell, W., Scheftner, W., Keller, M., Endicott, J., Maser, J., & Klerman, G. L. (1993). The enduring psychosocial consequences of mania and depression. *American Journal of Psychiatry, 150,* 720–727.

Coyne, J. C. (1976). Depression and the response of others. *Journal of Abnormal Psychology, 85,* 186–193.

Cuijpers, P. (2005). Depressive disorders in caregivers of dementia patients: A systematic review. *Aging and Mental Health, 9,* 325–330.

Cummings, E. M., Keller, P. S., & Davies, P. T. (2005). Towards a family process model of maternal and paternal depressive symptoms: Exploring multiple relations with child and family functioning. *Journal of Child Psychology and Psychiatry, and Allied Disciplines, 46,* 479–489.

Cumsille, P. E., & Epstein, N. (1994). Family cohesion, family adaptability, social support, and adolescent depressive symptoms in outpatient clinic families. *Journal of Family Psychology, 8,* 202–214.

Daley, S. E., & Hammen, C. (2002). Depressive symptoms and close relationships during the transition to adulthood: Perspectives from dysphoric women, their best friends, and their romantic partners. *Journal of Consulting and Clinical Psychology, 70,* 129–141.

Davila, J., & Bradbury, T. N. (2001). Attachment insecurity and the distinction between unhappy spouses who do and do not divorce. *Journal of Family Psychology, 15,* 371–393.

Davila, J., Bradbury, T. N., Cohan, C. L., & Tochluk, S. (1997). Marital functioning and depressive symptoms: Evidence for a stress generation model. *Journal of Personality and Social Psychology, 73,* 849–861.

Davila, J., Karney, B. R., Hall, T., & Bradbury, T. N. (2003). Depressive symptoms and marital satisfaction: Within-subject associations and the moderating effects of gender and neuroticism. *Journal of Family Psychology, 17,* 557–570.

Davila, J., Ramsay, M., Stroud, C. B., & Steinberg, S. J. (2006). Attachment as vulnerability to the development of psychopathology. In B. L. Hankin & J. R. Z. Abela (Eds.), *Development of psychopathology: A vulnerability–stress perspective* (pp. 215–242). Thousand Oaks, CA: Sage.

Davila, J., Steinberg, S. J., Kachadourian, L., Cobb, R., & Fincham, F. (2004). Romantic involvement and depressive symptoms in early and late adolescence: The role of preoccupied relational style. *Personal Relationships, 11,* 161–178.

DePaulo, B. (2006). *Singled out: How singles are stereotyped, stigmatized, and ignored, and still live happily ever after.* New York: St. Martins Press.

D'Onofrio, B. M., Turkheimer, E., Emery, R. E., Slutske, W. S., Heath, A. C., Madden, P. A., et al. (2005). A genetically informed study of marital instability and its association with offspring psychopathology. *Journal of Abnormal Psychology, 4,* 570–586.

Donovan, W. L., Leavitt, L. A., & Walsh, R. O. (1998). Conflict and depression predict maternal sensitivity to infant cries. *Infant Behavior and Development, 21,* 505–517.

Dore, G., & Romans, S. E. (2001). Impact of bipolar affective disorder on family and partners. *Journal of Affective Disorders, 67,* 147–158.

Downey, G., & Coyne, J. C. (1990). Children of depressed parents: An integrative review. *Psychological Bulletin, 108,* 50–76.

Elgar, F. J., Curtis, L. L., McGrath, P. J., Waschbusch, D. A., & Stewart, S. H. (2003). Antecedent–consequence conditions in maternal mood and child adjustment: A four-year cross-lagged study. *Journal of Clinical Child and Adolescent Psychology, 32,* 362–374.

Elgar, F. J., Waschbusch, D. A., McGrath, P. J., Stewart, S. H., & Curtis, L. J. (2004). Temporal relations in daily-reported maternal mood and disruptive child behavior. *Journal of Abnormal Child Psychology, 32*(3), 237–247.

El-Sheikh, M., & Elmore-Staton, L. (2004). The link between marital conflict and child adjustment: Parent–child conflict and perceived attachments as mediators, potentiators, and mitigators of risk. *Development and Psychopathology, 16,* 631–648.

Emery, R. E., Weintraub, S., & Neale, J. M. (1982). Effects of marital discord on the school behavior of children with schizophrenic, affectively disordered, and normal parents. *Journal of Abnormal Child Psychology, 10,* 215–228.

Essex, M. J., Klein, M. H., Cho, E., & Kraemer, H. C. (2003). Exposure to maternal depression and marital conflict: Gender differences in children's later mental health symptoms. *Journal of the American Academy of Child and Adolescent Psychiatry, 42,* 728–737.

Faraone, S. V., Kremen, W. S., & Tsuang, M. T. (1990). Genetic transmission of major affective disorders: Quantitative models and linkage analyses. *Psychological Bulletin, 108,* 109–127.

Fauber, R., Forehand, R., Thomas, A. M., & Wierson, M. (1990). A mediational model of the impact of marital conflict on adolescent adjustment in intact and divorced families: The role of disrupted parenting. *Child Development, 61,* 1112–1123.

Fendrich, M., Warner, V., & Weissman, M. M. (1990). Family risk factors, parental depression, and psychopathology in offspring. *Developmental Psychology, 26,* 40–50.

Field, T., Diego, M., Dieter, J., Hernandez-Reif, M., Schanberg, S., Kuhn, C., et al. (2004). Prenatal depression effects on the fetus and the newborn. *Infant Behavior and Development, 27,* 216–229.

Frank, E., Targum, S. D., Gershon, E. S., Anderson, C., Stewart, B. D., Davenport, Y., et al. (1981). A comparison of nonpatient with bipolar patient–well spouse couples. *American Journal of Psychiatry, 138,* 764–768.

Galliher, R. V., Rostosky, S. S., Welsh, D. P., & Kawaguchi, M. C. (1999). Power and psychological well-being in late adolescent romantic relationships. *Sex Roles, 40,* 689–710.

Garber, J., Robinson, N. S., & Valentiner, D. (1997). The relation between parenting and adolescent depression: Self-worth as a mediator. *Journal of Adolescent Research, 12,* 12–33.

Gartstein, M. A., & Sheeber, L. (2004). Child behavior problems and maternal symptoms of depression: A mediational model. *Journal of Child and Adolescent Psychiatric Nursing, 17,* 141–150.

Ge, X., Natsuaki, M. N., & Conger, R. D. (2006). Trajectories of depressive symptoms and stressful life events among male and female adolescents in divorced and nondivorced families. *Development and Psychopathology, 18,* 253–273.

Geller, B., Bolhofner, K., Craney, J. L., Williams, M., DelBello, M. P., & Gundersen, K. (2000). Psychosocial functioning in a prepubertal and early adolescent bipolar disorder phenotype. *Journal of the American Academy of Child and Adolescent Psychiatry, 39,* 1543–1548.

Geller, B., Craney, J. L., Bolhofner, K., Nickelsburg, M. J., Williams, M., & Zimerman, B. (2002). Two-year prospective follow-up of children with prepubertal and early onset bipolar disorder phenotype. *American Journal of Psychiatry, 159,* 927–933.

Geller, B., Tillman, R., Craney, J. L., & Bolhofner, K. (2004). Four-year prospective outcome and natural history of mania in children with prepubertal and early adolescent bipolar disorder phenotype. *Archives of General Psychiatry, 61,* 459–467.

Gilman, S. E., Kawachi, I., Fitzmaurice, G. M., & Buka, S. L. (2003). Family disruption in childhood and risk of adult depression. *American Journal of Psychiatry, 160,* 939–946.

Goodman, S. H., & Gotlib, I. H. (1999). Risk for psychopathology in the children of depressed mothers: A developmental model for understanding mechanisms of transmission. *Psychological Review, 106,* 458–490.

Goodwin, F. K., & Jamison, K. R. (2007). *Manic–depressive illness: Bipolar disorders and recurrent depression* (2nd ed.). New York: Oxford University Press.

Gordon, K. C., Friedman, M. A., & Miller, I. W. (2005). Marital attributions as moderators of the marital discord–depression link. *Journal of Social and Clinical Psychology, 24,* 876–893.

Gotlib, I. H., & Goodman, S. H. (1999). Children of parents with depression. In W. K. Silverman & T. H. Ollendick (Eds.), *Developmental issues in the clinical treatment of children* (pp. 415–432). Boston: Allyn & Bacon.

Gotlib, I. H., Lewinsohn, P. M., & Seeley, J. R. (1998). Consequences of depression during adolescence: Marital status and marital functioning in early adulthood. *Journal of Abnormal Psychology, 107,* 686–690.

Gotlib, I. H., & Robinson, L. A. (1982). Responses to depressed individuals: Discrepancies between self-report and observer-rated behavior. *Journal of Abnormal Psychology, 91,* 231–240.

Gotlib, I. H., Traill, S. K., Montoya, R. L., Joormann, J., & Chang, K. (2005). Attention and memory biases in the offspring of parents with bipolar disorder: Indications from a pilot study. *Journal of Child Psychology and Psychiatry, and Allied Disciplines, 46,* 84–93.

Gotlib, I. H., Whiffen, V. E., Wallace, P. M., & Mount, J. H. (1991). Prospective investigation of postpartum depression: Factors involved in onset and recovery. *Journal of Abnormal Psychology, 100,* 122–132.

Graham, C. A., & Easterbrooks, M. A. (2000). School-aged children's vulnerability to depressive symptomatology: The role of attachment security, maternal depressive symptomatology, and economic risk. *Development and Psychopathology, 12,* 201–213.

Greenberger, E., Chen, C., Tally, S. R., & Dong, Q. (2000). Family, peer, and individual correlates of depressive symptomatology among U.S. and Chinese adolescents. *Journal of Consulting and Clinical Psychology, 68,* 209–219.

Grych, J. H., Jouriles, E. N., Swank, P. R., McDonald, R., & Norwood, W. D. (2000). Patterns of adjustment among children of battered women. *Journal of Consulting and Clinical Psychology, 68,* 84–94.

Gutierrez-Lobos, K., Wolfl, G., & Scherer, M. (2000). The gender gap in depression reconsidered: The influence of marital employment status on the female/male ratio of treated incidence rates. *Social Psychiatry and Psychiatric Epidemiology, 35,* 145–156.

Haley, W. E., Levine, E. G., Brown, S. L., & Bartolucci, A. A. (1987). Stress, appraisal, coping, and social support as predictors of adaptational outcome among dementia caregivers. *Psychology and Aging, 2,* 323–330.

Hammen, C. (1991). Generation of stress in the course of unipolar depression. *Journal of Abnormal Psychology, 100,* 555–561.

Hammen, C., & Brennan, P. A. (2002). Interpersonal dysfunction in depressed women: Impairments independent of depressive symptoms. *Journal of Affective Disorders, 72,* 145–156.

Hammen, C., & Brennan, P. A. (2003). Severity, chronicity, and timing of maternal depression and risk for adolescent offspring diagnoses in a community sample. *Archives of General Psychiatry, 60,* 253–258.

Hammen, C., Burge, D., Burney, E., & Adrian, C. (1990). Longitudinal study of diagnoses in children of women with unipolar and bipolar affective disorder. *Archives of General Psychiatry, 47,* 1112–1117.

Hammen, C., Shih, J. H., & Brennan, P. A. (2004). Intergenerational transmission of depression: Test of an interpersonal stress model in a community sample. *Journal of Consulting and Clinical Psychology, 72,* 511–522.

Hankin, B. L. (2005). Childhood maltreatment and psychopathology: Prospective tests of attachment, cognitive vulnerability, and stress as mediating processes. *Cognitive Therapy and Research, 29,* 645–671.

Henin, A., Biederman, J., Mick, E., Sachs, G. S., Hirshfeld-Becker, D. R., Siegel, R. S., et al. (2005). Psychopathology in the offspring of parents with bipolar disorder: A controlled study. *Biological Psychiatry, 58,* 554–561.

Hillegers, M. H., Reichart, C. G., Wals, M., Verhulst, F. C., Ormel, J., & Nolen, W. A. (2005). Five-year prospective outcome of psychopathology in the adolescent offspring of bipolar parents. *Bipolar Disorders, 7,* 344–350.

Hipwell, A. E., Goossens, F. A., Melhuish, E. C., & Kumar, R. (2000). Severe maternal psychopathology and infant–mother attachment. *Development and Psychopathology, 12,* 157–175.

Hipwell, A. E., & Kumar, R. (1996). Maternal psychopathology and prediction of outcome based on mother–infant interaction ratings (BMIS). *British Journal of Psychiatry, 169,* 655–661.

Hooley, J. M., Richters, J. E., Weintraub, S., & Neale, J. M. (1987). Psychopathology and marital distress: The positive side of positive symptoms. *Journal of Abnormal Psychology, 96,* 27–33.

Hooley, J. M., & Teasdale, J. D. (1989). Predictors of relapse in unipolar depressives: Expressed emotion, marital distress, and perceived criticism. *Journal of Abnormal Psychology, 98,* 229–235.

Hoover, C. F., & Fitzgerald, G. (1981). Marital conflict of manic–depressive patients. *Archives of General Psychiatry, 38,* 65–67.

Horesh, N., & Fennig, S. (2000). Perception of spouses and relationships: A matched control study of patients with severe affective disorder in remission and their spouses. *Journal of Nervous and Mental Disease, 188,* 463–466.

Inaba, A., Thoits, P. A., & Ueno, K. (2005). Depression in the United States and Japan: Gender, marital status, and SES patterns. *Social Science and Medicine, 61,* 2280–2292.

Ingram, R. E. (1990). Self-focused attention in clinical disorders: Review and a conceptual model. *Psychological Bulletin, 107,* 156–176.

Jackman-Cram, S., Dobson, K. S., & Martin, R. (2006). Marital problem-solving behavior in depression and marital distress. *Journal of Abnormal Psychology, 115,* 380–384.

Johnson, L., Lundstrom, O., Aberg-Wistedt, A., & Mathe, A. A. (2003). Social support in bipolar disorder: Its relevance to remission and relapse. *Bipolar Disorders, 5,* 129–137.

Joyner, K., & Udry, R. (2000). You don't bring me anything but down: Adolescent romance and depression. *Journal of Health and Social Behavior, 41,* 369–391.

Kane, P., & Garber, J. (2004). The relations among depression in fathers, children's psychopathology, and father–child conflict: A meta-analysis. *Clinical Psychology Review, 24,* 339–360.

Kaslow, N. J., Deering, C. G., & Racusin, G. R. (1994). Depressed children and their families. *Clinical Psychology Review, 14,* 39–59.

Kaslow, N. J., Jones, C. A., & Palin, F. (2005). A relational perspective on depressed children: Family patterns and interventions. In W. M. Pinsof & J. L. Lebow (Eds.), *Family psychology: The art of the science* (pp. 215–242). New York: Oxford University Press.

Kelly, J. B. (2000). Children's adjustment in conflicted marriage and divorce: A decade review of research. *Journal of the American Academy of Child and Adolescent Psychiatry, 39,* 963–973.

Kenney-Benson, G. A., & Pomerantz, E. M. (2005). The role of mothers' use of control in children's perfectionism: Implications for the development of children's depressive symptoms. *Journal of Personality, 73,* 23–46.

Kenny, M. E., Moilanen, D. L., Lomax, R., & Brabeck, M. M. (1993). Contributions of parental attachments to view of self and depressive symptoms in early adolescents. *Journal of Early Adolescence, 13,* 408–430.

Kessing, L. V., Agerbo, E., & Mortensen, P. B. (2004). Major stressful life events and other risk factors for first admission with mania. *Bipolar Disorders, 6,* 122–129.

Kessler, R. C., Berglund, P., Demler, O., Jin, R., Koretz, D., Merikangas, K. R., et al. (2003). The epidemiology of major depressive disorder: Results for the National Comorbidity Survey Replication (NCS-R). *Journal of the American Medical Association, 289,* 3095–3105.

Kessler, R. C., Walters, E. E., & Forthofer, M. S. (1998). The social consequences of psychiatric disorders: III. Probability of marital stability. *American Journal of Psychiatry, 155,* 1092–1096.

Kim, E. Y., Miklowitz, D. J., Biuckians, A., & Mullen, K. (2007). Life stress and the course of early-onset bipolar disorder. *Journal of Affective Disorders, 99,* 37–44.

Klein, D. N., Depue, R. A., & Krauss, S. P. (1986). Social adjustment in the offspring of parents with bipolar affective disorder. *Journal of Psychopathology and Behavioral Assessment, 8,* 355–366.

Klimes-Dougan, B., Ronsaville, D., Wiggs, E. A., & Martinez, P. E. (2006). Neuropsychological functioning in adolescent children of mothers with a history of bipolar or major depressive disorders. *Biological Psychiatry, 60,* 957–965.

Kochanska, G., Kuczynski, L., Radke-Yarrow, M., & Welsh, J. D. (1987). Resolutions of control episodes between well and affectively ill mothers and their young children. *Journal of Abnormal Child Psychology, 15,* 441–456.

La Greca, A. M., & Harrison, H. M. (2005). Adolescent peer relations, friendships, and romantic relationships: Do they predict social anxiety and depression? *Journal of Clinical Child and Adolescent Psychology, 34,* 49–61.

Lam, D., Donaldson, C., Brown, Y., & Malliaris, Y. (2005). Burden and marital and sexual satisfaction in partners of bipolar patients. *Bipolar Disorders, 7,* 431–440.

Lapalme, M., Hodgins, S., & LaRoche, C. (1997). Children of parents with bipolar disorder: A metaanalysis of risk for mental disorders. *Canadian Journal of Psychiatry, 42,* 623–631.

Leff, J., & Vaughn, C. (1985). *Expressed emotion in families.* New York: Guilford Press.

Levkovitz, V., Fennig, S., Horesh, N., Barak, V., & Treves, I. (2000). Perception of ill spouse and dyadic relationship in couples with affective disorder and those without. *Journal of Affective Disorders, 58,* 237–240.

Levkovitz, V., Lamy, D., Ternachiano, P., Treves, I., & Fennig, S. (2003). Perceptions of dyadic relationship and emotional states in patients with affective disorder. *Journal of Affective Disorders, 75,* 19–28.

Lewinsohn, P. M., Olino, T. M., & Klein, D. N. (2005). Psychosocial impairment in offspring of depressed parents. *Psychological Medicine, 35,* 1493–1503.

Lovejoy, M. C., Graczyk, P. A., O'Hare, E., & Neuman, G. (2000). Maternal depression and parenting behavior: A meta-analytic review. *Clinical Psychology Review, 20,* 561–592.

Maciejewski, P. K., Prigerson, H. G., & Mazure, C. M. (2001). Sex differences in event-related risk for major depression. *Psychological Medicine, 31,* 593–604.

Margolese, S. K., Markiewicz, D., & Doyle, A. B. (2005). Attachment to parents, best friend, and romantic partner: Predicting different pathways to depression in adolescence. *Journal of Youth and Adolescence, 34,* 637–650.

Martins, C., & Gaffan, E. A. (2000). Effects of early maternal depression on patterns of infant–mother attachment: A meta-analytic investigation. *Journal of Child Psychology and Psychiatry, and Allied Disciplines, 41,* 737–746.

Mathews, C., & Reus, V. (2001). Assortative mating in the affective disorders: A systematic review and meta-analysis. *Comprehensive Psychiatry, 42,* 257–262.

McCabe, S. B., & Gotlib, I. H. (1993). Interaction of couples with and without a depressed spouse: Self-report and observations of problem-solving situations. *Journal of Social and Personal Relationships, 10,* 589–599.

McCleary, L., & Sanford, M. (2002). Parental expressed emotion in depressed adolescents: Prediction of clinical course and relationship to comorbid disorders and social functioning. *Journal of Child Psychology and Psychiatry, and Allied Disciplines, 43,* 587–595.

McGuffin, P., Rijsdijk, F., Andrew, M., Sham, P., Katz, R., & Cardno, A. (2003). The heritability of bipolar affective disorder and the genetic relationship to unipolar depression. *Archives of General Psychiatry, 60,* 497–502.

Merikangas, K. R., & Spiker, D. G. (1982). Assortative mating among in-patients with primary affective disorder. *Psychological Medicine, 12,* 753–764.

Meyer, S. E., Carlson, G. A., Wiggs, E. A., Ronsaville, D. S., Martinez, P. E., Klimes-Dougan, B., et al. (2006). A prospective high-risk study of the association among maternal negativity, apparent frontal lobe dysfunction, and the development of bipolar disorder. *Development and Psychopathology, 18,* 573–589.

Miklowitz, D. J. (2004). The role of family systems in severe and recurrent psychiatric disorders: A developmental psychopathology view. *Development and Psychopathology, 16,* 667–688.

Miklowitz, D. J., Biuckians, A., & Richards, J. A. (2006). Early-onset bipolar disorder: A family treatment perspective. *Development and Psychopathology, 18,* 1247–1265.

Monroe, S. M., Bromet, E. J., Connell, M. M., & Steiner, S. C. (1986). Social support, life events, and depressive symptoms: A 1-year prospective study. *Journal of Consulting and Clinical Psychology, 54,* 424–431.

Monroe, S. M., Rohde, P., Seeley, J. R., & Lewinsohn, P. M. (1999). Life events and depression in adolescence: Relationship loss as a prospective risk factor for first onset of major depressive disorder. *Journal of Abnormal Psychology, 108,* 606–614.

Mundt, C., Kronmuller, K., & Backenstrass, M. (2000). Interactional styles in bipolar disorder. In A. Marneros & J. Angst (Eds.), *Bipolar disorders: 100 years after manic–depressive insanity* (pp. 201–213). London: Kluwer Academic.

Neeren, A., Alloy, L. B., & Abramson, L. Y. (in press). History of parenting and bipolar spectrum disorders. *Journal of Social and Clinical Psychology.*

Perlick, D., Clarkin, J., Sirey, J., Raue, P., Greenfield, S., Struening, E., et al. (1999). Burden experienced by care-givers of persons with bipolar affective disorder. *British Journal of Psychiatry, 175,* 56–62.

Perlick, D. A., Rosenheck, R. R., Clarkin, J. F., Raue, P., & Sirey, J. (2001). Impact of family burden and patient symptom status on clinical outcome on bipolar affective disorder. *Journal of Nervous and Mental Disease, 189,* 31–37.

Pineda, A. Q., Cole, D. A., & Bruce, A. E. (2007). Mother–adolescent interactions and adolescent depressive symptoms: A sequential analysis. *Journal of Social and Personal Relationships, 24,* 5–19.

Pinquart, M., & Duberstein, P. R. (2005). Optimism, pessimism, and depressive symptoms in spouses of lung cancer patients. *Psychology and Health, 20,* 565–578.

Pinquart, M., & Sörensen, S. (2005). Caregiving distress and psychological health of caregivers. In K. V. Oxington (Ed.), *Psychology of stress* (pp. 165–206). Hauppauge, NY: Nova Biomedical.

Quatman, T., Sampson, K., Robinson, C., & Watson, C. M. (2001). Academic, motivational, and emotional correlates of adolescent dating. *Genetic, Social, and General Psychology Monographs, 127,* 211–234.

Radke-Yarrow, M. (1998). *Children of depressed mothers: From early childhood to maturity.* Cambridge, UK: Cambridge University Press.

Reichart, C. G., van der Ende, J., Wals, M., Hillegers, M. H. J., Nolen, W. A., Ormel, J., et al. (2007). Social functioning of bipolar offspring. *Journal of Affective Disorders, 98,* 207–213.

Reuter, M. A., Scaramella, L., Wallace, L. E., & Conger, R. D. (1999). First onset of depressive or anxiety disorders predicted by the longitudinal course of internalizing symptoms and parent–adolescent disagreements. *Archives of General Psychiatry, 56,* 726–732.

Rice, F., Harold, G. T., Shelton, K. H., & Thapar, A. (2006). Family conflict interacts with genetic liability in predicting childhood and adolescent depression. *Journal of the American Academy of Child and Adolescent Psychiatry, 45,* 841–848.

Rohde, P., Lewinsohn, P. M., Klein, D. N., & Seeley, J. R. (2005). Association of parental depression with psychiatric course from adolescence to young adulthood among formerly depressed individuals. *Journal of Abnormal Psychology, 114,* 409–420.

Romanoski, A. J., Folstein, M. F., Nestadt, G., Chahal, R., Merchant, A., Brown, C. H., et al. (1992). The epidemiology of psychiatrist-ascertained depression and DSM-III depressive disorders: Results from the Eastern Baltimore Mental Health Survey clinical reappraisal. *Psychological Medicine, 22,* 629–655.

Rose, A. J. (2002). Co-rumination in the friendships of girls and boys. *Child Development, 73,* 1830–1843.

Sacco, W. P., Dumont, C. P., & Dow, M. G. (1993). Attributional, perceptual, and affective responses to depressed and nondepressed marital partners. *Journal of Consulting and Clinical Psychology, 61,* 1076–1082.

Sayers, S. L, Kohn, C. S., & Fresco, D. M. (2001). Marital cognitions and depression in the context of marital discord. *Cognitive Therapy and Research, 25,* 713–732.

Schwartz, C. E., Dorer, D. J., Beardslee, W. R., Lavori, P. W., & Keller, M. B. (1990). Maternal expressed emotion and parental affective disorder: Risk for childhood depressive disorder, substance abuse, or conduct disorder. *Journal of Psychiatric Research, 24,* 231–250.

Sheeber, L., Hops, H., Alpert, A., Davis, B., & Andrews, J. (1997). Family support and conflict: Prospective relations to adolescent depression. *Journal of Abnormal Child Psychology, 25,* 333–344.

Sheeber, L., Hops, H., Andrews, J., Alpert, T., & Davis, B. (1998). Interactional processes in families with depressed and non-depressed adolescents: Reinforcement of depressive behavior. *Behaviour Research and Therapy, 36,* 417–427.

Sheeber, L., Hops, H., & Davis, B. (2001). Family processes in adolescent depression. *Clinical Child and Family Psychology Review, 4,* 19–35.

Sheeber, L. B., Davis, B., Leve, C., Hops, H., & Tildesley, E. (2007). Adolescents' relationships with their mothers and fathers: Associations with depressive disorder and subdiagnostic symptomatology. *Journal of Abnormal Psychology, 116,* 144–154.

Silk, J. S., Shaw, D. S., Forbes, E. E., Lane, T. L., & Kovacs, M. (2006). Maternal depression and child internalizing: The moderating role of child emotion regulation. *Journal of Clinical Child and Adolescent Psychology, 35,* 116–126.

Starr, L. R., & Davila, J. (2007). *Differentiating interpersonal correlates of depressive symptoms and social anxiety in adolescence: Implications for models of comorbidity.* Manuscript under review.

Starr, L. R., & Davila, J. (in press). Clarifying co-rumination: Association with internalizing symptoms and romantic involvement among adolescent girls. *Journal of Adolescence.*

Steinberg, S. J., & Davila, J. (2007). *Adolescent romantic functioning and depression: The moderating role of parental emotional availability.* Manuscript submitted for publication.

Storksen, I., Roysamb, E., Holmen, T. L., & Tambs, K. (2006). Adolescent adjustment and well-being: Effects of parental divorce and distress. *Scandinavian Journal of Psychology, 47,* 75–84.

Strohschien, L. (2005). Parental divorce and child mental health trajectories. *Journal of Marriage and Family, 67,* 1286–1300.

Stroud, C. B., & Davila, J. (in press). Pubertal timing and depressive symptoms in early adolescents: The roles of romantic competence and romantic experiences. *Journal of Youth and Adolescence.*

Sund, A. M., & Wichstrom, L. (2002). Insecure attachment as a risk factor for future depressive symptoms in early adolescence. *Journal of the American Academy of Child and Adolescent Psychiatry, 41,* 1478–1486.

Suppes, T., Leverich, G. S., Keck, P. E., Nolen, W. A., Denicoff, K. D., Altshuler, L. L., et al. (2001). The Stanley Foundation Bipolar Treatment Outcome Network II: Demographics and illness characteristics of the first 261 patients. *Journal of Affective Disorders, 67,* 45–59.

Tannenbaum, L., & Forehand, R. (1994). Maternal depressive mood: The role of the father in preventing adolescent problem behaviors. *Behaviour Research and Therapy, 32,* 321–325.

Targum, S. D., Dibble, E., Davenport, Y. B., & Gershon, E. S. (1981). The Family Attitudes Questionnaire: Patients' and spouses' views of bipolar illness. *Archives of General Psychiatry, 38,* 562–568.

Terry, D. J., Mayocchi, L., & Hynes, G. J. (1996). Depressive symptomatology in new mothers: A stress and coping perspective. *Journal of Abnormal Psychology, 105,* 220–231.

Teti, D. M., & Gelfand, D. M. (1991). Behavioral competence among mothers of infants in the first year: The mediational role of maternal self-efficacy. *Child Development, 62,* 918–929.

Toth, S. L., & Cicchetti, D. (1996). Patterns of relatedness, depressive symptomatology, and perceived competence in maltreated children. *Journal of Consulting and Clinical Psychology, 64,* 32–41.

Tsuchiya, K. J., Byrne, M., & Mortensen, P. B. (2003). Risk factors in relation to an emergence of bipolar disorder: A systematic review. *Bipolar Disorders, 5,* 231–242.

Turner, H. A., & Kopiec, K. (2006). Exposure to interparental conflict and psychological disorder among young adults. *Journal of Family Issues, 27,* 131–158.

Uebelacker, L. A., Courtnage, E. S., & Whisman, M. A. (2003). Correlates of depression and marital dissatisfaction: Perceptions of marital communication style. *Journal of Social and Personal Relationships, 20,* 757–769.

Uehara, T., Yokoyama, T., Goto, M., & Ihda, S. (1996). Expressed emotion and short-term treatment outcome of outpatients with major depression. *Comprehensive Psychiatry, 37,* 299–304.

Umberson, D., & Williams, K. (1999). Family status and mental health. In C. S. Aneshensel & J. C. Phelan (Eds.), *Handbook of the sociology of mental health* (pp. 225–253). New York: Kluwer Academic/Plenum Press.

van IJzendoorn, M. H., Schuengel, C., & Bakermans-Kranenburg, M. J. (1999). Disorganized attachment in early childhood: Meta-analysis of precursors, concomitants, and sequelae. *Development and Psychopathology, 11,* 225–249.

Vendlinski, M., Silk, J. S., Shaw, D. S., & Lane, T. J. (2006). Ethnic differences in relations between family process and child internalizing problems. *Journal of Child Psychology and Psychiatry, and Allied Disciplines, 47,* 960–969.

Wade, T. D., & Kendler, K. S. (2000). The relationship between social support and major depression: Cross-sectional, longitudinal, and genetic perspectives. *Journal of Nervous and Mental Disease, 188,* 251–258.

Webster-Stratton, C., & Hammond, M. (1988). Maternal depression and its relationship to life stress, perceptions of child behavior problems, parenting behaviors, and child conduct problems. *Journal of Abnormal Child Psychology, 16,* 299–315.

Weissman, M. M., & Olfson, M. (1995). Depression in women: Implications for health care research. *Science, 269,* 799–801.

Whiffen, V. E. (2005). Disentangling causality in the associations between couple and family processes and depression. In W. M. Pinsof & J. L. Lebow (Eds.), *Family psychology: The art of the science* (pp. 375–398). Oxford, UK: Oxford University Press.

Whiffen, V. E., Kallos-Lilly, V., & MacDonald, B. J. (2001). Depression and attachment in couples. *Cognitive Therapy and Research, 25,* 421–434.

Whisman, M. A. (1999). Marital dissatisfaction and psychiatric disorders: Results from the national comorbidity survey. *Journal of Abnormal Psychology, 108,* 701–706.

Whisman, M. A. (2001). The association between depression and marital dissatisfaction. In S. R. H. Beach (Ed.), *Marital and family processes in depression: A scientific foundation for clinical practice* (pp. 3–24). Washington, DC: American Psychological Association.

Whisman, M. A. (2007). Marital distress and DSM-IV psychiatric disorders in a population-based national survey. *Journal of Abnormal Psychology, 116,* 638–643.

Whisman, M. A., & Bruce, M. L. (1999). Marital dissatisfaction and incidence of major depressive episode in a community sample. *Journal of Abnormal Psychology, 108,* 674–678.

Whisman, M. A., Uebelacker, L. A., Tolejko, N., Chatav, Y., & McKelvie, M. (2006, November). *Marital dissatisfaction and depression in older adults: Is the association confounded by personality?* Paper presented at the 40th annual convention of the Association for Behavioral and Cognitive Therapies, Chicago.

Whisman, M. A., Weinstock, L. M., & Tolejko, N. (2006). Marriage and depression. In C. L. M. Keyes & S. H. Goodman (Eds.), *Women and depression: A handbook for the social, behavioral, and biomedical sciences* (pp. 219–240). New York: Cambridge University Press.

Whisman, M. A., Weinstock, L. M., & Uebelacker, L. A. (2002). Mood reactivity to marital conflict: The influence of marital dissatisfaction and depression. *Behavior Therapy, 33,* 299–314.

Whitbeck, L. B., Hoyt, D. R., Simons, R. L., & Conger, R. D. (1992). Intergenerational continuity of parental rejection and depressed affect. *Journal of Personality and Social Psychology, 63,* 1036–1045.

Williams, S., Connolly, J., & Segal, Z. V. (2001). Intimacy in relationships and cognitive vulnerability to depression in adolescent girls. *Cognitive Therapy and Research, 25,* 477–496.

Yan, L. J., Hammen, C., Cohen, A. N., Daley, S. E., & Henry, R. M. (2004). Expressed emotion versus relationship quality variables in the prediction of recurrence in bipolar patients. *Journal of Affective Disorders, 83,* 199–206.

Yazici, O., Kora, K., Ucok, A., Tunali, D., & Turan, N. (1999). Predictors of lithium prophylaxis in bipolar patients. *Journal of Affective Disorders, 55,* 133–142.

Yoneda, A., & Davila, J. (2008). *Emotional and sexual attractions: Differing implications for the psychological health of early adolescent females.* Manuscript submitted for publication.

CHAPTER 21

Depression in Later Life

Epidemiology, Assessment, Impact, and Treatment

Dan G. Blazer *and* Celia F. Hybels

"**I** am old and getting older. There's absolutely nothing that will stop me becoming frail and debilitated. No one cares about me. I forget what day of the week it is, because each day is just like the next. I'm disgusted with my life. Some people my age did everything exactly as they wanted and got everything they desired. I did everything wrong and got nothing." Older adults are sometimes heard to make such statements. Depression, hopelessness, helplessness, uselessness, and loneliness are considered ubiquitous as people become older. In her book *The Coming of Age*, Simone de Beauvoir relates the story of the young Buddha, Prince Siddhartha. One day he left his beautiful palace and traveled in his chariot through the countryside. There he saw a tottering, wrinkled, white-haired, decrepit old man who was bent over and gradually moving forward, mumbling something incomprehensible. The young prince told his charioteer, "It's the world's pity, that weak and ignorant beings, drunk with the vanity of youth, do not behold old age. Let us hurry back to the palace. What is the use of pleasures and delights in life, since I myself am the future dwelling-place of old-age?" (de Beauvoir, 1973, p. 7).

Despite this discouraging perception of old age, most older adults experience good life satisfaction, especially if they are not plagued by excessive physical illness and functional incapacity (Gatz & Zarit, 1999). Even so, depression is the most frequent cause of emotional suffering in later life and, when present, significantly reduces the quality of life among older adults (Berkman et al., 1986; Blazer, 2002a; Doraiswamy, Khan, Donahue, & Richard, 2002; Schneider, Reynolds, Lebowitz, & Friedhoff, 1994). Interest in late-life depression has increased considerably among investigators over the past 20 years. Many gaps in our understanding of the phenomenology, diagnosis, and prognosis have been filled (Alexopoulos, Meyers, Young, Mattis, & Kakuma, 1993; Beekman et al., 2002; Schulz, Drayer, & Rollman, 2002). We have learned much about the etiology of depression in older adults (Blazer & Hybels, 2005). Finally, the evidence base for therapies used to treat late-life depression has increased dramatically (Arean & Cook, 2002; Reynolds et al., 1999, 2006; Unutzer et al., 2002).

In this chapter, we explore late-life depression from a clinical and investigative perspective, identifying the significant increase in what we know and the gaps that remain. We first address case definitions of late-life depression, because existing nomenclature does not capture the vicissitudes of late-life mood disorders. We review the epidemiology of mood disorders, both studies of symptom frequency and those that use diagnostic categories, such as those found in the fourth, text revision edition of the *Diagnostic and Statistical Manual of Mental Disorders* (DSM-IV-TR; American Psychiatric Association, 2000) We follow this discussion with a review of the longitudinal course and outcomes of late-life depressive disorders, then review the biological, psychological, and social origins of late-life depression. We next review the elements of a thorough diagnostic workup, including screening and laboratory tests, the diagnostic interview, and treatment approaches, with a brief section on bipolar disorder. Finally, we review future directions for research into late-life mood disorders.

CASE DEFINITIONS OF LATE-LIFE DEPRESSION

The diagnostic criteria for late-life depression are neither simple nor straightforward. First, investigators to date have found no biological markers for the most common depressive syndromes in later life (though many biological correlates have been identified). In addition, symptoms do not easily cluster into mutually exclusive categories that permit easy classification. For example, there is considerable overlap between symptoms of depression and symptoms of anxiety. Finally, neither clinicians nor clinical investigators agree as to what constitutes a clinically significant episode of depression (regardless of age). For example, do mild but persistent depressive symptoms constitute a pathological condition or a normal variant of mood in the population? Therefore, we present some clinically useful case definitions of late-life depression, some which are included in DSM-IV-TR and some of which are not. *Major depression* is the core diagnosis for clinical depression. To meet criteria for a diagnosis, the older adult must exhibit at least one of two basic symptoms (depressed mood and/or lack of interest) for 2 weeks or more. Older adults are more likely to complain of a loss of interest than to present with an overt expression of a depressed mood. In addition, to be diagnosed with major depression, the older adult must exhibit at least four or more of the following symptoms for at least 2 weeks. Older adults tend to differ somewhat from middle-age adults in the presentation of these criteria symptoms (Blazer, Bachar, & Hughes, 1987):

- Feelings of worthlessness or inappropriate guilt (guilt is less frequent among older adults than among younger adults as a symptom of depression).
- Diminished ability to concentrate or to make decisions (older adults are no more likely than younger adults to complain of difficulty with concentration and memory, but they are more likely than younger adults to exhibit positive findings on psychological testing in the midst of an episode of depression).
- Fatigue (a common symptom regardless of age in the moderate to severely depressed).
- Psychomotor agitation or retardation (either can be seen in late life).
- Increase or decrease in weight or appetite (older adults rarely gain weight in the midst of a depression, whereas even a weight loss of 5 pounds is a cardinal symptom of late-life depression if no other explanation can be found for the weight loss).

- Recurrent thoughts of death or suicide (older adults are less likely to express suicidal ideation, though they may frequently ruminate about death in the midst of an episode of depression) (American Psychiatric Association 2000).

Even so, the diagnosis of major depression in an older adult without comorbid physical illness or cognitive impairment should be no more difficult than it is in a younger adult.

Minor, subsyndromal, or subthreshold depression is not at present an accepted diagnosis in DSM-IV-TR, though symptoms for minor depression are suggested in the manual's Appendix. The diagnosis is made when the core symptoms are present, along with one to three additional symptoms for at least 2 weeks. A number of additional definitions of *subthreshold* or *subsyndromal* depression have emerged. In epidemiological studies, the most common definition is a score of 16 or greater on the Center for Epidemiologic Studies Depression Scale (CES-D)(Radloff, 1977), yet not meeting criteria for major depression. Still others have suggested a diagnosis of subthreshold depression below the usual cut point on the CES-D (Hybels, Blazer, & Pieper, 2001). A further variant that is thought to be more common in older adults is *depression without sadness* (i.e., depressive symptoms but no complaint of being sad or depressed) (Gallo, Rabins, & Lyketsos, 1997). *Dysthymic disorder* is a less severe but more chronic variant of depression. To meet criteria the older adult must experience symptoms most of the time for at least 2 years (American Psychiatric Association, 2000). This disorder does not usually begin in late life, but it can persist from midlife into late life (Blazer, 1994; Devenand et al., 1994).

Some differences between early-onset (a first episode prior to the age of 60) and *late-onset* (first episode at age 60 years or later) depression have been reported in addition to symptom presentation. For example, personality problems, a family history of psychiatric disorder, and stressful ongoing events, such as a dysfunctional marriage, are more common in early-onset depression. Interest in differentiating an early- versus late-onset episode of depression derives in part from recent interest in the etiology of first-onset depressions in late life.

Vascular depression, a depression proposed to be secondary to vascular lesions in the brain, appears to present with slightly different symptoms than typical episodes of major depression in late life. For example, these older adults experience problems with executive cognitive function, such as verbal fluency, recognition memory, and forward planning (Krishnan, Hays, & Blazer, 1997). Some investigators have recently proposed criteria for a *depression of Alzheimer's disease*. In persons who meet criteria for a dementing disorder of the Alzheimer's type, the appearance of three symptoms, such as depressed mood, anhedonia, social isolation (not a symptom criterion for major depression), poor appetite, poor sleep, psychomotor changes, irritability (not a symptom of major depression), fatigue and loss of energy, feelings of worthlessness, and suicidal thoughts, would qualify for the diagnosis (Olin et al., 2002). Finally, *psychotic depression* (in contrast to nonpsychotic depression) may occur in as many as 20–45% of hospitalized older adult patients but is much less frequent in the community (Kivela, Pahkala, & Laippala, 1988; Meyers, 1992).

EPIDEMIOLOGY OF LATE-LIFE DEPRESSION

Table 21.1 lists the prevalence of depression reported in selected studies of older adults in community populations. The lifetime prevalence of major depression in these studies ranges from 2.6 to 10.6% (Hasin, Goodwin, Stinson, & Grant, 2005; Kessler et al., 2005; Lee et

TABLE 21.1. Prevalence of Depression in Older Adults Reported from Selected Community Studies

Authors	Study	Location	n^a	Age	Instrument	Period	Outcome	Prevalence
Regier et al. (1988)	ECA	5 U.S. cities	5,702 (18,571)	65+	DIS	1-month	Major depression Dysthymia	0.7% 1.8%
Beekman et al. (1995)	LASA	Netherlands	3,056	55–85	DIS CES-D	1-month Current	Major depression Minor depression	2.02% 12.9%
Hasin et al. (2005)	NESARC	U.S.	(43,093)	65+	AUDADIS-IV	12-month Lifetime	Major depression Major depression	2.69% 8.19%
Kessler et al. (2005)	NCS-R	U.S.	(9,282)	60+	WMH-CIDI	Lifetime Lifetime	Major depression Dysthymia	10.6% 1.3%
Patten et al. (2006)	CCHS	Canada	(36,984)	65+	CIDI	12-month Current	Major depression Major depression	1.9% 0.9%
Lee et al. (2007)	WMH-China	Beijing and Shanghai	(5,201)	65+	WMH-CIDI	Lifetime	Major depression	2.6%
Williams et al. (2007)	NSAL	U.S.	1,084 (6,082)	60+	CIDI	Lifetime	Major depression	4.5% AAs 7.6% CBs 9.3% whites
Blazer et al. (1991)	EPESE	NC	3,998	65+	CES-D		Depressive Sx	9.0%
Black et al. (1998)	Hispanic EPESE	5 states	2,823	65+	CES-D		Depressive Sx	17.3% males; 31.9% females

Note. ECA, Epidemiologic Catchment Area; DIS, Diagnostic Interview Schedule (Robins et al., 1981); LASA, Longitudinal Aging Study Amsterdam; CES-D, Center for Epidemiologic Studies—Depression Scale (Radloff, 1977); NESARC, National Epidemiologic Survey on Alcoholism and Related Conditions; AUDADIS-IV, Alcohol Use Disorder and Associated Disabilities Interview Schedule—DSM-IV Version (Grant et al., 2001); NCS-R, National Comorbidity Study—Replication; CIDI, Composite International Diagnostic Interview (Kessler & Ustun, 2004); WMH, World Mental Health Survey; CCHS, Canadian Community Health Survey; NSAL, National Survey of American Life; AAs, African Americans; CBs, Caribbean Blacks; EPESE, Established Populations for Epidemiologic Studies of the Elderly; Sx, symptoms.
^{a}Number of age eligible with (total sample size) provided, if available.

al., 2007; Williams, Gonzalez, & Neighbors, 2007), whereas the lifetime prevalence of dysthymia may be 1 to 3% (Kessler et al., 2005). Current or 1-month prevalence of major depression in this age group may be less than 1% (Patten, Wang, & Williams, 2006; Regier et al., 1988), although a higher prevalence has been reported (Beekman et al., 1995). Among community-dwelling older adults, the prevalence of clinically significant depressive symptoms or minor depression is much higher than that of major depression (Blazer, Hughes, & George, 1987), and may range to 9% (Blazer, Burchett, Service, & George, 1991) or more in selected population subgroups, such as Hispanic older adults (Black, Goodwin, & Markides, 1998). Both major depression and depressive symptoms are more common in older adult females than in males (Black et al., 1998), and may be lower in African Americans than in European Americans (Williams et al., 2007).

The prevalence of major and minor depression is generally higher in clinical populations. Lyness, King, Cox, Yoediono, and Caine (1999) reported that the current prevalence of subsyndromal depression in a primary care sample was 9.9% compared to a prevalence of 6.5% for major depression, 5.2% for minor depression, and 0.9% for dysthymia. Among hospitalized patients, the prevalence of major or minor depression ranges from 11 to 23% (Koenig, Meador, Cohen, & Blazer, 1988). Finally, in a study of institutionalized older adults, 12.4% of residents met criteria for major depression, whereas 30.5% had minor depression or clinically significant depressive symptomatology (Parmelee, Katz, & Lawton, 1989).

The annual incidence of major depressive disorder (MDD) per 100 person-years of risk reported from the Epidemiologic Catchment Area (ECA) study was 1.25 among those 65 or older (0.90 for males and 1.48 for females) (Eaton et al., 1989), a lower incidence than that observed in younger adults. The incidence of depression follows the same female:male ratio in the very old, and the incidence of first-onset depression may increase with age among persons ages 70–85 (Palsson, Ostling, & Skoog, 2001).

OUTCOME OF LATE-LIFE DEPRESSION

Though episodes of depression across the life cycle, especially episodes of more severe depression, almost always remit, or at least partially remit, depression is a chronic and recurrent illness. Data from a community study of older adults from the Netherlands illustrate this chronicity. Among subjects with clinically significant depressive symptoms, 23% improved, 44% experienced an unfavorable but fluctuating course, and 33% experienced a severe and chronic course over a 6-year period (Beekman et al., 2002).

Studies that have focused on older adults in clinic settings reveal similar chronicity (Alexopoulos et al., 1996; Baldwin & Jolley, 1986; Murphy, 1983). Elaine Murphy (1983) followed a group of older adult depressed subjects (many of whom were medically ill) over 1 year. She found that 35% experienced a good outcome, 48% experienced a fluctuating course or remain continuously ill, and 14% died. In one study, only 12% of a group of older adult patients experiencing depression, who had been followed for 25 years and had experienced severe depression earlier in life, remained continuously well over the follow-up period (Brodaty, Luscombe, Peisah, Anstey, & Andrews, 2001). The prognosis from clinical studies of depressed older adults with late-life depression, however, is similar to that of younger adults when the older adults are not plagued with comorbid medical illness, functional impairment, or cognitive impairment (Keller, Shapiro, Lavori, & Wolfe, 1982a, 1982b). Comorbid depression is associated with a less favorable prognosis. When major depression is comorbid with dysthymic disorder, the prognosis is poor. Factors predicting partial remission were similar to those predicting no remission, and poor social support and functional limitations increased the risk for poor outcome in these subjects (Hybels, Blazer, & Steffens, 2005).

More severe depression in late life is often associated with cognitive impairment. When the depression improves, the cognitive impairment often improves as well. Nevertheless, the interaction of comorbid depression and cognitive impairment is a risk for the later emergence of Alzheimer's disease (Alexopoulos et al., 1993). Therefore, early depressive symptoms associated with mild cognitive impairment may represent a preclinical sign and should be considered a risk for impending Alzheimer's disease or vascular dementia (Li, Meyer, & Thornby, 2001). Depression can further complicate Alzheimer's disease over time by increasing disability and physical aggression, thereby contributing to depression among caregivers (Gonzales-Salvador, Aragano, Lyketsos, & Barba, 1999). Depressive symptoms in patients with Alzheimer's disease resolve spontaneously at a greater frequency, without requiring intensive therapy (e.g., medication therapy) than those among older adults with depression and vascular dementia, in whom depressive symptoms tend to be persistent and refractory to drug treatment (Li et al., 2001).

Depression and medical problems often coexist, and the causal pathway is bidirectional. For example, depression is a frequent and important contributing cause of weight loss in late life (Morley & Kraenzle, 1994). Frailty, leading to profound weight loss, can in turn contribute to clinically important depressive symptoms (Fried, 1994). Depression is also associated with many chronic medical illnesses, including cardiovascular disease and diabetes (Blazer, Moody-Ayers, Craft-Morgan, & Burchett, 2002; Williams et al., 2002). The mechanisms that underlie the association between depression and physical illness in older adults are not well understood. Perhaps the best established association between depression and physical problems is that between depression and functional impairment (Blazer et al., 1991; Bruce, 2001). For example, in one study, depressed older adults were 67% more likely to experience impairment in activities of daily living and 73% more likely to experience mobility restrictions 6 years after initial evaluation than were those who were not depressed (Penninx, Leveille, Ferrucci, van Eijk, & Guralnik, 1999). Disability, in turn, can increase the risk for depressive symptoms (Kennedy, Kelman, & Thomas, 1990). Explanations for this bidirectional association include the propensity for physical disability to lead to a higher frequency of negative life events, which in turn increases the risk for depression; restricted social and leisure activities secondary to physical disability; and the isolation and reduced quality of social support often inherent in physical disability (Blazer, 1983).

Suicide is the most tragic consequence of late-life depression. The association of depression and suicide across the life cycle has been well documented (Conwell, Duberstein, & Caine, 2002). In recent years, however, late-life suicide rates have declined. From World War II until about 1980, suicide rates declined among older adults, especially among white males (who have a much higher suicide rate than do other age, sex, and racial/ethnic groups; National Center for Health Statistics, 2001). During the decade of the 1980s, suicide rates increased in white males. Suicide rates once again have declined since the latter 1980s. From 1987 to 2002 (15 years), the rates among persons 65 years of age and older declined from 21.7 to 15.6 per 100,000 (McKeown, Cuffe, & Schulz, 2006).

Despite their confined environment, hospitalized patients with mood disorders are also at risk for suicide. In a study of older inpatients hospitalized for psychiatric disorders in Denmark, those with mood disorders were twice as likely to commit suicide. More than one-half of the suicides occurred either within the first week of admission or discharge

(Erlangsen, Zarit, Tu, & Conwell, 2006). Suicide rates in hospitalized depressed older adults may be 10 times as high as rates for the community at large. Despite the potential for widespread use of antidepressant medication in older adults to reduce the burden of depression (and therefore suicide), one group found a fivefold higher risk of completed suicide during the first month in older adults treated with selective serotonin reuptake inhibitors (SSRIs) compared with other antidepressants, independent of a recent diagnosis of depression or the receipt of psychiatric care, and suicide of a violent nature was clearly more frequent (Juurlink, Mamdani, Kopp, & Redelmeier, 2006).

ORIGINS OF LATE-LIFE DEPRESSION

Older adults present a paradox to clinicians and investigators who seek to understand the origins of depression (Blazer & Hybels, 2005). On the one hand, older adults appear to be at greater biological vulnerability than are people in midlife. As documented earlier, however, the frequency of severe depression (except in institutional settings) is lower in late life than in midlife, suggesting that psychological and social factors may offer protection.

Biological Origins

Twin studies of older adults in Scandinavia document the relative contribution of hereditary and environmental factors to self-reported depressive symptoms. In one study from Sweden, genetic influences accounted for 16% of the variance in depressive symptoms and 19% in symptoms specific to biological factors, such as sleep. On the other hand, genetic influences contributed only minimally to expressions of depressed mood and positive affect (Gatz, Pedersen, Plomin, Nesselroade, & McClearn, 1992). Therefore, not all depressive symptoms are equally influenced by heredity. Virtually every study of major depression has documented a relative greater frequency among women than among men (Krause, 1986), potentially due to selective survival (men die earlier than women) or to a greater likelihood that women report symptoms more frequently than men (Hinton, Zweifach, Oishi, Tang, & Unutzer, 2006); it is uncertain whether genetic factors contribute to this sex difference.

Though no single genetic marker has yet been identified for depression at any age, two are of some interest and represent the type of findings that may lead to significant changes in the way depression is conceptualized and treated in the future. In one study, older adults with late-onset depression presented a higher frequency of the *C677T* mutation of the MTHFR (methylenetetrahydrofolate reductase) enzyme than did patients with early-onset depression (Hickie et al., 2001). In a second study, investigators found that older adults with a homozygous short allele polymorphism in the serotonin transporter gene (*5-HTT*) were less likely to respond to SSRI treatment than were their long allele counterparts (Zhang et al., 2005).

In studies of depression across the life cycle, underactivity of serotonin neurotransmission has been a key focus of research into the pathophysiology of depression. Although serotonin activity, namely, 5-HT_{2A} receptor binding, decreases in a variety of brain regions throughout the life cycle, there is less decrease from midlife to late life than from young adulthood to midlife (Sheline, Mintun, Moerlein, & Snyder, 2002).

Yet another biological correlate of depression across the life cycle is hypersecretion of corticotropin-releasing factor (CRF). CRF, however, also declines as age advances (Gottfries, 1990). Other endocrine abnormalities have been associated with late-life depression, including high levels of cortisol (Yaffe, Ettinger, & Pressman, 1998), which may be associated with anatomical changes, specifically, atrophy of the hippocampus (Sapolsky, 2001). In a vicious cycle, depressive symptoms can lead to increased cortisol secretion, which inhibits neurogenesis, leading to hippocampal volume loss that may in turn mediate symptoms of depression.

Investigators have long noted the association of depressive symptoms and vascular risk factors. Hypertension has also been associated with an increased risk of depression, although results of studies have not been consistent (Lyness, King, Conwell, Cox, & Caine, 2000). Brain scans, especially those using magnetic resonance imaging (MRI), have revealed white matter hyperintensities in the subcortical region, suggesting disruption of neural circuits associated with depression (Taylor et al., 2003). As we noted earlier, these findings indicate depressive symptoms in concert with reduced executive cognitive function.

Psychological Origins

Many different psychological theories have been postulated to explain depression across the life cycle. Older depressed individuals with a personality disorder are much more likely than those without a personality disorder to experience reemergence of depressive symptoms, hopelessness, and ambivalence regarding emotional expression (Morse & Lynch, 2004). Personality may also interact with factors such as life events to increase risk for depression, for example, adjusting to physical illness or reduced physical function (Mazure, Maciejewski, Jacobs, & Bruce, 2002). In several studies, late-life depression has also been associated with neuroticism (Henderson, Jorm, & MacKinnon, 1993).

By far the most frequent psychological construct applied to depressive disorders across the life cycle is cognitive distortions (Beck, 1987; see Joormann, Chapter 13, this volume). In a study of the experience and impact of adverse life events, older patients with dysthymia were more likely to report recent live events with greater negative impact, particularly interpersonal conflicts (Devenand, Kim, Paykina, & Sackeim, 2002). In a community-based study, older adult subjects who endorsed more depressive symptoms used rumination and catastrophizing more frequently, and positive reappraisal less frequently, than did those with fewer symptoms (Kraaij & de Wilde, 2001). Perceived loss of internal locus of control has also been found to be associated with both the onset and persistence of depressive symptoms in a community sample (Beekman, Deeg, & Geerlings, 2001).

Two factors are worth considering in understanding the psychological (as well as social and biological) risk for depression in late life (Blazer & Hybels, 2005). The first is socioemotional selectivity theory (Carstensen, Mayr, Pasupathi, & Nesselroade, 2000). According to this theory, older persons perceive time and past experience differently than do younger persons. Specifically, younger adults prioritize the pursuit of knowledge, recognizing they have much to learn and relatively long futures, even if this requires suppressing emotional well-being. In contrast, older adults perceive time as relatively limited, leading them to deemphasize negative experiences and to prioritize emotionally meaningful goals. Older adults selectively recall and attend to positive information, termed the *positivity effect*, which may confer benefits on well-being.

Second, adults are postulated to acquire more wisdom as they grow older. Although wisdom can be a nebulous concept, investigators in Germany have operationalized this construct in community samples (Baltes & Staudinger, 2000). *Wisdom* is defined as an expert knowledge system focused on the fundamental pragmatics of life, such as knowledge and judgment about the meaningful conduct of life, the orchestrating of human development toward optimal goals, while simultaneously attending to personal and collective well-being.

These investigators identified five criteria associated with wisdom: rich factual knowledge; rich procedural knowledge (i.e., knowing how to develop strategies for addressing problems); relativism of values and life priorities (e.g., developing tolerances for differences in society); lifespan contextualization (i.e., integrating life experiences that are seemingly conflicting); and the recognition and management of uncertainty (recognizing that the feature cannot be known with certainty). Individuals possessing wisdom, therefore, can more easily address problems and respond to life stresses, reducing the risk of depression.

Social Origins

Many social factors have been associated with the onset and persistence of late-life depression. There is a strong association between severe stressful events, such as bereavement and life-threatening illnesses, and the onset of major depression in later life (Murphy, 1982). Older adults lacking a confidant are especially vulnerable to live stressors. Given that certain devastating life events are more common in late life, it is tempting to assume that older adults are at increased risk for experiencing stressful events that may be associated with depression. Yet most stressful events that lead to depression are predictable, that is, "on time," events. For example, the death of a sibling is a severe and perhaps catastrophic event that can frequently lead to depression. During midlife, such a death is unexpected, and the adjustment is more difficult. In contrast, although a loss in late life may be severe, the death is usually not unexpected. In addition, many events that lead to depression actually occur more frequently earlier than later in life, such as divorce and difficulties with the law (Hughes, Blazer, & George, 1988).

DIAGNOSTIC WORKUP

Older adults are much less likely than younger adults to use mental health services when they are depressed (Unutzer et al., 1997). Most older adults who do see a clinician for their late-life depression usually are seen in a primary care physician's office (Gallo & Coyne, 2000). Therefore, the diagnostic workup and initiation of therapy usually begins in this setting. Although many psychological tests are available to screen for and identify cases of late-life mood disorders, such as major depression and dysthymia, the diagnosis ultimately derives from a careful history. In obtaining information necessary to make a diagnosis, the clinician should focus on present symptoms, past history (especially a history of previous episodic symptoms similar to those presenting at the time of the interview), family history, recent life events, changes in social and economic status, recent medical problems, and family history. In the absence of comorbid disorders, such as Alzheimer's disease or significant physical dysfunction, the diagnostic criteria for major depression in DSM-IV-TR are applicable as described earlier (Hinton et al., 2006).

A number of available scales have been used to screen for late-life depression in both clinical and community settings. These include the Geriatric Depression Scale (GDS; Yesavage, Brink, & Rose, 1983) and the CES-D (Radloff, 1977). A screen for depressive symptoms should be augmented with a screen for cognitive functioning, with a scale such as the Mini-Mental State Examination (MMSE) (Folstein, Folstein, & McHugh, 1975). Investigators have reported sex differences in symptoms in the presentation of depression in late life. Specifically, older men are not only less likely than older women to be referred for depressive symptoms but also less likely to endorse core depressive symptoms and to have received treatment for depression (Blazer et al., 1991). Diagnostic instruments used for case finding include the Structured Clinical Interview for DSM (SCID; Robins, Helzer, & Croughan, 1981) and the Diagnostic Interview Schedule (DIS; Spitzer, Williams, Gibbon, & First, 1990) (see Nezu, Nezu, Friedman, & Lee, Chapter 3, this volume).

In addition, the clinician should screen for suicidal thoughts or behaviors. The older adult can be asked a series of questions to determine progressive potential risk. As is the case with younger individuals, if the older depressed patient has considered a specific means for harming him- or herself (e.g., taking pills or hanging oneself), then the risk for suicide is increased. These questions, however, are probably of less value in evaluating risk for suicide than an assessment of known risk factors, such as white race, male sex, lower income, social isolation, divorced or widowed, bereaved, suffering from comorbid medical illness, diagnosed with depression in the past, abuse of alcohol or other substances, and a history of previous suicide attempts (Blazer, 2002a).

TREATMENT OF LATE-LIFE DEPRESSION

There are no true biological markers for any of the subtypes of late-life depression; therefore, no definitive laboratory tests assist the clinician in designing therapies for older depressed patients. The one exception is brain scanning in vascular depression, where the presence of subcortical white matter hyperintensities can assist in the diagnosis. Routine laboratory tests, such as a chemistry screen or an electrocardiogram, are employed as a baseline for determining the biological effects of biological therapies. If a medical illness is suspected to contribute to the depressive disorder, a number of elective laboratory tests can be ordered, including a thyroid screen for undiagnosed thyroid dysfunction, vitamin B_{12} and folate assays, as well as polysomnography, if sleep abnormalities cannot be explained.

Biological Therapies

The foundation for the treatment of moderate to severe depression in late life is antidepressant medication (Jacobson, Pies, & Katz, 2007; Nezu, 1987). All of the currently available antidepressant medications are virtually equal in efficacy. Therefore, clinicians usually choose an antidepressant based on the side effects that they hope to avoid. SSRIs have become the preferred antidepressant medication of most clinicians. Side effects from earlier generations of antidepressants (specifically the tricyclic antidepressants), such as dry mouth, constipation, occasional confusion, postural hypotension, and urinary retention, are avoided with the SSRIs. Even so, the SSRIs can lead to side effects such as weight loss, agitation, sleep loss, and, in some rare situations, a potential increased risk for suicidal behavior. Currently available SSRI medications include citalopram, paroxetine, fluoxetine, fluvoxamine, and escitalopram. Other "new generation" antidepressants include mirtazapine, venlafaxine, bupropion, and duloxetine.

Clinicians treating older adults with medication (whether alone or in combination with current psychotherapeutic approaches) must be realistic regarding the prognosis for recovery from a moderate to severe episode of depression. Most antidepressants exhibit efficacy within 4–6 weeks. Yet the actual time from the initiation of therapy to a subjective report that the older adult truly feels "like my old self" may take months and even up to a year for those experiencing a severe depressive episode. Biological symptoms, such as sleep difficulties, may improve more quickly with antidepressant therapy; subjective well-being and an interest in life requires a much longer time to reemerge. One reason is that older adults who recover from a moderate to severe episode of depression require time to reintegrate into their usual life activities, because they often hesitate to return to past social activities for fear of embarrassment after a prolonged episode of depression.

Some depressive episodes do not respond to antidepressant medication and are severe enough to require electroconvulsive therapy (ECT) (Flint & Rifat, 1998). Severe depressive symptoms, psychotic symptoms, a potential for suicide, and a history of responding to ECT in the past are indications for ECT. The primary adverse reaction to ECT in late life is memory problems during the few weeks during and following treatment, and though this symptom most always remits with time, it can be very disturbing to older adults. The ability to administer ECT to older adults as outpatients has greatly reduced both the cost and the inconvenience and stigma of receiving the treatment.

Psychological Therapies

Many different psychotherapies have been used with depressed older adults. An increasing body of literature supports the value of psychotherapy in the treatment of mild to moderate depressive disorders (Lynch & Aspnes, 2004). Cognitive-behavioral therapies (CBTs) have been studied most frequently (Arean & Cook, 2002) and address problematic thoughts that initiate and perpetuate depressive symptoms. The goal of therapy is to change the thoughts and dysfunctional attitudes that initiate symptoms and may lead to a relapse. The process by which cognitive therapy works is not entirely clear (see Hollon & Dimidjian, Chapter 25, this volume). For example, some data suggest that the most important mechanism of change in cognitive therapy is altered thought attribution, such as reevaluation of events. Another aspect of CBT that is thought to be effective is actual change of behavior itself. Depressive symptoms lead to activities that in turn perpetuate the depression. The goal of therapy, therefore, is to change behaviors through, for example, skills training (problem solving and interpersonal skills) and even exercise. Older people with lifelong habits may be less inclined to change behavior, but this type of therapy can be effective (Lynch & Aspnes, 2004).

A variant of CBT is social problem-solving therapy (PST). Ineffective coping in stressful situations is thought to lead to a breakdown of problem-solving abilities and, consequently, to an increase in the propensity to become depressed in late life (Nezu, 1987). The therapist teaches the patient a structured format for solving problems that includes problem details, goals, solutions, specific solution advantages, and an assessment of the final solution within context. In other words, PST refines and augments the usual strategies employed by older adults to handle day-to-day problems.

Interpersonal psychotherapy (IPT), a popular manualized treatment, focuses on four factors that are thought to initiate and perpetuate depressive symptoms (Frank, Frank, & Cornes, 1993; see Beach, Jones, & Franklin, Chapter 27, this volume). Similar to CBT, IPT focuses on social context. Grief, interpersonal disputes, role transitions, and interpersonal deficits (e.g., the lack of ability to assert oneself in social situations) comprise the treatment focus. IPT utilizes role playing, communication analysis, clarification of the patients wants and needs, and connections between the affect of the patient and environmental events. IPT has been found to be effective in preventing short-term relapse of major depression but not long-term outcome. One advantage of IPT is that older patients are less likely to drop out of treatment than is the case with many other psychotherapeutic approaches (Reynolds et al., 1999, 2006).

Family Intervention

A clinician can rarely treat older adults without some interaction with family members, whether spouses, children, or siblings. Family members almost always accompany the older depressed patient to the office for an initial evaluation, and the patient rarely prohibits the clinician from discussing the depression with a family member. Clinicians should take advantage of this opportunity. Family members can provide valuable information to complement the interview with the older adult about the duration and severity of symptoms, about differences they witness in the older adult during the depression compared to his or her usual state, and about information concerning life events that may have contributed to the depressive episode. In addition, the clinician should address concerns of the family (whether these concerns are verbalized or not). Family members often benefit from an explanation by the clinician of the symptoms of depression (e.g., addressing the question, "Why does Mom sit in the chair all day?"). They also benefit from guidance for addressing disturbing behaviors, such as inactivity and negative ruminations. Finally, families should be warned of the risk for suicide (despite the best efforts of families and clinicians, suicide cannot be absolutely prevented) and instructed about means for reducing the risk of suicide, such as removing weapons from the house.

PREVENTION

Can late-life depression be prevented? From the perspective of public health, both secondary prevention (early detection and treatment) and tertiary prevention (rehabilitation) are the heart and soul of our current therapeutic approach (see Muñoz, Le, Clarke, Barrera, & Torres, Chapter 23, this volume). Yet this leaves unanswered the question of whether the onset of an episode of major depression can be prevented in the first place. In a recent review, Blazer (2002b) proposed that targeting symptoms of sadness and loneliness through an enhancement of self-efficacy may prevent depressive symptoms from evolving into a full-blown episode of major depression. *Self-efficacy* is the belief that one can organize and execute the courses of action required to develop and enhance a person's belief that he or she can act in ways that lead to a desired goal.

Self-efficacy is strengthened not by some general or abstract instruction, but by the experience of successfully dealing with and overcoming specific problems. A number of skills appear to increase self-efficacy: maintaining and promoting physical health (e.g., controlling blood glucose levels in borderline diabetes); enhancing cognitive performance (e.g., through the creative use of life review); enhancing physical functioning (e.g., age appropriate exercise); developing a greater sense of personal control and mastery (e.g., developing coping strategies); improving social skills (e.g., through social skills training); and enhancing a sense of personal and existential integrity (e.g., working through past traumatic events).

There are few empirical studies to inform the clinician and investigator of the usefulness of developing these skills. Nevertheless, there is ample reason to consider these interventions, so that adverse consequences of precursors of late-life depression, such as sadness and loneliness, can be prevented from becoming more serious outcomes.

BIPOLAR DISORDERS

In this chapter we have focused on late-life depression, because this disorder occurs far more frequently than bipolar disorder in older adults. Nevertheless, a few words are in order about the latter. First, older adults with recurrent unipolar depression are less likely than younger adults to experience bipolar disorder. When bipolar disorder does emerge in late life, the symptoms are often atypical. Older adults in late life who do experience an episode of mania may be more irritable than happy. Anger, rather than excessive spending or expansive ideas, may dominate the clinical picture. At times, racing thoughts may be misinterpreted as a problem with memory or information processing. Once the diagnosis is made, however, the management is similar across the life cycle, and pharmacological management is the centerpiece of management. Lithium carbonate and valproic acid are the drugs of choice. Fortunately, they are often effective in doses much lower than those used when treating younger adults. For example, an older adult with bipolar disorder may be managed on 300 mg of lithium per day, with serum lithium levels between 0.2 and 0.5 mEq/L in comparison to a younger patient treated with 1,200 mg per day, with levels between 0.8 and 1.2 mEq/L. Working with the family of the older bipolar patient can often assist in identifying an episode early and adjusting medications, so that hospitalization can be avoided.

CONCLUSIONS AND FUTURE DIRECTIONS

Basic scientists and clinical investigators have increased the extant empirical data on late-life depression at an almost dizzying pace over the past 30 years. For example, the neurobiological substrate of late-life depression has emerged in increasing detail through both structural and functional scanning techniques. Studies of the phenomenology of late-life depression have enabled investigators to disaggregate the construct into potentially valuable subtypes, such as subthreshold depression, for future research. Therapies have been studied in much greater detail, especially the value of combined pharmacotherapy and psychotherapy over time. In summary, the diagnosis and treatment of late-life depression is now buttressed by an evidence base that was virtually absent three decades ago, except for the occasional clinical report.

Clinicians are therefore armed with a veritable textbook of important knowledge about the characteristics, origins, outcomes, and therapies for this most disabling and potentially fatal condition. Nevertheless, knowledge alone cannot render a clinician competent to care for a depressed older adult. That can only come through experience, and the experience needed is very clear. Clinicians must talk with their patients, and with their patient's families. And they must talk with them through time. No journal article or review chapter can replace the living textbook of the client/patient who sits with the observant and caring clinician.

Despite the significant advances in our empirical understanding of the epidemiology, etiology, diagnosis, and treatment of late-life depression, many topics require further research. Three areas are illustrative. First, the subtypes of late-life depression must be better refined, so that therapies can be tailored better to phenotypes that more closely reflect neuro- and psychopathology. For example, the construct of vascular depression has emerged. Given the combined diagnostic requirements of clinical symptoms and signs on the MRI scan, this construct permits a more focused exploration of genetic predisposition, as well as potential environmental factors that may contribute to the cause of the disorder. Yet vascular depression is most certainly not a single, unitary construct; instead, it interacts with brain changes secondary to stress (e.g., hippocampal shrinkage), and perhaps other brain changes, such as those found with Alzheimer's disease.

Second, new pharmacotherapies and psychotherapies must be developed, and existing therapies must be studied so they can be applied optimally to increase both time to remission and achievement of as complete a remission as possible. Although the advent of the new generation of antidepressants has been a boon in treating late-life depression, the initial promise of a more potent therapy virtually without side effects has not stood the test of time. Many side effects that prevented treatment in the past have been alleviated through the use of the new medications, yet new side effects have emerged, some quite serious (e.g., the syndrome of inappropriate antidiuretic hormone secretion). We are far from having identified optimal agents for the pharmacological treatment of late-life depression. New psychotherapies currently being tested with older adults could lead to incremental yet important improvements or flexibility.

Third, the predictors of persistent depression must be studied further, for evidence has emerged that depression in late life can lead to many adverse outcomes, such as increased mortality secondary to cardiovascular disease and dementing disorders. There is no question that late-life depression has adverse effects on both short- and long-term physical and mental health. Yet the nuances of these adverse outcomes have yet to be discovered. These nuances could have major implications clinically in terms of managing the depressed older adult who is experiencing a chronic disease over time. In summary, we have learned much, but we still have much to learn.

REFERENCES

Alexopoulos, G., Meyers, B., Young, R., Kakuma, T., Feder, M., Einhorn, A., et al. (1996). Recovery in geriatric depression. *Archives of General Psychiatry, 53*, 305–312.

Alexopoulos, G., Meyers, B., Young, R., Mattis, S., & Kakuma, T. (1993). The course of geriatric depression with "reversible dementia": A controlled study. *American Journal of Psychiatry, 150*, 1693–1699.

American Psychiatric Association (2000). *Diagnostic and statistical manual of mental disorders* (4th ed., text rev.). Washington, DC: Author.

Arean, P., & Cook, B. (2002). Psychotherapy and combined psychotherapy/pharmacotherapy for late life depression. *Biological Psychiatry, 52*, 293–303.

Baldwin, R., & Jolley, D. (1986). The prognosis of depression in old age. *British Journal of Psychiatry, 149*, 574–583.

Baltes, P., & Staudinger, U. (2000). Wisdom: A metahuerastic (pragmatic) to orchestrate mind and virtue toward excellence. *American Psychologist, 55*, 122–136.

Beck, A. (1987). Cognitive model of depression. *Journal of Cognitive Psychotherapy, 1*, 2–27.

Beekman, A., Deeg, D., & Geerlings, R. (2001). Emergence and persistence of late life depression: A 3-year follow-up of the Longitudinal Aging Study Amsterdam. *Journal of Affective Disorders, 65*, 131–138.

Beekman, A., Deeg, D., van Tilberg, T., Smit, J., Hooijer, C., & van Tilberg, W. (1995). Major and minor depression in later life: A study of prevalence and risk factors. *Journal of Affective Disorders, 36*, 65–75.

Beekman, A., Geerlings, S., Deeg, D., Smit, J., Scoevers, R., de Beurs, E., et al. (2002). The natural history of late-life depression. *Archives of General Psychiatry, 59*, 605–611.

Berkman, L., Berkman, C., Kasl, S., Freeman, D., Leo, L., Ostfeld, A., et al. (1986). Depressive symptoms in relation to physical health and functioning in the elderly. *American Journal of Epidemiology, 124*, 372–388.

Black, S., Goodwin, J., & Markides, K. (1998). The association between chronic diseases and depressive symptomology in older Mexican Americans. *Journals of Gerontology: Medical Sciences, 53,* M118–M194.

Blazer, D. (1983). Impact of late-life depression on the social network. *American Journal of Psychiatry, 140,* 162–166.

Blazer, D. (1994). Dysthymia in community and clinical samples of older adults. *American Journal of Psychiatry, 151,* 1567–1569.

Blazer, D. (2002a). *Depression in late life* (3rd ed.). New York: Springer.

Blazer, D. (2002b). Self-efficacy and depression in late life: A primary prevention proposal. *Aging and Mental Health, 6,* 319–328.

Blazer, D., Bachar, J., & Hughes, D. (1987). Major depression with melancholia: A comparison of middle-aged and elderly adults. *Journal of the American Geriatrics Society, 35,* 927–932.

Blazer, D., Burchett, B., Service, C., & George, L. (1991). The association of age and depression among the elderly: An epidemiologic exploration. *Journals of Gerontology: Medical Sciences, 46,* M210–M215.

Blazer, D., Hughes, D., & George, L. (1987). The epidemiology of depression in an elderly community population. *Gerontologist, 27,* 281–287.

Blazer, D., & Hybels, C. (2005). Origins of depression in later life. *Psychological Medicine, 35,* 1241–1252.

Blazer, D., Moody-Ayers, S., Craft-Morgan, J., & Burchett, B. (2002). Depression in diabetes and obesity: Racial/ethnic/gender issues in older adults. *Journal of Psychosomatic Research, 52,* 1–4.

Brodaty, J., Luscombe, G., Peisah, C., Anstey, K., & Andrews, G. (2001). A 25-year longitudinal, comparison study of the outcome of depression. *Psychological Medicine, 31,* 1347–1359.

Bruce, M. (2001). Depression and disability in late life: Directions for future research. *American Journal of Geriatric Psychiatry, 9,* 102–112.

Carstensen, L., Mayr, U., Pasupathi, M., & Nesselroade, J. (2000). Emotional experience in everyday life across the adult life span. *Journal of Personality and Social Psychology, 79,* 644–655.

Conwell, Y., Duberstein, P., & Caine, E. (2002). Risk factors for suicide in later life. *Biological Psychiatry, 52,* 193–204.

de Beauvoir, S. (1973). *The coming of age* (P. O'Brian, Trans.). New York: Warner Paperback Library.

Devenand, D., Kim, M., Paykina, N., & Sackeim, H. (2002). Adverse life events in elderly patients with major depression or dysthymia and in healthy-control subjects. *American Journal of Geriatric Psychiatry, 10,* 265–274.

Devenand, D., Noble, M., Singer, T., Kiersky, J., Turret, N., Roose, S., et al. (1994). Is dysthymia a different disorder in the elderly? *American Journal of Psychiatry, 151,* 1592–1599.

Doraiswamy, P., Khan, Z., & Donahue, R., & Richard, N. E. (2002). The spectrum of quality-of-life impairments in recurrent geriatric depression. *Journals of Gerontology: Medical Sciences, 57,* M134–M137.

Eaton, W., Kramer, M., Anthony, J., Dryman, A., Shapiro, S., & Locke, B. (1989). The incidence of specific DIS/DSM-III mental disorders: Data from the NIMH Epidemiologic Catchment Area program. *Acta Psychiatrica Scandinavica, 79,* 109–125.

Erlangsen, A., Zarit, S., Tu, X., & Conwell, Y. (2006). Suicide among older psychiatric inpatients: An evidence-based study of a high risk group. *American Journal of Geriatric Psychiatry, 14,* 734–741.

Flint, A., & Rifat, S. (1998). The treatment of psychotic depression in later life: A comparison of pharmacotherapy and ECT. *Journal of Geriatric Psychiatry, 13,* 23–28.

Folstein, M., Folstein, S., & McHugh, P. (1975). Mini-Mental State: A practical method for grading the cognitive state of patients for the clinician. *Journal of Psychiatric Research, 12,* 189–198.

Frank, E., Frank, N., & Cornes, C. (1993). Interpersonal psychotherapy in the treatment of late life depression. In G. Klerman & M. Weissman (Eds.), *New applications of interpersonal psychotherapy* (pp. 167–198). Washington, DC: American Psychiatric Press.

Fried, L. (1994). Frailty. In W. Hazzard, E. Bierman, J. Blass, W. Ettinger, Jr., & J. Halter (Eds.), *Principles of geriatric medicine and gerontology* (3rd ed., pp. 1149–1156). New York: McGraw-Hill.

Gallo, J., & Coyne, J. (2000). The challenge of depression in late life: Bridging science and service in primary care. *Journal of the American Medical Association, 284,* 1570–1572.

Gallo, J., Rabins, P., & Lyketsos, C. (1997). Depression without sadness: Functional outcomes of nondysphoric depression in later life. *Journal of the American Geriatrics Society, 45,* 570–578.

Gatz, M., Pedersen, N., Plomin, R., Nesselroade, J., & McClearn, G. (1992). Importance of shared genes and shared environments for symptoms of depression in older adults. *Journal of Abnormal Psychology, 101,* 701–708.

Gatz, M., & Zarit, S. (1999). A good old age: Paradox or possibility. In V. Bengtson, J. Ruth, & K. Schaie (Eds.), *Theories of gerontology* (pp. 396–416). New York: Springer.

Gonzales-Salvador, T., Aragano, C., Lyketsos, C., & Barba, A. (1999). The stress and psychological morbidity of the Alzheimer patient caregiver. *International Journal of Geriatric Psychiatry, 14,* 701–710.

Gottfries, C. (1990). Neurochemical aspects on aging and diseases with cognitive impairment. *Journal of Neuroscience Research, 27,* 541–547.

Grant, B. F., Dawson, D. A., & Hasin, D. S. (2001). *The Alcohol Use Disorder and Associated Disabilities Interview Schedule DSM-IV.* Bethesda, MD: National Institute on Alcohol Abuse and Alcoholism.

Hasin, D., Goodwin, R., Stinson, F., & Grant, B. (2005). Epidemiology of major depressive disorder. *Archives of General Psychiatry, 62,* 1097–1106.

Henderson, A., Jorm, A., & MacKinnon, A. (1993). The prevalence of depressive disorders and the distribution of depressive symptoms in later life: A survey using draft ICD-10 and DSM-III-R. *Psychological Medicine, 23,* 719–729.

Hickie, I., Scott, E., Naismith, S., Ward, P., Turner, K., Parker, G., et al. (2001). Late-onset depression: Genetic, vascular and clinical contributions. *Psychological Medicine, 31,* 1403–1412.

Hinton, L., Zweifach, M., Oishi, S., Tang, L., & Unutzer, J. (2006). Gender disparities in the treatment of late-life depression: Qualitative and quantitative findings from the IMPACT trial. *American Journal of Geriatric Psychiatry, 14,* 884–892.

Hughes, D., Blazer, D., & George, L. (1988). Age differences in life events: A multivariate controlled analysis. *International Journal of Aging and Human Development, 127,* 207–220.

Hybels, C., Blazer, D., & Pieper, C. (2001). Toward a threshold for subthreshold depression: An analysis of correlates of depression by severity of symptoms using data from an elderly community survey. *Gerontologist, 41,* 357–365.

Hybels, C., Blazer, D., & Steffens, D. (2005). Predictors of partial remission in older patients treated for major depression: The role of comorbid dysthymia. *American Journal of Geriatric Psychiatry, 13,* 713–721.

Jacobson, S., Pies, R., & Katz, I. (2007). *Clinical manual of geriatric pharmacology.* Washington, DC: American Psychiatric Publishing.

Juurlink, D., Mamdani, M., Kopp, A., & Redelmeier, D. (2006). The risk of suicide with selective serotonin reuptake inhibitors in the elderly. *American Journal of Psychiatry, 163,* 813–821.

Keller, M., Shapiro, R., Lavori, P., & Wolfe, N. (1982a). Recovery in major depressive disorder: Analyses with the life table. *Archives of General Psychiatry, 39,* 905–910.

Keller, M., Shapiro, R., Lavori, P., & Wolfe, N. (1982b). Relapse in major depressive disorder: Analysis with the life table. *Archives of General Psychiatry, 39,* 911–915.

Kennedy, G., Kelman, H., & Thomas, C. (1990). The emergence of depressive symptoms in late life: The importance of declining health and increasing disability. *Journal of Community Health, 15,* 93–104.

Kessler, R., Berglund, P., Demler, O., Jin, R., Merikangas, K., & Walters, E. (2005). Lifetime prevalence and age-of-onset distributions of DSM-IV disorders in the National Comorbidity Survey Replication. *Archives of General Psychiatry, 62,* 593–602.

Kessler, R. E., & Ustün, T. B. (2004). The World Mental Health (WMH) Survey Initiative version of the World Health Organization (WHO) Composite International Diagnostic Interview (CIDI). *International Journal of Methods in Psychiatric Research, 13,* 93–121.

Kivela, S., Pahkala, K., & Laippala, P. (1988). Prevalence of depression in an elderly Finnish population. *Acta Psychiatrica Scandinavica, 78,* 401–413.

Koenig, H., Meador, K., Cohen, H., & Blazer, D. (1988). Depression in elderly hospitalized patients with medical illness. *Archives of Internal Medicine, 148,* 1929–1936.

Kraaij, V., & de Wilde, E. (2001). Negative life events and depressive symptoms in the elderly: A life span perspective. *Aging and Mental Health, 5,* 84–91.

Krause, N. (1986). Stress and sex differences in depressive symptoms among older adults. *Journal of Gerontology, 41,* 727–731.

Krishnan, K. R., Hays, J., & Blazer, D. (1997). MRI-defined vascular depression. *American Journal of Psychiatry, 154,* 497–501.

Lee, S., Tsang, A., Zhang, M. Y., Huang, Y. O., He, Y. L., Liu, Z. R., et al. (2007). Lifetime prevalence and inter-cohort variation in DSM-IV disorders in metropolitan China. *Psychological Medicine, 37,* 61–73.

Li, Y., Meyer, J., & Thornby, J. (2001). Longitudinal follow-up of depressive symptoms among normal versus cognitively impaired elderly. *International Journal of Geriatric Psychiatry, 16,* 718–727.

Lynch, T., & Aspnes, A. (2004). Individual and group psychotherapy. In D. Blazer, D. Steffens, & E. Busse (Eds.), *American Psychiatric Press textbook of geriatric psychiatry* (pp. 443–458). Washington DC: American Psychiatric Press.

Lyness, J., King, D., Conwell, Y., Cox, E., & Caine, E. (2000). Cerebrovascular risk factors and 1-year depression outcome in older primary care patients. *American Journal of Psychiatry, 157,* 1499–1501.

Lyness, J., King, D., Cox, C., Yoediono, Z., & Caine, E. (1999). The importance of subsyndromal depression in older primary care patients: Prevalence and associated functional disability. *Journal of the American Geriatrics Society, 47,* 647–652.

Mazure, C., Maciejewski, P., Jacobs, S., & Bruce, M. (2002). Stressful life events interacting with cognitive/personality styles to predict late-onset major depression. *American Journal of Geriatric Psychiatry, 10,* 297–304.

McKeown, R., Cuffe, S., & Schulz, R. (2006). U.S. suicide rates by age group, 1970–2002: An examination of recent trends. *American Journal of Public Health, 96,* 1744–1751.

Meyers, B. (1992). Geriatric delusional depression. *Clinics in Geriatric Medicine, 8,* 299–308.

Morley, J., & Kraenzle, D. (1994). Causes of weight loss in a community nursing home. *Journal of the American Geriatrics Society, 42,* 583–585.

Morse, J., & Lynch, T. (2004). A preliminary investigation of self-reported personality disorders in late life: Prevalence, predictors of depressive severity, and clinical correlates. *Aging and Mental Health, 8,* 307–315.

Murphy, E. (1982). Social origins of depression in old age. *British Journal of Psychiatry, 141,* 135–142.

Murphy, E. (1983). The prognosis of depression in old age. *British Journal of Psychiatry, 142,* 111–119.

National Center for Health Statistics. (2001). *Death rates for 72 selected causes by 5-year age groups, race, and sex: United States, 1979–1998.* Washington, DC: Author.

Nezu, A. (1987). A problem-solving formulation of depression: A literature review and proposal of a pluralistic model. *Clinical Psychological Reviews, 7,* 121–144.

Olin, J., Schneider, L., Katz, I., Meyers, B., Alexopoulos, G., Breitner, J., et al. (2002). Provisional diagnostic criteria for depression of Alzheimer disease. *American Journal of Geriatric Psychiatry, 10,* 125–128.

Palsson, S., Ostling, S., & Skoog, I. (2001). The incidence of first-onset depression in a population followed from the age of 70 to 85. *Psychological Medicine, 31,* 1159–1168.

Parmelee, P., Katz, I., & Lawton, M. (1989). Depression among institutionalized aged: Assessment and prevalence estimation. *Journals of Gerontology: Medical Sciences, 44,* M22–M29.

Patten, S., Wang, J., & Williams, J. (2006). Descriptive epidemiology of major depression in Canada. *Canadian Journal of Psychiatry, 51,* 84–90.

Penninx, B., Leveille, S., Ferrucci, L., van Eijk, J., & Guralnik, J. (1999). Exploring the effect of depression on physical disability: Longitudinal evidence from the established populations for epidemiologic studies of the elderly. *American Journal of Public Health, 89,* 1346–1352.

Radloff, L. (1977). The CES-D Scale: A self-report depression scale for research in the general population. *Applied Psychological Measures, 1,* 385–401.

Regier, D., Boyd, J., Burke, J., Rae, D., Myers, J., Kramer, M., et al. (1988). One-month prevalence of mental disorders in the United States: Based on five Epidemiologic Catchment Area sites. *Archives of General Psychiatry, 45,* 977–986.

Reynolds, C., Dew, M., Pollock, B., Mulsant, B., Frank, E., Miller, M., et al. (2006). Maintenance treatment of major depression in old age. *New England Journal of Medicine, 354,* 1130–1138.

Reynolds, C., Frank, E., Perel, J., Imber, S., Cornes, C., Miller, M., et al. (1999). Nortriptyline and interpersonal psychotherapy as maintenance therapies for recurrent major depression: A randomized controlled trial in patients older than 59 years. *Journal of the American Medical Association, 281,* 39–45.

Robins, L., Helzer, J., & Croughan, J. (1981). Diagnostic Interview Schedule: Its history, characteristics and validity. *Archives of General Psychiatry, 38,* 381–389.

Sapolsky, R. (2001). Depression, antidepressants, and the shrinking hippocampus. *Proceedings of the National Academy of Sciences USA, 98,* 12320–12323.

Schneider, L., Reynolds, C., Lebowitz, B., & Friedhoff, A. (1994). *Diagnosis and treatment of depression in late life.* Washington, DC: American Psychiatric Press.

Schulz, R., Drayer, R., & Rollman, B. (2002). Depression as a risk factor for non-suicide mortality in the elderly. *Biological Psychiatry, 52,* 205–225.

Sheline, Y., Mintun, M., Moerlein, S., & Snyder, A. (2002). Greater loss of 5-HT$_{2A}$ receptors in midlife than in late life. *American Journal of Psychiatry, 159,* 430–435.

Spitzer, R., Williams, J., Gibbon, M., & First, M. (1990). *Structured Clinical Interview for DSM-III-R.* New York: New York State Psychiatric Institute, Biometrics Research.

Taylor, W., Steffens, D., MacFall, J., McQuoid, D., Payne, M., Provenzale, J., et al. (2003). White matter hyperintensity progression and late-life depression outcomes. *Archives of General Psychiatry, 60,* 1090–1096.

Unutzer, J., Katon, W., Callahan, C. M., Williams, J., Hunkeler, E., Harpole, L., et al. (2002). Collaborative care management of late-life depression in the primary care setting. *Journal of the American Medical Association, 288,* 2836–2845.

Unutzer, J., Patrick, D., Simon, G., Grembowski, D., Walker, E., Rutter, C., et al. (1997). Depressive symptoms and the cost of health services in HMO patients 65+ years and older. *Journal of the American Medical Association, 277,* 1618–1623.

Williams, D., Gonzalez, H., & Neighbors, H. (2007). Prevalence and distribution of major depressive disorder in African Americans, Caribbean blacks, and non-Hispanic whites. *Archives of General Psychiatry, 64,* 305–315.

Williams, S., Kasl, S., Heiat, A., Abramson, J., Krumholz, H., & Vaccarino, V. (2002). Depression and risk of heart failure among the elderly: A prospective community-based study. *Psychosomatic Medicine, 64,* 6–12.

Yaffe, K., Ettinger, B., & Pressman, A. (1998). Neuropsychiatric function and dehydroepiandrosterone sulfate in elderly women: A prospective study. *Biological Psychiatry, 43,* 694–700.

Yesavage, J., Brink, T., & Rose, T. (1983). Development and validation of a geriatric depression screening scale: A preliminary report. *Journal of Psychiatric Research, 17,* 37–49.

Zhang, X., Gainetdinov, R., Beaulieu, J., Sotnikova, T., Uhrch, L., Williams, R., et al. (2005). Loss-of-function mutation in tryptophan hydroxilae-2 identified in unipolar major depression. *Neuron, 45,* 11–16.

CHAPTER 22

Depression and Suicide

Alan L. Berman

Patient suicide and nonfatal suicidal behaviors are occupational hazards for mental health professionals, because they reflect the major life-threatening complications of mental disorders, notably depression. Suicide is an outcome that requires that several things go wrong all at once. The patient must be biologically or psychologically vulnerable (i.e., must have perpetuating and predisposing risk), must have proximal and contributing factors that facilitate or trigger suicidal behavior at its particular timing, and must have a weakening of protective factors that otherwise serve to sustain him or her in times of crisis or great emotional pain.

Mental disorders represent the most significant category of predisposing risk for suicide. The relative risk of suicide is exacerbated significantly among those with diagnosed psychiatric syndromes when compared to those without diagnoses, with more than 90% of suicides studied by psychological autopsy having a retrospectively diagnosed mental disorder (Tanney, 2000). Mental disorders impair coping abilities and resilience, amplify distress, and decrease protections; their role in establishing suicidal vulnerability, therefore, is readily understandable.

The risk of suicide and suicidal behavior is intimately tied to depressive disorders. Suicide ideation or attempt is one of the nine criteria that define major depression. Indeed, 40% of clinically depressed patients over the age of 17 have suicidal thoughts (Substance Abuse and Mental Health Services Administration, 2006b). Disturbances of mood are implicated in almost all suicidal acts, and risk of suicide is elevated in all forms of mood disorder. In some jurisdictions, medical examiners and coroners will readily (and some will *only*) conclude a self-inflicted death to be a suicide when it is noted that the decedent was depressed, as if depressed individuals never die an unintentional death.

It has been proposed (Brent, 2007) that there was a direct causal connection between a decade of declining suicide rates (particularly among adolescents) observed internationally between 1995 and 2003, and contemporaneously increased rates of prescription of selective serotonin reuptake inhibitors (SSRIs). Consequent to the U.S. Food and Drug Administration (FDA) black box warnings regarding observed suicidality among those taking SSRIs, reductions in rates of diagnosis and treatment (with SSRIs) of pediatric depression have been observed (Libby et al., 2007) and, concurrently, rates of adolescent suicide have increased. Although these observations are correlational and not evidence of causation, the implication that better acute and long-term treatment of depression result in decreased suicidality among patients receiving that treatment is clearly a preventive effort worthy of support and evaluation.

To that end, the goals of this chapter are to update the reader on the empirical link between suicide risk and depression, and to delineate clinical and public health implications in assessing and treating depression as an approach to suicide prevention.

EPIDEMIOLOGY OF SUICIDE AND SUICIDAL BEHAVIORS

In the United States suicide is the 11th leading cause of death, accounting for 32,439 deaths across all ages in 2004.[1] The prevalence of suicide is nearly twice that of homicide. More than 75% of all suicides are completed by males, and 90% are completed by European Americans; indeed, suicide is the eighth leading cause of death among males and the 10th leading cause of death among European Americans. Among European Americans ages 15–34, suicide is ranked second as a leading cause of death; among Native Americans and Alaskan Natives, suicide is the second leading cause of death among 10- to 34-year-olds.

The ratio of male to female suicide increased by more than one-third between 1940 and the end of the last century, marked by increasing rates of suicide among males and declining rates of suicide among females. Given that depression is more frequently diagnosed among women than among men (see Nolen-Hoeksema & Hilt, Chapter 17, this volume), these findings are consistent with the hypothesis that depression is relatively underdetected among men and overdetected among women. Alternatively, these gender differences support the fact that suicide is multidetermined and cannot be explained simply as a consequence of depression.

Nonfatal suicide attempts are much more frequently self-reported and observed among females, by a ratio, after childhood, of about 3:1 (Moscicki, 1994). Epidemiological data regarding nonfatal suicide attempts rely on hospital discharge and trauma registry data. These data are only available for a select number of states and generally reflect a female to male ratio of about 3:2, with hospital admissions peaking for 15- to 24-year-olds (*www.sprc.org/ stateinformation/pdf/statedatasheets.asp*). Although lifetime rates of nonfatal suicide attempt for blacks are estimated at about 60% those of whites (Kessler, Borges, & Walters, 1999), a recent study estimated the lifetime prevalence of attempts among blacks at 4.1%, almost double that of earlier reported estimates.

In 2003, there were 348,830 nonfatal emergency department admissions of adults age 18 or older who had harmed themselves (CDC, 2005, *http://webappa.cdc.gov/sasweb/ncipc/ nfirates2001.html*). It is important to note, however, that because the majority of people who attempt suicide never reach medical care facilities, it is inappropriate to use this data source as a measure of the prevalence of these behaviors in the community. In fact, self-report data from large surveys of community respondents suggest much higher rates of annual and lifetime suicidal behaviors (see below).

High school-based surveys of adolescent risk-taking behaviors are conducted biannually by the CDC and consistently report a predominance of females in self-reported nonfatal attempts (MMWR [*Morbidity and Mortality Weekly Report*] Surveillance Summaries,

2006). The prevalence of self-reported suicide attempts in this cohort is in the range of 8–9% per year, with about 1 in 3 persons reporting that his or her attempt required medical intervention.

Kessler and colleagues (1999) reported on the prevalence of lifetime suicide attempts based on almost 6,000 respondents to the National Comorbidity Survey. Of these respondents, with 13.5% reporting lifetime suicide ideation and 4.6% reporting an attempt, more than one-third stated that the attempt was serious, and that they survived only because of luck. The risk of an attempt was high among ideators if they had formed a plan to act. Risk of an attempt was significantly related to being female by a ratio of 2.2:1.0 (vs. male), and having been previously married. Cross-national comparisons of rates of suicide attempts are reasonably consistent with variations associated with being currently divorced/separated and rates of psychiatric disorder (Weissman et al., 1999). Risk for attempt is high among other groups as well. Paul and colleagues (2002), for example, reporting results of a telephone probability sample of nearly 3,000 men who have sex with men, found the lifetime prevalence of suicide attempt to be 12%, with more than 70% of these occurring before the age of 25.

Suicide rates vary by age, peaking among those age 75 and older, where undiagnosed and untreated depression is most often observed to be a major risk factor. Suicide is the second leading cause of death among 25- to 34-year-olds, particularly in males. Among women, rates of suicide peak in midlife. That said, among 15- to 24-year-old females suicide is the second leading cause of death in this age group.

Suicide rates vary geographically across the United States, with the highest rates consistently found among residents of the intermountain states of the West. In 2004, the top 10 state suicide rates were observed in Alaska, Montana, Nevada, New Mexico, Wyoming, Colorado, Idaho, Utah, Oregon, and, in the only exception to this Western tilt, West Virginia. Interestingly, among persons age 18 and older, seven of these states ranked in the top 10 in episodes of major depressive episode in 2004–2005 (*www.oas.samhsa.gov/2k5state/appb.htm*). That said, however, those jurisdictions rounding out the top 10 in major depressive episodes rank among those lowest in suicide rates (Washington, D.C.—51st, Massachusetts—49th, and Maine—21st). Spearman's rank correlation between rankings of all states is only r_s = .44, thus accounting for only about one-fifth the variance.[2]

SUICIDE AND MENTAL DISORDERS

Psychological autopsy studies document that a mental disorder[3] is the most strongly associated variable of risk for completed suicide, with approximately 90% of completed suicides being diagnosed retrospectively (Cavanaugh, Carson, Sharpe, & Lawrie, 2003; Conwell et al., 1996; Fleischman, Bertolote, Belfer, & Beautrais, 2005; Goldsmith, Pellmar, Kleinman, & Bunney, 2002). Concurrently, strong associations between psychiatric disorders and self-reported nonfatal suicide attempts have been demonstrated (Kessler et al., 1999). In the general population, suicide accounts for approximately 1–2% of all deaths annually; in clinical populations, mortality by suicide in persons with mental disorders is variously estimated as three to five times this number (Tanney, 2000). Of course, because the former proportion already includes those with mental disorders, the estimated comparative mortality would be even greater. That said, however, more than 95% of those affected with a mental disorder do not complete suicide (Goldsmith et al., 2002).

These findings have both clinical and public health implications. First, lifetime rates of contact with mental health services among those who later completed suicide averaged 53%, with an average of 32% doing so in the 12 months prior to their death (Luoma, Martin, & Pearson, 2002). Thus, a great number of persons at risk for suicide, the overwhelming proportion of whom have one or more mental disorders in need of treatment, simply do not seek or get that treatment. The public health implication is that programs designed to reduce stigma about being a mental health consumer, to educate the public about mental disorders and suicide, to decrease barriers to care, and/or to increase case finding are crucial to get people in need into treatment. That said, surveys of psychiatrists and psychologists who have been in practice approximately 20 years indicate that approximately 50 and 75%, respectively, have lost at least one patient to suicide (Chemtob et al., 1998a, 1998b). Thus, as noted earlier, suicide is a significant occupational risk for mental health practitioners. Of interest, mental health professionals, in stark contrast to medical professionals, rarely make statements of risk estimates to new patients, despite clear evidence that having a mental disorder, especially a mood disorder, is associated with significantly increased suicide risk. It may behoove the clinical practitioner to so inform patients and family members as a standard of care intervention, and as a good risk management strategy, of patients' significantly increased risk of suicide. As well, this strategy is designed to alert patient support systems to align with the therapist to monitor their loved one collaboratively and report any observed acute risk factors for suicide (see below).

Second, a substantial majority (two-thirds) of adults with a diagnosable mental disorder does not receive treatment (U.S. Department of Health and Human Services, 1999), with most believing their problems will abate without professional help (Kessler et al., 1997). A recent Canadian study (Cheung & Dewa, 2007) found that roughly 40% of adolescents and young adults with depression, and 50% of those with suicidality, had not used any mental health services. Although most people with a mental disorder eventually seek treatment (an estimated 80%), it is well known that delayed treatment is associated with more frequent and more severe episodes, as well as treatment resistance (Kessler et al., 2005; Wang et al., 2005). Thus, among those with mental disorders, early identification, referral, and enhanced help-seeking/help-receiving behaviors are important for effective treatment and a presumed preventive effect on suicide and suicidal behaviors.

Of those persons who complete suicide, a greater proportion contact their primary care provider within 1 year before suicide than contact mental health specialists (77 vs. 32%; Luoma et al., 2002). Primary care physicians (PCPs) generally are first contacted for mental health problems and often are the source of care for depression preferred by community residents (Goldman, Nielsen, & Champion, 1999). Moreover, PCPs are the most frequent prescribers of psychotropic medications, especially for children and adolescents (Olfson, Marcus, Weissman, & Jensen, 2002). Consequently, the Institute of Medicine has appropriately and strongly recommended that tools for screening suicide risk and training in suicide risk assessment be widely disseminated to PCPs (Goldsmith et al., 2002).

SUICIDE AND DEPRESSIVE DISORDERS

A large number of reports underscore the importance of disturbances of mood in all suicidal behaviors. An average 60% of completed suicides studied by psychological autopsy have been diagnosed with a depressive disorder (Tanney, 2000), by far the single most prevalent class of mental disorders associated with suicide. Harris and Barraclough (1997) conducted a meta-analysis of the literature on mental disorders and suicide, and found that mood disorders had a standardized mortality ratio of 20.4 (persons with mood disorders vs. general population). Beautrais and colleagues (1996) compared 302 consecutive individuals who made medically serious suicide attempts to more than 1,000 random controls, and found an odds ratio (OR) of 33.4 for individuals with mood disorders.

Among the mood disorders, a gradient of risk for suicide appears to extend from primary unipolar depression to bipolar depression. Harris and Barraclough (1997) reported a 20-fold increased risk for patients with unipolar depression versus a 15-fold increased risk for those with bipolar disorder. Ösby, Brandt, Correiia, Ekbom, and Sparén (2001) similarly found greater risk for suicide in Swedish patients with unipolar disorder, as well as a greater risk for females with either diagnosis. Angst, Angst, Gerber-Werder, and Gamma (2005) prospectively followed 406 patients with unipolar and bipolar depression over a 40- to 44-year period after psychiatric hospitalization in Zurich, and reported that 14.5% of patients with unipolar depression and 8.2% of patients with bipolar disorder had died by suicide. The majority of suicides occurred in the first 10 years after admission. Tondo and Baldessarini (2005) analyzed the relevant literature and concluded that the jury was still out on this issue, because 10 studies reported higher risks of suicidal behavior among unipolar depressives, 11 studies reported higher risks of suicidal behavior among bipolar depressives, and 1 study reported no differences. Dysthymic disorders, found to have a lower suicide risk than either unipolar or bipolar disorders (Guze & Robins, 1970), appear to involve more significant risk when there is early onset of the disorder (Szadocky & Fazekas, 1994).

An estimate reported by Guze and Robins (1970) that 15% of patients with severe depressive disorder died by suicide was for years an accepted fact. This proportion was bolstered years later by Goodwin and Jamison (1990), who suggested that 19% of depressed patients die by suicide. Blair-West, Mellsop, and Eyeson-Anan (1997), however, argued that the lifetime risk of suicide in major depression was greatly overestimated due to sampling bias, because both these reports focused primarily on hospitalized inpatients with major depression, followed during years of greatest risk, and were not representative of all depressed patients. Their recalculated lifetime risk of suicide for all patients with major depression was 3.4%. More recently, Bostwick and Pankratz (2000) estimated lifetime risk for suicide among those hospitalized for suicidality (9%) and for depression without suicidality (4%), and those treated mainly as outpatients (2.2%). Simon and Von Korff (1998) similarly reported a fourfold increased rate of suicide for persons treated as psychiatric inpatients versus outpatients.

Rhimer (2005) reviewed 10 published studies involving more than 3,000 patients and concluded that patients with bipolar II disorder, relative to those with bipolar I disorder, were overrepresented among both completed and attempted suicides. Focusing only on nonfatal suicide attempts, Tanney (2000) reported that unipolar and bipolar disorders were about equally involved, with suicide attempt rates of patients with bipolar II disorder appearing to be equal to rates of those with bipolar I disorder. Similarly, Ruggero, Chelminski, Young, and Zimmerman (2007) found similar rates of suicide attempts among patients with bipolar I and II disorders. Overall, Jamison (2000) suggests that between 25 and 50% of patients with bipolar disorder will make at least one suicide attempt. Valtonen and colleagues (2006) found that 20% of psychiatric inpatients and outpatients diagnosed with bipolar (I and II) disorder in Finland attempted suicide in an 18-month follow-up.

Suicidality in bipolar disorder varies by the severity, course, and phase of the disorder. Both prospective and retrospective studies (Isometsä, Henrikkson, Aro, & Lönnqvist, 1994; Tondo et al., 1999; Valtonen et al., 2007) provide support for the observation that suicide and suicidal behaviors among patients with major mood disorders are more likely to occur during a major depressive episode or, secondarily, during dysphoric–irritable mixed (vs. pure manic or euthymic) states (Baldessarini, Pompili, & Tondo, 2006).

COMORBIDITY

Comorbidity is a significant risk factor for suicide and suicidal behaviors, generally increasing risk over that found when there is only one psychiatric diagnosis (cf. Kessler et al., 1999). For example, Beautrais and colleagues (1996) found that 57% of persons who made serious suicide attempts had two or more disorders. Moreover, they reported that the risk of attempt increased with psychiatric comorbidity: Attempters with two or more disorders had 90 times the odds of a medically serious attempt compared with those with no disorder. Hawton, Houston, Haw, Townsend, and Harriss (2003) reported that 44% of 111 hospitalized suicide attempters had comorbid Axis I and Axis II diagnoses; the most common comorbid Axis I diagnosis was depression.

Henriksson and colleagues (1993) conducted a psychological autopsy of every sixth suicide in a 1-year sample of 1,397 consecutive suicides in Finland and found that some form of mood disorder was present in 59% of cases. Eighty-five percent of suicides with major depression were comorbid; 28% were comorbid with alcohol dependence or abuse (more likely in males); 31% had a comorbid personality disorder (more likely younger persons); and 49% had significant comorbid Axis III physical illness (more likely among older adults). Cheng (1995) reported on a case–control study of Chinese and aboriginal suicides. One-half of those diagnosed with major depressive disorder (MDD) had comorbid substance abuse, 66% had comorbid personality disorder, and 33% had a double depression. Vuorilehto, Melartin, and Isometsä (2006) also reported that lifetime suicidal behavior was strongly predicted by comorbid depressive and personality disorder diagnoses.

Eighty-five percent of those suicides with MDD in a 1-year psychological autopsy study in Finland (Isometsä et al., 1994) were comorbid cases, including 71% of bipolar cases, of which more than half of the males were alcohol-dependent. Numerous other studies (see Rhimer, 2007) support this finding, with particular comorbid association with substance use disorders, anxiety disorders, and Axis III medical illnesses. In addition, a systematic review of risk factors for deliberate self-harm in schizophrenia, itself a strong predictor of suicide, found a depressive episode to be associated with suicide attempts (Haw, Hawton, Sutton, Sinclair, & Deeks, 2005).

Although clearly established, it is difficult to evaluate the impact of comorbidity on suicide risk. How much risk may be attributed independently to each disorder? Is risk cumulative or interactive? Which disorder is primary and which is secondary in its contribution to suicide risk? With regard to the most frequently observed comorbid disorders, substance abuse and depression, the hypothesis that alcohol dependence may be part of the depressive spectrum is intriguing. Here, it is assumed that mood disorders preexist and are exacerbated in severity (as is suicide risk) by the disinhibiting effects of substance abuse intoxication (Tanney, 2000). That said, the National Survey on Drug Use and Health (Substance Abuse Mental Health Services Administration, 2006b) recently estimated that 2.7 million Americans age 18 or older had a co-occurring major depressive episode and alcohol use disorder in the last 12 months, making this a cohort at significant risk for suicide. With regard to comorbid MDD and generalized anxiety disorder, a study in New Zealand found that for one-third of the comorbid patients, depression onset occurred first; for one-third, anxiety onset occurred first; and for one-third, depression and anxiety began concurrently (Moffitt et al., 2007). Whatever the sequence of onset, comorbidity between depression and anxiety is significant and, in turn, increases risk of suicidal behavior.

SYMPTOM COMPONENTS AND SUICIDE RISK

Another significant phenomenon concerns the role of specific symptoms (diagnostic components) in elevating risk for suicide. Three symptom clusters—anhedonia, hopelessness, and anxiety; agitation and panic; and aggression and impulsivity—have been hypothesized to increase risk for suicide (Fawcett, Busch, Jacobs, Kravitz, & Fogg, 1997). Others have suggested that severity of symptoms (degree of psychic pain, number of criteria symptoms, or duration), global insomnia, agitation, hopelessness, and self-neglect (cf. Fawcett, 2006; Tanney, 2000) are linked to elevated risk. We will say more about these symptoms in our discussion of acute suicide risk.

ASSESSING VERSUS PREDICTING RISK
FOR SUICIDE OR SUICIDAL BEHAVIORS

If 60% of persons who engage in suicidal behavior have a diagnosable depression, can we similarly estimate the proportion of those with a diagnosable depression who engage in suicidal behavior? In any given 1-year period, 8.7% of the population, or about 19.75 million American adults, has a major depression (Vasiliadis, Lesage, Adair, Wang, & Kessler, 2007; the number is even greater if we rely on Kessler et al.'s [1994] finding of a 12-month major depressive episode prevalence of 10.3%; see also Kessler & Wang, Chapter 1, this volume). Correspondingly, there are an estimated 380,000 combined suicide completions and medically serious attempts annually. It appears, therefore, that fewer than 2% of depressed adults in the United States engage in suicidal behavior annually. Given that major depression is a significant predisposing risk factor for suicide, it remains readily apparent that *predicting* which depressed patients will be among this 2% in the next 12 months, much less in the next few days, is equivalent to searching for the proverbial needle in a haystack.

The clinician's responsibility, therefore, is not to predict suicide or suicidal behavior for an individual patient. Suicidal behaviors have a low base rate, even among vulnerable populations, such that a prediction of a suicidal act would most often be wrong. We simply cannot reasonably predict who will act at what time and in what way, with what outcome. Our task, instead, is to assess risk (potential) for suicidal behavior and to formulate a judgment about a patient's risk level for engaging in suicidal behavior leading to an unpredictable outcome (nonfatal or lethal). Correspondingly, that formulation of level of risk (chronic [low to high] and/or acute [low to high]) should inform treatment planning and implementation. To accomplish this process with a patient with a mood disorder, the clinician first needs to be reasonably informed regarding empirically defined risk factors for suicide and any that are specifically related to mood disorders, to have an interview strategy designed to elicit necessary information from and about the patient, and to articulate a rationale to evaluate risk and to formulate the patient's potential to act in a life-threatening manner in the near term.

RISK FACTORS FOR SUICIDE

Risk factors may be classified as perpetuating, predisposing, or precipitating. Predisposing risk factors may be subclassified as chronic or acute. Furthermore, there are associated contributing risk factors that increase otherwise existing risk.

Perpetuating risk factors associated with suicide are historic and/or enduring, but are not subject to change through intervention, clinical or otherwise. For example, a family history of suicide or suicidal behavior, violence (including sexual abuse), or major mental or substance use disorder, especially one that required inpatient hospitalization, increases risk among offspring. The pathways for this transmitted risk may be biological (genetic, biochemical) or psychological (social modeling, deprivation of nurturing parenting) (Mann, Waternaux, Haas, & Malone, 1999; Maris, 1997).

Notably, a prior suicide attempt significantly increases risk of future suicidal behavior and the possibility of completed suicide. Owens, Horrocks, and House (2002), in a systematic review of 90 studies of persons who had made a suicide attempt, reported that 16% made another attempt within 12 months and 21% made an attempt 1–4 years after the index attempt. The estimated proportion of attempters who go on to complete suicide at any point in their life is 10–15% (Fremouw, de Perczel, & Ellis, 1990). Beautrais (2006) followed 302 medically serious suicide attempters hospitalized in Christchurch, New Zealand, 40% of whom had a diagnosed mood disorder. After 5 years, 74% of all deaths in this group were by suicide or suspected suicide (single-vehicle motor vehicle accidents [MVAs]), and the majority of these occurred within 18 months of the index attempt. Beautrais reported that the risk of completed suicide increased in proportion to the number of observed risk factors. In addition, risk of near-term suicide increases if the prior history of suicide is relatively recent, involved multiple past attempts, and/or the outcome of past attempts was not positive (e.g., leading to a good alliance with a therapist and a positive therapeutic experience; see section on intent, motivation, and lethality below). The risk of suicide among patients with bipolar disorder is highest among those with a history of prior attempt (Simpson & Jamison, 1999). As evidence of this, Valtonen and colleagues (2006) reported a 3.8 OR with regard to previous suicide attempts as a predictor of a subsequent attempt among patients with bipolar disorder studied prospectively for 18 months.

Predisposing risk factors are those attributes, traits, and/or other characteristics associated with suicide. Because they are more clinical and dynamic in nature, they are amenable to intervention and potential change. Here, for example, mental disorders, and mood disorders in particular, are significant predisposing risk factors. For adolescents, conduct disorders and substance use disorders are the other most significant predisposing Axis I diagnoses associated with suicide. Data from a large New York City area psychological autopsy study of adolescent suicides indicate that the rate of suicide in males with antisocial behavior is more than three times the base rate for the age group (Gould, Shaffer, Fisher, Kleinman, & Morishima, 1992). In a Pittsburgh area psychological autopsy study of 67 adolescent suicide completers, 40% had a substance use diagnosis, often comorbid with a mood disorder (Brent et al., 1993).

Alcoholism is implicated in about 25% of all suicides in the United States (Lester, 2000). A diagnosis of a substance use disorder is a chronic predisposing risk factor for suicide. In contrast, increased or excessive current drinking to intoxication is an *acute* predisposing risk factor for suicide (see below).

A comorbid Axis III disorder is another example of a predisposing risk factor. Various serious medical conditions are associated with different levels of increased risk; for example, a diagnosis of HIV/AIDS has an OR of 6.6, a diagnosis of malignant neoplasms of the head or neck has an OR of 11.4, and a diagnosis of multiple sclerosis has an OR of 2.4 (Kelly, Mufson, & Rogers, 1999).

Social isolation, or lack of attachment to others, increases suicide risk, with risk increasingly conferred by acute and traumatic loss of relationship (see precipitating factors below). The literature on marital status and its relation to suicide risk, for example, describes a gradient of risk (higher to lower) from acute loss (divorce and separation, and young widowhood) to expected loss (widowhood in older age), to single, never-married to married (least risk, except in adolescence, when early marriage typically signals family and/or other problems) (Maris, Berman, & Silverman, 2000).

Precipitating risk factors, otherwise known as triggering events, are stressors associated with the timing of suicidal behavior. In the context of *vulnerability* (predisposing risk), acute stressors—typically, losses (real, anticipated, or fantasized)—represent the clichéd straw that breaks the camel's back. These might involve losses of attachment (e.g., relationship, job), identity (e.g., career, persona), autonomy (e.g., debilitating and burdensome illness), or function (e.g., caused by acute psychiatric symptoms). They may take the form of acute disappointments, humiliations, threats of legal action or incarceration, unemployment, and so on, but always they signal an ego-dystonic event that is experienced as stressful, intolerable, and/or challenging to the individual's usual repertoire of coping skills (see Monroe, Slavich, & Georgiades, Chapter 15, this volume). Precipitating events are particularly significant in cueing the need for a suicide risk evaluation in a vulnerable patient.

Contributing risk factors are contextual characteristics that, when in evidence, are known to be associated with increased suicide risk. These factors include, for example, an available and accessible firearm (e.g., in the home) (Brent & Bridge, 2003) or recent discharge from inpatient psychiatric hospitalization, particularly after brief hospitalization for mood disorder, of a patient with limited external resources, which has been found to increase risk of suicide in the first 7 days after discharge by a factor of 288 (Qin & Nordentoft, 2005). Another example of a contributing risk factor is exposure to another's suicide, which can have a contagious effect on vulnerable others (Agerbo, Nordentoft, & Mortensen, 2003).

The number of risk factors identified from case–control and psychological autopsy research with suicidal individuals is too great to review thoroughly here. The reader is referred to any of several major texts in suicidology (Berman, Jobes, & Silverman, 2006; Hawton & van Heeringen, 2000; Jacobs, 1999; Maris et al., 2000) for a more thorough discussion and greater understanding of these risk factors.

Acute Risk Factors (Warning Signs)

Most important in signaling near-term risk and the immediate demand to evaluate and document suicide risk are risk factors more proximately associated with completed suicide (i.e., occurring within 6 to 12 months of the suicidal act). These have been captured by the mnemonic *Is Path Warm* (*www.suicidology.org*):

• *I: Ideation.* Suicide ideation is a significant precursor to suicidal behavior, especially if suicidal thoughts are persistent and intrusive, lead to planning, and are associated with intent (see below). Ideation may be expressed verbally through threats, in written form, or it may be translated into behavior, such as looking for ways to kill oneself. This said, the majority of patients who go on to complete suicide may not report suicide ideation (Busch,

Fawcett, & Jacobs, 2003) when seen immediately before their deaths; thus, learning how to ask about and confront denied ideation in the context of other risk factors is crucial to preventing suicidal acts (see below).

- *S: Substance use.* Increasing or excessive substance use (alcohol or drugs, e.g., binge drinking), especially in conjunction with episodes of depression, is common. Alcohol intoxication, common at the time of the suicidal act (Bartels et al., 2002; Lester, 2000), facilitates suicidal behavior by reducing inhibitions, increasing impulsivity, and so on. In addition, substance use often is an attempt to self-medicate depression and/or anxiety.

- *P: Purposelessness.* Seeing no purpose in living or having no sense of purpose in life is a risk factor. Suicidal people have low self-esteem, and reasons for dying may overwhelm reasons for living. Suicidal people also perceive a sense of burdensomeness (Joiner, 2005).

- *A: Anxiety.* Symptoms include severe anxiety, agitation, or insomnia (or *hypersomnia*, sleeping all the time) (Fawcett et al., 1990). Emotional turmoil (psychic anxiety) and insomnia are key symptoms of both anxiety and mood disorders, and are strongly linked to cognitive confusion (diminished concentration, indecision) and poor regulation of emotions and behavior (impulsivity). Agitation may be observed as a form of depressive turmoil.

- *T: Feeling Trapped,* like there is no way out. Suicidal people think differently about themselves and their world. Their cognitions constrict and they become less adaptable in their problem solving, dissolving into seemingly black-and-white choices (dichotomous thinking) as if they are trapped and suicide is the only escape from their psychic pain (Ellis, 2006; Shneidman, 1996). Associated with this feeling is the affect of *desperation*, which, according to therapists who have lost a patient to suicide, is particularly intense among these patients shortly before their deaths (Hendin, Maltsberger, & Szanto, 2007).

- *H: Hopelessness.* One of the enduring findings in the suicidology literature is the significance of hopelessness as the best clinical predictor of suicide among depressed patients (Beck, 1987; Brown, Beck, Steer, & Grisham, 2000; Mann et al., 1999). Hopelessness, a chronic and acute risk factor for suicide, manifests itself clinically in its relation both to suicide ideation, even in the absence of depression (Elliott & Frude, 2001), and to feeling trapped (discussed earlier). Valtonen and colleagues (2007) found hopelessness to be related to suicidal behavior during the depressed phase of bipolar disorder.

- *W: Withdrawal,* from society, friends, and usual activities, occurs. Severe *anhedonia*, a loss of pleasure or interest (discussed earlier), manifests itself in behavioral avoidance of usual and sustaining attachments, work, school, friends, and hobbies. Such withdrawal makes one feel intolerably alone, which further fuels suicidal thinking.

- *A: Anger, rage, or seeking revenge.* Rage signals the potential for violent behavior and impulsive acts, and has been linked, in the form of reactive aggression, to suicidal acts (Conner, Duberstein, Conwell, & Caine, 2003). Suicidal people often feel wronged by others (not nurtured, teased, abused, unloved), which affects their self-esteem and engenders feelings of anger in response to deep psychic pain. Some seek revenge through taking their own lives ("They'll be sorry"); a few kill others before taking their own lives (Berman, 1996; Marzuk, Tardiff, & Hirsch, 1992).

- *R: Recklessness.* Suicidal behavior is strongly related to other risk-taking and life-threatening behaviors, signaling a disregard for oneself and a passive wish to let fate decide whether one lives or dies. Sudden and dramatic changes in behavior toward less self-care and self-regard signal potential danger.

- *M: Dramatic mood changes.* Mood cycling, one of the symptoms associated with short-term risk (Fawcett et al., 1987), may indicate the worsening of a mood or other disorder (Cavanaugh, Owens, & Johnstone, 2002).

In addition, although empirical support is inconclusive, anecdotal evidence of the presence of auditory hallucinations in the context of suicidal vulnerability (e.g., a history of prior attempt) should be taken seriously (Harkavy-Friedman et al., 2003), and delusions, particularly in the context of bipolar disorders or schizophrenia, may signal acute risk for suicide.

PROTECTIVE FACTORS

Suicidal patients who do not die as a result of a suicidal act may be ambivalent about dying; that is, they still have some will to live in spite of their reason or urge to die. It is widely believed (and there are ecological-level supporting data) that other factors, such as the availability of supportive others, access to healthy social supports, short-term plans for the future, a strong therapeutic alliance, religiosity, problem-solving skills, and so on, protect people from acting on suicidal urges. That said, in the presence of acute suicide risk and intolerable psychic pain, protective factors may be overwhelmed. After all, married people, clergypersons, physicians, and attorneys all have completed suicide.

INTENT, MOTIVATION, AND LETHALITY

A thorough evaluation of suicide risk entails an understanding and exploration of the patient's intent, motivation, and relative and potential lethality. *Intent* refers to the patient's aim, purpose, or goal in acting upon suicidal thoughts. Even when ideation is denied, evidence of high acute risk should suggest the need for attention to defining the reward value that suicide might convey for the patient versus a pained continuation of life. Seeking a solution to unendurable pain through ending consciousness (Shneidman, 1996) is a primary aim of most suicidal patients. Some may have different goals to reunite with a deceased loved one in afterlife, to be reborn, to punish others, and so forth. *Motivation* refers to the thwarted or frustrated needs that drive the urge to suicide. Patients are driven to suicide when they feel helpless (suicide is a form of mastery and taking control) and want to hurt others (suicide is a hostile act against both the self and others). This inquiry establishes one potential target for treatment planning. *Lethality* refers to the medical–biological danger or threat to life were an individual to act on a planned method of suicide. Firearms, for example, have a greater than 90% chance of resulting in death. Overdoses of available prescribed medications have different levels of lethality based on each medication's specific toxicity and the patient's body weight (Berman, Shepherd, & Silverman, 2003).

Of particular note is the significance of a patient's reaction to having survived a medically serious, nonfatal suicide attempt. Patients who report regret at having survived, who still harbor thoughts of wanting to die, and/or who state that they are intent on making another attempt, should be considered to be at very high and immediate risk (Beautrais, 2006).

ELICITING SUICIDE IDEATION

Patients communicating suicidal thoughts and evidence of impulsivity or suicidal thoughts with evidence of planning need to be thoroughly evaluated. Patients who deny suicidal thoughts in a context of other signs of acute and chronic risk (vulnerability) should be directly, yet gently, confronted with the contradiction posed by their clinical presentation and their denial of suicidal thinking, and asked to make sense of the apparent contradiction. The clinician should be wary of a patient's statements to the contrary when and if so much other behavioral data speak to the reasonability that he or she may have considered suicide.

An excellent guide to help elicit suicide ideation, including illustrations of validity techniques and a strategy for placing current risk in the context of past suicide risk, is found in Shea (2004).

STRATEGIES FOR SUICIDE RISK FORMULATION

There is no valid actuarial system for formulating risk for suicide—no questionnaire with a minimum cutoff score, for example. Formulating level of risk is a clinical art based on the empirical science of understanding suicide risk factors and how they dynamically interact. There are currently three models upon which the clinical practitioner might base level of risk decision making.

The Recognizing and Responding to Suicide Risk (RRSR) model, taught and rehearsed in an applied clinical skills training program (*www.suicidolgy.org/trainingrrsr*), formulates level of risk on the basis of interplay between judgments of chronic risk (low to high vulnerability) and acute risk (low to high). When any level of acute risk exists in a context of moderate to high chronic risk, overall suicide risk, at a minimum, is judged to be moderate. When several acute risk factors are evident in that same level of chronic vulnerability, suicide risk is judged to be high and demands immediate precautionary treatment planning and implementation.

The National Suicide Prevention Lifeline (NSPL) model (Joiner et al., 2007) clusters observations in four facets of suicidality, influenced by *Is Path Warm* warning signs: *suicidal desire* (including, e.g., ideation, hopelessness, perceived burdensomeness, feeling trapped), *suicide capability* (including, e.g., history of past attempts, rage, anxiety, available means), *suicide intent* (including, e.g., an available plan, expressed intent to die, preparatory behaviors), and the absence of *buffers against suicidality* (protective factors). In this model, *high risk* is defined by the presence of all three core factors (desire, capability, and intent), regardless of the presence of buffers.

The third model may be intuited from defining criteria outlined by Tanney (2000). Here, risk factors are clustered to define *readiness* (presence of stressors, evidence of arousal [anxiety, anger], and evidence of lethality [planning and means]), *acceptability* (hopelessness [constricted problem-solving ability] and ambivalence), *lack of support* (intolerable aloneness, worthlessness, lack of help seeking/receiving), and *failed protections* (disinhibition [impulsivity, acute intoxication, rage] and lack of attachments).

Whatever model the clinician prefers or uses,[4] the standard of care requires that he or she make a reasonable assessment and overall judgment of risk based on a reasonable dataset of both historical and current mental status and symptoms (diagnosis). With that formulation, treatment planning and management of suicide risk comprise the next step.

TREATMENT PLANNING AND THE STANDARD OF CARE

Once the degree of suicide risk has been evaluated and documented, inclusive of the clinician's rationale for the judged level of risk, a treatment plan must be designed first to reduce any evaluated short-term risk for suicide or suicidal behaviors, then, in the longer-term, to decrease the patient's vulnerability once again to be suicidal. The evaluation, if reasonable, both meets the standard of care, which requires consideration that a depressed patient already has some level of chronic risk for suicide, and allows development of a targeted treatment plan. The standard of care establishes an obligation (a duty) to care for the patient. That duty is optimally met by a targeted plan establishing, first and foremost, that treatment is directed to reduce acute (heightened, short-term) risk. This translates into a multipronged approach that focuses treatment not just on management of depression, for example, by treating the patient with an antidepressant, but also on those acute psychiatric symptoms that destabilize and inform the patient's elevated risk potentially to act as a danger to him- or herself. This is especially important, because it is well established that "antidepressant therapy typically involves a substantial delay before clinically obvious improvements occur" (American Psychiatric Association, 2003, p. 38).

The need to protect an acutely at-risk patient from his or her own impulses should motivate the clinician to consider short-term inpatient care (including the need for close observation and monitoring). The clinician should be aware of relevant state statutes regarding criteria for involuntary hospitalization, because the worst time to search for these criteria is in the heat of a suicidal crisis. Inpatient units need to be suicide-proofed, and staff should be thoroughly trained on the unit's policies and procedures regarding patients deemed to be at risk for suicide. A patient at risk for suicide should be placed on closer levels of observation than 15-minute checks during periods of heightened acute risk; Busch and colleagues (2003) reported that 42% of the 76 inpatient suicides they reviewed were on 15-minute checks at the time of their suicide. *No-suicide contracts*, used in the great majority of inpatient psychiatric facilities, have no documented clinical value with suicidal patients, and consideration should be given to an alternative *commitment to treatment* (Rudd, Mandrusiak, & Joiner, 2006), which is an agreement between the patient and clinician to engage in treatment and to integrate a collaboratively developed crisis response plan that the patient agrees to follow if and when he or she is in suicidal crisis. In contrast to a no-suicide contract, it does not restrict the patient's option to consider suicide.

Given the heightened risk of suicide immediately after discharge, suicide risk should be reevaluated before discharge. Careful consideration needs to be given to continuity of care issues following discharge, with maximum awareness to ensuring, as much as is possible, compliance with recommendations for follow-up outpatient care. A meeting with family members is strongly recommended to review warning signs of suicide risk that should be reported if observed, and to discuss adherence with medication and other recommended treatments, and so on. In this regard, the American Association of Suicidology has prepared the Recommendations for Inpatient and Residential Patients Known to Be at Elevated Risk for Suicide (*www.suicidology.org/displaycommon.cfm?an=4*).

Treatment of the suicidal, depressed patient is facilitated by establishing a collaborative alliance and attempting to maximize the patient's adherence to treatment recommendations. Reviews of treatment studies of patients who have attempted suicide (Arensman et al., 2001; Linehan, 1998), based on randomized clinical trials (RCTs), reveal that there are relatively few such trials; consequently, there are few empirically demonstrated effective treatments. These reviews suggest that more intensive interventions, including outreach, where possible, cognitive-behavioral (e.g., problem-solving therapy, dialectical behavior therapy, and interpersonal psychotherapy [IPT]) interventions, and antidepressant medications have some degree of demonstrated effectiveness. These findings, of course, are tempered by the fact that most treatment studies are relatively short-term and are therefore limited to readily measured behavioral outcomes, and that high-risk patients generally have been excluded from these trials. It should be noted that, as yet, no clinical trial has shown inpatient hospitalization to be effective with suicidal patients (Comtois & Linehan, 2006). Suicides do occur in psychiatric hospitals, even when patients are on high-level suicide watch (Busch et al., 2003). Yet there simply is no suitable alternative when a patient needs close monitoring and observation during a period of acute risk. Accordingly, a number of risk management decisions and specific treatment interventions should be guided by both best practices and standards of care guidelines available in the literature (American Psychiatric Association, 2003; Berman, 2006).

Psychological autopsy studies of completed suicides reveal remarkable undertreatment of mentally disordered patients who complete suicide (Isometsä, 2001). Medications are found in as few as 3% of suicides in postmortem toxicology analyses (Baldessarini et al., 2006). Two relatively recent examples regarding antidepressant treatment of adolescents who completed suicide are telling in this regard. In Utah, Moskos, Olson, Halbern, Keller, and Gray (2005) studied 151 consecutive suicides of youth ages 13–21 during a 28-month period. Among decedents with a psychiatric diagnosis, less than one-half (44%) were reported to have been prescribed medication (most frequently an antidepressant). Yet, at autopsy, toxicology reports indicated that none of these youth had any detectable level of psychotropic medication in his or her blood.

Similarly, Leon and colleagues (2006) reported on 41 youth suicides in New York City between 1999 and 2002. Out of 36 serum toxicological analyses conducted, only one decedent was found to have detectable antidepressants at autopsy. It should be noted that all these deaths occurred well before the FDA issued its black box warning regarding suicide risk and antidepressants.

Thus, we have more than incidental data to suggest that depressed patients at risk for suicide are less than optimally involved in treatment and that even when they are, their treatment is less than optimal.

A NOTE ON PHARMACOTHERAPY

Evidence that specific pharmacological interventions reduce suicide risk is limited and "largely inconclusive" (Baldessarini, Pompili, & Tondo, 2006). Ecological-level studies have generally noted an inverse relation between rates of prescription of nontricyclic antidepressants, notably SSRI antidepressants, and contemporaneously observed rates of suicide (cf. Grunebaum, Ellis, Li, Oquendo, & Mann, 2004; Olfson, Shaffer, Marcus, & Greenberg, 2003), but these data do not imply causation. Recent studies (Gibbons et al., 2007; Simon & Savarino, 2007) offer encouraging findings that antidepressants may play a protective role against emergent suicidal behavior. Studies that led to the FDA's black box warning about the role antidepressants may play in causing suicide are limited to an aggregate increase (4 vs. 2% in placebos) of suicide ideation and attempt in patients under age 25 taking antidepressants; there has been no evidence, however, that these antidepressants play any role in causing completed suicides in this age group. Moreover, there is compelling evidence that these same antidepressants play a protective role in older patients (U.S. Food and Drug Administration, 2006).

A Task Force report (Mann, Emslie, et al., 2005) by the American College of Neuropsychopharmacology evaluated the safety and efficacy of SSRI antidepressants for depressed youth under age 18 and determined that two of five SSRIs (fluoxetine and citalopram) were significantly more effective than placebos on primary outcome variables studied in pediatric RCTs. Moreover, the Task Force report noted that speculations in the literature that SSRIs cause akathisia, which, in turn, may increase the risk of suicide, have not been systematically tested.

In contrast to the debate on the efficacy and safety of antidepressants, there is considerable case–control evidence of lower rates of suicide and suicide attempts during lithium maintenance treatment of bipolar disorder (Baldessarini, Tondo, et al., 2006) and recent evidence of a significant effect on suicide risk in recurrent MDD (Guzzetta, Tondo, Centorrino, & Baldessarini, 2007).

CONCLUSIONS AND FUTURE DIRECTIONS

Suicide and suicidal behaviors are the most anxiety-provoking complications of mood disorders. Effective management of the risk of these behaviors by reasonable and frequent assessments and implementation of treatment plans designed to reduce assessed risk is the best antianxiety agent we have.

Mann, Apter, and colleagues (2005) examined evidence for a range of suicide prevention interventions and strategies, and concluded that depression education of PCPs is one of the two most promising strategies for lowering rates of suicide. The premise for this finding was that PCPs lack knowledge about, or fail to screen patients for, depression, and that these factors contribute to the relatively low rate of treatment found in the months before a suicide. Similarly, the Surgeon General of the United States concluded that mental health professionals overall are "not adequately trained to provide adequate assessment, treatment, and management of suicidal persons" (U.S. Public Health Service, 2001, p. 79). The Institute of Medicine (Goldsmith et al., 2002) in its landmark report *Reducing Suicide: A National Imperative*, strongly recommended that medical and mental health professional organizations "should encourage (or require, when appropriate) their memberships to increase their skills in suicide risk detection and intervention" (p. 436). Accordingly, the American Association of Suicidology, under contract to the Suicide Prevention Resource Center, convened a Task Force of Clinical Suicidologists who in turn defined 24 core competencies (knowledge, skills, and abilities) that comprise a skills set for more effective clinical work with at-risk patients. These competencies have now been incorporated into two training programs, one primarily knowledge-based (Assessing and Managing Suicide Risk: *www.sprc.org/featured_resources/trainingandevents/index.asp*), and the other more skills-rehearsal and case application–based (Recognizing and Responding to Suicide Risk: (*www.suicidology.org/trainingrrsr*).

A number of other suicide prevention strategies (e.g., depression screening, and public and gatekeeper education approaches) were described by Mann, Apter, and colleagues (2005) as needing more efficacy and effectiveness data. These approaches, widely implemented across the United States in spite of the need for more consistent outcome data, have as their defined goal the better identification and referral of patients at risk for suicide. An effectively trained clinical professional is the logical endpoint to which these case-finding prevention programs will need to refer identified, at-risk patients. Clinical caregivers who understand and can effectively assess and treat patients with mood disorders having suicide risk are our most important link in the suicide prevention chain.

To make this task more reasonable, a great deal more research is needed to focus clinical signs of suicide risk that are age-specific (adolescent vs. adult vs. geriatric) and subdiagnosis-specific (unipolar vs. bipolar I vs. bipolar II vs. dysthymia vs. double depression). Both psychosocial and biological markers need to be refined, especially as they may relate to assessments of more acute risk based on observations over the suicidal patient's last hours and days rather than months. Treatment and prevention studies, particularly those based on well-controlled clinical trials among diverse populations, need to be funded and carried out. To accomplish these ends, better surveillance of suicidal behaviors is needed, and more reliable classification of cases for study of homogeneous and high-risk groups is essential.

At the turn of this century, both the Surgeon General's National Strategy (U.S. Public Health Service, 2001) and the report of the Institute of Medicine (Goldsmith et al., 2002) laid out ambitious, but reasonable, national goals and objectives for reducing the rate and impact of suicide. Since these reports were published, more than 150,000 Americans have died by suicide. Accomplishing these objectives, as noted in the subtitle of the Institute of Medicine report, must be "a national imperative."

ACKNOWLEDGMENT

With my deepest gratitude, background research for this chapter was developed by Rachel Shapiro.

NOTES

1. U.S. mortality data are obtained from the Web-Based Injury Statistics Query and Reporting System (WISQARS), available through the Centers for Disease Control and Prevention (CDC) website for the years 1981 to the latest year available at the time of writing (currently 2004): *www.cdc.gov/sasweb/ncipc/motrate.html.*

2. A number of other factors have been hypothesized to explain these observed geographic variations in suicide rates in the United States (e.g., more significant barriers to receiving care given distances between person at risk and agency of help, greater prevalence of acute alcoholic intoxication, less help-seeking behavior given the "frontier character" of those living in the West), but none has any substantial evidence to be explanatory of these variations.

3. Those most commonly observed among adults are mood disorders, alcoholism, and schizophrenia; and among adolescents are mood disorders, substance use disorders, and conduct disorders.

4. To date, these models have not been tested empirically.

REFERENCES

Agerbo, E., Nordentoft, M., & Mortensen, P. B. (2003). Familial, psychiatric, and socioeconomic risk factors for suicide in young people: Nested case–control study. *British Medical Journal, 325*, 74–77.

American Psychiatric Association. (2003). *Practice guidelines for the assessment and treatment of patients with suicidal behaviors.* Washington, DC: Author.

Angst, J., Angst, F., Gerber-Werder, R., & Gamma, A. (2005). Suicide in 406 mood-disorder patients with and without long-term medication: A 40 to 44 year follow-up. *Archives of Suicide Research, 9*(3), 279–300.

Arensman, E., Townsend, E., Hawton, K., Bremer, S., Feldman, E., Goldney, R., et al. (2001). Psychosocial and pharmacological treatment of patients following deliberate self-harm: The methodological issues involved in evaluating effectiveness. *Suicide and Life-Threatening Behavior, 31*(2), 169–180.

Baldessarini, R. J., Pompili, M., & Tondo, L. (2006). Suicide in bipolar disorders: Risks and management. *CNS Spectrums, 11*(6), 465–471.

Baldessarini, R. J., Tondo, L., Davis, P., Pompili, M., Goodwin, F. K., & Hennen, J. (2006). Decreased risk of suicides and attempts during long-term lithium treatment: A meta-analytic review. *Bipolar Disorders, 8*(5, Pt. 2), 625–639.

Bartels, S. J., Coakley, E., Oxman, T. E., Constantino, G., Oslin, D., Chen, H., et al. (2002). Suicidal and death ideation in older primary care patients with depression, anxiety, and at-risk alcohol use. *American Journal of Geriatric Psychiatry, 10,* 417–427.

Beautrais, A. (2006, April). *Is suicidal behaviour a chronic condition?* Presentation made to the annual meeting of the American Association of Suicidology, Seattle, WA.

Beautrais, A. L., Joyce, P. R., Mulder, D. M., Fergusson, B. J., Deavoll, B. J., & Nightengale, S. K. (1996). Prevalence and comorbidity of mental disorders in persons making serious suicide attempts: A case–control study. *American Journal of Psychiatry, 153,* 1009–1014.

Beck, A. T. (1987). Hopelessness as a predictor of eventual suicide. *Annals of the New York Academy of Sciences, 487,* 90–96.

Berman, A. L. (1996). Dyadic death: A typology. *Suicide and Life-Threatening Behavior, 26*(4), 342–350.

Berman, A. L. (2006). Risk management with suicidal patients. *Journal of Clinical Psychology, 62*(2), 171–184.

Berman, A. L., Jobes, D. A., & Silverman, M. M. (2006). *Adolescent suicide: Assessment and intervention* (2nd ed.). Washington, DC: American Psychological Association.

Berman, A. L., Shepherd, G., & Silverman, M. M. (2003). The LSARS-II: Lethality of suicide attempts rating scale—updated. *Suicide and Life-Threatening Behavior, 33*(3), 261–276.

Blair-West, G. W., Mellsop, G. W., & Eyeson-Anan, M. L. (1997). Down-rating lifetime suicide risk in major depression. *Acta Psychiatrica Scandinavica, 95,* 259–263.

Bostwick, J. M., & Pankratz, S. (2000). Affective disorders and suicide risk: A reexamination. *American Journal of Psychiatry, 157,* 1925–1932.

Brent, D. A. (2007). Antidepressants and suicidal behavior: Cause or cure? *American Journal of Psychiatry, 164*(7), 989–991.

Brent, D. A., & Bridge, J. (2003). Firearms availability and suicide: A review of the literature. *American Behavioral Scientist, 46,* 1192–1210.

Brent, D. A., Perper, J. A., Moritz, G., Allman, C., Friend, A., Roth, C., et al. (1993). Psychiatric risk factors for adolescent suicide: A case–control study. *Journal of the American Academy of Child and Adolescent Psychiatry, 32,* 521–529.

Brown, G. K., Beck, A. T., Steer, R. A., & Grisham, J. R. (2000). Risk factors for suicide in psychiatric outpatients: A 20 year prospective study. *Journal of Consulting and Clinical Psychology, 68,* 371–377.

Busch, K. A., Fawcett, J., & Jacobs, D. G. (2003). Clinical correlates of inpatient suicide. *Journal of Clinical Psychiatry, 64,* 14–19.

Cavanaugh, J. T., Carson, J. T., Sharpe, M., & Lawrie, S. M. (2003). Psychological autopsy studies of suicide: A systematic review. *Psychological Medicine, 33*(3), 395–405.

Cavanaugh, J. T., Owens, D. G., & Johnstone, E. C. (2002). Suicide and undetermined death in southeast Scotland: A case–control study using the psychological autopsy method. *Psychological Medicine, 29,* 1141–1149.

Chemtob, C., Hamada, R., Bauer, G., Kinney, B., & Torigoe, R. (1988a). Patients' suicides: Frequency and impact on psychiatrists. *American Journal of Psychiatry, 145,* 224–228.

Chemtob, C., Hamada, R., Bauer, G., Torigoe, R., & Kinney, B. (1988b). Patient suicide: Frequency and impact on psychologists. *Professional Psychology: Research and Practice, 19*(4), 416–420.

Cheng, A. T. (1995). Mental illness and suicide: A case–control study in east Taiwan. *Archives of General Psychiatry, 52*(7), 594–603.

Cheung, A. H., & Dewa, C. S. (2007). Mental health service use among adolescents and young adults with major depressive disorder and suicidality. *Canadian Journal of Psychiatry, 52*(4), 228–232.

Comtois, K. A., & Linehan, M. M. (2006). Psychosocial treatments of suicidal behaviors: A practice-friendly review. *Journal of Clinical Psychology, 62*(2), 161–170.

Conner, K. R., Duberstein, P. R., Conwell, Y., & Caine, E. D. (2003). Reactive aggression and suicide: Theory and evidence. *Aggression and Violent Behavior, 8*(4), 413–432.

Conwell, Y., Duberstein, P. R., Cox, C., Herrmann, J. H., Forbes, N. T., & Caine, E. D. (1996). Relationship of age and Axis I diagnoses in victims of completed suicide: A psychological autopsy study. *American Journal of Psychiatry, 153*, 1001–1008.

Elliott, J., & Frude, N. (2001). Stress, coping styles, and hopelessness in self-poisoners. *Crisis, 22*(1), 20–26.

Ellis, T. (Ed.). (2006). *Cognition and suicide: Theory, research, and therapy.* Washington, DC: American Psychological Association.

Fawcett, J. (2006). Depressive disorders. In R. I. Simon & R. E. Hales (Eds.), *Textbook of suicide assessment and management* (pp. 255–275). Washington, DC: American Psychiatric Publishing.

Fawcett, J., Busch, K., Jacobs, D., Kravitz, H., & Fogg, L. F. (1997). Suicide: A four-pathway clinical biochemical pathway. In D. Stoff & J. J. Mann (Eds.), *The neurology of suicide: From the bench to the clinic* (pp. 286–301). New York: New York Academy of Sciences.

Fawcett, J., Scheftner, W., Clark, D., Hedeker, D., Gibbons, R., & Coryell, W. (1987). Clinical predictors of suicide in patients with major affective disorders: A controlled prospective study. *American Journal of Psychiatry, 144*(1), 35–40.

Fawcett, J., Scheftner, W. A., Fogg, L., Clark, D. C., Young, M. A., Hedeker, D., et al. (1990). Time-related predictors of suicide in major affective disorder. *American Journal of Psychiatry, 147*, 1189–1194.

Fleischman, A., Bertolote, J. M., Belfer, M., & Beautrais, A. (2005). Completed suicide and psychiatric diagnoses in young people: A critical examination of the evidence. *American Journal of Orthopsychiatry, 75*(4), 676–683.

Fremouw, W. J., de Perczel, M., & Ellis, T. (1990). *Suicide risk: Assessment and response guidelines.* Elmsford, NY: Pergamon Press.

Gibbons, R. D., Borwn, C. H., Hur, K., Marcus, S. M., Bhaumik, D. K., & Mann, J. J. (2007). Relationship between antidepressants and suicide attempts: An analysis of the Veterans Administration data sets. *American Journal of Psychiatry, 164*, 1044–1049.

Goldman, L. S., Nielsen, N. H., & Champion, H. C. (1999). Awareness, diagnosis, and treatment of depression. *Journal of General Internal Medicine, 14*(9), 569–580.

Goldsmith, S. K., Pellmar, T. C., Kleinman, A. M., & Bunney, W. E. (Eds.). (2002). *Reducing suicide: A national imperative.* Washington, DC: National Academies Press.

Goodwin, F. K., & Jamison, K. R. (1990). *Manic-depressive illness.* New York: Oxford University Press.

Gould, M. S., Shaffer, D., Fisher, P., Kleinman, M., & Morishima, A. (1992). The clinical predication of adolescent suicide. In R. W. Maris, A. L. Berman, J. T. Maltsberger, & R. I. Yufit (Eds.), *Assessment and prediction of suicide* (pp. 130–143). New York: Guilford Press.

Gruenbaum, M. F., Ellis, S. P., Li, S., Oquendo, M. A., & Mann, J. J. (2004). Antidepressants and suicide risk in the United States, 1985–1999. *Journal of Clinical Psychiatry, 65*(11), 1456–1462.

Guze, S. B., & Robins, E. (1970). Suicide and primary affective disorders. *British Journal of Psychiatry, 117*, 437–438.

Guzzetta, F., Tondo, L., Centorrino, F., & Baldessarini, R. J. (2007). Lithium treatment reduces suicide risk in recurrent major depressive disorder. *Journal of Clinical Psychiatry, 68*(3), 380–383.

Harkavy-Firedman, J. M., Kimhy, D., Nelson, E. A., Venarde, D. F., Malaspina, D., & Mann, J. J. (2003). Suicide attempts in schizophrenia: The role of command hallucinations for suicide. *Journal of Clinical Psychiatry, 64*(8), 871–874.

Harris, E. C., & Barraclough, B. (1997). Suicide as an outcome for mental disorders: A meta-analysis. *British Journal of Psychiatry, 170*, 205–228.

Haw, C., Hawton, K., Sutton, L., Sinclair, J., & Deeks, J. (2005). Schizophrenia and deliberate self-harm: A systematic review of risk factors. *Suicide and Life-Threatening Behavior, 35*(1), 50–62.

Hawton, K., Houston, K., Haw, C., Townsend, E., & Harriss, L. (2003). Comorbidity of Axis I and Axis II disorders in patients who attempted suicide. *American Journal of Psychiatry, 160*(8), 1494–1500.

Hawton, K., & van Heeringen, K. (Eds.). (2000). *Suicide and attempted suicide.* Chichester, UK: Wiley.

Hendin, H., Maltsberger, J. T., & Szanto, K. (2007). The role of intense affective states in signaling a suicidal crisis. *Journal of Nervous and Mental Disorders, 195*(5), 363–368.

Henriksson, M. M., Aro, H. M., Marttunen, M. J., Heikkinen, M. E., Isometsä, E. T., Kuoppasalmi, K. I., et al. (1993). Mental disorders and comorbidity in suicide. *American Journal of Psychiatry, 150*, 935–940.

Isometsä, E. T. (2001). Psychological autopsy studies: A review. *European Psychiatry, 16*(7), 379–385.

Isometsä, E. T., Henrikkson, M. M., Aro, H. M., & Lönnqvist, J. K. (1994). Suicide in bipolar disorder in Finland. *American Journal of Psychiatry, 151,* 1020–1024.

Jacobs, D. (Ed.). (1999). *The Harvard Medical School guide to suicide assessment and intervention.* San Francisco: Jossey-Bass.

Jamison, K. R. (2000). Suicide and bipolar disorder. *Journal of Clinical Psychiatry, 61*(Suppl. 9), 47–51.

Joiner, T. (2005). *Why people die by suicide.* Cambridge, MA: Harvard University Press.

Joiner, T., Kalafat, J., Draper, J., Stokes, H., Knudson, M., Berman, A. L., et al. (2007). Establishing standards for the assessment of suicide risk among callers to the National Suicide Prevention Lifeline. *Suicide and Life-Threatening Behavior, 37*(3), 353–365.

Kelly, M. J., Mufson, M. J., & Rogers, M. P. (1999). Medical settings and suicide. In D. G. Jacobs (Ed.), *The Harvard Medical School guide to suicide assessment and intervention* (pp. 491–519). San Francisco: Jossey-Bass.

Kessler, R. C., Bergland, P., Demier, O., Jin, R., Merikangas, K. R., & Walters, E. E. (2005). Lifetime prevalence and age-of-onset distributions of DSM-IV disorders in the National Comorbidity Survey Replication. *Archives of General Psychiatry, 62*(6), 593–602.

Kessler, R. C., Borges, G., & Walters, E. E. (1999). Prevalence of and risk factors for lifetime suicide attempts in the National Comorbidity Study. *Archives of General Psychiatry, 56,* 617–626.

Kessler, R. C., Frank, R. G., Edlund, M., Katz, S. J., Lin, E., & Leaf, P. (1997). Differences in the use of psychiatric outpatient services between the United States and Ontario. *New England Journal of Medicine, 336,* 551–557.

Kessler, R. C, McGonagle, K. A., Zhao, S., Nelson, C. B., Hughes, M., Eshlerman, S., et al. (1994). Lifetime and 12-month prevalence of DSM-III-R psychiatric disorders in the United States. *Archives of General Psychiatry, 51*(1), 8–19.

Leon, A. C., Marzuk, P. M., Tardiff, K., Bucciarwlli, A., Markham Piper, T., & Galea, S. (2006). Antidepressants and youth suicide in New York City, 1999–2002. *Journal of the American Academy of Child and Adolescent Suicide, 45*(9), 1054–1058.

Lester, D. (2000). Alcoholism, substance abuse, and suicide. In R. W. Maris, A. L. Berman, & M. M. Silverman (Eds.), *Comprehensive textbook of suicidology* (pp. 357–375). New York: Guilford Press.

Libby, A. M., Brent, D. A., Morrato, E., Orton, H. D., Allen, R., & Valuck, R. J. (2007). Decline in treatment of pediatric depression after FDA advisory on risk of suicidality with SSRIs. *American Journal of Psychiatry, 164*(6), 884–891.

Linehan, M. M. (1998, April). *A review of treatment studies of attempted suicide patients.* Paper presented at the 31st Annual Conference of the American Association of Suicidology, Bethesda, MD.

Luoma, J., Martin, C. E., & Pearson, J. L. (2002). Contact with mental health and primary care providers before suicide: A review of the evidence. *American Journal of Psychiatry, 159*(6), 909–916.

Mann, J. J., Apter, A., Bertolote, J., Beautrais, A., Currier, D., Haas, A., et al. (2005). Suicide prevention strategies. *Journal of the American Medical Association, 294*(16), 2064–2074.

Mann, J. J., Emslie, G., Baldessarini, R. J., Beardslee, W., Fawcett, J. A., Goodwin, F. K., et al. (2005). ACNP Task Force report on SSRIs and suicidal behavior in youth. *Neuropsychopharmacology, 31,* 473–492.

Mann, J. J., Waternaux, C., Haas, G. L., & Malone, K. M. (1999). Toward a clinical model of suicidal behavior in psychiatric patients. *American Journal of Psychiatry, 156,* 181–189.

Maris, R. W. (1997). Social and familial risk factors in suicidal behavior. *Psychiatric Clinics of North America, 20,* 519–550.

Maris, R. W., Berman, A. L., & Silverman, M. M. (2000). *Comprehensive textbook of suicidology,* New York: Guilford Press.

Marzuk, P. M., Tardiff, K., & Hirsch, C. J. (1992). The epidemiology of murder–suicide. *Journal of the American Medical Association, 267*(23), 3179–3183.

MMWR Surveillance Summaries. (2006). Youth Risk Behavior Surveillance—United States, 2005. *Morbidity and Mortality Weekly Report, 55*(SS-5), 1–108.

Moffitt, T. E., Harrington, H., Caspi, A., Kim-Cohen, J., Goldberg, D., Gregory, A. M., et al. (2007). Depression and generalized anxiety disorder: Cumulative and sequential comorbidity in a birth cohort followed prospectively to age 32 years. *Archives of General Psychiatry, 64*(6), 651–660.

Moscicki, E. K. (1994). Gender differences in completed and attempted suicides. *Annals of Epidemiology, 4*, 152–158.

Moskos, M., Olson, L., Halbern, S., Keller, T., & Gray, D. (2005). Utah Youth Suicide Study: Psychological autopsy. *Suicide and Life-Threatening Behavior, 35*(5), 525–536.

Olfson, M., Marcus, S. C., Weissman, M. M., & Jensen, P. S. (2002). National trends in the use of psychotropic medications by children. *Journal of the American Academy of Child and Adolescent Psychiatry, 41*(5), 514–521.

Olfson, M., Shaffer, D., Marcus, S. C., & Greenberg, T. (2003). Relationship between antidepressant medication treatment and suicide in adolescents. *Archives of General Psychiatry, 60*(10), 978–982.

Ösby, U., Brandt, L., Correiia, N., Ekbom, A., & Sparén, P. (2001). Excess mortality in bipolar and unipolar disorder in Sweden. *Archives of General Psychiatry, 58*, 844–850.

Owens, D., Horrocks, J., & House, A. (2002). Fatal and non-fatal repetition of self-harm: Systematic review. *British Journal of Psychiatry, 181*, 193–199.

Paul, J. P., Catania, J., Pollack, L., Moskowitz, J., Canchola, J., Mills, T., et al. (2002). Suicide attempts among gay and bisexual men: Lifetime prevalence and antecedents. *American Journal of Public Health, 92*, 1338–1345.

Qin, P., & Nordentoft, M. (2005). Suicide risk in relation to psychiatric hospitalization: Evidence on longitudinal registers. *Archives of General Psychiatry, 62*, 427–432.

Rhimer, Z. (2005). Prediction and prevention of suicide in bipolar disorders. *Clinical Neuropsychiatry, 2*, 48–54.

Rhimer, Z. (2007). Suicide risk in mood disorders. *Current Opinion in Psychiatry, 20*(1), 17–22.

Rudd, M. D., Mandrusiak, M., & Joiner, T. (2006). The case against no-suicide contracts: The commitment to treatment statement as a practice alternative. *Journal of Clinical Psychology, 62*(2), 243–251.

Ruggero, C. J., Chelminski, I., Young, D., & Zimmerman, M. (2007). Psychosocial impairment associated with bipolar II disorder. *Journal of Affective Disorders, 104*, 53–60.

Shea, S. (2004). The delicate art of eliciting suicidal ideation. *Psychiatric Annals, 34*(5), 385–400.

Shneidman, E. S. (1996). *The suicidal mind.* Oxford, UK: Oxford University Press.

Simon, G. E., & Savarino, J. (2007). Suicide attempts among patients starting depression treatment with medications or psychotherapy. *American Journal of Psychiatry, 164*(7), 1029–1034.

Simon, G. E., & Von Korff, M. (1998). Suicide mortality among patients treated for depression in an insured population. *American Journal of Epidemiology, 147*, 155–160.

Simpson, S. G., & Jamison, K. R. (1999). The risk of suicide in bipolar patients. *Journal of Clinical Psychiatry, 60*(Suppl. 2), 53–56.

Substance Abuse Mental Health Services Administration. (2006a). *Results from the National Survey on Drug Use and Health: National findings* (NDCUH Series H-30, DHHS Publication No. SMA 06-4194). Rockville, MD: Office of Applied Studies.

Substance Abuse Mental Health Services Administration. (2006b). Suicidal thoughts, suicide attempts, major depressive episode, and substance abuse among adults. *OAS Report, 34*, 1–8.

Szadocky, E., & Fazekas, I. (1994). The role of psychological and biological variables in separating chronic and non-chronic major depression and early/late-onset dysthmia. *Journal of Affective Disorders, 32*, 1–11.

Tanney, B. L. (2000). Psychiatric diagnoses and suicidal acts. In R. W. Maris, A. L. Berman, & M. M. Silverman (Eds.), *Comprehensive textbook of suicidology* (pp. 311–341). New York: Guilford Press.

Tondo, L., & Baldessarini, R. J. (2005). Suicide risk in bipolar disorder. *Clinical Neuropsychiatry, 2*, 55–65.

Tondo, L., Baldessarini, R. J., Hennen, J., Minnai, G., Salis, P., Scamonatti, L., et al. (1999). Suicide attempts in major affective disorder patients with comorbid substance abuse disorders. *Journal of Clinical Psychiatry, 60*(Suppl.), 63–69.

U.S. Department of Health and Human Services. (1999). *Mental health: A report of the Surgeon General—Executive Summary.* Rockville, MD: U.S. Department of Health and Human Services, Substance Abuse and Mental Health Services Administration, Center for Mental Health Services, National Institutes of Health, National Institute of Mental Health.

U. S. Food and Drug Administration. (2006, November 16). *Clinical review: Relationship between antidepressant drugs and suicidality in adults.* Washington, DC: Author.

U.S. Public Health Service. (2001). *National strategy for suicide prevention: Goals and objectives for action.* Washington, DC: Department of Health and Human Services.

Valtonen, H. M., Suominen, K., Mantere, O., Leppämäki, S., Arvilommi, P., & Isometsä, E. T. (2006). Prospective study of risk factors for attempted suicide among patients with bipolar disorder. *Bipolar Disorders, 8*(5, Pt. 2), 576–585.

Valtonen, H. M., Suominen, K., Mantere, O., Leppämäki, S., Arvilommi, P., & Isometsä, E. T. (2007). Suicidal behavior during different phases of bipolar disorder. *Journal of Affective Disorders, 97*(1–3), 101–107.

Vasiliadis, H.-M., Lesage, A., Adair, C., Wang, P. S., & Kessler, R. C. (2007). Do Canada and the United States differ in prevalence of depression and utilization of services? *Psychiatric Services, 58,* 63–71.

Vuorilehto, M. S., Melartin, T. K., & Isometsä, E. T. (2006). Suicidal behavior among primary care patients with depressive disorders. *Psychological Medicine, 36*(2), 203–210.

Wang, P. S., Bergland, P., Olfson, M., Pincus, H. A., Wells, K. B., & Kessler, R. C. (2005). Failure and delay in initial treatment contact after first onset of mental disorders in the National Comorbidity Survey Replication. *Archives of General Psychiatry, 62*(6), 603–613..

Weissman, M. M., Bland, R. C., Canino, G. J., Greenwald, S., Hwo, H.-G., Joyce, P. R., et al. (1999). Prevalence of suicide ideation and suicide attempts in nine countries. *Psychological Medicine, 29,* 9–17.

PART IV

PREVENTION
AND TREATMENT
OF DEPRESSION

In recent years there have been significant developments in interventions for depression. This section includes six chapters that review the methods and evidence for the effectiveness of both prevention and treatment efforts. Muñoz, Le, Clarke, Barrera, and Torres (Chapter 23) discuss prevention, its importance, and the diverse ways in which investigators have attempted to prevent development of depression or to reduce its impact in adults and children. Among typical treatments, pharmacotherapy is the most widely disseminated approach; in this context, both standard and innovative approaches to acute, continuation, and maintenance treatment are discussed by Gitlin (Chapter 24). Three of the most effective and well-validated psychotherapies for depression and bipolar disorder are discussed by authors who have contributed to its development and empirical evaluation. Cognitive-behavioral treatment is presented and reviewed by Hollon and Dimidjian (Chapter 25). Miklowitz (Chapter 26) reviews the literature on pharmacological and psychosocial interventions for bipolar disorder. Marital and family therapies, as well as interpersonal psychotherapy for depression, are discussed by Beach, Jones, and Franklin (Chapter 27). Finally, Kaslow, Davis, and Smith (Chapter 28) review the unique issues and treatment methods applied to the treatment of depression in children and adolescents.

PART V

PREVENTION
AND TREATMENT
OF DISEASE

CHAPTER 23

Preventing First Onset and Recurrence of Major Depressive Episodes

Ricardo F. Muñoz, Huynh-Nhu Le, Gregory N. Clarke,
Alinne Z. Barrera, *and* Leandro D. Torres

Depression is a major public health problem. In the United States, 17% of adults experience at least one episode of major depression during their life (Kessler et al., 1994, 2005). The World Health Organization (WHO) reports that major depression (1) is the leading cause of disability in the world; (2) was the fourth most important disorder in 1990; and (3) will become the second most important disorder by the year 2020 in terms of the burden of disease in the world, taking into account both disability and mortality (Murray & Lopez, 1996). When there is an epidemic of this type, treatment is not enough (Le, Muñoz, Ghosh Ippen, & Stoddard, 2003). It is necessary to dedicate a substantial portion of our resources to prevention (Albee, 1985).

Most mental health resources are currently dedicated to treatment. In the case of major depression, however, there are serious limits to treatment. For example, treatment reaches very few persons in need. This is especially true for diverse populations; depressed African American and Latino adults are often less likely than their non-Hispanic white counterparts to use outpatient mental health services (Hough et al., 1987; Ojeda & McGuire, 2006). Among patients who adhere to treatment as directed (and most do not) about one-third recover (e.g., full remission), one-third have some moderate response but are not fully remitted, and one-third do not respond (Depression Guideline Panel, 1993a; Rush, Trivedi, et al., 2006). And even when treatment is effective, the chance of recurrence of a major depressive episode (MDE) is 50% after one episode, 70% after two episodes, and 90% after three episodes (Depression Guideline Panel, 1993b; Judd, 1997). Therefore, preventing new episodes of major depression and, ideally, the first episode, is essential.

DELINEATING THE SCOPE OF PREVENTIVE INTERVENTIONS

The Institute of Medicine (IOM) Report on Preventing Mental Disorders (Mrazek & Haggerty, 1994) was a spirited call for increased research on preventive interventions. The IOM Committee felt that the traditional, three-level public health definitions (primary, secondary, or tertiary prevention) confused preventive and treatment interventions. Therefore, the Committee proposed a more categorical definition (see Figure 2.1, p. 23, in Mrazek & Haggerty, 1994). *Prevention* refers to interventions occurring *before the onset* of the disorder and is designed to prevent the occurrence of the disorder. *Treatment* refers to interventions occurring after the onset of the disorder to bring a quick end to the clinical episode. Treatment can be provided after early case-finding outreach efforts or as traditional treatment services, in which patients bring themselves, or are brought into treatment once they have the disorder. *Maintenance* refers to interventions that occur after the acute episode has abated to reduce likelihood of relapse, recurrence, or disability in a patient who has received treatment.

Within prevention interventions, three sublevels were defined: *universal* (targeted at the general public or community regardless of risk), *selective* (targeted at community individuals or groups demonstrating a higher than average risk), and *indicated* (targeted at high-risk individuals with early signs or symptoms but not meeting diagnostic criteria for the disorder) (Mrazek & Haggerty, 1994).

In this chapter, we follow the IOM definitions. Specifically, we review randomized controlled trials (RCTs) designed to prevent MDEs—those trials that recruit participants who do not meet criteria for MDEs at trial entry, and that specifically compare rates of incidence in the experimental and comparison or control conditions. The outcome of interest is whether interventions yield significantly lower rates of new MDEs. We consider studies of populations of both high-risk individuals identified in nonclinical settings (i.e., in an attempt to prevent the onset of major depression), and individuals with past major depression who have recovered for a long enough period (e.g., more than 8 weeks below criteria for full remission; Frank et al., 1991; Rush, Kraemer, et al., 2006) that recurrence of clinical depression would be considered the onset of a new episode.

We acknowledge that the prevention field is not yet advanced enough to provide a large number of such RCTs. Many investigators in the area of prevention are studying the feasibility of reducing depressive symptoms in at-risk populations, with the explicit or implicit expectation that doing so will eventually reduce incidence of clinical MDEs. Several studies have used traditional group or individually administered preventive interventions focusing on symptom reduction, with most demonstrating effectiveness in reducing depressive symptoms. Prevention efforts aimed at symptom reduction (vs. MDE incidence) among vulnerable children and adolescents have not consistently produced significant, long-term effects (Horowitz & Garber, 2006). From this body of literature, researchers have suggested expanding preventive efforts so that multiple factors (e.g., being female, family history) that increase the risk for depression are targeted in prevention trials (Garber, 2006). We believe these important studies are on the road to preventing clinical depression, but reduction in symptoms may or may not lead to reduction in incidence. We exclude from consideration in this chapter studies focused on depressive symptom reduction. For a more detailed discussion of prevention intervention investigations focused on reducing depressive symptoms in children and adolescents, see Horowitz and Garber (2006), and in adults, see Barrera, Torres, and Muñoz (2007), Cuijpers, Van Straten, and Smit (2005), and Muñoz, Le, Clarke, and Jaycox (2002).

SPECIAL ISSUES IN PREVENTION RESEARCH

In treatment research trials, upon entry into the study, all participants meet diagnostic criteria for the disorder being treated. They either volunteer for treatment trials or seek psychological services; therefore, they are fairly motivated seekers of treatment. In contrast, participants in prevention of first-onset trials, by definition, have not developed, or are not currently experiencing, the disorder to be prevented. Thus, as part of outreach, it is crucial to provide prevention participants a convincing rationale for attending the intervention, using the methods taught, and allowing researchers to interview them over an extended period of time. This generally requires added attention to issues of recruitment and retention—in particular for minority groups, who heavily underutilize treatment services (Alegría et al., 2007; Hough et al., 1987). Therefore, it is particularly important to provide preventive services that are accessible and acceptable to such groups. In addition, individuals who have been treated successfully for major depression are at high risk for recurrent episodes. Thus, they are a reasonable high-risk group to target for prevention of new episodes. For further discussions of issues in prevention research, see Muñoz and Ying (1993); for issues with women and minorities, see Mendelson and Muñoz (2006), and with Latino populations, see Pérez and Muñoz (2008).

EMPIRICALLY TESTED PREVENTIVE INTERVENTIONS THROUGH THE LIFE CYCLE

We now address three stages in the life cycle: adulthood, the school years, and the beginning of life. We begin with adulthood, because the first depression prevention trials were conducted with adults and gradually moved to younger groups. See Table 23.1 for specific details concerning the 13 trials designed to examine whether interventions reduce incidence of MDEs.

Preventing Depression in Adulthood

Strategies to prevent depression have often come from what we already know about the treatment of depression. We have much evidence that mood regulation skills are as effective as antidepressants to treat major depression and reduce the likelihood of relapse/recurrence (Hollon, Stewart, & Strunk, 2006; Paykel et al., 1999; Teasdale et al., 2000). Why wait until someone has a clinical depression to teach him or her these methods? The idea is logical. But is it practical? How do we reach the person ahead of time, for example, before he or she experiences a full major depressive episode and seeks traditional care?

Randomized Trials Designed to Prevent Major Depressive Episodes

The San Francisco Depression Prevention Research Project, conducted from 1983 to 1986, was the first randomized controlled prevention trial intended to examine whether an intervention could prevent new clinical episodes of major depression (Muñoz & Ying, 1993; Muñoz, Ying, Armas, Chan, & Gurza, 1987). Participants were 150 English- and Spanish-speaking, predominantly minority, primary care patients without any psychiatric disorder. Those in the intervention condition received 8 weekly group sessions of the Depression Prevention Course (Muñoz, 1984), focusing on cognitive-behavioral approaches

TABLE 23.1. Randomized Trials Designed to Test Reduction of Incidence of Major Depressive Episodes

Study	Muñoz et al. (1987), Muñoz & Ying (1993), Muñoz et al. (1995)	Clarke et al. (1995)	Seligman et al. (1999)	Elliott et al. (2000)	Clarke et al. (2001)	Zlotnick et al. (2001)
Participants	150 Spanish- and English-speaking adult public sector primary care patients	150 high school students with elevated depression symptoms	231 college freshmen	99 women pregnant with 1st or 2nd child	94 adolescent offspring of depressed parents	35 low-income pregnant women on public assistance
Condition assignment	Random (78 control, 72 exp)	Random (74 control, 76 exp)	Random (124 control, 109 exp)	Random (52 control, 47 exp)	Random (49 control, 45 exp)	Random (18 control, 17 exp)
Intervention	8 weekly 2-hour group sessions teaching cognitive-behavioral self-control methods	15 hourlong group sessions teaching cognitive restructuring skills	8 weekly 2-hour group sessions teaching cognitive-behavioral skills; 6 individual	11 monthly group sessions separately for 1st- and 2nd-time mothers; one midpregnancy visit	15 hourlong group sessions teaching cognitive restructuring skills	4 hourlong group sessions teaching interpersonal skills
Manual	Depression Prevention Course	Coping with Stress Course	Apex Project Manual for Group Leaders	Preparation for parenthood (1st-time mothers); surviving parenthood (2nd-time mothers)	Coping with Stress Course (modified)	Survival Skills for New Moms
Control/comparison condition	No intervention and 40-minute videotape version of CBT skills	Usual care (very little)	No intervention; assessments only	Usual care	HMO usual care	Usual antenatal care
Assessment intervals	Pre, post, 6, 12 months	Pre, post, 6, 12 months	Pre, post, 6, 12, 18, 24, 30, 36 months; 36 monthly symptom ratings	Pre (pregnancy), 3- and 12-months postpartum	Pre, post, 12, 24 months	Pre, post, 3 months

Assessment instruments Incidence	DIS	K-SADS, LIFE	SCID; LIFE	Present State Examination	K-SADS, LIFE	SCID
Other	Depression: BDI, CES-D	Other: CES, PAS, PBI, SAQ, SPQ	Depression: CES-D, Hamilton Anxiety Scale	Depression Scale Other: GAF	Depression: BDI, Hamilton Depression Scale Anxiety: BAI, Hamilton Anxiety Scale	Depression, anxiety, and somatic subscales of the CCEI; EPDS; Self-Rating Questionnaire
Findings Incidence	MDE incidence at 12-month FU: control, 5.5%; exp, 3.0%	Total depression[a] incidence at 12-month FU: control, 25.7%; exp, 14.5%	MDE incidence at 3 years: control, 10.9%; exp, 13.2%	MDE incidence over 3-month FU: control, 39%; exp, 19%, only 1st-time mothers	MDE incidence at 12-month FU: control, 28.8%; exp, 9.3%	MDE incidence at 3-month FU: control, 33%; exp, 0%
Significant difference in incidence	N.S.	Yes ($p < .05$)	N.S.	Yes ($p < .05$)	Yes ($p < .005$)	Yes ($p = .02$)
Depressive symptoms	BDI: Significant CES-D: N.S.	CES-D: N.S.	BDI, BAI: Significant Hamilton Depression Scale: N.S. Hamilton Anxiety Scale: N.S.	EPDS, CCEI scales, SRQ: Significant 1st-time mothers only at 3 months	CES-D: Significant	BDI: Significant
Other findings	Significant changes in cognitions, pleasant activities, social activities. Changes related to reductions in depressive symptoms.	GAF: N.S.	Significant changes in explanatory style, hopelessness, dysfunctional attitudes. Changes mediated the depressive symptoms in exp group		GAF: Significant CBCL: N.S.	

(continued)

TABLE 23.1. (continued)

Study	Spence et al. (2003)	Gillham et al. (2006)	Sheffield et al. (2006)	Young et al. (2006)	Zlotnick et al. (2006)	Muñoz et al. (2007)
Participants	1,500 12- to 14-year-olds from 16 high schools in Australia	271 11- to 12-year-olds with elevated depressive symptoms	2,479 13- to 15-year-old Australians with elevated symptoms of depression	Forty-one inner-city 7th- to 10th-grade mostly Latino adolescents	Ninety-nine low-income pregnant women on public assistance	Forty-one low-income pregnant women at high risk for MDEs based on Le et al. (2004)
Condition assignment	Random (749 control, 751 exp)	Random (124 control, 147 exp)	Random (614 control, 634 exp-U, 722 exp-I, 636 exp-U + I)	Random (14 school counselor, 27 exp)	Random (46 control, 53 exp)	Random (20 control, 21 exp)
Intervention	Eight weekly 50-minute class sessions teaching cognitive restructuring and problem-solving skills	Twelve 90-minute group sessions teaching cognitive-behavioral skills	Exp-U: 8 weekly 50-minute sessions delivered over school term; Exp-I: 8 weekly 90-minute sessions; all were group sessions teaching cognitive restructuring and problem-solving skills	Two initial individual and 8 weekly 90-minute group sessions teaching how to identify and resolve interpersonal conflicts	Four hourlong group session teaching interpersonal skills; one 50-minute individual booster session	Twelve weekly 2-hour group sessions teaching how to use thoughts, activities, and contacts with others; psychoeducation related to pregnancy, parenting, and child development
Manual	Problem Solving for Life Program	PRP	Problem Solving for Life Program	IPT—Adolescent Skills Training	Survival Skills for New Moms and a booster session	Mothers and Babies Course
Control/comparison condition	No intervention—assessment only	Usual care	No intervention—assessment only	School counselor or social worker	Usual antenatal care	Usual care
Assessment intervals	Pre, post, 12 months	Pre, post, 6, 12, 18, 24 months	Pre, post, 6, 12 months	Pre, post, 3, 6 months	Pre, post, 3 months	Pre, post, 1, 3, 6, 12 months

	ADIS-C, DY, LIFE	Obtained from HMO database	ADIS-C, LIFE	K-SADS-PL	LIFE	Maternal Mood Screener (for DSM MDEs)
Assessment instruments Incidence						
Other	Depression: BDI Other: YSR, CASAFS, SPSI-R, CASQ-R, LER, CSRFFI, PSFL	Depression: CDI Other: CASQ,	Depression: CDI, CES-D, BHS Other: SCAS, YSR, SPSI-R, CATS, CASAFS	Depression: CES-D Other: CGAS	Depression: BDI Other: Range of Impaired Functioning Tool	Depression: CES-D; EPDS
Findings Incidence	MDE incidence for high symptom over 12-month FU: control, 8.4%; exp, 9.9%	MDE incidence at 2-year FU, high symptom: control, 36%; exp, 21%; low-symptom: control, 13%; exp, 19%	Total depressive disorder in high symptom over 18 month FU: control, 20.4%; exp-U, 18.1%; exp-I, 21.4; exp-U + I, 17.8%	Total depression[a] incidence at 6-month FU: SC, 28.6%; exp, 3.7%	MDE incidence at 3- months at FU: control, 20%; exp, 4%	MDE incidence at 12-month FU: control, 25%; exp, 14% ($b = 0.28$)
Significant differences in incidence	N.S.	N.S.	N.S.	Yes ($p = .08$)	Yes ($p = .04$)	N.S.
Depressive symptoms	BDI: N.S.	CDI: N.S.	CDI, CES-D, BHS: N.S.	CES-D: Significant	BDI: N.S.	CES-D: N.S. EPDS: N.S.
Other findings	YSR, SPSI-R, CASQ-R: N.S.	Improved explanatory style for positive events for PRP ($p < .01$)	SCAS, YSR, SPSI-R, CATS, CASAFS: N.S.	CGAS: Significant	Range of Impaired Functioning Tool: N.S.	Participant ratings of course were positive.

Note. ADIS-C, Anxiety Disorders Interview Schedule for Children; BAI, Beck Anxiety Inventory; BDI, Beck Depression Inventory; BHS, Beck Hopelessness Scale; CASAFS, Children and Adolescent Social and Adaptive Functioning Scale; CASQ, Cleveland Adolescent Sleepiness Questionnaire; CATS, Children's Automatic Thoughts Scale; CBCL, Child Behavior Checklist; CBT, cognitive-behavioral therapy; CCEI, Crown Crisp Experimental Index; CDI, Children's Depression Inventory; CES-D, Center for Epidemiologic Studies Depression Scale; CGAS, Children's Global Assessment Scale; CSRFFI, Colorado Self-Report of Family Functioning Inventory; DSI, Diagnostic Interview Schedule; DY, Four questions to screen for dysthymia based on DSM-IV; EPDS, Edinburgh Postnatal Depression Scale; exp, experimental condition; FU, follow-up; GAF, Global Assessment of Functioning Scale; I, indicated condition; K-SADS-PL, Schedule for Affective Disorders and Schizophrenia for School-Age Children—Present and Lifetime version; LER, Life Events Record; LIFE, Longitudinal Interval Follow-Up Examination; N.S., not significant; PAS, Pleasant Activities Schedule; PBI, Personal Beliefs Inventory; PRP, Penn Resiliency Program; PSFL, Problem Solving for Life; SAQ, Self-Assessment Questionnaire; SCAS, Spence Children's Anxiety Scale; SCID, Structured Clinical Interview for DSM-IV; SPQ, Subjective Probability Questionnaire; SPSI-R, Social Problem-Solving Inventory—Revised; SRQ, Self Rating Questionnaire; YSR, Youth Self-Report form of the Child Behavior Checklist; U, universal condition.

[a]Includes major depression and dysthymia.

based on social learning theory (Bandura, 1977; Lewinsohn, Muñoz, Youngren, & Zeiss, 1986). At the 1-year follow-up, six patients met DSM criteria for MDE during the last year: four in the control group, and two in the experimental condition (both of the latter dropped out of the intervention early). Although results were in the desired direction, the low incidence did not allow sufficient power to test whether the rate of new cases was significantly reduced. Depressive symptoms measured by the Beck Depression Inventory (BDI), but not the Center for Epidemiologic Studies Depression Scale (CES-D), were significantly lower in the intervention condition than in the control condition. There was also evidence of mediation of cognitive-behavioral variables on the reduction in symptoms (Muñoz et al., 1995).

Seligman, Schulman, DeRubeis, and Hollon (1999) conducted a randomized controlled prevention trial that focused on college freshmen. The intervention tested was the Apex Program (Gillham et al., 1991), which includes cognitive restructuring and problem-solving components. Participants were 231 college students who scored in the most pessimistic quartile on a measure of explanatory style. At 3-year follow-up, 11% of controls and 13% of prevention group participants had experienced an MDE, a nonsignificant difference. The investigators reported a significantly lower rate of moderate generalized anxiety in the prevention group. No effects were found for academic achievement, but effects were significant for health factors (Gillham, Shatté, & Freres, 2000). There were significant reductions in both depressive and anxiety symptoms, and evidence that changes in explanatory style, dysfunctional attitudes, and hopelessness partially mediated changes in depressive symptoms.

In summary, preventive interventions for adults have promise but have yet to yield significant reduction in incidence of MDEs. The key will be the combination of identifying groups with higher incidence, increasing the potency of the preventive interventions, and including samples large enough to detect expected effects (generally, sample sizes must be larger in prevention than in treatment trials). We must ask ourselves, however, whether it might be more effective to intervene earlier. Thus, in the next section, we focus on interventions for children in school.

Interventions during the School Years

Epidemiological studies indicate a point prevalence between 0.4% and 2.5% for depressive disorders among prepubertal children (Birmaher et al., 1996). Moreover, the number of children who are experiencing depressive symptoms is much larger (Smucker, Craighead, Craighead, & Green, 1986), and having even a few symptoms of depression is associated with psychosocial impairment and multiple comorbidities (Coyle et al., 2003).

Late childhood or early adolescence may be a particularly fruitful period in which to mount preventive efforts. Depression rates clearly begin to rise in early adolescence, especially for girls, at about age 12 (reviewed by Birmaher et al., 1996), with older adolescents reporting rates of depression close to those seen in adults (Lewinsohn, Hops, Roberts, Seeley, & Andrews, 1993; Weissman, Fendrich, Warner, & Wickramaratne, 1992). Some studies have found that, by age 18, as many as 20% of high school students report experiencing at least one episode of unipolar depression (Lewinsohn et al., 1993), which significantly increases the risk of repeated depressive episodes later in life (Lewinsohn, Rohde, Klein, & Seeley, 1999; Pine, Cohen, Gurley, Brook, & Ma, 1998). Thus, the school years are an important period during which to attempt to prevent and treat depression.

Preventing Depression in Adolescence

INDICATED PREVENTION IN YOUTH WITH ELEVATED SUBDIAGNOSTIC
DEPRESSIVE SYMPTOMS

Clarke and colleagues (1995) administered a self-report depression scale (CES-D) to 1,652 youth in either universal prevention health class curricula or control classrooms. "Demoralized" youth above the 75th percentile on the CES-D, without current affective disorders, were invited to take part in a subsequent indicated prevention study. These demoralized adolescents were randomly assigned to either a 15-session cognitive group prevention intervention (n = 76) or a usual care control condition (n = 74). The prevention program (Clarke & Lewinsohn, 1995) focused on teaching adolescents to identify and challenge irrational or highly negative thoughts (for details, see Clarke, 2000). Prevention subjects reported significantly lower total incidence of MDEs over the 12-month follow-up period (14.5 vs. 25.7%, respectively). A four-site RCT, led by Judy Garber of Vanderbilt University, has recently replicated and extended these findings in a sample of 316 at-risk youth, using enrollment criteria and an intervention similar to Clarke and colleagues. In this replication study (Garber et al., 2007), adolescents were randomly assigned to either the prevention group (8 weekly, 90-minute group sessions followed by 6 monthly sessions), or to treatment as usual (TAU). Youth in both conditions were free to use nonstudy mental health services. There was a significant prevention effect through the 8-month follow-up. The hazard of depression onset was significantly lower in the prevention condition compared to the TAU group (HR = .62, 95% CI .397–.985). Youth in the prevention program showed a lower rate of incident depression (22%) compared to those in TAU (33%; risk difference 11%, Wald chi-square = 4.10; P = .043). Current parental depression at baseline also significantly moderated the effectiveness of the prevention program. Among participants whose parents were not in an active depressive episode at baseline, outcomes for youth in the prevention program (n = 77, 12%) were superior to those for youth in TAU (n = 77, 41%; risk difference = 29%), whereas outcomes for youth whose parents were currently depressed were not significantly different for those in the prevention program (n = 77, 32%) versus TAU (n = 74, 25%; risk difference = 7%).

A recent trial compared an interpersonal psychotherapy—adolescent skills training (IPT-AST) intervention to school counseling (SC) in a sample of inner-city adolescents with elevated depressive symptoms (Young, Mufson, & Davies, 2006). IPT-AST, a modified version of the original IPT—adolescent group intervention (Mufson, Gallagher, Dorta, & Young, 2004), focuses on teaching and practicing skills that can be applied to interpersonal problem areas. There was a significant prevention effect throughout the 6-month follow-up period: 3.7% of the adolescents in the intervention group (1 out of 27) were diagnosed with depression, compared to 28.6% of the comparison group (4 out of 14).

Gillham, Hamilton, Freres, Patton, and Gallop (2006) examined the effectiveness of the Penn Resiliency Program (PRP) delivered by therapists in a health management organization (HMO) primary care setting. At the 2-year follow-up, the intervention yielded a lower incidence of MDEs among high-symptom participants assigned to the PRP (n = 56) than among those in the usual care (n = 57) condition (21 vs. 36%, respectively), but this difference did not reach statistical significance.

Two large-scale, school-based, indicated prevention trials by a team of Australian researchers also failed to produce desired effects on the incidence of MDEs. The first trial examined a cognitive-behavioral therapy (CBT) and problem-solving, teacher-led intervention versus a monitoring control condition (Spence, Sheffield, & Donovan, 2003). Twelve-month findings revealed that high-risk youth assigned to the intervention (n = 111) reported a nonsignificant lower incidence of MDE than did their control (n = 113) counterparts (8.4 vs. 9.9%, respectively); by the 4-year follow-up, there were no significant differences between conditions, because 25% of all participants reported a depressive episode (Spence, Sheffield, & Donovan, 2005). The authors later examined a universal, indicated and combined universal, indicated–CBT intervention approach in a sample (n = 2,479) of 13- to 15-year-olds from 36 schools (Sheffield et al., 2006). Students with "high symptoms" (n = 521) were randomized to one of the four conditions; there were no significant group differences in MDE incidence throughout the 18-month period of investigation.

INDICATED PREVENTION IN YOUTH WITH DEPRESSED PARENTS

Another indicated prevention study was completed with adolescent children of depressed parents (Clarke et al., 2001). Index parents were recruited from HMO-enrolled adults being treated for depression, who had offspring ages 13–18. Youth classified as "demoralized" (i.e., depressive symptoms did not meet full criteria for a DSM-III-R affective disorder, CES-D score greater than 24, and/or with a past MDE) were randomized either to usual HMO care (n = 49) or a 15-session group prevention program using cognitive therapy methods (n = 45). Significant prevention effects were found for self-reported depressive symptoms, as well as global functioning. Survival analyses indicated a significantly lower incidence of MDEs for the experimental condition (9.3% cumulative MDE incidence) compared to the usual care control condition (28.8%) at 14-month follow-up.

Preventing Depression during the Grammar School Years

Prevention work for school-age children is still in the preliminary stages. To date, there have been no universal or selected prevention studies published that focus on the prevention of depressive disorders. Instead, preliminary work falls into the "indicated" category, where studies focus on high-risk populations but only assess changes in depressive symptoms, and not incidence of depressive episodes.

Many sequelae of perinatal depression and other risk factors are already present long before school starts (O'Hara & Swain, 1996). Ideally, one would begin before birth, or even before conception, by reducing the proportion of unintended pregnancies (see Brown & Eisenberg, 1995). We now turn to work that focuses on the beginning of life.

Preventing Perinatal Depression and Depression in Early Childhood

INCIDENCE AND PREVALENCE OF MAJOR DEPRESSION IN THE PRESCHOOL YEARS

The incidence of major depression for children younger than age 6 is not known (Luby, 2000). It is challenging to assess this incidence, because it is uncertain whether symptoms that resemble depression are actually due to depression or are merely developmentally transient and normative difficulties.

To understand the development of emotion dysregulation processes during early childhood, investigators have studied infants and children of depressed parents and the parents themselves (although the majority of these studies focus on mothers; for reviews, see Le & Boyd, 2006; Shafii & Shafii, 1992). Much of this research has documented that perinatal depression has detrimental consequences for the mother, her developing child, and the quality of the mother–infant relationship (Beck, 2006). Moreover, children of depressed parents are at increased risk of becoming depressed themselves in their lifetime (Beardslee, Versage, & Gladstone, 1998; Downey & Coyne, 1990) and, typically, with an earlier onset of first MDE compared to depressed youth whose parents are not depressed (Weissman et al., 2006). Thus, in early childhood, the focus in prevention of depression should begin with mothers-to-be who are at risk for developing depression during pregnancy and the early postpartum period.

PRELIMINARY WORK TOWARD PREVENTION OF PERINATAL MDEs

Few rigorous studies have focused on preventing perinatal depression, most often studied as postpartum depression (PPD). Austin (2003) reviewed five studies that evaluated the efficacy of prenatal interventions aimed at preventing PPD in high-risk women. These interventions varied in terms of sample characteristics, sample size, selection of risk factors, intervention content and characteristics, facilitator background and training, and outcome measures. Two of these studies (Elliott et al., 2000; Zlotnick, Johnson, Miller, Pearlstein, & Howard, 2001) found that the intervention groups had significantly lower depressive symptoms and incidence of PPD than did the control groups at 3-month follow-up; the other three studies did not find differences in outcomes (Brugha et al., 2000; Buist, Westley, & Hill, 1999; Stamp, Williams, & Crowther, 1995). Specifically, Elliott and colleagues (2000) reported that an 11-session psychoeducational group intervention resulted in significantly lower PPD rates in women expecting their first child (39% in the control condition vs. 19% in the intervention). Zlotnick and colleagues (2001; Zlotnick, Miller, Pearlstein, Howard, & Sweeny, 2006) found this effect using two brief interventions based on the IPT approach, which taught women about the transition to motherhood, identifying and resolving interpersonal conflicts, and seeking social support; booster sessions were added to reinforce skills and to problem-solve challenges associated with a newborn child. An initial investigation revealed that the IPT-based approach prevented the onset of PPD in a small sample (n = 37) of pregnant women with at least one risk factor for PPD compared to women assigned to the treatment-as-usual (TAU) condition (0 vs. 33%, respectively; Zlotnick et al., 2001), whereas in a larger (n = 99) investigation, the intervention was associated with a 4% PPD rate at 3-month follow-up compared to a 20% PPD rate in the TAU control condition (Zlotnick et al., 2006).

Recently, Muñoz and colleagues (2007) conducted a randomized pilot trial to evaluate a 12-session weekly cognitive-behavioral group intervention during pregnancy and four booster sessions in the first year postpartum in a sample of 41 predominantly low-income Latinas at high risk for postpartum depression (i.e., history of major depression and/or high depressive symptoms, but not meeting criteria for a current MDE; Le, Muñoz, Soto, Delucchi, & Ghosh Ippen, 2004). The intervention was adapted from the Depression Prevention Course (Muñoz, 1984) for use with pregnant young women (Mothers and Babies Course; Muñoz et al., 2001). Results at 1-year postpartum indicated that 14% of women in the intervention condition developed a new onset of major depression compared to 25% in the usual care condition (not significant; effect size, h = 0.28), with no differences in depressive symptoms (Muñoz et al., 2007).

From the data presented thus far, there is some evidence that the incidence of MDEs can be reduced in women postpartum. Nevertheless, treatment is warranted for those high-risk participants who do go on to develop an MDE. Chabrol and colleagues (2002) addressed this need by designing and testing a two-stage prevention and treatment program for 258 women with elevated symptoms of depression. The prevention intervention was delivered during days 2–5 postpartum, while the women were still hospitalized. Participants reporting elevated depressive symptoms 4–6 weeks postpartum were invited to participate in the treatment intervention, which comprised five to eight 1-hour weekly home visits. The prevention intervention significantly reduced the incidence of *probable* depression, defined as having elevated symptom scores on the Edinburgh Postnatal Depression Scale, a widely used screening measure of risk for PPD (30.2% in the intervention condition vs. 48.2% in the control condition).

Taken together, these investigations provide limited evidence that brief preventive interventions are effective in preventing and reducing the incidence of PPD during the initial period following childbirth, and that such interventions are effective for ethnically diverse women at risk for depression. The available evidence remains equivocal, however, given the inconsistency in demonstrating the positive impact of prevention interventions (Le & Boyd, 2006), the dearth of evidence regarding the long-term impact of such interventions, and the limited number of investigations that have assessed the incidence of MDE meeting full diagnostic criteria versus *probable* cases (e.g., Chabrol et al., 2002). At a broader level, successful RCTs have at least two characteristics. First, they identify groups at high imminent risk (25% or more in 1 year) instead of only lifetime risk. Second, they utilize brief and effective mood management self-help interventions, such as those based on CBT or IPT methods.

PREVENTING DEPRESSION RELAPSE AND RECURRENCE

As stated previously, if the first onset of depression is not prevented, then individuals are at high risk for recurrence after the initial episode resolves (Judd et al., 2000). The same epidemiological evidence that demonstrates an increasing risk of recurrence with each additional episode (Solomon et al., 2000), however, also indicates that recurrence is not inevitable, suggesting that it may be avoidable. Clinical trials that have been careful to distinguish between *relapse* (a resurgence of the episode being treated) and *recurrence* (the emergence of a new episode) have clearly demonstrated that continuing antidepressant medication at the same dose used to resolve the acute episode of depression reduces the likelihood of recurrence (e.g., Frank et al., 1990). Indeed, maintenance medication can reduce the likelihood of subsequent episodes by as much as 70% (Geddes et al., 2003). By definition, all strategies to prevent new episodes of depression following a first onset are considered *maintenance* (Mrazek & Haggerty, 1994), with medication as the primary maintenance strategy in psychiatric practice (American Psychiatric Association, 2000; Geddes et al., 2003).

A primary limitation is that maintenance medication does not extend protection against recurrence once medication use ceases; thus, it is more prophylactic than protective. One study estimated that the risk of recurrence is 11 times greater in those who are withdrawn from maintenance medication (Kupfer et al., 1992), with approximately 40% of individuals experiencing a recurrence within 6 months of withdrawal (Hollon et al., 2005; Kupfer et al., 1992). Thus, although such prophylactic treatment can clearly be effective, it requires the continuous expenditure of resources—in terms of medication costs, clinician time for medication management, and patient exposure to medication-mediated adverse effects—to confer its beneficial effects against recurrence. Follow-up studies of individuals who responded to acute treatment with cognitive therapy (CT) have revealed that once treatment ends, these individuals tend to have lower relapse rates than do those who responded to acute treatment with pharmacotherapy, suggesting that CT may function as an enduring *protective interven-*

tion, and not merely as prophylaxis (Evans et al., 1992; Hollon et al., 2005, 2006). In contrast to prophylactic treatment, protective interventions would be time- and resource-limited, yet still confer protection against recurrence. These studies, however, were subject to a potential "differential sieve" that could have confounded a protective effect of CT with the initial response to treatment (Hollon et al., 2005). Strong tests of protective interventions against recurrence would require, at minimum, randomization either to the protective intervention or to a control condition *after* participants have recovered from the acute episode of major depression, following the classic designs used to test maintenance medication (e.g., Frank et al., 1990).

Although, to our knowledge, no RCT has tested a protective intervention specifically targeting recurrence, findings from a handful of studies have suggested such protective effects. Two trials tested the effectiveness of individual CT in protecting against subsequent episodes after participants had responded to acute treatment with CT (Jarrett et al., 1998) or antidepressant medication (Fava, Rafanelli, Grandi, Conti, & Belluardo, 1998; Fava et al., 2004). Jarrett and colleagues (1998) found that over a 16-month follow-up period, continuing with a brief course of CT reduced relapse rates from 67% in a repeated assessment control to 16% in the CT condition, but only for those with a history of early-onset major depressive disorder. Fava and colleagues (1998, 2004) found that individuals receiving CT, compared to controls receiving clinical management, had a lower likelihood of experiencing a subsequent episode of depression over both 2-year (25 vs. 80%, respectively) and 6-year (40 vs. 90%, respectively) follow-up periods. Two other trials found evidence for the protective effect of group interventions compared to TAU following remission from an acute episode of recurrent depression (Bockting et al., 2005; Teasdale et al., 2000). Compared to TAU, a group CT intervention reduced the rate of subsequent episodes over a 2-year follow-up period from 72 to 46% in individuals with a history of five or more previous episodes of depression (Bockting et al., 2005). Among persons with a history of three or more previous episodes of depression, only 37% of those who received mindfulness-based CT had a subsequent episode of depression over a 60-week follow-up period, compared to the 66% of those who received TAU (Teasdale et al., 2000).

Although none of these trials required participants to have attained recovery prior to randomization and none could specifically test the effectiveness of their interventions against recurrence, the reduction of relapse rates for periods of as much as 6 years increases the likelihood that these protective interventions are not confined to relapse but also extend to recurrence; conservative definitions of recovery currently require at most 6 months of sustained remission (Frank et al., 1991; Rush, Kraemer, et al., 2006). Interestingly, Teasdale and colleagues (2000) found no difference in relapse rates between individuals whose remission was less than 1 year and those whose remission was more than 1 year (and is therefore likely a recovery), further bolstering the implication that recurrence may be prevented by a protective intervention. Thus, although the data to date are not conclusive, they are encouraging that time- and resource-limited interventions can be developed to protect individuals from recurrence once they have attained recovery from an episode of recurrent depression.

To date, these protective effects have been demonstrated only in adults; it is also essential that protective interventions be developed for younger populations given that a recurrent course of depression may begin in earlier stages of life (Beardslee, 2002). Prevention of recurrence in younger populations is an understudied area, but recent demonstrations of the effectiveness of maintenance medication in children increase confidence that maintenance strategies can also be developed for children and adolescents (Emslie et al., 2004).

RECOMMENDATIONS FOR FUTURE RESEARCH AND PRACTICE

In summary, we have identified 13 published RCTs designed to test whether interventions reduced incidence of MDEs. The state of the science as of 2008 is encouraging, because seven of these trials have reported significant reductions in MDE incidence. Successful trials generally identify populations at risk for a high incidence of MDEs and provide interventions that have been shown to be effective in preventing MDEs. It appears that these interventions, such as techniques used in IPT and CBT approaches, can have a preventive effect. Moreover, published studies to date show stronger preventive effects for adolescents than for adults.

Below are five further recommendations that attempt to enhance research in the prevention of depression.

1. Future studies should maximize the ability to clearly detect the prevention of new MDEs by utilizing methods that (a) have successfully identified participants at high imminent risk; and (b) provide a standardized measurement of new MDEs that adhere to current diagnostic criteria. To provide a reasonable test of whether rates of onset of MDEs can be reduced, preventive RCTs need to include a sufficiently long follow-up period (at least 1 year). Prevention studies should test specific, well-defined interventions, so that either positive or negative outcomes can inform the field about the impact of the intervention. Brown and Liao (1999), for example, discuss design issues for prerandomization, intervention, and postintervention, focusing on different examples of prevention research as a primary strategy to prevent mental health problems.

2. The preventive intervention ideally should address healthy development, as well as prevent psychopathology (Muñoz, 1998), by evaluating its impact on associated outcomes that are relevant to the populations of interest. Therefore, studies should also explicitly measure effects on collateral public health problems, such as smoking, other substance abuse, unplanned pregnancies, marital problems, school performance, job performance, and physical health (Muñoz, 2005). Given that depression is highly comorbid, prevention studies should also be designed to evaluate effects on disorders in addition to depression (see, e.g., Seligman et al., 1999). In addition, prevention studies should consciously target varied specific populations, including ethnically diverse and specific age groups. We must avoid a major weakness of the treatment outcome literature, in which few studies test efficacy of depression treatment with ethnic/minority groups. Furthermore, we must address differences in developmental stage: The literature is sorely lacking in the area of prevention of depression among the very young and the old (Le & Boyd, 2006). Finally, prevention studies are more likely to reach their intended audiences if they involve collaboration with community settings, such as the home, schools, health systems, and religious networks, and if their evaluation assesses dimensions such as reach, efficacy, adoptions, implementation, and maintenance (Glasgow, Vogt, & Boles, 1999).

3. Preventive interventions need to be adapted for implementation with innovative methods, not just delivered by licensed professionals (Christensen, Miller, & Muñoz, 1978; Hollon et al., 2002). For example, an intervention provided via television (Muñoz, Glish, Soo-Hoo, & Robertson, 1982) or the Internet (Christensen & Griffiths, 2002; Muñoz et al., 2006) can reach many more people per year than can face-to-face interventions by doctoral-level professionals. Given the need to reach larger groups with preventive interventions, we must develop and test interventions in which the usual ratio of professionals to consumers is significantly smaller. Otherwise, we will have the same shortage of personnel as we do now in terms of providing treatment interventions.

4. The distinction between *relapse* and *recurrence* is an important consideration when evaluating the impact of protective interventions; the first implies that the previous episode has not fully resolved, whereas the second indicates that a new episode has developed (Rush, Kraemer, et al., 2006; Segal, Pearson, & Thase, 2003). Given the mounting evidence that incomplete recovery from depression generally portends a higher risk of subsequent episodes (e.g., Judd et al., 2000; Tranter, O'Donovan, Chandarana, & Kennedy, 2002), full remission should be the optimal target of treatment (Israel, 2006; Keller, 2003; Thase, 2003). It is becoming clearer, however, that a significant proportion of individuals who meet criteria for current definitions of *remission* still have significant symptoms and psychosocial dysfunction (Zimmerman, Posternak, & Chelminski, 2005, 2007). It is quite possible, therefore, that some individuals who achieve remission may still be ill and require additional treatment before prevention strategies are applied. Indeed, given the current state of knowledge, it is unclear whether protective interventions achieve their effects through a sort of psychological inoculation, or whether they merely help individuals achieve a more complete remission. Refinement in the definitions of *remission* and *recovery* that are tied to clinical outcomes clearly are desirable (e.g., see Riso et al., 1997), because such refinements would provide clearer clinical targets for evaluating both treatment and prevention strategies. RCTs to prevent recurrence in participants specifically selected for having achieved strict recovery criteria would contribute significantly to this important and relatively neglected area.

5. Just as it has been demonstrated that we can prevent MDEs within unipolar major depression, is it possible to prevent bipolar disorder? Can interventions aimed at preventing manic or hypomanic episodes be guided by CBT approaches just as they have been in the prevention of unipolar depression? CBT, family-focused therapy, and psychoeducation treatment interventions have demonstrated the most robust effects toward relapse prevention of bipolar disorder (Zaretsky, Rizvi, & Parikh, 2007) and are appropriate as adjunct psychosocial treatments to pharmacotherapy in preventing and prolonging intervals between relapses of bipolar disorder (Miklowitz, 2006; Satterfield, 1999). However, this is clearly an area of research that would benefit from further investigation (for conceptual directions, see Akiskal, 1987).

CONCLUDING REMARKS

Developing methods to prevent the onset of major depression is the next great challenge for the mental health field. The WHO has identified unipolar major depression as the number one cause of disability worldwide (Murray & Lopez, 1996). According to the IOM, major depression is most likely the first mental disorder that we will be able to prevent (Mrazek & Haggerty, 1994). It is time to start the journey toward a world without depression (Muñoz, 2001).

ACKNOWLEDGMENTS

We gratefully acknowledge support from the University of California Office of the President Committee on Latino Research for the University of California, San Francisco (UCSF)/San Francisco General Hospital (SFGH) Latino Mental Health Research Program; Drs. Cloyce Duncan and Gwendolyn Evans for their generous support of the Mothers and Babies Project; and the National Institute of Mental Health (NIMH) (Grant Nos. MH 37992 and MH 596056) for support of the Depression Prevention

Research Project and the Mothers and Babies Intervention Development Project (Ricardo F. Muñoz, Principal Investigator). Huynh-Nhu Le's work was supported by a UCSF/SFGH Clinical Psychology Training Program (CPTP) Fellowship, an NIMH-funded Psychology and Medicine Postdoctoral Fellowship (Nancy Adler, Principal Investigator), the Department of Psychiatry at UCSF, and the Health Resources and Services Administration/Maternal Child Health Bureau (Grant No. R40 MC02497). Alinne Z. Barrera was supported by a CPTP Fellowship and an NIMH National Research Service Award Individual Postdoctoral Fellowship (No. MH 07771). Leandro D. Torres was supported by a CPTP Fellowship.

REFERENCES

Akiskal, H.S. (1987). Overview of biobehavioral factors in the prevention of mood disorders. In R.F. Muñoz (Ed.), *Depression prevention: Research directions* (pp. 263–277). Washington, DC: Hemisphere.

Albee, G. (1985). The argument for primary prevention. *Journal of Primary Prevention, 5,* 213–219.

Alegría, M., Mulvaney-Day, N., Woo, M., Torres, M., Gao, S., Oddo, V., et al. (2007). Correlates of past year mental health service use among Latinos: Results from the National Latino and Asian American Study. *American Journal of Public Health, 97*(1), 76–83.

American Psychiatric Association. (2000). Practice guideline for the treatment of patients with major depressive disorder (revision). *American Journal of Psychiatry, 157*(Suppl. 4), 1–45.

Austin, M. P. (2003). Targeted group antenatal prevention of postnatal depression: A review. *Acta Psychiatrica Scandinavica, 107*(4), 244–250.

Bandura, A. (Ed.). (1977). *Social learning theory.* Englewood Cliffs, NJ: Prentice-Hall.

Barrera, A. Z., Torres, L. D., & Muñoz, R. F. (2007). Prevention of depression: The state of the science at the beginning of the 21st century. *International Review of Psychiatry, 19*(6), 655–670.

Beardslee, W. R. (2002). *Out of the darkened room: When a parent is depressed: Protecting the children and strengthening the family.* New York: Little, Brown.

Beardslee, W. R., Versage, E. M., & Gladstone, T. R. G. (1998). Children of affectively ill parents: A review of the past 10 years. *Journal of the American Academy of Child and Adolescent Psychiatry, 37*(11), 1134–1141.

Beck, C. T. (2006). Postpartum depression: It isn't just the blues. *American Journal of Nursing, 106,* 40–50.

Birmaher, B., Ryan, N. D., Williamson, D. E., Brent, D. A., Kaufman, J., Dahl, R. E., et al. (1996). Childhood and adolescent depression: A review of the past 10 years, Part I. *Journal of the American Academy of Child and Adolescent Psychiatry, 35*(11), 1427–1439.

Bockting, C. L., Schene, A. H., Spinoven, P., Koeter, M. W. J., Wouters, L., Huyser, J., et al. (2005). Preventing relapse/recurrence in recurrent depression with cognitive therapy: A randomized controlled trial. *Journal of Consulting and Clinical Psychology, 73,* 647–657.

Brown, C. H., & Liao, J. (1999). Principles for designing randomized preventive trials in mental health: An emerging developmental epidemiology paradigm. *American Journal of Community Psychology, 27*(5), 673–710.

Brown, S. S., & Eisenberg, L. (Eds.). (1995). *The best intentions: Unintended pregnancy and the well-being of children and families.* Washington, DC: National Academy Press.

Brugha, T. S., Wheatley, S., Taub, N. A., Culverwell, A., Friedman, T., Kirwan, P., et al. (2000). Pragmatic randomized trial of antenatal intervention to prevent post-natal depression by reducing psychosocial risk factors. *Psychological Medicine, 30,* 1273–1281.

Buist, A. E., Westley, D., & Hill, C. (1999). Antenatal prevention of postnatal depression. *Archives of Women's Mental Health 1*(4), 167–173.

Chabrol, H., Teissedre, F., Saint-Jean, M., Teisseyre, N., Rogé, B., & Mullet, E. (2002). Prevention and treatment of post-partum depression: A controlled randomized study on women at risk. *Psychological Medicine, 32,* 1039–1047.

Christensen, A., Miller, W. R., & Muñoz, R. F. (1978). Paraprofessionals, partners, peers, paraphernalia, and print: Expanding mental health service delivery. *Professional Psychology, 9*, 249–270.

Christensen, H., & Griffiths, K. M. (2002). The prevention of depression using the Internet. *Medical Journal of Australia, 177*, S122–S125.

Clarke, G. N. (2000). Prevention of depression in at-risk samples of adolescents. In C. A. Essau & F. Petermann (Eds.), *Depressive disorders in children and adolescents: Epidemiology, risk factors, and treatment* (8th ed., pp. 341–360). Northvale, NJ: Jason Aronson.

Clarke, G. N., Hawkins, W., Murphy, M., Sheeber, L. B., Lewinsohn, P. M., & Seeley, J. R. (1995). Targeted prevention of unipolar depressive disorder in an at-risk sample of high school adolescents: A randomized trial of a group cognitive intervention. *Journal of the American Academy of Child and Adolescent Psychiatry, 34*, 312–321.

Clarke, G. N., Hornbrook, M. C., Lynch, F. L., Polen, M., Gale, J., Beardslee, W. R., et al. (2001). A randomized trial of a group cognitive intervention for preventing depression in adolescent offspring of depressed parents. *Archives of General Psychiatry, 58*, 1127–1134.

Clarke, G. N., & Lewinsohn, P. M. (1995). *Instructor's manual for the Adolescent Coping with Stress Course*. Unpublished manuscript, Center for Health Research, Portland, OR.

Coyle, J. T., Pine, D. S., Charney, D. S., Lewis, L., Nemeroff, C. B., Carlson, G. A., et al. (2003). The Depression and Bipolar Support Alliance Consensus Development Panel: Depression and Bipolar Support Alliance consensus statement on the unmet needs in diagnosis and treatment of mood disorders in children and adolescents. *Journal of the American Academy of Child and Adolescent Psychiatry, 42*(12), 1494–1503.

Cuijpers, P., Van Straten, A., & Smit, F. (2005) Preventing the incidence of new cases of mental disorders: A meta-analytic review. *Journal of Nervous and Mental Disease, 193*(2), 119–125.

Depression Guideline Panel. (1993a). *Depression in primary care: Detection, diagnosis and treatment: Quick reference guide for clinicians* (Clinical Practice Guideline No. 5, AHCPR Publication No. 93-0552). Rockville, MD: Department of Health and Human Services, Public Health Service, Agency for Health Care Policy and Research.

Depression Guideline Panel. (1993b). *Depression in primary care: Vol. 2. Treatment of major depression* (Clinical Practice Guideline No. 5, AHCPR Publication No. 93-0551). Rockville, MD: Department of Health and Human Services, Public Health Service, Agency for Health Care Policy and Research.

Downey, G., & Coyne, J. C. (1990). Children of depressed parents: An integrative review. *Psychological Bulletin, 108*(1), 50–76.

Elliott, S. A., Leverton, T. J., Sanjack, M., Turner, H., Cowmeadow, P., Hopkins, J., et al. (2000). Promoting mental health after childbirth: A controlled trial of primary prevention of postnatal depression. *British Journal of Clinical Psychology, 39*(3), 223–241.

Emslie, G. J., Heiligenstein, J. H., Hoog, S. L., Dineen Wagner, K., Findling, R. L., & McCracken, J. T. (2004). Fluoxetine treatment for prevention of relapse of depression in children and adolescents: A double-blind, placebo-controlled study. *Journal of the American Academy of Child and Adolescent Psychiatry, 43*, 1397–1405.

Evans, M. D., Hollon, S. D., DeRubeis, R. J., Piasecki, J. M., Grove, W. M., Garvery, M. J., et al. (1992). Differential relapse following cognitive therapy and pharmacotherapy for depression. *Archives of General Psychiatry, 49*, 802–808.

Fava, G. A., Rafanelli, C., Grandi, S., Conti, S., & Belluardo, P. (1998). Prevention of recurrent depression with cognitive behavioral therapy: Preliminary findings. *Archives of General Psychiatry, 55*(9), 816–820.

Fava, G. A., Ruini, C., Rafanelli, C., Finos, L., Conti, S., & Grandi, S. (2004). Six-year outcome of cognitive behavior therapy for prevention of recurrent depression. *American Journal of Psychiatry, 161*, 1872–1876.

Frank, E., Kupfer, D. J., Perel, J. M., Cornes, C., Jarret, D. B., Mallinger, A. G., et al. (1990). Three-year outcomes for maintenance therapies in recurrent depression. *Archives of General Psychiatry, 47*, 1093–1099.

Frank, E., Prien, R. F., Jarrett, R. B., Keller, M. B., Kupfer, D. J., Lavori, P. W., et al. (1991). Conceptualization and rationale for consensus definitions of terms in major depressive disorder: Remission, recovery, relapse, and recurrence. *Archives of General Psychiatry, 48*, 851–855.

Garber, J. (2006). Depression in children and adolescents: Linking risk, research, and prevention. *American Journal of Preventive Medicine, 31*(6), 104–125.

Garber, J., Brent, D., Clarke, G., Beardslee, W., Weersing, V. R., Gladstone, T., et al. (2007, October). *Prevention of depression in at-risk adolescents: Rationale, design, and preliminary results.* Paper presented at the annual conference of the American Academy of Child and Adolescent Psychiatry, Boston.

Geddes, J. R., Carney, S. M., Davies, C., Furukawa, T. A., Kupfer, D. J., Frank, E., et al. (2003). Relapse prevention with antidepressant drug treatment in depressive disorders: A systematic review. *Lancet, 361*, 653–661.

Gillham, J. E., Hamilton, J., Freres, D. R., Patton, K., & Gallop, R. (2006). Preventing depression among early adolescents in the primary care setting: A randomized controlled study of the Penn Resiliency Program. *Journal of Abnormal Child Psychology, 34*(2), 203–219.

Gillham, J. E., Jaycox, L., Reivich, K., Hollon, S. D., Freeman, A., DeRubeis, R. J., et al. (1991). *The Apex Project manual for group leaders.* Unpublished manuscript, University of Pennsylvania, Philadelphia.

Gillham, J. E., Shatté, A. J., & Freres, D. R. (2000). Preventing depression: A review of cognitive-behavioral and family interventions. *Applied and Preventive Psychology, 9*(2), 63–88.

Glasgow, R. F., Vogt, T. M., & Boles, S. M. (1999). Evaluating the public health impact of health promotions interventions: The RE-AIM framework. *American Journal of Public Health, 89*, 1322–1327.

Hollon, S. D., DeRubeis, R. J., Shelton, R. C., Amsterdam, J. D., Salomon, R. M., O'Reardon, J. P., et al. (2005). Prevention of relapse following cognitive therapy versus medication in moderate to severe depression. *Archives of General Psychiatry, 62*, 417–422.

Hollon, S. D., Muñoz, R. F., Barlow, D. H., Beardslee, W. R., Bell, C. C., Bernal, G., et al. (2002). Psychosocial intervention development for the prevention and treatment of depression: Promoting innovation and increasing access. *Biological Psychiatry, 52*, 610–630.

Hollon, S. D., Stewart, M. O., & Strunk, D. (2006). Enduring effects for cognitive behavior therapy in the treatment of depression and anxiety. *Annual Review of Psychology, 57*, 285–315.

Horowitz, J. L., & Garber, J. (2006). The prevention of depressive symptoms in children and adolescents: A meta-analytic review. *Journal of Consulting and Clinical Psychology, 74*(3), 401–415.

Hough, R. L., Landsverk, J. A., Karno, M., Burnam, M. A., Timbers, D. M., Escobar, J. I., et al. (1987). Utilization of health and mental health services by Los Angeles Mexican-Americans and non-hispanic whites. *Archives of General Psychiatry, 44*(8), 702–709.

Israel, J. A. (2006). Remission in depression: Definition and initial treatment approaches. *Journal of Psychopharmacology, 20*(Suppl. 3), 5–10.

Jarrett, R. B., Baco, M. R., Risser, R. C., Ramanan, J., Marwill, M., Kraft, D., et al. (1998). Is there a role for continuation phase cognitive therapy for depressed outpatients? *Journal of Consulting and Clinical Psychology, 66*, 1036–1040.

Judd, L. L. (1997). The clinical course of unipolar major depressive disorders. *Archives of General Psychiatry, 54*, 989–991.

Judd, L. L., Paulus, M. J., Schettler, P. J., Akiskal, H. S., Endicott, J., Leon, A. C., et al. (2000). Does incomplete recovery from first lifetime major depressive episode herald a chronic course of illness? *American Journal of Psychiatry, 157*, 1501–1504.

Keller, M. B. (2003). Past, present and future directions for defining optimal treatment outcomes in depression: Remission and beyond. *Journal of the American Medical Association, 289*, 3152–3160.

Kessler, R. C., Berglund, P., Demler, O., Jin, R., Merikangas, K. R., & Walters, E. E. (2005). Lifetime prevalence and age-of-onset distributions of DSM-IV disorders in the National Comorbidity Survey Replication. *Archives of General Psychiatry, 62*, 593–602.

Kessler, R. C., McGonagle, K. A., Shanyang, Z., Nelson, C. B., Hughes, M., Eshleman, S., et al. (1994). Lifetime and 12-month prevalence of DSM-III-R psychiatric disorders in the United States: Results from the National Comorbidity Survey. *Archives of General Psychiatry, 51*(1), 8–19.

Kupfer, D. J., Frank, E., Perel, J. M., Cornes, C., Mallinger, A. G., Thase, M. E., et al. (1992). Five-year outcome for maintenance therapies in recurrent depression. *Archives of General Psychiatry, 49*, 769–773.

Le, H. N., & Boyd, R. C. (2006). Prevention of major depression: Early detection and early intervention in the general population. *Clinical Neuropsychiatry, 3*(1), 6–22.

Le, H. N., Muñoz, R. F., Ghosh Ippen, C., & Stoddard, J. (2003). Treatment is not enough: We must prevent major depression in women. *Prevention and Treatment, 6*, Article 10. Retrieved February 24, 2007, from *psycnet.apa.org/fa=main.doiLanding&doi=10.1037/1522-3736.6.1.6102*

Le, H. N., Muñoz, R. F., Soto, J., Delucchi, K., & Ghosh Ippen, C. (2004). Identifying risk for onset of major depressive episodes in a low-income Latinas during pregnancy and postpartum. *Hispanic Journal of Behavioral Sciences, 26*, 463–482.

Lewinsohn, P. M., Hops, H., Roberts, R. E., Seeley, J. R., & Andrews, J. A. (1993). Adolescent psychopathology: I. Prevalence and incidence of depression and other DSM-III-R disorders in high school students. *Journal of Abnormal Psychology, 102*, 133–144.

Lewinsohn, P. M., Muñoz, R. F., Youngren, M. A., & Zeiss, A. M. (1986). *Control your depression.* New York: Prentice Hall.

Lewinsohn, P. M., Rohde, P., Klein, D. N., & Seeley, J. R. (1999). Natural course of adolescent major depressive disorder: I. Continuity into young adulthood. *Journal of the American Academy of Child and Adolescent Psychiatry, 38*, 56–63.

Luby, J. L. (2000). Depression. In C. H. Zeanah (Ed.), *Handbook of infant mental health* (2nd ed., pp. 382–396). New York: Guilford Press.

Mendelson, T., & Muñoz, R. F. (2006). Prevention of depression in women. In C. L. M. Keyes & S. H. Goodman (Eds.), *Women and depression: A handbook for the social, behavioral, and biomedical sciences* (pp. 450–478). New York: Cambridge University Press.

Miklowitz, D. J. (2006). A review of evidence-based psychosocial interventions for bipolar disorder. *Journal of Clinical Psychiatry, 67*(Suppl. 11), 28–33.

Mrazek, P., & Haggerty, R. (1994). *Reducing risks for mental disorders: Frontiers for preventive intervention research.* Washington, DC: National Academy Press.

Mufson, L., Gallagher, T., Dorta, K. P., & Young, J. F. (2004). Interpersonal psychotherapy for adolescent depression: Adaptation for group therapy. *American Journal of Psychotherapy, 58*, 220–237.

Muñoz, R. F. (1984). *The Depression Prevention Course.* Retrieved May 9, 2007, from *www.medschool. ucsf.edu/latino/manuals.aspx*.

Muñoz, R. F. (1998). Preventing major depression by promoting emotion regulation: A conceptual framework and some practical tools. *International Journal of Mental Health Promotion* (Inaugural Issue), 23–40.

Muñoz, R. F. (2001). On the road to a world without depression. *Journal of Primary Prevention, 21*, 325–338.

Muñoz, R. F. (2005). *La depresión y la salud de nuestros pueblos* [Depression and the health of our communities]. *Salud Mental, 28*(4), 1–9. Retrieved February 24, 2007, from *www.inprf-cd.org.mx/pdf/ sm2804/sm280401.pdf*

Muñoz, R. F., Ghosh-Ippen, C., Le, H. N., Lieberman, A. F., Diaz, M. A., & La Plante, L. (2001). *The Mothers and Babies Course: A reality management approach* [Participant manual]. Retrieved May 9, 2007, from *www.medschool.ucsf.edu/latino/manuals.aspx*

Muñoz, R. F., Glish, M., Soo-Hoo, T., & Robertson, J. L. (1982). The San Francisco Mood Survey Project: Preliminary work toward the prevention of depression. *American Journal of Community Psychology, 10*, 317–329.

Muñoz, R. F., Le, H. N., Clarke, G., & Jaycox, L. (2002). Preventing the onset of major depression. In I. H. Gotlib & C. L. Hammen (Eds.), *Handbook of depression* (pp. 343–359). New York: Guilford Press.

Muñoz, R. F., Le, H. N., Ghosh Ippen, C., Diaz, M. A., Urizar, G. G., Soto, J., et al. (2007). Prevention of postpartum depression in low-income women: Development of the Mothers and Babies Course. *Cognitive and Behavioral Practice, 14*, 70–83.

Muñoz, R. F., Lenert, L. L., Delucchi, K., Stoddard, J., Pérez, J. E., Penilla, C., et al. (2006). Toward evidence-based Internet interventions: A Spanish/English web site for international smoking cessation trials. *Nicotine and Tobacco Research, 8*, 77–87.

Muñoz, R. F., & Ying, Y. (1993). *The prevention of depression: Research and practice.* Baltimore: Johns Hopkins University Press.

Muñoz, R. F., Ying, Y. W., Armas, R., Chan, F., & Gurza, R. (1987). The San Francisco Depression Prevention Research Project: A randomized trial with medical outpatients. In R. F. Muñoz (Ed.), *Depression prevention: Research directions* (pp. 199–215). Washington, DC: Hemisphere.

Muñoz, R. F., Ying, Y. W., Bernal, G., Pérez-Stable, E. J., Sorensen, J. L., Hargreaves, W. A., et al. (1995). Prevention of depression with primary care patients: A randomized controlled trial. *American Journal of Community Psychology, 23*(2), 199–222.

Murray, C. J. L., & Lopez, A. D. (1996). *The global burden of disease: Summary.* Boston: Harvard University Press.

O'Hara, M. W., & Swain, A. M. (1996). Rates and risk of postpartum depression: A meta-analysis. *International Review of Psychiatry, 8*(1), 37–54.

Ojeda, V. D., & McGuire, T. G. (2006). Gender and racial/ethnic differences in use of outpatient mental health and substance use services by depressed adults. *Psychiatric Quarterly, 77,* 211–222.

Paykel, E. S., Scott, J., Teasdale, J. D., Johnson, A. L., Garland, A., Moore, R., et al. (1999). Prevention of relapse in residual depression by cognitive therapy: A controlled trial. *Archives of General Psychiatry, 56*(9), 829–835.

Pérez, J., & Muñoz, R. F. (2008). Prevention of Depression in Latinos. In S. Aguilar-Gaxiola & T. Gullotta (Eds.), *Depression in Latinos: Assessment, treatment, and prevention* (pp. 117–139). New York: Springer.

Pine, D. S., Cohen, P., Gurley, D., Brook, J., & Ma, Y. (1998). The risk for early-adulthood anxiety and depressive disorders in adolescents with anxiety and depressive disorders. *Archives of General Psychiatry, 55,* 56–64.

Riso, L. P., Thase, M. E., Howland, R. H., Friedman, E. S., Simons, A. D., & Tu, X. M. (1997). A prospective test of criteria for response, remission, relapse, recovery, and recurrence in depressed patients treated with cognitive behavior therapy. *Journal of Affective Disorders, 43,* 131–142.

Rush, A. J., Kraemer, H. C., Sackelm, H. A., Fava, M., Trivedi, M. H., Frank, E., et al. (2006). Report by the ACNP task force on response and remission in major depressive disorder. *Neuropsychopharmacology, 31,* 1841–1853.

Rush, A. J., Trivedi, M. H., Wisniewski, S. R., Nierenberg, A. A., Stewart, J. W., Warden, D., et al. (2006). Acute and longer-term outcomes in depressed outpatients requiring one or several treatment steps: A STAR*D report. *American Journal of Psychiatry, 163*(11), 1905–1917.

Satterfield, J. M. (1999). Adjunctive cognitive-behavioral therapy for rapid-cycling bipolar disorder: An empirical case study. *Psychiatry, 62,* 357–369.

Segal, Z. V., Pearson, J. L., & Thase, M. E. (2003). Challenges in preventing relapse in major depression: Report of a National Institute of Mental Health Workshop on the state of the science of relapse prevention in major depression. *Journal of Affective Disorders, 77,* 97–108.

Seligman, M. E. P., Schulman, P., DeRubeis, R. J., & Hollon, S. D. (1999). The prevention of depression and anxiety. *Prevention and Treatment, 2,* Article 8.

Shafii, M., & Shafii, S. L. (1992). Clinical manifestations and developmental psychopathology of depression. In *Clinical guide to depression in children and adolescents* (pp. 3–42). Washington, DC: American Psychiatric Press.

Sheffield, J. K., Spence, S. H., Rapee, R. M., Kowalenko, N., Wignall, A., Davis, A., et al. (2006). Evaluation of universal, indicated, and combined cognitive-behavioral approaches to the prevention of depression among adolescents. *Journal of Consulting and Clinical Psychology, 74*(1), 66–79.

Smucker, M. R., Craighead, W. E., Craighead, L. W., & Green, B. J. (1986). Normative and reliability data for the Children's Depression Inventory. *Journal of Abnormal Child Psychology, 14*(1), 25–39.

Solomon, D. A., Keller, M. B., Leon, A. C., Mueller, T. I., Lavori, P. W., Shea, M. T., et al. (2000). Multiple recurrences of major depressive disorder. *American Journal of Psychiatry, 157,* 229–233.

Spence, S. H., Sheffield, J. K., & Donovan, C. L. (2003). Preventing adolescent depression: An evaluation of the Problem Solving for Life Program. *Journal of Consulting and Clinical Psychology, 71*(1), 3–13.

Spence, S. H., Sheffield, J. K., & Donovan, C. L. (2005). Long-term outcome of a school-based, universal approach to prevention of depression in adolescents. *Journal of Consulting and Clinical Psychology, 73*(1), 160–167.

Stamp, G. E., Williams, A. S., & Crowther, C. A. (1995). Evaluation of antenatal and postnatal support to overcome postnatal depression: A randomized, controlled trial. *Birth*, *22*(3), 138–143.

Teasdale, J. D., Segal, Z. V., Williams, J. M. G., Ridgeway, V. A., Soulsby, J. M., & Lau, M. A. (2000). Prevention of relapse/recurrence in major depression by mindfulness-based cognitive therapy. *Journal of Consulting and Clinical Psychology*, *68*(4), 615–623.

Thase, M. E. (2003). Achieving remission and managing relapse in depression. *Journal of Clinical Psychiatry*, *64*(Suppl. 18), 3–7.

Tranter, R., O'Donovan, C., Chandarana, P., & Kennedy, S. (2002). Prevalence and outcome of partial remission in depression. *Journal of Psychiatry and Neuroscience*, *27*, 241–247.

Weissman, M. M., Fendrich, M., Warner, V., & Wickramaratne, P. (1992). Incidence of psychiatric disorder in offspring at high and low risk for depression. *Journal of the American Academy of Child and Adolescent Psychiatry*, *31*, 640–648.

Weissman, M. M., Wickramaratne, P., Nomura, Y., Warner, V., Pilowsky, D., & Verdeli, H. (2006). Offspring of depressed parents: 20 years later. *American Journal of Psychiatry*, *163*, 1001–1008.

Young, J. F., Mufson, L., & Davies, M. (2006). Efficacy of Interpersonal Psychotherapy—Adolescent Skills Training: An indicated prevention intervention for depression. *Journal of Child Psychology and Psychiatry, and Allied Disciplines*, *47*(12), 1254–1262.

Zaretsky, A. E., Rizvi, S., & Parikh, S. V. (2007). How well do psychosocial interventions work in bipolar disorder? *Canadian Journal of Psychiatry*, *52*(1), 14–21.

Zimmerman, M., Posternak, M. A., & Chelminski, I. (2005). Is the cutoff to define remission on the Hamilton Rating Scale for Depression too high? *Journal of Nervous and Mental Disease*, *193*, 170–175.

Zimmerman, M., Posternak, M. A., & Chelminski, I. (2007). Heterogeneity among depressed outpatients considered to be in remission. *Comprehensive Psychiatry*, *48*, 113–117.

Zlotnick, C., Johnson, S. L., Miller, I. W., Pearlstein, T., & Howard, M. (2001). Postpartum depression in women receiving public assistance: Pilot study of an interpersonal-therapy-oriented group intervention. *American Journal of Psychiatry*, *158*(4), 638–640.

Zlotnick, C., Miller, I. W., Pearlstein, T., Howard, M., & Sweeny, P. (2006). A preventive intervention for pregnant women on public assistance at risk for postpartum depression. *American Journal of Psychiatry*, *163*(8), 1443–1445.

CHAPTER 24

Pharmacotherapy and Other Somatic Treatments for Depression

Michael J. Gitlin

Antidepressants have been available for over half a century. Preceded by insulin shock and then electroconvulsive therapy (ECT), the first antidepressants—imipramine, a tricylic agent, and iproniazid, a monoamine oxidase (MAO) inhibitor—were first demonstrated as effective in the 1950s. After 30+ years of very slow progress in the area, in 1987, the first agent of the second generation of antidepressants, fluoxetine (Prozac), was released. Within a brief period of time, clinicians and patients alike realized that the new agents "felt" different than the older agents. Their side effect profiles differed, compliance rates were higher, and their efficacy in a wider spectrum of disorders was apparent. In the last two decades, 11 antidepressants (and a unique delivery system of an older agent) with a variety of biological effects, chemical structures and differing side effects have been released, representing a minor explosion of treatment options. Yet there is no substantial evidence that any of our newer agents are more effective (as defined by response or remission rates; see below for details) than imipramine, our original 1950s prototype.

At this point, antidepressants are absolute mainstays of modern psychopharmacology, prescribed liberally by primary care physicians and other physician specialists, in addition to psychiatrists. However, conflict and concern about whether antidepressants are overprescribed, or whether their risks have been minimized, continue. The best example of this is the mixture of thoughtful discussion and unreasonable hysteria surrounding the issue of antidepressants and their potential for causing new-onset suicidality in children/adolescents and, to a lesser degree, adults (see Berman, Chapter 22, this volume, for details). These polarized opinions have obscured both the knowledge gained and the knowledge gaps in antidepressant therapies. In this chapter, a middle ground approach will be presented. It reviews the phases of treatment for depression with antidepressants; the choices of available agents; the advantages and disadvantages of the antidepressant classes and agents; the choices for treating nonresponsive patients; the use of somatic, nonpharmacological treatments for de-

pression; the use of antidepressants for special populations; and continuation and maintenance treatments. The chapter concludes with a summary of some of the current critical,
clinical research questions in the area.

PHASES OF PHARMACOTHERAPY OF DEPRESSION

Antidepressants can be prescribed for any one of three goals or phases described as *acute*,
continuation, and *maintenance* treatment. The goal of acute treatment is to alleviate the
symptoms of an active depression. The goal of continuation treatment is to prevent a relapse
into the same episode for which treatment was begun. By definition, *continuation* treatment
begins at the time of remission from the acute depressive episode. The reasons for the longer
length of time—typically measured in months, not weeks—needed for continuation treatment (as opposed to acute treatment) are unknown. This may reflect simply protecting a patient from relapse until spontaneous remission might have occurred without treatment. Another possibility is that, as with other disorders in medicine, clinical remission precedes
biological remission. Longer time may be needed for the therapeutic effects of antidepressants on brain function to become more permanent. Maintenance therapy is considered to
begin when the goal is to prevent future recurrences of depressive episodes (or to prevent a
recurrence of depressive symptoms following the successful treatment of a chronic depression). Given the recent data on the natural history of depression (see Thase, Chapter 9, this
volume), consideration of maintenance treatment with antidepressants should commonly be
discussed with patients.

   These phases of treatment follow naturally from one to another. This chapter focuses
intensively on acute treatment, following which both the data and current clinical practice
on continuation and maintenance treatment are presented.

ACUTE PHARMACOLOGICAL TREATMENT OF DEPRESSION

Currently Available Agents

Table 24.1 shows the 26 antidepressants available at the beginning of 2007, divided into
pharmacological classes, with typical dose ranges. Table 24.2 lists the antidepressants by
their side effect profiles. No classification scheme is either consistent or comprehensive; each
class is defined by different unifying characteristics. The tricyclic antidepressants share a
similar chemical structure and a relatively similar side effect profile, but differ in their neurotransmitter effects. Selective serotonin reuptake inhibitors (SSRIs) vary widely in chemical
structure but share similar neurotransmitter effects and side effect profiles. The two dual-
action agents share the effect of enhancing both serotoninergic and noradrenergic function.
MAO inhibitors also share both biological effects and a common side effect profile, although the recent release of selegiline in a skin patch form provides an option unique in its
delivery system and somewhat different in its side effect profile (see below). The other
agents, listed as novel agents, are each dissimilar from each other and from other classes.
Conceptually, each novel agent should be listed as a separate class of antidepressants containing only one currently available medication.

   All currently available antidepressants alter the function of either central nervous system serotonin or norepinephrine, or both. The mechanisms of action by which antidepressants precipitate mood changes are still obscure. Yet explaining antidepressant efficacy by

TABLE 24.1. Antidepressants

Class[a]	Typical starting dose (mg)	Usual dosage range (mg daily)
Selective serotonin reuptake inhibitors (SSRIs)		
Citalopram (Celexa)	10–20	20–60
S-citalopram (Lexapro)	5–10	10–30
Fluoxetine (Prozac)	10–20	10–80
Fluvoxamine (Luvox)	25–50	100–300
Paroxetine (Paxil)	10–20	20–60
Sertraline (Zoloft)	25–50	50–200
Novel antidepressants		
Bupropion (Wellbutrin)	100–150	300–450
Mirtazapine (Remeron)	15–30	15–60
Nefazodone (Serzone)	50	400–600
Trazodone[b] (Desyrel)	50	150–400
Dual-action agents		
Venlafaxine (Effexor)	37.5–75	150–300
Duloxetine (Cymbalta)	20–30	60–120
Tricyclics + related compounds		
Amitriptyline (Elavil, Endep)	25–50	100–300
Amoxapine (Asendin)	50–100	150–400
Clomipramine (Anafranil)	25–50	100–250
Desipramine (Norpramin, Pertofrane)	25–50	100–300
Doxepin (Sinequan, Adapin)	25–50	100–300
Imipramine (Tofranil)	25–50	100–300
Maprotiline(Ludiomil)	25–50	100–225
Nortriptyline (Aventyl, Pamelor)	10–25	50–150
Protriptyline (Vivactil)	10	15–60
Trimipramine (Surmontil)	25–50	100–300
Monoamine oxidase inhibitors (MAOIs)		
Isocarboxazid (Marplan)	10–20	30–60
Phenelzine (Nardil)	15–30	30–90
Selegiline (Eldepryl)	10	20–60
Selegiline transdermal (Emsam patch)	6	6–12
Tranylcypromine (Parnate)	10–20	30–60

[a]Trade name is in parentheses.

[b]Rarely used as antidepressant; prescribed more in low dose as hypnotic.

initial effects on these neurotransmitters is naive and likely to be incorrect. As an example, tricyclics and SSRIs block the reuptake of norephinephrine and/or serotonin into the presynaptic neuron, thereby allowing more of the neurotransmitter to be available to the postsynaptic neuron. This effect is relatively immediate after a first antidepressant dose, yet patients do not improve immediately. The temporal dissociation of a biological effect from a clinical effect implies that another set of biological effects may be more relevant. Thus, a second set of hypotheses examine the "downstream" effects of antidepressants (i.e., the effects beyond the cell surface receptor sites). Areas of active investigation are the intracellular second messenger systems and more specific effects on intracellular protein synthesis. A third and most recent set of hypotheses focuses on the effects of antidepressants in enhancing neuronal growth—both *neurogenesis*, the production of new neurons in adults, and enhancing neuronal function by the sprouting of dendrites, called *dendritic arborization*. These effects are regulated in part by a brain peptide, brain-derived neurotropic factor (BDNF). Of note, antidepressants have been shown to increase neurogenesis in rats. Furthermore, the antidepressant classes that have shown these positive effects include SSRIs, tricyclic antidepressants, and MAO inhibitors (Duman & Monteggia, 2006). The positive effects on neuronal remodeling and neurogenesis seem to require 2–4 weeks of treatment, similar to the overall time frame of clinical response to these agents in depressed individuals. ECT, with its well-documented antidepressant effects, also increases BDNF expression, as does transcranial magnetic stimulation (TMS), a more recently described antidepressant treatment (see below for details).

Selective Serotonin Reuptake Inhibitors

The antidepressants in this class still dominate the treatment of depression in the United States. Their popularity reflects their relatively benign side effect profile and the fact that the initial dose is close to the therapeutic dose, thereby making careful, slow dose titration unnecessary. Additionally, because all the SSRIs except S-citalopram are now available as generic preparations, their cost is relatively low. Although all SSRIs strongly block the presynaptic reuptake of serotonin, which increases its availability to the postsynaptic neuron, thereby enhancing serotoninergic function, the individual agents are not biologically identical, merely similar. As examples, citalopram (Celexa) is the most selective of the SSRIs, fluoxetine the least; sertraline (Zoloft) additionally blocks the reuptake of dopamine (albeit weakly). The clinical significance of these differences is unclear. Some experts hypothesize that these biological differences may explain the study results and clinical observation that one individual patient may respond better to one SSRI than to another, but no data address this question. The most recently released of the SSRIs, S-citalopram (Lexapro), is the "S" or left isomer (referring to the direction of the molecules of a compound, analogous to left vs. right hands). Although its side effect profile is minimally different from citalopram (it is slightly less sedating), it is very similar in most characteristics.

All SSRIs share a relatively similar side effect profile (see Table 24.2). The common side effects potentially seen with all SSRIs are nausea, activation (insomnia, nervousness), sedation, and sexual side effects. Nausea and activation effects are seen maximally in the beginning of treatment and diminish over the first few days to weeks of treatment. In contrast, tolerance does not typically develop to sedation and sexual side effects, making these more problematic side effects in the long term. In general, rates of nausea and sexual side effects are relatively similar across individual SSRI agents. Rates of sedation and activation, however, differ. Fluoxetine and sertraline are most commonly associated with activation effects, whereas paroxetine and fluvoxamine are more likely to cause sedation.

Another difference between the individual SSRI antidepressants is their capacity to alter the metabolism of other medications through the cytochrome P450 system, the group of hepatic (liver) enzymes that metabolize foods, toxins, and medications (Spina, Scordo, & D'Arrigo, 2003). Because the P450 system comprises many different enzymes, each of which metabolize different medications, and each SSRI has a different profile of P450 effects, simple generalizations are impossible. With healthy patients on no other medications (thereby precluding drug–drug interactions), these effects are irrelevant. For medically complicated depressed persons who may be on many other medications, the possibility of interactions may be important. Although interindividual variability is large, fluoxetine, paroxetine, and

TABLE 24.2. Common Side Effects of Antidepressants

Name[a]	Sedation	Stimulation hypotension	Postural effects	Anticholinergic	Other side effects
Selective serotonin reuptake inhibitors (SSRIs)					
Citalopram (Celexa)	+	+	0	0	Sexual
S-citalopram (Lexapro)	0+	+	0	0	Sexual
Fluoxetine (Prozac)	0+	+++	0	0	Sexual
Fluvoxamine (Luvox)	+	+	0	0	Sexual
Paroxetine (Paxil)	+	+	0	+	Sexual, weight gain
Sertraline (Zoloft)	0+	++	0	0	Sexual
Novel antidepressants					
Bupropion (Wellbutrin)	0	++	0	0	
Mirtazapine (Remeron)	+++	0	0	0	Weight gain
Nefazodone (Serzone)	+++	0	++	0	
Trazodone (Desyrel)	+++	0	+++	0	
Dual-action agents					
Venlafaxine (Effexor)	+	+	0	0	Dose-related hypertension
Duloxetine (Cymbalta)	0+	0+	0	0	Nausea, dry mouth, constipation
Tricyclics and related compounds					
Amitriptyline (Elavil, Endep)	+++	0	+++	+++	
Amoxapine (Asendin)	+	0	++	+	
Clomipramine (Anafranil)	+++	0	+++	+++	
Desipramine (Norpramin, Pertofrane)	+	+	++	+	
Doxepin (Sinequan, Adapin)	+++	0	++	++	
Imipramine (Tofranil)	++	+	+++	++	
Maprotiline (Ludiomil)	++	+	+	+	
Nortriptyline (Aventyl, Pamelor)	++	0	+	+	
Protriptyline (Vivactil)	+	+	++	+++	

(*continued*)

TABLE 24.2. (continued)

Name[a]	Sedation	Stimulation hypotension	Postural effects	Anticholinergic	Other side effects
Trimipramine (Surmontil)	+++	0	++	+++	
Monoamine oxidase inhibitors (MAOIs)					
Isocarboxazid (Marplan)	++	+	+++	+	Weight gain, insomnia, sexual
Phenelzine (Nardil)	++	+	+++	+	Weight gain, insomnia, sexual
Selegiline (Eldepryl)	+	+	++	+	
Selegiline transdermal (Emsam)	0	+	+	0+	Skin reaction to patch
Tranylcypromine (Parnate)	+	+	+++	+	Insomnia, sexual

[a]Trade name is in parentheses.

fluvoxamine have greater potential for P450 interactions than do citalopram, S-citalopram, and sertraline.

Bupropion

Bupropion (Wellbutrin), available in an immediate release (IR) preparation, sustained release (SR), and a once daily more extended release (XL), is a novel agent with effects on norepinephrine and dopamine and no serotoninergic effects (Asher et al., 1995). Bupropion is a stimulating antidepressant, with the most common side effects of insomnia, anxiety, tremor, and headache. It is never sedating and is associated with virtually no sexual side effects and no weight gain. The IR and SR forms should be administered in divided dose, whereas the XL form can be taken once daily. All three preparations are available in generic form. The major safety concern is bupropion's propensity to cause seizures at a slightly higher rate than the other new antidepressants (Davidson, 1989). Bupropion is contraindicated in patients with seizure disorders or active eating disorders, such as bulimia nervosa or anorexia nervosa (which lower the seizure threshold, presumably via electrolyte abnormalities).

Dual-Action Agents: Venlafaxine and Duloxetine

At a low to moderate dose (up to 125 mg or so), venlafaxine (Effexor) is an SSRI with strong, selective effects on serotonin. As the dose is increased beyond that level, reuptake blockade of norepinephrine begins, giving venlafaxine a dual effect (Harvey, Rudolph, & Preskorn, 2000). Some studies indicate that, especially at higher doses, venlafaxine may show greater efficacy than the SSRIs, especially for more severely depressed individuals. The side effect profile of venlafaxine is almost identical to that of the SSRIs. As venlafaxine doses increase, a dose-related hypertension may emerge, affecting up to 9% of treated patients at high dose (Thase, 1998). Therefore, at daily doses of 150 mg or above, blood pressure monitoring is required. Venlafaxine XR is usually prescribed because of its lower rate of nausea compared to venlafaxine IR.

Duloxetine (Cymbalta), released in 2004, also blocks the reuptake of both norepinephrine and serotonin, but it does so in a more balanced manner, affecting both neurotransmitter systems at all prescribed doses. The clinical significance of this is unclear. Aside from its antidepressant efficacy (Kornstein, Wohlreich, Mallinckrodt, Watkin, & Stewart, 2006), duloxetine is both effective and commonly prescribed for neuropathic pain (e.g., diabetic neuropathy and postherpetic neuralgia) (Goldstein, Lu, Detke, Lee, & Iyengar, 2005). Its side effect profile differs somewhat from both the SSRIs and venlafaxine, in that its most common side effects are nausea early in treatment, dry mouth, and constipation. For unclear reasons, it may have a somewhat lower sexual side effect liability compared to the SSRIs (Delgado et al., 2005). In contrast to venlafaxine, duloxetine does not confer any consistent risk of hypertension (Thase et al., 2005).

Nefazodone

Nefazodone has a unique biological profile, in that it only weakly blocks the reuptake of serotonin, has weak noradrenergic activity, and strongly blocks the serotonin (5-HT$_2$) receptor (Taylor et al., 1995). It is unclear how this translates into antidepressant activity. Nefazodone can be highly sedating, thereby making its use preferable in anxious, agitated, insomniac patients. Nefazodone's full antidepressant efficacy is seen at higher doses (400–600 mg) than originally thought (Keller et al., 2000). Many patients have difficulty achieving these doses because of the sedation. Advantages of nefazodone are the lack of sexual side effects and lack of weight gain associated with its use. Unfortunately, nefazodone has more recently been demonstrated to cause rare but potentially fatal hepatic (liver) toxicity (Lucena, Carvajal, Andrade, & Velasco, 2003). Because of this, the proprietary preparation, Serzone, was voluntarily withdrawn from the market, and few new patients are prescribed generic nefazodone.

Mirtazapine

The presumed mechanism of antidepressant activity of mirtazapine (Remeron) is complex, with presynaptic noradrenergic blocking (thereby enhancing noradrenergic function) and secondary enhancement of serotoninergic activity (Gorman, 1999). Because its most common side effects are sedation and weight gain, mirtazapine is most commonly prescribed to depressed patients, especially older adults with anorexia, agitation, and insomnia.

Tricyclics

As the oldest class of antidepressants, the tricyclics, so designated because of their three-ring structure, are still prescribed for depression but virtually never as first-line agents. These changes in prescribing practices reflect the relative side effect profiles of the tricyclics versus the newer agents, not efficacy, because no newer antidepressant has shown greater efficacy than the tricyclics. Advantages of the tricyclics include their long track record of efficacy; once-daily dosing for all agents; relatively inexpensive cost, because they are available in generic preparations; and the ability to measure their concentration in blood, which, for some agents, correlates with efficacy and potential toxicity (Perry, Zeilmann, & Arndt, 1994). (In contrast, levels of SSRI or other newer antidepressants are available but do not correlate with either efficacy or side effects.) The disadvantages of tricyclics include the need to increase the dose gradually to achieve full effect, a process that may take weeks; a substantial side effect profile, including dry mouth, blurry vision, constipation, urinary hesitation, dizziness upon standing up, sedation, weight gain and others; greater likelihood of exacerbating a number of coexisting medical disorders; and high lethality in overdose. Tricyclic antidepressants are especially difficult and potentially dangerous medications in the presence of cardiac disease, because agents of this antidepressant class alter cardiac conduction and may either cause or exacerbate cardiac arrhthymias (Roose & Spatz, 1999).

Despite sharing many basic similarities, individual tricyclic agents differ in both biological effects and side effects. Biologically, some tricyclics, such as desipramine, are relatively selective in their effects on norepinephrine, whereas others are more mixed in their effects. Clomipramine (Anafranil) differs from all other tricyclics in its powerful serotoninergic properties, akin to the SSRIs, which allows it to be used as a first-line agent to treat obsessive–compulsive disorder. In side effects profiles, desipramine, nortriptyline, and imipramine are much less sedating than are amitriptyline, clomipramine, and doxepin.

MAO Inhibitors

In general, MAO inhibitors have been relegated to third- or fourth-line antidepressants despite their unique utility for a subset of depressed patients. Their disfavor among clinicians and patients is due partly to their side effect profile but more because the use of oral MAO inhibitors requires strict dietary restrictions, without which severe, potentially life-threatening hypertensive reactions may occur. Because of these dangers, only responsible, compliant patients should take oral MAO inhibitors. Although early studies seemed to indicate that MAO inhibitors were not as effective as the tricyclics for severe, classic depression, this observation was due to the low, inadequate doses used in these studies. In later studies using higher doses, the MAO inhibitors are equivalent in effectiveness to other antidepressant classes (Davis, Wang, & Janicak, 1993).

The dietary restrictions are predicated on the need to avoid certain amines in foods, especially tyramine, which can raise blood pressure to dangerous levels in the presence of an MAO inhibitor. The mechanism by which MAO inhibitors cause hypertension in association with certain foods has been well elucidated. In the absence of MAO inhibitors, ingested tyramine is metabolized by the enzyme MAO, which exists in both the lining of the intestinal tract and the liver. Additionally, tyramine releases norepinephrine intracellularly. The amount of norepinephrine available is increased in the presence of an MAO inhibitor. Both of the mechanisms independently contribute to the food-related hypertension. By far, aged cheeses are the most dangerous foods for patients taking MAO inhibitors and should be strictly forbidden. Any competent psychopharmacologist will have a written list of proscribed foods to be given to any patient taking an MAO inhibitor (Gardner, Shulman, Walker, & Tailor, 1996).

By somewhat different mechanisms, certain medications are also contraindicated for use with an MAO inhibitor. Most important among these are over-the-counter cold preparations containing pseudoephedrine, certain opiates such as meperidine (Demerol), and all strongly serotoninergic antidepressants, such as the SSRIs and venlafaxine. The combination of a strongly serotoninergic agent with an MAO inhibitor provokes a serotonin syndrome, a potentially fatal syndrome characterized by fever, muscle rigidity, low blood pressure, and mental status changes.

MAO inhibitors are also characterized by nondangerous but problematic side effects that further limit their acceptance by patients and severely decrease compliance with their use. These include postural dizziness, weight gain (especially with phenelzine), insomnia, daytime fatigue, and sexual dysfunction.

In 2006, transdermal selegiline (Emsam) was released. Its active ingredient, selegiline, is available as an oral MAO inhibitor. The transdermal preparation is administered as a daily patch. Because a transdermal preparation bypasses both gut and hepatic effects, the hypertensive effects of dietary tyramine are markedly diminished. Therefore, in low but still effective doses (6 mg patch), transdermal selegiline does not require any dietary restrictions and is the only MAO inhibitor preparation available in the United States without these requirements. At 9 and 12 mg patch doses, dietary restrictions are required, although the risk of hypertensive reactions is still less than with oral MAO inhibitors. Additionally, the nondangerous MAO inhibitor side effects noted earlier are, in general, less common with transdermal selegiline compared to the oral MAO inhibitors. The major concerns about transdermal selegiline are its high cost and whether it is as effective as the oral MAO inhibitors (Feiger, Rickels, Rynn, Zimbroff, & Robinson, 2006).

Rational Selection of an Antidepressant

Table 24.3 shows the classic factors used by skillful clinicians to choose a specific antidepressant. As can be seen, issues relating to side effect profiles, which, it is assumed, relate partially to compliance, dominate the decision. Experienced clinicians use the differences among antidepressants of sedation–activation to benefit patients by typically prescribing activating agents to lethargic, psychomotor-retarded, depressed patients and sedating agents to more anxious, agitated, insomniac individuals. In controlled trials, there is little evidence that pretreatment anxiety ratings predict response to less or more sedating antidepressants (Zimmerman et al., 2005). Nonetheless, clinical decisions are dominated by these considerations (Zimmerman et al., 2004). Depressive subtypes are those that may predict response to one class of antidepressant more than another, such as atypical depression (see below). For many patients, cost continues to be an important factor in antidepressant choice. As of early 2008, all the SSRIs except S-citalopram are generic medications, as are nefazodone, the non-XR form of venlafaxine, mirtazapine, and all forms of bupropion.

Among the secondary factors that determine choice of medications, no consistent data have shown that depressions can be subtyped by neurotransmitter effects (i.e., clinicians cannot categorize a patient as having a serotoninergic vs. noradrenergic depression). Although family history of response is a commonsense approach to choosing a specific antidepressant, data supporting this approach are remarkably sparse (Malhotra, Murphy, & Kennedy, 2004). Blood levels, as noted earlier, are useful only in monitoring some of the tricyclic agents. Safety/medical considerations were especially relevant in the gradual shift away from the tricyclics and MAO inhibitors toward the newer antidepressants, which are medically safer. Among the newer agents, the only safety considerations are the relative P450 effects (described in the SSRI section earlier) and the seizure concerns with bupropion for patients with preexisting seizure disorders and eating disorders. Given how infrequently older agents are prescribed for depression, safety/medical considerations are less primary concerns than in the past.

Although no single antidepressant is more or less effective than the others in double-blind studies of unselected patients with major depression, some clinical features or clinical subtypes (depression with psychotic features, atypical features and seasonal patterns) may predict differential responses and/or require different approaches.

Psychotic depression (DSM-IV major depression with psychotic features) has been shown in a number of studies to respond less well to an antidepressant than to an antidepressant plus an antipsychotic or to ECT. Some recent studies have indicated that SSRIs may be beneficial for psychotic depressions (Wijkstra, Lijmer, Balk, Geddes, & Nolen, 2006).

TABLE 24.3. Considerations in Choosing a Specific Antidepressant

Primary	Secondary
• History of past response	Neurotransmitter specificity
• Side effect profile	Family history of response
• Depressive subtype (e.g., atypical depression)	Blood-level considerations
• Cost	Safety and medical issues

Current recommendations allow for single-agent treatment or antidepressant plus antipsychotic for milder psychotic depression, whereas combination treatment or ECT should be used as the first line in more severe cases.

Atypical depression (DSM-IV depression with atypical features) responds preferentially to MAO inhibitors over tricyclics, although both are significantly more effective than placebo (Liebowitz et al., 1988). Although some studies using either post hoc analyses or small sample sizes also found SSRIs to also be effective, the best controlled study found fluoxetine to be equivalently effective to imipramine for atypical depression, with response rates lower than those found in other studies with MAO inhibitors (McGrath et al., 2000). However, given the differential side effect profiles, SSRIs are typically prescribed first for those with atypical depression. Additionally, many clinicians have observed (without consistent supporting data) that depressed patients with marked irritability and/or rejection sensitivity, but without meeting full criteria for atypical depression, respond very well to SSRIs.

Seasonal (winter) depression, which typically emerges between October and December, and spontaneously remits in the late winter or early spring, responds both to light therapy and to antidepressants (Lam et al., 2006). Lights used to treat winter depression are full frequency, similar to indoor grow lights or to sunlight. With the use of high-intensity (6,000–10,000 lux) light boxes for 30 minutes daily, usually in the morning, light therapy is significantly more effective than control treatment (typically nonbright lights) (Golden et al., 2005). Side effects seen with light therapy are typically mild, and include headaches and eye or vision problems (Kogan & Guilford, 1998).

General Principles of Pharmacotherapy of Depression

Classic response rates to a single antidepressant, derived from earlier studies, are 60+% compared to a placebo response rate of 30%, a difference of 30% (Klein, Gittelman-Klein, Quitkin, & Rifkin, 1980). However, analyzing studies since 1980, drug–placebo differences have diminished to 19%, due primarily to an increase in placebo response rates (Walsh, Seidman, Sysko, & Gould, 2002). This probably reflects the type of patients entering clinical trials in the last few decades. Regardless of how we understand these placebo response rates, they are real and have their own characteristic biology, which may differ from that in medication responses (Leuchter, Cook, Witte, Morgan, & Abrams, 2002). (Absolute response rates are somewhat inflated compared to what might be seen in clinical practice, because they exclude those who fail to complete the trial [typically estimated as 10–15% even with the newer agents].) In clinical trials, response is usually defined as a 50% or more decrease in the Hamilton Depression Scale (HAMD) and a Clinical Global Improvement score of 1 or 2 (which equates to *very much improved* or *much improved*). Many antidepressant responders are substantially better, but still show many residual depressive signs and symptoms. Because of this, many recent studies have utilized remission as the primary outcome variable.

Typically, *remission* is defined as a HAMD score < 7 or a parallel score on other rating scales. At this symptom level, patients feel substantially well, although not necessarily asymptomatic. In recent studies, remission rates range between 25 and 40%, clearly indicating treatment outcome that is inadequate for the majority of treated patients. As an example, in the largest and among the best recent studies on depression, STAR*D (Sequenced Treatment Alternatives to Relieve Depression), based on 2,876 patients in 41 sites, the remission rate to the first antidepressant prescribed was 28% after up to 14 weeks of treatment (Trivedi, Rush, et al., 2006). Aside from the obvious goal of having patient feel as well as possible, remission from an acute depressive episode predicts lower relapse rates (Paykel et al., 1995; Rush, Trivedi, Wisniewski, Nierenberg, et al., 2006).

In general, all antidepressants and antidepressant classes can be considered equivalent in efficacy. Some meta-analyses have suggested a somewhat higher remission rate with venlafaxine compared to SSRIs (theoretically, because of its effect on two neurotransmitters rather than the single effect on serotonin seen with SSRIs) (Smith, Dempster, Glanville, Freemantle, & Anderson, 2002; Thase, Entsuah, & Rudolph, 2001). However, recent head-to-head studies have not demonstrated this difference (Bielski, Ventura, & Chang, 2004), and the STAR*D study did not show a differential efficacy between sertraline (an SSRI) and venlafaxine (see below; Rush, Trivedi, Wisniewski, Stewart, et al., 2006).

Two obvious, important areas of clinical interest in which recent data and analyses have cast doubt on long-accepted conclusions include when an antidepressant begins to work and how long it takes to see a full response.

Classically, antidepressants were thought to work after at least 2 weeks. Indeed, early responses were often considered—with some research backing (Quitkin, Rabkin, Ross, & Stewart, 1984)—to be placebo responses. However, over the last decade, meta-analyses have demonstrated that antidepressant effects—regardless of the antidepressant class—are seen early, with continuing improvement over subsequent weeks (Posternak & Zimmerman, 2005; Taylor, Freemantle, Geddes, & Bhagwagar, 2006). Over 60% of the improvement occurs within the first 2 weeks of treatment and drug–placebo differences are the most pronounced during this time. An earlier study showed that a partial response at 2–4 weeks of treatment is a relatively robust predictor of a full antidepressant effect at 6 weeks (Nierenberg et al., 2000).

The proper length of a full antidepressant trial has similarly undergone revisionist thinking. Classically, a full antidepressant trial was considered to be 6 weeks. However, in the STAR*D trial of 2,876 depressed outpatients, mean time to remission was 6.7 weeks, with 40% of patients achieving remission between weeks 8 and 14 (Trivedi, Rush, et al., 2006). Because STAR*D was not placebo controlled (it was meant to mimic real-world settings), it is difficult to interpret fully the time to remission data. Nonetheless, this is significantly longer than the 6-week trials typical of both research and clinical treatment.

Finally, a number of studies have recently examined whether antidepressants are associated with suicidality in adults (see Berman, Chapter 22, this volume, for a more in-depth discussion about this issue in children and adolescents). A full discussion of this issue is beyond the scope of this chapter. Nonetheless, there is no evidence that, in adults over age 25, the use of antidepressants is associated with completed suicide or serious suicide attempts (Olfson, Marcus, & Shaffer, 2006; Simon, Savarino, Operskalski, & Wang, 2006). Furthermore, undertreatment of depression poses a much great risk for suicide than excessive use of antidepressants, as exemplified by the low rate of antidepressant concentrations in the blood of patients who have committed suicide (Isacsson, Holmgren, & Ahlner, 2005).

Treatment-Resistant Depression

With antidepressant response rates of 65% at best, and with many of those persons called responders still having residual symptoms, suggested approaches to the 35–40% of nonresponders and the 60–75% of nonremitters are multiple and varied. Unfortunately, the field still lacks a data-based approach to antidepressant treatment failures, because the vast majority of studies in this area typically describe a pharmacotherapeutic approach compared to a placebo condition (Gitlin, 2005). Studies evaluating comparative approaches to treatment-resistant depression, which mimic clinical decision making, are unusual, and no consensus approach exists.

In evaluating treatment resistance, it must first be established that the patient has a potentially treatable depression and not just dysphoric mood based solely on a personality disorder or another psychiatric disorder associated with depressive mood (Gitlin, 2005). Comorbid medical and psychiatric disorders (including comorbid drug/alcohol abuse) may also predict a negative antidepressant response and should be vigorously treated when present. The presence of severe psychosocial factors has been reported to be associated with a poorer antidepressant response. Finally, noncompliance should always be considered with antidepressant treatment failure.

Pharmacological options for treatment resistance have been conceptually divided into optimization, switching, augmentation, or combination (Price, 1990). *Optimization* describes continuing to prescribe the original antidepressant, but at higher dose or for a longer trial (e.g., the 14 weeks utilized in the STAR*D trial). Dose escalation beyond medium doses is more likely to be helpful for patients taking tricyclic antidepressants and venlafaxine, and for some patients on MAO inhibitors, and is unlikely to be helpful with SSRIs (Adli, Baethge, Heinz, Langlitz, & Bauer, 2005). Switching to another antidepressant is a self-evident option. *Augmentation* is defined as adding a second agent that itself is not an antidepressant but that might augment the effect of the original medication. In *combination* treatment, a second agent that is itself an antidepressant is added.

The relative merits of switching within versus across an antidepressant class continues to be controversial. Practically, the usual clinical question is whether to switch to a second SSRI if a depressed patient has failed an adequate trial of the first SSRI or switch to an agent from a different class, such as bupropion, venlafaxine, or others. (Failure to respond must be distinguished from inability to tolerate the first agent, in which case, most clinicians would continue to pursue other agents within the same class.) Only a handful of well-designed, placebo-controlled studies have addressed this question and, overall, no conclusive evidence suggests switching across versus within class (Ruhe, Huyser, Swinkels, & Schene, 2006). In the largest, random assignment, but non-blinded, non–placebo controlled study, 727 patients who had failed to remit and/or could not tolerate citalopram as part of the STAR*D study were prescribed sertraline (another SSRI), venlafaxine, or bupropion. Remission rates were essentially identical—25–27% across the three treatments (Rush, Trivedi, Wisniewski, Stewart, et al., 2006). Thus, in the largest trial of its type, switching within and across antidepressant classes were equally effective strategies, contrary to many expert opinions. In practice, only rarely will a clinician prescribe a third SSRI if a patient has failed two prior agents of that class.

Once a *full trial* (i.e., adequate dose for an adequate period of time) has been achieved, the clinical question is whether to switch to another antidepressant or to add another agent, whether an adjunctive agent or another antidepressant. Although the usual recommendations are to switch antidepressants in the case of nonresponse and to add a second agent when a patient is a partial responder, data on this question are inconclusive, and actual pre-scribing practices are dictated by local customs and individual practitioner experiences and treatment philosophies.

Options for adding a second agent are listed in Table 24.4. Lithium is the most well-studied agent, with 10 double-blind studies published. A meta-analysis of these studies dem-onstrates clear evidence of efficacy compared to placebo (Crossley & Bauer, 2007). Re-sponse typically occurs within 2 weeks and at doses that tend to be lower than those used in treating bipolar disorder. In the STAR*D study, patients randomly assigned to adjunctive lithium, after failing an initial antidepressant, and either a second agent or a different aug-mentation agent showed only a 16% remission rate (Nierenberg et al., 2006). This may be due to the low doses used, poor tolerability, or the fact that patients had failed two prior an-tidepressant treatments. Despite the overall strength of the research evidence, many clini-cians feel negatively toward adjunctive lithium because of both a poorer observed response than is seen in published studies and the lack of patient acceptance due to side effects and the need for blood tests with lithium use (Valenstein et al., 2006).

T_3 (tri-iodothyronine, marketed as Cytomel), a thyroid hormone, has been tested in five double-blind studies as an adjunctive antidepressant treatment, with positive response seen in some, but not all, studies (Aronson, Offman, Joffe, & Naylor, 1996). In the STAR*D study comparing adjunctive lithium to adjunctive T_3, the latter was well tolerated but only modestly effective (25% remission rate; Nierenberg et al., 2006). Its mechanism of action is not well understood, but it is unlikely that it is simply supplementing thyroid hormone to patients who are hypothyroid (low thyroid), because pretreatment thyroid function does not predict T_3 response. Prescribing T_3 as an adjunctive agent is simple, with doses relatively low compared to situations in which it is prescribed for overt thyroid disease. T_3 is associ-ated with few side effects. Despite its simplicity, clinicians tend to use other adjunctive ap-proaches before T_3, because of a general clinical sense that it is often not effective enough.

Combining two antidepressants is a commonly employed strategy for refractory depres-sion. Almost always, the second agent prescribed is from a different class than is the first an-tidepressant. Thus, combining fluoxetine and paroxetine makes little sense; combining an SSRI with bupropion or mirtazapine is more common and is theoretically more reasonable. Only one randomly assigned, controlled treatment trial has demonstrated greater efficacy of combination treatment (desipramine plus fluoxetine) compared to either drug given alone (Nelson et al., 2004). In the STAR*D study, 565 patients who had failed to remit with citalopram were randomly assigned to bupropion (a combination treatment) or buspirone (see below) (Trivedi, Fava, et al., 2006). Using HAMD scores, 30% of patients remitted with combination treatment.

Adjunctive stimulants such as methylphenidate (Ritalin), d-amphetamine (Dexedrine) and, more recently, modafinil (Provigil), are popular choices as adjunctive agents. Modest evidence for modafinil has been published (DeBattista et al., 2003; Fava, Thase, & DeBattista, 2005). In neither of the two published studies examining the adjunctive efficacy of classic stimulants (extended-release methylphenidate in both studies) did drug separate from placebo (Patkar et al., 2006; Ravindran et al., 2008). Nonetheless, stimulants are often prescribed as the first adjunctive treatment. When stimulants work as adjunctive agents, they do so within a few days at most, which adds to their popularity

Second-line treatments for treatment refractory depression are also listed in Table 24.4. Adding a second-generation antipsychotic, typically at low dose, has become a relatively commonly used adjunctive treatment approach. Both a recent meta-analysis examining all controlled trials and a recent large-scale double-blind study of aripiprazole demonstrated

TABLE 24.4. Adjunctive/Combination Strategies for Treatment-Resistant Depression

First line	Second line	Other
Lithium	Second-generation antipsychotic	St. John's wort
T$_3$	Buspirone	Electroconvulsive therapy (ECT)
Combination of two antidepressants[a]	Lamotrigine	Vagal nerve stimulation (VNS)
Stimulant		Transcranial magnetic stimulation (TMS)

[a]Except for a strongly serotoninergic antidepressant plus MAO inhibitor.

clear efficacy of this approach (Berman et al., 2007; Papakostas, Shelton, Smith, & Fava, 2007).

Buspirone (Buspar) is an antianxiety agent that enhances serotonin. As with other approaches, open studies tended to be positive, whereas the two double-blind studies showed minimal evidence of efficacy (Appelberg et al., 2001; Landén, Björling, & Fahlén, 1998). In the STAR*D study described earlier, adjunctive buspirone showed some efficacy (30% remission rates) but poorer tolerability and less effect in secondary analyses compared to combination treatment with bupropion (Trivedi, Fava, et al., 2006). The lack of placebo in this study precludes evaluating whether the relatively comparable efficacy for adjunctive bupropion and buspirone can be interpreted as positive or negative for both approaches.

Lamotrigine (Lamictal), an anticonvulsant with some antidepressant properties (Calabrese et al., 1999), commonly prescribed for bipolar depression, has become another second adjunctive (or solo agent) treatment for refractory depression. No substantial database supports this practice, but many practitioners report its efficacy in some patients.

Studies comparing any of these approaches are few. In one study, both lithium and T$_3$ were significantly more effective augmenting agents of a tricyclic compared to placebo, and equivalent in effectiveness (Joffe, Singer, Levitt, & MacDonald, 1993). In another study, nonresponders or partial responders to fluoxetine 20 mg were randomly assigned in a double-blind fashion to increased fluoxetine dose (optimization), adjunctive desipramine, or adjunctive lithium (Fava, Alpert, Nierenberg, Worthington, & Rosenbaum, 2000). Response rates for the three groups ranged between 27 and 38%, with no significant differences between the approaches. Partial responders were more likely to respond than were nonresponders. In a third study with patients who had failed to respond to sertraline 50–100 mg, longer time on sertraline and addition of mianserin (an antidepressant available in Europe, but not in the United States) were somewhat more effective than increasing the sertraline dose (Licht & Qvitzau, 2002).

Finally, the STAR*D study, which was randomized but not blinded or placebo-controlled, found equivalent and only modest remission rates (<20%) for mirtazapine versus nortriptyline and tranylcypromine versus venlafaxine plus mirtazapine in patients who had failed either two or three prior treatments, respectively (Fava et al., 2006; McGrath et al., 2006). These relatively poor results assuredly reflect patients' higher grades of treatment refractoriness (based on having failed two or more treatments as opposed to one treatment) rather than the inherent lack of efficacy of these treatments compared to treatments given earlier in the algorithm (e.g., the bupropion vs. buspirone adjunctive study noted above) (Trivedi, Fava, et al., 2006) or the switch study (Rush, Trivedi, Wisniewski, Stewart, et al., 2006). This is consistent with a naturalistic study demonstrating that depressed patients who had failed two to five prior antidepressant regimens showed only 18% response and 8% remission over 2 years with continued naturalistic treatment (Dunner et al., 2006).

In the area of augmentation–combination approaches to treatment-resistant depression, actual clinical practices do not necessarily follow the research literature. Whereas lithium and T_3 are the best documented treatments, surveys indicate that the most commonly used approaches among expert clinicians are combinations (especially SSRIs and bupropion), adjunctive stimulants (Fava, Mischoulon, & Rosenbaum, 1998), and adjunctive antipsychotics (Valenstein et al., 2006).

Complementary and Other Somatic Therapies

In the last 5 years, nonprescription (i.e., over the counter) and nonpharmacological somatic treatments for depression have become areas of increasing clinical research and practice. Among the nonprescription treatments, St. John's wort and omega-3 fatty acids are the most commonly prescribed. For somatic, nonpharmacological treatments, ECT, available for decades, still dominates, but two newer treatments, vagal nerve stimulation (VNS) and transcranial magnetic stimulation (TMS) have now been added to the list.

St. John's wort (*Hypericum perforatum*) has been the subject of many trials and even more controversy. Initial studies were marred by poor methodology. More recently, however, a number of reasonably designed studies have generally, but not always, demonstrated efficacy in typical doses of 900–1,200 mg daily compared to either placebo or to standard antidepressant (Linde, Berner, Egger, & Mulrow, 2005; Werneke, Horn, & Taylor, 2004). St. John's wort should be considered as an alternative option for mild to moderate depression. It is generally not perceived as a serious consideration for moderate to severe or treatment-resistant depression.

Omega-3 fatty acids have been evaluated as antidepressant treatments using three rationales (Parker, Gibson, et al., 2006): (1) Lipids play an important role in neuronal signal transduction processes; (2) omega-3 fatty acid levels, or the ratio of omega-3 to omega-6 fatty acids, have been shown to be abnormal in depressed patients; and (3) there is a strong inverse relationship between the consumption of omega-3 fatty acids in a population and the prevalence of depression. A meta-analysis of the few studies in both bipolar and unipolar depression demonstrated efficacy (Freeman et al., 2006). It is still unclear whether one omega-3 fatty acid (eicosapentanoic acid [EHA] vs. docosahexaenoic acid [DHA]) is better than another (or whether a combination is optimal) and what comprises optimal doses.

Electroconvulsive Therapy

Although it is, of course, a somatic treatment rather than a pharmacotherapy, ECT remains the most important approach for treatment-resistant depression. Despite its recent (many decades) track record of consistent safety and efficacy, it still retains a reputation in many parts of the country as a barbaric and dangerous treatment. ECT is rarely used as a first-line treatment for depression. Typically, it is recommended for patients who have failed multiple antidepressant therapies, especially if the depression is severe and associated with significant suicidal ideation and/or functional impairment. ECT may be the treatment of choice for depression with psychotic features (Wheeler Vega, Mortimer, & Tyson, 2000).

Classic remission rates with ECT, derived from clinical trial data, are usually given as 70–90% (Husain et al., 2004). However, recent naturalistic data from community settings suggest lower remission rates of 30–47% (Prudic, Olfson, Marcus, Fuller, & Sackeim, 2004) and a high relapse rate in 6 months for those who responded acutely. Predictors of a lower remission rate to ECT were comorbid personality disorders and inadequate length of treatment (i.e., treating to response instead of remission).

The major side effects of ECT are cognitive (American Psychiatric Association Committee on Electroconvulsive Therapy, 2001). Patients can expect to have post-ECT confusion, especially after the later treatments. Anterograde and retrograde memory deficits are common, and are maximal for the time close to the ECT. Memory improves over many weeks, typically, but not always to normal levels (with the exception of the time around the ECT itself), although the evaluation of memory in ECT patients is confounded by the cognitive disturbances associated with the depression. A few patients complain of long-term cognitive disturbances.

ECT is given as a series of treatments, two to three times weekly, with a total of 6–12 treatments (American Psychiatric Association Committee on Electroconvulsive Therapy, 2001). It may be given to inpatients or outpatients. Safety is ensured by the use of short-acting anesthesia, a muscle relaxant (to prevent broken bones, as in the past) and, in the better settings, electroencephalographic (EEG) monitoring. Technical considerations primarily include whether to use bilateral or unilateral placement (i.e., passing the electrical current through both hemispheres of the brain vs. the nondominant hemisphere only) and the dose of electricity used. Bilateral placement and higher voltage are both associated with greater cognitive side effects but may be more effective for some patients. Results of the most systematic study suggested that high-voltage, unilateral ECT may be the best compromise to achieve efficacy with fewer cognitive side effects (Sackeim et al., 2000).

The major problem with ECT is its high relapse rate after successful acute treatment. Data on strategies to prevent post-ECT relapse are described below in the section on continuation treatment.

Vagal Nerve Stimulation

VNS, an established treatment for treatment-resistant epilepsy, has recently been approved by the U.S. Food and Drug Administration (FDA) as a treatment for refractory depression. Originally suggested by reports of mood improvement in VNS-treated patients with epilepsy, VNS is applied by a pulse-generating device implanted subcutaneously in the patient's chest (like a cardiac pacemaker), with a wire attached to the patient's left vagus nerve. The stimulator is then programmed externally. VNS's efficacy in depression is generally considered weak compared to other established treatments. However, VNS studies in depression have addressed only individuals with treatment-resistant depression (i.e., those whose naturalistic prognoses are poor). Three-month data comparing VNS to sham VNS (in which the device is inserted but never turned on) show only marginal benefit for active treatment (Rush et al., 2005). However, comparing VNS to treatment as usual showed increasing efficacy for VNS over 1 year (George et al., 2005). By the end of 1 year, VNS-treated patients showed 27% response rates compared to 13% for treatment as usual. Improvement plateaus after 1 year, with sustained but not greater responses at 2 years compared to 1 year (Nahas et al., 2005). Side effects with VNS are hoarseness (because the vagal nerve innervates the vocal chords), cough, and mild shortness of breath.

VNS has been infrequently utilized since its approval by the FDA. This reflects both its relatively weak database, need for surgical implantation, and its very high cost and uncertain approval by insurance companies. Because its efficacy is apparent only after a number of months, it is probably not a reasonable treatment option for acute depression. Yet it is a reasonable consideration for those patients who are severely and chronically treatment resistant.

Transcranial Magnetic Stimulation

Initially developed as a research tool for investigating cortical function and nerve conduction, TMS has evolved into a potential treatment alternative for depression. It was reviewed by the FDA and not approved in 2007 due to insufficient efficacy. It is already in clinical use in a number of other countries, including Canada. TMS is administered by placing an electromagnetic coil over the scalp and creating a rapidly changing magnetic field that induces an electric current, stimulating the local underlying cortex. Because of the localized effect (typically placed over the left dorsolateral prefrontal cortex), many of the side effects seen with ECT, such as cognitive disturbance, are nonexistent with TMS. Additionally, TMS does not require anesthesia, providing another safety advantage. As expected, the mechanism of action by which TMS may benefit depression is unknown.

Over 30 relatively small-scale controlled studies examining antidepressant effects of TMS have been published (Herrmann & Ebmeier, 2006; Schutter, in press) with marked differences in methods and results. (The control treatment in these studies is sham ECT, in which the coil is placed at an angle to the skull, thereby markedly reducing the effect on the cortex.) These differing methods include, in part, the many variables for which optimal parameters still have not been established, such as stimulation frequency, stimulation intensity, train duration (length of a burst of pulses), number of trains per session, and so forth (Holtzheimer & Avery, 2005). Nonetheless, meta-analyses of these studies indicates clear efficacy with a moderate-to-large effect size (Herrmann & Ebmeier, 2006; Schutter, in press). In the largest controlled study, however, TMS showed only a trend difference from placebo ($p = .057$) in the primary outcome variable, although secondary analyses showed significant differences (O'Reardon et al., 2007). Preliminary evidence has shown that predictors of response to acute TMS are younger age and less treatment resistance (Fregni et al., 2006), suggesting that TMS may be an alternative to antidepressants rather than to ECT and VNS, which are reserved for treatment-resistant depressions. Data comparing TMS to ECT are conflicted, but a number of studies show greater efficacy with ECT, especially with psychotic or severe depression (Eranti et al., 2007; Rachid & Bertschy, 2006).

Overall, then, TMS may become a viable, alternative somatic treatment for depression. Its strengths lie in its safety, because it neither requires anesthesia nor causes cognitive side effects. However, its efficacy data are still not robust, its use in treatment-resistant depression is uncertain, and it is likely to be far more expensive than antidepressants and more cumbersome (requiring administration in an office with the TMS machine).

TREATING SPECIAL POPULATIONS

Three populations of depressed patients warrant separate discussions because of the unique considerations associated with their treatment: bipolar depression; dysthymic disorder and chronic major depression; and depression during pregnancy and the postpartum period.

Bipolar Depression

Bipolar depression is associated with patients who have had one or more manias or hypomanias. A number of naturalistic studies have clearly demonstrated that depression is the dominant pole in bipolar disorder, with persons with bipolar I and II disorders spending substantially more time depressed than manic or hypomanic (Judd et al., 2002, 2003).

Ironically, then, compared to the treatment of major depression, for which there are hundreds of double-blind studies, bipolar depression has until recently been relatively ignored as a topic of clinical research. This assuredly reflects the ethical and clinical concerns about potentially inducing manic–hypomanic episodes by antidepressants. Nonetheless, we know far less about how to treat the dominant pole of bipolar disorder than we do about the less common pole (mania–hypomania).

Conceptually, in contrast to treating major depression, deciding how best to treat bipolar depression requires both safety and efficacy considerations (i.e., Will the antidepressant provoke mania–hypomania or induce rapid cycling between depression and mania [a notoriously treatment-resistant phase of bipolar disorder]?). All antidepressant treatments (including ECT) have the capacity to provoke manic–hypomanic switches in some individuals. (Although some patients with unipolar major depression will become manic de novo with antidepressants, the risk is relatively small. These individuals are usually presumed to have latent bipolar disorder that simply did not express itself until provoked by the antidepressant.) Studies published in the pre-SSRI era demonstrated the capacity of the tricyclic antidepressants to cause mania and/or to induce rapid cycling relatively commonly, leading to a notion of avoiding antidepressants in bipolar patients whenever possible. A difficulty in quantifying this risk is the natural course of bipolar disorder, in which many patients become manic after a depression, regardless of whether antidepressants are prescribed. Despite this caveat, one retrospective review estimated that (predominantly tricyclic) antidepressants provoked manias in 35% of treatment-resistant patients and a more rapid cycling pattern in 26% (Altshuler et al., 1995). The newer antidepressants may be associated with fewer pharmacological manias–hypomanias compared to the older agents, but these data are not definitive. Thus, there is enormous controversy in the field as to overall treatment principles for bipolar depression. One school recommends that bipolar depression be treated aggressively with mood stabilizers (e.g., lithium, valproate [Depakote], or lamotrigine [Lamictal], because these medications do not cause pharmacological manias/hypomanias), with antidepressants prescribed only much later in the treatment, and only if absolutely necessary (Ghaemi, Hsu, Soldani, & Goodwin, 2003). The other school points to the demonstrated efficacy of antidepressants in bipolar depression and lower switch rates with newer antidepressants, and suggests their use earlier in treatment (albeit typically added to a mood stabilizer) (Gijsman, Geddes, Rendell, Nolen, & Goodwin, 2004; Möller, Grunze, & Broich, 2006). A recent large (n = 366) study of bipolar depression, however, found no efficacy in two antidepressants, paroxetine and bupropion, compared to placebo when added to a mood stabilizer (Sachs et al., 2007).

Among the mood stabilizers, lithium and lamotrigine are prescribed most frequently to treat acute bipolar depression. Lithium shows some efficacy but almost no recent data (Souza & Goodwin, 1991). Lamotrigine demonstrated clear efficacy in one study (Calabrese et al., 1999), although results of later studies were more equivocal. A pooled analysis, however, did demonstrate efficacy (Geddes et al., 2006). However, regardless of the controlled data, lamotrigine, is commonly prescribed in the community for acute bipolar depression. The second-generation antipsychotic quetiapine has also demonstrated efficacy as a treatment for acute bipolar depression (Calabrese et al., 2005; Thase et al., 2006).

Recent studies using the newer antidepressants—especially SSRIs and bupropion—seem to indicate a relatively larger measure of safety compared to the tricyclics, although this conclusion must still be considered tentative, because of the paucity of controlled studies. One important recent study compared sertraline (an SSRI), bupropion, and venlafaxine prescribed in a blinded, but not placebo-controlled, fashion to 174 patients with bipolar I and

II depression who were all taking mood stabilizers. Different switch rates depending on definitions have been presented, but using a conservative definition of a Young Mania Rating Scale > 13, switch rates were 7, 4, and 15%, respectively, with a significantly higher switch rate with venlafaxine (Post et al., 2006). This result agrees with an earlier study that also showed higher switch rates with venlafaxine compared to an SSRI (Vieta et al., 2002). It has been suggested that this may reflect a higher switch rate with dual-action agents (e.g., tricyclics, which also have predominantly dual action). In the previously cited double-blind study of bipolar depression, in which bupropion and paroxetine were not more effective than placebo, switch rates into mania or hypomania also did not differ between drug and placebo (10 vs. 11%), providing further evidence of safety with the newer antidepressants (Sachs et al., 2007).

Dysthymic Disorder and Chronic Depressions

Dysthymic disorder should be considered a mild chronic depression, not a disorder distinct and separate from major depression. Following this conceptualization, dysthymic disorder should be treated in a manner indistinguishable from that of major depression. Consistent with this notion, many, but not all, of the relatively few pharmacotherapy studies in this area have combined chronic major depression, dysthymic disorder, and double depression in their inclusion criteria. Response rates to antidepressants of chronic major depression versus double depression versus dysthymia are comparable (De Lima, Hotoph, & Wessely, 1999). A diverse range of antidepressants has been found to be superior to placebo in the treatment of chronic depression, with no single agent more consistently effective than any other, similar to results in classic major depression. As expected from the acute depression studies, two large studies comparing an SSRI to a tricyclic have found similar efficacy but difference in tolerability, with tricyclic-treated patients showing higher dropout rates (Keller et al., 1998; Thase et al., 1996). Nefazodone has also demonstrated a robust effect in treating chronic depression (Keller et al., 2000). These studies also suggest that antidepressant response rates with chronic depression are generally similar to those seen in acute depression studies, although direct comparison studies are limited. At this point, although chronicity itself is a negative predictor of antidepressant response, it should not preclude a thorough set of antidepressant trials.

Depression during Pregnancy or the Postpartum Period

Because the mean age of onset of depression and the age at which women are most likely to become pregnant coincide, the problem of how to manage depression and antidepressants in preparation for, during, and following pregnancy is a critical issue in psychopharmacology. The central concern in considering the use of antidepressants during pregnancy is their potential effects on fetal, then infant, development. The three main areas of potential concern are *physical teratogenicity*, *neonatal toxicity*, and *behavioral teratogenicity*. These terms refer, respectively, to physical malformations present at birth; abnormalities present at birth that are due to the active presence of the medication (or withdrawal effects) and are typically reversible; and longer term abnormalities, such as cognitive effects, activity levels, and propensity for development of psychiatric disorders later in life. All conclusions in this area must be tempered by three methodological considerations: (1) the lack of controlled studies in this area, which are ethically impossible; (2) maternal anxiety, distress, and depression during pregnancy that may affect some aspects of neonatal development (Field, Diego, & Hernandez-Reif, 2006); and (3) the marked disparity seen in results across studies.

An important factor to be considered for optimal clinical decisions is, of course, the potential risk in *not* treating a woman with a depressive disorder during pregnancy. Earlier reports suggested that pregnancy is a time of unusually good psychiatric health for women, and that there might be less need for antidepressants during this time. The best recent study, however, demonstrates that women with depressive disorders who discontinue antidepressants around the time of conception or soon thereafter in pregnancy relapse significantly more frequently than do those who continue their treatment (68 vs. 26%, $p < .001$; Cohen et al., 2006).

For the SSRIs, the initial data showed consistent safety and no evidence of teratogenicity. Neither fluoxetine nor citalopram (available in Europe for many years before its release in the United States) seem to be associated with major fetal malformations (Hallberg & Sjoblom, 2005). Data for sertraline are similarly reassuring. However, in one database, cardiac ventricular septal defects have been reported to be associated with intrauterine paroxetine exposure (GlaxoSmithKline, unpublished data). Two recent studies found rare increased specific defects but the absolute risks were small (Alwan, Reefhuis, Rasmussen, Olney, & Friedman, 2007; Louik, Lin, Werler, Hernández-Díaz, & Mitchell, 2007). Among the older agents, whereas tricyclics show no clear association with fetal malformations, MAO inhibitors are generally avoided during pregnancy because of both blood pressure concerns and the results of animal studies (Kalra & Einarson, 2006).

The major recent concerns surround the question of safety of the SSRIs with regard to later exposure (second half of pregnancy or third trimester) being associated with potential neonatal toxicity (Austin, 2006). One area of concern has been the observation of a neonatal behavioral syndrome characterized by respiratory distress, irritability, feeding difficulties, and, less commonly, seizures, which have been attributed to either excessive serotoninergic effect or, conversely, a withdrawal syndrome (Moses-Kolko et al., 2005; Sanz, De las Cuevas, Kiuru, Bate, & Edwards, 2005). Another study suggested higher rates of primary pulmonary hypertension in infants exposed to SSRIs in the second half of pregnancy (Chambers et al., 2006). For any of these syndromes, distinguishing the effects of antepartum depression from pharmacological effects on infant outcome has been difficult in most of these databases. However, two recent studies compared outcomes in infants of depressed mothers treated with SSRIs, infants of depressed mothers not treated, and a control population (Oberlander, Warburton, Misri, Aghajanian, & Hertzman, 2006; Suri et al., 2007). After controlling for other variables (including maternal illness severity), infants exposed to antidepressants still showed significantly higher rates of respiratory distress and low birthweight rates in one study, and lower gestational age at birth and higher rates of admission to the special care nursery in the other study. It is important to acknowledge that many of these findings have not been replicated, that other findings (e.g., lower gestational age at birth) may have no long-term consequences, and that the absolute risk of some of the abnormalities seen, even if increased, is still very small. As an example, in one study, the absolute rate of primary pulmonary hypertension in SSRI-exposed fetuses was increased compared to the control population, but was only 1% (Chambers et al., 2006).

Data on behavioral teratogenicity are exceedingly sparse, because studies in this area require long-term follow-up. Thus far, no evidence of cognitive, temperamental, or behavioral developmental abnormalities has been demonstrated in children exposed *in utero* to tricyclic antidepressants or SSRIs (Misri et al., 2006; Nulman et al., 1997, 2002). Data on development into adolescence and young adulthood do not exist.

Given the current conflicting data regarding SSRI safety, there is no clear consensus on treatment recommendations for pregnant depressed women. The ultimate decision on how best to manage depression for any individual woman is, of course, discussed between the prescribing physician, the pregnant woman (preferably in anticipation of pregnancy), the father (if present), and the therapist. In these discussions, the potential and, in many cases, unknown risk of treatment must be balanced against the risk of no treatment, with the potential for depression during pregnancy. Possible strategies include withdrawing the antidepressant before conception, discontinuing the antidepressant when pregnancy is confirmed, avoiding medication during the first trimester, discontinuing the antidepressant midway through pregnancy (given the concerns about late pregnancy effects), or continuing the medication throughout the pregnancy. Severity of the depression, its recurrent nature, whether the woman has previously been able to withdraw from antidepressants without depressive relapse for some time, and the availability and efficacy of psychotherapeutic intervention are all important factors to weigh in the decision.

Whether to breast-feed is another issue for depressed women on antidepressants. The context of this decision is the high risk of postpartum depression in women with a prior history of depression (O'Hara, 1995). In contrast to the ingestion of medications during pregnancy, infant and maternal exposure to antidepressants can, of course, be separated after birth. All psychotropic medications are secreted in breast milk in variable amounts. Infant plasma levels of the antidepressant are usually extremely low or undetectable by current assay techniques, indicating little risk for harm (Eberhard-Gran, Eskild, & Opjordsmoen, 2006). However, a few case reports suggest that an occasional breast-feeding neonate either accumulates relatively higher amounts of medications or is unusually susceptible to side effects and may show negative effects. Effects of long-term exposure to antidepressants from breast-feeding are unknown.

Although no controlled studies have yet demonstrated the efficacy of antidepressants in preventing or treating postpartum depression, clinically, antidepressants are prescribed in this situation in a manner analogous to that in nonpostpartum depressions, with proper discussion and informed consent if the woman elects to breast-feed.

CONTINUATION TREATMENT

The previous sections are based on treatment of depression in the acute phase. The goal of continuation treatment is, as noted earlier, to prevent a relapse soon after improvement from the acute depressive episode. Clinically, continuation treatment begins when patient and clinician agree that the former is conclusively better, and that further changes in medications to control symptoms are not needed. Continuation treatment with antidepressants, using the acute treatment dose, is associated with reduced relapse rates compared to switching to placebo. Only two studies—one evaluating a tricyclic and the other, an SSRI—have specifically examined the optimal length of continuation period (Prien & Kupfer, 1986; Reimherr et al., 1998). In both studies, continuation therapy was more effective than placebo in preventing relapse. The usual recommendation for 4–9 months of continuation treatment fits the available data.

If long-term maintenance treatment is clinically unnecessary (see next section) and the antidepressant is to be discontinued, common sense dictates that it be tapered rather than stopped suddenly. Should depressive symptoms return during tapering, they are typically milder and treatment can be more easily reinstated compared to a full, sudden recurrence, which is more likely to occur if the antidepressant is stopped precipitously. Additionally, discontinuation/withdrawal symptoms may be seen with a variety of antidepressants and are also avoided with medication tapering. The only reasonable exception to these recommendations is fluoxetine, which, because of its long half-life, is essentially self-tapering. The optimal time period for medication tapering after continuation therapy is unstudied, but a reasonable time period is 4–8 weeks.

MAINTENANCE TREATMENT

Because, in the majority of patients, depression is either a recurrent or chronic disorder (see Muñoz, Le, Clarke, Barrera, & Torres, Chapter 23, this volume), long-term preventive treatment should be commonly considered. Factors in deciding which depressed individuals are appropriate candidates for maintenance therapy are based more on common sense than on data. They include the number of depressive episodes over a lifetime, the frequency of depressive episodes, the severity of the depressions (including both symptom severity and functional consequences), the responsiveness of episodes to prior treatments, the speed with which episodes have emerged, and insight into emerging depressive symptoms (Gitlin, 1996).

Many patients are concerned about potential long-term side effects of antidepressants on body organs, such as liver, kidney, and especially brain. Although definitive studies do not exist, there is no evidence whatsoever that antidepressants as a class (available for over 50 years) or SSRIs specifically (available for 20 years), are associated with any long-term negative effects on organ function or physiology. It is also important to remind patients that untreated depression may have long-term medical consequences (e.g., see Freedland & Carney, Chapter 6, this volume, on depression and medical health). As with the decision about antidepressants and pregnancy, the potential risks of treating must always be balanced against the risks of not treating.

Because of the length of time needed for proper study of maintenance treatment, no truly long-term studies have examined the efficacy of antidepressants in preventing depressive recurrences. Only one controlled maintenance study extended beyond 2 years (Frank et al., 1990). Nonetheless, virtually all maintenance studies with tricyclic or SSRI antidepressants have demonstrated greater efficacy of active agents compared to placebo in preventing depressive recurrences. There is no evidence that any single antidepressant prevents future episodes better than any other. Additionally, although not commonly used in the United States, lithium has been demonstrated to be an effective preventive antidepressant therapy (Souza & Goodwin, 1991).

Few studies have addressed the question of optimal antidepressant doses in maintenance treatment. Based on extrapolation from two studies that were not designed specifically to answer this question (Frank et al., 1993; Prien et al., 1984), the current consensus is that patients in maintenance treatment should remain on their acute treatment doses. The only exception to this would be a patient for whom the side effects are sufficiently distressing that adherence to treatment is jeopardized.

The efficacy of antidepressants as maintenance treatment for chronic depressions has also been shown in two studies examining a tricyclic and an SSRI, respectively (Kocsis et al., 1996; Keller et al., 1998). In both studies, after successful acute and continuation treatment, the antidepressant was associated with significantly lower recurrence rates compared to placebo over 2 years and 1½ years, respectively.

A final area of inquiry concerns proper continuation/maintenance treatment for patients who respond successfully to ECT. It has long been known that without prophylactic treatment after successful ECT, relapse rates are very high. More recent studies, however, have indicated that relapse rates are still high despite preventive antidepressant therapies, especially with those patients who had not responded to antidepressants prior to ECT (as opposed to those given ECT because of psychotic features or clinical urgency) (Sackeim et al., 1990). Therefore, many patients are treated with combination treatment (e.g., with an antidepressant plus a mood stabilizer) to prevent relapse following acute ECT (Sackeim et al., 2001). Another option that is commonly considered is continuation/maintenance in which the frequency of ECT is gradually reduced to once-monthly treatments. In the only random assignment study, continuation ECT was as effective as lithium–nortriptyline combination (Kellner et al., 2006). However, neither treatment was very effective or acceptable to patients, because 54% in each group either relapsed or dropped out over 6 months.

FUTURE DIRECTIONS FOR RESEARCH

When the first edition of this textbook was published 7 years ago, a series of "future directions for research" was suggested. These included the need for antidepressants with greater efficacy; novel biological approaches in developing new antidepressants; more systematic assessment and demonstrated efficacy of approaches to treatment-resistant depression; enhanced capacity to predict antidepressant response; more data on bipolar depression; and more information of the basics of antidepressant prescribing, such as optimal doses, time to efficacy, and so forth. Despite a number of important studies addressing these issues, definitive answers to these questions still lie in the future.

No new agent has demonstrated efficacy beyond that seen with imipramine, the first tricyclic, released over one-half century ago. We certainly have more selectively acting antidepressants, such as SSRIs, and dual-action agents (similar to the tricyclics) with significantly fewer side effects, and greater patient and physician acceptance. But enhanced efficacy with a single agent continues to be out of reach.

With 7 more years of data on the basics of prescribing antidepressants—when antidepressants begin to work, and the length of a full trial, beyond which further improvement is unlikely to occur—we know more but have neither definitive data nor consensus conclusions. As reviewed earlier, antidepressants may work faster than was assumed and, according to the STAR*D study, a full trial may take up to 14 weeks. Yet STAR*D had no placebo condition, and it has certainly not changed prescribing practices; few, if any, clinicians provide antidepressant trials for 3 months or more. Thus, the impact of these more recent data and their translation into optimal clinical practice remains to be clarified in the future.

Of the three antidepressants released during these last 7 years, one was another SSRI (the sixth S-citalopram), another was a second dual-action agent (duloxetine), and still another was an MAO inhibitor in a patch form (selegiline transdermal patch). Thus, no new mechanism of action, or even a new class of antidepressants, has appeared, nor is any on the immediate horizon. However, preliminary evidence has suggested the potential efficacy of quetiapine, a second-generation antipsychotic, as a solo agent treatment or as an adjunctive treatment for major depression (Cutler et al., 2007). If confirmed, this would indicate a new use of an already available class of medications. Whether this effect would generalize to other second-generation antipsychotics is not known. The antiglucocorticoid agents discussed 7 years ago are still under investigation. Modest efficacy has been demonstrated in studies in psychotic depression (DeBattista et al., 2006), but no large-scale data have emerged to support these agents as the next important class of antidepressants. Despite this, ongoing work is exploring the development of agents that alter the function of the hypothalamic–pituitary–adrenal (HPA) system, especially agents that block the effects of corticotropin-releasing hormone (CRH), which is presumed to underlie dysfunction in the HPA system. Additionally, current and future research is actively pursuing the development of agents that will stimulate BDNF.

Switch strategies, adjunctive agents, and antidepressant combination strategies—the mainstay treatments for treatment resistant depression—have a bit more data in support of their use, but not much more. The STAR*D study demonstrated that all of these options are successful with some patients, but more importantly, that if the first few approaches fail, later approaches are increasingly unsuccessful (i.e., treatment failure predicts treatment failure). Additionally, because of the design of the STAR*D study, it is not possible to make meaningful comparisons between the different treatments in the algorithm, because different subpopulations were used in each phase of the trial. What STAR*D did show, however, is the ability to evaluate various treatment strategies with "real" patients, similar to those seen in clinical work, as opposed to the more rarefied patients in usual placebo-controlled studies, who do not resemble depressed patients seen in the community. This points the way to future studies in which representative patients can be evaluated and treated, generating data that are applicable to all depressed patients.

One area of real progress, although the impact of these options is still unclear, has been the approval of VNS and the possible approval in the near future for TMS. Given the expense and cumbersome nature of both these treatments, it is unlikely that they will revolutionize the area of antidepressant treatments. Nonetheless, they represent novel alternatives for patients who are either treatment-resistant or -intolerant. In the near future, the roles of these somatic therapies and their place in the algorithm of antidepressant treatments will be clarified.

The goal of dividing depression into hoped for separate and distinct biological subtypes that allow accurate predictions of responses to different biological agents (e.g., SSRIs vs. dual-action antidepressants) has been the Holy Grail of depression pharmacotherapy. The quest continues. No validated predictor has emerged, although preliminary work has suggested the use of quantitative EEGs to predict antidepressant responses and responses to different antidepressant classes (Cook et al., 2002).

Bipolar depression has finally become an area of active research. The first good studies have now been published, and a number of others will be available in the next few years, promising data-based recommendations for treatment instead of passionate clinical beliefs dominating the discussion. The relative role of mood stabilizers versus antidepressants—even the question of whether antidepressants alone can be prescribed for bipolar II depressions—is beginning to be addressed in thoughtful studies (Parker, Tully, Olley, & Hadzi-Pavlovic, 2006).

Overall, then, although no extraordinary breakthroughs have radically altered the pharmacotherapy of depressive disorders, important and highly relevant clinical data are emerging. For now, and in the foreseeable future, however, we continue as we have in the past—treating depressed patients as best we can with the optimal combination of data-based treatments, clinical experience, and as much wisdom as we can muster.

REFERENCES

Adli, M., Baethge, C., Heinz, A., Langlitz, N., & Bauer, M. (2005). Is dose escalation of antidepressants a rational strategy after a medium-dose treatment has failed?: A systematic review. *European Archives of Psychiatry and Clinical Neuroscience, 255*(6), 387–400.

Altshuler, L. L., Post, R. M., Leverich, G. S., Mikalauskas, K., Rosoff, A., & Ackerman, L. (1995). Antidepressant-induced mania and cycle acceleration: A controversy revisited. *American Journal of Psychiatry, 152*(8), 1130–1138.

Alwan, S., Reefhuis, J., Rasmussen, S. A., Olney, R. S., & Friedman, J. M. (2007). Use of selective serotonin-reuptake inhibitors in pregnancy and the risk of birth defects. *New England Journal of Medicine, 356*, 2684–2692.

American Psychiatric Association Committee on Electroconvulsive Therapy. (2001). *The practice of electroconvulsive therapy: Recommendations for treatment, training, and privileging* (2nd ed.). Washington, DC: American Psychiatric Association.

Appelberg, B. G., Syvalahti, E. K., Koskinen, T. E., Mehtonen, O. P., Muhonen, T. T., & Naukkarinen, H. H. (2001). Patients with severe depression may benefit from buspirone augmentation of selective serotonin reuptake inhibitors: Results from a placebo-controlled, randomized, double-blind, placebo wash-in study. *Journal of Clinical Psychiatry, 62*(6), 448–452.

Aronson, R., Offman, H. J., Joffe, R. T., & Naylor, C. D. (1996). Triiodothyronine augmentation in the treatment of refractory depression. *Archives of General Psychiatry, 53*, 842–848.

Asher, J. A., Cole, G. O., Colin, J. N., Feighner, J. P., Ferris, R. M., Fibiger, H. C., et al. (1995). Bupropion: A review of its mechanisms of antidepressant activity. *Journal of Clinical Psychiatry, 56*, 395–401.

Austin, M. P. (2006). To treat or not to treat: Maternal depression, SSRI use in pregnancy and adverse neonatal effects. *Psychological Medicine, 36*(12), 1663–1670.

Berman, R. M., Marcus, R. N., Swanink, R., McQuade, R. D., Carson, W. H., Corey-Lisle, P. K., et al. (2007). The efficacy and safety of aripiprazole as adjunctive therapy in major depressive disorder: A multicenter, randomized, double-blind, placebo-controlled study. *Journal of Clinical Psychiatry, 68*, 843–853.

Bielski, R. J., Ventura, D., & Chang, C. C. (2004). A double-blind comparison of escitalopram and venlafaxine extended release in the treatment of major depressive disorder. *Journal of Clinical Psychiatry, 65*(9), 1190–1196.

Calabrese, J. R., Bowden, C. L., Sachs, G. S., Ascher, J. A., Monaghan, E., & Rudd, G. D. (1999). A double-blind placebo-controlled study of lamotrigine monotherapy in outpatients with bipolar I depression. *Journal of Clinical Psychiatry, 60*(2), 79–88.

Calabrese, J. R., Keck, P. E., Jr., Macfadden, W., Minkwitz, M., Ketter, T. A., Weisler, R. H., et al. (2005). A randomized, double-blind, placebo-controlled trial of quetiapine in the treatment of bipolar I or II depression. *American Journal of Psychiatry, 162*(7), 1351–1360.

Chambers, C. D., Hernandez-Diaz, S., Van Marter, L. J., Werler, M. M., Louik, C., Jones, K. L., et al. (2006). Selective serotonin reuptake inhibitors and risk of persistent pulmonary hypertension of the newborn. *New England Journal of Medicine, 354*(6), 579–587.

Cohen, L. S., Altshuler, L. L., Harlow, B. L., Nonacs, R., Newport, D. J., Viguera, A. C., et al. (2006). Relapse of major depression during pregnancy in women who maintain or discontinue antidepressant treatment. *Journal of the American Medical Association, 295*(5), 499–507.

Cook, I. A., Leuchter, A. F., Morgan, M., Witte, E., Stubbeman, W. F., Abrams, M., et al. (2002). Early changes in prefrontal activity characterize clinical responders to antidepressants. *Neuropsychopharmacology, 27*(1), 120–131.

Crossley, N. A., & Bauer, N. (2007). Acceleration and augmentation of antidepressants with lithium for depressive disorders: Two meta-analyses of randomized, placebo-controlled trials. *Journal of Clinical Psychiatry, 68*, 935–940.

Cutler, A. J., Montomery, S., Feifel, D., Lazarus, A., Schollin, M., & Brecher, M. (2007, December). *Extended release quetiapine fumarate (quetiapine XR) monotherapy in patients with major depressive disorder (MDD): Results from a double-blind, randomized Phase III study.* Paper presented at the 46th annual meeting of the American College of Neuropsychopharmacology, Boca Raton, FL.

Davidson, J. R. T. (1989). Seizures and bupropion: A review. *Journal of Clinical Psychiatry, 50*, 256–261.

Davis, J. M., Wang, Z., & Janicak, P. G. (1993). A quantitative analysis of clinical drug trials for the treatment of affective disorders. *Psychopharmacological Bulletin, 29*, 175–181.

DeBattista, C., Belanoff, J., Glass, S., Khan, A., Horne, R. L., Blasey, C., et al. (2006). Mifepristone versus placebo in the treatment of psychosis in patients with psychotic major depression. *Biological Psychiatry, 60*(12), 1343–1349.

DeBattista, C., Doghramji, K., Menza, M. A., Rosenthal, M. H., Fieve, R. R., & the Modafinil in Depression Study Group. (2003). Adjunct modafinil for the short-term treatment of fatigue and sleepiness in patients with major depressive disorder: A preliminary double-blind, placebo-controlled study. *Journal of Clinical Psychiatry, 64*(9), 1057–1064.

De Lima, M. S., Hotoph, M., & Wessely, S. (1999). The efficacy of drug treatments for dysthymia: A systematic review and meta-analysis. *Psychological Medicine, 29*, 1273–1289.

Delgado, P. L., Brannan, S. K., Mallinckrodt, C. H., Tran, P. V., McNamara, R. K., Wang, F., et al. (2005). Sexual functioning assessed in four double-blind placebo- and paroxetine-controlled trials of duloxetine for major depressive disorder. *Journal of Clinical Psychiatry, 66*(6), 686–692.

Duman, R. S., & Monteggia, L. M. (2006). A neurotrophic model for stress-related mood disorders. *Biological Psychiatry, 59*(12), 1116–1127.

Dunner, D. L., Rush, A. J., Russell, J. M., Burke, M., Woodard, S., Wingard, P., et al. (2006). Prospective, long-term, multicenter study of the naturalistic outcomes of patients with treatment-resistant depression. *Journal of Clinical Psychiatry, 67*(5), 688–695.

Eberhard-Gran, M., Eskild, A., & Opjordsmoen, S. (2006). Use of psychotropic medications in treating mood disorders during lactation: Practical recommendations. *CNS Drugs, 20*(3), 187–198.

Eranti, S., Mogg, A., Pluck, G., Landau, S., Purvis, R., Brown, R. G., et al. (2007). A randomized, controlled trial with 6-month follow-up of repetitive transcranial magnetic stimulation and electroconvulsive therapy for severe depression. *American Journal of Psychiatry, 164*(1), 73–81.

Fava, M., Alpert, J. E., Nierenberg, A. A., Worthington, J. J., & Rosenbaum, J. F. (2000, May). Double-blind study of high-dose fluoxetine versus lithium or desipramine augmentation of fluoxetine in partial and nonresponders to fluoxetine. In *Syllabus of American Psychiatric Association annual meeting* (pp. 35–36). Chicago: American Psychiatric Press.

Fava, M., Mischoulon, D., & Rosenbaum, J. (1998). Augmentation strategies for failed SSRI treatment. *American Society of Clinical Psychopharmacology Progress Notes, 9*, 7.

Fava, M., Rush, A. J., Wisniewski, S. R., Nierenberg, A. A., Alpert, J. E., McGrath, P. J., et al. (2006). A comparison of mirtazapine and nortriptyline following two consecutive failed medication treatments for depressed outpatients: A STAR*D report. *American Journal of Psychiatry, 163*(7), 1161–1172.

Fava, M., Thase, M. E., & DeBattista, C. (2005). A multicenter, placebo-controlled study of modafinil augmentation in partial responders to selective serotonin reuptake inhibitors with persistent fatigue and sleepiness. *Journal of Clinical Psychiatry, 66*(1), 85–93.

Feiger, A. D., Rickels, K., Rynn, M. A., Zimbroff, D. L., & Robinson, D. S. (2006). Selegiline transdermal system for the treatment of major depressive disorder: An 8-week, double-blind, placebo-controlled, flexible-dose titration trial. *Journal of Clinical Psychiatry, 67*(9), 1354–1361.

Field, T., Diego, M., & Hernandez-Reif, M. (2006). Prenatal depression effects on the fetus and newborn: A review. *Infant Behavior and Development, 29*(3), 445–455.

Frank, E., Kupfer, D. J., Perel, J. M., Cornes, C., Jarrett, D. B., Mallinger, A. G., et al. (1990). Three-year outcomes for maintenance therapies in recurrent depression. *Archives of General Psychiatry, 47*, 1093–1099.

Frank, E., Kupfer, D. J., Perel, J. M., Cornes, C., Mallinger, A. G., Thase, M. E., et al. (1993). Comparison of full-dose versus half-dose pharmacotherapy in the maintenance treatment of recurrent depression. *Journal of Affective Disorders, 27*, 139–145.

Freeman, M. P., Hibbeln, J. R., Wisner, K. L., Davis, J. M., Mischoulon, D., Peet, M., et al. (2006). Omega-3 fatty acids: Evidence basis for treatment and future research in psychiatry. *Journal of Clinical Psychiatry, 67*(12), 1954–1967.

Fregni, F., Marcolin, M. A., Myczkowski, M., Amiaz, R., Hasey, G., Rumi, D. O., et al. (2006). Predictors of antidepressant response in clinical trials of transcranial magnetic stimulation. *International Journal of Neuropsychopharmacology, 9*(6), 641–654.

Gardner, D. M., Shulman, K. I., Walker, S. E., & Tailor, S. A. N. (1996). The making of a user friendly MAOI diet. *Journal of Clinical Psychiatry, 57*(3), 99–104.

Geddes, J., Nierenberg, A., Bourne, E., Adams, B., White, R., Nanry, K., et al. (2006, May). *Lamotrigine for acute treatment of bipolar depression: A retrospective pooled analysis of response rates in three trials.* Presented at the annual meeting of the American Psychiatric Association, Toronto, Canada.

George, M. S., Rush, A. J., Marangell, L. B., Sackeim, H. A., Brannan, S. K., Davis, S. M., et al. (2005). A one-year comparison of vagus nerve stimulation with treatment as usual for treatment-resistant depression. *Biological Psychiatry, 58*(5), 364–373.

Ghaemi, S. N., Hsu, D. J., Soldani, F., & Goodwin, F. K. (2003). Antidepressants in bipolar disorder: The case for caution. *Bipolar Disorders, 5*(6), 421–433.

Gijsman, H. J., Geddes, J. R., Rendell, J. M., Nolen, W. A., & Goodwin, G. M. (2004). Antidepressants for bipolar depression: A systematic review of randomized, controlled trials. *American Journal of Psychiatry, 161*(9), 1537–1547.

Gitlin, M. (1996). *The psychotherapist's guide to psychopharmacology* (2nd ed.). New York: Free Press.

Gitlin, M. (2005). Treatment of refractory depression. In J. Licinio & M. Wong (Eds.), *Biology of depression* (pp. 387–412). Weinheim, Germany: Wiley-VCH.

Golden, R. N., Gaynes, B. N., Ekstrom, R. D., Hamer, R. M., Jacobsen, F. M., Suppes, T., et al. (2005). The efficacy of light therapy in the treatment of mood disorders: A review and meta-analysis of the evidence. *American Journal of Psychiatry, 162*(4), 656–662.

Goldstein, D. J., Lu, Y., Detke, M. J., Lee, T. C., & Iyengar, S. (2005). Duloxetine vs. placebo in patients with painful diabetic neuropathy. *Pain, 116*(1–2), 109–118.

Gorman, J. M. (1999). Mirtazapine: Clinical overview. *Journal of Clinical Psychiatry, 60*(Suppl. 17), 9–13.

Hallberg, P., & Sjoblom, V. (2005). The use of selective serotonin reuptake inhibitors during pregnancy and breast-feeding: A review and clinical aspects. *Journal of Clinical Psychopharmacology, 25*(1), 59–73.

Harvey, A. T., Rudolph, R. L., & Preskorn, S. H. (2000). Evidence of the dual mechanisms of action of venlafaxine. *Archives of General Psychiatry, 57*, 503–509.

Herrmann, L. L., & Ebmeier, K. P. (2006). Factors modifying the efficacy of transcranial magnetic stimulation in the treatment of depression: A review. *Journal of Clinical Psychiatry, 67*(12), 1870–1876.

Holtzheimer, P. E., & Avery, D. H. (2005). Focal brain stimulation for treatment-resistant depression: Transcranial magnetic stimulation, vagus-nerve stimulation, and deep-brain stimulation. *Primary Psychiatry, 12*(2), 57–64.

Husain, M. M., Rush, A. J., Fink, M., Knapp, R., Petrides, G., Rummans, T., et al. (2004). Speed of response and remission in major depressive disorder with acute electroconvulsive therapy (ECT): A Consortium for Research in ECT (CORE) report. *Journal of Clinical Psychiatry, 65*(4), 485–491.

Isacsson, G., Holmgren, P., & Ahlner, J. (2005). Selective serotonin reuptake inhibitor antidepressants and the risk of suicide: A controlled forensic database study of 14,857 suicides. *Acta Psychiatrica Scandinavica, 111*, 286–290.

Joffe, R. T., Singer, W., Levitt, A. J., & MacDonald, C. (1993). A placebo-controlled comparison of lithium and tri-iodothyronine augmentation in tricyclic antidepressants in unipolar refractory depression. *Archives of General Psychiatry, 50*, 387–393.

Judd, L. L., Akiskal, H. S., Schettler, P. J., Coryell, W., Endicott, J., Maser, J. D., et al. (2003). A prospective investigation of the natural history of the long-term weekly symptomatic status of bipolar II disorder. *Archives of General Psychiatry, 60*(3), 261–269.

Judd, L. L., Akiskal, H. S., Schettler, P. J., Endicott, J., Maser, J., Solomon, D. A., et al. (2002). The long-term natural history of the weekly symptomatic status of bipolar I disorder. *Archives of General Psychiatry, 59*(6), 530–537.

Kalra, S., & Einarson, A. (2006). Prevalence, clinical course, and management of depression during pregnancy. In V. Hendrick (Ed.), *Psychiatric disorders in pregnancy and the postpartum* (pp. 13–40). Totowata, NJ: Humana Press.

Keller, M. B., Gelenberg, A. J., Hirschfeld, R. M. A., Rush, A. J., Thase, M. E., Kocsis, J. H., et al. (1998). The treatment of chronic depression, Part 2: A double-blind, randomized trial of sertraline and imipramine. *Journal of Clinical Psychiatry, 59*(11), 598–606.

Keller, M. B., McCullough, J. P., Klein, D. N., Arnow, B., Dunner, D. L., Gelenberg, A. J., et al. (2000). Nefazodone, psychotherapy, and their combination for the treatment of chronic depression: A comparison of nefazodone, the cognitive behavioral-analysis system of psychotherapy, and their combination for the treatment of chronic depression. *New England Journal of Medicine, 342*, 1462–1470.

Kellner, C. H., Knapp, R. G., Petrides, G., Rummans, T. A., Husain, M. M., Rasmussen, K., et al. (2006). Continuation electroconvulsive therapy vs. pharmacotherapy for relapse prevention in major depression: A multisite study from the Consortium for Research in Electroconvulsive Therapy (CORE). *Archives of General Psychiatry, 63*(12), 1337–1344.

Klein, D. F., Gittelman-Klein, R., Quitkin, F. M., & Rifkin, A. (1980). *Diagnosis and drug treatment of psychiatric disorders.* Baltimore: Williams & Wilkins.

Kocsis, J. H., Friedman, R. A., Markowitz, J. C., Leon, A. C., Miller, N. L., Gniwesch, L., et al. (1996). Maintenance therapy for chronic depression: A controlled clinical trial of desipramine. *Archives of General Psychiatry, 53*, 769–774.

Kogan, A. O., & Guilford, P. M. (1998). Side effects of short-term 10,000-lux light therapy. *American Journal of Psychiatry, 155*(2), 293–294.

Kornstein, S. G., Wohlreich, M. M., Mallinckrodt, C. H., Watkin, J. G., & Stewart, D. E. (2006). Duloxetine efficacy for major depressive disorder in male vs. female patients: Data from seven randomized, double-blind, placebo-controlled trials. *Journal of Clinical Psychiatry, 67*(5), 761–770.

Lam, R. W., Levitt, A. J., Levitan, R. D., Enns, M. W., Morehouse, R., Michalak, E. E., et al. (2006). The Can-SAD study: A randomized controlled trial of the effectiveness of light therapy and fluoxetine in patients with winter seasonal affective disorder. *American Journal of Psychiatry, 163*(5), 805–812.

Landén, M., Björling, G., & Fahlén, T. (1998). A randomized, double-blind placebo-controlled trial of buspirone in combination with an SSRI in patients with treatment-refractory depression. *Journal of Clinical Psychiatry, 59*, 664–668.

Leuchter, A. F., Cook, I. A., Witte, E. A., Morgan, M., & Abrams, M. (2002). Changes in brain function of depressed subjects during treatment with placebo. *American Journal of Psychiatry, 159*(1), 122–129.

Licht, R. W., & Qvitzau, S. (2002). Treatment strategies in patients with major depression not responding to first-line sertraline treatment: A randomised study of extended duration of treatment, dose increase or mianserin augmentation. *Psychopharmacology, 161*(2), 143–151.

Liebowitz, M. R., Quitkin, F. M., Stewart, J. W., McGrath, P. J., Harrison, W. M., Markowitz, J. S., et al. (1988). Antidepressant specificity in atypical depression. *Archives of General Psychiatry, 45*, 129–137.

Linde, K., Berner, M., Egger, M., & Mulrow, C. (2005). St John's wort for depression: Meta-analysis of randomised controlled trials. *British Journal of Psychiatry, 186*, 99–107.

Louik, C., Lin, A. E., Werler, M. M., Hernández-Díaz, S., & Mitchell, A. A. (2007). First-trimester use of selective serotonin-reuptake inhibitors and the risk of birth defects. *New England Journal of Medicine, 356*, 2675–2683.

Lucena, M. I., Carvajal, A., Andrade, R. J., & Velasco, A. (2003). Antidepressant-induced hepatotoxicity. *Expert Opinion on Drug Safety, 2*(3), 249–262.

Malhotra, A. K., Murphy, G. M., Jr., & Kennedy, J. L. (2004). Pharmacogenetics of psychotropic drug response. *American Journal of Psychiatry, 161*(5), 780–796.

McGrath, P. J., Stewart, J. W., Fava, M., Trivedi, M. H., Wisniewski, S. R., Nierenberg, A. A., et al. (2006). Tranylcypromine versus venlafaxine plus mirtazapine following three failed antidepressant medication trials for depression: A STAR*D report. *American Journal of Psychiatry, 163*(9), 1531–1541.

McGrath, P. J., Stewart, J. W., Janal, M. N., Petkova, E., Quitkin, F. M., & Klein, D. F. (2000). A placebo-controlled study of fluoxetine versus imipramine in the acute treatment of atypical depression. *American Journal of Psychiatry, 157*(3), 344–350.

Misri, S., Reebye, P., Kendrick, K., Carter, D., Ryan, D., Grunau, R. E., et al. (2006). Internalizing behaviors in 4-year-old children exposed in utero to psychotropic medications. *American Journal of Psychiatry, 163*(6), 1026–1032.

Möller, H. J., Grunze, H., & Broich, K. (2006). Do recent efficacy data on the drug treatment of acute bipolar depression support the position that drugs other than antidepressants are the treatment of choice?: A conceptual review. *European Archives of Psychiatry and Clinical Neuroscience, 256*, 1–16.

Moses-Kolko, E. L., Bogen, D., Perel, J., Bregar, A., Uhl, K., Levin, B., et al. (2005). Neonatal signs after late *in utero* exposure to serotonin reuptake inhibitors: Literature review and implications for clinical applications. *Journal of the American Medical Association, 293*(19), 2372–2383.

Nahas, Z., Marangell, L. B., Husain, M. M., Rush, A. J., Sackeim, H. A., Lisanby, S. H., et al. (2005). Two-year outcome of vagus nerve stimulation (VNS) for treatment of major depressive episodes. *Journal of Clinical Psychiatry, 66*(9), 1097–1104.

Nelson, J. C., Mazure, C. M., Jatlow, P. I., Bowers, M. B., Jr., & Price, L. H. (2004). Combining norepinephrine and serotonin reuptake inhibition mechanisms for treatment of depression: A double-blind, randomized study. *Biological Psychiatry, 55*(3), 296–300.

Nierenberg, A. A., Farabaugh, A. H., Alpert, J. E., Gordon, J., Worthington, J. J., Rosenbaum, J. F., et al. (2000). Timing of onset of antidepressant response with fluoxetine treatment. *American Journal of Psychiatry, 157*(9), 1423–1428.

Nierenberg, A. A., Fava, M., Trivedi, M. H., Wisniewski, S. R., Thase, M. E., McGrath, P. J., et al. (2006). A comparison of lithium and T(3) augmentation following two failed medication treatments for depression: A STAR*D report. *American Journal of Psychiatry, 163*(9), 1519–1530.

Nulman, I., Rovet, J., Stewart, D. E., Wolpin, J., Gardner, H. A., Theis, J. G. W., et al. (1997). Neurodevelopment of children exposed in utero to antidepressant drugs. *New England Journal of Medicine, 336*(4), 258–262.

Nulman, I., Rovet, J., Stewart, D. E., Wolpin, J., Pace-Asciak, P., Shuhaiber, S., et al. (2002). Child development following exposure to tricyclic antidepressants or fluoxetine throughout fetal life: a prospective, controlled study. *American Journal of Psychiatry, 159*(11), 1889–1895.

Oberlander, T. F., Warburton, W., Misri, S., Aghajanian, J., & Hertzman, C. (2006). Neonatal outcomes after prenatal exposure to selective serotonin reuptake inhibitor antidepressants and maternal depression using population-based linked health data. *Archives of General Psychiatry, 63*(8), 898–906.

O'Hara, M. (1995). *Postpartum depression: Causes and consequences.* New York: Springer-Verlag.

Olfson, M., Marcus, S. C., & Shaffer, D. (2006). Antidepressant drug therapy and suicide in severely depressed children and adults: A case–control study. *Archives of General Psychiatry, 63*(8), 865–872.

O'Reardon, J. P., Solvason, H. B., Janicak, P. G., Sampson, S., Isenberg, K. E., Nahas, Z., et al. (2007). Efficacy and safety of transcranial magnetic stimulation in the acute treatment of major depression: A multisite randomized controlled trial. *Biological Psychiatry, 62*, 1208–1216.

Papakostas, G. I., Shelton, R. C., Smith, J., & Fava, M. (2007). Augmentation of antidepressants with atypical antipsychotic medications for treatment-resistant major depressive disorder: A meta-analysis. *Journal of Clinical Psychiatry, 68*, 826–831.

Parker, G., Gibson, N. A., Brotchie, H., Heruc, G., Rees, A. M., & Hadzi-Pavlovic, D. (2006). Omega-3 fatty acids and mood disorders. *American Journal of Psychiatry, 163*(6), 969–978.

Parker, G., Tully, L., Olley, A., & Hadzi-Pavlovic, D. (2006). SSRIs as mood stabilizers for bipolar II disorder?: A proof of concept study. *Journal of Affective Disorders, 92*(2–3), 205–214.

Patkar, A. A., Masand, P. S., Pae, C. U., Peindl, K., Hooper-Wood, C., Mannelli, P., et al. (2006). A randomized, double-blind, placebo-controlled trial of augmentation with an extended release formulation of methylphenidate in outpatients with treatment-resistant depression. *Journal of Clinical Psychopharmacology, 26*, 653–656.

Paykel, E. S., Ramana, R., Cooper, Z., Hayhurst, H., Kerr, J., & Barocka, A. (1995). Residual symptoms after partial remission: An important outcome in depression. *Psychological Medicine, 25*(6), 1171–1180.

Perry, P. J., Zeilmann, C., & Arndt, S. (1994). Tricyclic antidepressant concentrations in plasma: An estimate of their sensitivity and specificity as a predictor of response *Journal of Clinical Psychopharmacology, 14*, 230–240.

Post, R. M., Altshuler, L. L., Leverich, G. S., Frye, M. A., Nolen, W. A., Kupka, R. W., et al. (2006). Mood switch in bipolar depression: Comparison of adjunctive venlafaxine, bupropion and sertraline. *British Journal of Psychiatry, 189*, 124–131.

Posternak, M. A., & Zimmerman, M. (2005). Is there a delay in the antidepressant effect?: A meta-analysis. *Journal of Clinical Psychiatry, 66*(2), 148–158.

Price, L. H. (1990). Pharmacological strategies in refractory depression. In A. Tasman, S. Goldfinger, & C. Kaufmann (Eds.), *Review of psychiatry* (Vol. 9, pp. 116–131). Washington, DC: American Psychiatric Press.

Prien, R. F., & Kupfer, D. J. (1986). Continuation drug therapy for major depressive episodes: How long should it be maintained? *American Journal of Psychiatry, 143*(1), 18–23.

Prien, R. F., Kupfer, D. J., Mansky, P. A., Small, J. G., Tuason, U. B., Voss, C. B., et al. (1984). Drug therapy in the prevention of recurrences in unipolar and bipolar affective disorders: A report of the NIMH Collaborative Study Group comparing lithium carbonate, imipramine and a lithium carbonate–imipramine combination. *Archives of General Psychiatry, 41,* 1096–1104.

Prudic, J., Olfson, M., Marcus, S. C., Fuller, R. B., & Sackeim, H. A. (2004). Effectiveness of electroconvulsive therapy in community settings. *Biological Psychiatry, 55*(3), 301–312.

Quitkin, F. M., Rabkin, J. G., Ross, D., & Stewart, J. W. (1984). Identification of true drug response to antidepressants: Use of pattern analysis. *Archives of General Psychiatry, 41*(8), 782–786.

Rachid, F., & Bertschy, G. (2006). Safety and efficacy of repetitive transcranial magnetic stimulation in the treatment of depression: A critical appraisal of the last 10 years. *Neurophysiologie Clinique, 36*(3), 157–183.

Ravindran, A. V., Kennedy, S., O'Donovan, C., Fallu, A., Camacho, F., & Binder, C. E. (2008). Osmotic-release oral system methylphenidate augmentation of antidepressant monotherapy in major depressive disorder: Results of a double-blind randomized, placebo-controlled trial. *Journal of Clinical Psychiatry, 69,* 87–94.

Reimherr, F. W., Amsterdam, J. D., Quitkin, F. M., Rosenbaum, J. F., Fava, M. F., Zajecka, J., et al. (1998). Optimal length of continuation therapy in depression: A prospective assessment during long-term fluoxetine treatment. *American Journal of Psychiatry, 155*(9), 1247–1253.

Roose, S. P., & Spatz, E. (1999). Treating depression in patients with ischemic heart disease. *Drug Safety, 20,* 459–465.

Ruhe, H. G., Huyser, J., Swinkels, J. A., & Schene, A. H. (2006). Switching antidepressants after a first selective serotonin reuptake inhibitor in major depressive disorder: A systematic review. *Journal of Clinical Psychiatry, 67*(12), 1836–1855.

Rush, A. J., Marangell, L. B., Sackeim, H. A., George, M. S., Brannan, S. K., Davis, S. M., et al. (2005). Vagus nerve stimulation for treatment-resistant depression: A randomized, controlled acute phase trial. *Biological Psychiatry, 58*(5), 347–354.

Rush, A. J., Trivedi, M. H., Wisniewski, S. R., Nierenberg, A. A., Stewart, J. W., Warden, D., et al. (2006). Acute and longer-term outcomes in depressed outpatients requiring one or several treatment steps: A STAR*D report. *American Journal of Psychiatry, 163*(11), 1905–1917.

Rush, A. J., Trivedi, M. H., Wisniewski, S. R., Stewart, J. W., Nierenberg, A. A., Thase, M. E., et al. (2006). Bupropion-SR, sertraline, or venlafaxine-XR after failure of SSRIs for depression? *New England Journal of Medicine, 354*(12), 1231–1242.

Sachs, G. S., Nierenberg, A. A., Calabrese, J. R., Marangell, L. B., Wisniewski, S. R., Gyulai, L., et al. (2007). Effectiveness of adjunctive antidepressant treatment for bipolar depression. *New England Journal of Medicine, 356,* 1711–1722.

Sackeim, H. A., Haskett, R. F., Mulsant, B. H., Thase, M. E., Mann, J. J., Pettinati, H. M., et al. (2001). Continuation pharmacotherapy in the prevention of relapse following electroconvulsive therapy: A randomized controlled trial. *Journal of the American Medical Association, 285*(10), 1299–1307.

Sackeim, H. A., Prudic, J., Devanand, D. P., Decina, P., Kerr B., & Malitz, S. (1990). The impact of medication resistance and continuation pharmacotherapy on relapse following response to electroconvulsive therapy in major depression. *Journal of Clinical Psychopharmacology, 10,* 96–104.

Sackeim, H. A., Prudic, J., Devanand, D. P., Nobler, M. S., Lisanby, S. H., Peyser, S., et al. (2000). A prospective, randomized, double-blind comparison of bilateral and right unilateral electroconvulsive therapy at different stimulus intensities. *Archives of General Psychiatry, 57,* 425–434.

Sanz, E. J., De las Cuevas, C., Kiuru, A., Bate, A., & Edwards, R. (2005). Selective serotonin reuptake inhibitors in pregnant women and neonatal withdrawal syndrome: A database analysis. *Lancet, 365,* 482–487.

Schutter, D. J. (in press). Antidepressant efficacy of high-frequency transcranial magnetic stimulation over the left dorsolateral prefrontal cortex in double-blind sham-controlled designs: A meta-analysis. *Psychological Medicine.*

Simon, G. E., Savarino, J., Operskalski, B., & Wang, P. S. (2006). Suicide risk during antidepressant treatment. *American Journal of Psychiatry, 163*(1), 41–47.

Smith, D., Dempster, C., Glanville, J., Freemantle, N., & Anderson, I. (2002). Efficacy and tolerability of venlafaxine compared with selective serotonin reuptake inhibitors and other antidepressants: A meta-analysis. *British Journal of Psychiatry, 180,* 396–404.

Souza, F. G. M., & Goodwin, G. M. (1991). Lithium treatment and prophylaxis in unipolar depression: A meta-analysis. *British Journal of Psychiatry, 158,* 666–675.

Spina, E., Scordo, M. G., & D'Arrigo, C. (2003). Metabolic drug interactions with new psychotropic agents. *Fundamental and Clinical Pharmacology, 17*(5), 517–538.

Suri, R., Altshuler, L., Hellemann, G., Burt, V. K., Aquino, A., & Mintz, J. (2002). Effects of antenatal depression and antidepressant treatment on gestational age at birth and risk of preterm birth. *American Journal of Psychiatry, 164*(7), 1206–1213.

Taylor, D. P., Carter, R. B., Eison, A. S., Mullins, U. L., Smith, H. L., Torrente, J. R., et al. (1995). Pharmacology and neurochemistry of nefazodone, a novel antidepressant drug. *Journal of Clinical Psychiatry, 56*(Suppl. 6), 3–11.

Taylor, M. J., Freemantle, N., Geddes, J. R., & Bhagwagar, Z. (2006). Early onset of selective serotonin reuptake inhibitor antidepressant action: Systematic review and meta-analysis. *Archives of General Psychiatry, 63*(11), 1217–1223.

Thase, M. E. (1998). Effects of venlafaxine on blood pressure: A meta-analysis of original data from 3,744 depressed patients. *Journal of Clinical Psychiatry, 59*(10), 502–508.

Thase, M. E., Entsuah, A. R., & Rudolph, R. L. (2001). Remission rates during treatment with venlafaxine or selective serotonin reuptake inhibitors. *British Journal of Psychiatry, 178,* 234–241.

Thase, M. E., Fava, M., Halbreich, U., Koscis, J. H., Koran, L., Davidson, J., et al. (1996). A placebo-controlled, randomized clinical trial comparing sertraline and imipramine for the treatment of dysthymia. *Archives of General Psychiatry, 53,* 777–784.

Thase, M. E., Macfadden, W., Weisler, R. H., Chang, W., Paulsson, B., Khan, A., et al. (2006). Efficacy of quetiapine monotherapy in bipolar I and II depression: A double-blind, placebo-controlled study (the BOLDER II study). *Journal of Clinical Psychopharmacology, 26*(6), 600–609.

Thase, M. E., Tran, P. V., Wiltse, C., Pangallo, B. A., Mallinckrodt, C., & Detke, M. J. (2005). Cardiovascular profile of duloxetine, a dual reuptake inhibitor of serotonin and norepinephrine. *Journal of Clinical Psychopharmacology, 25*(2), 132–140.

Trivedi, M. H., Fava, M., Wisniewski, S. R., Thase, M. E., Quitkin, F., Warden, D., et al. (2006). Medication augmentation after the failure of SSRIs for depression. *New England Journal of Medicine, 354*(12), 1243–1252.

Trivedi, M. H., Rush, A. J., Wisniewski, S. R., Nierenberg, A. A., Warden, D., Ritz, L., et al. (2006). Evaluation of outcomes with citalopram for depression using measurement-based care in STAR*D: Implications for clinical practice. *American Journal of Psychiatry, 163*(1), 28–40.

Valenstein, M., McCarthy, J. F., Austin, K. L., Greden, J. F., Young, E. A., & Blow, F. C. (2006). What happened to lithium?: Antidepressant augmentation in clinical settings. *American Journal of Psychiatry, 163*(7), 1219–1225.

Vieta, E., Martinez-Aran, A., Goikolea, J. M., Torrent, C., Colom, F., Benabarre, A., et al. (2002). A randomized trial comparing paroxetine and venlafaxine in the treatment of bipolar depressed patients taking mood stabilizers. *Journal of Clinical Psychiatry, 63*(6), 508–512.

Walsh, B. T., Seidman, S. N., Sysko, R., & Gould, M. (2002). Placebo response in studies of major depression: Variable, substantial, and growing. *Journal of the American Medical Association, 287*(14), 1840–1847.

Werneke, U., Horn, O., & Taylor, D. M. (2004). How effective is St John's wort?: The evidence revisited. *Journal of Clinical Psychiatry, 65*(5), 611–617.

Wheeler Vega, J. A., Mortimer, A. M., & Tyson, P. J. (2000). Somatic treatment of psychotic depression: Review and recommendations for practice. *Journal of Clinical Psychopharmacology, 20*(5), 504–519.

Wijkstra, J., Lijmer, J., Balk, F. J., Geddes, J. R., & Nolen, W. A. (2006). Pharmacological treatment for unipolar psychotic depression: Systematic review and meta-analysis. *British Journal of Psychiatry*, *188*, 410–415.

Zimmerman, M., Posternak, M., Friedman, M., Attiullah, N., Baymiller, S., Boland, R., et al. (2004). Which factors influence psychiatrists' selection of antidepressants? *American Journal of Psychiatry*, *161*(7), 1285–1289.

Zimmerman, M., Posternak, M. A., Attiullah, N., Friedman, M., Boland, R. J., Baymiller, S., et al. (2005). Why isn't bupropion the most frequently prescribed antidepressant? *Journal of Clinical Psychiatry*, *66*(5), 603–610.

CHAPTER 25

Cognitive and Behavioral Treatment of Depression

Steven D. Hollon *and* Sona Dimidjian

The cognitive and behavioral therapies are among the most widely used treatments for depression. These approaches have been shown to be as efficacious as medications in the reduction of acute distress and quite possibly longer lasting (Hollon, Thase, & Markowitz, 2002). There are even indications that they can prevent first episodes in at-risk persons who have never been depressed (Gillham, Shatte, & Freres, 2000).

This chapter focuses on the nature and efficacy of the various cognitive and behavioral interventions. These include not only cognitive therapy and related cognitive-behavioral interventions but also behavioral activation (BA), a newly articulated approach, and other, related behavioral interventions. These approaches overlap to some extent in their procedures of operation but differ in other respects with regard to both theory and practice. Whether these differences matter remains to be seen, but they have implications for the nature of the patients treated and the ease with which the respective treatments can be disseminated.

COGNITIVE THERAPY AND RELATED INTERVENTIONS

Cognitive therapy (CT) is one of the earliest and best established of the cognitive behavioral interventions (Hollon & Beck, 2004). The cognitive interventions are based on the notion that the way people interpret life experiences influences how they feel about those events and what they attempt to cope with them behaviorally (A. T. Beck, 1991). According to cognitive theory, people who are prone to depression are unduly negative in their perceptions of themselves, their worlds, and their futures (the negative cognitive triad), and are susceptible to a host of information-processing distortions that makes it difficult for them to benefit from positive experience. Their thinking is seen as being dominated by negative *cognitive schemas*, organized knowledge systems that contain both core beliefs and underlying assumptions, and that dictate the operation of biases in information processing. These schemas often function as "silent" *diatheses* (risk factors) that are activated by negative life events; for patients with more chronic distress, the schemas may be in a state of continuous activation (see Joormann, Chapter 13, this volume, for an extended discussion of this theory).

Cognitive Model and Theory of Change

CT is predicated on the notion that teaching patients to recognize and examine their negative beliefs and maladaptive information-processing proclivities can help produce relief from distress and enable them to cope more effectively with life's challenges (Beck, Rush, Shaw, & Emery, 1979). The primary role of the therapist is to teach patients a set of skills that help them learn how to examine the accuracy of their beliefs and to modify their own behaviors. The ultimate goal of therapy is to help clients learn to use these tools independently. Such skills are not only important for symptom relief but may also minimize the chances of future recurrence of symptoms.

A successful course of CT accomplishes its goals through a structured, collaborative process that includes three distinct but interrelated components. The first component comprises a thorough *exploration* of the patient's dysfunctional beliefs, or more generally, the patient's personal meaning system. A careful *examination* of that well-articulated belief system comprises the second component of the therapy process. In this process, evidence speaking for and against the belief is reviewed, alternative explanations or interpretations are considered, and the consequences that might ensue if the belief were true are considered and put in a realistic perspective. Finally, active *experimentation*, designed specifically to "test" the validity of the maladaptive belief systems, is the third component of the therapeutic endeavor. These three components are not necessarily incorporated in a linear fashion; patients are often encouraged to engage in behavioral experiments to test specific predictions before they are trained to examine the accuracy of those beliefs or to explore the larger meaning systems in which they are embedded. Nonetheless, these components always are incorporated in an integrated fashion, and other forms of experimentation are used to examine the accuracy of underlying core beliefs in even the latest parts of therapy.

The Structure of CT within and across Sessions

Individual sessions typically begin with the therapist and patient working together to set an agenda to prioritize matters of importance and ensure that their time together is spent efficiently. Once areas of difficulty are delineated, the therapist uses a series of gentle, thoughtful questions to help bring to light the dysfunctional thoughts and beliefs that may be driving the patient's distress and maladaptive behaviors. This process of exploring maladaptive automatic thoughts and their underlying core beliefs has been referred to as *Socratic questioning* and is assumed to be critical to successful CT. By its very nature, it avoids confrontation, because the goal is to discover whether certain thoughts and beliefs are not serving the patient well rather than to expose him or her as a "faulty thinker." A failure to fully understand the patient's personal meaning system could hinder progress. In particular, it is often important to "follow the affect." To the extent that the theory is correct, any strong affect should be associated with thoughts and beliefs that would make the reaction understandable if they were true. If the therapist cannot imagine feeling what the patient feels if he or she believed what the patient believes, then still more of the meaning system needs to be explored.

From the first session on, therapist and patient collaboratively generate assignments for the patient to complete between sessions. These assignments, which can be written or behavioral, often incorporate the experimental component of the therapeutic process. They allow the patient and therapist to test the patient's negative beliefs and predictions, and to gather evidence necessary for cognitive change.

As therapy continues, the therapist and the patient work collaboratively to examine whether the patient's interpretations of events and beliefs about self, world, and future are accurate and/or adaptive. Progress is regularly and systematically assessed in terms of concrete behavioral outcomes. As patient and therapist gain a better understanding of the patient's worldview, and as problematic core beliefs and underlying assumptions begin to change, they may revisit goals. New techniques are introduced throughout therapy, but all serve to address the same concept: the testing of negative beliefs and expectations.

CT emphasizes the links among belief, mood, and behavior. As a result, many effective techniques incorporate behavioral interventions in the service of testing specific automatic negative thoughts and underlying beliefs or assumptions (Bennett-Levy et al., 2004). For example, depressed patients often feel overwhelmed and unable to cope with life's demands. In fact, patients may indeed be facing serious demands in a number of different areas, including problems in relationships, financial difficulties, and difficulties at work. Such patients might be encouraged to list what they need to do, then to break large tasks into smaller constituent steps.

Patients are then encouraged to run an experiment to see whether they can get things done by focusing on accomplishing just one step at a time. After doing this graded task assignment, patients often find that they more easily complete the larger tasks they set for themselves, because they are less likely to be overwhelmed by their own negative thinking. This experience of success is used to disconfirm patients' negative expectation and to question underlying beliefs in their own incompetence.

Use of the various techniques depends on patients' goals and symptoms. Some techniques, such as the graded task assignment described earlier or a detailed schedule of activities to complete across a given period of time (activity schedule), are particularly useful early in therapy. Such concrete behavioral assignments allow patients to learn the observational and problem-solving skills they will be used throughout therapy and motivate them to take an active approach to problem solving and the pursuit of goals.

Other techniques emphasize more cognitive strategies. For example, patients typically are taught to ask themselves a series of questions to examine the accuracy of their negative beliefs:

1. What is the *evidence* for and against that belief?
2. Are there *alternative explanations* for that event other than the one that first occurred to me?
3. What are the real *implications* if that belief is true?

The Dysfunctional Thoughts Record (DTR) is a formalized way for the patient to identify, evaluate, and respond to negative automatic thoughts in a written format. The DTR comprises separate columns for recording the specific event that triggered a negative belief and the consequent feelings. The patient is encouraged to record each aspect of the problematic situation, to explore the larger meaning system in which that negative belief is embedded, then to examine the accuracy of the belief using the three questions just described, and perhaps collecting more information or running a behavioral experiment to test those beliefs. Additional techniques include teaching problem-solving and decision-making skills, developing flash cards with important phrases as patient self-reminders, and employing in-session role play to practice real-life interactions.

The Course of CT and Schema-Focused Modifications

CT is designed to be an efficient, structured, short-term form of treatment. For patients with uncomplicated depressions—that is, for people who have an essentially adaptive view of themselves, the world, and the future when they are not depressed—this might mean a treatment length of 10–20 sessions over 12–16 weeks (J. Beck, 1995). In contrast, however, patients with long-standing histories of rigid dysfunctional beliefs may need a considerably longer course of treatment. For such a patient, the inaccurate beliefs and related maladaptive behaviors are deeply entrenched, because the individual has had little experience questioning those beliefs and behaviors. As a result, more exploration and examination of the faulty belief system, and more experimentation designed to modify those beliefs, often are required. Thus, regardless of the persistence of depressive symptoms, it is the patient's particular set of maladaptive or dysfunctional beliefs that is the primary target of CT.

In recent years, CT has evolved with respect to its approach to the treatment of long-standing symptoms and personality disorders (Beck, Freeman, Davis, & Associates, 2003). The process of providing a cognitive conceptualization was always a central organizing principle of the approach, but early efforts with episodically depressed patients focused more exclusively on applying cognitive and behavioral techniques to the resolution of negative thoughts and maladaptive behaviors in response to life difficulties "in the here and now." Attention to earlier life events and childhood antecedents that contributed to the development of these underlying schemas was reserved for later sessions, after the patient was largely free of symptoms. In a similar fashion, attention was paid to the therapeutic relationship only when problems arose in the working alliance.

Over the last two decades, it has become clear that patients with histories of chronic depression, or depressions superimposed on long-standing character disorders, have no other way of thinking about themselves and often need help to construct completely new schemas to guide thinking and behavior. For these patients, Beck uses the metaphor of a "three-legged stool" to describe his approach to the implementation of CT. According to this metaphor, the three "legs" include exploring (1) the thoughts and feelings that surround some particular current life concern; (2) the historical antecedents that gave rise to those beliefs; and (3) the way in which those beliefs manifest themselves in the ongoing therapeutic relationship.

This process seems to help the patient recognize that much of his or her distress stems from these long-standing maladaptive beliefs (and not just from events). Moreover, it further helps to recognize that these beliefs often were acquired early in life, before the patient developed the capacity to make the kinds of reasoned judgments that came with greater maturity. Most importantly, it often helps to make sense out of habitual and self-defeating patterns of behavior that often represent misguided strategies to compensate for perceived limitations and dangers specified by those beliefs. Dealing with the manifestations of these attitudes and beliefs, and the maladaptive behaviors they engender in the context of the therapeutic relationship, provides an opportunity to try out new behaviors in a somewhat safer interpersonal context. Although many of these strategies are reminiscent of more dynamic therapies, the discussion is always brought back around to just how these beliefs can be tested in current life situations, and no presumption is made that unconscious sexual or aggressive drives are at the core of the patient's difficulties.

Evidence for Efficacy and Comparisons to Medication

CT has been one of the most extensively studied of the psychosocial interventions and it has typically fared well in comparisons to minimal treatment controls and other psychosocial interventions (DeRubeis & Crits-Christoph, 1998). Early studies suggested that CT was superior to medications, but they were flawed with respect to the way that pharmacotherapy was implemented (Blackburn, Bishop, Glen, Whalley, & Christie, 1981; Rush, Beck, Kovacs, & Hollon, 1977). Subsequent studies that did a better job of adequately implementing both interventions typically found that CT was about as efficacious as medications (Hollon, DeRubeis, Evans, et al., 1992; Murphy, Simons, Wetzel, & Lustman, 1984). In the National Institute of Mental Health (NIMH) Treatment of Depression Collaborative Research Project (TDCRP), however, CT was found to be less efficacious than medications and no more efficacious than pill-placebo among patients with more severe depressions (Elkin et al., 1995). Given the size of this study and the fact that it was the first placebo-controlled comparison to medication, the TDCRP had a major impact on the field and led to the recommendation that CT not be used alone in the treatment of severely depressed patients (American Psychiatric Association, 2000).

It is important to note, however, that differences among the sites in their prior experience with CT mirrored differences in efficacy of the approach (Jacobson & Hollon, 1996a). At the two sites with less prior experience with the modality, CT did no better than pill-placebo, whereas at a third site, with greater prior experience in the approach, CT did as well as medications (Jacobson & Hollon, 1996b). This suggests that the TDCRP may have failed to implement CT in an adequate fashion at each of its sites, just as some of the earlier comparative trials may have failed to implement drug treatment adequately.

It now appears that the TDCRP was something of an anomaly; again, subsequent studies have suggested that CT is as efficacious as medications when both are adequately implemented. For example, Jarrett and colleagues (1999) found CT to be as efficacious as medications and that each was superior to a pill-placebo control in the treatment of atypical depression. Similarly, DeRubeis and colleagues (2005) found CT to be as efficacious as medications and that each was superior to pill-placebo in the treatment of severely depressed outpatients. In both instances, considerable care was taken to ensure that both modalities were well implemented by experienced, highly trained, and closely supervised therapists.

Does CT Have an Enduring Effect?

There are consistent indications that CT has an enduring effect that lasts beyond the end of treatment (Hollon, Stewart, & Strunk, 2006). Several studies have shown that patients treated to remission with CT are about half as likely as patients treated to remission with medications to relapse following treatment termination (Blackburn, Eunson, & Bishop, 1986; Kovacs, Rush, Beck, & Hollon, 1981; Simons, Murphy, Levine, & Wetzel, 1986), and that the magnitude of this enduring effect is about as great as that when patients are kept on continuation medications (Evans et al., 1992; Hollon et al., 2005). The only study to date that has not found enduring effect was the NIMH TDCRP, and its apparent nonsignificant differences did favor prior CT (Shea et al., 1992).

Klein (1996) has argued that such findings could be an artifact of differential attrition, because high-risk patients may need medications to improve, and low-risk patients may be unable to tolerate medications side effects, therefore dropping out of treatment at a differential rate. Such proclivities could lead acute treatment to serve as a "differential sieve" that systematically biases subsequent comparisons against medication treatment if a greater proportion of high-risk patients completed and responded to medication than to CT. It is noteworthy, however, that several studies that first treated patients to remission or recovery with medications and subsequently randomized patients to CT or related interventions also have shown an enduring effect that could not be attributed to differential attrition (Bockting et al., 2005; Fava, Rafanelli, Grandi, Conti, & Belluardo, 1998; Paykel et al., 1999; Teasdale et al., 2002). Moreover, there are even indications that CT can be used to prevent the onset of symptoms in at-risk people who are not currently depressed (Seligman, Schulman, DeRubeis, & Hollon, 1999).

Who Responds to CT?

There is currently little good evidence to support the notion that certain types of patients do better or worse in CT than in other types of treatments. Although it has long been assumed that patients with endogenous or melancholic depressions respond better to medications than they do to psychosocial interventions such as CT, there is little evidence to support this position (Blackburn et al., 1981; DeRubeis et al., 2005; Hollon, DeRubeis, Evans, et al., 1992; Kovacs et al., 1981; Murphy et al., 1984; Sotsky et al., 1991). Thase and colleagues (1994) have suggested that more severely depressed women respond less well than more severely depressed men to CT and might do better still in interpersonal psychotherapy (Thase, Frank, Kornstein, & Yonkers, 2000), but these conclusions were based on comparisons between treatments across studies and not on direct experimental comparisons. Conversely, CT has been said to be superior to either interpersonal psychotherapy (IPT) or medication treatment in patients with underlying personality disorders (American Psychiatric Association, 2000), but this claim was based on a misreading of findings from the TDCRP. What that study actually found was that absence of a personality disorder did not predict better response to CT, as it did in the other conditions (Shea et al., 1990). In the recent study by DeRubeis and colleagues, patients with Axis II personality disorders actually did better on medications than in CT, whereas patients without Axis II disorders showed the opposite pattern of response (Fournier et al., 2008). A reanalysis of data from the TDCRP found that patients who engage in interpersonal avoidance do better in CT than in IPT, whereas patients with a more obsessive style show the opposite pattern of response, but these findings have not yet been replicated (Barber & Muenz, 1996).

MECHANISMS OF CHANGE AND PREVENTION

It is unclear precisely how CT produces its effects. Early studies suggest that CT may work (at least in part) through processes and mechanisms specified by theory. For example, in a pair of studies, DeRubeis and colleagues found that the extent to which therapists utilize concrete behavioral and cognitive change strategies in early sessions predicts subsequent change in depression (DeRubeis & Feeley, 1990; Feeley, DeRubeis, & Gelfand, 1999). On the other hand, the quality of the helping alliance (a nonspecific aspect of the therapeutic relationship) was more a consequence than a cause of symptomatic change. This suggests that it may not be necessary to build the relationship before trying to produce change; rather, working to produce change may in turn build a sense of trust and collaboration.

Similarly, cognitive theory suggests that whereas disconfirming negative expectations may be the most efficient way to reduce existing distress, changing underlying explanatory style or self-concept may be more central to the prevention of future episodes (Abramson, Metalsky, & Alloy, 1989). Several early studies examining change in beliefs over time found that patients treated with drugs alone showed as much change in hopelessness as did patients treated to remission with CT. The patterns of change in the two modalities, however, were quite different, in that change in expectations appeared to drive change in depression in CT, whereas change in depression appeared to drive change in expectations in medication treatment (DeRubeis et al., 1990). This suggests that whereas disconfirming negative expectations may play a causal role in reducing distress in CT, the reduction of distress via biological means leads to a change in expectations in medication treatment.

At the same time, changes in core beliefs and information-processing proclivities may be central to the prevention of subsequent relapse and recurrence. For example, in an earlier trial, change in explanatory style was specific to CT and predictive of subsequent freedom from relapse following treatment termination (Hollon, Evans, & DeRubeis, 1990). Whereas change in expectations was nonspecific and occurred in conjunction with change in depression (whether cause or consequence), change in explanatory style occurred only in CT and happened later in the course of therapy, well after the bulk of the change in depression. This suggests that change in these underlying proclivities is not necessary for initial symptom reduction, but it may be central to the prevention of subsequent symptom return. The acquisition of cognitive skills in recognizing and disputing negative beliefs predicted subsequent freedom from relapse in the trial by DeRubeis and colleagues (Strunk, DeRubeis, Chiu, & Alvarez, 2007), and similar changes in information-processing proclivities appeared to mediate the preventive effects observed in one study with a nonclinical high-risk sample (Seligman et al., 1999). These are the same processes targeted by theory and shown in longitudinal designs to confer risk for depression. The fact that drugs do little to reduce these purported diatheses or underlying risk suggests convergence across different types of evidence regarding possible mediation. Although it is unclear whether patients change in some way that redresses underlying vulnerabilities, or whether they merely develop compensatory skills, it is apparent that risk is reduced (Barber & DeRubeis, 1989).

Others have suggested that changing the content of negative thoughts and beliefs does not prevent relapse; rather, it is changing one's relationship to negative thoughts and beliefs that confers protection (Teasdale et al., 2002). Specifically, it has been proposed that during CT, patients learn to "decenter" from their negative thoughts and develop the ability to experience internal events from a stance of metacognitive awareness. From this stance, patients are less personally identified with thoughts and can experience them as events arising and passing in the mind.

Recent studies suggest that differences between CT and pharmacotherapy in the processes of change may be reflected in underlying neural mechanisms. Depressed patients typically show hyperactivity in the limbic regions that are important to perceiving emotional aspects of information (especially the amygdala), and hypoactivity in areas of the prefrontal cortex that exert inhibitory control over those limbic regions (Drevets, 2000; Gotlib & Hamilton, in press). Direct comparisons are still few, but antidepressant medications appear to target the limbic system directly (Mayberg, 2003), whereas cognitive therapy appears to have more of an effect on cortical functions (Siegle, Carter, & Thase, 2006). Findings have not always been consistent with initial expectations; for example, in one trial, CT led to a further decrease in resting metabolism in the prefrontal cortex (Goldapple et al., 2004); this finding, however, could reflect lowering of tonic resting-state activity that allows for greater reactivity when executive control is recruited. The general sense to date is that medications work from the "bottom up" through their effects on the limbic system, whereas CT works from the "top down" by bolstering higher-order executive processes centered in the cortex (Seminowicz et al., 2004).

PROBLEMS IN DISSEMINATION AND ROBUSTNESS ACROSS TRIALS

Despite its apparent efficacy and evidence of enduring effects, CT has not always been easy to disseminate and has suffered from a lack of robustness across trials. The TDCRP stands as one clear example of a study in which experienced therapists had trouble learning to apply CT; a recent comparison to BA, discussed below, may represent another example (Dimidjian et al., 2006). In each of these studies, CT was outperformed by medications and at least one other psychosocial intervention (IPT in the first instance and BA in the second) in the treatment of more severely depressed patients. Similarly, DeRubeis and colleagues (2005) found a significant site × treatment interaction in which CT did better relative to medications at the site at which it was first developed than it did at the other site in the study. Thus, questions can be raised as to how easy or difficult it is for even experienced psychotherapists to learn to use the approach, especially with more complicated patients (Coffman, Martell, Dimidjian, Gallop, & Hollon, 2007). We return to these issues when we discuss the more purely behavioral interventions in the sections that follow.

OTHER COGNITIVE-BEHAVIORAL INTERVENTIONS

Several other types of cognitive-behavioral interventions differ from CT with respect to both underlying theory and actual procedures of intervention. The cognitive-behavioral analysis system of psychotherapy (CBASP) was designed specifically for working with patients with long-standing affective distress, who are presumed to have arrested emotional development that prevents their learning from experience (McCullough, 2000). CBASP represents an amalgamation of cognitive, behavioral, and interpersonal strategies designed to motivate chronically depressed persons to change and to help them develop needed problem-solving and relationship skills. Although its underlying theoretical rationale is rich and complex, its actual operational procedures are relatively straightforward and concrete: Patients are trained to apply a simple algorithm in problematic interpersonal situations to guide their choice of specific behaviors that are most likely to help them get what they want. In a trial in patients with chronic depression, adding CBASP to medications worked better than did either single modality alone, with drugs working faster and psychotherapy producing more change in the later stages of therapy (Keller et al., 2000). It remains to be seen whether this approach will live up to its initial promise, but it has generated considerable enthusiasm in the field and has proven to be particularly attractive to therapists trained in more traditional approaches.

Mindfulness-based cognitive therapy (MBCT) represents an integration of meditation with more conventional cognitive therapy. In this approach, patients are trained to observe their thoughts without responding to them affectively, in addition to more conventional training in cognitive restructuring found in CT (Segal, Williams, & Teasdale, 2002). MBCT has mostly been applied to patients already brought to remission with medication treatment, but it has been found to prevent subsequent relapse or recurrence in patients withdrawn from medications in a pair of randomized controlled trials (Ma & Teasdale, 2004; Teasdale et al., 2000). Curiously, in both studies, the magnitude of the effect produced by MBCT was greatest for patients with three or more prior episodes, a pattern of moderation quite distinct from that typically found for CT. Recent studies also have begun to explore the value of MBCT for the treatment of acute depression, with preliminary data suggesting that treatment-resistant depressed patients who receive MBCT experience substantial improvement over the course of treatment (Kenny & Williams, 2007).

Well-being therapy (WBT) is a variation of cognitive therapy that focuses on efforts to develop a sense of purpose in life and to enhance a subjective sense well-being (Fava, 1999). Unlike more conventional CT, which emphasizes the amelioration of negative thinking, WBT seeks to balance this approach with specific activities and strategies that promote a sense of accomplishment and purpose. Although it is not widely known in the larger treatment community and has not been directly compared to more conventional CT, the application of WBT was found to prevent subsequent recurrence following medication withdrawal in patients first treated to recovery with drugs alone (Fava et al., 1998).

Finally, Seligman, Rashid, and Parks (2006) have developed an approach called positive psychotherapy (PPT) that focuses almost wholly on the pursuit of a sense of meaning and positive regard in life. The approach is an outgrowth of positive psychology and is based on a careful examination of those strategies that seem to contribute most to a sense of meaning and purpose in living (Seligman & Csikszentmihalyi, 2000). Participants are encouraged to engage in a series of specific activities that may range from doing something nice for random others to expressing their appreciation to people who have made an important contribution to their lives. Although it has not yet been tested in a clinical population, PPT has generated considerable interest in the field and appears to lead to reductions in distress and dysphoria almost as an incidental by-product of gains in a sense of purpose in life (Seligman, Steen, Parks, & Peterson, 2005).

MORE PURELY BEHAVIORAL INTERVENTIONS

There also exist a number of related interventions that are considered to be more purely behavioral, such as problem-solving therapy, training in self-control, skills training, contingency management, and BA and other activation approaches to depression. Although cognitive and behavioral approaches can be differentiated theoretically, they are often combined in actual clinical practice, and a precise taxonomy is sometimes hard to maintain. Certainly, problem-solving therapy and training in self-control may have important cognitive elements, as may skills training (depending on how it is done). Conversely, contingency management is typically conducted in accordance with a more purely behavioral conceptualization, although it may be argued that the strategy of highlighting contingent relations is a cognitive one. Although they have not been tested as extensively as cognitive therapy, each generally has fared well in controlled trials (American Psychiatric Association, 2000).

For example, problem-solving therapy is predicated on the notion that deficits in coping skills contribute to the onset and maintenance of depression (D'Zurilla & Nezu, 1982). It seeks to teach patients how to define life problems in ways that facilitate finding a solution, and helps them to generate and to choose among several possible alternatives. Problem-solving therapy has been found to be superior to minimal treatment and to nonspecific controls in a pair of studies with symptomatic community volunteers (Nezu, 1986; Nezu & Perri, 1989). More recently, investigators in England have found a brief version of problem-solving therapy to be comparable to drugs and superior to placebo in the treatment of depression in a general practice sample (Mynors-Wallace, Gath, Day, & Baker, 2000; Mynors-Wallace, Gath, Lloyd-Thomas, & Tomlinson, 1995). These studies suggest that problem-solving approaches have considerable merit.

Self-control therapy involves teaching patients to monitor and to evaluate their own actions more positively, and to reward themselves when they meet reasonable standards of behavior (Rehm, 1977). Although typically classified as a behavioral intervention, because it draws so heavily on reinforcement theory, self-control therapy clearly contains some cognitive elements in terms of the attention devoted to the standards that patients use for self-evaluation. Self-control therapy has been evaluated in a number of controlled trials, most involving less severely depressed community volunteers. In these studies, it typically has been found to be superior to minimal treatment controls and comparable to other treatment interventions (Fuchs & Rehm, 1977; Kornblith, Rehm, O'Hara, & Lamparski, 1983; Rabin, Kaslow, & Rehm, 1984; Rehm, Fuchs, Roth, Kornblith, & Romano, 1979; Rehm et al., 1981; Rude, 1986). Studies in fully clinical populations have been few but generally supportive. For example, Roth, Bielski, Jones, Parker, and Osborn (1982) found that adding drugs did little to enhance the efficacy of self-control therapy alone in an outpatient sample. Similarly, Van den Hout, Arntz, and Kunkels (1995) found that the addition of self-control therapy enhanced response relative to usual care in a day treatment sample.

More purely behavioral interventions based on operant theory typically also have fared well in controlled trials, although, once again, they have not been extensively tested. Hersen, Bellack, Himmelhoch, and Thase (1984) found no differences between social skills training (combined with either drugs or pill-placebo) and drugs alone or a brief dynamic psychotherapy in a sample of depressed female outpatients. McLean and Hakstian (1979) found a modest advantage for a behavioral intervention based on contingency management relative to either medications alone or a brief dynamic psychotherapy in the treatment of depressed outpatients. O'Leary and Beach (1990) found that behavioral marital therapy was as efficacious as CT and superior to a wait-list control in the treatment of depression in couples with marital distress. Similarly, Jacobson, Dobson, Fruzetti, Schmaling, and Salusky (1991) found that behavioral marital therapy was as efficacious as CT in reducing depression in women with marital distress, but less efficacious than CT for women without such marital problems.

BEHAVIORAL ACTIVATION AND OTHER ACTIVATION-ORIENTED TREATMENTS

Work on purely behavioral treatments for depression had stagnated somewhat before publication of a component analysis by Jacobson and colleagues (1996). In this study, the BA component of CT produced as much change as did the full treatment package. Moreover, there were no differences in subsequent rates of relapse following treatment termination (Gortner, Gollan, Dobson, & Jacobson, 1998). These findings were so unexpected that Jacobson, Martell, and Dimidjian (2001) developed a more comprehensive version of the approach rooted in the work of Lewinsohn (1974) and Ferster (1973, 1981), both of whom highlighted the centrality of context and activity in understanding depression.

The rationale for treatment that informs BA emphasizes the role of life contexts that are characterized by low levels of positive reinforcement and high levels of aversive control in precipitating or maintaining depression. In addition, an individual's tendency to respond to such contexts with avoidance and withdrawal is highlighted. The BA approach to treatment emphasizes that such responses are natural and understandable; they also, however, prevent contact with experiences that could improve mood and prevent active problem solving to improve life context. Guided activation is proposed as a general approach to help to disrupt the context–activity–mood relations that maintain depression.

The implementation of BA is highly idiographic; thus, a careful assessment of the factors that maintain a particular patient's depression helps a therapist to individualize the general model and guides the selection of treatment strategies. Therapists work with clients to define and to describe key problems specifically, and to examine the behavioral patterns that prompt or maintain such problems. Self-monitoring is a key tool used in the assessment process. A substantial amount of treatment is focused on helping patients identify contingent relations among situations, activities, and moods.

Like cognitive therapy, BA is a highly structured approach. Therapists work collaboratively with patients to set and to follow an agenda each session. Therapists also clearly review progress since previous sessions, frequently using patient ratings on the Beck Depression Inventory to assess change. Assigning and reviewing homework is a major focus of BA, and therapists spend considerable time anticipating and troubleshooting potential barriers and working with clients to maximize their commitment to action.

Over the course of treatment, therapists utilize a small set of strategies and maintain an overriding focus on activation. Primary strategies include developing activation assignments that increase pleasure and mastery, and approach behavior (as opposed to avoidance behavior). Therapists work with clients to schedule activities and frequently structure activities to break larger activities down into their constituent parts and sequence them to increase likelihood of success. BA therapists frequently work with patients to generate and to evaluate solutions to problems, and may teach skills as appropriate (e.g., assertiveness). Therapists in BA do not target the direct modification of thoughts or beliefs as do cognitive therapists. Although BA therapists may assess negative or ruminative thinking patterns, treatment strategies emphasize highlighting the consequences of ruminative thinking, practice in engaging with direct and immediate experience, and refocusing on immediate goals. In general, a primary treatment goal of BA is to encourage patients to act proactively instead of engaging in avoidance behaviors. This strategy is similar in many respects to the one that forms the core of the CBASP, described earlier in this chapter (McCullough, 2000).

BA was recently compared to cognitive therapy and to pharmacotherapy (paroxetine) in a randomized, placebo-controlled clinical trial (Dimidjian et al. 2006). Results suggest that BA has considerable promise. Among more severely depressed patients, it was comparable in outcomes to pharmacotherapy and significantly outperformed CT; among less severely depressed patients, no differences among the treatments were observed. Patients treated with BA also did as well with respect to the prevention of relapse as those treated with CT or continued on their medication over the follow-up period, although only those previously treated with CT demonstrated significant advantage compared to those whose medication was discontinued (Dobson et al., 2008). These findings suggest that BA also has promise with respect to enduring effects.

The encouraging findings associated with BA are consistent with other trials investigating related activation approaches to depression. An early dismantling study among older adults, for instance, also found no differences between a purely behavioral and a cognitive bibliotherapy intervention, with both significantly outperforming a control intervention (Scogin, Jamison, & Gochneaur, 1989). A related behavioral activation model has shown promise in the treatment of depression among cancer patients (Hopko, Bell, Armento, Hunt, & Lejuez, 2005) and among psychiatric inpatients (Hopko, Lejuez, LePage, Hopko, & McNiel, 2003). Exercise-based interventions have also accumulated increasing support in the treatment of depression (Stathopoulou, Powers, Berry, Smits, & Otto, 2006).

In summary, if the early findings on BA hold, they may go a long way toward reviving interest in more purely behavioral interventions (Hollon, 2001). Such interventions may be considerably easier to apply, and may lend themselves more readily to dissemination, than either CT or more traditional psychotherapeutic approaches. If these conditions hold, the potential benefits of such an approach may be significant.

CONCLUSIONS AND FUTURE DIRECTIONS

Cognitive and behavioral interventions are clearly efficacious in the treatment of depression and, moreover, appear to have enduring effects that prevent subsequent risk. CT may work by teaching patients to identify and to test their negative beliefs and information-processing strategies, although the success of more purely behavioral interventions raises the question of whether focusing on change in beliefs is truly necessary to produce symptom change. At the least, it seems that the provision of a set of strategies that patients can use to relieve their own distress produces lasting change. It does appear that these strategies can be extended to patients with more severe and complicated depressions, although questions remain about how robust CT is in that regard. It is possible that more purely behavioral approaches will prove to be easier to disseminate that CT.

Recent studies further suggest that simpler and more concrete behavioral interventions are efficacious for many patients with affective distress, including those with severe or chronic depression. To the extent that this is true, it may facilitate the dissemination of these approaches to the clinical practice community, which is increasingly coming to rely on less extensively trained practitioners and shorter treatment intervals. Combined with indications that the cognitive and behavioral interventions may have enduring effects that can be used to prevent the onset of both initial and subsequent episodes, these findings should create real enthusiasm for these approaches in the field.

Despite all that we have learned in recent years, there is clearly much that we still need to know. Although cognitive and behavioral interventions are clearly efficacious in the treatment of depression, it is still not clear which patients respond best to which interventions. There are recurring suggestions that certain types of patients may do better on some medications than on others, and the same may prove true for other types of psychosocial treatments (Hollon, Thase, et al., 2002). These "indications," however, are hard to pin down and sometimes seem more firmly entrenched in clinical lore than in empirical data. Nonetheless, it is easier to determine whether something works in general than it is to determine the best treatment for a particular type of patient.

Even more critically, it remains to be seen whether the enduring effect produced by cognitive and behavioral interventions extends to the prevention of recurrence. That these interventions have an enduring effect seems to be clear, but this effect would be more interesting theoretically and more important pragmatically if it worked to prevent the onset of wholly new episodes. As effective as medications are (and they are largely safe and effective), there is no evidence that they do anything to reduce subsequent risk once their use is discontinued

(Hollon, 1996). Because depression tends to be a chronic episodic disorder, any treatment that can reduce subsequent risk would be a real boon to the field, both in terms of the reduction of human misery and the savings in costs to society. Clearly, more work is needed to determine whether cognitive-behavioral interventions really reduce risk for subsequent episodes (recurrence).

Closely related is the notion of primary prevention. Not only do the cognitive and behavioral interventions appear to have an enduring effect, but there is also reason to believe that they may have a preventive effect in at-risk persons who have yet to have their first episode. Throughout the history of medical science, major public health advances have occurred more as a consequence of prevention than of treatment (Hollon, DeRubeis, & Seligman, 1992). Much of this work will need to take place outside of traditional service delivery settings, most likely in schools and in general practice settings. Nonetheless, it is clear that the technology already exists both to detect persons at risk and to provide them with strategies and tools that can protect them against subsequent risk (Gillham et al., 2000; see Muñoz, Le, Clarke, Barrera, & Torres, Chapter 23, this volume).

Much of this progress has occurred in conjunction with a growing understanding of the basic processes that underlie the nature and expression of depression. Depression is a disorder that is clearly affected by biological, psychological, and sociological factors, and important advances in treatment both draw upon and feed back to advances in basic research (Hollon, Muñoz, et al., 2002). The cognitive-behavioral interventions in particular have benefited from advances in understanding of basic cognitive processes and our growing understanding of information processing (Hollon & Garber, 1990; see Joormann, Chapter 13, this volume). Advances in basic attachment theory have informed the development of interpersonal psychotherapy, and the development of new drug therapies clearly has benefited from and contributed to the growth in knowledge about the basic neurological processes underlying affective distress (Shelton, Hollon, Purdon, & Loosen, 1991). The direct links between basic and applied research rarely are clear, but they are important.

In this regard, several questions seem particularly important. For example, depression often involves disruptions in social bonds, yet drugs and cognitive-behavioral therapy are among its most efficacious interventions (along with IPT). Similarly, biological processes often trigger affective distress, and both genes and environmental events appear to confer risk for subsequent distress (Caspi et al., 2003; see Levinson, Chapter 8, this volume). Maladaptive beliefs and attitudes appear to be acquired through either route and further amplify risk for those who are so predisposed. Nonetheless, we have little clear understanding of how these various processes relate to one another, or exactly how our treatments work when they do indeed work. The brain is an organ designed to mediate interaction with the environment, and there is reason to believe that it is capable of responding to external contingencies within the constraints set by biology (Davidson, Pizzagalli, Nitschke, & Putnam, 2002). Clearly, more needs to be done to explore the ways in which cognitive and interpersonal processes interface with basic biology in determining the nature and expression of depression.

ACKNOWLEDGMENTS

Preparation of this chapter was supported by a research grant (No. MH55875) and independent scientist award (No. MH01697) from the National Institute of Mental Health to Steven D. Hollon.

REFERENCES

Abramson, L. Y., Metalsky, G. I., & Alloy, L. B. (1989). Hopelessness depression: A theory-based subtype of depression: A metatheoretical analysis with implications for psychopathology research. *Psychological Review, 96,* 358–372.

American Psychiatric Association. (2000). Practice guideline for the treatment of patients with major depressive disorder (revision). *American Journal of Psychiatry, 157*(Suppl. 4), 1–45.

Barber, J. P., & DeRubeis, R. J. (1989). On second thought: Where the action is in cognitive therapy for depression. *Cognitive Therapy and Research, 13,* 441–457.

Barber, J. P., & Muenz, L. R. (1996). The role of avoidance and obsessiveness in matching patients to cognitive and interpersonal psychotherapy: Empirical findings from the Treatment for Depression Collaborative Research Program. *Journal of Consulting and Clinical Psychology, 64,* 951–958.

Beck, A. T. (1991). Cognitive therapy: A 30-year retrospective. *American Psychologist, 46,* 368–375.

Beck, A. T., Freeman, A., Davis, D. D., & Associates. (2003). *Cognitive therapy of personality disorders* (2nd ed.). New York: Guilford Press.

Beck, A. T., Rush, A. J., Shaw, B. F., & Emery, G. (1979). *The cognitive therapy of depression.* New York: Guilford Press.

Beck, J. S. (1995). *Cognitive therapy: Basics and beyond.* New York: Guilford Press.

Bennett-Levy, J., Butler, G., Fennell, M., Hackmann, A., Mueller, M., & Westbrook, D. (2004). *Oxford guide to behavioural experiments in cognitive therapy.* Oxford, UK: Oxford University Press.

Blackburn, I. M., Bishop, S., Glen, A. I. M., Whalley, L. J., & Christie, J. E. (1981). The efficacy of cognitive therapy in depression: A treatment trial using cognitive therapy and pharmacotherapy, each alone and in combination. *British Journal of Psychiatry, 139,* 181–189.

Blackburn, I. M., Eunson, K. M., & Bishop, S. (1986). A two-year naturalistic follow-up of depressed patients treated with cognitive therapy, pharmacotherapy and a combination of both. *Journal of Affective Disorders, 10,* 67–75.

Bockting, C. L., Schene, A. H., Spinhoven, P., Koeter, M. W. J., Wouters, L. F., Huyser, J., et al. (2005). Preventing relapse/recurrence in recurrent depression with cognitive therapy: A randomized controlled trial. *Journal of Consulting and Clinical Psychology, 73,* 647–657.

Caspi, A., Sugden, K., Moffitt, T. E., Taylor, A., Craig, I. W., Harrington, H., et al. (2003). Influence of life stress on depression: Moderation by a polymorphism in the 5-HTT gene. *Science, 301,* 386–389.

Coffman, S., Martell, C. R., Dimidjian, S., Gallop, R., & Hollon, S. D. (2007). Extreme non-response in cognitive therapy: Can behavioral activation succeed where cognitive therapy fails? *Journal of Consulting and Clinical Psychology, 75,* 531–541.

Davidson, R. J., Pizzagalli, D., Nitschke, J. B., & Putnam, K. (2002). Depression: Perspectives from affective neuroscience. *Annual Review of Psychology, 35,* 545–574.

DeRubeis, R. J., & Crits-Christoph, P. (1998). Empirically supported individual and group psychological treatments for adult mental disorders. *Journal of Consulting and Clinical Psychology, 66,* 37–52.

DeRubeis, R. J., Evans, M. D., Hollon, S. D., Garvey, M. J., Grove, W. M., & Tuason, V. B. (1990). How does cognitive therapy work?: Cognitive change and symptom change in cognitive therapy and pharmacotherapy for depression. *Journal of Consulting and Clinical Psychology, 58,* 862–869.

DeRubeis, R. J., & Feeley, M. (1990). Determinants of change in cognitive therapy for depression. *Cognitive Therapy and Research, 14,* 469–482.

DeRubeis, R. J., Hollon, S. D., Amsterdam, J. D., Shelton, R. C., Young, P. R., Salomon, R. M., et al. (2005). Cognitive therapy vs. medications in the treatment of moderate to severe depression. *Archives of General Psychiatry, 62,* 409–416.

Dimidjian, S., Hollon, S. D., Dobson, K. S., Schmaling, K. B., Kohlenberg, R. J., Addis, M. E., et al. (2006). Behavioral activation, cognitive therapy, and antidepressant medication in the acute treatment of major depression. *Journal of Consulting and Clinical Psychology, 74,* 658–670.

Dobson, K. S., Hollon, S. D., Dimidjian, S., Schmaling, K. B., Kohlenberg, R. J., Gallop, R., et al. (2008). Behavioral activation, cognitive therapy, and anti-depressant medication in the treatment of major depression: Prevention of relapse effects. *Journal of Consulting and Clinical Psychology, 76,* 468–477.

Drevets, W. C. (2000). Neuroimaging studies of mood disorders. *Biological Psychiatry, 48,* 813–829.

D'Zurilla, T. J., & Nezu, A. (1982). Social problem solving in adults. In P. C. Kendall (Ed.), *Advances in cognitive-behavioral research and therapy* (Vol. 1, pp. 202–274). New York: Academic Press.

Elkin, I., Gibbons, R. D., Shea, T., Sotsky, S. M., Watkins, J. T., Pilkonis, P. A., et al. (1995). Initial severity and differential treatment outcome in the National Institute of Mental Health Treatment of Depression Collaborative Research Program. *Journal of Consulting and Clinical Psychology, 63*, 841–847.

Evans, M. D., Hollon, S. D., DeRubeis, R. J., Piasecki, J., Grove, W. M., Garvey, M. J., et al. (1992). Differential relapse following cognitive therapy and pharmacotherapy for depression. *Archives of General Psychiatry, 49*, 802–808.

Fava, G. A. (1999). Well-being therapy: Conceptual and technical issues. *Psychotherapy and Psychosomatics, 68*(4), 171–179.

Fava, G. A., Rafanelli, C., Grandi, S., Conti, S., & Belluardo, P. (1998). Prevention of recurrent depression with cognitive behavioral therapy. *Archives of General Psychiatry, 55*, 816–820.

Feeley, M., DeRubeis, R. J., & Gelfand, L. A. (1999). The temporal relation of adherence and alliance to symptom change in cognitive therapy for depression. *Journal of Consulting and Clinical Psychology, 67*, 578–582.

Ferster, C. B. (1973). A functional analysis of depression. *American Psychologist, 28*, 857–870.

Ferster, C. B. (1981). A functional analysis of behavior therapy. In L. P. Rehm (Ed.), *Behavior therapy for depression: Present status and future directions* (pp. 181–196). New York: Academic Press.

Fournier, J. C., DeRubeis, R. J., Shelton, R. C., Gallop, R., Amsterdam, J. D., & Hollon, S. D. (2008). Cognitive therapy vs. antidepressant medications in the treatment of depressed patients with and without personality disorder. *British Journal of Psychiatry, 192*, 124–129.

Fuchs, C. Z., & Rehm, L. P. (1977). A self-control behavior therapy program for depression. *Journal of Consulting and Clinical Psychology, 45*, 206–215.

Gillham, J. E., Shatte, A. J., & Freres, D. R. (2000). Preventing depression: A review of cognitive-behavioral and family interventions. *Applied and Preventive Psychology, 9*, 63–88.

Goldapple, K., Segal, Z., Garson, C., Lau, M., Bieling, P., Kennedy, S., et al. (2004). Modulation of cortical–limbic pathways in major depression: Treatment-specific effects of cognitive behavior therapy. *Archives of General Psychiatry, 61*, 34–41.

Gortner, E. T., Gollan, J. K., Dobson, K. S., & Jacobson, N. S. (1998). Cognitive-behavioral treatment for depression: Relapse prevention. *Journal of Consulting and Clinical Psychology, 66*, 377–384.

Gotlib, I. H., & Hamilton, J. P. (in press). Neuroimaging and depression: Current status and unresolved issues. *Psychological Science.*

Hersen, M., Bellack, A. S., Himmelhoch, J. M., & Thase, M. E. (1984). Effects of social skill training, amitriptyline, and psychotherapy in unipolar depressed women. *Behavior Therapy, 15*, 21–40.

Hollon, S. D. (1996). The efficacy and effectiveness of psychotherapy relative to medications. *American Psychologist, 51*, 1025–1030.

Hollon, S. D. (2001). Behavioral activation treatment for depression: A commentary. *Clinical Psychology: Science and Practice, 8*, 271–273.

Hollon, S. D., & Beck, A. T. (2004). Cognitive and cognitive behavioral therapies. In M. J. Lambert (Ed.), *Garfield and Bergin's handbook of psychotherapy and behavior change: An empirical analysis* (5th ed., pp. 447–492). New York: Wiley.

Hollon, S. D., DeRubeis, R. J., Evans, M. D., Wiemer, M. J., Garvey, M. J., Grove, W. M., et al. (1992). Cognitive therapy and pharmacotherapy for depression: Singly and in combination. *Archives of General Psychiatry, 49*, 774–781.

Hollon, S. D., DeRubeis, R. J., & Seligman, M. E. P. (1992). Cognitive therapy and the prevention of depression. *Applied and Preventive Psychology, 1*, 89–95.

Hollon, S. D., DeRubeis, R. J., Shelton, R. C., Amsterdam, J. D., Salomon, R. M., O'Reardon, J. P., et al. (2005). Prevention of relapse following cognitive therapy versus medications in moderate to severe depression. *Archives of General Psychiatry, 62*, 417–422.

Hollon, S. D., Evans, M. D., & DeRubeis, R. J. (1990). Cognitive mediation of relapse prevention following treatment for depression: Implications of differential risk. In R. E. Ingram (Ed.), *Psychological aspects of depression* (pp. 114–136). New York: Plenum Press.

Hollon, S. D., & Garber, J. (1990). Cognitive therapy of depression: A social-cognitive perspective. *Personality and Social Psychology Bulletin, 16*, 58–73.

Hollon, S. D., Muñoz, R. F., Barlow, D. H., Beardslee, W. R., Bell, C. C., Bernal, G., et al. (2002). Psychosocial intervention development for the prevention and treatment of depression: Promoting innovation and increasing access. *Biological Psychiatry, 52,* 610–630.

Hollon, S. D., Stewart, M. O., & Strunk, D. (2006). Cognitive behavior therapy has enduring effects in the treatment of depression and anxiety. *Annual Review of Psychology, 57,* 285–315.

Hollon, S. D., Thase, M. E., & Markowitz, J. C. (2002). Treatment and prevention of depression. *Psychological Science in the Public Interest, 3,* 39–77.

Hopko, D. R., Bell, J. L., Armento, M. E. A., Hunt, M. K., & Lejuez, C. W. (2005). Behavior therapy for depressed cancer patients in primary care. *Psychotherapy: Theory, Research, Practice and Training, 42,* 236–243.

Hopko, D. R., Lejuez, C. W., LePage, J. P., Hopko, S. D., & McNeil, D. W. (2003). A brief behavioral activation treatment for depression: A randomized pilot trial within an inpatient psychiatric hospital. *Behavior Modification, 27,* 458–469.

Jacobson, N. S., Dobson, K., Fruzzetti, A. E., Schmaling, K. B., & Salusky, S. (1991). Marital therapy as a treatment for depression. *Journal of Consulting and Clinical Psychology, 59,* 547–557.

Jacobson, N. S., Dobson, K. S., Truax, P. A., Addis, M. E., Koerner, K., Gollan, J. K., et al. (1996). A component analysis of cognitive-behavior treatment for depression. *Journal of Consulting and Clinical Psychology, 64,* 295–304.

Jacobson, N. S., & Hollon, S. D. (1996a). Cognitive-behavior therapy versus pharmacotherapy: Now that the jury's returned its verdict, its time to present the rest of the evidence. *Journal of Consulting and Clinical Psychology, 64,* 74–80.

Jacobson, N. S., & Hollon, S. D. (1996b). Prospects for future comparisons between drugs and psychotherapy: Lessons from the CBT-versus-pharmacotherapy exchange. *Journal of Consulting and Clinical Psychology, 64,* 104–108.

Jacobson, N. S., Martell, C., & Dimidjian, S. (2001). Behavioral activation treatment for depression: Returning to contextual roots. *Clinical Psychology: Science and Practice, 8,* 255–270.

Jarrett, R. B., Schaffer, M., McIntire, D., Witt-Browder, A., Kraft, D., & Risser, R. C. (1999). Treatment of atypical depression with cognitive therapy or phenelzine: A double-blind, placebo-controlled trial. *Archives of General Psychiatry, 56,* 431–437.

Keller, M. B., McCullough, J. P., Klein, D. N., Arnow, B., Dunner, D. L., Gelenberg, A. J., et al. (2000). A comparison of nefazodone, the cognitive behavioral-analysis system of psychotherapy, and their combination for the treatment of chronic depression. *New England Journal of Medicine, 342,* 1462–1470.

Kenny, M. A., & Williams, J. M. G. (2007). Treatment-resistant depressed patients show a good response to mindfulness-based cognitive therapy. *Behaviour Research and Therapy, 43,* 617–625.

Klein, D. F. (1996). Preventing hung juries about therapy studies. *Journal of Consulting and Clinical Psychology, 64,* 81–87.

Kornblith, S. J., Rehm, L. P., O'Hara, M. W., & Lamparski, D. M. (1983). The contribution of self-reinforcement training and behavioral assignments to the efficacy of self-control therapy for depression. *Cognitive Therapy and Research, 7,* 499–527.

Kovacs, M., Rush, A. J., Beck, A. T., & Hollon, S. D. (1981). Depressed outpatients treated with cognitive therapy or pharmacotherapy. *Archives of General Psychiatry, 38,* 33–39.

Lewinsohn, P. M. (1974). A behavioral approach to depression. In R. M. Friedman & M. M. Katz (Eds.), *The psychology of depression: Contemporary theory and research* (pp. 157–185). New York: Wiley.

Ma, S. H., & Teasdale, J. D. (2004). Mindfulness-based cognitive therapy for depression: Replication and exploration of differential relapse prevention effects. *Journal of Consulting and Clinical Psychology, 72*(1), 31–40.

Mayberg, H. S. (2003). Modulating dysfunctional limbic-cortical circuits in depression: Towards development of brain-based algorithms for diagnosis and optimised treatment. *British Medical Bulletin, 65,* 193–207.

McCullough, J. P., Jr. (2000). *Treatment for chronic depression: Cognitive behavioral analysis system for psychotherapy (CBASP).* New York: Guilford Press.

McLean, P. D., & Hakstian, A. R. (1979). Clinical depression: Comparative efficacy of outpatient treatments. *Journal of Consulting and Clinical Psychology, 47,* 818–836.

Murphy, G. E., Simons, A. D., Wetzel, R. D., & Lustman, P. J. (1984). Cognitive therapy and pharmacotherapy, singly and together, in the treatment of depression. *Archives of General Psychiatry, 41*, 33–41.

Mynors-Wallis, L. M., Gath, D., Day, A., & Baker, F. (2000). Randomised controlled trial of problem-solving treatment, antidepressant medication and combined treatment for major depression in primary care. *British Medical Journal, 320*, 26–30.

Mynors-Wallis, L. M., Gath, D. H., Lloyd-Thomas, A. R., & Tomlinson, D. (1995). Randomised controlled trial comparing problem solving treatment with amitriptyline and placebo for major depression in primary care. *British Medical Journal, 310*, 441–445.

Nezu, A. M. (1986). Efficacy of a social problem-solving therapy approach for unipolar depression. *Journal of Consulting and Clinical Psychology, 54*, 196–202.

Nezu, A. M., & Perri, M. G. (1989). Social problem-solving therapy for unipolar depression: An initial dismantling investigation. *Journal of Consulting and Clinical Psychology, 57*, 408–413.

O'Leary, K. D., & Beach, S. R. H. (1990). Marital therapy: A viable treatment for depression and marital discord. *American Journal of Psychiatry, 147*, 183–186.

Paykel, E. S., Scott, J., Teasdale, J. D., Johnson, A. L., Garland, A., Moore, R., et al. (1999). Prevention of relapse in residual depression by cognitive therapy. *Archives of General Psychiatry, 56*, 829–835.

Rabin, A. S., Kaslow, N. J., & Rehm, L. P. (1984). Changes in symptoms of depression during course of therapy. *Cognitive Therapy and Research, 8*, 479–488.

Rehm, L. P. (1977). A self-control model of depression. *Behavior Therapy, 8*, 787–804.

Rehm, L. P., Fuchs, C. Z., Roth, D. M., Kornblith, S. J., & Romano, J. M. (1979). A comparison of self-control and assertion skills treatments of depression. *Behavior Therapy, 10*, 429–442.

Rehm, L. P., Kornblith, S. J., O'Hara, M. W., Lamparski, D. M., Romano, J. M., & Volkin, J. (1981). An evaluation of major components in a self-control behavior therapy program for depression. *Behavior Modification, 5*, 459–490.

Roth, D., Bielski, R., Jones, M., Parker, W., & Osborn, G. (1982). A comparison of self-control therapy and combined self-control therapy and antidepressant medication in the treatment of depression. *Behavior Therapy, 13*, 133–144.

Rude, S. S. (1986). Relative benefits of assertion or cognitive self-control treatment for depression as a function of proficiency in each domain. *Journal of Consulting and Clinical Psychology, 54*, 390–394.

Rush, A. J., Beck, A. T., Kovacs, M., & Hollon, S. D. (1977). Comparative efficacy of cognitive therapy and pharmacotherapy in the treatment of depressed outpatients. *Cognitive Therapy and Research, 1*, 17–38.

Scogin, F., Jamison, C., & Gochneaur, K. (1989). Comparative efficacy of cognitive and behavioral bibliotherapy for mildly and moderately depressed older adults. *Journal of Consulting and Clinical Psychology, 57*, 403–407.

Segal, Z. V., Williams, J. M. G., & Teasdale, J. D. (2002). *Mindfulness-based cognitive therapy for depression.* New York: Guilford Press.

Seligman, M. E. P., & Csikszentmihalyi, M. (2000). Positive psychology: An introduction. *American Psychologist, 55*(1), 5–14.

Seligman, M. E. P., Rashid, T., & Parks, A. C. (2006). Positive psychotherapy. *American Psychologist, 61*(8), 774–788.

Seligman, M. E. P., Schulman, P., DeRubeis, R. J., & Hollon, S. D. (1999). Primary prevention of depression and anxiety with cognitive therapy. *Prevention and Treatment, 2*, Article 8. Available online at *journals.apa.org/prevention/volume2/pre002008a.html*

Seligman, M. E. P., Steen, T. A., Parks, N., & Peterson, C. (2005). Positive psychology progress: Empirical validation of interventions. *American Psychologist, 60*(5), 410–421.

Seminowicz, D. A., Mayberg, H. S., McIntosh, A. R., Goldapple, K., Kennedy, S., Segal, Z., et al. (2004). Limbic–frontal circuitry in major depression: A path modeling meta-analysis. *NeuroImage, 22*, 409–418.

Shea, M. T., Elkin, I., Imber, S. D., Sotsky, S. M., Watkins, J. T., Collins, J. F., et al. (1992). Course of depressive symptoms over follow-up: Findings from the National Institute of Mental Health Treatment of Depression Collaborative Research Program. *Archives of General Psychiatry, 49*, 782–787.

Shea, M. T., Pilkonis, P. A., Beckham, E., Collins, J. F., Elkin, I., Sotsky, S. M., et al. (1990). Personality disorders and treatment outcome in the NIMH Treatment of Depression Collaborative Research Program. *American Journal of Psychiatry, 147*, 711–718.

Shelton, R. C., Hollon, S. D., Purdon, S. E., & Loosen, P. T. (1991). Biological and psychological aspects of depression. *Behavior Therapy, 22*, 201–228.

Siegle, G. J., Carter, C. S., & Thase, M. E. (2006). Use of fMRI to predict recovery from unipolar depression with cognitive behavior therapy. *American Journal of Psychiatry, 163*, 735–738.

Simons, A. D., Murphy, G. E., Levine, J. E., & Wetzel, R. D. (1986). Cognitive therapy and pharmacotherapy for depression: Sustained improvement over one year. *Archives of General Psychiatry, 43*, 43–49.

Sotsky, S. M., Glass, D. R., Shea, M. T., Pilkonis, P. A., Collins, J. F., Elkin, I., et al. (1991). Patient predictors of response to psychotherapy and pharmacotherapy: Findings in the NIMH Treatment of Depression Collaborative Research Program. *American Journal of Psychiatry, 148*, 997–1008.

Stathopoulou, G., Powers, M. B., Berry, A. C., Smits, J. A. J., & Otto, M. W. (2006). Exercise interventions for mental health: A quantitative and qualitative review. *Clinical Psychology: Science and Practice, 13*, 179–193.

Strunk, D. R., DeRubeis, R. J., Chiu, A. W., & Alvarez, J. (2007). Patients' competence in and performance of cognitive therapy skills: Relation to the reduction of relapse risk following treatment for depression. *Journal of Consulting and Clinical Psychology, 75*, 523–529.

Teasdale, J. D., Moore, R. G., Hayhurst, H., Pope, M., Williams, S., & Segal, Z. V. (2002). Metacognitive awareness and prevention of relapse in depression: Empirical evidence. *Journal of Consulting and Clinical Psychology, 70*, 275–287.

Teasdale, J. D., Segal, Z., Williams, J. M. G., Ridgeway, V. A., Soulsby, J. M., & Lau, M. A. (2000). Prevention of relapse/recurrence in major depression by mindfulness-based cognitive therapy. *Journal of Consulting and Clinical Psychology, 68*(4), 615–623.

Thase, M. E., Frank, E., Kornstein, S., & Yonkers, K. A. (2000). Gender differences in response to treatments of depression. In E. Frank (Ed.), *Gender and its effects on psychopathology* (pp. 103–129). Washington, DC: American Psychiatric Press.

Thase, M. E., Reynolds, C. F., Frank, E., Simons, A. D., McGeary, J., Fasiczka, A. L., et al. (1994). Do depressed men and women respond similarly to cognitive behavior therapy? *American Journal of Psychiatry, 151*, 500–505.

Van den Hout, J. H., Arntz, A., & Kunkels, F. H. (1995). Efficacy of a self-control therapy program in a psychiatric day-treatment center. *Acta Psychiatrica Scandinavica, 92*, 25–29.

CHAPTER 26

Pharmacotherapy and Psychosocial Treatments for Bipolar Disorder

David J. Miklowitz

Bipolar disorder is a reasonably common and highly debilitating illness. Bipolar I and II disorder affects as many as 1 in 50 persons; when its spectrum variants are included, the rate goes up to 4.5% in epidemiological samples (Merikangas et al., 2007). Between 50 and 67% of patients have their illness onset before age 18, and between 13 and 28%, before age 13 (Perlis et al., 2004). The disorder is highly recurrent and disabling, leading to unemployment or lost days of work, high rates of divorce, legal problems, and low quality of life. In the year 2020, bipolar disorder is projected to be the sixth leading cause of disability worldwide (Murray & Lopez, 1996).

The evidence that lithium, and, more recently, the anticonvulsants and atypical antipsychotics are effective in controlling manic or depressive episodes is substantial (Tondo, Baldessarini, & Floris, 2001; Yatham et al., 2005). However, full and rapid recovery from episodes, notably bipolar depressive episodes, are often unattainable with pharmacotherapy alone. In a 26-week randomized trial involving 22 sites (the Systematic Treatment Enhancement Program for Bipolar Disorder, or STEP-BD), recovery from a bipolar depressive episode occurred in only 21–27% of patients receiving optimal pharmacotherapy with mood stabilizers (Sachs et al., 2007). In a 4-year follow-up of children with bipolar I disorder (mean age, 10.8 years) with manic episodes, most of whom were undergoing pharmacotherapy, Geller, Tillman, Craney, and Bolhofner (2004) found that the duration of episodes (without recovery) averaged 79 weeks. The effectiveness of pharmacotherapy alone is even more questionable when one examines the long-term course of the disorder. In Geller and colleagues' 4-year follow-up, children with bipolar disorder spent an average of 57% of their total weeks with diagnosable mania or hypomania, and 47% of the total weeks with major or minor depression or dysthymia. Rates of recurrence among adults average 40% in 1 year, 60% over 2 years, and 73% over 5 years (Gitlin, Swendsen, Heller, & Hammen, 1995). In a study of 1,469 bipolar I and II adults followed over 1 year, 49% had recurrences of their disorder; twice as many of these recurrences were for depressive episodes as for manic episodes (Perlis et al., 2006).

Thus, the longitudinal course of bipolar disorder is marked by recurrences, residual symptoms, and functional impairments. Two integrated treatment avenues are essential to providing optimal outcomes for bipolar patients—flexible pharmacotherapy (allowing for changes in drug or dosage patterns as patients relapse or remit) and psychosocial interventions. This biopsychosocial approach to treatment is gaining traction and is now favored in the majority of treatment guidelines for bipolar disorder in the United States, Canada, and Europe (e.g., Goodwin, 2003; Keck et al., 2004; Suppes et al., 2005; Yatham et al., 2005).

This chapter reviews the literature on drug and psychosocial treatments. Because there are comprehensive reviews of the pharmacotherapy literature (e.g., Thase, 2006a, 2006b), this chapter places greater emphasis on psychosocial intervention trials. A final section offers recommendations for future research.

PHARMACOTHERAPY FOR BIPOLAR DISORDER

Pharmacological studies have generally been focused on the acute stabilization of manic or depressive episodes, whereas psychosocial studies have generally focused on maintenance treatment (prevention of recurrence and mitigation of residual symptoms). These different emphases reflect in part the more rapid response of patients to pharmacotherapy than to psychotherapy, and that psychotherapy often involves the incorporation of skills before effects can be observed. In the following sections, recent findings from large-scale clinical trials are reviewed, and gaps in the literature are highlighted.

Proper Diagnosis

The effectiveness of drug or psychosocial treatment can be undermined when patients are misdiagnosed with other conditions or have unrecognized comorbid disorders. The most straightforward example is the misdiagnosis of bipolar depression as unipolar depression. Patients with depression who have unrecognized bipolar syndromes are often given antidepressants alone, which can precipitate treatment-emergent affective switches or cycle acceleration (Thase, 2006a, 2006b). The consequences can be dire for adolescent patients who, due to unnecessary antidepressant treatment, develop an earlier onset of mania than they might have without antidepressants. Likewise, young patients who are bipolar but are misdiagnosed with attention-deficit/hyperactivity disorder (ADHD) may develop behavioral disinhibition in response to psychostimulants. Until biomarkers specific to the pathophysiology of bipolar disorder are identified, accurate diagnoses through structured clinical interviews and personal histories are essential to successful treatment (Thase, 2006b).

What Is a Mood Stabilizer?

Mood stabilizers are drugs that are effective in treating or preventing manic, mixed, and/or depressive episodes, without triggering new episodes of the opposite polarity (Keck et al., 2004). Psychiatrists increasingly are substituting divalproex sodium, lamotrigine, or the atypical antipsychotics for lithium, or combining these agents to control acute manic or mixed episodes, to alleviate depressive symptoms, and/or to prevent recurrences. This change in practice is generally attributed to the more tolerable side effect profiles among anticonvulsant or atypical antipsychotic agents in contrast to lithium. There is, however, little evidence that these alternative agents are more effective than lithium.

The following medications have been approved by the Food and Drug Administration (FDA) for the treatment of bipolar disorder: lithium; the anticonvulsants divalproex sodium (valproate, Depakote, Depakene, or Depakon), lamotrigine (Lamictal), and carbamazepine (Tegretol); the atypical antipsychotics (olanzapine [Zyprexa], aripiprazole [Abilify], quetiapine [Seroquel], risperidone [Risperdal], and ziprasidone [Geodon]); the combination of olanzapine and fluoxetine (Prozac), also called OFC or Symbiax; and the traditional antipsychotic chlorpromazine (Thorazine). These medications are often combined with antipressants or anxiolytic agents. Lithium, risperidone, and aripiprazole are approved for use in the treatment of mania among adolescents.

These drugs have multiple mechanisms of action. Lithium and valproate both inhibit the protein kinase C signal transduction pathway. Lithium also has inhibitory effects on calcium, glutamate, and guanine nucleotide-binding proteins (G-proteins), all components of the intracellular signaling cascade (Manji et al., 2003). Lithium and the selective serotonin reuptake inhibitors (SSRIs) have neuroprotective effects in preventing *apoptosis* (cell death). The atypical antipsychotics selectively block dopamine and serotonin receptors, thus having broad effects on mood and anxiety, as well as psychosis (Tohen et al., 2002). The various antidepressants alleviate depression primarily through serotoninergic, dopaminergic, and noradrenergic mechanisms. They may also reduce the output of glucocorticoids, which, if overproduced, can lead to the destruction of hippocampal cells (Sapolsky, 2000).

Anticonvulsants such as divalproex may have "antikindling" effects through diminishing excitation and enhancing inhibition in the mesolimbic system and other neural circuits responsible for emotion regulation (Goldberg, 2004). Lamotrigine and carbamazepine reduce the outflow, the presynaptic release, or the postsynaptic uptake of excitatory amino acids such as glutamate.

Evidence for Drug Efficacy in Randomized Clinical Trials

Treatment of Mania

Lithium remains the mainstay of treatment for adults, although its use in children is overshadowed by prescriptions for divalproex sodium. Approximately 60–70% of persons with bipolar disorder show a remission of manic symptoms on lithium (for review, see Keck et al., 2004). The benefits of lithium do not come without costs: Common side effects include somnolence, nausea, diarrhea, cognitive dulling, weight gain, stomach irritation, thirst, motor tremors, acne, and a long-term risk of kidney clearance problems and hypothyroidism.

Lithium is impressive as a prophylactic agent in maintenance treatment. One review of studies between 1970 and 1990 concluded that lithium reduced rates of hospitalization by 82%. However, patients still had an average of about one manic or depressive episode per year (Tondo et al., 2001). A meta-analysis of long-term lithium usage, which included 770 participants in five placebo-controlled, randomized trials, concluded that lithium was effective in reducing manic relapses (average of 14 vs. 24% placebo relapse rate), but its effects in preventing depressive relapses failed to reach statistical significance (25 vs. 32%) (Geddes, Burgess, Hawton, Jamison, & Goodwin, 2004). Thus, lithium significantly reduces overall rates of relapse, but patients continue to have "breakthrough" depressive and, to a lesser extent, manic recurrences.

Divalproex sodium appears to be as effective as lithium in controlling manic episodes but may have a milder side effect profile. Side effects of divalproex include nausea, stomach pain, fatigue, weight gain, elevated liver enzymes, and depression of platelet counts. It is not clear which patient characteristics moderate the efficacy of lithium versus divalproex. Data from six open trials have shown that patients who are unresponsive to lithium often respond to divalproex (Schneck, 2006). However, head-to-head comparisons of lithium and divalproex in maintenance treatment find no significant difference in time to recurrence among bipolar adults with rapid cycling (Calabrese, Shelton, et al., 2005) or bipolar children followed over 18–20 months (Findling et al., 2005).

Carbamazepine (Tegretol) appears to be comparable to lithium in controlling mania and is an effective adjunct to lithium in treating rapid cycling (Denicoff et al., 1997). However, there is less enthusiasm for carbamazepine because of its side effect profile, which can include neurotoxicity, elevation of liver enzymes, hyponatremia, and a depression of white blood cells.

A meta-analysis of 24 studies ($n = 6,187$) examined the use of atypical antipsychotics in the treatment of mania (Scherk, Pajonk, & Leucht, 2007). Atypicals were significantly superior to placebo in treating mania, and were just as effective as mood stabilizers. The most efficacious treatment for mania was found to be the combination of atypicals and mood stabilizers (e.g., quetiapine plus divalproex).

It is unclear whether certain atypicals are more effective than others in treating mania. The most well-studied atypical is olanzapine (Zyprexa), which has particularly strong effects on mania, mixed states, and rapid cycling. Its efficacy in preventing manic or mixed-episode recurrences appears to be comparable to or better than divalproex (Tohen et al., 2005), and provides additional prophylaxis when used adjunctively to lithium or divalproex (Tohen et al., 2002). Unfortunately, most atypical antipsychotics are associated with significant weight gain, metabolic disturbances, extrapyramidal symptoms, somnolence, and sedation (DelBello et al., 2006; Kowatch et al., 2005; Tohen et al., 2003).

Treatment of Depression

Lithium and divalproex are the recommended first-line options for mild-to-moderate episodes of bipolar depression. Lithium did as well as the combination of lithium and antidepressants in one study, especially when patients were maintained on blood levels of 0.8 mEq/L or higher (Nemeroff et al., 2001). Also, lithium appears to have strong antisuicide benefits. A study of over 21,000 patients with bipolar disorder found that patients treated with lithium were less likely to attempt or to complete suicide than patients who received divalproex or carbamazepine (Goodwin et al., 2003).

Depression generally has a slower recovery trajectory than mania, and mood stabilizers more effectively treat and prevent manic than depressive episodes (Moller, Grunze, & Broich, 2006). As a result, many clinicians augment mood stabilizers with other agents to enhance recovery. There is considerable debate about whether mood stabilizers should be augmented with antidepressants given their propensity to cause affective switches or rapid cycling. When used alone, antidepressants can induce mania and accelerate mood cycling in 20–40% of patients (Goldberg, 2004). However, there is less evidence that antidepressants cause cycle acceleration when used in combination with adequate dosages of mood stabilizers.

A naturalistic study from the Stanley Foundation Network (Altshuler et al., 2003) found that bipolar patients ($n = 84$) successfully treated for depression with mood stabilizers and SSRIs were less likely to develop depression if they continued antidepressants for 6 months after remission. In contrast, the STEP-BD study found no differences in time to recovery among 366 bipolar depressed patients randomly assigned to mood stabilizers plus antidepressants (buproprion or paroxetine) or mood stabilizers plus placebo (Sachs et al., 2007). However, neither study found an association between antidepressant usage and the likelihood of treatment-emergent mania or hypomania.

One implication of these findings is that antidepressants should be continued among patients who have shown a positive response during an acute depressive episode. However, antidepressants may be neither necessary nor sufficient adjuncts to mood stabilizers in the initial treatment of bipolar depressive episodes. Current treatment guidelines generally only recommend adjunctive antidepressants if other agents have failed in the treatment of bipolar depression, and then only in combination with a mood stabilizing or atypical antipsychotic agent (e.g., Yatham et al., 2005).

Lamotrigine, the only agent other than lithium approved by the FDA as a maintenance agent in bipolar I disorder, appears to be efficacious in the acute and preventive treatment of bipolar depression (Bowden et al., 2003). Somewhat paradoxically, it has no greater effect than placebo in stabilizing manic episodes, but it has some effects in preventing manic relapses (Goodwin et al., 2004). Lamotrigine was found to be effective in preventing relapse in a 6-month study of rapid-cycling patients with bipolar II disorder, most of whom had recurrent depressions (Calabrese et al., 2000). Whereas lamotrigine appears to be more robust than lithium in stabilizing depressive episodes, lithium may be stronger than lamotrigine in stabilizing manic episodes (Goodwin et al., 2004).

A randomized trial involving patients with bipolar depression who had failed on at least two antidepressants found that patients treated with lamotrigine had lower depression severity ratings over 16 weeks than patients treated with inositol or risperidone (Nierenberg et al., 2006). Adverse reactions to lamotrigine can include a serious skin rash in about 5–10% of patients, and in about 0.1% of cases can progress into Stevens–Johnson syndrome, a potentially fatal dermatological reaction (Thase, 2006b).

A new fixed-dose preparation combining olanzapine and fluoxetine appears to be more effective than olanzapine alone (Tohen et al., 2003). OFC also had faster depression response rates and a greater reduction in mania scores than lamotrigine in one 7-week trial (Brown et al., 2006). Neither treatment caused treatment-emergent affective switches, although tolerability was generally better for lamotrigine than for OFC.

Finally, evidence is building for the efficacy of the atypical antipsychotic quetiapine (Seroquel) in recovery from bipolar depression. Quetiapine may have a more favorable side effect profile than olanzapine or OFC. Among patients with bipolar I and II depressions, quetiapine was clearly superior to placebo at both 300 and 600 mg dosages (Calabrese, Keck, et al., 2005; Thase, 2006b).

Issues in the Pharmacotherapy of Bipolar Disorder in Childhood and Adolescence

Child and adolescent bipolar disorder is particularly difficult to assess, diagnose, and treat, in part because of the lack of consensus on its boundaries (Kowatch et al., 2005). Mania in preschool or school-age children may present as chronic and nonepisodic, and/or with mixed features or rapid cycling. Preadolescent and adolescent mania is characterized by lengthy episodes, a high rate of psychosis, and a highly recurrent course (Geller et al., 2004; Pavuluri, Birmaher, & Naylor, 2005).

Because full coverage of the childhood pharmacotherapy literature is beyond the scope of this chapter, the reader is referred to recent comprehensive reviews (e.g., Kowatch et al., 2005; Pavuluri et al., 2005). The best evidence is for lithium, divalproex, and atypical antipsychotics in the treatment of adolescent mania. For example, quetiapine is effective alone or in conjunction with divalproex (DelBello et al., 2002, 2006). Few data exist on the treatment of bipolar depression in children.

The possible risk of polycystic ovary syndrome associated with divalproex—although not yet proven to exist—has diminished enthusiasm for the use of this drug in treating bipolar disorder among female adolescents (Thase, 2006a). Likewise, weight gain and other metabolic side effects from atypical antipsychotics pose unacceptable health risks to younger patients. Even more worrisome is the possibly increased risk of suicidal behaviors among youth treated with antidepressants.

The difficulty in balancing effective treatment and side effects has prompted the development of treatment guidelines for bipolar children and teens (Kowatch et al., 2005). These guidelines favor beginning with a mood-stabilizing agent and/or adding an atypical antipsychotic, and augmenting with another mood stabilizer or atypical antipsychotic, if response is only partial. Later stages of the algorithms include combination of two mood stabilizers and an atypical agent, or, in the case of intractable depressions among adolescents, electroconvulsive therapy (ECT). Treatment of comorbid disorders with psychostimulants (for ADHD) or SSRIs (for anxiety disorders) is acceptable, but only after the child's mood has been fully stabilized.

Methodological Limitations of Pharmacological Treatment Studies

Two issues stand out as methodological shortcomings of the existing studies of pharmacotherapy for bipolar disorder. These shortcomings generally characterize psychosocial treatment studies as well. First is the near-exclusive focus on symptomatic improvement to the neglect of functional (i.e., vocational, relationship) improvement or quality of life. Bipolar patients have ongoing problems in social and occupational functioning even once they are symptomatically remitted (Coryell et al., 1993). In a 12-month follow-up of patients initially hospitalized for a manic or mixed episode, Keck and colleagues (1998) found that 48% recovered symptomatically by 12 months, but only 24% showed full recovery of function.

Second, few drug or psychosocial studies examine medication adherence as a mediator of treatment outcomes. One of the major reasons for the ineffectiveness of drug treatment for bipolar disorder is inconsistency in patients' usage patterns. Laboratory-based drug efficacy and effectiveness trials often differ in results due to the high rate of medication discontinuation in everyday practice (Colom et al., 2000). Unfortunately, patients who rapidly discontinue medications are at an increased risk for recurrence and suicide (Tondo & Baldessarini, 2000).

Rates of medication nonadherence are reported differently across studies. For example, Strakowski and colleagues (1998) reported that up to 60% of patients discontinued medications or were partially nonadherent in the year after a manic or mixed episode. Patients in a community clinic study took lithium for an average of only 76 days (Johnson & McFarland, 1996). In a bipolar adolescent sample, only 35% of the patients took all of their medications as prescribed (Coletti, Leigh, Gallelli, & Kafantaris, 2005).

Nonadherence is a serious problem for all long-lasting medical conditions with intermittent symptoms. Beyond this, medication issues specific to bipolar disorder include side effects (e.g., weight gain, fatigue, cognitive dulling), dislike of having one's mood controlled by a medication, lack of family or social supports, poor doctor–patient relationship, and lack of information about the disorder. The patients at highest risk for nonadherence are younger, have more severe illnesses, and are more likely to have comorbid personality disorders or substance use disorders (Colom et al., 2000).

Thus, future drug or psychosocial studies would benefit from including functional improvement as a key outcome criterion. Examining the mediating effects of medication adherence is critical to determining the effectiveness of both classes of treatments.

PSYCHOSOCIAL TREATMENTS FOR BIPOLAR DISORDER

The majority of existing randomized trials have considered psychotherapy to be a maintenance treatment (oriented toward relapse prevention and management of residual symptoms), but more recent studies have also considered its value in stabilizing acute episodes of depression. Modern psychosocial approaches are based in research showing that psychosocial stressors have a role in eliciting episodes of bipolar disorder (for a review of this area, see Johnson, Cuellar, & Miller, Chapter 7, this volume). There is prognostic evidence for three types of psychosocial stress: (1) life events stress, notably events that engage the patient in goal pursuit (Johnson, 2005) or that disrupt sleep–wake cycles and other circadian rhythms (Malkoff-Schwartz et al., 1998); (2) high family expressed emotion (EE) or family discord (Kim & Miklowitz, 2004; Miklowitz, Goldstein, Nuechterlein, Snyder, & Mintz, 1988; Miklowitz et al., 2000; Yan, Hammen, Cohen, Daley, & Henry, 2004); and (3) early childhood adversity in the form of sexual or physical abuse or parental neglect (Dienes, Hammen, Henry, Cohen, & Daley, 2006; Post & Leverich, 2006). Among preadolescent and adolescent patients with bipolar disorder, life stressors (Kim, Miklowitz, Biuckians, & Mullen, 2007), family EE (Miklowitz, Biuckians, & Richards, 2006), and low parental warmth (Geller et al., 2004) are prospectively associated with symptom severity and recurrence.

Moderators of the effects of life stress, which would be quite informative for the development of psychosocial interventions, have not been identified. In two studies of college undergraduates with a history of hypomanic or depressive symptoms, negative life events predicted increases in depressive symptoms only among students with negative cognitive styles (Reilly-Harrington, Alloy, Fresco, & Whitehouse, 1999). Despite theories of kindling (Post & Leverich, 2006), life events do not appear to be more potent in provoking initial episodes than later episodes in either adult (Hammen & Gitlin, 1997; Hlastala et al., 2000) or adolescent samples (Hillegers et al., 2004). There is better evidence for a stress reactivity hypothesis, in which certain subgroups of patients become more vulnerable to stress with repeated episodes or due to antecedent vulnerabilities (Hammen & Gitlin, 1997). For example, one study found that early childhood adversity moderated the relationship between life stress and recurrence among bipolar adults, such that patients with more severe early adversity (particularly parental neglect) reported lower levels of stress prior to recurrences than did patients with less severe early adversity (Dienes et al., 2006).

Many of the existing psychotherapy studies cite these stress–outcome studies as justifications for their approach. However, few studies have examined interactions between psychotherapy and stress factors in alleviating bipolar symptoms, or the extent to which the effects of psychotherapy are mediated by changes in the patients' ability to cope with stress. The examination of moderators and mediators is a major gap in this literature, as elaborated below.

Cognitive-Behavioral Therapy

Cognitive-behavioral therapy (CBT) approaches to bipolar disorder are similar to the models used in major depression and comprise behavioral activation (i.e., scheduling of pleasurable life events) followed by cognitive restructuring and modifying core dysfunctional beliefs. CBT for bipolar disorder also includes disorder-specific elements, such as restructuring hyperpositive thinking and monitoring daily activities to reduce overstimulation.

Early CBT approaches focused on cognitions related to medications (e.g., "Taking lithium means giving up my creativity"). The first randomized, controlled trial of CBT for remitted bipolar patients found benefits of a six-session treatment over medication alone in enhancing compliance with medications and reducing rehospitalization over a 6-month period (Cochran, 1984). There have been two randomized, controlled relapse prevention studies of CBT since then (the Systematic Treatment Enhancement Program [STEP-BD] multisite trial, which focused on depression recovery, is covered later). Lam, Hayward, Watkins, Wright, & Sham (2005) randomly assigned 103 bipolar patients to CBT (12–18 sessions) plus pharmacotherapy versus usual care and pharmacotherapy. Importantly, patients had been in remission for at least 6 months but had had three or more episodes in the past 5 years. The 1-year results were positive: 44% of the patients in CBT relapsed versus 75% of those in usual care; patients in CBT also spent fewer days in mood episodes. The results were weakened over 30 months: Patients in CBT no longer differed from patients in usual care in time to recurrence, although patients in CBT still had fewer days in mood episodes and an increased ability to recognize early warning signs of recurrence.

In secondary reanalyses, Lam, Wright, and Sham (2005) showed that patients who rated themselves high on "hyperpositive self" had high rates of relapse even if they received CBT. This finding suggests an avenue for enhancing CBT for bipolar disorder: developing techniques to identify and challenge manic or grandiose cognitions (e.g., overestimation of benefits and underestimation of risks of impulsive behaviors; beliefs that one can control the disorder through conscious effort). There may be a brief window of opportunity during the initial manic escalation in which this kind of cognitive restructuring is still possible.

The largest trial of CBT to date ($n = 253$) examined a 22-session CBT versus treatment as usual (TAU) in five mental health centers in the United Kingdom (Scott et al., 2006). The patients had been in various clinical states before entry into the trial. Over an 18-month follow-up, no effects were found for CBT on time to recurrence. However, a post hoc analysis revealed that patients with < 12 episodes had fewer recurrences if treated with CBT than with TAU. Patients with 12 or more episodes were more likely to have recurrences in CBT than in TAU. These results suggest two possibilities: CBT is best suited to the earlier phases of the disorder (before it becomes highly chronic), or CBT may be unsettling and agitating to patients who have had numerous episodes.

Future studies of CBT should consider the addition of mindfulness meditation strategies for highly chronic patients. A mindfulness-based form of group CBT was more effective than TAU in preventing recurrences among patients with unipolar depression with three or more prior depressive episodes, but not among patients with fewer than three episodes (Segal, Williams, & Teasdale, 2002).

Interpersonal and Social Rhythm Therapy

Interpersonal and social rhythm therapy (IPSRT), a descendent of the interpersonal psychotherapy of depression, consists of interpersonal problem-solving, clarification, and interpretation to help patients resolve issues related to grief, role transitions, role disputes, or interpersonal deficits. IPSRT emphasizes the role of social and circadian rhythm dysregulation in the onset of manic episodes. The IPSRT is based on the Ehlers, Kupfer, Frank, and Monk (1993) notions of social zeitgebers (timekeepers) and zeitstorers (time disturbers). Life events that disrupt social zeitgebers are believed to precipitate episodes of depression or mania, whereas treatments or lifestyle changes that help strengthen zeitgebers are expected to help stabilize moods. Direct tests of this model have established a role for social rhythm disruption in the onset of manic episodes, but not in the onset of depressive episodes (Malkoff-Schwartz et al., 1998).

Unlike CBT, IPSRT has been tested primarily with bipolar patients who began treatment shortly after an acute episode of mania or depression. In the Pittsburgh Maintenance Therapies for Bipolar Disorder (MTBD) trial (Frank et al., 2005), 175 patients were randomly assigned during an acute treatment phase to weekly IPSRT plus protocol pharmacotherapy or active clinical management plus protocol pharmacotherapy. Once patients had recovered, according to research criteria, they were rerandomized at the beginning of a maintenance phase to IPSRT or active clinical management on a monthly basis for up to 2 years. The results were complex but generally supported the efficacy of the social rhythm approach: IPSRT in the acute phase was associated with longer survival time prior to recurrences in the maintenance phase than clinical management. However, continued treatment with IPSRT during the maintenance phase did not affect recurrence rates during maintenance treatment.

In a nonrandomized study, Miklowitz, Richards, and colleagues (2003) examined the combined effects of individual IPSRT sessions and family-focused treatment sessions among 30 bipolar patients who had had an episode of mania, hypomania, or depression in the prior 3 months. All patients received pharmacotherapy from study-affiliated psychiatrists. The rationale for combining IPSRT with family therapy was that family members would assist patients in learning to stabilize social rhythms and sleep–wake cycles. Over 1 year of treatment, patients in the combined treatment had longer periods of remission prior to recurrence and less severe depressive symptoms than patients in an historical comparison group ($n = 70$) who received medication, two sessions of family education, and crisis management. The combined treatment did not affect manic symptoms.

Family-Focused Therapy

Family-focused therapy (FFT) is a 9-month, 21-session outpatient treatment for patients and their immediate family members (spouse, parents, siblings). It consists of psychoeducation about bipolar disorder, communication enhancement training, and problem-solving skills training (Miklowitz & Goldstein, 1997). Given in conjunction with pharmacotherapy during the postepisode period, FFT aims to hasten stabilization and reduce the likelihood of early recurrences. It seeks to (1) increase the family's understanding of mood disorder episodes, (2) acknowledge the patient's vulnerability to future episodes and the early signs of recurrence, (3) enhance the patient's adherence to medications, (4) help the patient and family members distinguish personality variables from signs of the disorder, (5) assist the patient and family members in coping with stressors that may precipitate episodes, and (6) increase the protective effects of family relationships during the stabilization period.

FFT has been tested in one open trial with a historical comparison group ($n = 32$; Miklowitz & Goldstein, 1990), two randomized trials focusing on relapse prevention (Miklowitz, George, Richards, Simoneau, & Suddath, 2003; Rea et al., 2003), and one randomized trial involving stabilization of bipolar depressive episodes (Miklowitz et al., 2007). The results are depicted in Table 26.1. Overall, FFT is associated with a 35–40% reduction in recurrence rates over 2 years, and a 48% increase in recovery rates over 1 year.

Exploratory analyses in two of these trials identified possible moderators and mediators of the effects of FFT. In a randomized trial at UCLA (Rea et al., 2003), being in family treatment decreased threefold the likelihood of relapse among poor premorbid patients (patients with low social and sexual adjustment during adolescence) in comparison with individual therapy. In a trial at the University of Colorado, FFT was more effective than crisis management in stabilizing mania symptoms among patients in high-EE critical families (Kim & Miklowitz, 2004). Although these treatment × moderator interactions were not strong enough to warrant limiting FFT to poor premorbid patients in high-EE families, they generate hypotheses for future trials about which subgroups of patients show a greater or lesser response to family intervention.

FFT was associated with an increase in the use of positive verbal and nonverbal communication in family interactions measured at a pretreatment baseline and again at 9 months. These improvements were correlated with symptomatic improvements of the patient over the same interval (Simoneau, Miklowitz, Richards, Saleem, & George, 1999). Patients in FFT were also more likely than patients in crisis management to be consistent with their lithium and/or anticonvulsant regimens, which in turn predicted the stabilization of mania symptoms over 2 years. Because of the design of the study, it was not possible to establish the direction of these associations (e.g., whether patients improved symptomatically first and, therefore, communicated better with their relatives, or the reverse).

There have been recent applications of FFT and similar treatments to child and adolescent bipolar patients. In a small-scale open trial, Miklowitz and colleagues (2006) found that adolescents with bipolar episodes who received FFT and pharmacotherapy stabilized over 24 months in terms of mania symptoms (Cohen's d = 1.19), depressive symptoms (d = 0.87), and Child Behavior Checklist Problem Behavior subtest scores (d = 0.99). The 21-session FFT, which was revised to address the developmental requirements of adolescents, is now being examined in a three-site, randomized trial. In an open trial of FFT in combination

TABLE 26.1. Recovery, Relapse, and Rehospitalization Rates in Family-Focused Treatment versus Comparison Groups

Study	Sample	Clinical state at entry	Comparison group	Recovery rate over 1 year	Relapse rate over 1 year	Relapse rate over 2 years
Miklowitz & Goldstein (1990)	23	Manic episode in prior 3 months	Treatment as usual	—	FFT, 11%; comparison, 61%	—
Miklowitz, George, et al. (2003)	101	Depressed or manic episode in prior 3 months	Crisis management	—	FFT, 26%; comparison, 39%	FFT, 35%; comparison, 54%
Rea et al. (2003)	53	Manic episode in prior 3 months	Individual therapy	—	FFT, 29%; comparison, 40%	FFT, 36%; comparison, 60%[a]
Miklowitz et al. (2007)	293	Acute depressive episode	Brief psychoeducation	FFT, 77%; Comparison, 52%[b]	—	—

[a]Based on rehospitalization rates.

[b]Based on recovery rates lasting ≥ 8 weeks during a 1-year study.

with individual CBT, West, Henry, and Pavuluri (2007) observed improvements in symptoms (mania, aggression, psychosis, depression) and global functioning among bipolar children ages 5–17. These improvements were observed immediately following the 12-session treatment and at 1, 2, and 3 years. Thus, FFT may enhance symptom stabilization in adult and child bipolar samples.

Group Treatments

Group psychoeducation appears to be a highly effective adjunct to pharmacotherapy in relapse prevention. Colom and associates (2003) randomly assigned bipolar patients to a 21-session structured psychoeducation group or an unstructured support group, both with standard pharmacotherapy. The inclusion criteria were similar to the Lam, Hayward, and colleagues (2005) study of CBT: The 120 patients had been in remission for at least 6 months. Results at the end of 2 years indicated a lower relapse rate in the psychoeducation group (67%) than in the unstructured group (92%). Patients in the psychoeducation group also had fewer (and shorter) hospitalizations, and maintained higher and more stable lithium levels. A strength of the study is the matching of the treatment and comparison arms on the number of sessions. Rates of attrition were somewhat higher (27%) in the structured than in the unstructured groups (19%).

Two large-scale, randomized trials have examined the effectiveness of group psychoeducation within the context of multicomponent care management plans. Bauer and colleagues (2006) examined a "collaborative care" program for bipolar patients at 11 Veterans Administration (VA) sites. The intervention included enhanced access to psychiatric care through a nurse coordinator, medication practice guidelines for the psychopharmacologist, and a group psychoeducational treatment to improve patients' self-management skills. Over a 3-year period, patients in the collaborative care treatment spent fewer weeks in manic episodes than did patients who received continued VA care (*n* = 306). Improvements in the collaborative care group were also observed in social role function, mental quality of life, and treatment satisfaction, especially in the second and third treatment years. There were no significant effects of collaborative care on mean manic and depressive symptoms over the 3-year period. Because the group psychoeducation was only one component of a larger collaborative care program, dismantling studies will be necessary to determine its unique contribution to clinical outcomes.

In the largest randomized trial of a psychosocial treatment for bipolar disorder (*n* = 441) to date, Simon Ludman, Bauer, Unutzer, and Operskalski (2006) compared a 2-year multicomponent care management intervention to TAU among patients in a health care network. Like the Bauer and colleagues (2006) study, the experimental intervention included pharmacotherapy, monthly telephone monitoring by a nurse care manager, relapse prevention planning, crisis intervention, and group psychoeducation. Over 2 years, patients in the multicomponent program had significantly lower mania scores and spent less time in manic or hypomanic episodes than those in the comparison group. There were no effects on depressive symptoms. Interestingly, the program only had effects among patients who had clinically significant symptoms upon entering the program. So it may be best to target patients who do not achieve full remission for this kind of multicomponent intervention. Indeed, patients with mood disorder who do not achieve full remission with pharmacotherapy are highly recurrence-prone (Perlis et al., 2006; Rush, 2007).

Group treatment has also been examined in highly relapse-prone patients with comorbid substance abuse disorders (Weiss et al., 2007). A total of 62 patients with bipolar disorder and substance or alcohol dependence received 20 weeks of "integrated group therapy" or group drug counseling. The integrated group used a CBT model focused on the similarities between bipolar disorder and substance dependence disorder in cognitions and behaviors during the recovery and relapse periods. Group drug counseling focused exclusively on encouraging abstinence and acquiring coping skills to address substance craving.

Over an 8-month period of treatment and follow-up, patients in the integrated groups had half as many days of substance use as patients receiving only drug counseling. The results were only significant for days of alcohol use, not drug use. No differences were observed in relapses of bipolar disorder; in fact, patients in the integrated groups had higher depression and mania scores during treatment and follow-up than patients in drug counseling. The authors concluded that the dual-diagnosis focus of the groups increased the likelihood that patients would recognize and report mood disorder symptoms. The possibility that decreasing alcohol abuse "unmasks" subsyndromal mood disorder symptoms deserves further study.

Overall, group psychoeducation appears to be a viable and possibly cost-effective alternative to individual or family approaches in the stabilization of manic and, in one study, depressive symptoms. The absence in these models of traditional psychological methods for treating depression—cognitive restructuring, behavioral activation, interpersonal problem solving, and increasing family or marital support—may limit their effectiveness in stabilizing depressive episodes. Research on the processes that mediate the effectiveness of group psychoeducation—decreased social isolation, medication adherence, the ability to recognize oncoming episodes, or support against the stigma of the disorder—may contribute to the development of group models with greater longevity of effects.

Comparison of Psychosocial Approaches: The STEP-BD Study

Many of the studies cited earlier were single-center studies at the universities in which the treatments were developed. The STEP-BD study examined pharmacological and psychosocial interventions in a practical clinical trial across 22 U.S. treatment centers (Sachs et al., 2007). In one part of the program, 293 patients with bipolar I and II disorder from 15 sites were randomly assigned to one of three intensive psychosocial treatments (30 sessions over 9 months of FFT, IPSRT, or CBT) in conjunction with best-practice medication treatment or a control treatment called collaborative care (CC). CC involved three psychotherapy sessions over 6 weeks and focused on developing a relapse prevention plan. All patients were in an acute episode of bipolar depression at the time of treatment randomization. Over 1 year, being in any of the intensive psychotherapies was associated with a higher recovery rate from depression (105/163, or 64.4%) than being in CC (67/130, or 51.5%; hazard ratio = 1.47) (Miklowitz, Otto, Frank, Reilly-Harrington, Wisniewski, et al., 2007). On average, patients in intensive treatment recovered within 169 days, compared to 279 days in the CC condition. Patients in intensive treatment were also 1.6 times more likely than patients in CC to be clinically well in any given month of the study. Rates of recovery over 1 year were as follows: FFT, 77% (20/26); IPSRT, 65% (40/62); CBT, 60% (45/75); and CC, 52%. The differences between the intensive modalities were not significant.

The positive effects of intensive psychosocial intervention extended to functional outcomes, as measured by the interview-based Range of Impaired Functioning Tool administered every 3 months (Miklowitz, Otto, Frank, Reilly-Harrington, Kogan, et al., 2007). Patients in FFT, IPSRT, or CBT had better total functioning, relationship functioning, and life satisfaction scores over 9 months than patients in CC, even after controlling baseline functioning scores and concurrent depression scores. No effects of psychosocial intervention were observed on work/role functioning or recreation scores over the 9-month treatment period. Possibly, psychosocial interventions that focus on the specific skills needed for vocational success (e.g., cognitive remediation, social skills training) will be necessary to enhance job functioning in the year after an acute depressive episode.

The STEP-BD study suggests that psychotherapy is a vital part of the effort to stabilize episodes of depression in bipolar illness, and that acutely depressed patients may require more intensive psychotherapy than is typically offered in community mental health centers. Further analyses of the STEP-BD dataset will consider moderators of treatment outcome which, hypothetically, might include baseline levels of cognitive distortions, perceptions of family conflict, or irregularity of daily or nightly routines.

Psychosocial Treatment for Bipolar Disorder: Common Ingredients

The STEP-BD study may have been statistically underpowered to identify differences between the intensive modalities in hastening clinical stabilization or enhancing functional recovery. Alternatively, the common elements of these treatments may have accounted for the majority of the variance in patient outcomes. Indeed, the commonalities among the existing psychosocial treatments for bipolar disorder are more striking than their differences. Miklowitz, Goodwin, Bauer, and Geddes (2008) designed a Therapist Strategies Questionnaire to tabulate common and specific elements of psychotherapies in the 14 randomized trials of bipolar disorder conducted to date. In analyses of data obtained from 31 clinicians who participated in the trials, several common and specific factors were identified, as summarized in Table 26.2.

Research has not established whether these common or specific elements are more or less important in bringing about therapeutic change. Possibly, future randomized trials might use dismantling strategies to identify the most effective components of these treatments, and develop "hybrid" models of psychotherapy that contain these most effective elements.

CONCLUSIONS AND FUTURE DIRECTIONS

Many questions remain to be resolved in future studies of drug and psychosocial treatments for bipolar disorder. First, pharmacotherapy trials and psychosocial treatment trials have largely developed independently. What is needed are large-scale "practical trials," such as the algorithm-testing approach used for treatment-resistant depression in the Sequenced Treatment Alternatives to Relieve Depression (STAR*D) trial (Rush, 2007), which combine pharmacotherapy decisions with psychotherapy decisions at different phases of the illness cycle. For example, is psychotherapy best introduced after one failed antidepressant trial? When attempting to stabilize bipolar depression, should psychotherapy be considered an alternative to adding a second mood stabilizer or atypical antipsychotic? If a patient does well in psychotherapy during an acute treatment phase, can one or more of his or her medications be safely tapered during the maintenance phase? Can certain forms of depression—notably, the moderate depressions that sometimes accompany bipolar II disorder—be treated with psychotherapy alone, with the option of introducing pharmacotherapy if there is no response?

TABLE 26.2. Common and Specific Factors in the Psychosocial Treatment of Bipolar Disorder

Structure

- Individual therapy
  - CBT (four randomized trials)
  - IPSRT (two trials)
  - Individual psychoeducation (three trials)
- Group psychoeducation (five trials)
- Family (five trials)

Common Elements (present in all or most of the experimental modalities)

- Psychoeducation: didactic information about the symptoms and diagnosis of bipolar disorder; its etiology, course, and treatment
- Education about medications and side effects
- Resolving key interpersonal and family problems
- Enhancing coping with the stigma of mental illness
- Community advocacy (assisting patient in obtaining needed services)

Specific Elements (present in some modalities more than others)

- Keeping a self-rated mood chart
- Relapse prevention planning: intervening early with prodromal symptoms
- Enhancing adherence with mood-stabilizing medications
- Behavioral activation/pleasant events scheduling
- Cognitive restructuring
- Tracking and regularization of sleep/wake cycles and daily routines
- Use of written psychoeducational materials
- Communication training
- Treatment for comorbid disorders

Second, considerable work is needed to identify moderators and mediators of treatment effects (Kraemer, Wilson, Fairburn, & Agras, 2002). Few moderators of effects have been identified for the various psychosocial modalities. Frank and colleagues (2005) found that patients without medical comorbidities did better with IPSRT than with active clinical management, whereas the reverse was true of patients who had medical comorbidities. Scott and colleagues (2006) found that CBT was more effective in preventing recurrences among patients with < 12 episodes. Finally, analyzing data from two trials of FFT, Kim and Miklowitz (2004) found that the association between EE-criticism in relatives and poor outcomes of mania among patients was stronger in control treatments than in FFT, suggesting that FFT may have "blunted" the impact of EE on subsequent patient outcomes.

The end goal of moderator analyses is to provide pragmatic clinical data on who will be most likely to benefit from which treatments. Nonetheless, studies of moderators must be powered with adequate sample sizes to identify treatment by moderator interactions reliably. Typically, clinical trials—notably, pharmacotherapy trials—have not been designed with moderators in mind, and exploratory examinations of moderators have sometimes capitalized on chance. Thus, replication of treatment by moderator interactions in subsequent trials, or meta-regression models that examine interactions across studies, will be necessary to translate subgroup findings into clinical recommendations.

Mediators typically refer to "change variables" that are measured before, during, and after treatment, and that explain how treatments work (Kraemer et al., 2002). In studies of FFT, treatment-associated changes in mania scores were mediated by improvements in medication adherence, whereas treatment-associated improvements in depressive symptoms were related to improvements in patient–relative interactions (Miklowitz, George, et al., 2003; Simoneau et al., 1999). In the Pittsburgh MTBD trial, stabilization of sleep–wake rhythms during an acute treatment phase mediated the success of IPSRT in delaying recurrences during a maintenance phase (Frank et al., 2005). It is less clear the degree to which the interpersonal part of IPSRT influences outcomes (e.g., whether patients resolve the interpersonal problem that brought them into treatment). To date, no treatment mediators have been identified in studies of CBT or group psychoeducation.

As noted earlier, patients with early-onset bipolar disorder are at risk for a host of adverse outcomes, including frequent cycling, mixed episodes, multiple comorbid disorders, suicidality, and treatment resistance. Given the disadvantages of polypharmacy for the younger age groups (e.g., significant weight gain, rash, possibly increased suicide risk), the importance of developing effective psychosocial interventions is critical. Possibly, effective psychosocial agents could reduce the number of medications needed to stabilize patients with early-onset bipolar disorder. The development of structured psychosocial approaches to childhood bipolar disorder is just beginning to receive attention (e.g., Fristad, Gavazzi, & Mackinaw-Koons, 2003).

Extending this rationale further, psychosocial interventions may have a role in staving off the initial onset of bipolar disorder. A study of FFT as an early preventive intervention is currently underway at the University of Colorado (Miklowitz, Principal Investigator) and at Stanford University School of Medicine (K. Chang, Principal Investigator). This study will examine the effects of a modified form of FFT for children who have subsyndromal symptoms of bipolar disorder and at least one first-degree relative with bipolar disorder. Theoretically, early intervention could reduce the likelihood, or perhaps delay the onset, of the initial episode of mania. In turn, preventing or delaying the initial episode may arrest the neurotoxic effects of repeated episodes of mood disorder on the developing brain.

Finally, there is a significant gap in the treatment dissemination literature. How does one teach pharmacological strategies or psychosocial interventions to practicing clinicians and make their use sustainable in community mental health settings? The appearance of practice parameters and multisite effectiveness trials, such as STEP-BD, are a move in the right direction. However, more needs to be done to ensure that training materials are widely available, training seminars are convenient and of low cost, and incentives are given to clinicians who use these empirically supported strategies. This "bench-to-bedside" approach will be essential in maintaining the recent gains of research on effective management strategies for this highly debilitating disorder.

REFERENCES

Altshuler, L., Suppes, T., Black, D., Nolen, W. A., Keck, P. E. J., Frye, M. A., et al. (2003). Impact of antidepressant discontinuation after acute bipolar depression remission on rates of depressive relapse at 1-year follow-up. *American Journal of Psychiatry, 160,* 1252–1262.

Bauer, M. S., McBride, L., Williford, W. O., Glick, H., Kinosian, B., Altshuler, L., et al. (2006). Cooperative Studies Program 430 Study Team: Collaborative care for bipolar disorder: Part II. Impact on clinical outcome, function, and costs. *Psychiatric Services, 57,* 937–945.

Bowden, C. L., Calabrese, J. R., Sachs, G., Yatham, L. N., Asghar, S. A., Hompland, M., et al. (2003). A placebo-controlled 18-month trial of lamotrigine and lithium maintenance treatment in recently manic or hypomanic patients with bipolar I disorder. *Archives of General Psychiatry, 60,* 392–400.

Brown, E. B., McElroy, S. L., Keck, P. E. J., Deldar, A., Adams, D. H., Tohen, M., et al. (2006). A 7-week, randomized, double-blind trial of olanzapine/fluoxetine combination versus lamotrigine in the treatment of bipolar I depression. *Journal of Clinical Psychiatry, 67*(7), 1025–1033.

Calabrese, J. R., Keck, P. E. J., Macfadden, W., Minkwitz, M., Ketter, T. A., Weisler, R. H., et al. (2005). A randomized, double-blind, placebo-controlled trial of quetiapine in the treatment of bipolar I or II depression. *American Journal of Psychiatry, 162*(7), 1351–1360.

Calabrese, J. R., Shelton, M. D., Rapport, D. J., Youngstrom, E. A., Jackson, K., Bilali, S., et al. (2005). A 20-month, double-blind, maintenance trial of lithium versus divalproex in rapid-cycling bipolar disorder. *American Journal of Psychiatry, 162*(11), 2152–2161.

Calabrese, J. R., Suppes, T., Bowden, C. L., Sachs, G. S., Swann, A. C., McElroy, S. L., et al. (2000). A double-blind, placebo-controlled, prophylaxis study of lamotrigine in rapid-cycling bipolar disorder: Lamictal 614 Study Group. *Journal of Clinical Psychiatry, 61*, 841–850.

Cochran, S. D. (1984). Preventing medical noncompliance in the outpatient treatment of bipolar affective disorders. *Journal of Consulting and Clinical Psychology, 52*, 873–878.

Coletti, D. J., Leigh, E., Gallelli, K. A., & Kafantaris, V. (2005). Patterns of adherence to treatment in adolescents with bipolar disorder. *Journal of Child and Adolescent Psychopharmacology, 15*(6), 913–917.

Colom, F., Vieta, E., Martinez-Aran, A., Reinares, M., Benabarre, A., & Gasto, C. (2000). Clinical factors associated with treatment noncompliance in euthymic bipolar patients. *Journal of Clinical Psychiatry, 61*, 549–555.

Colom, F., Vieta, E., Martinez-Aran, A., Reinares, M., Goikolea, J. M., Benabarre, A., et al. (2003). A randomized trial on the efficacy of group psychoeducation in the prophylaxis of recurrences in bipolar patients whose disease is in remission. *Archives of General Psychiatry, 60*, 402–407.

Coryell, W., Scheftner, W., Keller, M., Endicott, J., Maser, J., & Klerman, G. L. (1993). The enduring psychosocial consequences of mania and depression. *American Journal of Psychiatry, 150*, 720–727.

DelBello, M. P., Kowatch, R. A., Adler, C. M., Stanford, K. E., Welge, J. A., Barzman, D. H., et al. (2006). A double-blind randomized pilot study comparing quetiapine and divalproex for adolescent mania. *Journal of the American Academy of Child and Adolescent Psychiatry, 45*(3), 305–313.

DelBello, M. P., Schwiers, M. L., Rosenberg, H. L., & Strakowski, S. M. (2002). A double-blind, randomized, placebo-controlled study of quetiapine as adjunctive treatment for adolescent mania. *Journal of the American Academy of Child and Adolescent Psychiatry, 41*, 1216–1223.

Denicoff, K. D., Smith-Jackson, E. E., Disney, E. R., Ali, S. O., Leverich, G. S., & Post, R. M. (1997). Comparative prophylactic efficacy of lithium, carbamazepine, and the combination in bipolar disorder. *Journal of Clinical Psychiatry, 58*, 470–478.

Dienes, K. A., Hammen, C., Henry, R. M., Cohen, A. N., & Daley, S. E. (2006). The stress sensitization hypothesis: Understanding the course of bipolar disorder. *Journal of Affective Disorders, 95*(1–3), 43–49.

Ehlers, C. L., Kupfer, D. J., Frank, E., & Monk, T. H. (1993). Biological rhythms and depression: The role of zeitgebers and zeitstorers. *Depression, 1*, 285–293.

Findling, R. L., McNamara, N. K., Youngstrom, E. A., Stansbrey, R. J., Gracious, B. L., Reed, M. D., et al. (2005). Double-blind 18-month trial of lithium versus divalproex maintenance treatment in pediatric bipolar disorder. *Journal of the American Academy of Child and Adolescent Psychiatry, 44*(5), 409–417.

Frank, E., Kupfer, D. J., Thase, M. E., Mallinger, A. G., Swartz, H. A., Fagiolini, A. M., et al. (2005). Two-year outcomes for interpersonal and social rhythm therapy in individuals with bipolar I disorder. *Archives of General Psychiatry, 62*(9), 996–1004.

Fristad, M. A., Gavazzi, S. M., & Mackinaw-Koons, B. (2003). Family psychoeducation: An adjunctive intervention for children with bipolar disorder. *Biological Psychiatry, 53*, 1000–1009.

Geddes, J. R., Burgess, S., Hawton, K., Jamison, K., & Goodwin, G. M. (2004). Long-term lithium therapy for bipolar disorder: Systematic review and meta-analysis of randomized controlled trials. *American Journal of Psychiatry, 161*(2), 217–222.

Geller, B., Tillman, R., Craney, J. L., & Bolhofner, K. (2004). Four-year prospective outcome and natural history of mania in children with a prepubertal and early adolescent bipolar disorder phenotype. *Archives of General Psychiatry, 61*, 459–467.

Gitlin, M. J., Swendsen, J., Heller, T. L., & Hammen, C. (1995). Relapse and impairment in bipolar disorder. *American Journal of Psychiatry*, 152(11), 1635–1640.

Goldberg, J. F. (2004). The changing landscape of psychopharmacology. In S. L. Johnson & R. L. Leahy (Eds.), *Psychological treatment of bipolar disorder* (pp. 109–138). New York: Guilford Press.

Goodwin, F. K., Fireman, B., Simon, G. E., Hunkeler, E. M., Lee, J., & Revicki, D. (2003). Suicide risk in bipolar disorder during treatment with lithium and divalproex. *Journal of the American Medical Association*, 290(11), 1467–1473.

Goodwin, G. M. (2003). Evidence-based guidelines for treating bipolar disorder: Recommendations from the British Association for Psychopharmacology. *Journal of Psychopharmacology*, 17, 149–173.

Goodwin, G. M., Bowden, C. L., Calabrese, J. R., Grunze, H., Kasper, S., White, R., et al. (2004). A pooled analysis of 2 placebo-controlled 18-month trials of lamotrigine and lithium maintenance in bipolar I disorder. *Journal of Clinical Psychiatry*, 65(3), 432–441.

Hammen, C., & Gitlin, M. J. (1997). Stress reactivity in bipolar patients and its relation to prior history of the disorder. *American Journal of Psychiatry*, 154, 856–857.

Hillegers, M. H., Burger, H., Wals, M., Reichart, C. G., Verhulst, F. C., Nolen, W. A., et al. (2004). Impact of stressful life events, familial loading and their interaction on the onset of mood disorders. *British Journal of Psychiatry*, 185, 97–101.

Hlastala, S. A., Frank, E., Kowalski, J., Sherrill, J. T., Tu, X. M., Anderson, B., et al. (2000). Stressful life events, bipolar disorder, and the "kindling model." *Journal of Abnormal Psychology*, 109, 777–786.

Johnson, R. E., & McFarland, B. H. (1996). Lithium use and discontinuation in a health maintenance organization. *American Journal of Psychiatry*, 153, 993–1000.

Johnson, S. L. (2005). Life events in bipolar disorder: Towards more specific models. *Clinical Psychology Review*, 25(8), 1008–1027.

Keck, P. E., Jr., McElroy, S. L., Strakowski, S. M., West, S. A., Sax, K. W., Hawkins, J. M., et al. (1998). Twelve-month outcome of patients with bipolar disorder following hospitalization for a manic or mixed episode. *American Journal of Psychiatry*, 155, 646–652.

Keck, P. E., Jr., Perlis, R. H., Otto, M. W., Carpenter, D., Docherty, J. P., & Ross, R. (2004, December). Expert Consensus Guideline Series: Treatment of bipolar disorder. *Postgraduate Medicine Special Report*, pp. 1–108.

Kim, E. Y., & Miklowitz, D. J. (2004). Expressed emotion as a predictor of outcome among bipolar patients undergoing family therapy. *Journal of Affective Disorders*, 82, 343–352.

Kim, E. Y., Miklowitz, D. J., Biuckians, A., & Mullen, K. (2007). Life stress and the course of early-onset bipolar disorder. *Journal of Affective Disorders*, 99(1), 37–44.

Kowatch, R. A., Fristad, M., Birmaher, B., Wagner, K. D., Findling, R. L., Hellander, M., et al. (2005). Treatment guidelines for children and adolescents with bipolar disorder. *Journal of the American Academy of Child and Adolescent Psychiatry*, 44(3), 213–235.

Kraemer, H. C., Wilson, T., Fairburn, C. G., & Agras, W. S. (2002). Mediators and moderators of treatment effects in randomized clinical trials. *Archives of General Psychiatry*, 59, 877–883.

Lam, D., Wright, K., & Sham, P. (2005). Sense of hyper-positive self and response to cognitive therapy in bipolar disorder. *Psychological Medicine*, 35(1), 69–77.

Lam, D. H., Hayward, P., Watkins, E. R., Wright, K., & Sham, P. (2005). Relapse prevention in patients with bipolar disorder: Cognitive therapy outcome after 2 years. *American Journal of Psychiatry*, 162, 324–329.

Malkoff-Schwartz, S., Frank, E., Anderson, B., Sherrill, J. T., Siegel, L., Patterson, D., et al. (1998). Stressful life events and social rhythm disruption in the onset of manic and depressive bipolar episodes: A preliminary investigation. *Archives of General Psychiatry*, 55, 702–707.

Manji, H. K., Quiroz, J. A., Payne, J. L., Singh, J., Lopes, B. P., Viegas, J. S., et al. (2003). The underlying neurobiology of bipolar disorder. *World Psychiatry*, 2(3), 136–146.

Merikangas, K. R., Akiskal, H. S., Angst, J., Greenberg, P. E., Hirschfeld, R. M. A., Petukhova, M., et al. (2007). Lifetime and 12-month prevalence of bipolar spectrum disorder in the National Comorbidity Survey Replication. *Archives of General Psychiatry*, 64, 543–552.

Miklowitz, D. J., Biuckians, A., & Richards, J. A. (2006). Early-onset bipolar disorder: A family treatment perspective. *Development and Psychopathology, 18*(4), 1247–1265.

Miklowitz, D. J., George, E. L., Richards, J. A., Simoneau, T. L., & Suddath, R. L. (2003). A randomized study of family-focused psychoeducation and pharmacotherapy in the outpatient management of bipolar disorder. *Archives of General Psychiatry, 60,* 904–912.

Miklowitz, D. J., & Goldstein, M. J. (1990). Behavioral family treatment for patients with bipolar affective disorder. *Behavior Modification, 14,* 457–489.

Miklowitz, D. J., & Goldstein, M. J. (1997). *Bipolar disorder: A family-focused treatment approach.* New York: Guilford Press.

Miklowitz, D. J., Goldstein, M. J., Nuechterlein, K. H., Snyder, K. S., & Mintz, J. (1988). Family factors and the course of bipolar affective disorder. *Archives of General Psychiatry, 45,* 225–231.

Miklowitz, D. J., Goodwin, G. M., Bauer, M. S., & Geddes, J. (2008). Common and specific elements of psychosocial treatments for bipolar disorder: A survey of clinicians participating in randomized trials. *Journal of Psychiatric Practice, 14,* 1–9.

Miklowitz, D. J., Otto, M. W., Frank, E., Reilly-Harrington, N. A., Kogan, J. N., Sachs, G. S., et al. (2007). Intensive psychosocial intervention enhances functioning in patients with bipolar depression: Results from a 9-month randomized controlled trial. *American Journal of Psychiatry, 164,* 1340–1347.

Miklowitz, D. J., Otto, M. W., Frank, E., Reilly-Harrington, N. A., Wisniewski, S. R., Kogan, J. N., et al. (2007). Psychosocial treatments for bipolar depression: A 1-year randomized trial from the Systematic Treatment Enhancement Program. *Archives of General Psychiatry, 64,* 419–427.

Miklowitz, D. J., Richards, J. A., George, E. L., Suddath, R. L., Frank, E., Powell, K., et al. (2003). Integrated family and individual therapy for bipolar disorder: Results of a treatment development study. *Journal of Clinical Psychiatry, 64,* 182–191.

Miklowitz, D. J., Simoneau, T. L., George, E. L., Richards, J. A., Kalbag, A., Sachs-Ericsson, N., et al. (2000). Family-focused treatment of bipolar disorder: 1-year effects of a psychoeducational program in conjunction with pharmacotherapy. *Biological Psychiatry, 48,* 582–592.

Moller, H. J., Grunze, H., & Broich, K. (2006). Do recent efficacy data on the drug treatment of acute bipolar depression support the position that drugs other than antidepressants are the treatment of choice?: A conceptual review. *European Archives of Psychiatry and Clinical Neuroscience, 256*(1), 1–16.

Murray, C. J. L., & Lopez, A. D. (1996). *The global burden of disease: A comprehensive assessment of mortality and disability from diseases, injuries, and risk factors in 1990 and projected to 2020.* Cambridge, MA: Harvard University Press.

Nemeroff, C. B., Evans, D. L., Gyulai, L., Sachs, G. S., Bowden, C. L., Gergel, I. P., et al. (2001). Double-blind, placebo-controlled comparison of imipramine and paroxetine in the treatment of bipolar depression. *American Journal of Psychiatry, 158*(6), 906–912.

Nierenberg, A. A., Ostacher, M. J., Calabrese, J. R., Ketter, T. A., Marangell, L., Miklowitz, D. J., et al. (2006). Treatment-resistant bipolar depression: A STEP-BD equipoise randomized effectiveness trial of antidepressant augmentation with lamotrigine, inositol or risperidone. *American Journal of Psychiatry, 163*(2), 210–216.

Pavuluri, M. N., Birmaher, B., & Naylor, M. W. (2005). Pediatric bipolar disorder: A review of the past 10 years. *Journal of the American Academy of Child and Adolescent Psychiatry, 44*(9), 846–871.

Perlis, R. H., Miyahara, S., Marangell, L. B., Wisniewski, S. R., Ostacher, M., DelBello, M. P., et al. (2004). Long-term implications of early onset in bipolar disorder: Data from the first 1,000 participants in the Systematic Treatment Enhancement Program for Bipolar Disorder (STEP-BD). *Biological Psychiatry, 55,* 875–881.

Perlis, R. H., Ostacher, M. J., Patel, J., Marangell, L. B., Zhang, H., Wisniewski, S. R., et al. (2006). Predictors of recurrence in bipolar disorder: Primary outcomes from the Systematic Treatment Enhancement Program for Bipolar Disorder (STEP-BD). *American Journal of Psychiatry, 163*(2), 217–224.

Post, R. M., & Leverich, G. S. (2006). The role of psychosocial stress in the onset and progression of bipolar disorder and its comorbidities: The need for earlier and alternative modes of therapeutic intervention. *Development and Psychopathology, 18*(4), 1181–1211.

Rea, M. M., Tompson, M., Miklowitz, D. J., Goldstein, M. J., Hwang, S., & Mintz, J. (2003). Family focused treatment vs. individual treatment for bipolar disorder: Results of a randomized clinical trial. *Journal of Consulting and Clinical Psychology, 71,* 482–492.

Reilly-Harrington, N. A., Alloy, L. B., Fresco, D. M., & Whitehouse, W. G. (1999). Cognitive styles and life events interact to predict bipolar and unipolar symptomatology. *Journal of Abnormal Psychology, 108,* 567–578.

Rush, A. J. (2007). STAR*D: What have we learned? *American Journal of Psychiatry, 164*(2), 201–204.

Sachs, G. S., Nierenberg, A. A., Calabrese, J. R., Marangell, L. B., Wisniewski, S. R., Gyulai, L., et al. (2007). Effectiveness of adjunctive antidepressant treatment for bipolar depression. *New England Journal of Medicine, 356,* 1–12.

Sapolsky, R. M. (2000). The possibility of neurotoxicity in the hippocampus in major depression: A primer on neuron death. *Biological Psychiatry, 48,* 755–765.

Scherk, H., Pajonk, F. G., & Leucht, S. (2007). Second-generation antipsychotic agents in the treatment of acute mania: A systematic review and meta-analysis of randomized controlled trials. *Archives of General Psychiatry, 64*(4), 442–455.

Schneck, C. D. (2006). Treatment of rapid-cycling bipolar disorder. *Journal of Clinical Psychiatry, 67*(Suppl. 11), 22–27.

Scott, J., Paykel, E., Morriss, R., Bentall, R., Kinderman, P., Johnson, T., et al. (2006). Cognitive behaviour therapy for severe and recurrent bipolar disorders: A randomised controlled trial. *British Journal of Psychiatry, 188,* 313–320.

Segal, Z. V., Williams, J. M. G., & Teasdale, J. D. (2002). *Mindfulness-based cognitive therapy for depression: A new approach to preventing relapse.* New York: Guilford Press.

Simon, G. E., Ludman, E. J., Bauer, M. S., Unutzer, J., & Operskalski, B. (2006). Long-term effectiveness and cost of a systematic care program for bipolar disorder. *Archives of General Psychiatry, 63*(5), 500–508.

Simoneau, T. L., Miklowitz, D. J., Richards, J. A., Saleem, R., & George, E. L. (1999). Bipolar disorder and family communication: Effects of a psychoeducational treatment program. *Journal of Abnormal Psychology, 108,* 588–597.

Strakowski, S. M., Keck, P. E., McElroy, S. L., West, S. A., Sax, K. W., Hawkins, J. M., et al. (1998). Twelve-month outcome after a first hospitalization for affective psychosis. *Archives of General Psychiatry, 55,* 49–55.

Suppes, T., Dennehy, E. B., Hirschfeld, R. M., Altshuler, L. L., Bowden, C. L., Calabrese, J. R., et al. (2005). The Texas implementation of medication algorithms: Update to the algorithms for treatment of bipolar I disorder. *Journal of Clinical Psychiatry, 66*(7), 870–886.

Thase, M. E. (2006a). Bipolar depression: Diagnostic and treatment challenges. *Development and Psychopathology, 18*(4), 1213–1230.

Thase, M. E. (2006b). Pharmacotherapy of bipolar depression: An update. *Current Psychiatry Reports, 8*(6), 478–488.

Tohen, M., Chengappa, K. N., Suppes, T., Zarate, C. A. J., Calabrese, J. R., Bowden, C. L., et al. (2002). Efficacy of olanzapine in combination with valproate or lithium in the treatment of mania in patients partially nonresponsive to valproate or lithium monotherapy. *Archives of General Psychiatry, 59,* 62–69.

Tohen, M., Kryzhanovskaya, L., Carlson, G., DelBello, M. P., Wozniak, J., Kowatch, R., et al. (2005). Olanzapine in the treatment of acute mania in adolescents with bipolar I disorder: A 3-week randomized double-blind placebo-controlled study. *Neuopsychopharmacology, 30*(Suppl. 1), 176.

Tohen, M., Vieta, E., Calabrese, J., Ketter, T. A., Sachs, G., Bowden, C., et al. (2003). Efficacy of olanzapine and olanzapine–fluoxetine combination in the treatment of bipolar I depression. *Archives of General Psychiatry, 60,* 1079–1088.

Tondo, L., & Baldessarini, R. J. (2000). Reducing suicide risk during lithium maintenance treatment. *Journal of Clinical Psychiatry, 61*(Suppl. 9), 97–104.

Tondo, L., Baldessarini, R. J., & Floris, G. (2001). Long-term clinical effectiveness of lithium maintenance treatment in types I and II bipolar disorders. *British Journal of Psychiatry, 41*(Suppl.), S184–S190.

Weiss, R. D., Griffin, M. L., Kolodziej, M. E., Greenfield, S. F., Najavits, L. M., Daley, D. C., et al. (2007). A randomized trial of integrated group therapy versus group drug counseling for patients with bipolar disorder and substance dependence. *American Journal of Psychiatry, 164*(1), 100–107.

West, A. E., Henry, D. B., & Pavuluri, M. N. (2007). Maintenance model of integrated psychosocial treatment in pediatric bipolar disorder: A pilot feasibility study. *Journal of the American Academy of Child and Adolescent Psychiatry, 46*(2), 205–212.

Yan, L. J., Hammen, C., Cohen, A. N., Daley, S. E., & Henry, R. M. (2004). Expressed emotion versus relationship quality variables in the prediction of recurrence in bipolar patients. *Journal of Affective Disorders, 83*, 199–206.

Yatham, L. N., Kennedy, S. H., O'Donovan, C., Parikh, S., MacQueen, G., McIntyre, R., et al. (2005). Canadian Network for Mood and Anxiety Treatments (CANMAT) guidelines for the management of patients with bipolar disorder: Consensus and controversies. *Bipolar Disorders, 7*(Suppl. 3), 5–69.

CHAPTER 27

Marital, Family, and Interpersonal Therapies for Depression in Adults

Steven R. H. Beach, Deborah J. Jones, *and* Kameron J. Franklin

Recent estimates suggest that up to 20% of adults report significant depressive symptoms in the past 1 week to 6 months (Kessler, Avenevoli, & Merikangas, 2001). Given its incidence and prevalence across the lifespan, depression has considerable potential to disrupt the lives of both sufferers and family members, with tremendous social and familial costs, along with economic costs estimated at $83 billion annually in the United States alone (Greenberg et al., 2003). It is not surprising, therefore, that depressed individuals often report problems with family relationships, and that concerns about family relationships are prominent for many depressed persons (Whisman, 2006), as are concerns with other interpersonal problems (Joiner & Coyne, 1999) and with bereavement (Paykel, 2003). This has led to suggestions that depressed persons may often benefit from marital therapy, parent training, or other interpersonal approaches to treatment, and has created interest in several family and interpersonal approaches to intervention with depressed patients.

Are marital, family, or other interpersonally oriented interventions useful for persons with depression? In the current chapter, we briefly lay out the argument in favor of the use of marital, parenting, and interpersonal therapies in the treatment of depression, limiting our focus to those marital, family, and interpersonal approaches that have been examined in treatment outcome research. We begin with evidence that the close relationships of depressed persons, and particularly their marital and parenting relationships, are often in need of repair, placing difficulties in close relationships in the broader context of stress, support, and vulnerability to depression, and discussing stress generation as a framework for understanding the connection between problems in close relationships and depression. We then review evidence for the efficacy of treatment, paying particular attention to the efficacy of marital and parent training for depressed individuals, and assessing whether these interventions are appropriate and useful for depressed persons. We also note the importance of interpersonal psychotherapy (IPT) as an approach that can address relationship difficulties, and that can be delivered to individuals. After reviewing the case supporting the use of marital, parenting, and interpersonal interventions for depressed persons, we examine possible indications for intervention. In the final two chapter sections, we discuss future directions for research and highlight the importance of research on understudied populations, with a particular emphasis on issues involving the application of marital, family, and interpersonal approaches to understudied groups. We then discuss the role of family-based preventive interventions to strengthen families as one important component in the effort to decrease the intergenerational transmission of depression.

THE CASE FOR MARITAL AND PARENTING INTERVENTIONS FOR DEPRESSION

There Is a Link between Marital and Family Relationships and Depression

How strong is the link between marital distress and depression? Whisman (2001) reported a moderate (approximately .4), negative association between marital quality and depressive symptomatology for both women ($r = -.42$) and men ($r = -.37$), indicating a significant relationship overall, and a significant, albeit small, gender difference. He also reported that the average Dyadic Adjustment Scale (DAS) score for the diagnosed population was 93.7 ($SD = 25.2$), indicating that the average depressed individual scored in the maritally distressed range of the DAS (DAS cutoff = 97). Thus, the marital relationships of depressed men and women are often (but not always) distressed. This finding is consistent with work indicating that marital satisfaction is the strongest predictor across many specific domains of life satisfaction (Fleeson, 2004) and that marital dissolution is strongly associated with increases in depression and depressive symptoms for both men and women (Wade & Pevalin, 2004). In addition, marital dissolution by death of a partner is associated with a ninefold increase in major depression and a fourfold increase in depressive symptoms among recently bereaved older adults (Turvey, Carney, & Arndt, 1999). Underscoring the importance of the broader interpersonal realm, the effect of bereavement is especially pronounced for those lacking social support (Wortman, Wolff, & Bonanno, 2004).

There Is also a Link between Parenting and Depression

What is the nature of the link between parenting behavior and depression? It has long been noted clinically that depressed patients report considerable distress and difficulty in their parenting relationships; some have attributed depressed mothers' level of dysphoria, at least in part, to their belief that they are inadequate parents. Supplementing clinical observation and patient self-report is a large body of direct observation documenting problems in parenting behavior. In a review of 46 observational studies of the parenting behavior of depressed women, Lovejoy, Graczyk, O'Hare, and Neuman (2000) found evidence that depressed mothers display more withdrawn behavior, as well as more negative parenting behavior. Further evidence suggests that the link between depression and compromised parenting is reciprocal, such that depression not only predicts impairments in parenting behavior and the quality of the parent–child relationship, but also that difficulties in the parent–child relationship in turn increase parents' vulnerability to depressive symptomatology (e.g., Jones, Beach, & Forehand, 2001). Consistent with the literature on marital relationships, there is reason to believe that many, but not all, depressed persons experience difficulties in parenting and in the parent–child relationship.

Other Social Difficulties and Depression

Depression is also associated with more general aspects of social disadvantage, such that those with lower socioeconomic status (SES) are at elevated risk of being depressed (Lorant, Deliege, & Eaton, 2003). As might be expected, much of the risk attributable to low SES is conferred by financial disadvantage, unemployment, low education, and low material standard of living (Fryers, Melzer, & Jenkins, 2003). It appears, however, that at least some of the effect of low SES is conferred by decreased social support among those with low SES (Turner & Marino, 1994); indeed, the impact of the lack of high-quality social relationships may be stronger for those disadvantaged by low SES (Turner, Lloyd, & Roszell, 1999), suggesting the potential importance of implementing relationally oriented interventions in low-SES populations. Similarly, risk of onset of a depressive episode is greater among single mothers than among married mothers (Brown & Moran, 1997), perhaps reflecting the combined effect of several factors. These findings underscore the potential importance of working to strengthen coparenting and other close relationships among depressed, single mothers.

These findings also highlight the importance of situating the discussion of relatively specific social stressors, such as marital problems and parenting difficulties, in the broader context of social stressors in general, and in the even broader context of stress and depression (see Hammen, 2005). Severe stressors, some of which are social in nature, often confer a relatively rapid increase in risk of onset of depression (Kendler, Karkowski, & Prescott, 1998). Thus, severely stressful relational events may warrant particular attention. Illustrating this point, Cano and O'Leary (2000) found that humiliating events, such as partner infidelity and threats of marital dissolution, resulted in a sixfold increase in diagnosis of depression, and that this increased risk remained after they controlled for family and personal history of depression. Furthermore, Whisman and Bruce (1999) found that marital dissatisfaction increased risk of subsequent diagnosis of depression by 2.7-fold in a large, representative community sample, and again the increased risk remained significant after controlling for demographic variables and personal history of depression. Similarly, marital conflict with physical abuse predicted increased depressive symptoms over time after researchers controlled for earlier symptoms (Beach et al., 2004). As these studies suggest, marital distress characterized by severely stressful marital events may be sufficiently potent to precipitate a depressive episode or exacerbate existing depressive symptoms.

It is also important to distinguish between "dependent" and "independent" stressful events. So-called "dependent" events—those to which the person may have contributed—contribute more to the prediction of depression than do "independent" events (Kendler, Karkowski, & Prescott, 1999a). Dependent events are particularly likely to be relational in nature, and include most stressors in the marital and parenting domains, suggesting that events in these domains may be part of a larger vicious cycle that includes personal vulnerabilities. Similarly, "chronic" stressors—those that have continued for a year or more—are as predictive, or are more predictive, of depression than are brief, acute stressors (McGonagle & Kessler, 1990), and relationship problems often fall into the "chronic" category as well.

Stress Generation

The stress generation framework (Hammen, 1991) describes a particular bidirectional pattern of causation between family relationships and depression that is consistent with the predictive power of dependent and chronic social stressors. In addition to providing a useful framework for integrating the broad literature on stress, social support, and depression outlined earlier, the stress generation framework also illustrates the vicious cycles that may emerge between depressive symptoms and interpersonal or family problems. Documenting one such vicious cycle for marital difficulties, Davila, Bradbury, Cohan, and Tochluk (1997) found that, compared to persons with fewer symptoms of depression, individuals with more depression symptoms displayed more negative supportive behavior toward the spouse and in their expectations regarding partner support. These negative behaviors and expectations were in turn related to greater marital stress. Finally, closing the loop, level of marital stress predicted subsequent depressive symptoms (after researchers controlled for earlier symptoms). Likewise, in his review of self-propagating processes in depression, Joiner (2000) highlights the propensity for depressed persons to seek negative feedback, to engage in excessive reassurance seeking, to avoid conflict and, in turn, to withdraw, and to elicit changes in their partners' view of them. In each case, the behavior resulting from the individual's depression may carry the potential to generate increased interpersonal stress or to shift the response of others in a negative direction. Consistent with the stress generation model, Joiner suggests that increased interpersonal negativity in turn helps to maintain depressive symptoms.

Kindling and Vulnerability

Finally, the broader literature on stress and depression suggests a "kindling" relationship between stress and depression. Current theorizing about kindling suggests that an initial depressive episode may lead to changes in the functioning of neurotransmitters and the limbic system that make the individual more prone to developing future episodes of depression. If early episodes of depression make a person more sensitive to developing depression, even small stressors can lead to later depressive episodes. As a result, whereas early episodes of depression are more strongly associated with the occurrence of recent, stressful life events, later episodes may require little or no stress to precipitate onset of the episode (Kendler, Thornton, & Gardner, 2000). However, additional work is necessary to determine whether there are critical periods and the range of experiences that may produce a kindling effect. In addition, it appears that the kindling effect may be more pronounced for those with low genetic loading for depression (Kendler, Thornton, & Gardner, 2001), suggesting greater potential for relationally focused efforts to prevent kindling among those with low genetic loading.

Are all persons equally reactive or vulnerable to negative interpersonal events? A large literature suggests that this is not the case. Personality variables (Davila, 2001), interpersonal sensitivities (Joiner, 2000), various negative childhood experiences (Hammen et al., 2000), and other individual-difference variables, some of which may be genetically influenced and interact with family context (e.g., Caspi, Sugden, & Moffitt, 2003), have been linked to differential vulnerability. This literature suggests that everyone does not start with an equal chance of becoming depressed in response to negative interpersonal events. In particular, some individuals may have a lower threshold for a depressive response (e.g., Hammen, Henry, & Daley, 2000), or may need no environmental precipitant for the onset of depressive episodes (Kendler et al., 2001).

Genetic Factors

Interestingly, recent work in behavioral genetics, using genetically informed designs, suggests that some interpersonal environments, such as marital satisfaction, are best represented as "nonshared environmental effects" that are not well modeled as resulting from the same genetic factors that produce vulnerability for depressive symptoms (Reiss et al., 2001). This means that it is not simply the case that the same genetic diathesis that produces depression also produces conflicted marital relationships. At the same time, there is emerging evidence of genetic factors that contribute to marital problems (e.g., Jockin & McGue, 1996; Spotts et al., 2005). The apparent contradiction in the findings may reflect the independence of genetic contributions to marital discord and depression, combined with the nonindependence of partners' marital satisfaction, and the iterative processes that connect them. Independent genetic contributions, combined with dependence in marital outcomes, could allow genetic contributions to one partner's satisfaction to be manifested as a nonshared environmental effect for the other. For example, it may be that genetic variation contributing to marital outcomes, such as the possible influence of variation in gamma-aminobutyric acid receptor (GABRA2) on marital status (Dick et al., 2006), is not linked to the genetic influences on depression (e.g., variation in the serotonin 5-HTT promoter region) either within person or through assortative mating. If this is the case, it may be that some sources of social stress generation are partially dependent on partner characteristics, thereby expanding the stress generation model.

Loss events, most of which are social in nature, and which are also particularly common in depression, deserve particular attention. Whereas most social stressors are heritable to some degree (Kendler et al., 1999a), indicating good potential to fit within a stress generation model and the treatments derived from such a perspective, exposure to bereavement is not heritable, suggesting that depressive responses to bereavement might need to be treated somewhat differently. In addition, loss events may be processed more flexibly in an individual format than in dyadic or relationship-specific formats, suggesting good potential for those depressive episodes triggered by loss and bereavement to be addressed by individual approaches such as IPT or its derivatives (e.g., Shear, 2005).

Parenting

In the area of parenting relationships, the reciprocal relationships among depression, parenting behavior, and parenting stress are also clear when viewed broadly. The data reviewed earlier, for example, suggest that parental depression is associated with a shift toward more lax, detached, inconsistent, and ineffective child management. In turn, parenting styles characteristic of depressed parents increase the likelihood for disruptive behaviors in children (e.g., Conger, Patterson, & Ge, 1995), which exacerbate difficulties in the parent–child relationship (e.g., Webster-Stratton & Spitzer, 1996) and maintain the type of vicious cycle described in the stress generation model (Jones, Beach, & Forehand, 2001).

Intergenerational Transmission of Depression

Children and adolescents of depressed parents are up to six times more likely to develop an affective disorder than are other children, and are at greater risk for other psychiatric and psychosocial problems as well (Gotlib & Goodman, 1999). Consistent with the stress generation framework, however, the intergenerational transmission of depression and other psychosocial adjustment problems can be attributed in part to the effects of parental depression on parenting and family functioning, rather than to direct transmission of the depressive symptoms per se (e.g., Beardslee & Podorefsky, 1988). For example, negative changes in parenting lead children of depressed parents to use maladaptive coping strategies, including emotional overinvolvement, guilt, and withdrawal and avoidance, that set the stage for maladjustment (Beardslee & Podorefsky, 1988; Kaslow, Deering, & Racusin, 1994).

In a longitudinal study, Hammen, Shih, and Brennan (2004) examined 800 women and their 15-year-old offspring. These authors found that maternal depression contributed to adolescents' stressful life events. The mechanisms through which maternal depression appeared to influence stress generation for offspring included negative parent–child relationships, as well as dysfunctional relations with others who interacted with the adolescent, including romantic partners, friends, and extended family.

Prevention of Intergenerational Transmission

In an effort to interrupt the intergenerational transmission of depression, investigators have developed interventions to prevent depression and other psychosocial adjustment difficulties in the children of depressed parents. For example, Clarke and colleagues (2001), using both family- and group-based programs, as well as a videotape psychoeducation program, demonstrated significant effects of a cognitive intervention for the prevention of depression in adolescent offspring of depressed parents. These prevention programs focus primarily on psychoeducation for both children and parents regarding risks for depression, as well as on strategies for identifying and challenging irrational, unrealistic, or overly negative thoughts, particularly those related to having a depressed parent. Suggesting good potential for the interruption of stress generation processes, findings revealed that youth in the prevention program evidenced lower levels of depressive symptoms and higher overall adjustment than did youth in the usual care control group.

Also relevant to prevention efforts, Sandler, Wolchik, Winslow, and Schenck (2006) have focused on ways to prevent the intergenerational transmission of stress related to divorce. The custodial parent's, typically the mother's, postdivorce parenting effectiveness is a central vehicle for influence on children's postdivorce functioning (Wolchik, Tein, Sandler, & Doyle, 2002), so it is a natural target for intervention designed to interrupt intergenerational stress transmission. Using a randomized prevention design, these investigators showed not only positive prevention effects overall but also that the benefits were greatest for families who entered with the greatest problems. Mediational analyses indicated that program effects on internalizing problems among children were mediated by improved mother–child relationship quality, whereas program effects on externalizing scores were mediated by both relationship quality and more effective discipline. Effects were maintained over a 6-year follow-up, suggesting that the program had a number of lasting benefits for participants and was successful in reducing many of the stressors and negative outcomes that typically follow parental divorce (Wolchik et al., 2002). Combined with evidence we consider below, these results suggest that parenting interventions have considerable potential to interrupt a number of important stress generation processes associated with depression and may be a key element in interrupting the intergenerational transmission of stress-generating mechanisms.

WHICH INTERVENTIONS SHOULD BE USED TO INTERRUPT STRESS GENERATION?

The stress generation framework can be viewed as a call to action. If depressive symptoms are maintained by a vicious cycle in which symptoms lead to stress-generating interpersonal processes and vice versa, stress generation may be an appropriate target for intervention. In particular, if stress generation processes serve not only to maintain depression but also to stoke the kindling process for future episodes of depression among those who might otherwise be at relatively low risk, and if they further increase the risk of intergeneration transmission of depression, then stress generation may be an essential target of intervention to reduce the burden of depression at a population level. Similarly, interrupting the stress generation process may be an important target of intervention among those who are currently depressed.

For those in an initial episode of depression, marital and parenting relationships may provide excellent points of therapeutic intervention with depressed persons if (1) the stress-generating behaviors in each domain are amenable to change, (2) depressed persons can make the necessary changes in response to treatment, and (3) these changes can be maintained over time. Failure to resolve key marital, family, or other interpersonal issues may interfere with the recovery process and increase the risk for relapse (cf. Hooley & Gotlib, 2000; Whisman, 2006). Accordingly, the stress generation framework suggests that marital and parenting relationships may be particularly useful targets of intervention for depressed individuals, with attention to a broad range of interpersonal processes that are potentially important in maximizing the impact of family and interpersonal interventions. Likewise, given the importance of loss events, bereavement, and social difficulties at the individual level, there is also an important need for interpersonal therapies that can be delivered individually. More broadly applicable forms of interpersonal intervention that require the presence of only the depressed person, such as IPT, may be useful when more targeted, family-focused methods of intervention are not practical options, or the events triggering the episode seem more amenable to resolution using an individual approach.

There Are Well-Established Interventions for Relational Problems

Are there effective interventions for marital discord, parenting difficulties, and other interpersonal stressors? For both marital discord and for problems in parenting behavior, well-specified approaches already have been shown to be efficacious and easily accessible to clinicians. For example, several approaches to marital therapy have been found to be efficacious, including behavioral marital therapy, cognitive-behavioral marital therapy, emotion-focused therapy, and insight-oriented marital therapy (Snyder, Castellani, & Whisman, 2006). In addition, cumulative evidence indicates that marital therapy is successful in reducing depressive symptoms.

Parent management training (Patterson, Reid, & Dishion, 1992), which targets the coercive and maladaptive patterns of parent–child interaction characteristic of children presenting with oppositional behavior, has been identified as a well-established treatment for disruptive behavior disorders (e.g., oppositional defiant disorder, conduct disorder) in children (for a review, see Kazdin, 2005). In addition to modifying parent and child behavior, there is reason to believe that a welcome side effect of parent management training is the alleviation of parental depression, and these effects may be relatively lasting.

Interpersonal psychotherapy (IPT) provides an additional well-studied, interpersonal approach that focuses on conflicts or interpersonal transitions, but unlike marital and parenting interventions, it typically involves only the depressed patient in therapy (Elkin et al., 1989). This suggests that IPT may have important practical advantages as a vehicle for interpersonal intervention in many cases. In addition, IPT has the potential to prevent recurrence and relapse, if it is maintained (Frank, Kupfer, & Perel, 1990).

Well-Established Marital Therapy Approaches for Persons with Depression

Does marital therapy work when applied to depressed patients? Because stress generation theory suggests the value of modifying the stress generation process as a way of influencing symptoms of depression, we examine only those studies that assessed change in both marital satisfaction and depression, and that used a standard outcome design with an appropriate sample size. Three studies compared behavioral marital therapy (BMT) to individual therapy with similar results. In the first study, Jacobson, Dobson, Fruzzetti, Schmaling, and Salusky (1991) randomly assigned 60 married, depressed women to BMT, individual cognitive therapy (CT), or a treatment combining BMT and CT. Couples were not selected for the presence of marital discord, and so could be subdivided into those who were more and less maritally distressed. In the second study, Beach and O'Leary (1992) randomly assigned 45 couples in which the wife was depressed to one of three conditions: (1) conjoint BMT; (2) individual CT; or (3) a 15-week wait-list condition. To be included in the study, both partners had to score in the discordant range of the DAS and report ongoing marital discord. Finally, Emanuels-Zuurveen and Emmelkamp (1996) assigned 27 depressed outpatients to either individual cognitive-behavioral therapy or communication-focused marital therapy. The sample for this study included both depressed husbands ($n = 13$) and depressed wives ($n = 14$). Across the three studies, BMT and individual therapy yielded equivalent outcomes when the dependent variable was depressive symptoms; marital therapy was superior to individual therapy in improving marital functioning. In addition, marital therapy was found to be significantly better than the wait-list control (Beach & O'Leary, 1992).

In a recent study, Bodenmann and colleagues trained spouses of depressed patients to help them process stressful events more effectively, and contrasted this marital condition with both CT and individual IPT. As in other, similar studies, the marital condition was as effective as the alternative, individual approaches to therapy in reducing depressive symptoms (for an extended discussion of the approach, see Bodenmann, 2007).

Consistent with the stress generation framework, two of the studies we reviewed earlier indicate that the effect of marital therapy on level of symptoms of depression is mediated by changes in marital adjustment. Beach and O'Leary (1992) found that posttherapy marital satisfaction fully accounted for the effect of marital therapy on depression. Likewise, Jacobson and colleagues (1991) found that changes in marital adjustment and depression covaried for depressed individuals who received marital therapy, but not for those who received CT. Therefore, it appears that marital therapy influences depressive symptomatology by either enhancing marital satisfaction directly or producing changes in the marital environment that are associated with enhanced satisfaction.

Cast within a stress generation framework, the results of these studies are sufficient to suggest several important conclusions. First, it is clear that efficacious forms of marital therapy can be safely and usefully applied to a depressed population. Second, BMT emerges as a specific and efficacious treatment for marital discord, even when the marital discord is occurring in the context of depression; that is, BMT has been shown in three independent studies to produce significant change in marital distress in a discordant and depressed population, and in each case it has outperformed a control group and/or an alternative intervention. Third, because the marital relationship appears to be an important context for stress generation, successful intervention of this sort can be viewed as particularly promising and provides a strong rationale for recommending marital intervention, where appropriate, with depressed patients. Fourth, work focused on training partners to provide effective social support in the context of marriage (Bodenmann, 2007) suggests the potential to expand marital models and supplement the focus on the conflict reduction that has been characteristic of the later stages of marital therapy for depression. Given the promising effects on reduction of depressive symptoms to date, it is important that work continue to specify the conditions under which marital therapy may serve as a treatment for depression in its own right as a preventive intervention, and as a means of reducing the stress generation processes associated with depression.

Well-Established Approaches to Parent Training for Depressed Patients

Given that compromised parenting is typical of depressed parents, and that parent-focused intervention reduces a number of stress-generating processes (Sandler et al., 2006), it is likely that treatment approaches targeting parenting behavior and the quality of the parent–child relationship may also be an important point of intervention for depressed parents.

In an early, suggestive attempt to examine the effect of parent training on depressive symptoms, Forehand, Wells, and Griest (1980) examined the effects of a parent training program in a sample of 15 clinic-referred children and their mothers. Forehand and colleagues found that mothers in the clinic-referred, but not those in the nonclinic group, evidenced a significant reduction in depressive symptoms from pre- to posttreatment. Hutchings, Lane, and Kelly (2004) examined the efficacy of behavioral parent training ($n = 21$) compared to standard mental health service treatment ($n = 13$) for parents of 2- to 10-year-old children who presented for conduct problems. The parent training intervention included many of the same strategies utilized by Forehand and colleagues, including observation and coding of parent–child interactions, instruction and practice on more adaptive parenting strategies, and homework, and found that mothers in the parenting intervention reported significantly lower levels of depression at 6-month and 4-year follow-ups than did mothers in the standard treatment group (Hutchings et al., 2004). Likewise, the effect on depression of Triple P (Positive Parenting Program), a universal prevention program developed by researchers in Australia to enhance child behavior and parenting efficacy, was also found to be associated with significant declines in parental depressive symptoms pre- to posttreatment (Gallart & Matthey, 2005).

Building on these findings, Beach and colleagues (2008) examined the effects of a prevention-oriented parenting intervention on 163 mothers with elevated depression scores. Compared with participation in the control group, participation in the parenting program was associated with reduced depressive symptoms, enhanced parenting, and improvements in youth behavior. Changes in parenting (consistent discipline, child monitoring, open communication), but not in youth intrapersonal competencies, were found significantly to mediate intervention effects on mothers' depression. Results support the link between reduced depressive symptoms and stronger family relationships, particularly the importance of enhanced parenting efficacy in alleviating depressive symptoms.

Examining parenting at an earlier stage of development, Gelfand, Teti, Seiner, and Jameson (1996) evaluated a multicomponent intervention program in which registered nurses visited depressed mothers of infants at their homes to assess mothers' parenting skills, to enhance mothers' self-confidence, and to reinforce their existing parenting techniques. Mothers diagnosed with major depression were assigned to the parenting intervention group ($n = 37$; i.e., needs assessment, modeling of warm mother–infant interactions, reinforcement of positive parenting skills) or the usual mental health care group (i.e., $n = 36$; ongoing treatment with referral source). Gelfand and colleagues found that mothers in the intervention group demonstrated significantly greater improvement in depressive symptoms than did those in usual care.

Sanders and McFarland (2000) also examined behavioral parenting training for parental depression. Forty-seven families in which the mother met diagnostic criteria for major depression, and in which at least one child met diagnostic criteria for either conduct disorder or oppositional defiant disorder, were randomly assigned either to the traditional behavioral family intervention (BFI; n = 24; instruction, role playing, feedback, and coaching in the use of social learning principles) or a cognitively enhanced BFI condition (CBFI; n = 23; in addition to traditional BFI skills, focused on identifying and interrupting dysfunctional child-related cognitions and automatic thoughts, and increasing relaxation). Although both interventions were associated with significant change in child behavior problems, significantly more mothers in the CBFI condition (72%) than in the BFI condition (35%) were not depressed at follow-up. The studies reviewed here suggest that parenting approaches are promising for alleviating parental depressive symptoms, as well as enhancing child outcomes. In addition, Sanders and McFarland's results highlight the potential for powerful combinations of parenting with cognitive intervention.

Well-Established Individual Approaches to Interpersonal Intervention with Depressed Persons

There are likely to be depressed individuals who would benefit from attention to interpersonal problems or interpersonal stress generation processes, but who, nonetheless, are not good candidates for dyadically oriented therapies. Such individuals may be particularly good candidates for IPT. For example, some depressed persons may need to attend therapy as individuals for various practical reasons, ranging from scheduling difficulties to unavailability of a partner or other family member. IPT may also help to resolve a wider range of difficult interpersonal transitions and/or interpersonal losses than would typically be handled in parenting or couple-focused approaches. IPT has been reviewed elsewhere by Westen and Morrison (2001), who indicate that IPT may be an efficacious treatment for depression, and is probably best viewed as having effects that are not significantly different from the effects of alternative psychosocial interventions for depression (e.g., CT). In addition, IPT performed well in the National Institute of Mental Health (NIMH)–supported Treatment of Depression Collaborative Research Program (Elkin et al., 1989), with treatment effects similar to those of both imiprimine and CT. It is not currently known, however, whether IPT reliably changes interpersonal functioning, or whether it serves to interrupt interpersonal stress generation processes directly.

TOWARD TREATMENT GUIDELINES

Should we expect marital and parenting interventions to be useful for all depressed persons who are married or who have children? Predictors of response to marital therapy suggest that there are decision rules that may help to guide the application of marital therapy for depression. BMT, and perhaps other forms of marital intervention, appear to work best when the marital problems are salient to the depressed spouses (Beach & O'Leary, 1992) or when the depressed persons believe that their marital difficulties have caused their current episode of depression (O'Leary, Risso, & Beach, 1990). Likewise, although severity of depressive symptoms may influence the ease of treatment, moderate to severe depression does not appear to preclude the use of marital therapy as an adjunctive intervention strategy. It seems, therefore, that BMT can be a safe and effective alternative to individual therapy for depression. Similarly, although it is in need of additional direct examination, it seems likely that marital therapy may prove to be a useful adjunctive treatment to medication. Similar conclusions are likely to hold for IPT provided in a couple format (IPT-CM). Although predictors of response to treatment have not been examined empirically for IPT-CM, it is consistent with IPT to choose as targets those problem areas that are salient to the patient and may be related to the maintenance of the current depressive episode (Weissman, Markowitz, & Klerman, 2000). Given the loss of positive interactions that is common in depression, it may be that marital approaches focused on the enhancement of positive interactions would be more universally applicable to depressed patients (e.g., Bodenmann, 2007), suggesting the potential to develop marital approaches that interrupt stress-generating processes and are more universally applicable than current approaches.

Although the research on predictors of differential response is less well developed in the case of parent training as an intervention for the depressed, one might hypothesize that similar patterns will emerge as additional work accumulates. If so, one would expect to find better response to parent training when the child's behavior problems are salient and are seen as serious (e.g., Sanders & McFarland, 2000) or, alternatively, when the child's problem behavior, or conflict with the child, is viewed as a major source of dysphoria and agitation. This suggests the value of parent training when the child carries a diagnosis of a disruptive behavior disorder, including oppositional defiant disorder or conduct disorder, or when the depressed adult is at a key transition that might render the parent relationship more salient, such as the birth of a child or the child's transition to adolescence. An advantage of parent training over marital therapy is that it may lend itself more easily to combination with CT (e.g., Sanders & McFarland, 2000), because parent training is often conducted with only the depressed person in attendance, although the generalization of the parenting skills to the home is more successful if both parents attend the session. Parent training may also be easier to accept for some depressed parents than an offer of marital therapy. Accordingly, it may be a better point of entry into the stress generation process for some depressed patients.

FUTURE DIRECTIONS FOR RESEARCH

Some work has suggested that the families most in need of treatment for depression do not have access to, or they fail to seek, mental health services. Thus, the relevance of marital and family therapies for depression depends on further consideration of the diverse individuals and families that we serve, including families experiencing SES disadvantage, gay and lesbian families, as well as ethnic/minority families.

Socioeconomic Status

Socially and economically disadvantaged families may be less likely to self-refer, and may have higher attrition rates and less successful treatment outcomes than do middle-class populations (e.g., Dumas, 1986). Many disadvantaged families do not access services, and those who do tend to see the service as coercive and intrusive rather than as beneficial. Therefore, efforts to offer family treatments for depression to disadvantaged groups will likely involve special considerations and accommodations. One way to reach disadvantaged families may involve routine screenings by health care professionals trusted by the family members, such as family practice physicians or social workers (but see Coyne, Thompson, Palmer, Kagee, & Maunsell, 2000, for an argument against routine screening in the absence of adequate follow-up). Alternatively, information about family intervention services may be provided in a nonthreatening manner at nontreatment points of contact, such as community health care clinics, family practitioners, day care centers, or through public service announcements. Similarly, it may be possible to provide universal access programs through community or religious settings (Hurt et al., 2006). An additional challenge to widespread dissemination of efficacious interventions for marital and parenting difficulties, however, is that they must be low cost, easily accessible, and available on a continuing basis. Thus, an important challenge for future research is that of packaging efficacious interventions and developing delivery systems that can meet the expanding needs of a depressed population.

Sexual Orientation

Family interventions for depression must also begin to consider alternative family forms. The special needs of gay and lesbian couples remain largely unexamined in the empirical literature, limiting the generalizability of current efficacy research. This deficit in the literature remains despite the finding that gay, lesbian, and bisexual people seek mental health services at a rate that is two to four times higher than that of heterosexual people. In addition, issues related to dyadic relationships and parents, disclosure of sexual orientation, and social network development may be relevant points of therapeutic intervention among gay, lesbian, and bisexual families.

Race/Ethnicity

Access to marital therapy and parenting programs differs across regions of the country and among ethnic groups (Stanley, Amato, Johnson, & Markman, 2006). The preponderance of work on race/ethnicity within both the marital and family therapy areas has focused on African American families. Dissemination is a particularly important issue for African Americans, who are underserved by typical means of health care delivery, and who may be less likely to advocate for mental health services in their communities due to skepticism about the benefits of these services (Murry & Brody, 2004). Reluctance to be involved in research or to seek services including mistrust of medical researchers, contextual factors (e.g., a lack of transportation or means to pay for services), and the perception that programs are likely to be culturally irrelevant may contribute to African Americans' status as the group with the highest therapy dropout rate of all ethnic groups (Sue, Zane, & Young, 1994). For these reasons, establishing trust and offering marital therapy approaches and parenting programs that take into consideration the racial, socioeconomic, and regional characteristics of the populations served are critical to meet the needs of African Americans and members of other ethnic minorities experiencing depression.

Religiosity

To present marital, parenting, or other interpersonal interventions in a culturally sensitive manner for depressed African Americans, a greater consideration of religiosity may also be important. Among African American couples, religiosity and church involvement predict relationship quality (Brody, Stoneman, & Flor, 1996), suggesting that this population is more likely to respond favorably to relationship enhancement programs that encourage couples to draw upon their own religious practices.

Historically, religious participation has been an important survival strategy for African Americans. For example, during enslavement and in the challenging postemancipation environment, a strong religious orientation served as a framework for preserving family values and overcoming staggering experiences of injustice in a dehumanizing environment. This legacy of spirituality and religious involvement has been passed down through generations and remains a consistent part of the fabric of African American communities and family life. As a consequence, it is likely that modifying empirically established programs to render them more clearly "religion-friendly" will be important in tailoring programs for use in the African American community. Working with community groups to find the best avenues for the incorporation of spiritual values will be essential for long-term acceptance of psychologically based family and interpersonal approaches.

In addition to paying more attention to the role of religion in the lives of African American adults and their families, there is strong theoretical and empirical evidence to support the importance of defining "family" and "parent" more broadly when working with African American adults who present with depression. For example, a growing number of African American women are in nontraditional marital or coparenting relationships (U.S. Bureau of the Census, 2005), a phenomenon attributed to the disproportionate rates of pregnancy among African American girls, but that also has been created by declining rates of marriage and rising divorce rates in the African American community (for a review, see McLoyd, Cauce, Takeuchi, & Wilson, 2000). The important role of extended family networks in the African American community generally, and for African American single mothers in particular, has been documented extensively in the literature (e.g., Jones, Zalot, Foster, Sterrett, & Chester, 2007). The most recent census data suggest that African American single-mother families are more likely than two-parent families to reside in the home of a relative, including a grandparent, aunt or uncle, or siblings, as well as nonrelatives and friends (U.S. Bureau of the Census, 2005). Even when African American single mothers do own or rent their own homes, they are more likely than married mothers to invite other family members, as well as nonrelatives, to reside with them. This tendency may be driven largely by socioeconomic necessity (U.S. Bureau of the Census, 2005); a growing body of research suggests, however, that relationships with other adults who live in the home, as well as those who do not, serve other valuable roles as well. Accordingly, rather than exclude depressed women in nontraditional relationships from relationship-based approaches to the treatment of depression, growing evidence suggests the importance of attending to relationships with extended family members or others in the home (see Jones et al., 2007).

With regard to coparenting relationships in particular, Jones and colleagues have examined the role of nonmarried coparents on maternal and child psychosocial functioning in African American single-mother families (e.g., Jones, Dorsey, et al., 2005; Jones, Forehand, O'Connell, Brody, & Armistead, 2005). For example, African American single mothers were asked if another adult or family member assisted them with childrearing and, if so, to identify the most important person. Although only 3% of mothers failed to identify another adult or family member who assisted with childrearing, the majority identified the child's maternal grandmother (31%) or biological father (26%). Others identified a maternal aunt (11%), the child's older sister (11%), as well as diverse group of other relatives and nonrelatives, such as friends and neighbors. Of most relevance to this chapter, the quality of mothers' relationships with their identified coparent was associated with maternal depressive symptoms and with quality of parenting behavior (Jones, Dorsey, et al., 2005). Mothers who reported experiencing greater conflict regarding childrearing issues with their coparents reported greater depressive symptoms and more compromised parenting. Given the previously discussed importance of including both mothers and fathers in behavioral parent training in intact families, clinicians conducting parent training with depressed African American single mothers should consider the possibility of including nonmarital or nontraditional coparents in behavioral parent training programs as well.

CONCLUSIONS: THE FUTURE OF FAMILY THERAPY FOR DEPRESSION

We have come far in the study of effective ways to intervene with the families of depressed patients. Although the current level of success should not be oversold, a solid conceptual foundation grounded in a stress generation framework is emerging to guide and support family interventions with depressed patients. A large and robust literature indicates that marital and parenting relationships are often problematic for depressed persons. From the perspective of the stress generation framework, difficulties in the area of marital and parenting relationships, and the likelihood that these processes will continue even after successful individual treatment, are troubling. At the same time, there is good evidence that these problematic relationships can be repaired, and it seems appropriate to recommend an efficacious, targeted intervention to effect that repair.

The stress generation framework suggests that targeted, efficacious interventions have the potential to break the vicious cycles that may serve to maintain depression. If so, interventions that include attention to problematic family relationships may decrease future distress and the risk for, or severity of, future episodes. This promise, however, awaits a conclusive demonstration. Nevertheless, available evidence is promising, and continuing efforts to document the conditions under which marital and parenting interventions are efficacious in relieving an episode of depression are warranted. In the meantime, both marital and parenting interventions can claim to be efficacious interventions for important sources of stress generation in depression.

The stress generation framework also highlights the potential for particular areas of individual vulnerability to lead to problematic interpersonal processes. As the connection between particular areas of individual vulnerability and interpersonal stress generation is more clearly mapped, it may be possible to develop integrated approaches that combine attention to both individual vulnerabilities and problematic interpersonal relations. In particular, stress generation theory lends itself to increasingly refined models and corresponding refinement of intervention. The stress generation framework also provides an excellent "neutral" framework within which researchers of various backgrounds and orientations can share information and innovative suggestions for intervention. As we keep marital and family interventions for depression tightly focused on their empirical foundation, it may be increasingly useful to adopt stress generation theory as a way to summarize empirical findings and guide intervention.

REFERENCES

Beach, S. R. H., Kim, S., Cercone-Keeney, J., Gupta, M., Arias, I., & Brody, G. (2004). Physical aggression and depressive symptoms: Gender asymmetry in effects? *Journal of Social and Personal Relationships, 21*, 341–360.

Beach, S. R. H., Kogan, S. M., Brody, G. H., Chen, Y., Lei, M., & Murry, V. M. (2008). Change in caregiver depression as a function of the Strong African American Families Program. *Journal of Family Psychology, 22*, 241–252.

Beach, S. R. H., & O'Leary, K. D. (1992). Treating depression in the context of marital discord: Outcome and predictors of response for marital therapy versus cognitive therapy. *Behavior Therapy, 23*, 507–258.

Beardslee, W. R., & Podorefsky, D. (1988). Resilient adolescents whose parents have serious affective and other psychiatric disorders: The importance of self-understanding and relationships. *American Journal of Psychiatry, 145*, 63–69.

Bodenmann, G. (2007). Improving in marital distress prevention programs and marital therapy: Dyadic coping and the 3-phase-method in working with couples. In L. VandeCreek & J. Allen (Eds.), *Innovations in clinical practice: Focus on group and family therapy* (pp. 235–252). Sarasota, FL: Professional Resources Press.

Brody, G. H., Stoneman, Z., & Flor, D. (1996). Parental religiosity, family processes, and youth competence in rural, two-parent African American families. *Developmental Psychology, 32*(4), 696–706.

Brown, G. W., & Moran, P. M. (1997). Single mothers, poverty, and depression. *Psychological Medicine, 27*, 21–33.

Cano, A., & O'Leary, K. D. (2000). Infidelity and separations precipitate major depressive episodes and symptoms of non-specific depression and anxiety. *Journal of Consulting and Clinical Psychology, 68*, 774–781.

Caspi, A., Sugden, K., & Moffitt, T. E. (2003). Influence of life stress on depression: Moderation by a polymorphism in the *5-HTT* gene. *Science, 301*, 386–389.

Clarke, G. N., Hornbrook, M., Lynch, F., Polen, M., Gale, J., Beardslee, W., et al. (2001). A randomized trial of group cognitive intervention for preventing depression in adolescent offspring of depressed parents. *Archives of General Psychiatry, 58*, 1127–1134.

Conger, R., Patterson, G., & Ge, X. (1995). It takes two to replicate: A mediational model of the impact of parents' stress on adolescent adjustment. *Child Development, 66*, 80–97.

Coyne, J. C., Thompson, R., Palmer, S. C., Kagee, A., & Maunsell, E. (2000). Should we screen for depression?: Caveats and potential pitfalls. *Applied and Preventive Psychology, 9*, 101–122.

Davila, J. (2001). Paths to unhappiness: The overlapping courses of depression and romantic dysfunction. In S. Beach (Ed.), *Marital and family processes in depression* (pp. 71–87). Washington, DC: American Psychological Association Press.

Davila, J., Bradbury, T. N., Cohan, C. L., & Tochluk, S. (1997). Marital functioning and depressive symptoms: Evidence for a stress generation model. *Journal of Personality and Social Psychology, 73*, 849–861.

Dick, D. M., Agrawal, A., Schuckit, M. A., Bierut, L., Hinrichs, A., Fox, L., et al. (2006). Marital status, alcohol dependence, and *GABRA2*: Evidence for gene–environment correlation and interaction. *Journal of Studies on Alcohol, 67*(2), 185–194.

Dumas, J. E. (1986). Parental perception and treatment outcome in families of aggressive children: A causal model. *Behavior Therapy, 17*(4), 420–432.

Elkin, I., Shea, M. T., Watkins, J. T., Imber, S. D., Sotsky, S. M., Collins, J. M., et al. (1989). National Institute of Mental Health Treatment of Depression Collaborative Research Program: General effectiveness of treatments. *Archives of General Psychiatry, 46*, 971–982.

Emanuels-Zuurveen, L., & Emmelkamp, P. M. (1996). Individual behavioral-cognitive therapy vs. marital therapy for depression in maritally distressed couples. *British Journal of Psychiatry, 169*, 181–188.

Fleeson, W. (2004). The quality of American life at the end of the century. In O. G. Brim, C. D. Ryff, & R. C. Kessler (Eds.), *How healthy are we?: A national study of well-being at midlife* (pp. 252–272). Chicago: University of Chicago Press.

Forehand, R., Wells, K. C., & Griest, D. L. (1980). An examination of the social validity of a parent training program. *Behavior Therapy, 11*, 488–502.

Frank, E., Kupfer, D. J., & Perel, J. M. (1990). Three-year outcomes for maintenance therapies in recurrent depression. *Archives of General Psychiatry, 47*, 1093–1099.

Fryers, T., Melzer, D., & Jenkins, R. (2003). Social inequalities and the common mental disorders: A systematic review of the evidence. *Social Psychiatry and Psychiatric Epidemiology, 38*, 229–237.

Gallart, S. C., & Matthey, S. (2005). The effectiveness of group Triple P and the impact of four telephone contacts. *Behavior Change, 22*, 71–80.

Gelfand, D. M., Teti, D. M., Seiner, S. A., & Jameson, P. B. (1996). Helping Mother fight depression: Evaluation of a home-based intervention for depressed mothers and their infants. *Journal of Clinical Child Psychology, 24,* 406–422.

Gotlib, I. H., & Goodman, S. H. (1999). Children of parents with depression. In W. K. Silverman & T. H. Ollendick (Eds.), *Developmental issues in the clinical treatment of children* (pp. 415–432). Boston: Allyn & Bacon.

Greenberg, P. E., Kessler, R. C., Birnbaum, H. G., Leong, S. A., Lowe, S. W., Berglund, P., et al. (2003). The economic burden of depression in the United States: How did it change between 1990 and 2000? *Journal of Clinical Psychiatry, 64,* 1465–1475.

Hammen, C. (1991). *Depression runs in families: The social context of risk and resilience in children of depressed mothers.* New York: Springer-Verlag.

Hammen, C. (2005). Stress and depression. *Annual Review of Clinical Psychology, 1,* 293–319.

Hammen, C., Henry, R., & Daley, S. E. (2000). Depression and sensitization to stressors among young women as a function of childhood adversity. *Journal of Consulting and Clinical Psychology, 68,* 782–787.

Hammen, C., Shih, J. H., & Brennan, P. A. (2004). Intergenerational transmission of depression: Test of an interpersonal stress model in a community sample. *Journal of Consulting and Clinical Psychology, 72*(3), 511–522.

Hooley, J. M., & Gotlib, I. H. (2000). A diathesis–stress conceptualization of expressed emotion and clinical outcome. *Applied and Preventive Psychology, 9,* 135–152.

Hurt, T. R., Franklin, K. J., Beach, S. R. H., Murry, V. B., Brody, G. H., McNair, L. D., et al. (2006). Dissemination of couples interventions among African American populations: Experiences from ProSAAM. *Couples Research and Therapy Newsletter, 12,* 13–16.

Hutchings, J., Lane, E., & Kelly, J. (2004). Comparison of two treatments for children with severely disruptive behaviors: A four-year follow-up. *Behavioral and Cognitive Psychotherapy, 32,* 15–30.

Jacobson, N. S., Dobson, K., Fruzzetti, A. E., Schmaling, K. B., & Salusky, S. (1991). Marital therapy as a treatment for depression. *Journal of Consulting and Clinical Psychology, 59,* 547–557.

Jockin, V., & McGue, D. T. (1996). Personality and divorce: A genetic analysis. *Journal of Personality and Social Psychology, 71,* 288–299.

Joiner, T. E. (2000). Depression's vicious scree: Self-propogating and erosive processes in depression chronicity. *Clinical Psychology: Science and Practice, 7,* 203–218.

Joiner, T. E., & Coyne, J. C. (1999). *The interactional nature of depression.* Washington, DC: American Psychological Association.

Jones, D. J., Beach, S. R. H., & Forehand, R. (2001). Stress generation in intact community families: Depressive symptoms, perceived family relationship stress, and implications for adolescent adjustment. *Journal of Social and Personal Relationships, 18,* 443–462.

Jones, D. J., Dorsey, S., Forehand, R., Foster, S., Armistead, L., & Brody, G. (2005). Co-parent support and conflict in African American single mother-headed families: Associations with mother and child adjustment. *Journal of Family Violence, 20,* 141–150.

Jones, D. J., Forehand, R., O'Connell, C., Brody, G., & Armistead, L. (2005). Neighborhood violence and maternal monitoring in African American single mother-headed families: An examination of the moderating role of social support. *Behavior Therapy, 36,* 25–34.

Jones, D. J., Zalot, A., Foster, S. E., Sterrett, E., & Chester, C. (2007). A review of childrearing in African American single mother families: The relevance of a coparenting framework. *Journal of Child and Family Studies, 16,* 671–683.

Kaslow, N. J., Deering, C. G., & Racusin, G. R. (1994). Depressed children and their families. *Clinical Psychology Review, 14,* 39–59.

Kazdin, A. E. (2005). *Parent management training: Treatment for oppositional, aggressive, and antisocial behavior in children and adolescents.* New York: Oxford University Press.

Kendler, K. S., Karkowski, L. M., & Prescott, C. A. (1998). Stressful life events and major depression: Risk period, long-term contextual threat and diagnostic specificity. *Journal of Nervous and Mental Disease, 186*(11), 661–669.

Kendler, K. S., Karkowski, L. M., & Prescott, C. A. (1999a). The assessment of dependence in the study of stressful life events: Validation using a twin design. *Psychological Medicine, 29,* 1455–1460.

Kendler, K. S., Karkowski, L. M., & Prescott, C. A. (1999b). Causal relationship between stressful life events and the onset of major depression. *American Journal of Psychiatry, 156*(6), 837–848.

Kendler, K. S., Thornton, L. M., & Gardner, C. O. (2000). Stressful life events and previous episodes in the etiology of major depression in women: An evaluation of the "kindling" hypothesis. *American Journal of Psychiatry, 157*(8), 1243–1251.

Kendler, K. S., Thornton, L. M., & Gardner, C. O. (2001). Genetic risk, number of previous depressive episodes, and stressful life events in predicting onset of major depression. *American Journal of Psychiatry, 158,* 582–586.

Kessler, R., Avenevoli, S., & Merikangas, K. R. (2001). Mood disorders in children and adolescents: An epidemiologic perspective. *Biological Psychiatry, 49,* 1002–1014.

Lorant, V., Deliege, D., & Eaton, W. (2003). Socioeconomic inequalities in depression: A metanalysis. *American Journal of Epidemiology, 157,* 98–112.

Lovejoy, M. C., Graczyk, P. A., O'Hare, E., & Neuman, G. (2000). Maternal depression and parenting behavior: A meta-analytic review. *Clinical Psychology Review, 20,* 561–592.

McGonagle, K. A., & Kessler, R. C. (1990). Chronic stress, acute stress, and depressive symptoms. *American Journal of Community Psychology, 18*(5), 681–706.

McLoyd, V. C., Cauce, A. M., Takeuchi, D., & Wilson, L. (2000). Marital processes and parental socialization in families of color: A decade review of research. *Journal of Marriage and the Family, 62,* 1070–1093.

Murry, V. M., & Brody, G. H. (2004). Partnering with community stakeholders: Engaging rural African American families in basic research and the Strong African American Families Preventive Intervention program. *Journal of Marital and Family Therapy, 30*(3), 271–283.

O'Leary, K. D., Risso, L., & Beach, S. R. H. (1992). Beliefs about the marital discord/depression link: Implications for outcome and treatment matching. *Behavior Therapy, 21,* 413–422.

Patterson, G. R., Reid, J. B., & Dishion, T. J. (1992). *Antisocial boys.* Eugene, OR: Castilia.

Paykel, E. S. (2003). Life events and affective disorders. *Acta Psychiatrica Scandinavica, 108,* 61–66.

Reiss, D., Pedersen, N. L., Cederblad, M., Lichtenstein, P., Hansson, K., Neiderhiser, J. M., et al. (2001). Genetic probes of three theories of maternal adjustment: I. Recent evidence and a model. *Family Process, 40,* 247–259.

Rounsaville, B. J., Weissman, M. M., Prusoff, B. A., & Herceg-Baron, R. L. (1979). Marital disputes and treatment outcome in depressed women. *Comprehensive Psychiatry, 20,* 483–490.

Sanders, M. R., & McFarland, M. (2000). Treatment of depressed mothers with disruptive children: A controlled evaluation of cognitive behavioral family intervention. *Behavior Therapy, 31,* 89–112.

Sandler, I. N., Wolchik, S. A., Winslow, E. B., & Schenck, C. (2006). Prevention as the promotion of healthy parenting following parental divorce. In S. R. H. Beach, M. Z. Wamboldt, N. J. Kaslow, R. E. Heyman, M. B. First, L. G. Underwood, et al. (Eds.), *Relational processes and DSM-V: Neuroscience, assessment, prevention, and treatment.* Washington: DC: American Psychiatric Publishing.

Shear, K. (2005). Symposium monograph supplement: Bereavement-related depression in the elderly. *CNS Spectrums, 10*(8), 3–5.

Snyder, D. K., Castellani, A. M., & Whisman, M. A. (2006). Current status and future directions in couple therapy. *Annual Review of Psychology, 57,* 317–344.

Spotts, E. L., Lichenstein, P., Pedersen, N., Neiderhiser, J. M., Hansson, K., Cederblad, M., et al. (2005). Personality and marital satisfaction: A behavioral genetic analysis. *European Journal of Personality, 19,* 205–227.

Stanley, S. M., Amato, P. R., Johnson, C. A., & Markman, H. J. (2006). Premarital education, marital quality, and marital stability: Findings from a large random household survey. *Journal of Family Psychology, 20,* 117–126.

Sue, S., Zane, N., & Young, K. (1994). Research on psychotherapy with culturally diverse populations. In A. E. Bergin & S. L. Garfield (Eds.), *Handbook of psychotherapy and behavior change* (4th ed., pp. 783–817). Oxford, UK: Wiley.

Turner, J., Lloyd, D. A., & Roszell, P. (1999). Personal resources and the social distribution of depression. *American Journal of Community Psychology, 27,* 643–672.

Turner, R. J., & Marino, F. (1994). Social support and social structure: A descriptive epidemiology. *Journal of Health and Social Behavior, 35,* 193–212.

Turvey, C., Carney, C., & Arndt, S. (1999). Conjugal loss and syndromal depression in a sample of elders aged 70 years or older. *American Journal of Psychiatry, 156,* 1596–1601.

U.S. Bureau of the Census. (2005, June 29). Current Population Survey, 2004 Annual Social and Economic (ASEC) Supplement. Retrieved October 1, 2005, from *www.census.gov/population/www/socdemo/hh-fam/cps2004.html*

Wade, T. J., & Pevalin, D. J. (2004). Marital transitions and mental health. *Journal of Health and Social Behavior, 45,* 155–170.

Webster-Stratton, C., & Spitzer, A.(1996). Parenting a young child with conduct problems: New insights using qualitative methods. In T. H. Ollendick & R. H. Prinz (Eds.), *Advances in clinical child psychology* (Vol. 18., pp. 1–62). New York: Plenum Press.

Weissman, M. M., Markowitz, J. C., & Klerman, G. L. (2000). *Comprehensive guide to interpersonal psychotherapy.* New York: Basic Books.

Westen, D., & Morrison, K. (2001). A multidimensional meta-analysis of treatments for depression, panic, and generalized anxiety disorder: An empirical examination of the status of empirically supported therapies. *Journal of Consulting and Clinical Psychology, 69*(6), 875–899.

Whisman, M. A. (2001). The association between depression and marital dissatisfaction. In S. R. H. Beach (Ed.), *Marital and family processes in depression* (pp. 3–24). Washington, DC: American Psychological Association.

Whisman, M. A. (2006). Role of couples relationships in understanding and treating mental disorder. In S. R. H. Beach, M. Z. Wamboldt, N. J. Kaslow, R. E. Heyman, M. B. First, L. G. Underwood, et al. (Eds.), *Relational processes and DSM-V: Neuroscience, assessment, prevention, and treatment* (pp. 225–238). Washington: DC: American Psychiatric Publishing.

Whisman, M. A., & Bruce, M. L. (1999). Marital distress and incidence of major depressive episode in a community sample. *Journal of Abnormal Psychology, 108,* 674–678.

Wolchik, S. A., Tein, J.-Y., Sandler, I. N., & Doyle, K. W. (2002). Fear of abandonment as a mediator of the relations between divorce stressors and mother–child relationship quality and children's adjustment problems. *Journal of Abnormal Child Psychology, 30,* 401–418.

Wortman, C. B., Wolff, K., & Bonanno, G. A. (2004). Loss of an intimate partner through death. In D. J. Mashek & A. P. Aron (Eds.), *Handbook of closeness and intimacy* (pp. 305–320). Mahwah, NJ: Erlbaum.

CHAPTER 28

Biological and Psychosocial Interventions for Depression in Children and Adolescents

Nadine J. Kaslow, Shane P. Davis, *and* Chaundrissa Oyeshiku Smith

Depression in youth is a serious public health problem associated with risk of suicidal behavior (Mann et al., 2006) and greater use of health care, school, and other social services (Lyon & Clarke, 2006). It occurs frequently; causes psychosocial impairment; is painful for depressed youth and those in their environment; and creates burden for depressed youth, their families, and society. There has been increased attention to empirically supported, biopsychosocially oriented programs to treat and prevent depression in young people during the past two decades (David-Ferdon & Kaslow, 2008; McClure, Kubiszyn, & Kaslow, 2002). There is support for pharmacological, psychosocial, and combined pharmacological and psychosocial interventions (Coyle et al., 2003; David-Ferdon & Kaslow, 2008; Varley, 2006; Wu et al., 2001). A recent meta-analysis found a small effect size (M = 0.34) for psychotherapeutic interventions (Weisz, McCarty, & Valeri, 2006). Some interventions have been shown to be cost-effective (Lynch et al., 2005; Lyon & Clarke, 2006). Yet depression in youth is underdiagnosed and undertreated (Wu et al., 2001), few youth receive psychotherapy (Ma, Lee, & Stafford, 2005), and recent concerns by the U.S. Food and Drug Administration (FDA) regarding the possible link between selective serotonin reuptake inhibitors (SSRIs) and suicidality has led to a decline in the use of these medications in children and adolescents, and in the treatment of pediatric depression (Libby et al., 2007). There are concerns that this reduction in pharmacological treatment of depression in youth may be associated with recent increases in suicide rates among youth (*Morbidity and Mortality World Report* [MMWR], 2007).

This chapter reviews the biological and psychosocial evidence-based interventions for children and adolescents, and prevention programs. For details, the reader is referred to recent articles (David-Ferdon & Kaslow, 2008; Weisz et al., 2006) and to earlier reviews

(Chorpita, 2002; Compton et al., 2004; Curry, 2001; Kaslow & Thompson, 1998; Reinecke, Ryan, & DuBois, 1998; Weisz, Doss, & Hawley, 2005). Mediators, moderators, and predictors of treatment outcome are addressed. Existing treatment guidelines are presented, and guiding principles for treating depressed youth are proffered. Future research directions are provided.

INTERVENTIONS

Biological Treatments

Pharmacological Interventions

The past decade has witnessed over a fourfold increase in pharmacological interventions for depressed youth (Ma et al., 2005). Antidepressant medications often are prescribed, either alone or in combination with psychosocial treatments (Debar, Clarke, O'Connor, & Nichols, 2001; Delate, Gelenberg, Simmons, & Motheral, 2004; Olfson, Gameroff, Marcus, & Waslick, 2003; Rushton & Whitmire, 2001; Wagner & Ambrosini, 2001). An estimated 1.4 million children received antidepressant medication in 2002 (Vitiello, Zuvekas, & Norquist, 2006) and approximately 6% of outpatient physician visits for children in the United States involve prescriptions for antidepressants (National Center for Health Statistics, 2004).

Data on the efficacy and safety of tricyclic antidepressants (TCAs) are not favorable (Mann et al., 2006; Michael & Crowley, 2002); thus, there has been increased use of SSRIs in depressed youth (Brown & Sammons, 2002). SSRIs have fewer side effects than TCAs, although they are not without side effects. Safety data on SSRIs are mixed but more positive than data for the TCAs (Cheung, Emslie, & Mayes, 2005; Rynn et al., 2006; Whittington et al., 2004).

Reviews of safety and efficacy data led regulators in the United States, Canada, and United Kingdom to issue warnings about the increased risk for suicidal behavior in youth on SSRIs. There are mood-related adverse effects in youth on antidepressants (Mann et al., 2006; Varley, 2006). However, given that untreated depression is a problem, those data suggest that pharmacotherapy may be helpful, and that studies comparing pharmacological and psychosocial interventions are more favorable for medications, there continues to be a role for antidepressants, if youth are monitored closely (Cheung, Emslie, & Mayes, 2006; Varley, 2006).

EFFICACY TRIALS

Randomized controlled trials (RCTs) have examined the efficacy of SSRIs with adolescents. Recent reviews provide inconsistent evidence for their efficacy (Emslie, Findling, et al., 2002). The most incontrovertible efficacy evidence is for fluoxetine (Prozac) (Emslie, Heiligenstein, et al., 2002; Emslie et al., 1997; Treatment for Adolescents with Depression Study [TADS] Team, 2004). The FDA has only approved fluoxetine for children and adolescents with major depressive disorder (MDD). Analyses of the pros and cons of antidepressants lead to the conclusion that fluoxetine has a role in the treatment of pediatric depression (Kratochvil, Vitiello, et al., 2006; Ryan, 2005), and that it is safe for use with this population (Whittington, Kendall, & Pilling, 2005).

There is mixed evidence for the following SSRIs with regard to outcome variables and age of the youth: citalopram (Celexa) (von Knorring, Olsson, Thomsen, Lemming, &

Hulten, 2006; Wagner et al., 2004), sertraline (Zoloft) (Melvin et al., 2006; Wagner et al., 2003), paroxetine (Paxil) (Berard, Fong, Carpenter, Thomason, & Wilkinson, 2006; Emslie, Wagner, et al., 2006; Keller et al., 2001; Wagner, 2003), and escitalopram (Lexapro) (Wagner, Jonas, Findling, Ventura, & Saikali, 2006). There are mixed findings from RCTs regarding serotonin–norepinepherine reuptake inhibitors (SNRIs): nefazodone (Serzone), venlafaxine (Effexor), and mirtazapine (Remeron) (Cheung et al., 2005, 2006; Emslie, Findling, et al., 2002; Emslie, Findling, Yeung, Kunz, & Li, 2007; Mann et al., 2006). However, evidence for SNRIs is insufficient to support their use for pediatric MDD (Cheung et al., 2006).

Some medications prevent relapse of MDD (Emslie et al., 2004). Other medications (e.g., fluoxetine, bupropion sustained release [Wellbutrin]) effectively treat depression that co-occurs with other disorders (e.g., attention-deficit/hyperactivity disorder, alcohol abuse) (Cornelius et al., 2001; Daviss et al., 2001). There are differential remission and response rates between the various medications (Cheung et al., 2005). Children and adolescents have differential response patterns to SSRIs (Donnelly et al., 2006; Wagner et al., 2006). Some studies show that adolescents respond more favorably than do prepubertal youth (Wagner et al., 2006), and others suggest that children respond more quickly than do adolescents (Donnelly et al., 2006). Methodological issues and publication biases make it difficult to determine the efficacy of SSRIs for depressed youth (Jureidini et al., 2004; Whittington et al., 2004).

Combined Pharmacological and Psychosocial Interventions

TREATMENT FOR ADOLESCENTS WITH DEPRESSION STUDY

The Treatment for Adolescents with Depression Study (TADS), a multisite trial sponsored by the National Institutes of Mental Health (NIMH) (Curry et al., 2006; Emslie, Kratochvil, et al., 2006; Kennard et al., 2006; Kratochvil, Emslie, et al., 2006; March, Silva, Vitiello, & the TADS Team, 2006; TADS Team, 2003, 2004, 2005; Vitiello, Rohde, et al., 2006), offers compelling evidence that favors SSRIs for adolescents with MDD. This randomized, masked effectiveness trial evaluates the effectiveness of four interventions: cognitive-behavioral therapy (CBT) alone, fluoxetine alone, combined medication and CBT, and placebo-pill alone.

The 12-week, 15-session CBT skills-based psychoeducational program focuses on depression and its causes, goal setting, mood monitoring, increasing pleasant activities, social problem solving, cognitive restructuring, and enhancing social skills. Two parent sessions offer information, and conjoint sessions address parent and adolescent concerns. The SSRI condition uses a flexible dosing schedule for fluoxetine; youth may receive up to 40 mg per day of fluoxetine by Week 8. Adolescents meet for six visits over 12 weeks with a pharmacotherapist, who provides monitoring and encouragement. Adolescents in the combined treatment receive all components of CBT alone and medication alone. Youth in the placebo group receive a sugar pill, following the same dose and monitoring patterns as those in the fluoxetine alone group.

Following acute treatment, 71% of the teens no longer met diagnostic criteria (i.e., responders), 50% had residual symptoms, and 23% had reached remission. Results indicate that the combined treatment was the most effective method in ameliorating depressive symptoms (clinician reports) and reducing suicidal ideation (teen reports). The superiority of the combined intervention was further supported by effect sizes; endpoint data related to 16 outcome variables; levels of global functioning, health outcomes, and quality of life; remission rates; response rate times; and probability of sustained early response. In general the data also suggest that fluoxetine was superior to CBT alone, but CBT was not more effective than placebo. This overall pattern of effects held true for youth with mild to moderate depression; however, for severely depressed youth, there was no evidence that the addition of CBT was helpful.

A few additional findings are noteworthy. First, combined treatment was superior to fluoxetine for youth with high levels of cognitive distortions, but for adolescents with adaptive cognitive processing, combined treatment and fluoxetine only were equally effective, and both were more effective than CBT alone or placebo. Second, the one group for which combined treatment and CBT alone were equally effective was youth from high-income families. Third, suicidal events were twice as common in adolescents treated with fluoxetine alone as in youth in the combined or CBT alone groups, potentially indicating that CBT protects against suicidal behavior. Fourth, youth who received fluoxetine, alone or in combination, endorsed physical symptoms at a rate twice that of the placebo group. Fifth, CBT was associated with the fewest adverse physical and psychiatric events, and fluoxetine alone related to the most adverse events.

OTHER RELEVANT STUDIES

Other studies also have found combined SSRI and CBT treatment to be more effective than an SSRI alone (Clarke et al., 2005). However, this has not always been the case (Goodyer et al., 2007; Melvin et al., 2006). Goodyer and colleagues (2007) found no evidence to support the relative superiority of a combined SSRI and CBT intervention over SSRI with routine clinical care for adolescents with moderate to severe depression. Melvin and coworkers (2006) did not find combined CBT and SSRI to be superior to either treatment alone.

FDA Warning

Many are reluctant to consider antidepressants due to the potential link between SSRIs and suicidal behavior, and the development of mania in youth (Mann et al., 2006). Concerns have become more pronounced in reaction to FDA warnings about the possibility of increased depressive symptoms and suicide risk for young persons on antidepressants. In October 2004, the FDA required that manufacturers inform consumers about the increased risk of suicidal thinking and behavior in youth treated with antidepressants via a boxed warning (black box) and Patient Education Guide (Newman, 2004). The FDA has presented strategies for bolstering safeguards for children taking antidepressants and has a medication guide regarding the use of antidepressants in youth. The FDA has not contraindicated any antidepressant for pediatric use.

These recommendations emerged following an examination of data pooled from 24 short-term, placebo-controlled trials of antidepressants with over 4,500 youth that yielded elevated rates of suicidal ideation and behavior, and serious suicidal events for youth receiving antidepressants compared to youth in the placebo condition, despite the fact that no one died from suicide (Hammad, Laughren, & Racoosin, 2006; Mosholder & Willy, 2006). A reanalysis of these data using the Columbia Classification Algorithm of Suicide Assessment yielded more suicidal events overall but fewer suicide attempts (Posner, Oquendo, Gould, Stanley, & Davies, 2007). However, a number of studies have found that SSRI use has no significant effect on the likelihood of suicidal behavior (Valuck, Libby, Sills, Giese, & Allen, 2004), that adolescent suicide rates in the United States have declined as antidepressant prescriptions increased (Gibbons, Hur, Bhaumik, & Mann, 2006; Olfson et al., 2003), and that autopsies fail to find antidepressant medication in the serum toxicology in most adolescent suicide completers (Isacsson, Holmgren, & Ahlner, 2005; Leon et al., 2006; Leon, Marzuk, Tardiff, & Teres, 2004). An FDA analysis demonstrated that even though there may have been increased risk for suicidality, depression improved in youth on fluoxetine four times as frequently as suicidality developed, suggesting an acceptable risk:benefit ratio, with appropriate monitoring and multimodal treatment (Brent, 2004). It remains unclear whether the black box warning will do more harm than good, and it is indeed concerning that it appears to be associated with significant reductions in aggregate rates of diagnosis and treatment of pediatric depression (Libby et al., 2007).

Electroconvulsive Therapy

There is a relative dearth of empirical information about the efficacy and optimal use of electroconvulsive therapy (ECT) (Walter, Rey, & Mitchell, 1999), because of its controversial nature and infrequent use despite transient and minor side effects and mood disorder responsiveness (Rey & Walter, 1997; Walter & Rey, 1997). Potential adverse effects include impaired memory, problems with new learning, seizures, risks associated with anesthesia, headaches, nausea, confusion, and agitation (American Academy of Child and Adolescent Psychiatry, 2004).

Practice parameters (American Academy of Child and Adolescent Psychiatry, 2004) recommend that ECT be used for depressed adolescents when two or more pharmacological interventions have failed or when severity of symptoms precludes waiting for another intervention to work, because doing so may endanger the life of the adolescent. They underscore the necessity for incorporating only those ECT methods with the least number of adverse effects and greatest efficacy. Very little is written about ECT with children, and there are no practice parameters for its usage with this population.

Most research ECT with adolescents is retrospective and typically has small samples (American Academy of Child and Adolescent Psychiatry, 2004). Studies show a 60–100% response rate and no evidence of impaired cognitive or social functioning. ECT has comparable effectiveness for adolescents and adults (Bloch, Levcovitch, Bloch, Mendlovic, & Ratzoni, 2001).

Psychosocial Treatments

Evidence-Based Descriptions and Categorizations

Consistent with the recommendations from the American Psychological Association (2006) Presidential Task Force on Evidence-Based Practice in Psychology, interventions for depressed youth should be *evidence based*. This definition is broader than that of *empirically supported treatments* (ESTs), because it integrates the best available empirical evidence with clinical expertise in the context of the characteristics of the individual child/adolescent, the youth's culture, and the preferences of all concerned parties. Neither definition represents a higher standard, rather a different perspective on what should be counted as evidence.

Various guidelines have been used to evaluate the efficacy and effectiveness of interventions. For example, David-Ferdon and Kaslow (2008) categorized existing studies in accord with the guidelines proposed by the Task Force on the Promotion and Dissemination of Psychological Procedures (Chambless et al., 1998; Lonigan, Elbert, & Johnson, 1998) to determine whether interventions were well-established or probably efficacious, taking into account specific programs, modalities, and broad theoretical orientations.

The following sections describe psychosocial interventions separately for elementary school children and adolescents. Separate attention is paid to the evidence bases for specific programs, modalities, and broad theoretical orientations (David-Ferdon & Kaslow, 2008). See Table 28.1 for details of the studies.

Interventions for Elementary School Children

SPECIFIC PROGRAM CLASSIFICATION SCHEMA

There are no well-established specific programs for depressed children. However, self-control therapy (SCT) (Stark, Reynolds, & Kaslow, 1987; Stark, Rouse, & Livingston, 1991) and the Penn Prevention Program/Penn Resiliency Program/Penn Enhancement Program/ Penn Optimism Program (PPP/PRP/PEP/POP), which includes culturally relevant modifications (Cardemil, Reivich, Beevers, Seligman, & James, 2007; Cardemil, Reivich, & Seligman, 2002; Gillham, Hamilton, Freres, Patton, & Gallop, 2006; Gillham & Reivich, 1999; Gillham, Reivich, et al., 2006; Gillham, Reivich, Jaycox, & Seligman, 1995; Gillham et al., 2007; Jaycox, Reivich, Gillham, & Seligman, 1994; Pattison & Lynd-Stevenson, 2001; Roberts, Kane, Thomson, Bishop, & Hart, 2003; Yu & Seligman, 2002), are probably efficacious. See Table 28.1 for details of studies examining these specific programs.

SCT (Stark et al., 1987, 1991) is a school-based cognitive-behavioral group intervention program that teaches self-management skills. It includes training in self-control, social skills, assertiveness, relaxation and imagery, and cognitive restructuring. It also may involve monthly family meetings that encourage parents to aid their depressed youth in incorporating newly learned skills and to increase the number of positive family activities. PPP/PRP/ PEP/POP (Cardemil et al., 2002, 2007; Gillham, Hamilton, et al., 2006; Gillham & Reivich, 1999; Gillham, Reivich, et al., 2006; Gillham et al., 1995, 2007; Jaycox et al., 1994; Pattison & Lynd-Stevenson, 2001; Roberts et al., 2003; Yu & Seligman, 2002) is a CBT approach that targets depressive symptoms of at-risk 10- to 15- year-olds in schools and primary care settings. It is administered in a group format and includes two components: cognitive therapy and social problem solving. With regard to the cognitive component, children are taught to identify negative beliefs, to evaluate the evidence for these beliefs, to generate more realistic alternatives, and to develop adaptive attributions for successes and failures. In the social problem-solving component, youth learn goal setting, perspective taking, information gathering, generation of alternatives for action, decision making, self-instruction, and managing family conflict and other stressors. It has been modified for youth from different cultural backgrounds in the United States and internationally, as well as specifically for females.

Other specific psychosocial interventions (i.e., Coping with Depression, Primary and Secondary Control Enhancement Training Program, Stress-Busters, Bereavement Group Intervention, Wisconsin Early Intervention, ACT, ADAPT, ACTION, Taking Action), most of which have a cognitive-behavioral orientation, appear effective in reducing depressive symptoms relative to control conditions (Asarnow, Scott, & Mintz, 2002; Clarke, Lewinsohn, & Hops, 1990; De Cuyper, Timbremont, Braet, De Backer, & Wullaert, 2004; King & Kirschenbaum, 1990; Pfeffer, Jiang, Kakuma, Hwang, & Metsch, 2002; Stark et al., 2007; Stark, Hargrave, et al., 2006; Stark, Herren, & Fisher, in press; Stark, Sander, et al., 2006; Weisz, Thurber, Sweeney, Proffitt, & LeGagnoux, 1997). For the most part, these programs

TABLE 28.1. Review of Psychosocial Intervention Studies to Treat Child and Adolescent Depression

Intervention/study authors	Comparison group	Sample characteristics	Intervention/setting/modality	Main outcomes
SCT (Stark et al., 1987)	SCT vs. BPST vs. WLC	29 elementary school children (ages 9–12) w/elevated depressive symptoms	12 session SCT/school-based/group format	SCT and BPST > WLC in reducing anxiety and depressive symptoms; SCT had greater scores than BPST below depression cutoff at 8 weeks; SCT had greater scores on positive concept; BPST showed decreases in social withdrawal and internalizing symptoms, as rated by mothers.
SCT (Stark et al., 1991)	SCT vs. Traditional Counseling	Elementary/middle school children w/ elevated depressive symptoms	24–26 sessions SCT + monthly family meetings/family session	Both groups reduced depressive symptoms at postintervention and 7-month follow-up; SCT significantly reduced depressive symptoms and cognitions at postintervention.
PRP (Jaycox et al., 1994)	PRP vs. NTC	142 children (ages 10–13) w/depressive symptoms and presence of parental conflict	12 session PRP/school-based/group format	PRP significantly reduced depressive symptoms and improved classroom behavior; fewer self-reports of moderate/severe depressive symptoms; differences remained at 6- and 24-month follow-up; no differences in explanatory style and parent reports of internalizing and externalizing symptoms at post intervention, but emerged at 6-month follow-up
PRP (Gillham et al., 2007)	PRP vs. PEP vs. NTC	697 middle school children	12-session PRP delivered by school staff/school-based/group format	No intervention effects on averaged scores of depressive symptoms from each group.
PRP (Gillham, Hamilton, et al., 2006)	PRP vs. usual care	271 children (age 11–12) w/elevated depressive symptoms	12-session PRP/primary care center/group format	PRP showed more improvements in explanatory style for positive events at 24-month follow-up; more beneficial for girls than for boys in reducing depressive symptoms.
PRP-CA (Gillham, Reivich, et al., 2006)	PRP vs. NTC	44 middle school children	12-session PRP-CA + parent component/school-based/group format	PRP-CA reduced depressive and anxiety symptoms during follow-up periods.
PRP (Chaplin et al., 2006)	PRP (all girls) vs. PRP (coed) vs. NTC	208 middle school adolescents (ages 11–14)	12-session PRP/school-based/group format	Girls group reduced hopelessness and greater attendance than coed group; no difference in depressive symptoms between coed and girls' groups; coed group decreased depressive symptoms but did not differ by gender.

Study	Comparison	Sample	Format	Results
PRP (Cardemil et al., 2002, 2007)	PRP vs. NTC	168 minority (i.e., Latino and African American) middle school to students (5th to 8th grade; mean age, 11.2) at risk for depression based on low-income status	12-session PRP/school-based/group format	PRP had fewer depressive symptoms, negative automatic thoughts, and less hopelessness at postintervention, 6-month, and 24-month follow-up. PRP showed greater self-esteem at follow-up; PRP shown not effective for depressive symptoms in African American youth.
POP (Yu & Seligman, 2002)	POP vs. NTC	220 Chinese children (1st to 6th grade; mean age, 11.8) w/elevated depressive symptoms and family conflict	Culturally informed POP/school-based/group format	POP showed significant reductions in depressive symptoms and greater increases in explanatory style at postintervention, and 3- and 6-month follow-up.
PPP (Roberts et al., 2003)	PPP vs. usual care	189 Australian adolescents (7th grade; mean age, 11.9) w/ depressive symptoms	PPP/school-based/group format	Comparable reductions in depressive symptoms in both groups at postintervention; PPP reduced internalizing symptoms via parent report at postintervention; no group differences via self- or parent report at 6-month follow-up.
CWD-A (Lewinsohn et al., 1990)	CWD-A adolescent only; CWD-A + parent vs. WLC	69 Adolescents with MDD or minor or intermittent depression	15- to 16-session CWD-A/group format	Both CWD-A conditions showed greater reductions in depressive symptoms and were less likely to meet diagnostic criteria for depression; results maintained at 24-month follow-up.
CWD-A (Clarke et al., 1995)	CWD-A vs. usual care	150 adolescents w/ elevated depressive symptoms	15-session CWD-A/school based/group format	CWD-A showed greater improvements in depressive symptoms and global functioning at postintervention; reduction in depressive disorders at 12-month follow-up.
CWD-A (Clarke et al., 1999)	CWD-A vs. CWD-A + parent vs. WLC	123 adolescents w/MDD or DD	16 session CWD-A/group format	Both CWD-A conditions showed greater depression recovery rates and improvements in self-reported depressive symptoms.
CWD-A (Clarke et al., 2001)	CWD-A + HMO care vs. HMO usual care	94 adolescents (ages 13–18) of a parent w/MDD/DD	15 session CWD-A + HMO care/HMO clinic office/group format	CWD-A + HMO showed greater improvements in psychological functioning and self- and interviewer-reported depression; onset of depression lower for CWD-A + HMO at 12- and 18-month follow-up.

(continued)

TABLE 28.1. (continued)

Intervention/study authors	Comparison group	Sample characteristics	Intervention/setting/modality	Main outcomes
CWD-A (Rohde et al., 2004)	CWD-A + optional parent training vs. life skills/tutoring control group	93 nonincarcerated adolescents (ages 13–17) w/MDD and conduct disorder, referred from Department of Juvenile Justice	16-session CWD-A w/optional parent training/group format	CWD-A showed greater rates of depression recovery based on youth report; results not maintained at 6- and 12-month follow-up.
IPT-A (Mufson et al., 1999)	IPT-A vs. once a month clinical monitoring control group	48 adolescents (ages 12–18) w/MDD	12-session IPT-A + weekly phone contact/outpatient clinic/individual therapy	IPT-A showed greater improvements in self- and clinician-reported depressive symptoms, social functioning, and interpersonal problem solving; 75% of IPT-A met recovery criteria, and 88% were no longer depressed at postintervention.
IPT-A (Mufson et al., 2004)	IPT-A vs. individual support therapy control group	63 adolescents (mean age, 15.1) w/MDD	IPT-A delivered by school staff/school-based/individual therapy	Both groups reduced depressive symptoms; IPT-A showed more improvements in depression and social functioning; differences remained at 16 weeks via clinician report.
IPT (Rossello & Bernal, 1999)	IPT vs. CBT vs. WLC	71 Puerto Rican adolescents (ages 13–17; mean age, 14.7) w/MDD	12-session IPT/outpatient clinic/individual therapy	82% of IPT adolescents below cutoff for depressive symptoms vs. 59% of CBT; both groups better than control group in reducing depression and enhancing self-esteem.

Note. SCT, self-control therapy; BPST, behavioral problem-solving therapy, WLC, wait-list control, CBT, cognitive-behavioral therapy; CB, cognitive-behavioral; PEP, Penn Enhancement Program; NTC, no-treatment control; PRP, Penn Resiliency Program; PRP-CA, Penn Resiliency Program for Children and Adolescents; POP, Penn Optimism Program; CWD-A, Coping with Depression—Adolescent; MDD, major depressive disorder; DD, dysthymic disorder; HMO, health maintenance organization; IPT-A, interpersonal therapy for adolescents; IPT, interpersonal therapy.

are prevention-oriented for youth with elevated depressive symptoms and typically are administered in school settings. However, because little empirical attention has been paid to these protocols, or because the findings have yet to be published in peer-reviewed journals, these specific interventions are deemed experimental.

MODALITY CLASSIFICATION SCHEMA

"Modality" refers to whether the treatment is individual, group, parent only, parent–youth, or family based. There are two well-established intervention modalities for depressed children: CBT modalities of group therapy with children only (Gillham, Hamilton, et al., 2006; Gillham et al., 1995; Jaycox et al., 1994; Kahn, Kehle, Jenson, & Clark, 1990; Roberts et al., 2003; Stark et al., 1987; Weisz et al., 1997; Yu & Seligman, 2002) and child group therapy with a parent component (Asarnow et al., 2002; Gillham, Reivich, et al., 2006; Stark et al., 1991). Two additional CBT modalities can be classified as experimental: CBT parent–child modality (Nelson, Barnard, & Cain, 2003) and CBT individual video self-monitoring (Kahn et al., 1990). Furthermore, modalities associated with nondirected support/psychoeducational, behavior therapy, and various family theories (Asarnow et al., 2002; Fristad, Arnett, & Gavazzi, 1998; Fristad, Goldberg-Arnold, & Gavazzi, 2003; Goldberg-Arnold, Fristad, & Gavazzi, 1999) are considered experimental.

THEORETICAL ORIENTATION CLASSIFICATION SCHEMA

David-Ferdon and Kaslow (2008) concluded that CBT is a well-established theoretical approach for depressed children (Asarnow et al., 2002; Gillham, Hamilton, et al., 2006; Gillham, Reivich, et al., 2006; Gillham et al., 1995; Jaycox et al., 1994; Kahn et al., 1990; Nelson et al., 2003; Roberts et al., 2003; Stark et al., 1987, 1991; Weisz et al., 1997; Yu & Seligman, 2002). Behavior therapy is probably an efficacious theoretical approach (Kahn et al., 1990; King & Kirschenbaum, 1990; Stark et al., 1987). Although there is some empirical support for a nondirected support/psychoeducational theoretical approach relative to a control group (Pfeffer et al., 2002), limited research related to this theoretical model means that it is classified as an experimental approach.

Interventions for Adolescents

SPECIFIC PROGRAM CLASSIFICATION SCHEMA

No specific psychosocial intervention for depressed adolescents can be classified as well established (David-Ferdon & Kaslow, 2008). However, Coping with Depression—Adolescent (CWD-A) (Clarke et al., 1995, 2001, 2002; Clarke, Rohde, Lewinsohn, Hops, & Seeley, 1999; Kaufman, Rohde, Seeley, Clarke, & Stice, 2005; Lewinsohn, Clarke, Hops, & Andrews, 1990; Lewinsohn, Clarke, Rohde, Hops, & Seeley, 1996; Rohde, Clarke, Mace, Jorgensen, & Seeley, 2004) and interpersonal psychotherapy for adolescents (IPT-A) (Mufson et al., 2004; Mufson, Weissman, Moreau, & Garfinkel, 1999) are two specific programs that are probably efficacious (David-Ferdon & Kaslow, 2008).

CWD-A (Clarke et al., 1995, 1999, 2001, 2002; Kaufman et al., 2005; Lewinsohn et al., 1990, 1996; Rohde et al., 2004), shown to be effective in all but one trial, typically comprises 15–16 sessions of 45–120 minutes each. It includes relaxation training, cognitive restructuring, pleasant activity scheduling, communication, and conflict-reduction techniques.

Concurrent parent groups, in which parents are informed about the topics and skills focused on in the adolescent program, are incorporated into some of the CWD-A protocols. CWD-A has informed the development of protocols by other investigatory teams (Asarnow et al., 2005; Clarke et al., 2005; TADS Team, 2004), with mixed outcomes. IPT-A, the other probably efficacious intervention protocol, has been found to be more efficacious than control conditions in two RCTs in ameliorating symptoms of depression and enhancing interpersonal functioning (Mufson et al., 1999, 2004). IPT-A, a developmentally informed modification of an intervention initially developed for the treatment of adult depression, addresses interpersonal issues specific to adolescence, such as changes in the parent–adolescent relationship due to shifts in closeness and authority. IPT-A encourages teenagers to link their difficulties to one of five primary problem areas: grief, role disputes, role transitions, interpersonal deficits, and single-parent families. IPT-A helps youth develop adaptive strategies for communication, affect expression, and social support system development and utilization. The program conveys that effective coping strategies will assist youth in addressing the aforementioned problem areas. The IPT-A protocol includes 12 individual sessions and may incorporate weekly telephone contact between the therapist and adolescent (Mufson et al., 1999).

A number of other specific psychosocial interventions can be classified as experimental: attachment-based family therapy, Depression Treatment Programme, and Feeling Good, have been found to be efficacious in reducing depressive symptoms relative to control conditions (Ackerson, Scogin, McKendree-Smith, & Lyman, 1998; Diamond, Reis, Diamond, Siqueland, & Isaacs, 2002; Diamond, Siqueland, & Diamond, 2003; Wood, Harrington, & Moore, 1996). One protocol that technically meets criteria for an experimental treatment is a quality improvement intervention for adolescent depression in primary care clinics (Asarnow et al., 2005). However, given the methodologically sophisticated nature of the RCT describing this approach, it is a promising rather than established approach.

MODALITY CLASSIFICATION SCHEMA

In terms of CBT treatments, the modality of CBT group, adolescent only (Clarke et al., 1995, 1999; Lewinsohn et al., 1990, 1996; Reynolds & Coats, 1986) is well established; the modalities of individual (Melvin et al., 2006; Rossello & Bernal, 1999; Wood et al., 1996), individual plus parent/family component (Brent et al., 1997; TADS Team, 2004), and adolescent group plus parent component modality (Clarke et al., 1995, 1999, 2001; Lewinsohn et al., 1990, 1996; Rohde et al., 2004) are probably efficacious; and self-directed bibliotherapy (Ackerson et al., 1998) and enhanced primary care services (Asarnow et al., 2005) are experimental.

In terms of IPT, the modality of individual treatment is well-established (Mufson et al., 1999, 2004; Rossello & Bernal, 1999). Other treatment modalities are experimental: nondirected support provided through an adolescent-only group (Fine, Forth, Gilbert, & Haley, 1991), family systems-oriented approach offered with the parent–adolescent subsystem (Diamond et al., 2002), and family interventions (Sanford et al., 2006).

THEORETICAL ORIENTATION CLASSIFICATION SCHEMA

When considering broad theoretical orientation, CBT and IPT (Mufson et al., 1999, 2004; Rossello & Bernal, 1999) are well-established. The theoretical approaches of nondirected support (Fine et al., 1991), family systems theory (Diamond et al., 2002), and behavior therapy (Reynolds & Coats, 1986) are considered experimental.

MEDIATORS, MODERATORS, AND PREDICTORS OF TREATMENT OUTCOME

The term "mediators" refers to the question of what change processes underlie improvement (Kazdin & Nock, 2003). Treatment effects may be mediated by improvements in depressive symptoms and reductions in depressogenic thinking (Ackerson et al., 1998; Gillham et al., 1995; Kaufman et al., 2005; Vitiello, Rohde, et al., 2006; Yu & Seligman, 2002).

There is a burgeoning literature on moderators of treatment outcome (Curry et al., 2006; Weersing & Brent, 2006). The term "moderators" refers to those factors that interact with treatment in predicting outcome. Evidence supports the following variables as potential key moderating influences: gender, family income, severity of depression, severity of cognitive distortions, family conflict, maternal depression, and parent involvement in treatment (Brent et al., 1997; Clarke, DeBar, & Lewinsohn, 2003; Clarke et al., 1992, 1999; Michael & Crowley, 2002; Sander & McCarty, 2005; Weersing & Brent, 2003; Weisz et al., 2006). Data on gender as a moderator are inconclusive (Clarke et al., 1999; Jayson, Wood, Kroll, Fraser, & Harrington, 1998; Kolko, Brent, Baugher, Bridge, & Birmaher, 2000; Michael & Crowley, 2002).

A number of variables predict treatment outcome; the presence of these variables is associated with more positive or negative outcomes (Barbe, Bridge, Birmaher, Kolko, & Brent, 2004; Birmaher et al., 2000; Brent et al., 1997, 1998; Clarke et al., 1992, 2002; Curry et al., 2006; Jayson et al., 1998; Rohde, Clarke, Lewinsohn, Seeley, & Kaufman, 2001; Rohde, Seeley, Kaufman, Clarke, & Stice, 2006; Sander & McCarty, 2005; Weersing & Brent, 2003; Young, Mufson, & Davies, 2006). These include age, disease severity and symptom presentation, comorbidity, functional impairment, expectations for improvement, and levels of family conflict. Not all studies find the same patterns of predictor variables, however. There is some evidence about predictors of recurrence of depressive symptoms following treatment; recurrence is predicted by symptom severity and family difficulties at intervention conclusion (Brent, Birmaher, Kolko, Baugher, & Bridge, 2001).

PREVENTION PROGRAMS

Prevention programs are detailed by Muñoz, Le, Clarke, Barrera, and Torres, Chapter 23, this volume. Therefore, this chapter briefly highlights the literature on preventing depressive symptoms and disorders in youth (Barrett & Turner, 2004; Beardslee & Gladstone, 2001; Sutton, 2007). Meta-analyses demonstrate small but significant effect sizes in the short-term prevention of depression; however, the effects over time are less clear (Horowitz & Garber, 2006). There are larger effects when interventions are of relatively longer duration (Jane-Llopis, Hosman, Jenkins, & Anderson, 2003).

Prevention programs have targeted children from first grade through high school. For the most part, these efforts have been psychoeducational and cognitive-behavioral in nature (Sutton, 2007), and have been conducted in school settings. Some school-based programs have focused on at-risk youth not defined by their depressive symptom status (Cutuli, Chaplin, Gillham, Reivich, & Seligman, 2006; Kellam, Rebok, Mayer, Ialongo, & Kalodner, 1994; Thompson, Eggert, & Herting, 2000) and have provided academic enhancement training, personal growth classes that integrate social support and life skills training, and so forth. The PRP detailed earlier has been used preventively. Other efforts targeting at-risk youth have been undertaken in clinical settings, often with children of depressed parents

(Beardslee, Gladstone, Wright, & Cooper, 2003; Beardslee et al., 1993, 1997; Beardslee, Wright, Rothberg, Salt, & Versage, 1996; Cicchetti, Rogosch, & Toth, 2000; Clarke et al., 1995, 2001). These programs have offered cognitive psychoeducation provided by clinicians or via a lecture, cognitive-behavioral techniques and skills training, parent–child attachment based work, and massage therapy.

Some prevention-oriented studies incorporate universal interventions delivered to all members of a population, whereas others use targeted or selective interventions delivered to a subgroup of high-risk youth (e.g., individuals with early signs of a mood disorder; children of depressed parents), as noted earlier. Some of the best-studied universal programs include Problem Solving for Life (PSFL), a school-based problem-solving and cognitive restructuring program (Sheffield et al., 2006; Spence, Sheffield, & Donovan, 2003, 2005); Resourceful Adolescent Program (RAP), a CBT protocol that incorporates cognitive restructuring, problem solving, stress management, and accessing social support that can be conducted with or without family involvement (Merry, McDowell, Wild, Bir, & Cunliffe, 2004; Shochet et al., 2001; Shochet & Ham, 2004); Training the Ease of Handling Social Aspects in Everyday Life (LISA), a CBT program that targets cognitive and social aspects of depression (Possel, Baldus, Horn, Groen, & Hautzinger, 2005; Possel, Horn, Groen, & Hautzinger, 2004); and the FRIENDS program that targets symptoms of anxiety and depression (Barrett, Farrell, Ollendick, & Dadds, 2006; Barrett & Turner, 2001; Lock & Barrett, 2003; Lowry-Webster, Barrett, & Dadds, 2001; Lowry-Webster, Barrett, & Lock, 2003). A recent meta-analysis revealed that targeted or selective programs are more effective than universal programs at postintervention and follow-up (Horowitz & Garber, 2006).

In general, prevention programs for youth depression have a cognitive-behavioral orientation, with an emphasis on training in coping, social problem solving, social skills, and communication skills. Parenting is a focus in some of programs. A comprehensive prevention program for depressed youth optimally should incorporate multiple components that target reducing risk factors and enhancing protective factors (Garber, 2006). When such programs are designed for offspring of depressed parents, they should attend to the characteristics of the child and other family members, comorbid conditions, and the family and social environment (Avenevoli & Merikangas, 2006).

GUIDELINES FOR MANAGING DEPRESSION

A series of guidelines has been offered for managing depression in young people, and some examples of major guidelines are described below.

National Institute for Health and Clinical Excellence

The National Institute for Health and Clinical Excellence (NICE) in the United Kingdom (*www.nice.org.uk*) published guidelines for identifying and managing depression in young people in primary, community, and secondary care settings. These guidelines highlight conducting patient-centered care; taking into account child and family needs and preferences; actively engaging the child and family in decision making; communicating effectively, which includes conveying evidence-based information in a culturally appropriate fashion; performing comprehensive assessments; coordinating care; addressing comorbid diagnoses and developmental, social, and educational problems; and ascertaining the need for biopsychosocial interventions for other family members. A comprehensive, evidence-based approach that differs depending on the severity of the child's depression is delineated.

American Academy of Child and Adolescent Psychiatry Treatment Parameters

The American Academy of Child and Adolescent Psychiatry (AACAP, 1998) notes that a diagnosis of a depressive disorder in a child or adolescent should only be made after completion of a culturally informed, comprehensive psychiatric evaluation that involves multiple informants and a multimethod assessment approach. During the intervention phase, treatment should be provided in the least restrictive environment. A treatment plan should identify biological and environmental factors, frequency of treatment sessions, and roles of the treating clinician(s). Efforts to promote successful therapy should be guided by creation of a therapeutic alliance among the clinician, youth, and family. This effort can be enhanced by providing information about the disorder to form a collaborative partnership with all involved, and recognizing that the youth's depression impacts all family members. Appropriate developmental considerations should be discussed with the youth, family, and other informants. During acute treatment, psychotherapy (CBT, IPT, family therapy) may be effective for mild to moderate symptoms of depression. Furthermore, the guidelines recommend SSRIs for depressed adolescents. Best practices suggest integrating medication for the youth with psychosocial intervention with the youth, family members, and other supports. To decrease the likelihood of relapse or recurrence, youth should continue to receive psychotherapy at least monthly and medication (if prescribed and shown effective) for at least 6–12 months. Subsequent to this period, clinical judgment should be used with regard to the necessity of maintenance therapy. It is recommended that adolescents who have experienced two to three episodes of MDD receive maintenance treatment at least 1–3 years.

Texas Children's Medication Algorithm Project

Ten principles undergird the most current Texas Children's Medication Algorithm Project (Hughes et al., 2007). Stage 0 is diagnostic assessment and monitoring. Stage 1 is monotherapy with SSRIs. Stage 2 pertains to switching to an alternative SSRI but continuing with a monotherapy approach. Stage 3 includes switching from an SSRI to alternative antidepressant monotherapy.

FUTURE DIRECTIONS

Based on the extant empirical data and practice guidelines (American Academy of Child and Adolescent Psychiatry, 2004; Hughes et al., 2007; Mann et al., 2006), the following recommendations may be offered for the assessment and treatment of depressed youth.

1. A biopsychosocial framework is valuable for conceptualizing depression and its treatment (Kaslow et al., 2007; Reinecke & Simons, 2005) and recent interventions with depressed youth have built on this model (e.g., TADS). From a biological perspective, depression may be conceptualized with regard to brain morphology, neurochemical abnormalities, and genetic association. A thorough understanding of youth depression must take into account individual psychological factors (e.g., intelligence, temperament, personality, cognitive

processes, affective experience and regulation, interpretations of experience, motivation, social skills, self-esteem, personal identity, attachment, perceived stress, perceived social support). The social domain refers to physical environment, external stressors, family environment, peer relationships, social support–isolation, role models, social expectations, value system, sociocultural factors (e.g., race, ethnicity, socioeconomic status, sexual orientation, religion, and culture), school/work history, medical–legal/insurance issues, and treatment experience.

2. Interventions should be developmentally informed given etiological differences in depression in children versus adolescents with regards to genes and environment (Rice, Harold, & Thapar, 2002; Silberg, Rutter, & Eaves, 2001); differential risk factors for the onset of juvenile versus adult depression (Jaffee et al., 2002; Kaufman, Martin, King, & Charney, 2001; Scourfield et al., 2003); variations across the lifespan in the manifestation of depression dependent on level of social, cognitive, emotional, and physiological development (Weiss & Garber, 2002); and differential response to pharmacological (Donnelly et al., 2006; Wagner et al., 2006) and psychosocial (Michael & Crowley, 2002) treatments based on age. Fortunately, attention increasingly has been paid to developmental adaptations of treatments (Weersing & Brent, 2006).

3. Attention should be paid to gender in the future design and evaluation of interventions, given that gender differences in rates of depression vary by age (Garber, Keiley, & Martin, 2002; Hankin et al., 1998; Hoffmann, Baldwin, & Cerbone, 2003; Nolen-Hoeksema, 2001, 2002), a finding that is true cross-culturally (Galambos, Leadbeater, & Barker, 2004; Wade, Cairney, & Pevalin, 2002); and in different symptom presentation of depression by gender (Bennett, Ambrosini, Kudes, Metz, & Rabinovich, 2005; Richardson et al., 2003; Waller et al., 2006). Biological, psychological, and social theories have been proposed to explain the gender gap and pertain to differences in the timing of the onset of puberty, hormonal changes, rates of negative childhood experiences and maltreatment, body image perceptions, health status, cognitive vulnerability, coping styles (e.g., rumination), stress levels and responses, interpersonal stress levels and orientations, socialization experiences and sociocultural roles (Cyranowski, Frank, Young, & Shear, 2000; Hankin & Abramson, 2001, 2002; Marcotte, Fortin, Potvin, & Papillon, 2002; Nolen-Hoeksema, 2001, 2002; Piccinelli & Wilkinson, 2000; Shih, Eberhart, Hammen, & Brennan, 2006; Williams, Colder, Richards, & Scalzo, 2002). Some intervention programs find that females respond more positively than males (Gillham, Hamilton, et al., 2006; Petersen, Leffert, Graham, Alwin, & Ding, 1997), whereas other programs find the opposite (Clarke, Hawkins, Murphy, & Sheeber, 1993; Ialongo et al., 1999; Kellam et al., 1994). Girls may benefit more from interpersonally oriented treatments, and boys may respond better to CBT (Garber, 2006). Recently, one gender-sensitive intervention, the ACTION treatment program designed for depressed girls, can be offered alone or in combination with parent training, and promising results have been obtained (Stark, Hargrave, et al., 2006, 2007; Stark, Herren, et al., in press; Stark, Sander, et al., 2006). The PRP has been studied in various formats for early adolescent females (Chaplin et al., 2006), and findings indicate that depressed girls benefit more from girls-only groups than from coed groups, suggesting the potential value of same-sex groups.

4. Interventions need to take into account sociocultural variables and to be developed and implemented in a culturally competent fashion. Although depression is evident in youth in all cultures, there may be differential prevalence rates across ethnic groups (Chen, Roberts, & Aday, 1998; Cole, Martin, Peeke, Henderson, & Harwell, 1998; Kistner, David, & White, 2003; Leech, Larkby, Day, & Day, 2006; Roberts, Roberts, & Chen, 1997; Sen,

2004; Siegel, Aneshensel, Taub, Cantwell, & Driscoll, 2001; Twenge & Nolen-Hoeksema, 2002; Wight, Aneshensel, Botticello, & Sepulveda, 2005), a finding influenced by other risk factors (e.g., family structure, household income) (Wight et al., 2005) and social class status (Doi, Roberts, Takeuchi, & Suzuki, 2001). Rates of depression appear linked to cultural factors, barriers to detection and treatment, rates of service utilization, and differential cultural norms related to displays of emotion and ways to cope with distress (Chen et al., 1998; Das, Olfson, McCurtis, & Weissman, 2006; Gee, 2004; McCarty et al., 1999; Sen, 2004; Wu et al., 2001). Also, differences in the presentation of depressive symptoms need to be accounted for in assessments and in ascertaining treatment outcome (Das et al., 2006). Furthermore, there is evidence for the value of culture-specific interventions for depressed youth and their families (Breland-Noble, Bell, & Nicolas, 2006; Griffith, Zucker, Bliss, Foster, & Kaslow, 2001; McClure, Connell, Zucker, Griffith, & Kaslow, 2005), and the likelihood that such approaches facilitate treatment engagement (Breland-Noble et al., 2006). Interventions may be more effective for youth from some ethnic groups than for those from others (Cardemil et al., 2002, 2007), and interventions may be effective in some, but not all, cultures (Pattison & Lynd-Stevenson, 2001; Roberts et al., 2003; Yu & Seligman, 2002). Furthermore, evidence-based intervention protocols for depressed youth may be culturally transportable (Rossello & Bernal, 1999).

5. Future therapies that are strength-based and enhance protective and resilience factors are likely to be effective and to have good buy-in from all parties (Goldstein & Brooks, 2005; Luthar, Cicchetti, & Becker, 2000). Youth who are resilient when encountering adversity, and who do not develop depression, exhibit many of the following characteristics: easygoing temperament, self-confidence, appropriate self-reliance, average intellectual functioning, and secure intrafamilial and extrafamilial attachments (Cicchetti & Rogosch, 1997; Denny, Clark, Fleming, & Wall, 2004; Graham & Easterbrooks, 2000). In addition, average level of intellectual functioning, easygoing temperament, high self-esteem and self-confidence, age-appropriate self-reliance, adaptive problem-solving and coping strategies, secure attachments to parents and peers, family support and cohesion, maternal warmth, effective communication among family members, strong sibling bonds, high levels of social support, involvement in positive social and extracurricular activities, school connectedness, low economic risk, and high levels of religiosity are associated with lower levels of depression (Dallaire et al., 2006; Denny et al., 2004; Dumont & Provost, 1999; Galambos et al., 2004; Miller & Gur, 2002; Muris, Meesters, van Melick, & Zwambag, 2001; Richmond, Stocker, & Rienks, 2005; Samaan, 2000; Shochet, Dadds, Dadds, Ham, & Montague, 2006). High self-understanding, positive self-esteem, capacity for age-appropriate autonomy, parent–child bond, family support and warmth, appropriate levels of parental monitoring, low parental psychological control and overinvolvement, social support quality and availability, and ability to form meaningful intimate relationships serve as protective factors against depression in at-risk youth (Beardslee, Versage, & Gladstone, 1998; Brennan, Le Brocque, & Hammen, 2003; Cicchetti & Rogosch, 1997; Kaufman et al., 2004, 2006; Klein & Forehand, 2000; Leech et al., 2006; Sugawara et al., 2002). The more protective factors in the child's life, the less likely the child is to develop depression, and this is true irrespective of the presence of risk factors (Resnick et al., 1997). Interventions that strengthen protective factors are likely to be useful and associated with high levels of satisfaction.

6. Screening in schools and physicians' offices can help to identify depressed youth and youth at risk for depression. Screening is effective for reducing disease burden (Cuijpers, van Straten, Smits, & Smit, 2006). Quality improvement programs in schools and primary care settings can enhance access to evidence-based intervention (Asarnow et al., 2005).

7. Prior to initiating treatment, a thorough diagnostic evaluation must be conducted, with attention to co-occurring conditions, depression in other family members, and family conflict. This evaluation, as well as the later evaluation of intervention outcomes, should incorporate developmentally appropriate measurement tools, be attuned to developmental considerations, and take into account feedback from school personnel.

8. Recommendations for interventions with regard to modality and theoretical orientation should be guided by assessment findings, research data, and expert clinical consensus. Information on both pharmacological and nonpharmacological intervention options should be provided to depressed youth and their caregivers.

9. Treatment decisions should be made collaboratively, with the assent/consent of youth and their caregivers, and should take into account family preferences, clinician judgment, and the aforementioned recommendations and information regarding treatment alternatives.

10. Treatments should target comorbid conditions, and if there are no evidence-based interventions for specific combinations of conditions, multiple evidence-based approaches may be needed either concurrently or sequentially. Available interventions for comorbid conditions (Rohde et al., 2004; Wignall, 2006) and prevention protocols for comorbid sets of symptoms (Barrett et al., 2006; Barrett & Turner, 2001; Lock & Barrett, 2003; Lowry-Webster et al., 2001, 2003) or related disorders (Cutuli et al., 2006) could serve as the basis for such decision making.

11. Interventions must be conducted by well-trained personnel, and an emphasis should be placed on treatment engagement and building a trusting therapeutic alliance.

12. Interventions, regardless of the nature of the program, modality, or theoretical approach, should target reduction of risk factors and enhancement of protective factors (Sims, Nottelmann, Koretz, & Pearson, 2006).

13. For elementary school children, some form of CBT should be considered separately or in conjunction with antidepressant medications. This treatment should include some, or all, of the following components: psychoeducation, affective education and mood monitoring, behavioral activation, cognitive restructuring, problem solving (including social problem solving), and coping skills training. It should also involve at minimum a parent education and training program. Ideally, concurrent family intervention should be provided.

14. For depressed adolescents, both CBT, as described earlier, and IPT may be useful. Again, some family involvement may be advantageous. These psychosocial interventions are likely to be most beneficial when combined with pharmacotherapy (TADS, 2003, 2004, 2005).

15. Based on the available evidence, prior to initiating an antidepressant trial, youth and their caregivers must be informed about the risk:benefit ratio of these medications and receive education about the need for close monitoring.

16. Depressed youth treated with antidepressants need close monitoring for worsening of their depressive symptoms, emergence of suicidality, manic switching, and other indicators of psychological distress. These interventions must be accompanied by psychoeducation for depressed youth and their caregivers. Given that medications are effective, it is important to convey to youth and their families that the risk of doing nothing is likely to be greater than the risks associated with taking the medications (Brent, 2004). Until more efficacy data become available from RCTs, fluoxetine (Prozac) should be the first antidepressant used.

17. For youth with treatment-resistant depression, combined and alternative treatments should be considered, and second opinions and expert consultation should be obtained.

18. ECT may be indicated for severe and persistent depression, with or without psychotic features, in which symptoms are significantly disabling and life-threatening, and when there has been a lack of adequate response to prior psychopharmacological and/or psychosocial interventions. A decision to use ECT must take into account ethical considerations (Cohen, Flament, Taieb, Thompson, & Basquin, 2000).

19. Most depressed youth require some form of continuation therapy, and many may need maintenance treatment (Park & Goodyer, 2000).

20. Prevention efforts may be most effective if they combine attention to cognitive-behavioral and interpersonal skills, and include booster sessions.

The following are suggestions for research studies. More efficacy, effectiveness, and hybrid efficacy–effectiveness trials are needed. These trials should focus on interventions guided by a broad array of theoretical perspectives and include the full gamut of intervention modalities. Treatment trials should be more inclusive with regard to comorbid conditions and the presence of suicidal behavior (Mann et al., 2006), and must be focused more on youth with diagnosable depressive disorders (Weersing & Brent, 2006). It is important to gain a more comprehensive understanding of the mechanisms, mediators, and moderators that influence treatment outcome, and doing so will allow for greater matching between depressed youth and various intervention alternatives (Zalsman, Brent, & Weersing, 2006). Given that there are high rates of incomplete recovery and sustained impairment even with intervention (Brent et al., 2001), and that many of the interventions are not particularly effective with severely depressed youth, research needs to focus on sequences and combinations of treatments that may yield more complete improvements (Zalsman et al., 2006) or be helpful to those most in need (Weersing & Brent, 2006). More attention needs to be given to the length of interventions and the value of booster sessions (Sutton, 2007). Data, whether or not they support a given intervention, should be disseminated to the public, so that a more honest assessment can be made about the efficacy and safety of various interventions (Mann et al., 2006). Only recently have studies begun to examine the relative cost-effectiveness of various interventions and prevention programs for depressed youth (Haby, Tonge, Littlefield, Carter, & Vos, 2004; Lynch et al., 2005; Sutton, 2007), and there is a great need for more empirical attention to cost-effectiveness in terms of types of intervention and providers.

REFERENCES

Ackerson, J., Scogin, F., McKendree-Smith, N., & Lyman, R. D. (1998). Cognitive bibliotherapy for mild and moderate adolescent depressive symptomatology. *Journal of Consulting and Clinical Psychology, 66*, 685–690.

American Academy of Child and Adolescent Psychiatry. (1998). Summary of the practice parameters for the assessment and treatment of children and adolescents with depressive disorders. *Journal of the American Academy of Child and Adolescent Psychiatry, 37*, 1234–1239.

American Academy of Child and Adolescent Psychiatry. (2004). Practice parameter for use of electroconvulsive therapy with adolescents. *Journal of the American Academy of Child and Adolescent Psychiatry, 43*, 1521–1539.

American Psychological Association. (2006). Evidence-based practice in psychology: APA Presidential Task Force on Evidence-Based Practice in Psychology. *American Psychologist, 61*, 271–285.

Asarnow, J. R., Jaycox, L. H., Duan, N., LaBorde, A. P., Rea, M. M., Murray, P., et al. (2005). Effectiveness of a quality improvement intervention for adolescent depression in primary care clinics: A randomized controlled trial. *Journal of the American Medical Association, 293*, 311–319.

Asarnow, J. R., Scott, C. V., & Mintz, J. (2002). A combined cognitive-behavioral family education intervention for depression in children: A treatment development study. *Cognitive Therapy and Research, 26,* 221–229.

Avenevoli, S., & Merikangas, K. R. (2006). Implications of high-risk family studies for prevention of depression. *American Journal of Preventive Medicine, 31,* S126–S135.

Barbe, R. P., Bridge, J., Birmaher, B., Kolko, D., & Brent, D. A. (2004). Suicidality and its relationship to treatment outcome in depressed adolescents. *Suicide and Life-Threatening Behavior, 34,* 44–55.

Barrett, P. M., Farrell, L. J., Ollendick, T. H., & Dadds, M. R. (2006). Long-term outcomes of an Australian universal prevention trial of anxiety and depression symptoms in children and youth: An evaluation of the FRIENDS program. *Journal of Clinical Child and Adolescent Psychology, 35,* 403–411.

Barrett, P. M., & Turner, C. (2001). Prevention of anxiety symptoms in primary school children: Preliminary results from a universal school-based trial. *British Journal of Clinical Psychology, 40,* 399–410.

Barrett, P. M., & Turner, C. M. (2004). Prevention of childhood anxiety and depression. In P. M. Barrett & T. H. Ollendick (Eds.), *Handbook of interventions that work with children and adolescents: Prevention and treatment* (pp. 429–474). New York: Wiley.

Beardslee, W. R., & Gladstone, T. R. (2001). Prevention of childhood depression: Recent findings and future prospects. *Biological Psychiatry, 49,* 1101–1110.

Beardslee, W. R., Gladstone, T. R. G., Wright, E. J., & Cooper, A. B. (2003). A family-based approach to the prevention of depressive symptoms in children at risk: Evidence of parental and child change. *Pediatrics, 112,* 119–131.

Beardslee, W. R., Salt, P., Porterfield, K., Rothberg, P., Van de Velde, P., Swatling, S., et al. (1993). Comparison of preventive interventions for families with parental affective disorder. *Journal of the American Academy of Child and Adolescent Psychiatry, 32,* 254–263.

Beardslee, W. R., Salt, P., Versage, E. M., Gladstone, T. R. G., Wright, E. J., & Rothberg, P. C. (1997). Sustained change in parents receiving preventive interventions for families with depression. *American Journal of Psychiatry, 154,* 510–515.

Beardslee, W. R., Versage, E. M., & Gladstone, T. R. G. (1998). Children of affectively ill parents: A review of the past 10 years. *Journal of the American Academy of Child and Adolescent Psychiatry, 37,* 1134–1141.

Beardslee, W. R., Wright, E., Rothberg, P. C., Salt, P., & Versage, E. (1996). Response of families to two preventive intervention strategies: Long-term differences in behavior and attitude change. *Journal of the American Academy of Child and Adolescent Psychiatry, 35,* 774–782.

Bennett, D. S., Ambrosini, P. J., Kudes, D., Metz, C., & Rabinovich, H. (2005). Gender differences in adolescent depression: Do symptoms differ for boys and girls? *Journal of Affective Disorders, 89,* 35–44.

Berard, R., Fong, R., Carpenter, D. J., Thomason, C., & Wilkinson, C. (2006). An international, multicenter, placebo-controlled trial of paroxetine in adolescents with major depressive disorder. *Journal of Child and Adolescent Psychopharmacology, 16,* 59–75.

Birmaher, B., Brent, D. A., Kolko, D., Baugher, M., Bridge, J., Holder, D., et al. (2000). Clinical outcome after short-term psychotherapy for adolescents with major depressive disorder. *Archives of General Psychiatry, 57,* 29–36.

Bloch, Y., Levcovitch, Y., Bloch, A. M., Mendlovic, S., & Ratzoni, G. (2001). Electroconvulsive therapy in adolescents: Similarities to and differences from adults. *Journal of the American Academy of Child and Adolescent Psychiatry, 40,* 1332–1336.

Breland-Noble, A. M., Bell, C. C., & Nicolas, G. (2006). Family first: The development of an evidence-based family intervention for increasing participation in psychiatric clinical care and research in depressed African American adolescents. *Family Process, 45,* 153–169.

Brennan, P. A., Le Brocque, R., & Hammen, C. L. (2003). Maternal depression, parent–child relationships, and resilient outcomes in adolescence. *Journal of the American Academy of Child and Adolescent Psychiatry, 42,* 1469–1477.

Brent, D. A. (2004). Antidepressants and pediatric depression: The risk of doing nothing. *New England Journal of Medicine, 351,* 1598–1601.

Brent, D. A., Birmaher, B., Kolko, D., Baugher, M., & Bridge, J. (2001). Subsyndromal depression in adolescents after a brief psychotherapy trial: Course and outcome. *Journal of Affective Disorders, 63,* 51–58.

Brent, D. A., Holder, D., Kolko, D., Birmaher, B., Baugher, M., Roth, C., et al. (1997). A clinical psychotherapy trial for adolescent depression comparing cognitive, family, and supportive therapy. *Archives of General Psychiatry, 54,* 877–885.

Brent, D. A., Kolko, D. J., Birmaher, B., Baugher, M., Bridge, J., Roth, C., et al. (1998). Predictors of treatment efficacy in a clinical trial of three psychosocial treatments for adolescent depression. *Journal of the American Academy of Child and Adolescent Psychiatry, 37,* 906–914.

Brown, R. T., & Sammons, M. T. (2002). Pediatric psychopharmacology: A review of new developments and recent research. *Professional Psychology: Research and Practice, 33,* 135–147.

Cardemil, E. V., Reivich, K. J., Beevers, C. G., Seligman, M. E. P., & James, J. (2007). The prevention of depressive symptoms in low-income, minority children: Two-year follow-up. *Behaviour Research and Therapy, 45,* 313–327.

Cardemil, E. V., Reivich, K. J., & Seligman, M. E. P. (2002). The prevention of depressive symptoms in low-income minority middle school students. *Prevention and Treatment, 5.*

Chambless, D. L., Baker, M. J., Baucom, D. H., Beutler, L. E., Calhoun, K. S., Crits-Christoph, P., et al. (1998). Update on empirically validated therapies, II. *Clinical Psychologist, 51,* 3–16.

Chaplin, T. M., Gillham, J. E., Reivich, K., Elkon, A. G. L., Samuels, B., Freres, D. R., et al. (2006). Depression prevention for early adolescent girls: A pilot study of all girls versus co-ed groups. *Journal of Early Adolescence, 26,* 110–126.

Chen, I. G., Roberts, R. E., & Aday, L. A. (1998). Ethnicity and adolescent depression: The case of Chinese Americans. *Journal of Nervous and Mental Disease, 186,* 623–630.

Cheung, A. H., Emslie, G. J., & Mayes, T. L. (2005). Review of the efficacy and safety of antidepressants in youth depression. *Journal of Child Psychology and Psychiatry, 46,* 735–754.

Cheung, A. H., Emslie, G. J., & Mayes, T. L. (2006). The use of antidepressants to treat depression in children and adolescents. *Canadian Medical Association Journal, 174,* 193–200.

Chorpita, B. F. (2002). The tripartite model and dimensions of anxiety and depression: An examination of structure in a large school sample. *Journal of Abnormal Child Psychology, 30,* 177–190.

Cicchetti, D., & Rogosch, F. A. (1997). The role of self-organization in the promotion of resilience in maltreated children. *Development and Psychopathology, 9,* 799–817.

Cicchetti, D., Rogosch, F. A., & Toth, S. L. (2000). The efficacy of toddler–parent psychotherapy for fostering cognitive development in offspring of depressed mothers. *Journal of Abnormal Child Psychology, 28,* 135–148.

Clarke, G. N., DeBar, L., Lynch, F., Powell, J., Gale, J., O'Connor, E., et al. (2005). A randomized effectiveness trial of brief cognitive-behavioral therapy for depressed adolescents receiving antidepressant medication. *Journal of the American Academy of Child and Adolescent Psychiatry, 44,* 888–898.

Clarke, G. N., DeBar, L. L., & Lewinsohn, P. M. (2003). Cognitive-behavioral group treatment for adolescent depression. In A. E. Kazdin & J. R. Weisz (Eds.), *Evidence-based psychotherapies for children and adolescents* (pp. 120–147). New York: Guilford Press.

Clarke, G. N., Hawkins, W., Murphy, M., & Sheeber, L. (1993). School-based primary prevention of depressive symptomatology in adolescents: Findings from two studies. *Journal of Adolescent Research, 8,* 183–204.

Clarke, G. N., Hawkins, W., Murphy, M., Sheeber, L., Lewinsohn, P. M., & Seeley, J. (1995). Targeted prevention of unipolar depressive disorder in an at risk sample of high school adolescents: A randomized trial of a group cognitive intervention. *American Academy of Child and Adolescent Psychiatry, 34,* 312–321.

Clarke, G. N., Hops, H., Lewinsohn, P. M., Andrews, J., Seeley, J. R., & Williams, J. (1992). Cognitive-behavioral group treatment of adolescent depression: Prediction of outcome. *Behavior Therapy, 23,* 341–352.

Clarke, G. N., Hornbrook, M., Lynch, F., Polen, M., Gale, J., Beardslee, W. R., et al. (2001). A randomized trial of a group cognitive intervention for preventing depression in adolescent offspring of depressed parents. *Archives of General Psychiatry, 58,* 1127–1134.

Clarke, G. N., Hornbrook, M., Lynch, F., Polen, M., Gale, J., O'Connor, E., et al. (2002). Group cognitive-behavioral treatment for depressed adolescent offspring of depressed parents in a health maintenance organization. *Journal of the American Academy of Child and Adolescent Psychiatry, 41,* 305–313.

Clarke, G. N., Lewinsohn, P. M., & Hops, H. (1990). *Adolescent Coping with Depression Course.* Eugene, OR: Castalia.

Clarke, G. N., Rohde, P., Lewinsohn, P. M., Hops, H., & Seeley, J. (1999). Cognitive-behavioral treatment of adolescent depression: Efficacy of acute group treatment and booster sessions. *Journal of the American Academy of Child and Adolescent Psychiatry, 38,* 272–279.

Cohen, D., Flament, M.-F., Taieb, O., Thompson, C., & Basquin, M. (2000). Electroconvulsive therapy in adolescence. *European Child and Adolescent Psychiatry, 9,* 1–6.

Cole, D. A., Martin, J. M., Peeke, L., Henderson, A., & Harwell, J. (1998). Validation of depression and anxiety measures in Euro-American and African American youths: Multitrait-multimethod analyses. *Psychological Assessment, 10,* 261–276.

Compton, S. N., March, J. S., Brent, D. A., Albano, A. M., Weersing, V. R., & Curry, J. F. (2004). Cognitive-behavioral psychotherapy for anxiety and depressive disorders in children and adolescents: An evidence-based medicine review. *Journal of the American Academy of Child and Adolescent Psychiatry, 43,* 930–959.

Cornelius, J. R., Bukstein, O. G., Salloum, I. M., Lynch, K., Pollock, N. K., Gershon, S., et al. (2001). Fluoxetine in adolescents with major depression and an alcohol use disorder. *Addictive Behaviors, 26,* 735–739.

Coyle, J. T., Pine, D. S., Charney, D. S., Lewis, L., Nemeroff, C. B., Carlson, G. A., et al. (2003). Depression and Bipolar Support Alliance Consensus Statement on the Unmet Needs in Diagnosis and Treatment of Mood Disorders in Children and Adolescents. *Journal of the American Academy of Child and Adolescent Psychiatry, 42,* 1494–1503.

Cuijpers, P., van Straten, A., Smits, N., & Smit, F. (2006). Screening and early psychological intervention for depression in schools and meta-analysis. *European Child and Adolescent Psychiatry, 15,* 300–307.

Curry, J., Rohde, P., Simons, A., Silva, S., Vitiello, B., Kratochvil, C. J., et al. (2006). Predictors and moderators of acute outcome in the Treatment for Adolescents with Depression Study (TADS). *Journal of the American Academy of Child and Adolescent Psychiatry, 45,* 1427–1439.

Curry, J. F. (2001). Specific psychotherapies for childhood and adolescent depression. *Biological Psychiatry, 49,* 1091–1100.

Cutuli, J. J., Chaplin, T. M., Gillham, J. E., Reivich, K., & Seligman, M. E. P. (2006). Preventing co-occurring depression symptoms in adolescents with conduct problems: The Penn Resiliency Program. *Annals of the New York Academy of Science, 1094,* 282–286.

Cyranowski, J. M., Frank, E., Young, E., & Shear, K. (2000). Adolescent onset of the gender difference in lifetime rates of major depression: A theoretical model. *Archives of General Psychiatry, 57,* 21–27.

Dallaire, D. H., Pineda, A. Q., Cole, D. A., Ciesla, J. A., Jacquez, F. M., LaGrange, B., et al. (2006). Relation of positive and negative parenting to children's depressive symptoms. *Journal of Clinical Child and Adolescent Psychology, 35,* 313–322.

Das, A. K., Olfson, M., McCurtis, H. L., & Weissman, M. M. (2006). Depression in African Americans: Breaking barriers to detection and treatment. *Journal of Family Practice, 55,* 30–39.

David-Ferdon, C., & Kaslow, N. J. (2008). Evidence-based psychosocial interventions for child and adolescent depression. *Journal of Clinical Child and Adolescent Psychology, 37,* 62–104.

Daviss, W. B., Bentivoglio, P., Racusin, R., Brown, K. M., Bostic, J. Q., & Wiley, L. (2001). Bupropion sustained release in adolescents with comorbid attention-deficit/hyperactivity disorder and depression. *Journal of the American Academy of Child and Adolescent Psychiatry, 40,* 307–314.

De Cuyper, S., Timbremont, B., Braet, C., De Backer, V., & Wullaert, T. (2004). Treating depressive symptoms in school children: A pilot study. *European Child and Adolescent Psychiatry, 13,* 105–114.

DeBar, L., Clarke, G. N., O'Connor, E., & Nichols, G. A. (2001). Treated prevalence, incidence, and pharmacotherapy of child and adolescent mood disorders in an HMO. *Mental Health Services Research, 3,* 73–89.

Delate, T., Gelenberg, A. J., Simmons, V. A., & Motheral, B. R. (2004). Trends in the use of antidepressants in a national sample of commercially insured pediatric patients, 1998–2002. *Psychiatric Services, 55*, 387–191.

Denny, S., Clark, T. C., Fleming, T., & Wall, M. (2004). Emotional resilience: Risk and protective factors for depression among alternative education students in New Zealand. *American Journal of Orthopsychiatry, 74*, 137–149.

Diamond, G. S., Reis, B. F., Diamond, G. M., Siqueland, L., & Isaacs, L. (2002). Attachment-based family therapy for depressed adolescents: A treatment development study. *Journal of the American Academy of Child and Adolescent Psychiatry, 41*, 1190–1196.

Diamond, G. S., Siqueland, L., & Diamond, G. M. (2003). Attachment-based family therapy for depressed adolescents: Programmatic treatment development. *Clinical Child and Family Psychology Review, 6*, 107–127.

Doi, Y., Roberts, R. E., Takeuchi, K., & Suzuki, S. (2001). Multiethnic comparison of adolescent major depression based on the DSM-IV criteria in a U.S.–Japan study. *Journal of the American Academy of Child and Adolescent Psychiatry, 40*, 1308–1315.

Donnelly, C. L., Wagner, K. D., Rynn, M., Ambrosini, P., Landau, P., Yang, R., et al. (2006). Sertraline in children and adolescents with major depressive disorder. *Journal of the American Academy of Child and Adolescent Psychiatry, 45*, 1162–1170.

Dumont, M., & Provost, M. A. (1999). Resilience in adolescents: Protective role of social support, coping strategies, self-esteem, and social activities on experience of stress and depression. *Journal of Youth and Adolescence, 28*, 343–363.

Emslie, G. J., Findling, R. L., Rynn, M., Marcus, R. N., Fernandes, L. A., D'Amico, M. F., et al. (2002). Efficacy and safety of nefazodone in the treatment of adolescents with major depressive disorder (Abstract). *Journal of Child and Adolescent Psychopharmacology, 12*, 299.

Emslie, G. J., Findling, R. L., Yeung, P. P., Kunz, N. R., & Li, Y. (2007). Venlafaxine ER for the treatment of pediatric subjects with depression: Results of two placebo-controlled trials. *Journal of the American Academy of Child and Adolescent Psychiatry, 46*, 479–488.

Emslie, G. J., Heiligenstein, J. H., Hoog, S. L., Wagner, K. D., Findling, R. L., McCracken, J., et al. (2004). Fluoxetine treatment for prevention of relapse of depression in children and adolescents: A double-blind, placebo-controlled study. *Journal of the American Academy of Child and Adolescent Psychiatry, 43*, 1397–1405.

Emslie, G. J., Heiligenstein, J. H., Wagner, K. D., Hoog, S. L., Ernest, D. E., Brown, E., et al. (2002). Fluoxetine for active treatment of depression in children and adolescents: A placebo-controlled, randomized clinical trial. *Journal of the American Academy of Child and Adolescent Psychiatry, 41*, 1205–1215.

Emslie, G. J., Kratochvil, C. J., Vitiello, B., Silva, S., Mayes, T., McNulty, S., et al. (2006). Treatment for Adolescents with Depression Study (TADS): Safety results. *Journal of the American Academy of Child and Adolescent Psychiatry, 45*, 1440–1455.

Emslie, G. J., Rush, A. J., Weinberg, W. A., Kowatch, R. A., Hughes, C. W., Carmody, T., et al. (1997). A double-blind, randomized, placebo-controlled trial of fluoxetine in children and adolescents with depression. *Archives of General Psychiatry, 54*, 1031–1037.

Emslie, G. J., Wagner, K. D., Kutcher, S., Krulewicz, S., Fong, R., Carpenter, D. J., et al. (2006). Paroxetine treatment in children and adolescents with major depressive disorder: A randomized, multicenter, double-blind, placebo-controlled trial. *Journal of the American Academy of Child and Adolescent Psychiatry, 45*, 709–719.

Fine, S., Forth, A., Gilbert, M., & Haley, G. (1991). Group therapy for adolescent depressive disorder: A comparison of social skills and therapeutic support. *Journal of the American Academy of Child and Adolescent Psychiatry, 30*, 79–85.

Fristad, M. A., Arnett, M. M., & Gavazzi, S. M. (1998). The impact of psychoeducational workshops on families of mood-disordered children. *Family Therapy, 25*, 151–159.

Fristad, M. A., Goldberg-Arnold, J. S., & Gavazzi, S. M. (2003). Multi-family psychoeducation groups in the treatment of children with mood disorders. *Journal of Marital and Family Therapy, 29*, 491–504.

Galambos, N. L., Leadbeater, B. J., & Barker, E. T. (2004). Gender differences in and risk factors for depression in adolescence: A 4-year longitudinal study. *International Journal of Behavioral Development, 28*, 16–25.

Garber, J. (2006). Depression in children and adolescents: Linking risk research and prevention. *American Journal of Preventive Medicine, 31*, S104–S125.

Garber, J., Keiley, M. K., & Martin, N. C. (2002). Developmental trajectories of adolescents' depressive symptoms: Predictors of change. *Journal of Consulting and Clinical Psychology, 70*, 79–95.

Gee, C. B. (2004). Assessment of anxiety and depression in Asian American youth. *Journal of Clinical Child and Adolescent Psychology, 33*, 269–271.

Gibbons, R. D., Hur, K., Bhaumik, D. K., & Mann, J. J. (2006). The relationship between antidepressant prescription rates and rate of early adolescent suicide. *American Journal of Psychiatry, 163*, 1898–1904.

Gillham, J. E., Hamilton, J., Freres, D. R., Patton, K., & Gallop, R. (2006). Preventing depression among early adolescents in the primary care setting: A randomized controlled study of the Penn Resiliency Program. *Journal of Abnormal Child Psychology, 34*, 203–219.

Gillham, J. E., Reivich, K., Freres, D. R., Lascher, M., Litzinger, S., Shatte, A. J., et al. (2006). School-based prevention of depression and anxiety symptoms in early adolescence: A pilot of a parent intervention component. *School Psychology Quarterly, 21*, 323–348.

Gillham, J. E., Reivich, K., Jaycox, L., & Seligman, M. E. P. (1995). Prevention of depressive symptoms in school children: Two year follow-up. *Psychological Science, 6*, 343–351.

Gillham, J. E., & Reivich, K. J. (1999). Prevention of depressive symptoms in school children: A research update. *Psychological Science, 10*, 461–462.

Gillham, J. E., Reivich, K. J., Freres, D. R., Chaplin, T. M., Shatte, A. J., Samuels, B., et al. (2007). School-based prevention of depressive symptoms: A randomized controlled study of the effectiveness and specificity of the Penn Resiliency Program. *Journal of Consulting and Clinical Psychology, 75*, 9–19.

Goldberg-Arnold, J. S., Fristad, M. A., & Gavazzi, S. M. (1999). Family psychoeducation: Giving caregivers what they want and need. *Family Relations, 48*, 1–7.

Goldstein, S., & Brooks, R. B. (Eds.). (2005). *Handbook of resilience in children.* New York: Kluwer Academic/Plenum Press.

Goodyer, I. M., Dubicka, B., Wilkinson, P., Kelvin, R., Roberts, C., Byford, S., et al. (2007). Selective serotonin reuptake inhibitors (SSRIs) and routine specialist care with and without cognitive behaviour therapy in adolescents with major depression: Randomised controlled trial. *British Medical Journal, 335*, 142–150.

Graham, C. A., & Easterbrooks, M. A. (2000). School-aged children's vulnerability to depressive symptomatology: The role of attachment security, maternal depressive symptomatology, and economic risk. *Development and Psychopathology, 12*, 201–213.

Griffith, J., Zucker, M., Bliss, M., Foster, J., & Kaslow, N. J. (2001). Family interventions for depressed African American adolescent females. *Innovations in Clinical Practice, 19*, 159–173.

Haby, M. M., Tonge, B. J., Littlefield, L., Carter, R., & Vos, T. (2004). Cost-effectiveness of cognitive behavioural therapy and selective serotonin reuptake inhibitors for major depression in children and adolescents. *Australian and New Zealand Journal of Psychiatry, 38*, 579–591.

Hammad, T. A., Laughren, T., & Racoosin, J. (2006). Suicidality in pediatric patients treated with antidepressant drugs. *Archives of General Psychiatry, 63*, 323–329.

Hankin, B. L., & Abramson, L. Y. (2001). Development of gender differences in depression: An elaborated cognitive vulnerability–transactional stress theory. *Psychological Bulletin, 127*, 773–796.

Hankin, B. L., & Abramson, L. Y. (2002). Measuring cognitive vulnerability to depression in adolescence: Reliability, validity, and gender differences. *Journal of Clinical Child and Adolescent Psychology, 31*, 491–504.

Hankin, B. L., Abramson, L. Y., Moffitt, T. E., Silva, P. A., McGee, R., & Angell, K. E. (1998). Development of depression from preadolescence to young adulthood: Emerging gender differences in a 10-year longitudinal study. *Journal of Abnormal Psychology, 107*, 128–140.

Hoffmann, J. P., Baldwin, S. A., & Cerbone, F. G. (2003). Onset of major depressive disorder among adolescents. *Journal of the American Academy of Child and Adolescent Psychiatry, 42*, 217–224.

Horowitz, J. L., & Garber, J. (2006). The prevention of depressive symptoms in children and adolescents: A meta-analytic review. *Journal of Consulting and Clinical Psychology, 74*, 401–415.

Hughes, C. W., Emslie, G. J., Crismon, M. L., Posner, K., Birmaher, B., Ryan, N. D., et al. (2007). Texas Children's Medication Algorithm Project: Update from Texas Consensus Conference Panel on

Medication Treatment of Childhood Major Depressive Disorder. *Journal of the American Academy of Child and Adolescent Psychiatry, 46,* 667–686.

Ialongo, N. S., Werthamer, L., Kellman, S. G., Brown, C. H., Wang, S. S.-H., & Lin, Y. (1999). Proximal impact of two first-grade preventive interventions on the early risk behaviors for later substance abuse, depression, and antisocial behavior. *American Journal of Community Psychology, 27,* 599–641.

Isacsson, G., Holmgren, P., & Ahlner, J. (2005). Selective serotonin reuptake inhibitor antidepressants and the risk of suicide: A controlled forensic database study of 1,4857 suicides. *Acta Psychiatrica Scandinavica, 96,* 94–100.

Jaffee, S. R., Moffitt, T. E., Caspi, A., Fombonne, E., Poulton, R., & Martin, J. (2002). Differences in early childhood risk factors for juvenile-onset and adult-onset depression. *Archives of General Psychiatry, 59,* 215–222.

Jane-Llopis, E., Hosman, C. M. H., Jenkins, R., & Anderson, P. (2003). Predictors of efficacy in depression prevention programmes: Meta-analysis. *British Journal of Psychiatry, 183,* 384–397.

Jaycox, L., Reivich, K., Gillham, J. E., & Seligman, M. E. P. (1994). Prevention of depressive symptoms in school children. *Behavioral Research and Therapy, 32,* 801–816.

Jayson, D., Wood, A., Kroll, L., Fraser, J., & Harrington, R. (1998). Which depressed patients respond to cognitive-behavioral treatment? *Journal of the American Academy of Child and Adolescent Psychiatry, 37,* 35–39.

Jureidini, J. N., Doecke, C. J., Mansfield, P. R., Haby, M. M., Menkes, D. B., & Tonkin, A. L. (2004). Efficacy and safety of antidepressants for children and adolescents. *British Medical Journal, 328,* 879–883.

Kahn, J., Kehle, T., Jenson, W., & Clark, E. (1990). Comparison of cognitive behavioral, relaxation, and self-modeling interventions for depression among middle-school students. *School Psychology Review, 19,* 196–211.

Kaslow, N. J., Bollini, A. M., Druss, B., Glueckauf, R. L., Goldfrank, L. R., Kelleher, K. J., et al. (2007). Health care for the whole person: Research update. *Professional Psychology: Research and Practice, 38,* 278–289.

Kaslow, N. J., & Thompson, M. (1998). Applying the criteria for empirically supported treatments to studies of psychosocial interventions for child and adolescent depression. *Journal of Clinical Child Psychology, 27,* 146–155.

Kaufman, J., Martin, A., King, R. A., & Charney, D. (2001). Are child-, adolescent-, and adult-onset depression one and the same disorder? *Biological Psychiatry, 49,* 980–1001.

Kaufman, J., Yang, B., Douglas-Palumberi, H., Houshyar, S., Lipschitz, D., Krystal, J. H., et al. (2004). Social supports and serotonin transporter gene moderate depression in maltreated children. *Proceedings of the National Academy of Sciences USA, 101,* 17316–17321.

Kaufman, J., Yang, B.-Y., Douglas-Palumberi, H., Grasso, D., Liptschitz, D., Houshyar, S., et al. (2006). Brain-derived neurotrophic factors–5-HTTLPR gene interactions and environmental modifiers of depression in children. *Biological Psychiatry, 59,* 673–680.

Kaufman, N. K., Rohde, P., Seeley, J. R., Clarke, G., & Stice, E. (2005). Potential mediators of cognitive-behavioral therapy for adolescents with comorbid major depression and conduct disorder. *Journal of Consulting and Clinical Psychology, 73,* 38–46.

Kazdin, A. E., & Nock, M. K. (2003). Delineating mechanisms of change in child and adolescent therapy: Methodological issues and research recommendations. *Journal of Child Psychology and Psychiatry, 44,* 1116–1129.

Kellam, S. G., Rebok, G. W., Mayer, L. S., Ialongo, N., & Kalodner, C. R. (1994). Depressive symptoms over first-grade and their response to a developmental epidemiologically preventive trial aimed at improving achievement. *Development and Psychopathology, 6,* 463–481.

Keller, M. B., Ryan, N. D., Strober, M., Klein, R. G., Kutcher, S., Birmaher, B., et al. (2001). Efficacy of paroxetine in the treatment of adolescent major depression: A randomized, controlled trial. *Journal of the American Academy of Child and Adolescent Psychiatry, 40,* 762–772.

Kennard, B., Silva, S., Vitiello, B., Curry, J., Kratochvil, C. J., Simons, A., et al. (2006). Remission and residual symptoms after short-term treatment in the Treatment of Adolescents with Depression Study (TADS). *Journal of the American Academy of Child and Adolescent Psychiatry, 45,* 1404–1411.

King, C. A., & Kirschenbaum, D. S. (1990). An experimental evaluation of a school-based program for children at risk: Wisconsin Early Intervention. *Journal of Community Psychology, 18*, 167–177.

Kistner, J. A., David, C. F., & White, B. A. (2003). Ethnic and sex differences in children's depressive symptoms: Mediating effects of perceived and actual competence. *Journal of Clinical Child and Adolescent Psychology, 32*, 341–350.

Klein, K., & Forehand, R. (2000). Family processes as resources for African American children exposed to a constellation of sociodemographic risk factors. *Journal of Clinical Child Psychology, 29*, 53–65.

Kolko, D., Brent, D. A., Baugher, M., Bridge, J., & Birmaher, B. (2000). Cognitive and family therapies for adolescent depression: Treatment specificity, mediation, and moderation. *Journal of Consulting and Clinical Psychology, 68*, 603–614.

Kratochvil, C. J., Emslie, G. J., Silva, S., McNulty, S., Walkup, J., Curry, J., et al. (2006). Acute time to response in the Treatment for Adolescents with Depression Study (TADS). *Journal of the American Academy of Child and Adolescent Psychiatry, 45*, 1412–1418.

Kratochvil, C. J., Vitiello, B., Walkup, J., Emslie, G. J., Waslick, B. D., Weller, E. B., et al. (2006). Selective serotonin reuptake inhibitors in pediatric depression: Is the balance between benefits and risks favorable? *Journal of Child and Adolescent Psychopharmacology, 16*, 11–24.

Leech, S. L., Larkby, C. A., Day, R., & Day, N. L. (2006). Predictors and correlates of high levels of depression and anxiety symptoms among children at age 10. *Journal of the American Academy of Child and Adolescent Psychiatry, 45*, 223–230.

Leon, A. C., Marzuk, P. M., Tardiff, K., Bucciarelli, A., Piper, T. M., & Galea, S. (2006). Antidepressants and youth suicide in New York City, 1999–2002. *Journal of the American Academy of Child and Adolescent Psychiatry, 45*, 1054–1058.

Leon, A. C., Marzuk, P. M., Tardiff, K., & Teres, J. J. (2004). Paroxetine, other antidepressants, and youth suicide in New York City: 1993 through 1998. *Journal of Clinical Psychiatry, 65*, 915–918.

Lewinsohn, P. M., Clarke, G., Hops, H., & Andrews, J. (1990). Cognitive-behavioral treatment for depressed adolescents. *Behavior Therapy, 21*, 385–401.

Lewinsohn, P. M., Clarke, G., Rohde, P., Hops, H., & Seeley, J. (1996). A course in coping: A cognitive-behavioral approach to the treatment of adolescent depression. In E. D. Hibbs & P. S. Jensen (Eds.), *Psychosocial treatments for child and adolescent disorders: Empirically based strategies for clinical practice* (pp. 109–135). Washington, DC: American Psychological Association.

Libby, A. M., Brent, D. A., Morrato, E. H., Orton, H. D., Allen, R., & Valuck, R. J. (2007). Decline in treatment of pediatric depression after FDA advisory on risk of suicidality with SSRIs. *American Journal of Psychiatry, 164*, 884–891.

Lock, S., & Barrett, P. M. (2003). A longitudinal study of developmental differences in universal preventive intervention for child anxiety. *Behaviour Change, 20*, 183–199.

Lonigan, C. J., Elbert, J. C., & Johnson, S. B. (1998). Empirically supported psychosocial interventions for children: An overview. *Journal of Clinical Child Psychology, 27*, 138–145.

Lowry-Webster, H. M., Barrett, P. M., & Dadds, M. R. (2001). A universal prevention trial of anxiety and depressive symptomatology in childhood: Preliminary data from an Australian study. *Behaviour Change, 18*, 36–50.

Lowry-Webster, H. M., Barrett, P. M., & Lock, S. (2003). A universal prevention trial of anxiety symptomatology during childhood: Results at 1-year follow-up. *Behaviour Change, 20*, 25–43.

Luthar, S. S., Cicchetti, D., & Becker, B. (2000). The construct of resilience: A critical evaluation and guidelines for future work. *Child Development, 71*, 543–562.

Lynch, F. L., Hornbrook, M., Clarke, G. N., Perrin, N., Polen, M. R., O'Connor, E., et al. (2005). Cost-effectiveness of an intervention to prevent depression in at-risk teens. *Archives of General Psychiatry, 62*, 1241–1248.

Lyon, F. L., & Clarke, G. N. (2006). Estimating the economic burden of depression in children and adolescents. *American Journal of Preventive Medicine, 31*, 143–151.

Ma, J., Lee, K.-V., & Stafford, R. S. (2005). Depression treatment during outpatient visits by U.S. children and adolescents. *Journal of Adolescent Health, 37*, 434–442.

Mann, J. J., Graham, E., Baldessarini, R. J., Beardslee, W. R., Fawcett, J. A., Goodwin, F. K., et al. (2006). ACNP Task Force Report on SSRIs and suicidal behavior in youth. *Neuropsychopharmacology, 31*, 473–492.

March, J. S., Silva, S., Vitiello, B., & the TADS Team. (2006). The Treatment for Adolescents with Depression Study (TADS): Methods and message at 12 weeks. *Journal of the American Academy of Child and Adolescent Psychiatry, 45,* 1393–1403.

Marcotte, D., Fortin, L., Potvin, P., & Papillon, M. (2002). Gender differences in depressive symptoms during adolescence: Role of gender-typed characteristics, self-esteem, body image, stressful life events, and pubertal status. *Journal of Emotional and Behavioral Disorders, 10,* 29–42.

McCarty, C. A., Weisz, J. R., Wanitromanee, K., Eastman, K. L., Suwanlert, S., Chaisyasit, W., et al. (1999). Culture, coping, and context: Primary and secondary control among Thai and American youth. *Journal of Child Psychology and Psychiatry, and Allied Disciplines, 40,* 809–818.

McClure, E. B., Connell, A., Zucker, M., Griffith, J. R., & Kaslow, N. J. (2005). The Adolescent Depression Empowerment Project (ADEPT): A culturally sensitive family treatment for depressed, African American girls. In E. D. Hibbs & P. S. Jensen (Eds.), *Psychosocial treatments for child and adolescent disorders: Empirically based strategies for clinical practice* (2nd ed., pp. 149–164). Washington, DC: American Psychological Association.

McClure, E. B., Kubiszyn, T., & Kaslow, N. J. (2002). Advances in the diagnosis and treatment of childhood mood disorders. *Professional Psychology: Research and Practice, 33,* 125–134.

Melvin, G. A., Tonge, B. J., King, N. J., Heyne, D., Gordon, M. S., & Klimkeit, E. (2006). A comparison of cognitive-behavioral therapy, sertraline, and their combination for adolescent depression. *Journal of the American Academy of Child and Adolescent Psychiatry, 45,* 1151–1161.

Merry, S., McDowell, H., Wild, C. J., Bir, J., & Cunliffe, R. (2004). A randomized placebo-controlled trial of a school-based depression prevention program. *Journal of the American Academy of Child and Adolescent Psychiatry, 43,* 538–547.

Michael, K. D., & Crowley, S. L. (2002). How effective are treatments for child and adolescent depression?: A meta-analytic review. *Clinical Psychology Review, 22,* 247–269.

Miller, L. J., & Gur, M. (2002). Religiosity, depression, and physical maturation in adolescent girls. *Journal of the American Academy of Child and Adolescent Psychiatry, 41,* 206–214.

Morbidity and Mortality World Report. (2007). *Suicide trends among youths and young adults aged 10–24 years—United States, 1990–2004.* Retrieved September 6, 2007, from *www.cdc.gov/od/oc/media/pressrel/2007/r070906.htm*

Mosholder, A. D., & Willy, M. (2006). Suicidal adverse events in pediatric randomized, controlled clinical trials of antidepressant drugs are associated with active drug treatment: A meta-analysis. *Journal of Child and Adolescent Psychopharmacology, 16,* 25–32.

Mufson, L. H., Dorta, K. P., Wickramaratne, P., Nomura, Y., Olfson, M., & Weissman, M. M. (2004). A randomized effectiveness trial of interpersonal psychotherapy for depressed adolescents. *Archives of General Psychiatry, 61,* 577–584.

Mufson, L. H., Weissman, M. M., Moreau, D., & Garfinkel, R. (1999). Efficacy of interpersonal psychotherapy for depressed adolescents. *Archives of General Psychiatry, 56,* 573–579.

Muris, P., Meesters, C., van Melick, M., & Zwambag, L. (2001). Self-reported attachment style, attachment quality, and symptoms of anxiety and depression in young adolescents. *Personality and Individual Differences, 30,* 809–818.

National Center for Health Statistics. (2004). *Health, United States, 2004.* Hyattsville, MD: Centers for Disease Control and Prevention.

Nelson, E. L., Barnard, M., & Cain, S. (2003). Treating childhood depression over videoconferencing. *Telemedicine Journal and E-Health, 9,* 49–55.

Newman, T. B. (2004). A black-box warning for antidepressants in children? *New England Journal of Medicine, 351,* 1595–1598.

Nolen-Hoeksema, S. (2001). Gender differences in depression. *Current Directions in Psychological Science, 10,* 173–176.

Nolen-Hoeksema, S. (2002). Gender differences in depression. In I. H. Gotlib & C. L. Hammen (Eds.), *Handbook of depression* (pp. 492–509). New York: Guilford Press.

Olfson, M., Gameroff, M. J., Marcus, S. C., & Waslick, B. D. (2003). Outpatient treatment of child and adolescent depression in the United States. *Archives of General Psychiatry, 60,* 1236–1242.

Park, R. J., & Goodyer, I. M. (2000). Clinical guidelines for depressive disorders in childhood and adolescence. *European Child and Adolescent Psychiatry, 9,* 147–161.

Pattison, C., & Lynd-Stevenson, R. M. (2001). The prevention of depressive symptoms in children: The immediate and long-term outcomes of a school-based program. *Behaviour Change, 18,* 92–102.

Petersen, A. C., Leffert, N., Graham, B., Alwin, J., & Ding, S. (1997). Promoting mental health during the transition into adolescence. In J. Schulenberg, J. L. Muggs, & A. Hierrelmann (Eds.), *Health risks and developmental transitions during adolescence* (pp. 471–497). New York: Cambridge University Press.

Pfeffer, C., Jiang, H., Kakuma, T., Hwang, J., & Metsch, M. (2002). Group intervention for children bereaved by the suicide of a relative. *Journal of the American Academy of Child and Adolescent Psychiatry, 41,* 505–513.

Piccinelli, M., & Wilkinson, G. (2000). Gender differences in depression. *British Journal of Psychiatry, 177,* 486–492.

Posner, K., Oquendo, M. A., Gould, M., Stanley, B., & Davies, M. (2007). Columbia Classification Algorithm of Suicide Assessment (C-CASA): Classification of suicidal events in the FDA's pediatric suicidal risk analysis of antidepressants. *American Journal of Psychiatry, 164,* 1035–1043.

Possel, P., Baldus, C., Horn, A. B., Groen, G., & Hautzinger, M. (2005). Influence of general self-efficacy on the effects of a school-based universal primary prevention program of depression symptoms in adolescents: A randomized and controlled follow-up study. *Journal of Child Psychology and Psychiatry, and Allied Disciplines, 46,* 982–994.

Possel, P., Horn, A. B., Groen, G., & Hautzinger, M. (2004). School-based prevention of depressive symptoms in adolescents: A six-month follow-up. *Journal of the American Academy of Child and Adolescent Psychiatry, 43,* 1003–1010.

Reinecke, M., & Simons, A. (2005). Vulnerability to depression among adolescents: Implications for cognitive-behavioral treatment. *Cognitive and Behavioral Practice, 12,* 166–176.

Reinecke, M. A., Ryan, N. E., & DuBois, D. L. (1998). Cognitive behavioral therapy of depression and depressive symptoms during adolescence: A review and meta-analysis. *Journal of the American Academy of Child and Adolescent Psychiatry, 37,* 26–34.

Resnick, M. D., Bearman, P. S., Blum, R. W., Bauman, K. E., Harris, K. M., Jones, J., et al. (1997). Protecting adolescents from harm: Findings from the National Longitudinal Study of Adolescent Health. *Journal of the American Medical Association, 278,* 823–832.

Rey, J. M., & Walter, G. (1997). Half a century of ECT use in young people. *American Journal of Psychiatry, 154,* 595–602.

Reynolds, W. M., & Coats, K. (1986). A comparison of cognitive-behavioral therapy and relaxation training for the treatment of depression in adolescents. *Journal of Consulting and Clinical Psychology, 54,* 653–660.

Rice, F., Harold, G. T., & Thapar, A. (2002). Assessing the effects of age, sex, and shared environment on the genetic aetiology of depression in childhood and adolescence. *Journal of Child Psychology and Psychiatry, and Allied Disciplines, 43,* 1039–1051.

Richardson, L. P., Davis, R., Poulton, R., McCauley, E., Moffitt, T. E., Caspi, A., et al. (2003). A longitudinal evaluation of adolescent depression and adult obesity. *Archives of Pediatrics and Adolescent Medicine, 157,* 739–745.

Richmond, M. K., Stocker, C. M., & Rienks, S. L. (2005). Longitudinal associations between sibling relationship quality, parental differential treatment, and children's adjustment. *Journal of Family Psychology, 19,* 550–559.

Roberts, C., Kane, R., Thomson, H., Bishop, B., & Hart, B. (2003). The prevention of depressive symptoms in rural school children: A randomized controlled trial. *Journal of Consulting and Clinical Psychology, 71,* 622–628.

Roberts, R. E., Roberts, C. R., & Chen, Y. R. (1997). Ethnocultural differences in prevalence of adolescent depression. *American Journal of Community Psychology, 25,* 95–110.

Rohde, P., Clarke, G., Mace, D. E., Jorgensen, J. S., & Seeley, J. R. (2004). An efficacy/effectiveness study of cognitive-behavioral treatment for adolescents with comorbid major depression and conduct disorder. *Journal of the American Academy of Child and Adolescent Psychiatry, 43,* 660–668.

Rohde, P., Clarke, G. N., Lewinsohn, P. M., Seeley, J. R., & Kaufman, N. K. (2001). Impact of comorbidity on a cognitive-behavioral group treatment for adolescent depression. *Journal of the American Academy of Child and Adolescent Psychiatry, 40,* 795–802.

Rohde, P., Seeley, J. R., Kaufman, N. K., Clarke, G. N., & Stice, E. (2006). Predicting time to recovery among depressed adolescents treated in two psychosocial group interventions. *Journal of Consulting and Clinical Psychology, 74,* 80–88.

Rossello, J., & Bernal, G. (1999). The efficacy of cognitive-behavioral and interpersonal treatments for depression in Puerto Rican adolescents. *Journal of Consulting and Clinical Psychology, 67,* 734–745.

Rushton, J. L., & Whitmire, J. T. (2001). Pediatric stimulant and selective serotonin reuptake inhibitor prescription trends: 1992 to 1998. *Archives of Pediatrics and Adolescent Medicine, 155,* 560–565.

Ryan, N. D. (2005). Treatment of depression in children and adolescents. *Lancet, 366,* 933–940.

Rynn, M. R., Wagner, K. D., Donnelly, C. L., Ambrosini, P., Wohlberg, C. J., Landau, P., et al. (2006). Long-term sertraline treatment of children and adolescents with major depressive disorder. *Journal of Child and Adolescent Psychopharmacology, 16,* 103–116.

Samaan, R. A. (2000). The influences of race, ethnicity, and poverty on the mental health of children. *Journal of Health Care for the Poor and Underserved, 11,* 100–110.

Sander, J. B., & McCarty, C. A. (2005). Youth depression in the family context: Familial risk factors and models of treatment. *Clinical Child and Family Psychology Review, 8,* 203–219.

Sanford, M., Boyle, M., McCleary, L., Miller, J. G., Steele, M., Duku, E., et al. (2006). A pilot study of adjunctive family psychoeducation in adolescent major depression: Feasibility and treatment effect. *Journal of the American Academy of Child and Adolescent Psychiatry, 45,* 386–395.

Scourfield, J., Rice, F., Thapar, A., Harold, G. T., Martin, N., & McGuffin, P. (2003). Depressive symptoms in children and adolescents: Changing aetiological influences with development. *Journal of Child Psychology and Psychiatry, and Allied Disciplines, 44,* 968–976.

Sen, B. (2004). Adolescent propensity for depressed mood and help seeking: Race and gender differences. *Journal of Mental Health Policy and Economics, 7,* 133–145.

Sheffield, J. K., Spence, S. H., Rapee, R. M., Kowalenko, N., Wignall, A., Davis, A., et al. (2006). Evaluation of universal, indicated, and combined cognitive-behavioral approaches to the prevention of depression in adolescents. *Journal of Consulting and Clinical Psychology, 74,* 66–79.

Shih, J. H., Eberhart, N. K., Hammen, C. L., & Brennan, P. A. (2006). Differential exposure and reactivity to interpersonal stress predicts sex differences in adolescent depression. *Journal of Clinical Child and Adolescent Psychology, 35,* 103–115.

Shochet, I. M., Dadds, I. M., Dadds, M. R., Ham, D., & Montague, R. (2006). School connectedness is an underemphasized parameter in adolescent mental health: Results of a community prediction study. *Journal of Clinical Child and Adolescent Psychology, 35,* 170–179.

Shochet, I. M., Dadds, M. R., Holland, D., Whitefield, K., Harnett, P. H., & Osgarby, S. M. (2001). The efficacy of a universal school-based program to prevent adolescent depression. *Journal of Clinical Child Psychology, 30,* 303–315.

Shochet, I. M., & Ham, D. (2004). Universal school-based approaches to preventing adolescent depression: Past findings and future directions of the Resourceful Adolescent Program. *International Journal of Mental Health Promotion, 6,* 17–25.

Siegel, J. M., Aneshensel, C. S., Taub, B., Cantwell, D. P., & Driscoll, A. K. (2001). Adolescent depressed mood in a multi-ethnic sample. *Prevention Research, 8,* 4–6.

Silberg, J. L., Rutter, M., & Eaves, L. J. (2001). Genetic and environmental influences on the temporal association between earlier anxiety and later depression in girls. *Biological Psychiatry, 49,* 1040–1049.

Sims, B. E., Nottelmann, E., Koretz, D. S., & Pearson, J. (2006). Prevention of depression in children and adolescents. *American Journal of Preventive Medicine, 31,* S99–S103.

Spence, S. H., Sheffield, J. K., & Donovan, C. L. (2003). Preventing adolescent depression: An evaluation of the Problem Solving for Life Program. *Journal of Consulting and Clinical Psychology, 71,* 3–13.

Spence, S. H., Sheffield, J. K., & Donovan, C. L. (2005). Long-term outcome of a school-based, universal approach to prevention of depression in adolescents. *Journal of Consulting and Clinical Psychology, 73,* 160–167.

Stark, K. D., Hargrave, J., Hersh, B., Greenberg, M., Herren, J., & Fisher, M. (2007). Treatment of childhood depression: The ACTION treatment program. In J. R. Z. Abela & B. L. Hankin (Eds.), *Handbook of depression in children and adolescents* (pp. 224–249). New York: Guilford Press.

Stark, K. D., Hargrave, J., Sander, J., Schnoebelen, S., Simpson, J., & Molnar, J. (2006). Treatment of childhood depression: The ACTION treatment program. In P. C. Kendall (Ed.), *Child and adolescent therapy: Cognitive-behavioral procedures* (3rd ed., pp. 169–216). New York: Guilford Press.

Stark, K. D., Herren, J., & Fisher, M. (in press). Treatment of childhood depression. In M. J. Mayer, R. V. Acker, J. Lochman, & F. M. Gresham (Eds.), *Cognitive-behavioral interventions for students with emotional/behavioral disorders.* New York: Guilford Press.

Stark, K. D., Reynolds, W. M., & Kaslow, N. J. (1987). A comparison of the relative efficacy of self-control therapy and behavior problem-solving therapy for depression in children. *Journal of Abnormal Child Psychology, 15,* 91–113.

Stark, K. D., Rouse, L., & Livingston, R. (1991). Treatment of depression during childhood and adolescence: Cognitive behavioral procedures for the individual and family. In P. Kendall (Ed.), *Child and adolescent therapy* (pp. 165–206). New York: Guilford Press.

Stark, K. D., Sander, J., Hauser, M., Simpson, J., Schnoebelen, S., Glenn, R., et al. (2006). Depressive disorders during childhood and adolescence. In E. J. Mash & R. A. Barkley (Eds.), *Treatment of childhood disorders* (3rd ed., pp. 336–407). New York: Guilford Press.

Sugawara, M., Akiko, Y., Noriko, T., Tomoe, K., Haya, S., Kensuke, S., et al. (2002). Marital relations and depression in school-age children: Links with family functioning and parental attitudes toward child rearing. *Japanese Journal of Educational Psychology, 50,* 129–140.

Sutton, J. M. (2007). Prevention of depression in youth: A qualitative review and future suggestions. *Clinical Psychology Review, 27,* 552–571.

Thompson, E. A., Eggert, L. L., & Herting, J. R. (2000). Mediating effects of an indicated prevention program for reducing youth depression and suicide risk behaviors. *Suicide and Life-Threatening Behavior, 30,* 252–271.

Treatment for Adolescents with Depression Study Team. (2003). Treatment for Adolescents with Depression Study (TADS): Rationale, design, and methods. *Journal of the American Academy of Child and Adolescent Psychiatry, 42,* 531–542.

Treatment for Adolescents with Depression Study (TADS) Team. (2004). Fluoxetine, cognitive-behavioral therapy, and their combination for adolescents with depression: Treatment for Adolescents with Depression Study (TADS) randomized controlled trial. *Journal of the American Medical Association, 292,* 807–820.

Treatment for Adolescents with Depression Study Team. (2005). The Treatment for Adolescents with Depression Study (TADS): Demographic and clinical characteristics. *Journal of the American Academy of Child and Adolescent Psychiatry, 44,* 28–40.

Twenge, J. M., & Nolen-Hoeksema, S. (2002). Age, gender, race, socioeconomic status, and birth cohort differences on the Children's Depression Inventory: A meta-analysis. *Journal of Abnormal Psychology, 111,* 578–588.

Valuck, R. J., Libby, A. M., Sills, M. R., Giese, A. A., & Allen, R. R. (2004). Antidepressant treatment and risk of suicide attempt by adolescents with major depressive disorder: A propensity-adjusted retrospective cohort study. *CNS Drugs, 18,* 1119–1132.

Varley, C. K. (2006). Treating depression in children and adolescents: What options now? *CNS Drugs, 20,* 1–13.

Vitiello, B., Rohde, P., Silva, S., Wells, K. C., Casat, C., Waslick, B. D., et al. (2006). Functioning and quality of life in the Treatment for Adolescents with Depression Study (TADS). *Journal of the American Academy of Child and Adolescent Psychiatry, 45,* 1419–1426.

Vitiello, B., Zuvekas, S. H., & Norquist, G. S. (2006). National estimates of antidepressant use among U.S. children, 1997–2002. *Journal of the American Academy of Child and Adolescent Psychiatry, 45,* 271–279.

von Knorring, A., Olsson, G. I., Thomsen, P. H., Lemming, O. M., & Hulten, A. (2006). A randomized, double-blind, placebo-controlled study of citalopram in adolescents with major depressive disorder. *Journal of Clinical Psychopharmacology, 26,* 311–315.

Wade, T. J., Cairney, J., & Pevalin, D. J. (2002). Emergence of gender differences in depression during adolescence: National panel results from three countries. *Journal of the American Academy of Child and Adolescent Psychiatry, 41,* 190–198.

Wagner, K. D. (2003). Paroxetine treatment of mood and anxiety disorders in children and adolescents. *Psychopharmacology Bulletin, 37*, 167–175.

Wagner, K. D., & Ambrosini, P. (2001). Childhood depression: Pharmacological therapy/treatment (pharmacotherapy of childhood depression). *Journal of Clinical Child Psychology, 30*, 88–97.

Wagner, K. D., Ambrosini, P., Rynn, M., Wohlberg, C., Yang, R., Greenbaum, M. S., et al. (2003). Efficacy of sertraline in the treatment of children and adolescents with major depressive disorder: Two randomized controlled trials. *Journal of the American Medical Association, 290*, 1033–1041.

Wagner, K. D., Jonas, J., Findling, R. L., Ventura, D., & Saikali, K. (2006). A double-blind, randomized, placebo-controlled trial of escitalopram in the treatment of pediatric depression. *Journal of the American Academy of Child and Adolescent Psychiatry, 45*, 280–288.

Wagner, K. D., Robb, A. S., Findling, R. L., Jin, J., Gutierrez, M. M., & Heydorn, W. E. (2004). A randomized, placebo-controlled trial of citalopram for the treatment of major depression in children and adolescents. *American Journal of Psychiatry, 161*, 1079–1083.

Waller, M. W., Hallfors, D. D., Halpern, C. T., Iritani, B. J., Ford, C. A., & Guo, G. (2006). Gender differences in associations between depressive symptoms and patterns of substance use and risky sexual behavior among a nationally representative sample of U.S. adolescents. *Archives of Women's Mental Health, 9*, 139–150.

Walter, G., & Rey, J. M. (1997). An epidemiological study of the use of ECT in adolescents. *Journal of the American Academy of Child and Adolescent Psychiatry, 36*, 809–815.

Walter, G., Rey, J. M., & Mitchell, P. B. (1999). Practitioner review: Electronconvulsive therapy in adolescents. *Journal of Child Psychology and Psychiatry, and Allied Disciplines, 40*, 325–334.

Weersing, V. R., & Brent, D. A. (2003). Cognitive-behavioral therapy for adolescent depression: Comparative efficacy, mediation, moderation, and effectiveness. In A. E. Kazdin & J. R. Weisz (Eds.), *Evidence-based psychotherapies for children and adolescents* (pp. 135–147). New York: Guilford Press.

Weersing, V. R., & Brent, D. A. (2006). Psychotherapy for depression in children and adolescents. In D. J. Stein, D. J. Kupfer, & A. F. Schatzberg (Eds.), *The American Psychiatric Publishing textbook of mood disorders* (pp. 421–436). Washington, DC: American Psychiatric Publishing.

Weiss, B., & Garber, J. (2002). Developmental differences in the phenomenology of depression. *Development and Psychopathology, 15*, 403–430.

Weisz, J. R., Doss, A. J., & Hawley, K. M. (2005). Youth psychotherapy outcome research: A review and critique of the evidence base. *Annual Review of Psychology, 56*, 337–363.

Weisz, J. R., McCarty, C. A., & Valeri, S. M. (2006). Effects of psychotherapy for depression in children and adolescents: A meta-analysis. *Psychological Bulletin, 132*, 132–149.

Weisz, J. R., Thurber, C., Sweeney, L., Proffitt, V., & LeGagnoux, G. (1997). Brief treatment of mild to moderate child depression using primary and secondary control enhancement training. *Journal of Consulting and Clinical Psychology, 65*, 703–707.

Whittington, C. J., Kendall, T., Fonagy, P., Cottrell, D., Cotgrove, A., & Boddington, E. (2004). Selective serotonin reuptake inhibitors in childhood depression: Systematic review of published versus unpublished data. *Lancet, 363*, 1341–1345.

Whittington, C. J., Kendall, T., & Pilling, S. (2005). Are the SSRIs and atypical antidepressants safe and effective for children and adolescents? *Current Opinion in Psychiatry, 18*, 21–25.

Wight, R. G., Aneshensel, C. S., Botticello, A. L., & Sepulveda, J. E. (2005). A multilevel analysis of ethnic variation in depressive symptoms among adolescents in the United States. *Social Science and Medicine, 6*, 2073–2084.

Wignall, A. (2006). Evaluation of a group CBT early intervention program for adolescents with comorbid depression and behaviour problems. *Australia Journal of Guidance and Counseling, 16*, 119–132.

Williams, P. G., Colder, C. R., Richards, M. H., & Scalzo, C. A. (2002). The role of self-assessed health in relationship between gender and depressive symptoms among adolescents. *Journal of Pediatric Psychology, 27*, 509–517.

Wood, A., Harrington, R., & Moore, A. (1996). Controlled trial of a brief cognitive-behavioural intervention in adolescent patients with depressive disorders. *Journal of Child Psychology and Psychiatry, 37*, 737–746.

Wu, P., Hoven, C. W., Cohen, P., Liu, X., Moore, R. E., Tiet, Q., et al. (2001). Factors associated with use of mental health services for depression by children and adolescents. *Psychiatric Services, 52,* 189–195.

Young, J. F., Mufson, L., & Davies, M. (2006). Impact of comorbid anxiety in an effectiveness study of interpersonal psychotherapy for depressed adolescents. *Journal of the American Academy of Child and Adolescent Psychiatry, 45,* 904–912.

Yu, D. L., & Seligman, M. E. P. (2002). Preventing depressive symptoms in Chinese children. *Prevention and Treatment, 5,* Article 9.

Zalsman, G., Brent, D. A., & Weersing, V. R. (2006). Depressive disorders in childhood and adolescence: An overview: Epidemiology, clinical manifestation, and risk factors. *Child and Adolescent Psychiatric Clinics of North America, 15,* 827–841.

CHAPTER 29

Closing Comments and Future Directions

Constance L. Hammen *and* Ian H. Gotlib

Six years have passed since the first edition of this *Handbook*, in which most of the chapters were based on work conducted largely in the latter part of the 20th century. Many of the chapters described advances in the field that have continued to inform research programs and clinical activities. The chapters in the first edition also identified ideas and agendas for future research. Even in the few years since then, a remarkable amount of research has been conducted. In this brief, final chapter we reflect on some of those accomplishments, and on what lies ahead.

DESCRIPTIVE ASPECTS OF DEPRESSION

The opening four chapters of the book have reviewed the epidemiological features, clinical course and consequences, and assessment methods of depression, as well as methodological issues that affect the nature and quality of research on all aspects of this disorder. The initial section also contains a dedicated chapter focused on bipolar depression and its clinical features and correlates; indeed, throughout this volume, there is expanded coverage of bipolar disorders. The initial section also includes a chapter with a focus new to this second edition, depression and medical illness.

With new epidemiological data emerging not just in the United States but also in international studies, as well as recent, large-scale naturalistic studies of psychiatric patients and those in primary care, there is general agreement underscoring the conclusion of the Surgeon General's Report in 2000 that depression is a significant public health problem. Further research has accumulated documenting the enormous toll of depression, its extensive costs not only to the person but also to the family, community, and society, and its recurrent and sometimes chronic nature, with the most pernicious cases originating in youth. The descriptive data paint a clear picture of urgent need for effective care, with the hope that analyses of the impact of depression and its burdens will yield cost-effectiveness data to demonstrate the benefits of treatment. The reality, however, continues to be grim: Most people with depressive disorders are not receiving adequate treatment, and some of those at greatest need have a variety of adverse conditions that impede access or responsiveness to services (e.g., comorbid psychiatric and medical conditions, and adverse sociodemographic conditions such as poverty, young or older age, and disadvantaged social circumstances, including minority and unmarried status). Indeed, it continues to be clear that all models of the etiology of depression and interventions to treat this disorder must account for the reliable associations between depression and being female, poor, disadvantaged, and, in many cultures, young.

There have been improvements in existing methods for the assessment of depression, and more instruments are now available for a variety of purposes, from screening to diagnosis. Nevertheless, further work is needed to refine assessment instruments, particularly for use in special populations, such as the medically ill and those from different cultures. Fundamental concepts of what constitutes the syndrome of depression are, of course, constantly under scrutiny. An inescapable reality is that depression represents phenotypically heterogeneous manifestations and likely multiple etiologies; most research, however, still approaches the topic as if it were a single entity (the "uniformity myth"). Although some progress has been made in elucidating subtypes of depression that might signal different etiological and treatment alternatives, further work is needed—a task made even more difficult by the pervasiveness of comorbid conditions. Similarly, many investigators conceptualize depression as existing on a continuum, including personality features and subsyndromal forms that nevertheless signal impairment and risk for disorders. As noted by several researchers, however, there are limitations and choices associated with the study of subclinical depression, and care must be taken to draw appropriate conclusions about the meaning and generality of studies based on continuum models of depression. Early-appearing temperamental traits may be among risk factors that predict depression, and improved recognition and assessment of such features, and evaluation of their correlates over time, may greatly enhance our understanding of depression and increase the opportunities for early detection and intervention.

The chapter on bipolar depression is a reminder that many years have passed since research on depression commonly commingled unipolar and bipolar participants—a testament to the advantages of diagnostic refinements. Nevertheless, there are many similarities between unipolar and bipolar depression, at least in phenomenology, and perhaps in psychosocial risk factors that affect severity and course. Because most cases of bipolar disorder may present initially as depression, there is considerable incentive for trying to find reliable distinguishing factors to recognize and promptly treat bipolar conditions. A further challenge, perhaps the consequence of increasing attention to bipolar disorder in both the clinical and research communities, is development of valid diagnostic distinctions between milder forms of bipolar disorder and unipolar depression. Until conceptual and diagnostic issues are resolved, there remains a threat that "unipolar" depression samples may be infused with depression occurring in the context of bipolar disorder.

Research on the associations among depression and medical illnesses has expanded dramatically in recent years, with increasing evidence that depression may contribute to the onset, course, morbidity, mortality, and impairment associated with certain illnesses. Many intriguing questions remain to be answered about the biobehavioral mechanisms, and the impact on health of interventions to treat depression. Not surprisingly, to resolve such questions, methodological and assessment issues also require attention.

VULNERABILITY, RISK, AND MODELS OF DEPRESSION

The second section of the book contains chapters on genetic, neurobiological, developmental, and psychosocial approaches to depression vulnerability, including family, cognitive, interpersonal, and environmental perspectives. These chapters represent topics that have been especially active in the few years since the first edition, particularly those reflecting conceptual, empirical, and methodological advances in biological aspects of depression, in parallel to the tidal wave of studies of the "decade of the brain" in relation to psychopathology in general.

Advances in genetic studies of depression reflect new methods and designs, expanding the once-dominant role of statistical studies of twin-based samples to include linkage, association, and candidate gene studies. Thus far, findings are striking in terms of volume of output, general support for small effects of multiple genes, typical lack of support for "main effects" in contrast to the patterns of emerging gene–environment interactions, and widening focus on various candidate genes beyond the serotonin transporter (5-HTTLPR) polymorphisms. The chapter on genetics identifies not only cutting edge results but also the important advantages and pitfalls of different methodologies. Gene–environment studies increasingly show mixed support for stress–5-HTTLPR interactions to predict depression, but it is noteworthy that most such studies are considerably more sophisticated relative to the genetic methodology than to the use of consistently defined constructs and well-validated measures of "stress" or "environment." Expansion of gene–environment methods to include additional genetic candidates, as well as further explication of gene–environment associations, will likely play large roles in future developments. Moreover, rapidly emerging data from large-scale linkage studies increasingly underscore the importance of trying to refine the phenotypes and, indeed, the endophenotypes of depression to identify those individuals at risk for genetically influenced forms of depression. Future developments will include the contributions of genomewide association studies already conducted and soon to be published; such studies will certainly influence the next generation of models and mechanisms of depression vulnerability.

Genetic, biological, and neuroscience methods and findings will be increasingly integrated into models that explain the mechanisms of depression and predictors of risk, including those factors at the endophenotype level. The chapter on neurobiological aspects of depression illustrates well the exponential increase in understanding of the enormously complex processes of the brain, from intracellular and gene activity to neural pathways, structure, and function. The new developments in methods and findings in just a few short years are remarkable and largely support the view of depression as a disorder of dysfunctional responses to stress—and of the progressive effects of stress and neurobiological processes as depression recurs over a lifetime. Although it is a considerable challenge for readers to stay abreast of new developments, the prospect of development of new interventions to alter or reverse the course of depression is rewarding indeed. New directions in neurobiological aspects of depression also include advances in methods and understanding of normal processes of mood, cognition, and behavior—as well as processes affecting normal and maladaptive development. Indeed, considerable research focusing on the influence of early adverse experiences, including both prenatal influences and exposure to stress, trauma, and dysfunctional parenting, implicates both neurodevelopmental and psychosocial processes as contributors to risk for depression.

Several chapters have focused on topics that have been long-running themes in understanding vulnerability to depression, including cognitive, environmental, and interpersonal factors, and status as offspring of depressed parents. Compared to studies in the past decade, each of these topics has identified recent research and new themes. For instance, research on cognitive vulnerability increasingly emphasizes information-processing paradigms that do not rely on self-reported content that may be subject to the effects of mood state and of participants' whims and motivations. Such paradigms suggest that depression is associated not simply with selective attention to negative stimuli, but with deficits in the ability to disengage from negative material and in the inhibition of irrelevant negative material that in turn are linked to difficulties in recruiting cognitive "repair" processes. Environmental approaches to depression vulnerability have commonly emphasized the role that stressors play as triggering events in diathesis–stress models. Increasingly, however, it has been important to acknowledge the dynamic role of stress over the course of recurrent episodes, and the resulting need to be more specific in separating studies of onset versus recurrent episodes of depression. The transactional relations between depression and stress also are noted, with the observation that depression, as well as vulnerabilities to depression, contributes to the occurrence of stress, perpetuating a vicious downward cycle. More investigation of the mechanisms by which stress triggers depressive reactions is warranted, and many of the chapters in this section of the book offer glimpses of ways to conceptualize maladaptive stress processes in depression. Stress research relevant to depression, as reflected in several chapters, includes not only recent stressful life events but also chronic stressful conditions, lifetime exposure to stressors, early childhood trauma and adversity, and "allostatic load."

Depression occurs in a social context, reflecting both the consequences of depression on relationships and vulnerabilities to depression that arise in maladaptive ways of construing the self in relation to others, and in characteristics that affect the quality and supportiveness of relationships with others, such as dependency, attachment insecurity, and excessive reassurance seeking. As is indicated in several chapters, difficulties in social relationships, as evidenced by behavioral inhibition, shyness, social withdrawal, and related constructs, appear to be risk factors for depression. Indeed, such vulnerabilities raise a recurring issue in the etiological approaches to depression: Which vulnerabilities are specific to depression, and which are related to anxiety disorders?

One of the challenges of research on the etiology of depression is integration across biological, genetic, developmental, cognitive, interpersonal, and environmental domains. Each chapter has reviewed emerging approaches to such integration and has called for further cross-fertilization and model building. An area especially ripe for such integrative strategies is the study of offspring at risk for depression due to their parents' depression. The approach not only provides a methodologically efficient method of examining potentially causal factors in youth likely to develop depression but also, by its nature, requires simultaneous attention to genetic/biological, stress, family/interpersonal, and developmental features of symptom development, cognitive, emotion regulation, and interpersonal skills and styles, as well as factors that modify depressive outcomes over time.

DEPRESSION IN SPECIFIC POPULATIONS

This section of the *Handbook* is a dramatic reminder of the heterogeneity of depression—how its occurrence, features and manifestations, and even causal and treatment implications may vary considerably by gender, age, and culture. Gender differences are virtually universal despite enormous variation in cultural and environmental circumstances of women's lives. Considerable research has examined these factors, and investigators now routinely analyze for and report gender differences in aspects of depression. Nevertheless, many issues remain to be resolved, including the important question of whether males and females differ primarily in first onset of depression but not in course and recurrence—a pattern that underscores the need for greater specification of differences between factors involved in onset and those implicated in recurrence. Cultural differences in expression and attributions about the meaning and causes of depression have become topics of increased research focus. Such studies not only contribute to our expanding conceptualizations of depression but also have practical implications for developing and matching individuals to culturally accepted interventions.

Three separate chapters have presented research on depression in children, adolescents, and older adults. We chose to include distinct chapters on these topics because of both the enormous amount of research conducted over the past few years and emerging evidence of the differences among children, adolescents, and older adults in clinical features and course, as well as in likely risk factors and etiological processes. Recent findings support the premise that first-onset depression in each of these age groups has somewhat different etiological and course implications. Research on depression in children no longer reflects mostly downward extensions of adult models; instead, it attempts to explore depression in terms of developmental processes and challenges, including temperament, stress reactivity and emotion regulation processes, and pubertal events. Although the full syndrome of depression is rare in children, refinements in assessment and detection of possible endophenotypic expressions may help to clarify the course and etiology. Adolescent depression is virtually the prototypic form of depression, because a large proportion of depressed adults experience their first episode in the teenage decade. The intriguing questions of emergence of gender differences and the rapid rate increase in major depression, especially in recently born cohorts, continue to challenge the field. The need for multivariate, transactional models that include developmentally salient factors and mechanisms is clearly articulated in several chapters and presents a challenging, if not daunting, task. The issue of depression in older adults has stimulated an increasing amount of attention given its possibly unique features and implications for quality-of-life and public health considerations. Increasingly, depression in older adults is recognized variously as a potential early warning sign of dementing disorders, as a contributor to ill health, and as detriment to effective functioning in older persons and their families. Because many early epidemiological studies omitted the oldest members of the population, and because biased perceptions of older adults obscured the detection of depression, the increased research focus in recent years is a welcome addition.

The chapter on depression in couples and families reflects several key issues: the impairing consequences of depression and the detrimental effects on functioning in important roles; the importance of environmental context as a moderator and mediator of risk factors for depression; and unique and similar relationship factors in unipolar and bipolar disorder. Although depression may be characterized variously as a mood disorder, a disorder of negative cognition, or a disorder of emotion regulation, it is most decidedly an interpersonal disorder, in that relationships may play a central role in contributing to, or protecting from, depression. It is also an interpersonal disorder in the sense that those in close relationships with the depressed person are also affected, with transactions among members of the relationship serving to alter the course of depression for worse or better. Increasingly, research with couples or families with a bipolar member is reflecting similar patterns. Intergenerational transmission of depression associated with family processes indicates a modifiable risk factor greatly in need of intervention.

Suicidal individuals are also a special population that is closely but not exclusively entwined with depressive disorders. This is depression at its most lethal and tragic, and research continues to struggle with basic issues of detection and effective prevention, including the dissemination of such knowledge more widely in the caregiver population. The task is made even more challenging with an increasingly culturally and ethnically diverse population—not to mention the complexities associated with suicidality in different age groups.

PREVENTION AND TREATMENT OF DEPRESSION

The six chapters in this section represent the diverse forms of evidence-based treatment—and prevention—of depression in adults and children. A new chapter on pharmacotherapy and psychotherapy of bipolar disorders has been added in this edition of the *Handbook*. Because depression is so prevalent, and also because its treatment with medication or psychotherapy has largely set the standards for "success" in treatment research, an enormous volume of research on treatment and prevention contributes to refinements in interventions, research designs, outcomes assessment, and dissemination.

Despite its intrinsic appeal, the ideal of preventing major depressive disorder (MDD) in those at risk has not been realized; there is little evidence of success in preventing the first MDD in adults, and only limited success in preventing MDD in adolescents. Outcomes vary by methodological factors such as sample size, recruitment, and focus of the intervention, and results from larger scale studies are in progress. More targeted preventions, such as children of depressed mothers or women at risk for postpartum depression, suggest reasons for optimism, and the field as a whole will benefit from methodological improvements.

Pharmacotherapy and other somatic treatments for unipolar depression remain the most commonly used tools in the treatment bag. The interesting issues in this field are not the success of the treatments, for there have in recent years been no significant breakthroughs in advancing response rates despite proliferation of new antidepressants. Rather, some of the issues that warrant attention are the increasing recognition of continuing symptoms despite treatment and the more recent use of remission, rather than symptom reduction, as the measure of outcome. There are also efforts to evaluate combinations or sequences of medications systematically for their effects on outcomes, and increased recognition and concern with "treatment-resistant" depressions. In view of the vastly complex decisions that physicians need to make in treating the complex patients they see—a problem compounded by the extensive dispensing of antidepressants by nonspecialist physicians—the chapter is especially helpful as a guide to clinical decision making.

Empirically supported psychotherapies for depression have proliferated over the past two decades, as documented in chapters covering cognitive and behavioral, and marital/family/interpersonal approaches. Recent studies indicate that cognitive-behavioral (CBT) and behavioral activation, for example, are as efficacious as pharmacotherapy even for severe depression, thus offering alternatives for those who either decline or should not use medications. Nevertheless, substantial challenges remain. One is the issue of whether psychotherapy promotes an enduring effect, as it intends to do, by providing tools for the person to use to prevent relapses and recurrences. Limited data show promise, but studies with longer follow-ups are needed to learn whether the treatments truly reduce recurrences. Another issue is dissemination. In particular, CBT seems to be challenging to train to high standards of therapist adherence and competence; behavioral activation appears to be promising as a target of dissemination, because it is both simpler to learn and simpler to teach patients.

Family, couple, and interpersonal models of therapy have also expanded in scope and empirical support. Based on the clear evidence that depression occurs in an interpersonal context, these therapy approaches attempt to deal directly with the social context. Marital, parent-training, and individual–interpersonal models of therapy all show evidence of success in symptom reduction and improved functioning. Nevertheless, such approaches—in common with most evidence-based psychotherapies—face important challenges in understanding mechanisms, matching patients to treatment modalities, and dissemination to populations in need, including those disadvantaged by socioeconomic, ethnic/cultural, and sexual orientation status.

Children and adolescents are highly underserved populations when it comes to treatment of emotional and behavioral disorders, and their needs are compounded by developmental issues. Indeed, developmental differences yield confusing and perhaps discouraging evidence concerning what is effective for the treatment of depression. Studies of selective serotonin reuptake inhibitor (SSRI) efficacy, for instance, present a mixed picture—one that has been clouded by the issue of whether suicidality is a side effect of such medications. The largest investigation, the Treatment of Adolescent Depression Study, has been clear on the positive outcomes associated with fluoxetine, with mixed but generally supportive evidence for CBT, or for the combination of CBT and medication, depending on outcome measures and characteristics of the youth. Enthusiasm for efforts to prevent depression in children and youth is understandable, but the evidence suggests that interventions targeting those at risk are more beneficial than are universal efforts. Overall, given the importance of the family context of depression, especially for children, intensive multimodal treatments likely hold the most promise. The final chapter in this section presents valuable clinical guidelines both for treating children and for improving research on treatments for depression.

The new chapter on treatments for bipolar disorder attests to the importance of adding psychosocial interventions as options to the traditional pharmacotherapy for patients with bipolar disorder. Medication treatments alone have not proven to be sufficient, although they are critically important, especially for treatment and prevention of manias, and many patients remain substantially depressed, symptomatic, and impaired. Growing recognition of bipolar disorder in children and adolescents has further highlighted the limitations of medication treatment alone. Several studies, including the large Systematic Treatment Enhancement Program for Bipolar Disorder, provide clear evidence that the addition of intensive psychotherapy (e.g., family focused-therapy or CBT) to medication leads to better and faster clinical and functional outcomes. The authors note that a study is underway to test the utility of a preventive intervention in a high-risk sample—mildly symptomatic youngsters who have a first-degree relative with bipolar disorder. Bipolar disorder has long been neglected by researchers (other than pharmacologists and biological psychiatrists), and it is exciting to see the extent to which the chapters in this book document a new trend of applying information and methods of depression research, as well as new models, to studies with bipolar samples.

Author Index

Subject Index

Page numbers followed by *f* indicate figure, *t* indicate table